AMERICAN ACADEMY
OF OPHTHALMOLOGY®
Protecting Sight. Empowering Lives.

6

Pediatric Ophthalmology and Strabismus

小儿眼科与斜视

2019–2020

BCSC

Basic and Clinical
Science Course™

基础与临床科学教程 ™

美国眼科学会　编

石一宁　主译

石广礼　主审

陕西新华出版传媒集团
陕西科学技术出版社
Shaanxi Science and Technology Press
西　安

著作权登记号 25-2020-129。

图书在版编目（CIP）数据

小儿眼科与斜视：2019-2020 基础与临床科学教程 / 美国眼科学会编；石一宁主译．— 西安：陕西科学技术出版社，2020.8
书名原文：Pediatric Ophthalmology and Strabismus: 2019-2020 Basic and Clinical Science Course™
ISBN 978-7-5369-7462-3

Ⅰ．①小… Ⅱ．①美… ②石… Ⅲ．①儿科学—眼科学②小儿疾病—斜视—诊疗 Ⅳ．① R779.7

中国版本图书馆 CIP 数据核字 (2020) 第 112206 号

小儿眼科与斜视
美国眼科学会　编
石一宁　主译　石广礼　主审

责任编辑　付　琨　潘晓洁
封面设计　曾　珂

出 版 者　陕西新华出版传媒集团　陕西科学技术出版社
西安市曲江新区登高路1388号陕西新华出版传媒产业大厦B座
电话（029）81205187　传真（029）81205155　邮编710061
http://www.snstp.com
发 行 者　陕西新华出版传媒集团　陕西科学技术出版社
电话（029）81205180 81206809
印　　刷　陕西金和印务有限公司
规　　格　889mm × 1194mm　16开本
印　　张　56.25
字　　数　1230千字
版　　次　2020年8月第1版
2020年8月第1次印刷
书　　号　ISBN 978-7-5369-7462-3
定　　价　580.00元

This publication is a translation of a publication of the American Academy of Ophthalmology entitled Basic and Clinical Science Course™, Section 6: *Pediatric Ophthalmology and Strabismus* published in 2019. This translation reflects current practice in the United States of America as of the date of its original publication by the Academy. The American Academy of Ophthalmology did not translate this publication into the language used in this publication and disclaims any responsibility for any errors, omissions or other possible fault in the translation.

本书为美国眼科学会系列教程“基础与临床科学教程”第6册《小儿眼科与斜视》的出版物译本，于2019年出版。这一译本的内容反映美国眼科学会在出版时最新的临床实践。美国眼科学会没有将原始出版物翻译成此书中所用的语言，对翻译中的任何错误、遗漏或其他可能的错误不承担任何责任。

The American Academy of Ophthalmology is the world's largest association of eye physicians and surgeons. A global community of 32,000 medical doctors, we protect sight and empower lives by setting the standards for ophthalmic education and advocating for our patients and the public. We innovate to advance our profession and to ensure the delivery of the highest-quality eye care. Learn more at www.aao.org.

美国眼科学会是全球最大的眼科医师协会。作为一个拥有32 000名医生会员的全球组织，为了保护患者视力，使患者拥有更好的生活，我们制定眼科教育的准则，并向我们的患者和公众普及眼科知识。我们不断进取以提升我们的专业水平，确保提供最高品质的眼健康服务。如需了解更多信息请访问 www.aao.org。

For information on becoming a member of the Academy or attending the Academy's Annual Meeting, call +1 (415) 561 8500, visit aao.org, or write to us at 655 Beach Street, San Francisco, CA 94109, USA.

有关加入本学会或参加学会年会的信息，请致电 +1 (415) 561 8500，或访问网站 aao.org，或致信美国加利福尼亚州旧金山海滩街655号。

“2019-2020 基础与临床科学教程”《小儿眼科与斜视》一书由美国眼科学会（AAO）组织编写，是国际眼科联盟（WOC）和中国医学考试网都推荐全世界的眼科医生和专业研究生学习的眼科临床教程。现在我们组织石一宁等专家翻译了此书。本书主要介绍了基础的眼部解剖学和生理学知识，斜弱视、小儿葡萄膜炎、青光眼、白内障等眼部疾病的检查、诊断与治疗，视力矫正等。本书涵盖面广、内容权威、实用性强。除了配有大量清晰的病理图片、临床学习视频外，还配有大量的测试题，能帮助读者加深对前面所学知识的理解，非常适合自学使用。本书在儿童眼健康基础知识、临床处理及最新进展方面具有独特优势，有助于我国眼科医生拓宽医学诊疗视野，系统学习小儿眼病的相关知识，提升业务能力及专业英文水平，从而更好地服务患者。本书将会成为青年眼科医生参加住院医师规范化培训和进行继续教育的重要教材，引导更多的眼科医生关注并学习儿童眼病的相关知识，积极推动我国儿童眼病诊疗水平的发展。

中文版翻译组（以翻译顺序为序）

主译

石一宁

主审

石广礼

专业总审校

石广礼

审校组

布　娟　钱学翰　丁　娟　朱　丹　刘陇黔　刘　虎　方　严　蒋　宁

英文总审校

李　易　陈研明　陈　卓

翻译组

扉　　页　杨嘉嵩

引　　言　唐志萍

第一章　唐志萍　梅　颖　布　娟

第二章　梅　颖　布　娟

第三章　梅　颖　刘凤阳　布　娟

第四章　汪晓倩　布　娟

第五章　张　乐　刘　念　布　娟

第六章　刘　念　杨嘉嵩　钱学翰

第七章　杨嘉嵩　龚　慧　谭　薇　钱学翰

第八章　谭　薇　杨　乐　丁　娟

第九章　杨　乐　刘　建　丁　娟

第十章　刘　建　芮　莹　丁　娟

第十一章　芮　莹　马玉红　丁　娟

第十二章　孙西宇　张　哲　丁　娟

第十三章　张　哲　许志强

第十四章　许志强　王文军　姚　森
第十五章　姚　森　朱　丹　蒋　宁
第十六章　朱　丹　蒋　宁
第十七章　温龙波　白嘎丽　蒋　宁
第十八章　白嘎丽　吴　捷　叶　璐　蒋　宁
第十九章　叶　璐　王　昞　蒋　宁
第二十章　王　昞　陈　琳　何元浩　刘陇黔
第二十一章　何元浩　吴以凡　陈　娜　刘陇黔
第二十二章　陈　娜　李世金　张令仪　刘陇黔
第二十三章　张令仪　仁千格麦　刘陇黔
第二十四章　陈晓航　刘陇黔　袁立飞
第二十五章　赵晓燕　孙新成　马君鑫　刘　虎
第二十六章　张　宁　赵方宇　刘陇黔
第二十七章　赵方宇　朱晓鹃　刘陇黔
第二十八章　朱晓鹃　李　霞　黄　雪　刘添添　刘陇黔
测试练习　刘未择　方　严

主审专家简介

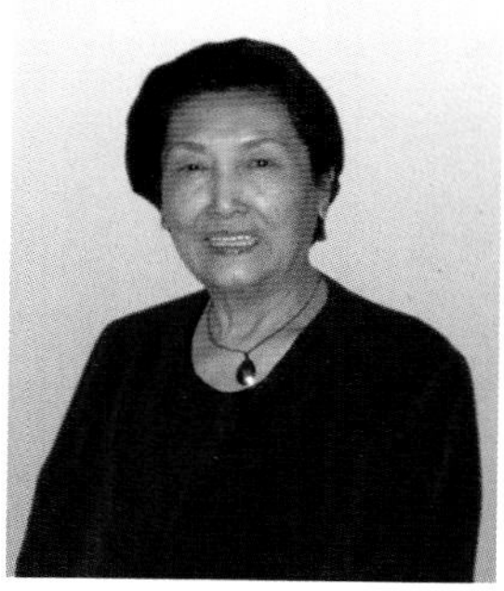

石广礼，教授，主任医师。1954年毕业于西北医学院，是新中国首批大学眼科本科医学生。在西安市中心医院眼科从事医疗教学及科研工作35年，迄今已从医70年（1951 ~ 2020年）。20世纪60年代，兼职西安市卫生局第二医学院及西安市卫生学校的教学工作。历任中华医学会陕西分会眼科学会第二届委员（1976 ~ 1986年）、第三届（1987 ~ 1992年）和第四届（1993 ~ 1997年）主任委员、第五届（1998 ~ 2002年）名誉主任委员，陕西医学会理事，中华医学会眼科学分会第四届（1988 ~ 1991年）、第五届（1992 ~ 1995年）、第六届（1996 ~ 1999年）常务委员。中华医学会资深会员及有突出贡献的专家，陕西省科普作家协会会员。

20世纪70年代中期，主持举办了陕西省眼科学习班，50多名来自陕西省各个地市区县的眼科专业人员参加了培训和学习，她克服了困难，自己刻蜡版，油印教材，组织编写出《眼科讲义（上、下）》，为陕西省基层医院培养出一批眼科专科医生，为基础医院眼科专科的建立和发展奠定了坚实的基础，这批医生中的许多人至今依然在为基层百姓贡献余热。

20世纪70 ~ 80年代初，医学会恢复学术交流工作后，积极开展学术活动，举办近10次五省区、省、市眼科学会年会，每月或季度进行省市学术及医疗经验的交流。组织编写了《眼科临床专题讲座》一书，为眼科学亚专科的形成建立与发展进行了初步探索。并在陕西省率先编写了《眼科医护常规》一书，此书首次提出了国内眼科医生规范化培训纲要和细则，制定了详细的各级医生的年度临床培训和继续教育学习目标、临床标准化操作要领，以及晋升考核计划、模块化及表格化亚专科病历，等等，成为高考恢复后第一批本科生的行医执业指南。

除了完成了繁重的教学和临床工作，还主持了多项科研项目和专利项目，均获省、市科技成果奖。发表论文70余篇，其中获省市论文奖12项。早在20世纪80年代初，就对儿童弱视与产式的关系进行了探讨，提出分娩产式对弱视影响的观点（见《弱视与分娩方式关系的调查分析》，《新医学》，1986年18期第15-16页）。与中国科学院陕西天文台联合，率先在国内开展儿童弱视研究，研制红光电子闪烁仪、三色光闪烁治疗仪、微型光刷弱视治疗仪及实体镜，减少患儿及家属长期往返医院的时间及经济负担，使弱视治疗家庭化，治疗仪器微型化，同时制定了以重建弱视立体视为终极目标的儿童弱视治疗的三部曲，并坚持对重度弱视及大龄弱视进行积极治疗的理念，被近期国际最新的研究成果，即脑中枢功能可塑性的论断所证实。

20世纪80年代中期，参与了国内首个角膜接触镜引进项目，此项目为陕西西北光学仪器厂与美国海昌角膜接触镜公司（为海昌隐形眼镜公司的前身）合作研发。开展了相关的科普教育工作，写出了国内首部关于隐形眼镜的著作《隐形眼镜 100 问》，此书先后 3 次修订发行，为国内角膜接触镜的安全应用和普及推广奠定了基础，获得了省、市科技成果奖。

在西北率先开展显微青光眼减压术、斜视矫正术，并在眼部美容手术方面有独特见地。师承陈达夫先生的中医眼科，对各种眼底病、近视眼底病变及顽固性角膜炎、干眼等主张联合中药治疗。作为“刘石氏饮®”“刘石氏贴®”“近释®”“泪释®”的研发人，与刘光汉、石一宁一起历经数十年研发，提出了独到的中药散剂临床应用方法，探讨出中药治疗眼底病及近视眼底改变的治疗组方，与陈卓、陈研明一起研发出无添加辅料的药食同源的中药新剂型。

从医 70 年来，花费大量时间和精力进行眼科医学的科学知识普及，编写科普书籍 10 余本，如《青光眼防治 100 问》《白内障防治 100 问》《近视眼防治 100 问》《常见眼病防治 100 问》《隐形眼镜 100 问》等，获陕西省 1996 年优秀科普作品奖。另外为现代家庭医疗保健出版的“十万个为什么”丛书撰写了眼科部分，受到家长们的欢迎。

在儿童青少年近视防控理念和措施方面，对初发近视，特别是调节性近视的儿童，应首选视功能的康复训练与应用中医等方法，来控制近视的发展速度，而不应该首次就诊即配发眼镜，即使配发眼镜后，依然要求家长树立近视控制的理念，追踪随访，这个观点现在依然是国家顶层设计的指导思想。

审校组专家简介（以翻译章节为序）

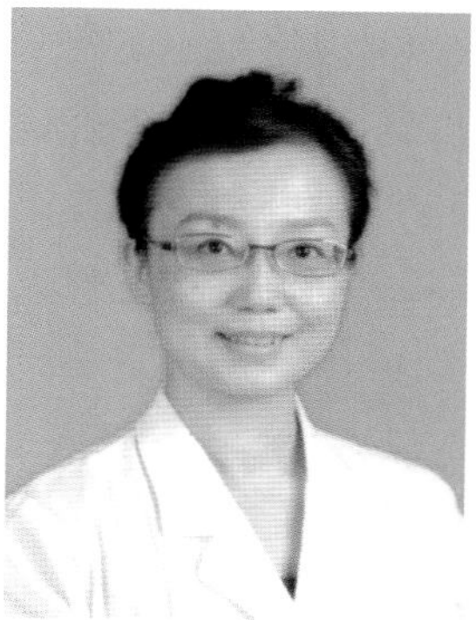

布娟，北京大学第三医院眼科，主任医师。中国医师协会眼科学分会斜视与小儿眼科专委会委员、中国医师协会青春期医学专业委员会青春期眼保健学组委员、北京眼科学会斜视与小儿眼科分委会常务委员、中国女医师协会眼科专委会斜弱视学组委员、北京市自然科学基金委员会评审专家、美国约翰霍普金斯医院威尔玛眼科研究所访问学者。主要从事成人斜视与儿童常见眼病的临床及科研教学工作，致力于青少年近视防控、弱视的个性化治疗、斜视微创手术、先天性眼球震颤的手术治疗等的研究。主持 1 项国家自然科学基金项目、1 项北京市科委创新课题项目、2 项北京大学林护基金项目、1 项北京大学第三医院种子基金项目。作为主要参加人员参与了 4 项国家自然科学基金项目和 1 项北京市自然科学基金项目的研究工作，以第一作者的身份在 The American Journal of Human Genetics、Molecular Vision、Indian J Ophthalmol 及国内核心期刊发表多篇文章。

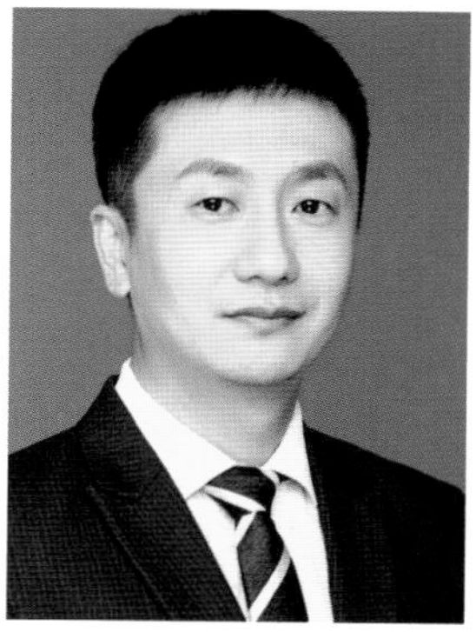

钱学翰，天津医科大学眼科医院，斜视与小儿眼科科主任，眼科学博士、硕士生导师，副主任医师。美国斜视与小儿眼科学会（AAPOS）国际委员，亚太斜视与小儿眼科（ASPOS) 委员，中华医学会眼科学分会斜视与小儿眼科学组委员。国家公派访问学者，赴美国进修斜视、弱视、近视等儿童眼科疾病，完成北美斜视与小儿眼科学会的中国培训项目，在美国期间，获优秀教学奖及社区眼科服务杰出贡献奖。回国后一直从事斜视与小儿眼科工作，有着数万余例门诊及手术治疗经历，经验丰富。带教国内外学生及进修医生 200 余人，发表学术论文 10 余篇，参加完成国家自然科学基金项目 2 项、市级科研课题项目多项。擅长成人与儿童的各种复杂性斜视及小儿常见眼病的诊断与治疗，自 2014 年起组建团队开展大规模儿童眼病筛查工作，建立了全国儿童眼病筛查网，将大数据、互联网及无纸化技术应用到儿童眼病筛查中，实现远程指导异地筛查数十万余人。创办“瞳心儿童眼病基金”，从事志愿服务近 20 年，组织大大小小 500 余次义诊活动，拥有丰富的团队培训管理经验，荣获第十一届中国优秀青年志愿者称号。连续 4 年组织并带领全国范围内首支赴西藏地区针对儿童眼病开展大规模筛查公益志愿服务团队圆满完成治疗及转诊服务，不仅为西藏地区儿童眼科提供了“精准帮扶”，也一举填补了西藏地区儿童眼病基础性数据的空白。

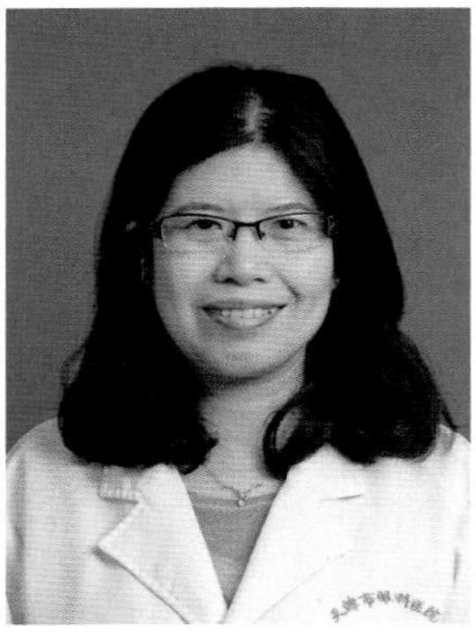

丁娟，天津市眼科医院，斜视与小儿眼科专业医学博士，副主任医师。中国医师协会神经修复专委会视觉修复学组委员，天津市生物医学工程学会眼科医学工程专业委员会委员。毕业于天津医科大学，师从我国著名眼科学专家赵堪兴教授。美国威斯康星大学眼科与视觉科学系任访问学者，接受国际著名小儿眼科专家 Bruton J Kushner 教授的系统专业指导。擅长小儿眼科斜视、弱视、视觉发育等疾病的诊断治疗。参与完成国家自然科学基金项目 2 项，天津市科委课题 1 项。发表国内外学术论文 10 余篇，其中 2 篇以第一作者身份被 SCI 收录。参编《眼科学》第七版、第八版，《斜视弱视学》（人民卫生出版社）。参译《斜视手术病例解析》《Harley 小儿眼科学》。

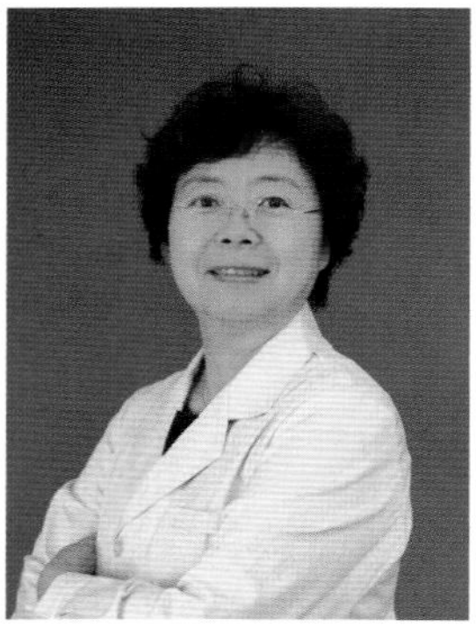

朱丹，主任医师、教授、医学博士，硕士研究生导师。内蒙古医科大学附属医院眼科主任，从事眼底病专业工作。在北京大学医学部获得硕士学位和博士学位；美国 TUFTS 大学医学院博士后，日本山梨大学医学院访问学者。任中华医学会眼科分会委员，眼底病学组委员，中国医师协会眼科学分会常委，内蒙古医学会眼科学会主任委员，内蒙古医师协会眼科学分会会长。任《中华眼科杂志》《中华眼底病杂志》《中华实验眼科杂志》《中华眼外伤职业眼病杂志》《中华眼科医学杂志》编委。承担国家自然科学基金项目 2 项，国家精准医学重大项目子课题 1 项，近 3 年发表 SCI 论文 10 篇，参编眼科学教材 3 部。“中华医学会奖”“草原英才”获得者。

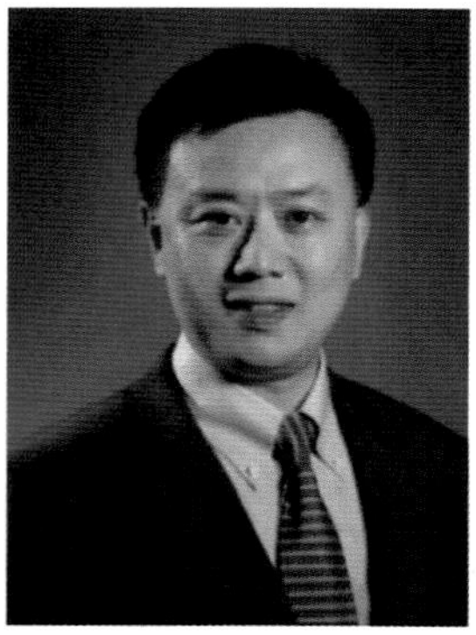

刘虎，医学博士、主任医师、教授、博士生导师，现任中华医学会眼科学分会斜视与小儿眼科学组副组长、中国医师协会眼科医师分会斜视与儿童眼病专业委员会副主任委员、江苏省医学会眼科学分会副主任委员。专业方向为斜视与小儿眼科。

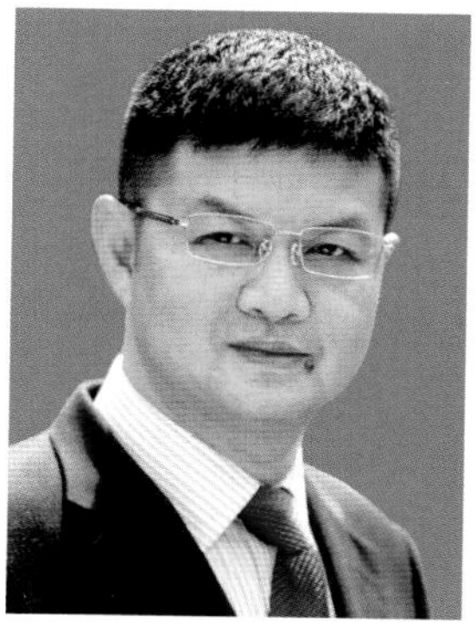

刘陇黔，教授，博士生导师，四川大学华西临床医学院眼视光学系主任兼眼科副主任。四川省学术技术带头人、四川省卫生健康首席专家，中华眼科学会视光学组、斜视与小儿眼科学组委员，中国医师协会委员兼视光学组委员，中国医促会眼视觉保健分会常委，四川省眼视光学学会会长，四川医学会眼科专委会前任主任委员及视光学组长，四川省医师协会眼科分会会长，四川预防医学会眼视觉保健分会主任委员、四川医促会眼视觉保健专委会主任委员，中国妇幼保健协会儿童眼保健专业委员会特邀专家组成员，中国眼镜行业 / 中国眼镜科技杂志高级视光学专家顾问；国际角膜塑形镜协会亚洲分会中国指导委员会专家委员，视觉发育视光师协会（COVD）中国第一个学术资深会员。《中华眼科杂志》《中国斜视与小儿眼科杂志》《Optometry and Vision Science》中文版等杂志编委。四川大学视光学教育和四川省视光学学科的创始人。培养研究生 70 多人，其中博士 18 人。承担科技部、省部级和国际合作多项课题，发表文章 180 多篇，被 SCI 收录 40 多篇，参编或主编专著教材 15 本。

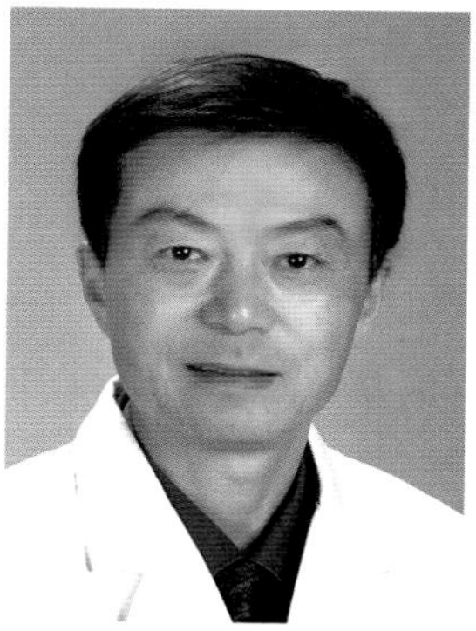

方严，安徽理工大学第一附属医院、第一临床学院名誉院长，安徽理工大学眼科研究所所长、研究员、教授、主任医师，安徽医科大学主办的《临床眼科杂志》执行主编，博士生导师。安徽省眼科学会主任委员，中华医学会眼科学分会青光眼学组委员，中国医师协会眼科医师分会常委。九三学社中央委员。主编《病理性近视眼眼底改变》(国家科学技术学术著作出版基金资助)等学术专著8部。

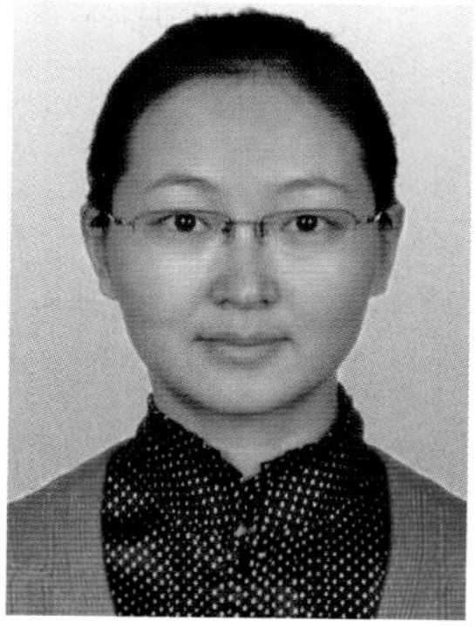

蒋宁，西北妇女儿童医院，儿科主治医师。2010 年毕业于四川大学华西临床医学院临床医学（7 年制）专业，2020 年毕业于西安交通大学医学部，获儿科学博士学位。在攻读博士学位期间参与完成国家自然科学基金项目 1 项，发表 SCI 论文 2 篇。目前从事儿科常见病与多发病的临床和科研工作，擅长儿童血液及消化系统疾病的诊断与治疗。

主译简介

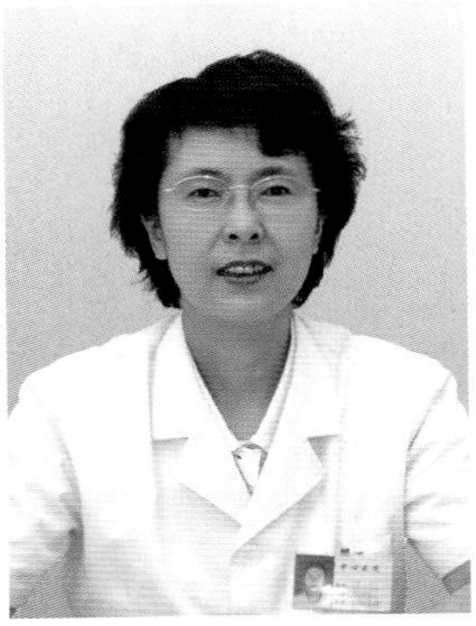

石一宁，教授，主任医师，西安交通大学研究生导师。陕西省有突出贡献专家、国务院特殊津贴专家。第十、十一、十二届政协西安市常委。

45 年来，一直从事眼科临床、科研及教学工作，共发表论文 100 余篇，参与及撰写专著 13 部，科技成果奖 14 项。

20 多年来，主要在儿童青少年近视的预测预警防控和高度近视及其严重并发症的防治 2 个方面进行了深入研究，并致力于中国近视防控的科普宣传。提出了中国儿童青少年近视形成机制的再认知——学前 3 ~ 6 岁的过度正视化过程的"二次发育理论"以及眼球过长的"眼内扩张理论"；梳理出近视形成的 5 大机制（生物几何光学机制、生物力学机制、生物光学机制、生物化学机制、生物学机制）；提出了近视控制关键点；提出了近视早发现、早控制、早治疗的创新性概念——"隐性近视"；首次提出综合评估眼生长发育的 11 项参数，根据 Gullsrand 模型眼进行逆向分解，制订出近视进展的量化预测系统和预警机制；量化描述了近视常见眼底改变，建立了临床简易可行的眼底观察指标；根据眼生物参数，提出了进展预测系统和预警机制，即眼健康的三级监测和近视防控的三级预警，以及七级眼健康档案和中国眼健康年度蓝皮书；提出了一揽子计划——近视防控体系，其中包括近视的连续性防控思想（3 阶段、5 要点、10 步曲）、近视的个性化防控设计（6 种状态、10 道防线）、其中包括近视的综合性防控理念（2 理论、4 要点、5 方面、10 项措施），以及模块化设计（儿童青少年眼健康 6 种状态和 6 道防线的 36 个模块化防控细则）。

5 年多来，以新的模式"眼健康工作室"作为实践基地，实现近视防控规范流程的完善和推广，探索近视防控体系的落实和发现和解决近视防控中的问题及解决方案。准备用 15 年时间追踪观察眼健康趋势、预测控制近视的形成和发展，从根本上有效遏制中国儿童青少年视觉健康的恶化现状。

于 1994 年起出版了《角膜接触镜 100 问》《隐形眼镜常识 100 问》《近视眼防治 100 问》（1998 年），《防治近视三岁抓起》（2010 年）和《拒绝近视，石一宁大夫有话说》（2016 年）等近视防控科普书。编辑和撰写《中国儿童青少年近视形成机制以及预测与防控》（2013 年）、《病理性近视眼眼底改变》（2014 年）、《中国儿童青少年近视防控流程的建议：近视防控共识》（2017 年）等近视防控专著。创新性采用中英文对照格式，翻译出版了德国 Klaus Schmid 的《近视手册 Myopia Manual 2017》（2018 年），以及美国眼科学会（AAO）的《基础与临床科学教程 BCSC——第 3 册 临床光学 Clinical Optics 2018–2019》（2019 年）和《第 6 册 小儿眼科学与斜视 Pediatric Ophthalmology and Strabismus 2019–2020》（2020 年）。

翻译组译者简介（以翻译章节为序）

翻译组

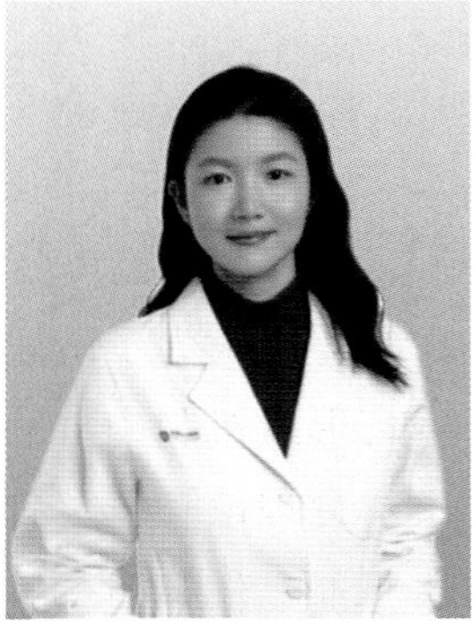

唐志萍，眼科学博士，副主任医师，就职于上海贝瞳眼科。1999年毕业于北京医科大学，主要从事眼科临床工作，对视网膜、视神经的损伤及保护进行了大量研究。上海市社会医疗机构眼科专委会委员，上海市长宁区社会医疗机构眼科专委会委员，云南省女医师协会眼科专业分委会委员，出版专著7本（人民卫生出版社），参译著作2本。获2015年云南科技厅科技一等奖，2016年云南省科技进步一等奖。

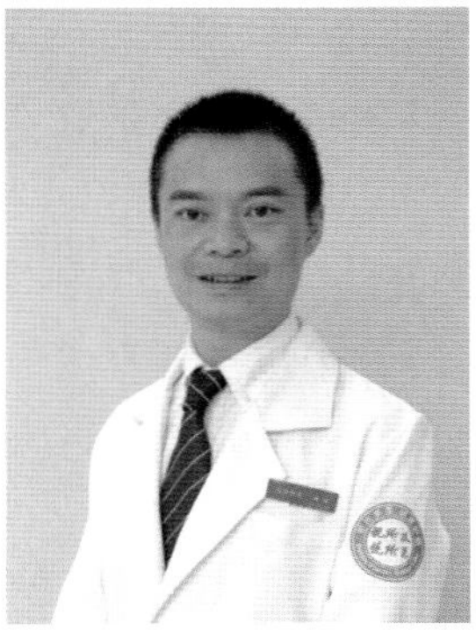

梅颖，上海新虹桥国际医学园区眼科中心业务院长，副主任医师。国际近视防控和角膜塑形学会资深会员（FIAOMC），国际角膜塑形学会亚洲分会资深会员（SIAOA），美国视觉训练和发展学会会员（COVD）。上海眼视光学研究中心学术委员，上海青少年近视眼防控专家联盟成员，中国标准化技术委员会眼镜验配服务分技术委员会委员，中国妇幼保健协会儿童眼保健分会委员。中国医学装备协会眼科专业委员，中山眼科中心技术培训中心客座讲师，中国卫生信息与健康医疗大数据学会委员，中国医师协会眼科分会青年后备人才。上海市社会医疗机构协会健康教育促进分会常务委员，《丁香园》特约作者，《中国眼镜科技杂志》专栏作者，眼视光英才计划“明日之星”成员，《中国临床医生杂志》特约编委。

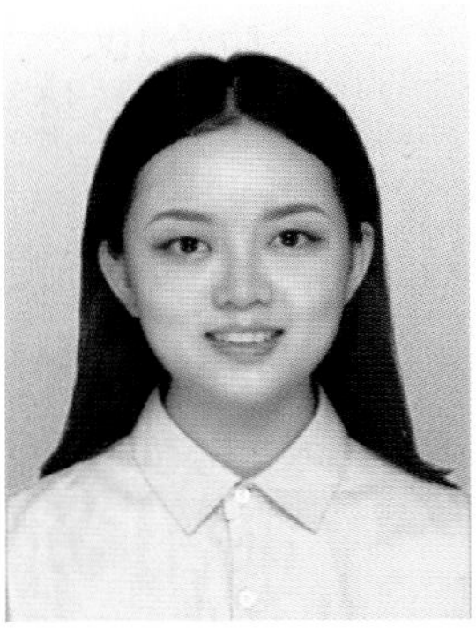

刘凤阳，就职于贵州省人民医院眼视光科。国际角膜塑形镜学会亚洲分会（IAOA）会员。2018年四川大学医学技术专业（眼视光学方向）硕士毕业，在校期间曾到香港理工大学眼科视光学院交流学习。发表SCI论文1篇，临床研究方向为近视、双眼视、角膜接触镜，师从我国知名眼科专家刘陇黔教授。参与翻译《临床光学》一书。

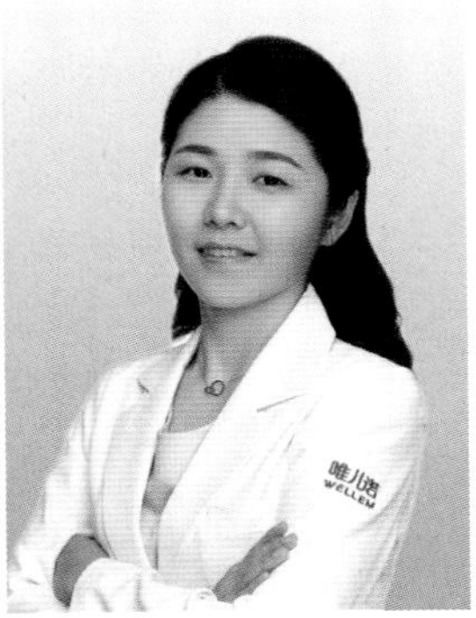

汪晓倩，复旦大学眼科学硕士，上海唯宜儿科诊所副院长，唯儿诺医疗集团医师委员会成员，江阴市中小学生近视眼防控中心主任，国际角膜塑形镜学会亚洲分会（IAOA）会员。既往执业于复旦大学附属眼耳鼻喉科医院、同济大学附属东方医院。师从褚仁远、瞿小妹教授，专业方向为近视防控、斜弱视非手术治疗、儿童常见眼病诊治。参与编写教材《眼病学》，参与翻译《临床光学》《近视手册》等。

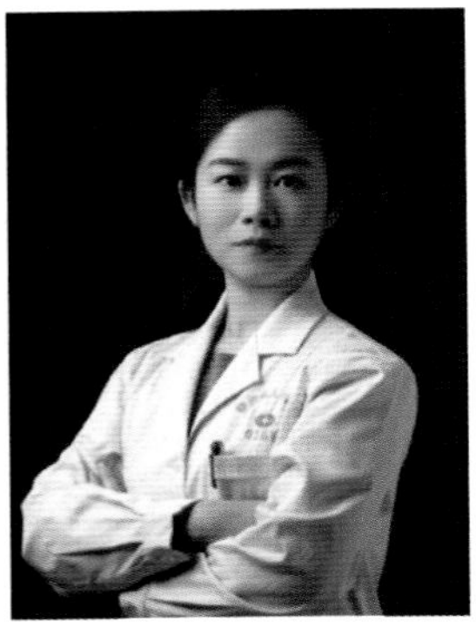

张乐，副主任医师，医学博士，硕士生导师。陕西省人民医院眼科住培基地教学主任，陕西省儿童福利会理事，西安医学会眼科学分会青年委员，西安医学会眼科学分会儿童眼病学组组员，国际角膜塑形术协会亚洲分会会员，陕西省保健协会青少年视力保健与视光学专业委员会委员。获英国格鲁斯特大学颁发的“国际糖网阅片师”资格。主要专业方向为斜弱视及小儿眼科、儿童视觉发育及复杂眼底疾病的诊治。主持省厅级自然科学基金及社会发展基金项目 2 项，参与完成国家自然科学基金项目 3 项。在 SCI 及中文核心期刊发表论文 10 余篇。

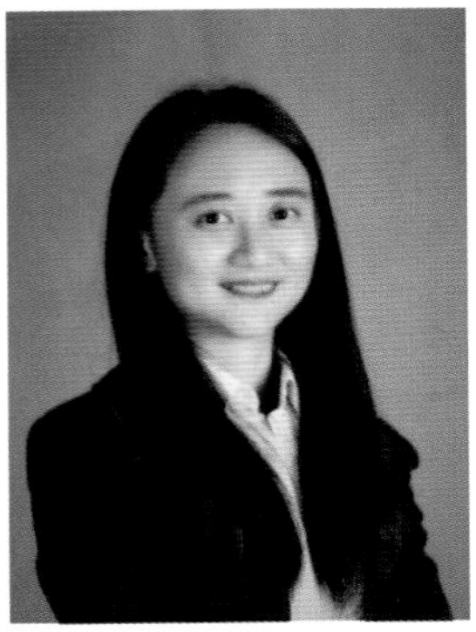

刘念，中山医科大学眼科视光学系首届毕业生，美国 Salus 大学宾西法尼亚视光学院临床视光学硕士。全国验光与配镜职业教育教学指导委员会委员，中国视光学发展教育计划教师，中国眼镜协会视光师分会会员，全国高职高专教材评审委员会委员，全国中职教材评审委员会主任委员，广东省视光学会常务委员，中山眼科培训中心客座讲师，IACLE 会员。现就职于广州市商贸职业学校，高级讲师，市级名师，市级专业带头人。主持制定全国中职眼视光与配镜专业教学标准，主编全国中职“十二五”规划教材，主持市级精品课程。

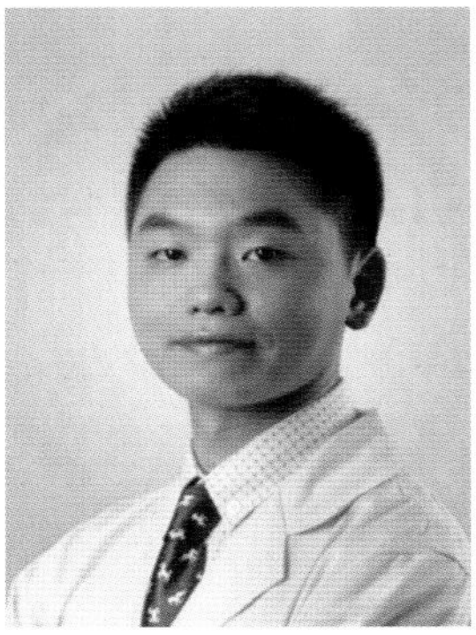

杨嘉嵩，主治医师，中南大学爱尔眼科学院博士研究生，师从国内著名眼科专家李文生教授。在高度近视眼底病变领域进行深入的研究。硕士师从于河南省眼科研究所院长著名眼底病专家宋宗明教授。开展各类玻璃体视网膜手术、白内障手术以及各类眼底疾病的诊治。多次应邀在全国会议发言交流，在国内外发表多篇专业论文。

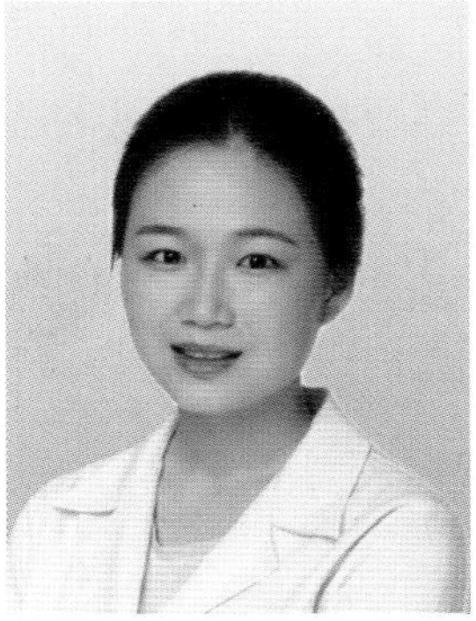

龚慧，中医眼科学硕士研究生，2017 年 6 月毕业于广州中医药大学，方向为眼视光学，目前工作于深圳市眼科医院，临床工作以小儿斜弱视诊治、青少年近视防控、视功能训练、低视力康复为主。

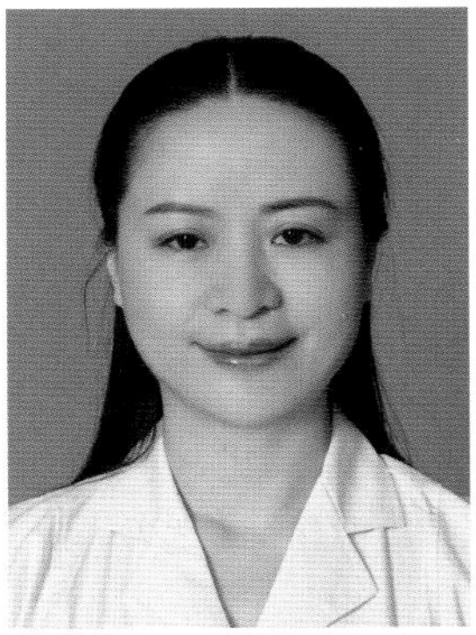

谭薇，遵义市第一人民医院（即遵义医科大学第三附属医院）副院长，医学博士，主任医师，硕士研究生导师。中国康复医学会视觉康复专委会常委，贵州省医学会毕业后医学教育分会常委，中华医学会贵州省分会眼科学专委会常委，遵义市医学会眼科学分会主任委员，遵义市眼科临床医学中心主任。从事眼科临床、教学、科研工作近 30 年，主要从事视光学和白内障的临床治疗和基础研究。擅长各种屈光手术及复杂性白内障的手术治疗。

作为项目负责人主持国家自然科学基金项目 1 项、省部级课题 2 项及地厅级课题项目 4 项。发表论文 40 余篇，其中被 SCI 收录 7 篇。

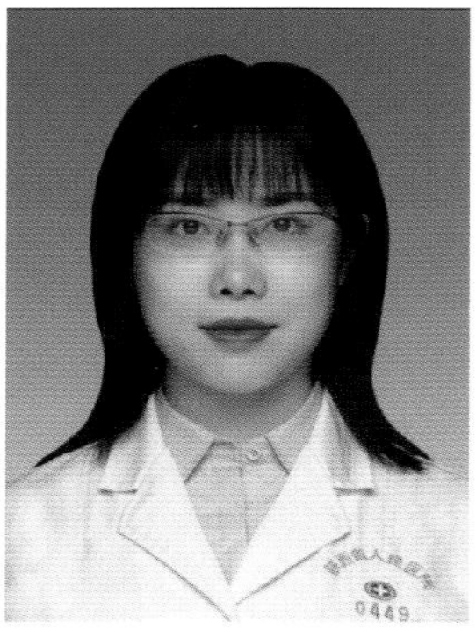

杨乐，医学硕士，陕西省人民医院眼科副主任医师，毕业于山东大学医学院。陕西省保健协会防盲专业委员会委员，陕西省医师协会眼科分会委员。擅长儿童及青少年近视防治，以及眼表疾病、葡萄膜炎、视网膜及视神经疾病、青光眼、白内障等眼科常见疾病的诊治。主持并参与省级科研基金项目 4 项。以第一作者及通讯作者身份在核心期刊发表论文 10 余篇。参编著作 2 部（《病理性近视眼眼底改变》《中国儿童青少年近视形成机制以及预测与防控》），参编翻译著作 1 部（《近视手册》）。

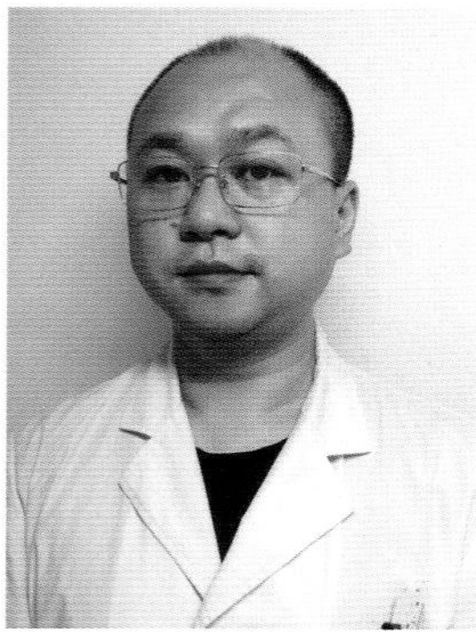

刘建，双本科学位，美国视光协会会员，一级视光师，现就职于成都爱眼坊视光有限公司。从事眼视光临床工作 10 余年，有丰富的临床眼视光及初级眼保健工作经验。擅长于儿童与青少年近视预防与控制、各类屈光不正的矫正、双眼视及视觉训练、角膜接触镜验配、低视力验配等。

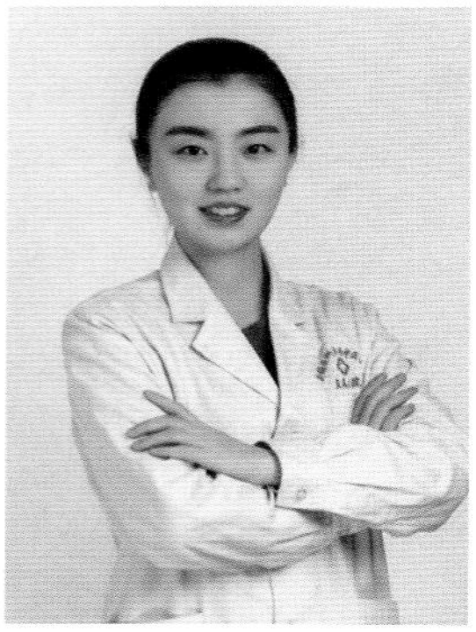

芮莹，擅长生物测量仪检测技术，从事儿童青少年视力康复工作 7 年。长年开展系统性近视防控工作，已帮助数万名中小学及高校在校学生建立眼健康档案。在视力筛查、近视发生年龄的预测、高度近视相关并发症预警等方面经验丰富。2017 年，采用中医诊治与新疆地域、饮食相结合疗法，在中小学生缓解视疲劳、预防近视产生等方面取得良好效果。2018 年参加全国首次儿童青少年近视调查工作，广受好评。

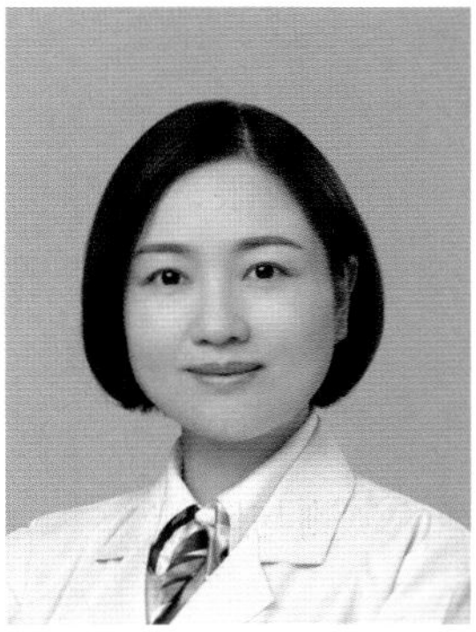

马玉红，硕士研究生，国家卫生部认证 PRK/LASIK 手术医师，高级验光师。曾任甘肃省武威医学科学院眼科主任，后兼任爱尔眼科医院屈光科主任、小儿眼科主任。从事眼科专业 17 年，先后师从国内小儿眼病专家赵堪兴、李丽华以及屈光手术专家王雁教授学习眼视光学、斜弱视及屈光手术。擅长白内障手术、斜视矫正手术、各类屈光矫正手术及眼视光技术应用。主持地市级科研课题 2 项，发表论文 6 篇。

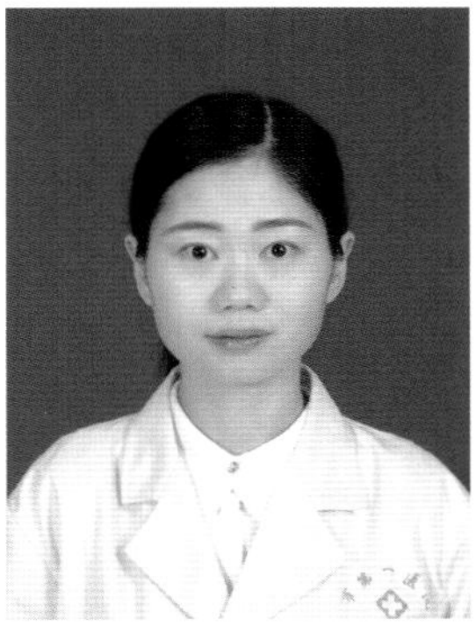

孙西宇，主治医师，眼科学硕士，毕业于温州医科大学附属眼视光学院。现任职于西安市第一医院眼科、激光近视治疗中心，主要从事角膜屈光手术及角膜胶原交联手术的相关研究，擅长近视、远视及散光的矫正与治疗，角膜塑形镜及硬性透氧性角膜接触镜（RGP）的验配，以及常见眼表疾病的诊断及治疗。

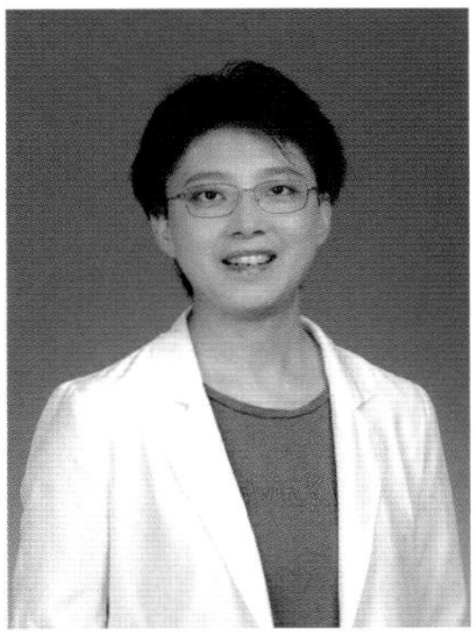

张哲，副主任医师，中国医师协会眼科医师分会青年委员，中国老年医学会眼科分会青年委员，山西省医学会眼科分会白内障学组委员，山西省医学会眼科分会青年委员，“三晋英才”青年优秀人才，美国白内障屈光手术学会会员。首都医科大学附属北京同仁医院眼科学硕士，天津医科大学天津市眼科医院博士，2011 年在日本埼玉县小儿医疗中心眼科研修。获得山西省科技进步二等奖 1 项、三等奖 1 项。发表 SCI 论文 5 篇、国家级论文 20 余篇。主持省级科研项目 2 项。先后在国际眼科会议进行大会发言交流 10 余次。

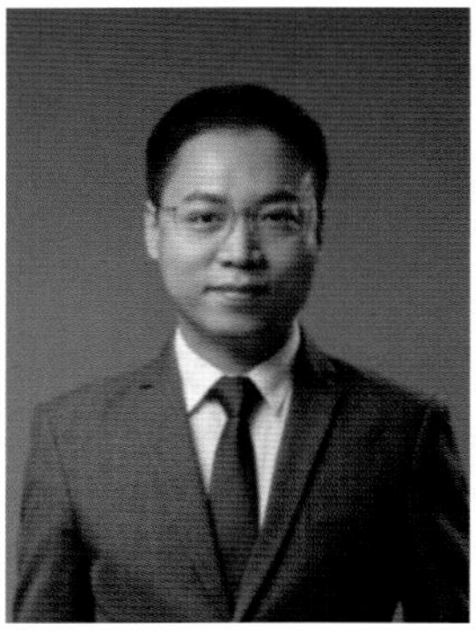

许志强，医师，验光技师，AOA会员，IAOA会员。目前就职于铂林眼科山西门诊，主要从事儿童青少年眼健康相关工作。曾先后就读于山西医科大学临床医学系、湖北科技学院眼视光系。曾赴美国伊利诺伊州立视光学院、加州大学伯克利分校视光学院交流学习。师从我国知名眼科专家石一宁教授、张丽军教授。参与编译视光学专著2部，通过各种平台发布科普文章多篇。

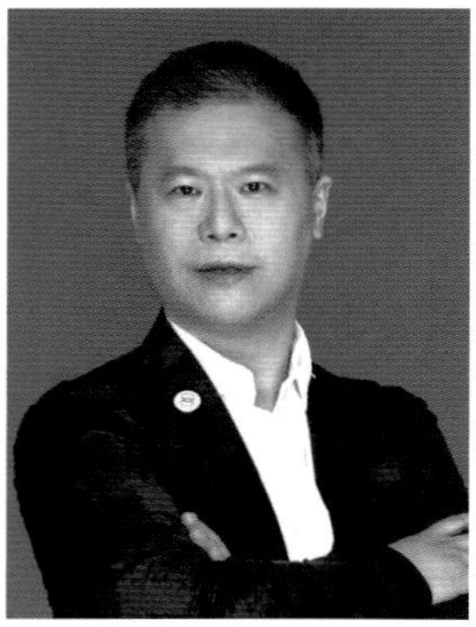

王文军，医学博士，西安市人民医院眼视光中心副主任医师。儿童眼科专家，专治各类儿童斜弱视、屈光不正。擅长早产儿视网膜病变筛查、诊断及治疗，青少年近视防控。曾获得陕西省科技进步二等奖，主持省、市级科技研究项目3项，参编专著3部，获得国家实用新型专利2项。西安医学院视光学专业特邀讲师。曾赴法国及美国短期研修。兼任国际角膜塑形镜学会亚洲分会资深会员，陕西省妇促会视光学分会理事兼秘书长，陕西省医学会新生儿分会早产儿学组委员，陕西省妇幼保健与优生优育协会儿童眼保健专业委员会委员，西安医学会眼科学分会常委，《中国妇幼健康》杂志编委。

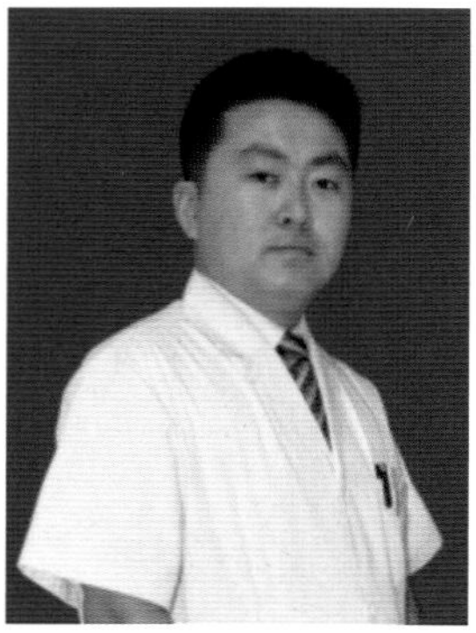

姚森，医师，AOA会员，IAOA会员，毕业于河北工程大学医学部。美国新英格兰视光学院和纽约州立大学视光学院访问学者，曾于河北省眼科医院（邢台眼科医院）完成3年眼科各亚专业进修学习，于天津医科大学及医大早稻田培训学校进行眼视光学相关培训学习。目前主要从事小儿眼科斜弱视及近视防治工作。

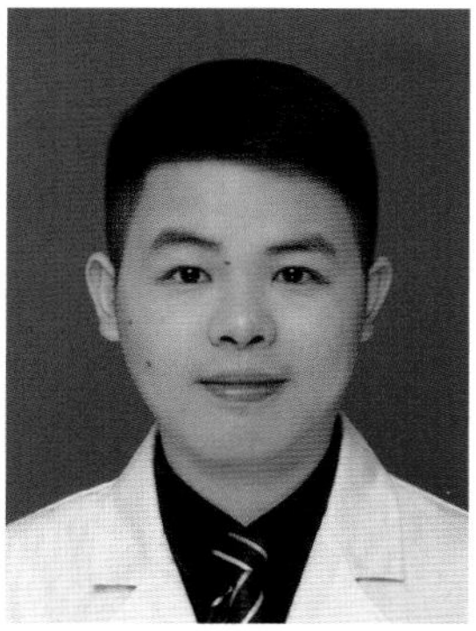

温龙波，眼科学博士，现就职于湖南爱尔眼视光研究所。全球首款近视防控智能可穿戴设备“云夹”的核心研发人员。主持“中南大学研究生自由探索”项目2项，参与多项省部级重点课题研究工作。连续4年获邀在ARVO年会上进行展示（2016~2019年），并荣获2019年ARVO International Travel Grant，连续两年获得“全国眼科年会优秀论文奖”（2017年、2018年），1篇研究论文入选2017年度眼视光学组十大科研亮点。参译专著《近视手册》，参编近视科普书籍《让孩子远离近视》。发表SCI论文4篇、CSCD论文2篇。作为共同发明人获国家发明专利5项、实用新型专利7项，荣获2018年“中国眼视光年度团队奖”。

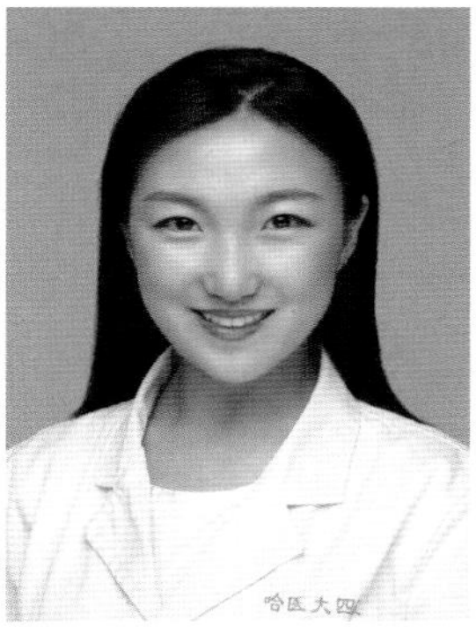

白嘎丽，医师，毕业于哈尔滨医科大学，在校期间曾赴俄罗斯阿穆尔医科大学附属医院交流学习，现就职于哈尔滨医科大学附属第四医院眼视光门诊部。

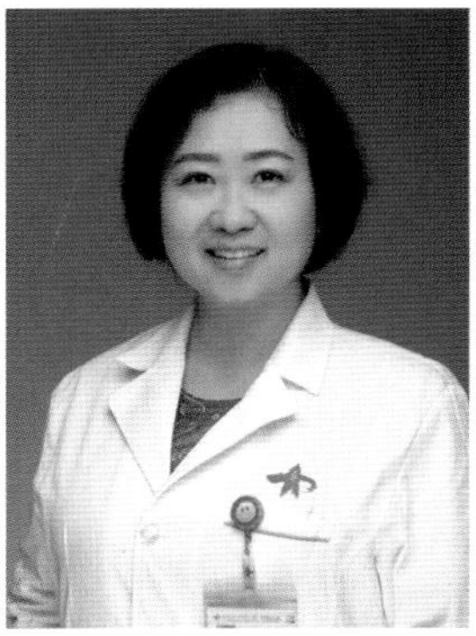

吴捷，眼科学博士，毕业于中山大学中山眼科中心。主要从事青少年近视眼防治、准分子激光屈光手术、硬性角膜接触镜、角膜塑形镜和弱视等视光学方面的研究。主持参与国家级、省市级、院校级科技攻关项目8项。发表SCI文章4篇、核心期刊文章8篇。开展“硬性角膜接触镜及角膜塑形镜”新医疗新技术研究项目2项，获发明专利1项。现为西安医学会第一届眼视光学分会常务委员，陕西省医学会眼科分会视光学与屈光手术学组委员，陕西省医学会激光医学分会青年委员，陕西省保健协会青少年视力保健与视光学专业委员会常务委员，国际角膜塑形学会资深会员（FIAO）国际角膜塑形学会亚洲分会资深会员（SIAOA）。

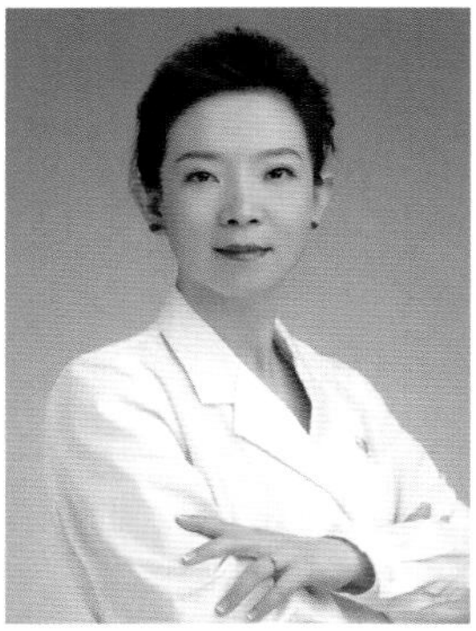

叶璐，女，主任医师。现任陕西省眼科医院、西安市第四医院眼科病院视光中心主任、眼屈光与眼保健专业主任，陕西省视光疾病临床医学研究中心常务副主任。陕西省妇促会视光与视觉健康专业委员会主任委员，陕西省医师协会眼科医师分会常务委员，西安市医学会眼视光学分会副主任委员，国际角膜塑形镜学会亚洲分会（IAOA）会员，中国女医师协会专委会视光学组委员，中国医学装备协会眼科专业委员会第二届委员，《中华眼科杂志》编委。

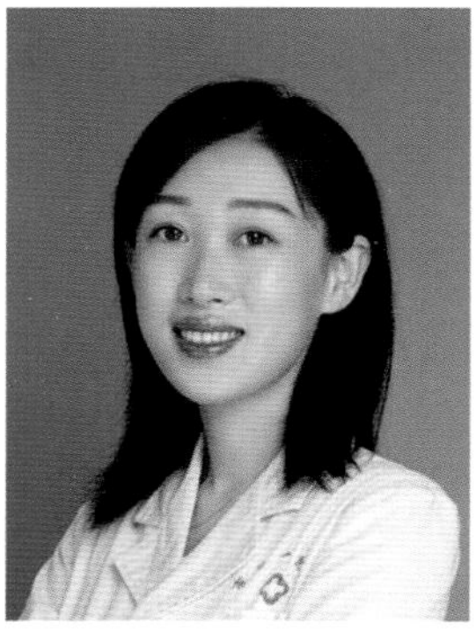

王昞，女，1986年，西安市第一医院眼科副主任医师，毕业于上海同济大学，眼科学硕士。从事眼科临床工作近10年，先后发表中文核心期刊论文4篇、SCI论文1篇，对小儿眼科及斜弱视相关疾病的诊断及治疗有丰富的经验。曾参加于加拿大举行的第23届虚拟医学及网络心理学会议，做大会发言《The relationship between amblypoia visual spatial resolution and binocular perceptual eye position in a pediatric population》。

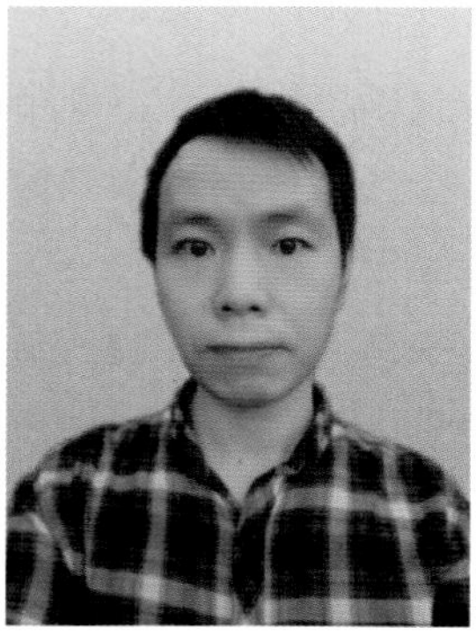

陈琳，主治医师，四川大学华西临床医学院与哈佛医学院联合培养博士在读，本科毕业于四川大学华西临床医学院，硕士研究生毕业于温州医科大学眼视光学院。现任遵义医科大学附属医院眼科暨贵州省眼科医院近视眼白内障治疗中心主治医师。主要从事眼科角膜疾病、青少年近视防控、屈光不正及白内障的诊断和治疗。

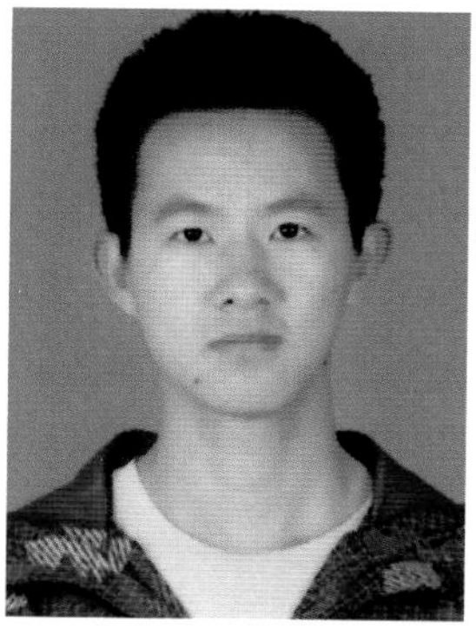

何元浩，本科毕业于四川大学眼视光学专业，现就读于四川大学华西临床医学院，眼视光学系硕士研究生在读，导师为刘陇黔教授。目前研究方向为角膜塑形镜。

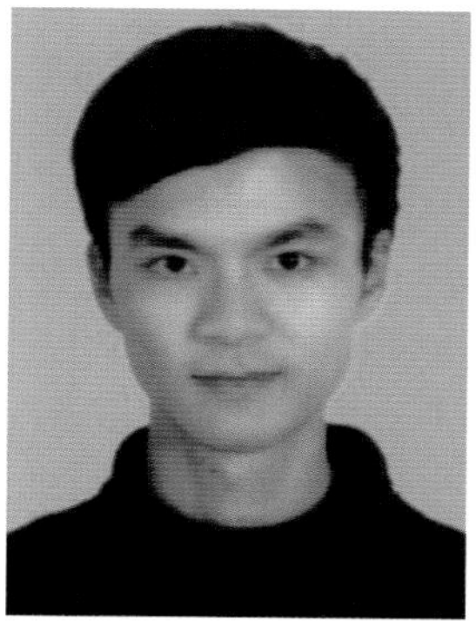

吴以凡，本科毕业于四川大学华西临床医学院眼视光学系，本科期间曾赴美国 Western University of Health and Science 交流学习。现通过推免于四川大学华西临床医学院眼视光学系硕博连读在读，为香港理工大学眼视光学院和四川大学联合培养博士，师从国内著名小儿眼科及斜弱视专家刘陇黔教授。目前的研究方向为近视、角膜接触镜。

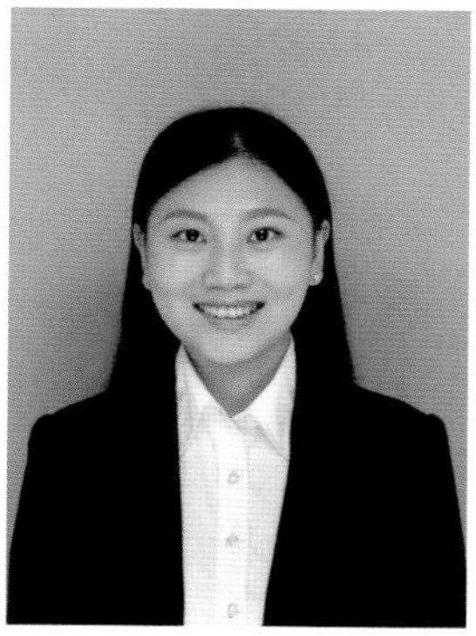

陈娜，本科毕业于四川大学眼视光学专业，2017 年经推免进入四川大学华西临床医学院攻读眼视光学硕士，导师为刘陇黔教授，研究方向主要为近视及双眼视。参与多项科研项目，发表 SCI 论文 1 篇。

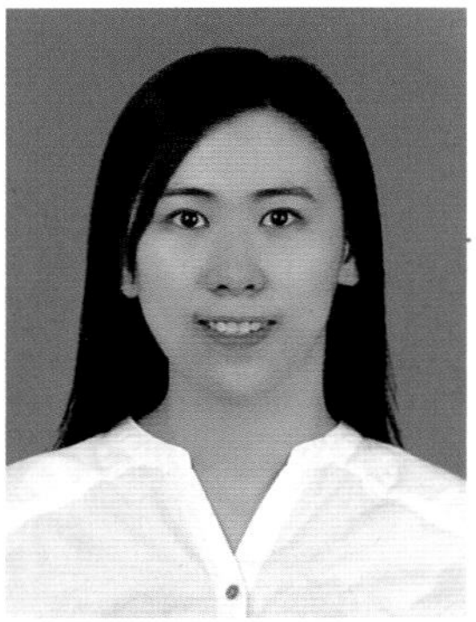

李世金，23 岁，2018 年本科毕业于天津医科大学眼视光学院，目前为四川大学华西临床医学院医技专业视光方向硕士研究生在读，师从刘陇黔教授，主要研究方向为双眼视。

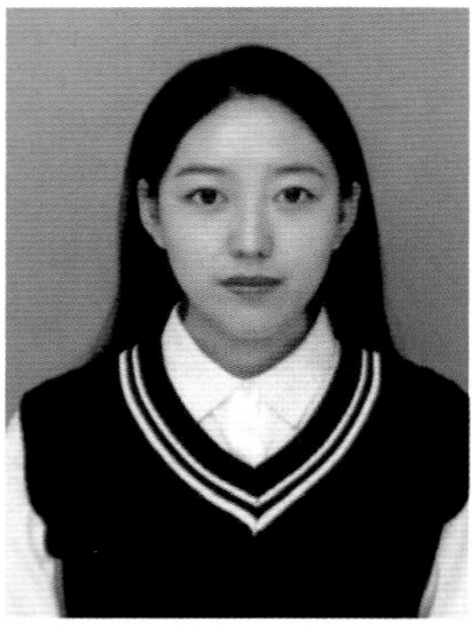

张令仪，女，本科毕业于天津医科大学，获得眼视光学和公共事业管理双学位。本科期间赴香港理工大学访问实习。曾多次获得校级奖学金，并于 2016 年获得豪雅一等奖学金。已有 1 篇论文被国内期刊收录。2017 年推免保送至四川大学华西临床医学院，师从国内著名小儿眼科专家刘陇黔教授，获得 2020 届“优秀研究生毕业生”称号。

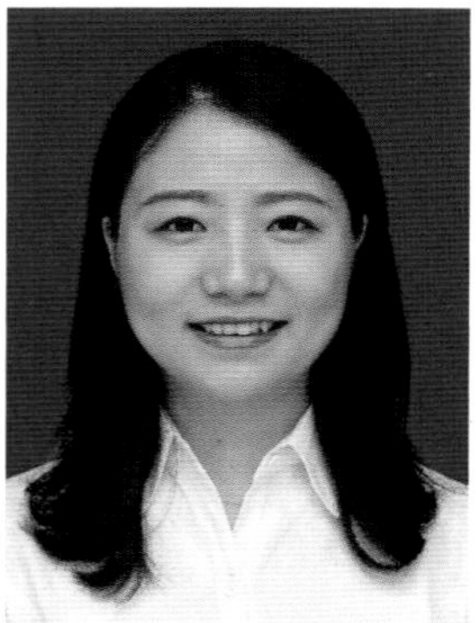

仁千格麦，女，现四川大学华西医院眼科技师。2012 年本科毕业于川北医学院眼视光学系。2020 年硕士毕业于四川大学华西临床医学院眼视光学系，师从国内著名小儿眼科专家刘陇黔教授。擅长各种疑难屈光不正的处理以及角膜塑形镜、RGP 的验配。发表 SCI 论文 1 篇。

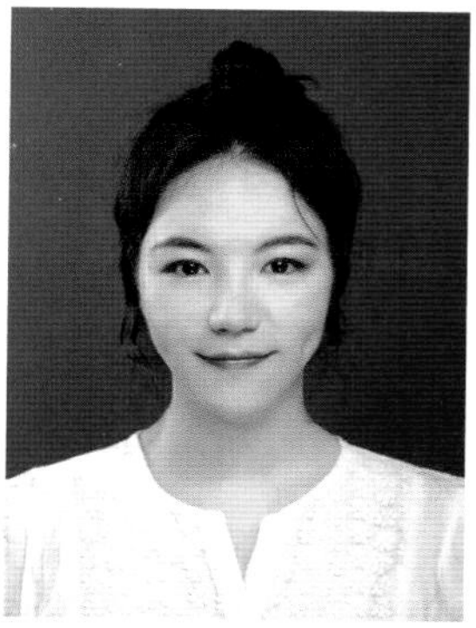

陈晓航，四川大学华西临床医学院眼视光博士，师从国内著名斜弱视与小儿眼科专家刘陇黔教授。研究方向为近视、斜视与弱视的临床表现及发病机制。截至 2020 年 7 月已参与发表文章 3 篇，参编书籍 1 部。近年来，积极参与国内大型斜弱视和视光学术会议，并做大会发言和壁报交流，曾多次参与重大科研项目申报及研究，担任大型眼视光类学术会议同声翻译、交替传译等，擅长视光专业知识的科普工作。

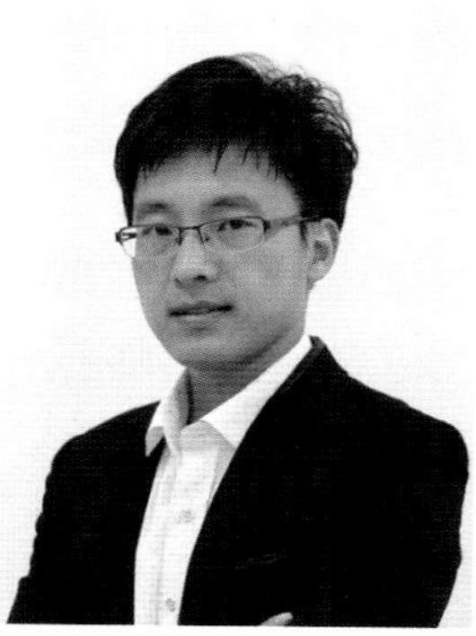

袁立飞，主治医师，眼科学硕士。毕业于天津医科大学，现就职于河北省眼科医院，主要从事眼底病、眼底影像诊断与激光治疗。参与省市级科研项目 3 项、国家自然基金项目 1 项，发表临床和科研论文 8 篇，其中 SCI 论文 3 篇。获河北省医学科技进步一等奖 1 项。现任中国民族医药学会眼科分会理事，河北省中西医结合学会眼科分会常务委员兼秘书，邢台市医学会眼科专业委员会委员兼秘书。2019 年被评为河北省“三三三人才工程”第三层次人选。

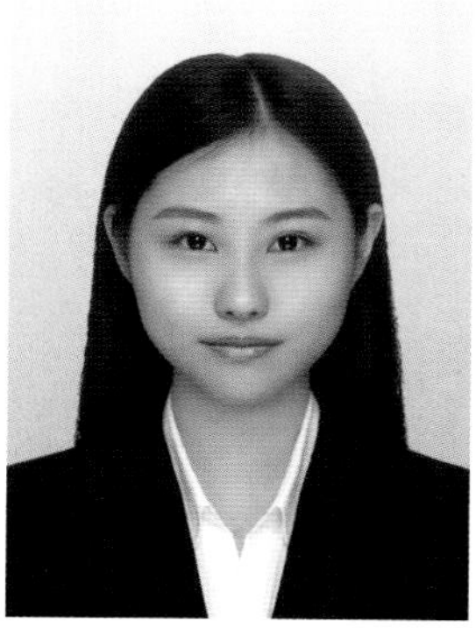

赵晓燕，江苏常州人，医学硕士。毕业于南京医科大学七学制临床医学眼科学专业斜视与小儿眼病方向，现就职于南京医科大学附属常州市第二人民医院。攻读硕士学位期间以第一作者身份发表 SCI 论文 1 篇，以共同作者身份发表 SCI 论文 3 篇。

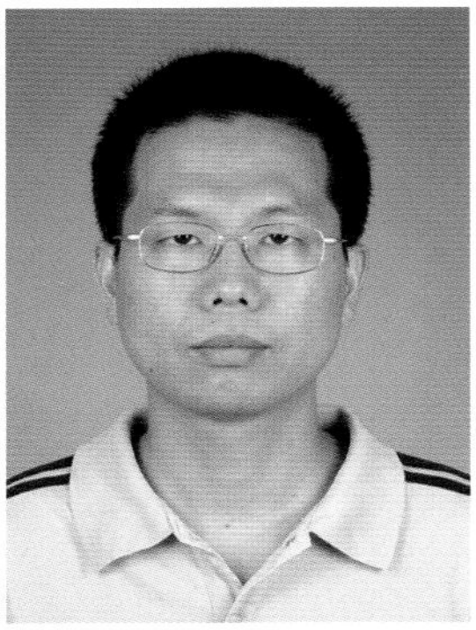

孙新成，医学硕士，副主任医师，硕士生导师。常州市医学会眼科分会委员兼秘书，江苏省医师协会眼科分会视光学组委员。

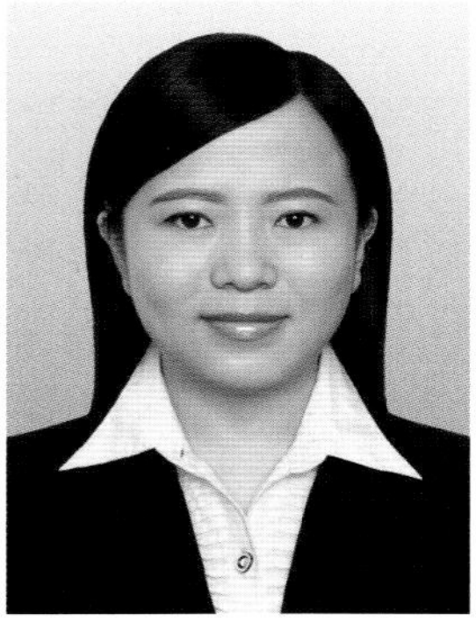

马君鑫，江苏南京人，医学硕士。眼科主治医生，南京医科大学本科、硕士毕业后就职于南京市第一医院眼科，现南京医科大学博士在读。近年来以第一作者身份发表 SCI 论文 1 篇，以共同作者身份发表 SCI 论文数篇。主持校级课题项目 1 项，多次参与省、市级课题及国家近视防控项目研究。专业方向为眼表疾病与小儿眼科。

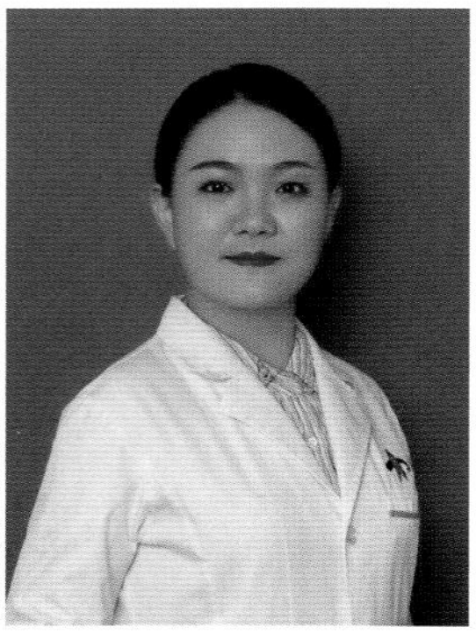

张宁，1988 年 12 月出生。现就职于西安交通大学第一附属医院。2017 年四川大学眼视光专业博士毕业，为香港理工大学眼视光学和四川大学联合培养博士。发表 SCI 论文 2 篇。临床与研究方向为弱视、近视及双眼视。

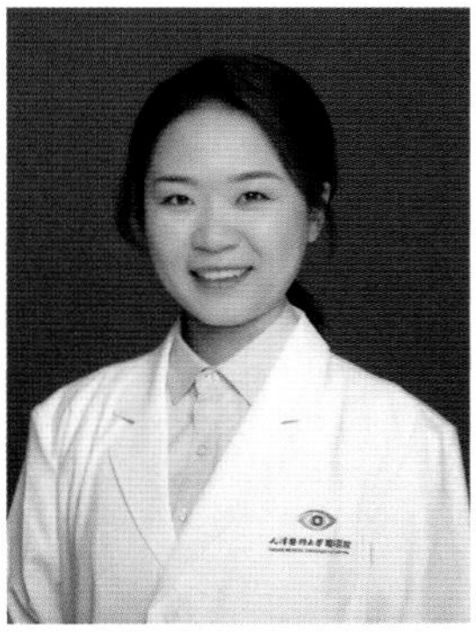

赵方宇，就职于天津医科大学眼科医院，2016 年于大连医科大学眼科学硕士毕业，于天津市眼科医院完成 3 年的住院医师规范化培训。临床与研究方向为白内障、青光眼及其他眼科的常见疾病。

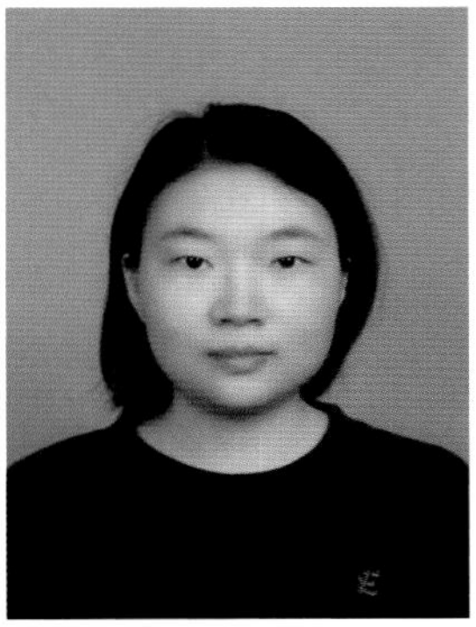

朱晓鹃，现就职于四川大学华西医院。硕士毕业于四川大学眼视光学专业，已获国家公派留学攻读博士学位资格。发表 SCI 论文 1 篇，研究方向为近视、高度近视等。

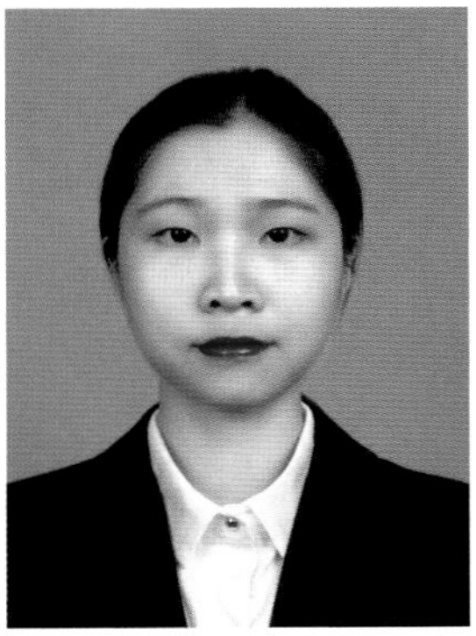

李霞，眼视光学硕士，本科就读于四川大学华西临床医学院眼视光专业，硕士由四川大学和香港理工大学联合培养，师从刘陇黔教授，研究方向为近视防控。在读期间多次参与全国眼科大会发言和壁报展示，并获得“优秀发言奖”，研究生毕业获得“优秀研究生干部”称号。熟练掌握角膜塑形镜验配技能，擅长青少年近视防控体系构建。

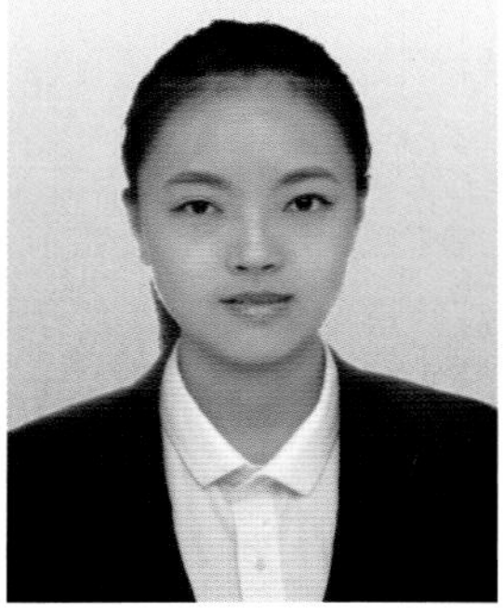

黄雪，四川大学华西临床医学院眼视光学硕士在读。2016 年本科毕业于四川大学华西临床医学院眼视光系，随后进入四川华西医院眼科完成了为期 2 年的眼科技师规范化培训。研究生期间的主要研究方向是获得性脑损伤患者双眼视功能的与康复训练。

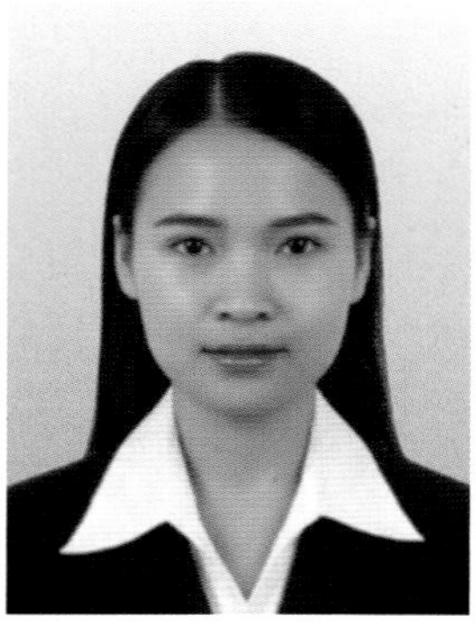

刘添添，四川大学华西临床医学院眼科学硕士在读，研究方向为视光学，研究生导师为刘陇黔教授。本科毕业于哈尔滨医科大学临床医学专业（5 年制），曾多次获得学校奖学金，多次参与“挑战杯”“大学生创新创业”等项目，并在四川大学“挑战杯”（2018~2019 年）中获得三等奖。

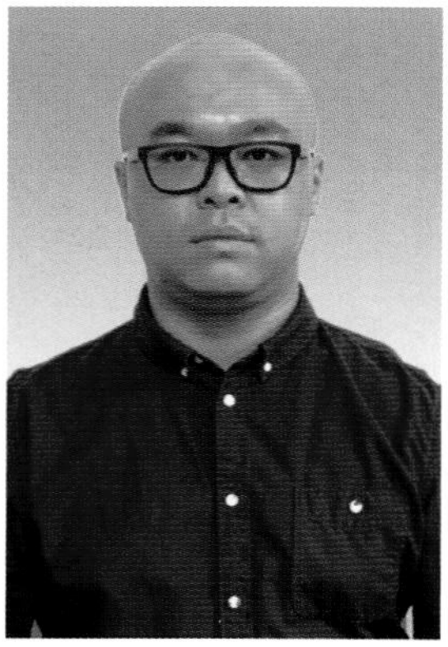

刘未择，毕业于西安交通大学临床医学专业，先后工作实习于西安交通大学第二附属医院（2016 年）、西安新城区石一宁眼科诊所（2018 年）、西安交通大学第一附属医院长安区医院（2019 年）。现在于西藏民族大学攻读骨科学硕士研究生专业学位。

英文总审校专家简介

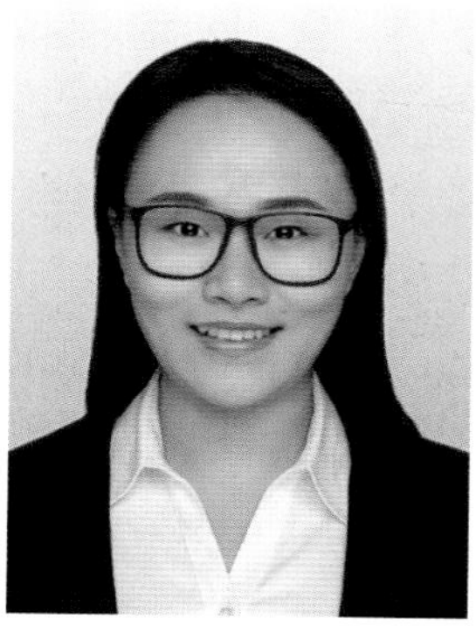

李易，主治医师，医学博士，现就职于天津医科大学眼科医院。美国德克萨斯大学医学院访问学者。本科就读于中国医科大学，临床医学专业（眼科与视光学方向）；硕博连读于中国医科大学，主要致力于青光眼视网膜神经节细胞凋亡机制及层粘连蛋白对视神经保护作用的研究。参与翻译多部眼科论著。

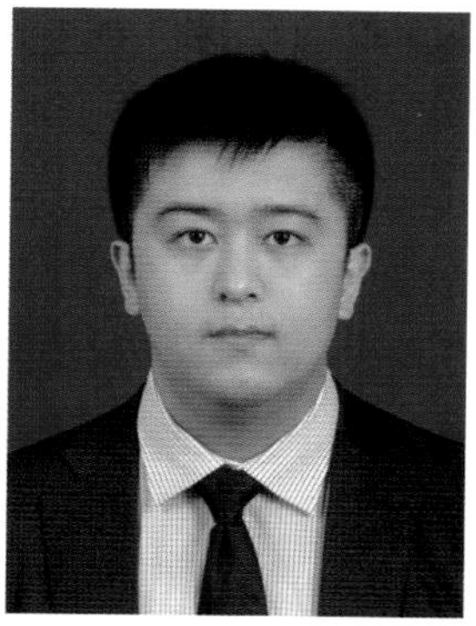

陈研明，2012 年毕业于西安交通大学医学院，2015 年毕业于中国医科大学眼科学研究院，2015 年作为美国纽黑文耶鲁大学医学院视觉科学交流访问学者进行临床研究至今。主要研究青光眼的分子和细胞学发病机制（视神经损伤机制、遗传学机制）及视盘星形胶质细胞蛋白组学分析。参与省级自然基金研究项目 5 项，发表论文 11 篇，参与专著撰写及翻译 4 部。

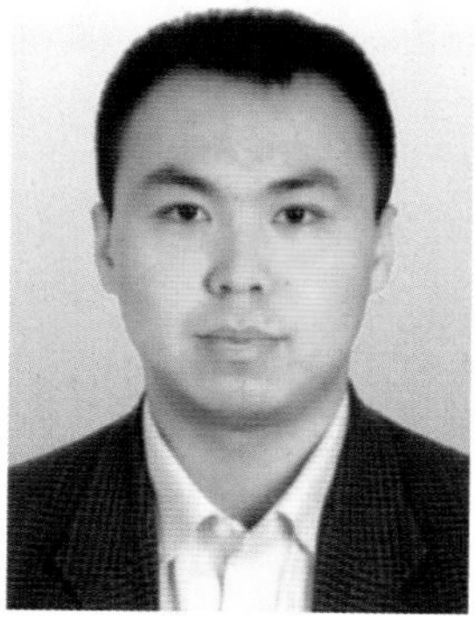

陈卓，副教授，西安医学院药物化学教研室主任。2010 年毕业于四川大学华西药学院药物化学专业。主讲“药物化学”“药物设计学”与“药物合成工艺学”课程。从事眼科新药的开发研究，主持完成多项自然科学基础研究项目。在抗翼状胬肉药物的研究中，获得的系列新颖化合物表现出良好的翼状胬肉抑制活性及相对现有药物较低的毒性。

序一

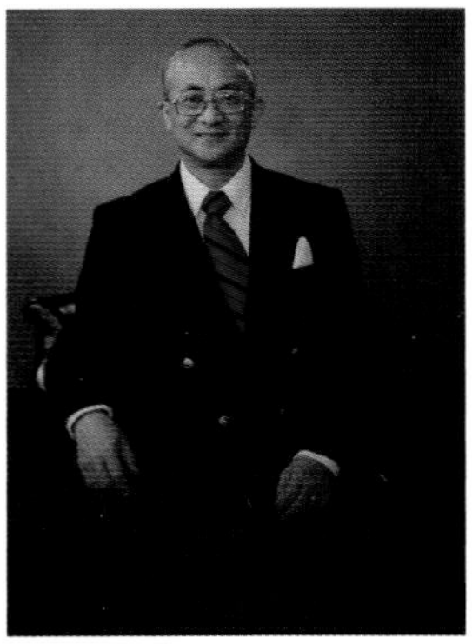

Preface Blooming of Eyecare for Children in China

序言：中国儿童眼科事业的蓬勃发展

From the Chinese translation of the section 6 of BCSC on *Pediatric Ophthalmology and Strabismus*

To a. the popularization of ICO Training Curricula in Pediatric Ophthalmology ,b. the establishment of Pediatric Ophthalmology as a Subspecialty in Ophthalmology and c. the definition of the Manpower Needs for Children Eyecare in China

推进“基础与临床科学教程”第6分册《小儿眼科与斜视》的中文翻译，是为了达到以下目的：① 普及儿科眼科 ICO 培训课程；② 建立儿科眼科学作为眼科学的分支学科；③ 明确中国儿童眼保健人力需求的界定。

Introduction

背景简介

In this Information Age, the quality of life is significantly linked to the quality of Vision Care in a community, and Vision Care must start in childhood. As such, childhood eyecare is one of the cornerstones of healthcare in a community.

在此资讯时代中，生活品质与社区视力保健品质息息相关，视力保健必须从儿童时期做起。因此，儿童眼保健是社区医疗保健的基石之一。

I write to congratulate the vigorous effort of a group of ophthalmic educators , headed by Prof. Shi Yi ning, with the strong support of Prof. Zhu Zhuangyong of the Shaanxi Science and Technology Press. They have reached an agreement with the American Academy of Ophthalmology, Inc. to translate and publish in Chinese the Section 6 of Basic and Clinical Science Course (BCSC) on *Pediatric Ophthalmology and Strabismus*. This important project will provide rich study material for the trainees and faculty of pediatric ophthalmology throughout China. This Herculean effort will long be remembered as a major step in improving eyecare for children in China.

石一宁教授为首的一群眼科教育工作者积极努力，获得原陕西科学技术出版社朱壮涌总编辑的大力支持，我谨向他们表示祝贺！他们与美国眼科学会达成协议，将“基础与临床科学教程”（英文名为 Basic and Clinical Science Course，简称 BCSC）第 6 分册《斜视与小儿眼科》翻译为中文并出版，将为中国儿童眼科的受训者和培训导师提供丰富的学习资料。这份艰巨的工作，作为中国改善儿童视力的重要措施，将会长久地被大家铭记不忘。

Historical Perspective

历史回顾

The Chinese translation of the 13 sections of the BCSC including the section 6 on *Pediatric Ophthalmology and Strabismus* was initiated by the leadership of the Chinese American Ophthalmological Society (CAOS) in the 1990s. The membership of CAOS consisted of ophthalmologists of Chinese Descent from all over the world. Their enthusiasm for improving eyecare in China led to the Chinese translation of the BCSC, and donations for this project came from the US, Singapore, Hong Kong and Taiwan. Dr. King Y Lee, then President of CAOS and the Undersigned obtained the right of Chinese translation of the BCSC from the American Academy of Ophthalmology and travelled to Beijing to establish an agreement with the Chinese Medical Society as the publisher. Prof. Li Zi-Liang was appointed the Editor-in- Chief and his most dedicated and tireless effort oversaw the completion of the project as the first complete translation of the BCSC into a foreign language.

20 世纪 90 年代，中美眼科学会发起并组织了 BCSC 一书共 13 个分册《小儿眼科与斜视》的中文翻译。中美眼科学会的成员，是来自世界各地的华裔眼科专家，他们怀着改善中国视力健康的热忱，在来自美国、新加坡、中国香港和中国台湾的捐赠资金支持及我的全力支持下，完成了 BCSC 一书的中文翻译。当时任中美眼科学会会长的李金义博士和我，从美国眼科学会获得了 BCSC 一书的中文翻译权，并前往北京与中华医学会签订了出版协议。当年李子良教授被任命为总编辑，经过他的多方协调和不懈努力，监督完成了该书的中文翻译工作，使其成为全套 BCSC 首个完整的外文翻译版本。

The Present Undertaking

目前工作

Decades have passed. The BCSC has been vigorously revised annually or biennially as the rapid progress of eyecare worldwide rolls on. I am pleased to be informed that Prof. Shi Yi ning and her colleagues have started a new Chinese translation of Section 6 of the BSCS. Furthermore they have improved the format to develop a bilingual version so that the trainees may not only learn new ophthalmic information but also develop English language as a skill to improve on international communication. It must be mentioned that while the current Section 6 is mostly written by American and Canadian experts, it is also reviewed by experts of the European Board of Ophthalmology . So the scope of teaching materials has included international input.

岁月如梭，随着全球眼保健事业的快速发展，BCSC 一书每年或每 2 年都会得到修订。我很高兴地获悉，石一宁教授和她的同事们已经开始了新版 BCSC 一书第 6 分册的中文翻译工作。他们将该书制作成双语版本，读者不仅可以学习新的眼科知识，而且可以提高英语使用水平、提升国际交流能力。尽管目前该书的第 6 分册主要由美国和加拿大专家所撰写，但同时也有欧洲眼科委员会专家参与相关内容的审校工作，因此该书融汇了多个国际专家的合作成果。

The Road Ahead

未来展望

While the BCSC provides study material for ophthalmology residents and faculty, the International Council of Ophthalmology has developed a definitive curriculum to incorporate these study materials into the training and clinical practice in the residency training process. The ICO residency training curriculum was published in 2006 under the Editorship of the Undersigned, and the curriculum has since been repeatedly revised. The 2012 version of the curriculum was translated into Chinese by Dr. Wang Ting of the Peking University Eye Center, Beijing, China. It is vitally important that the leadership of the pediatric ophthalmology in China will vigorously adopt the curriculum in their training program so that the trainees will apply the study material of BCSC into their clinical practice.

国际眼科学会开发了完整的培训大纲，把 BCSC 一书的学习材料融入住院医师的培训过程和临床实践中。该培训大纲在我任主编时已于 2006 年出版，此后不断得到修订。2012 年版的大纲由北京大学眼科中心王婷博士翻译成中文。中国儿童眼科事业的领导者应在培训项目中积极使用该大纲，以期帮助受训者将 BCSC 的学习内容应用于临床实践中。

Furthermore, in order to greatly improve eyecare for children, pediatric ophthalmology must be established as a definitive subspecialty in ophthalmology. To assist this goal worldwide, the International Council of Ophthalmology, establishes an ICO Subspecialty Curriculum for Training of post residency

Fellowship in pediatric ophthalmology in 2017. This subspecialty curriculum was drafted by experts from Hong Kong, Nigeria, Lebanon, Belgium, ,Australia, Germany, United States , United Kingdom and Argentina. In addition, a subspecialty Certificate Examination for pediatric ophthalmology has been conducted by the European Board of Ophthalmology (EBO),the European Strabismus Association (ESA) and the European Pediatric Ophthalmological Society.

为了进一步改善儿童眼保健状况，我们必须将儿童眼科建立为眼科学的亚专科。国际眼科学会为了协助在全世界范围内实现上述目标，于 2017 年设立了儿童眼科亚专科培训大纲，用于培训后住院医师的主治医师。该亚专科培训大纲由来自中国香港、尼日利亚、黎巴嫩、比利时、澳大利亚、德国、美国、英国和阿根廷的专家起草。此外，欧洲眼科学会、欧洲斜视学会和欧洲儿科眼科学会，已经开展了儿童眼科亚专科证书考试。

China has a big population. The need of manpower for children eyecare must be defined and the provision of resources must be carefully planned to carry out the anticipated blooming of children eyecare in the coming decades.

中国人口众多，必须确定儿童眼保健的人力需求，并且必须仔细规划资源供应，以实现儿童眼保健在未来几十年中的预期发展目标。

Conclusion

结论

June 6, 2020 was the 25thNational Eye Care day in China. It is a declaration that the Country focuses on the improvement of eyecare for its population in this information age. I plead with the leadership of hospitals and eyecare institutions to invest resources to develop the division of pediatric ophthalmology and to expand clinical activities such as Amblyopia Training Clinic, pediatric optometric center, ,myopia screening program for school children, Screening Clinic for retinopathy of prematurity, Retinal Imaging Center for Children, Clinic for Congenital Eye Diseases such as congenital cataract, congenital glaucoma and congenital ptosis and Molecular Genetic Laboratory.

2020 年 6 月 6 日是中国第 25 个全国护眼日，在这资讯发达的时代里，国家已明确宣布将聚焦于改善人民的眼保健水平。我恳请医院和眼科学院的领导们投入资源来发展儿童眼科，并且扩大临床活动，如弱视训练门诊，儿童验光中心，学龄儿童近视筛查项目，早产儿视网膜病变筛查门诊，儿童视网膜影像中心，先天性白内障、先天性青光眼以及先天性上睑下垂先天性眼病门诊和分子遗传学实验室，等等。

I am grateful to Prof. Bu Juan who translates this English draft into Chinese in order to be a bilingual version of this Preface.

最后，非常感谢布娟教授把本人的英文版序言翻译成中文，此书因而获得双语序言。

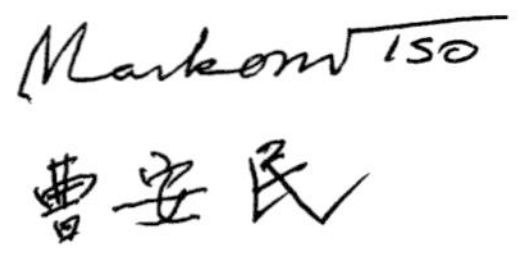

Mark O. M. Tso, M.D., D.Sc., FARVO.

Professor of Ophthalmology, Emeritus

Wilmer Eye Institute, The Johns Hopkins University.

Chair XI , Academia Ophthalmologica Internationalis

Former Vice President (1998–2006) and Director for Education (2006–2010), International Council of Ophthalmology

Founder and First Director, (2001–2010) Peking University Eye Center

曹安民，医学博士，理学博士，FARVO

约翰霍普金斯大学威尔玛眼科研究所荣休眼科教授

国际眼科科学院第十一任院士

国际眼科学会前副主席（1998~2006 年）和前教育总监（2006~2010 年）

北京大学眼科中心创始人并第一届主任（2001~2010 年）

序二

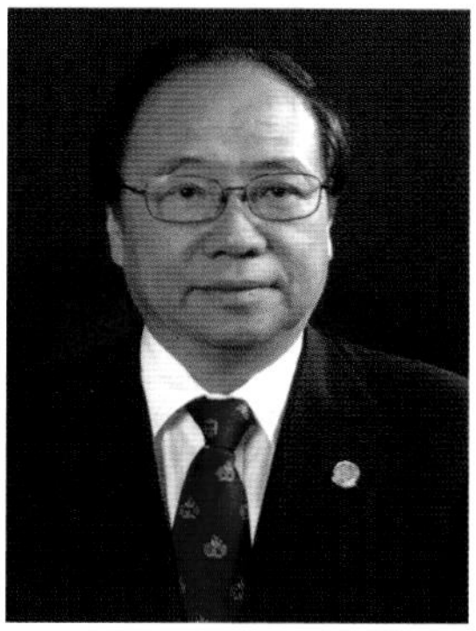

我祝贺石一宁教授组织和领衔翻译的美国眼科学会“基础与临床科学教程”（Basic and Clinical Science Course，BCSC）第 6 册《小儿眼科与斜视》（*Pediatric Ophthalmology and Strabismus, 2019–2020*）中英文对照版顺利出版。BCSC 是美国眼科学会为满足住院医师培训需要和临床医师的业务提高所组织编写的一套眼科学综合性简明教材。它从最初采用主要依靠课外阅读方式来学习的简单提纲格式，已经发展为使用方便、更能适用于眼科学教学的独立教材。美国眼科学会每年对其进行修改和更新，其目标是将眼科学的基础科学和临床实践整合起来，使眼科医师能了解眼科学各亚专科的最新进展。BCSC 还提供了一些选择的参考文献，读者可以在书本学习的基础上扩大学习范围。因此，BCSC 是当今世界上质量最高的住院医师培训教材，也是眼科临床医师不断提高自己的自学资料。BCSC 和美国眼科学会编制的《眼科临床指南》（Preferred Practice Pattern，PPP）是美国眼科住院医师培训的主要教材。BCSC 共有 13 册，除了第一册讲的是普通内科学的进展，第二册讲的是眼科学的基础和原则外，其余 11 册都是在讲述眼科学各亚专科的内容，包括临床光学，眼科病理学和与眼内肿瘤，神经眼科学，眼眶、眼睑和泪器，外眼疾病与角膜病，眼内炎症与葡萄膜炎，青光眼，晶状体与白内障，视网膜与玻璃体，屈光手术。而第 6 册则是小儿眼科学与斜视，内容十分丰富，包括可以获得最多的信息而且能将伤害和不适减低到最低限度的幼儿眼部评估技术，眼外肌的解剖和生理学，弱视的分类、诊断和治疗选择，斜视的诊断和检查技术、分类及其处理，斜视手术的并发症，眼球震颤的类型，儿童视力下降的诊断途径，儿童先天性和获得性眼部感染的鉴别诊断和处理，儿童常见的泪道系统的异常和处理，儿童角膜、眼前节和虹膜的异常，儿童青光眼的诊断和治疗选择，儿童白内障和其他晶状体异常的常见类型、诊断和治疗，儿童葡萄膜炎的诊断，儿童玻璃体视网膜疾病、视乳头和代谢性疾病的诊断和鉴别诊断，儿童眼部肿瘤的特点，儿童眼外伤的特点。所有这些内容对提高我国眼科医师，特别是小儿眼科亚专科医师诊治儿童眼病的水平具有重要的意义。因此石一宁教授及其团队的工作是值得赞赏的。本书采用中英文对照的方式，更能满足我国绝大多数眼科医师的自学需要。

优秀的眼科教材不仅方便教学，保证住院医师的培训质量，而且可以使我国眼科医师了解国际眼科诊疗的先进理念和实践，从而提高我国眼科的整体水平。从我国实行“改革开放”的政策以来，国内外的眼科学术交流日趋活跃，我们不仅关注国际眼科学的进展，而且也注意引进高质量的眼科学教材。1990 年 3 月时任中华医学会眼科学分会副主任委员嵇训传和袁佳琴教授参加了在新加坡召开的第 26 届国际眼科学会联盟（IFOS）国际眼科学术大会，在会议期间与美国中美眼科学会的理事，以及中国香港和台湾等地华裔眼科学者共同讨论了中国眼科的发展和教育前景，大家一致同意将美国眼科学会出版的 BCSC 译为中文在我国出版，为中国眼科医师的继续教育提供教材。这一意愿得到了美国眼科学会常务副主席 Bruce Spivey 教授的热诚支持。其后他与中华医学会副会长曹泽毅教授签署了版权转让同意书。中美眼科学会前主席 Mark Tso（曹安民）教授和时任主席 King Lee（李英尧）教授以及海内外华裔眼科学界慷慨捐助，积极筹措出版资金，交由中华眼科学会眼科学分会副主任委员李子良教授具体负责组织翻译，中华医学会出版社负责出版。1994 年 BCSC 第 8 册《外眼病和角膜病》中文版出版。为了促进中国的眼科教学工作和研究工作，中美国眼科学会设立金苹果奖和金钥匙奖，在 1992 年第五届中华医学会全国眼科学术大会上首次颁奖，授予在中国眼科教学和科学研究中做出杰出成就的人员。这一系列的国际眼科界交流活动和华裔眼科学者的支持，使中国眼科医师首次了解了 BCSC，促进了我国眼科教育工作的开展。此外，中华医学会眼科学分会还努力引进了美国眼科学会另一套优秀眼科教材 PPP。2003 年 9 月，作为中华医学会眼科学分会主任委员的我在参加世界卫生组织（WHO）召开的全球眼科研究工作会议期间，得知为了提高发展中国家的眼科临床水平，大会组委会鼓励将国际眼科理事会（International Council of Ophthalmology，ICO）认为的最好的临床服务指南转移到发展中国家去，当即就向 WHO 提出将 PPP 转移到中国的申请，此申请得到了批准，大会组委会委派一些专家来华开展工作。虽然当时我们大多数眼科医师并不熟悉 PPP，对其编制原则、方法、结构和内容有很多不了解的地方，但是感觉到这是眼科学应用循证医学的重要成果，代表了国际眼科学的最高水平，是缩短我国眼科学和国际眼科学差距的一次难得的契机。中华医学会眼科学分会的主要领导们也统一思想，认为这是规范我国眼科医疗服务，提高眼科医疗服务水平的一次极好的机会，为此开展了大量的工作。2004 年 9 月中华医学会眼科学分会召开第一次 PPP 工作会议，WHO、美国眼科学会和美国国家眼科研究所的专家介绍了 PPP 的基本原则、主要内容、编排结构，得到了良好的反应。2005 年中华医学会眼科学分会再次召开 PPP 工作会议，WHO 和美国眼科学会和美国国家眼科研究所的专家再次参加会议，并同国内专家一起就 PPP 在中国的适用性问题进行了认真讨论。此后根据 PPP 的内容，出版了 3 版 PPP 的中文版，使 PPP 在我国得到了极大的推广。正是这些引进优良眼科学教材的工作，使我国广大的眼科医师了解了国际最先进的眼科诊疗思想、理念和实践，从而提高了我国眼科的临床水平，促进了我国眼科学的发展。

小儿眼科学是眼科学的重要部分，涉及亿万儿童青少年的眼病防治和眼健康。从 1999 年 WHO 发起"视觉 2020，人人享有看见权利"行动以来，我国将儿童盲的防治列为防盲工作的重点之一，取得了很大的成绩。但是儿童的眼病还有很多，斜视、弱视、先天性白内障、儿童青光眼都是有可能导致严重视力损伤的眼病，需要我们积极防治。在我国，儿童青少年中近视眼的问题越来越严重，尚未得到根本性的改善，也需要我们积极研究，采取有效的措施进行防治。只有这样才能使我国的儿童青少年保持眼健康，使他们有一个光明的未来。儿童眼病的防治和眼健康，需要我们从婴幼儿抓起，更需要我们充分地了解儿童的眼部解剖和生理，了解小儿眼科学的进展。石一宁教授及其团队完成的 BCSC 第 6 册《小儿眼科与斜视》的中英文对照版将会有助于推动我国小儿眼科学的发展。

我期望本书的出版能为提高我国眼科住院医师的规范化培训水平和小儿眼科学的水平发挥积极的作用。我也希望参与编译本书的眼科医师们能继续关注 BCSC 的进展，定期地将小儿眼科学的新内容进行介绍和解读，使我们能够及时了解小儿眼科学的新进展。

中国医学科学院，北京协和医学院
北京协和医院眼科教授
国际眼科科学院院士和第一副主席
2020 年 7 月 12 日于北京

赵家良教授，曾任中国医学科学院眼科研究中心主任，北京协和医院眼科主任，中华医学会眼科学会主任委员、防盲学组组长，《中华眼科杂志》总编辑，中国医师协会眼科医师分会分长、防治视觉损伤委员会主任委员，亚太眼科学会理事会理事、副主席及防盲委员会主席，国际眼科理事会理事。现任中国残疾人联合会康复协会副理事长，中国非公立医疗机构眼科委员会主任委员。2004 年当选为国际眼科科学院院士、2018 年 6 月当选为国际眼科科学院副主席。

获北京市科技进步三等奖、Carl Kupfer 国际防盲奖、亚洲太平洋地区白内障屈光手术学会杰出成就奖、北京市科技进步二等奖、中华医学科技奖二等奖、亚洲太平洋地区眼科学会奖、中华眼科杰出成就奖、亚太眼科学会 Arthur Lim 奖、中美眼科学会金苹果奖、美国南加大 Doheny 眼科研究所“Doheny 学者”的称号、中国医师奖、亚太眼科学会最高奖 Jose Rizal 奖、国家科技奖二等奖、海外华人视觉和眼科研究会视觉和眼科研究杰出领导奖、中华医学会眼科学分会终身成就奖、美国眼科学会成就奖 2019 年北京协和医院杰出成就奖。在国内外学术杂志发表论文 200 多篇。

序三

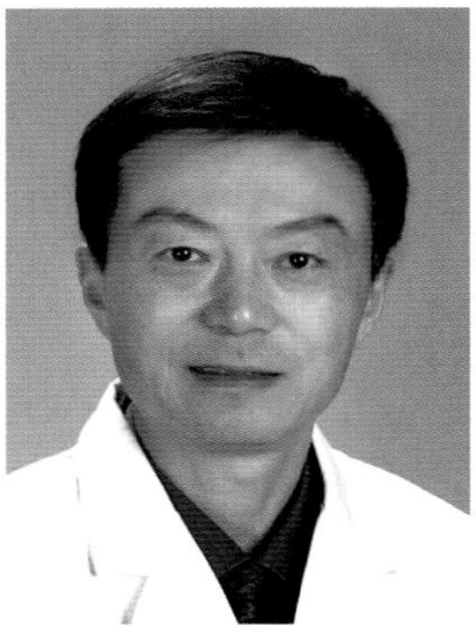

我国小儿眼科与斜视专业事业的发展方兴未艾，但在服务水平和专业能力建设上也存在着不均衡现象，因此，坚持知识更新和继续教育仍然十分重要。早在2009年，谢立信教授曾组织翻译出版了《Harley小儿眼科学 第5版》经典专著，对推动独立的小儿眼科专业的发展起到了推动促进作用。与成人眼科不同，小儿眼科表现出其特殊性，即从孕期、出生直至青春期的10余年间，儿童生长发育过程中异常与眼病。为此，对该专业的教材编写与教程设计安排十分重要。

我和石一宁教授前10年主要从事了儿童青少年近视的流行病学、发病机制、近视防控，以及病理性近视眼底改变等方面的探索和研究。石一宁教授近几年尤其注意到国内眼视光学专业人才的教育和培养问题，希望通过学习眼视光学的基础理论、基本知识，掌握儿童青少年生长发育过程中的异常与眼病的诊断、预防与治疗的基本技能，使中国有更多的了解和掌握小儿眼科专科基本知识的眼科医生和视光医师服务于社会。

2019年石一宁教授曾经组织国内从事眼视光学专业的人员翻译出版了由美国眼科学会（AAO）编写的《临床光学（2018–2019）》一书，是AAO编写的基础与临床科学教程（BCSC）第3册。此书的出版对中国视光医生和视光中心的培训提供了很大帮助，也是中国眼科医生的重要补充教材。本次翻译出版的《小儿眼科与斜视（2019–2020）》一书是BCSC系列的第6册，是前一册的继续，因为视光学在小儿眼科占有重要篇幅，只有对儿童青少年眼生长发育以及异常和疾病有了深入的了解，才能够理解儿童屈光的变化，探索其变化规律，寻找出解决的有效方法。

BCSC的目标是通过研究与回顾来增加医生的眼科知识，鼓励医生阅读课文，然后回答书后提出的问题，以此提升业务水平。这次石一宁教授再次组织学者翻译了BCSC中的《小儿眼科与斜视》这部教材，使国内从事小儿眼科医生能够看到原版国际眼科医生培养的基础教材，可以在这本翻译版图书中阅读到原文，有益于提升临床医生的专业英语水平，有利于中国眼科医生的国际化培训。希望《小儿眼科与斜视》这部教材的中英文双语译本的出版能够对小儿眼科与斜视专业医生的培训有所帮助，期望中国小儿眼科与斜视专业事业的发展日新月异，呵护好儿童眼健康。

安徽理工大学第一附属医院、第一临床学院名誉院长

2020.7.15

序四

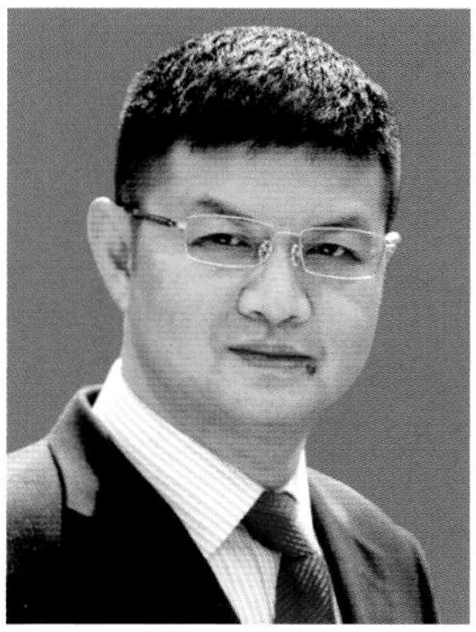

如果说 *General Ophthalmology* 带我进入眼科的大门，那么美国眼科学会（American academy of ophthalmology, AAO）的 *Basicand Clinical Science Course* 伴随了我早期眼科从医任教的生涯，这套书在我从眼科住院医师到成为眼科副教授的过程中，一直是我从图书馆反复循环借阅的读物，使我能够全面系统地掌握眼科知识和理论。以后又成为我向我的学生推荐的必须读物。我初次阅读的是该书的1982~1983 年版，最后接触的是 1996~1997 年版，该书一直在实时更新，以保持跟日新月异发展的眼科学同步。这套书籍只有 12 册，从 *Update on General Medicine Fundamentals and Principles of Ophthalmology* 到覆盖眼科所有的亚专业所有的内容。不像眼科其他亚专业那样形象直观，斜视与小儿眼科亚专业需要一定的抽象和逻辑思维能力，常常成为大多数眼科住院医师的不可逾越的障碍，该套书籍的第 6 册《小儿眼科与斜视》(*Pediatric Ophthalmology and Strabismus*)的翻译出版，将为他们的学习扫清障碍。同时，难得可贵的是该书为双语出版，使得学习者在学习知识的同时，也能获得相应专业英语的学习，以避免“oblique amblyopia”这样机器翻译的笑话。

该分册涵盖内容广泛，专业知识内容层层递进、深入浅出，便于读者加强对知识的理解和系统化知识体系的形成。书中基础部分包括基本术语、解剖知识、相关基本检查以及生理学和病理学；弱视、斜视部分讲解了其相关诊断、分类、评估与治疗，包括手术相关术式、注意事项等；小儿眼病方面囊括了眼部及其附属器各部分先天性异常或发育异常疾病，如眼睑、眼眶、泪道、眼表、视盘等；另外，还有对与小儿眼科相关的常见全身与系统性疾病的详尽阐述。实践和应用向来是检验学习效果的最好方式，本书籍讲解内容后附有习题与解析，也能让读者可以更加准确地了解自己对新鲜知识的掌握情况并从中发现问题，学以致用，才能更好地服务于读者的临床、教学工作。

我国斜视与小儿眼科亚专业草创建立至今已有 40 余载，历经了刘家琦、方谦逊、郭静秋、赵堪兴等教授几代人的奉献和努力，逐步完善学科建设，培养了一批批优秀的临床、教学、科研人才。此次由石一宁教授牵头开展的对《*Pediatric Ophthalmology and Strabismus 2019–2020*》的翻译工作，也是希望将国外该领域最新的临床经验、前沿技术作为借鉴引入国内，同时进一步推进斜视与小儿眼科的诊疗规范化，尽可能地消减国内在此领域的伪科学。该书的翻译出版将为我国更广大的小儿眼科与斜视亚专业团队提供学习的重要资料，为专业的发展继续添砖加瓦。翻译团队除了需要精准地译出原稿内容的基础知识之外，也需要对书籍中专业内容讲述的方式、语句习惯等进行了细细揣摩、推敲。经过翻译团队大量的讨论工作和专业审校团队、英语审校团队审校后，才最终为大家呈现出不仅仅是一本语言翻译图书，而是从根本上更加符合我国读者的阅读习惯，适合我国眼科医师，尤其立志从事斜视与小儿眼科医师阅读的中式教材。

为了保证本书翻译的专业准确性、语言的流畅性，石一宁教授领衔组织了庞大的翻译团队。团队中不仅具有刘虎、钱学翰、布娟等业界大咖，更有一批在知识方面嗷嗷待哺的青年才俊。感谢石一宁教授的信任和邀请，我的10多名学生得以参加翻译工作。尽管他们具有较强的语言能力，但其专业知识仍比较欠缺。通过此次翻译工作，使他们的专业理论知识水平大大提高。当然，必要的付出是必不可少。很多次组会，为了一个词、一个句子，查阅文献和数据，引经据典，直到达成共识为止。由此我能感受到此次翻译团队所付出的大量努力，尤其是石一宁教授的付出。

很荣幸受石一宁教授之托再为该书撰写序言，我也因此提前拿到了全书的手稿，先阅为快，阔别多年，再次相见，无比欣喜。在此对此书的顺利出版表示祝贺！

刘陇黔

四川大学华西临床医学院眼视光学系主任兼眼科副主任

2020年7月

序五

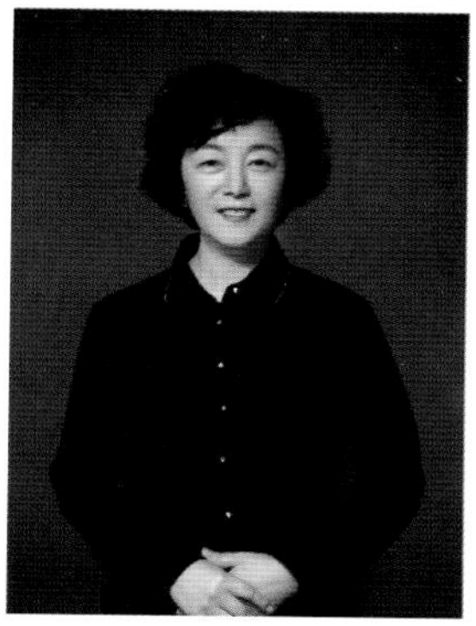

石一宁教授领衔的精英团队翻译的“2018 –2019 基础与临床科学教程”第 3 分册《临床光学》于 2019 年 7 月出版后，国内眼科医生尤其是视光从业者爱不释手、争相传阅，一时洛阳纸贵。仅时隔 1 年，第 6 分册《小儿眼科与斜视》的译著即将付梓，其热忱的学者情怀令人感动，敬业学术精神令人佩服，而作为一名眼科人，更多的是一份由衷的感谢——感谢一宁教授为眼科事业的辛勤耕耘、孜孜以求，感谢一宁教授为小儿眼科医生送出的一份宝贵礼物。

美国眼科学会编辑出版的学术期刊、专题手册、影像资料和幻灯片是美国眼科住院医师的必读教材，特别是“基础和临床科学教程”，内容详尽、结构精炼、系统性强，知识更新快，被世界各地眼科界广泛采用，也深受我国眼科人的推崇和欢迎。

追溯历史，我们的眼科前辈为了中国眼科发展、眼科医生的培养，高瞻远瞩、呕心沥血，能将全套教程翻译出版是他们的梦想。20 世纪的 90 年代，国际眼科学会在新加坡举行，当时的中美眼科学会理事及两岸三地的华裔眼科学界权威齐聚狮城，共同研讨中国眼科教育的前景和未来，大家一致决定要将美国眼科学会所编纂的眼科住院医师教育手册在中国翻译出版，该项工作由时任中华医学会副主任委员李子良教授负责。海内外华裔眼科前辈为此慷慨捐助，在众多前贤的倾心努力下，历时 4 年由中华医学会组织出版。此书简洁精湛、新颖卓越，为全球系统性眼科教育课程的最佳典范。全套分 11 册，此套中文版译本也成为中国眼科教育之骨干教材，本专业培训的“圣经”，培养了很多优秀的眼科医师，该书将永留史册。

时过境迁，中国眼科发生了翻天覆地的变化，逐渐与国际接轨，由于“基础和临床科学教程”每 2 年更新 1 次，每次都有新观点、新概念、新技术问世。加之 2019 年为最新版本大修之年，石一宁教授相时而动，翻译了 2019 年版的第 3 分册《临床光学》和第 6 分册《小儿眼科与斜视》，这 2 册都是小儿眼科医师的必修之课。而《临床光学》作为国际眼科医师考试（ICO）必考科目的指定教材，从视光理论知识和临床实践需求的角度，详尽介绍了眼科医生必须掌握的知识要点，为眼科医生提供了完整的视光学知识架构。第 6 分册《小儿眼科与斜视》译著则更是小儿眼科医生期盼已久的经典，其内容精炼、观点新颖、图文并茂，视频同步，涵盖面广，集发育性眼病、全身病、系统性疾病及综合征为一体。有助于小儿眼科医生由浅入深、循序渐进、系统地进行学习，将对国内小儿眼科医生培养起到积极的推动作用，为中国未来眼科教学注入新鲜血液。

石一宁教授译著的最大精彩与亮点是创造性地采取了双语版本的形式，以中英双语对照的格式排版，这样使读者不仅可以学习其中的临床知识，还可以阅读到“原汁原味”的基础教材，极大地帮助其专业英语水平的提高，为拓展更多的相关英文专著的学习及以后参与国际学术交流打下坚实的基础，同时为国外的眼科同道学习汉语开通了独特渠道。

小儿眼科专业独有的特殊性，体现在发育过程中不同年龄的特性及其发病的相关性，对疾病的治疗方法都与成人有诸多不同之处。我国斜视与小儿眼科专业虽然起步较晚，但发展迅速，斜视和小儿眼科专业领域已发生了巨大的变化。如今，该专业已成为眼科临床和科研领域的重要的组成部分。从业队伍不断壮大，但是依然供不应求。从业人员的培训和继续教育逐步规范，业务素质不断提升，但是业务能力和服务水平尚不均衡。所以，坚持专业队伍的继续教育与知识更新，培养合格的斜视与小儿眼科医生需要高质量的教材。

另一方面，小儿眼科专业新概念和新方法在快速发展，技术上不断更新。科技进步和知识更新还需要有与时俱进的教程同步相随，本译著将把国外最先进规范的理念和丰富的临床经验及时呈献给眼科同道。

青少年近视防控已经是石一宁教授执着的追求和目标。10 多年前，当她发现中国近视眼的发病率高速增长，毅然放弃了她喜爱的玻璃体视网膜专业，利用著书、讲学、研究、网络宣传、开设工作室等多种形式，踏上了专职防控近视之路，为此她已发表了 100 余篇论文和 5 本眼科书籍，积极开展科普宣传、专业培训、科研立项等相关工作。多年来，石一宁教授为青少年近视防控积极探索并奔走呼吁，为没有得力的防控措施而忧心忡忡，也为国家政府的高度重视和有力支持而欢欣鼓舞，其心之诚、其意之切，令人感佩。

在习近平总书记“共同呵护好孩子的眼睛，让他们拥有一个光明的未来”的重要指示引导下，儿童青少年的近视防控引起了全社会的重视。在这样的时代背景下，《临床光学》和《小儿眼科与斜视》的翻译出版，也是一名眼科医生实现近视防控初心的实现。在翻译工作中，一宁教授和她的团队为了一个概念、一个句子，反复推敲、几经斟酌、一再讨论，力求措辞精准、文笔流畅，其严谨、科学的态度和敬业、专注的精神值得我们学习和铭记。“看似寻常最奇崛，成如容易却艰辛”，一部好书凝结着所有人辛勤的付出和艰辛的努力。

第 6 分册《小儿眼科与斜视》译著的出版乃为译者和读者共同之幸事。我们相信，石一宁教授团队含辛茹苦地翻译出版的第 3 分册《临床光学》和第 6 分册《小儿眼科与斜视》将成为我国眼科学征途中的一个重要里程碑和记录。衷心祝贺本译著成功出版，希望斜视与小儿眼科医生从中获益，为呵护儿童眼健康发挥积极作用。

山西省眼科医院斜视与小儿眼科

2020 年 7 月 17 日

张丽军，主任医师，二级教授，硕士研究生导师。山西省“三晋英才”支持计划拔尖骨干人才，山西省委联系的高级专家，山西省优秀专家，山西省眼科医院斜视与小儿眼科主任。曾任中华医学会全国斜视与小儿眼科学组委员、山西省医学会眼科分会常委，现任山西省医学会斜视与小儿眼科学组组长、中国医师协会眼科医师分会第五届委员会儿童眼健康专业委员会委员。从事斜视与小儿眼科 30 余年，擅长斜视、弱视、儿童白内障、屈光不正、上睑下垂等小儿眼病。曾在日本、新加坡研修。

序六

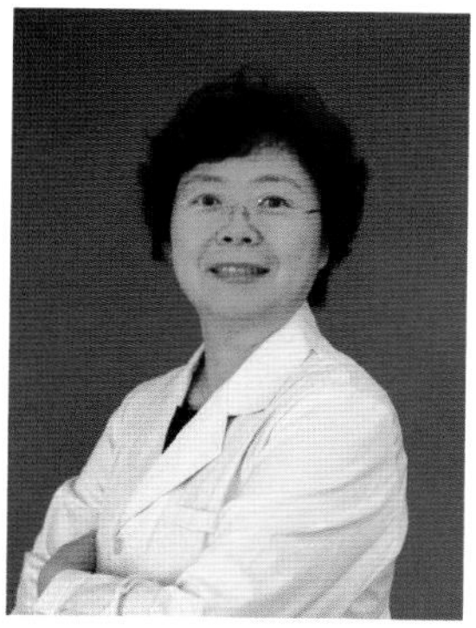

在临床医学的任何一个学科，儿童疾病都绝对不是成人疾病的缩微版，儿童眼病也是一样。儿童眼病除眼视光与斜弱视外，涉及眼科各个亚专科，还包括很多先天性眼病，同时儿童的不合作性和儿童眼球解剖结构的特殊性，使儿童眼病诊断和治疗的难度和复杂程度远远高于成人眼病。目前我国眼科界对儿童眼病的诊断和治疗已经接近国际先进水平，但还存在一些不足，如专门从事儿童眼科的医生比较少，对除视光、斜弱视等常见儿童眼病之外的其他疾病认识不足，以及广大西部地区的儿童眼科专业发展落后等问题。

以石一宁教授为主译的眼科医生团队，将美国眼科学会出版的继续教育课程中的《小儿眼科与斜视》一书翻译成中文版，就是希望通过他们的努力将儿童眼病的全貌呈现给广大眼科工作者。此书翻译工作的完成和出版，必将对我国儿童眼病的发展起到积极的推动作用，此书将会成为青年眼科医生继续教育和住院医师规范化培训的重要辅助教材，将会引导更多的眼科医生关注、学习和从事儿童眼病专业。

石一宁教授多年来一直从事儿童眼病的临床和研究，同时还是一位具有丰富经验的资深眼底病专家。退休后她仍笔耕不辍，发表了多部著作和译著，是我们中青年医生学习的榜样。本书的翻译工作由石一宁教授牵头，组织国内在儿童眼病的临床和研究方面具有丰富经验的专家团队共同完成，必将呈现给大家一部全面、实用、新颖的高水平译著。

关注儿童就是关注未来。

朱丹

内蒙古医科大学附属医院

2020 年 7 月 13 日

序七

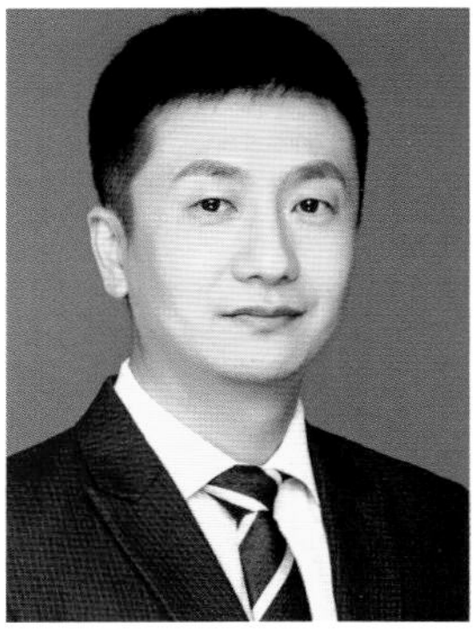

儿童是国家和民族的未来，呵护好儿童视觉健康才会带来国家和民族的光明未来，这一点已成为政府社会家庭的共识。儿童视觉健康关系到的基础知识有很多方面，临床处理手段多种多样，涉及相关研究领域的最新进展层出不穷。因此国外一些具有远见卓识的著名眼科学家将小儿眼科与斜视这 2 个亚专业融合，诞生了斜视与小儿眼科学。美国眼科学会都会定期将这些领域的研究成果浓缩为 BCSC 第 6 册，以推动斜视与小儿眼科临床水平的不断提升。从目录就可以看出，孩子不是成人的缩小版，而是处处体现了视觉发育过程中婴幼儿及儿童青少年眼病的特殊性。

我国斜视与小儿眼科的前辈们以宽广的视野和敏锐的眼光洞察到这一趋势。20 世纪中叶，赫雨时教授在国内首次成立专科，将斜视弱视作为独立的眼科亚专业发展，与此同时，其他儿童眼病的处理在大多数医院则由不同亚专业的医生承担。20 世纪 80 年代中期，刘家琦教授在国内综合医院率先创立小儿眼科。21 世纪以来，中华医学会眼科学会分会在赵堪兴教授的领导推动下，明确将眼肌学组改为斜视与小儿眼科学组，产生了巨大的导向作用。赵教授不遗余力地推动国内外学术交流，加强年轻医生培养，BCSC 第 6 册在其中扮演了重要角色。

目前斜视与小儿眼科形成了斜视、弱视、双眼视功能，其他儿童眼病，儿童屈光不正与近视防控，儿童眼保健 4 个方向。专业蓬勃发展，从业队伍不断壮大（但是依然供不应求），从业人员业务素质不断提高。但限于各地区经济社会发展水平能力不同，业务能力和服务水平尚不均衡，坚持专业队伍的继续教育，保持国际背景下的知识更新，培养合格的各层次人才等都需要高质量的教材。石一宁教授从事眼科临床实践多年，对儿童眼健康事业有很强的使命感。她慧眼识珠，发现了 BCSC 第 6 册在讲述儿童眼健康基础知识、临床处理及最新进展上的独特优势，特别是对边远欠发达地区的年轻从业人员培养，具有结构清晰、概念明确、重点突出、便于讲述的独特魅力。但由于各个地区对英文原著阅读能力的参差不齐，难免会造成对原著内容的不同理解。因此石教授投入大量精力，组织了国内众多既具有良好教育背景，又有临床实践经验的中青年专业医生，同时还聘请了国内具备国际学术交流背景的相关专家担任审译，精心地将这部书翻译成了中文，并以中英文对照的形式排版印刷。本书的翻译过程中，经历了新冠肺炎的严重影响，石教授逐一克服了重重困难，其精神令人钦佩。希望本书能将 BCSC 第 6 册的精彩内容用中文原汁原味地呈现给国内眼科同道，使我国众多斜视与小儿眼科从业者从中获益，为实现全社会共同呵护儿童眼健康、让他们拥有光明的未来而发挥积极的作用。

钱学翰

2020 年 7 月 12 日于天津

序八

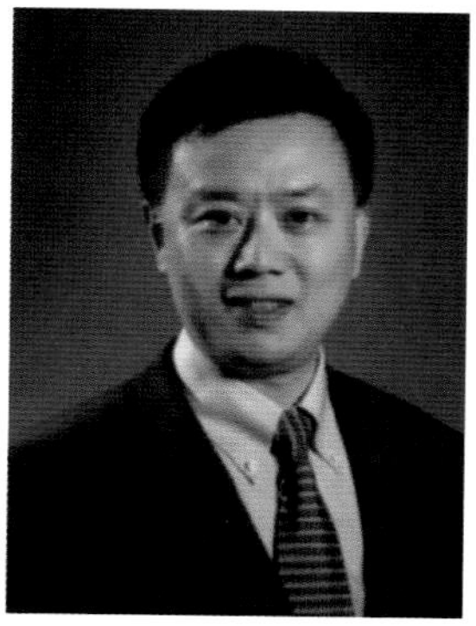

幸赖石一宁教授的信任，我和我的团队一起参与了她组织的“Basic and Clinical Science Course”分册之一*Pediatric Ophthalmology and Strabismus*的翻译工作，在石教授的精心组织下，经过近百位眼科同道的共同努力，*Pediatric Ophthalmology and Strabismus*中文版今得以顺利出版，谨在此表示祝贺！

斜视与小儿眼科是一门以眼球运动异常、双眼视发育和儿童眼病为主要研究内容的眼科亚专业。小儿眼科并非成人眼科的缩小版，由于视觉神经系统尚未发育成熟，儿童眼病的诊断和治疗与成人颇有差异，若处理不当，不仅影响儿童视觉神经系统的正常发育，严重者还会导致弱视、立体盲等难以逆转的视功能异常。作为小儿眼科大夫，临床诊治眼病的同时，应密切关注患儿的双眼视发育，并将促进双眼视发育的理念贯穿在眼病诊治的全过程。同样，儿童眼保健大夫和视光师也应将尽早地发现影响儿童双眼视发育的异常因素（知觉、运动和中枢等），促进双眼视的正常发育作为工作重点。

20年前，我有幸师从我国斜视与小儿眼科学科带头人赵堪兴教授，并自此成为斜视与小儿眼科专业的一员。在赵教授的教育与培养下，我逐渐对斜视与小儿眼科有所了解。回想学习之初，我也曾为双眼视理论的晦涩难懂而却步，也曾为斜视知觉和运动功能评估、手术设计的复杂而感到迷茫，也曾为与儿童患者的交流沟通不畅而感到苦恼……20世纪90年代，国内相关的专著并不多，1998年我第一次接触美国眼科学会出版的“Basic and Clinical Science Course”系列教程，其内容之新颖、文字之精炼、疾病诊治理念之先进令我耳目一新。尤其是*Pediatric Ophthalmology and Strabismus*分册，有别于其他专著，该分册从介绍如何与儿童沟通开始。众所周知，儿童患者就诊时多有恐惧情绪，且难以准确表述自身症状，检查多不配合，与患儿良好沟通是儿童眼科大夫面临的一大挑战。通过学习“Rapport With Children: Tips for a Productive Examination”一节，我不仅掌握了与患儿沟通的技巧，更重要的是改变了我对沟通的认识，而这些改变使我受益匪浅并影响我一生。

石教授主译的*Pediatric Ophthalmology and Strabismus*分册共有28个章节，其中第1~14章主要介绍小儿眼科检查、斜视术语、眼外肌解剖和各种不同类型的斜视，第15~16章着重介绍眼的生长与发育、视力发育，第17~28章则重点介绍儿童常见眼病和系统疾病在眼部表现。该分册的内容丰富新颖，且许多章节都在汲取最新临床研究成果和临床指南的基础上做了更新。经过该书各位译者的辛勤努力，译文力求“信、达、雅”。无疑，该书的出版将会进一步推动我国斜视与小儿眼科临床诊疗的规范化、标准化和国际化，也必将为提高我国斜视与小儿眼科大夫的专业水平发挥积极的作用。

“指穷于为薪，火传也，不知其尽也。”1984年中华医学会眼科学分会成立眼肌学组以来，在前辈们的引领下，我国斜视与小儿眼科专业在学科发展方面取得了不俗的成绩。尤其是近年来，国家卫健委颁布了一系列的政策法规，我国儿童眼保健专业蓬勃发展，以人群为基础的视力筛查和儿童眼病防治工作在基层妇幼系统已经逐步开展。妇幼系统三级网络的群体防治工作的开展，一方面给儿童眼病的早期发现和早期诊断提供可能，另一方面，也对我国斜视与小儿眼科大夫的临床诊治水平提出了新的要求。面对机遇和挑战，我国斜视与小儿眼科同道应在实践中不断提升临床诊治水平，通过继续教育学习国内外本专业的新理念和新技术，结合我国临床工作的现状，科学地应用国外的临床规范和指南，根据不同地区的特点，推广适宜技术。毋庸置疑，在国内儿童眼保健、儿童眼科和儿童眼视光工作者的共同努力下，我们一定能呵护好孩子的眼睛，让孩子们都能拥有一个光明的未来！

刘虎

2020 年 7 月 17 日

序九

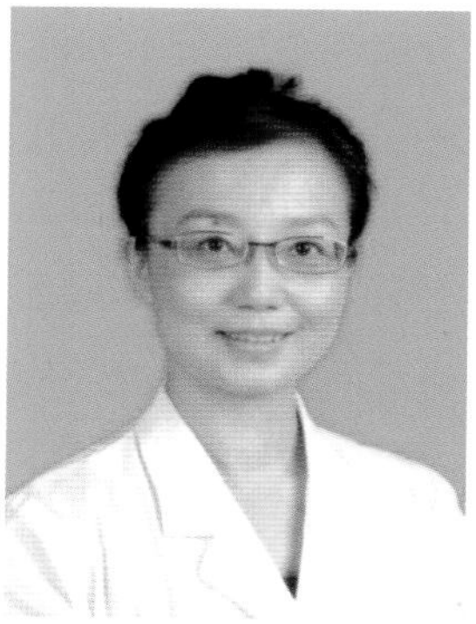

我国改革开放以来，诸多方面都需要与国际接轨，国内眼科界也不例外，需要与国际前沿眼科知识保持同步。1990 年国际眼科学会学术大会在新加坡举行，会议期间美国中美眼科学会理事与中国香港、台湾等各地的华裔眼科学者共同讨论中国眼科发展及教育前景，一致同意将美国眼科学会出版的 12 册继续教育课程的系列教材翻译为中文出版，为中国眼科医师的继续教育提供教材。这一主张得到了时任美国眼科学会执行副主席 Bruce E.Spivey 博士的热烈支持，并与时任中华医学会副会长曹泽毅教授签署了版权转让同意书。中美眼科学会前主席 Mark O.M.Tso 博士（曹安民教授）、时任主席 King Y.Lee 博士及海内外华裔眼科学界慷慨捐助积极筹资，由时任中华眼科学会副主任委员李子良具体负责组织翻译，中华医学会出版社负责出版。

第一次接触到上述系列教材中文版，是我本人准备参加国际眼科考试（ICO）时。该系列教材对提高复习效率和考试通过率起到较好的帮助作用，但由于当时复习时间紧，并未仔细深入地阅读这套教材的原版。曹安民教授一直致力于国内眼科专科医师的培训教育工作，我第二次接触到上述系列教材中文版，是曹教授组织我们北大眼科中心各亚专业组的专科医生赴国内一些地方医院进行教学培训前的课程准备时。曹安民教授殷切地希望能把美国眼科学会出版的眼科系列教材中的各种知识，通过专科培训活动传播给地方医院的年轻住院医生，他把制定小儿眼科培训大纲的任务交给了我。我因此有机会再次仔细对照阅读了该系列教材中文版与英文版中有关小儿眼科的部分，感觉从中得到许多收获。例如，国内的小儿眼科医生通常重点关注小儿的斜视和弱视 2 种疾病，实际上小儿眼科包括了许多跟儿童视觉发育息息相关的其他很多疾病，并不是所有成人的眼科疾病发生在小儿身上那么简单。在阅读英文原版时能更深刻地体会到翻译成中文后未被清晰表达的意思，并且在阅读英文原版时丰富和积累了眼科专业词汇，对提高与国外同行交流的能力非常有帮助。

20 多年过去了，国际眼科界不断发展创新，知识积累有了长足进步，这套系列教材也在不断更新中，石一宁教授再次组织国内各专业知名专家对上述英文系列教材的最新版本进行翻译，我有幸参与了该翻译文本的部分审校工作。这个版本的最大特色在于双语对照，因为通过阅读英文原版，可以帮助提升读者的双语认知能力，使其更好地理解某些细节知识，可以帮助提高临床医生的专业外语水平、与国际同行进行学术交流的能力。同时更为准确的中文翻译又为广大基层临床工作者提供了阅读的便利，本书还可以成为临床医生眼科综合知识学习的重要参考资料。

“后人总是站在前人的肩膀上远眺，人类才得以进步。”希望即将出版的这套眼科系列教材中英文对照版，能够帮助国内新一代眼科医生不断开阔视野、探究新知、创新前进。

布娟

2020 年 7 月 17 日

序十

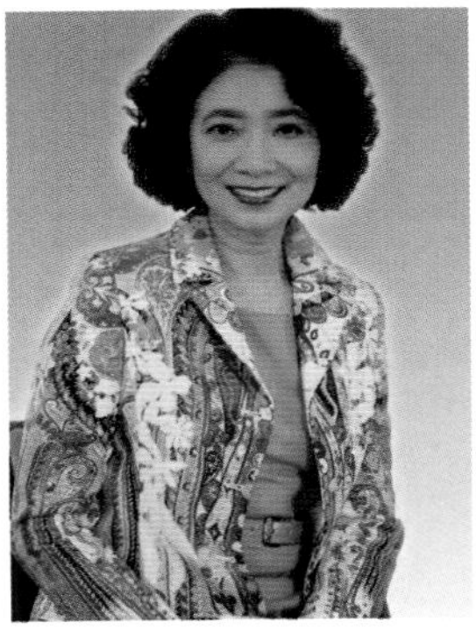

本书是美国眼科学会（AAO）的教材之一，同时是国际眼科医师（ICO）视光学和器械学考试部分的参考书之一，本书更关注于小儿眼科与斜视。2009 年，“健康快车”引入 ICO 考试的中文试卷，使英文欠佳的医生也可以参加这一国际考试。然而，由于考试的所有参考书目均为英文版，国内医生普遍反映备考存在很大困难。本书的中文翻译出版无疑是带给视光学和器械学考生们的一个大好消息。中国的眼科医生不仅能阅读原版的基础教材，通过阅读原文提升专业英文水平，更能对照中文版的内容，以更快地丰富知识及增进了解。感谢石一宁教授等人的倾力翻译。

自 1997 年成立以来，“健康快车”一直致力于中国内地的扶贫治盲及眼科医生的培训工作。石一宁教授曾担任“健康快车”陕西西安眼科中心（陕西省人民医院眼科）主任，且一直热心于眼科医生的培训与分享，“健康快车”对石一宁教授深存敬意。

方黄吉雯

健康快车创会主席

2020-8

方黄吉雯女士是一名特许会计师，2007 年退休之前担任普华永道中国业务主席。1983~1989 年，出任香港市政局和区议会议员；1988~1991 年，出任香港立法会议员；1992 年，成为首批中国政府的港事顾问之一；1993~1997 年，作为香港特别行政区筹委会委员，担任经济组召集人；1997~2002 年，担任香港行政会议成员。

方黄吉雯也因其慈善工作而闻名，其中尤以 1997 年香港回归之际创立的“健康快车”慈善项目影响最广。1997~2019 年，有超过 21 万名中国偏远地区的贫困白内障患者，在“健康快车”火车医院上接受了免费白内障手术并重获光明。“健康快车”还在内地偏远地区，成立了超过 80 间眼科中心。方黄吉雯还于 2012 年，在香港创立了艺育菁英基金会，并担任主席。

方黄吉雯于 1998 年荣获香港“太平绅士”称号，1999 年获得香港特区政府颁授的金紫荆星章。2008 年，方黄吉雯获得美国前总统克林顿颁发的克林顿全球倡议奖，此奖项以表彰她对慈善事业的贡献。2003 年、2008 年和 2013 年，方黄吉雯女士担任中国人民政治协商会议第十、十一、十二届全国委员会委员。

序十一

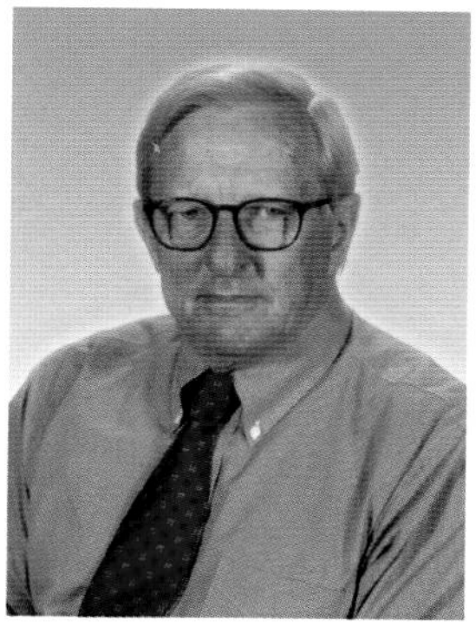

This is a brilliant book! The original book in English is a classic and it is wonderful that Prof Shi Yining has created this bilingual version which is not just translated from English to Chinese but it has the two languages side-by-side: English on the left and Chinese on the right. This is a book that will clearly help Chinese doctors to learn the vital basis of their practise. It will also help them to better their English and do we even dare hope that some English ophthalmologists will learn some Chinese!

这本书真是十分精彩！英文原版自是一部经典，另外石一宁教授更是创造性地做出了一个双语版本。这不仅仅是将英文翻译为汉语，而是2种语言并排显示：左边为英文，右边为汉语。毫无疑问，这本书将帮助中国医生认识行医中的重要理念并提高其专业技能。这也将有助于他们提升英语水平，甚至也能帮助一些使用英语的眼科医生学习一点汉语！

Professor Shi has had extensive experience in residency education, she has published a hundred scientific papers and 5 ophthalmic books, including other bilingual interpretations. This new bilingual version is poised to become a very significant part of Chinese ophthalmology' s rapid advances in learning and ultimately in improving patient care based on the scientific foundations of our profession.

石教授在培训住院医师方面有着丰富的经验，她已发表了100余篇论文，出版了5本眼科书籍，还有其他双语版本的书籍。这一新的双语版书籍必将成为快速发展的中国眼科学中的重要组成部分，并且在我们的科学研究基础之上最终能更好地服务于患者。

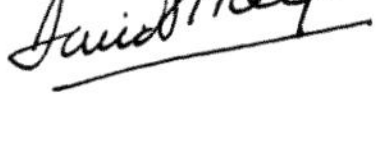

Prof David Taylor, FRCOphth. FRCPCH, DSc (Med)

Professor Emeritus, Paediatric Ophthalmology, Great Ormond Street Institute of Child Health, University College London. Previously, Director(Honorary), International Council of Ophthalmology Examinations

大卫泰勒教授，皇家眼科学院会员，皇家儿科与儿童健康学院会员，理学博士（医学）

小儿眼科荣誉教授，大奥蒙德街儿童健康研究所，伦敦大学学院。国际眼科考试委员会前荣誉主任

BCSC® volumes are designed to increase the physician's ophthalmic knowledge through study and review. Users of this activity are encouraged to read the text and then answer the study questions provided at the back of the book.

Cover image: From BCSC Section 9, *Uveitis and Ocular Inflammation*. Large mutton-fat keratic precipitates in a patient with sarcoidosis. (*Courtesy of Debra Goldstein, MD.*)

BCSC 旨在通过研究与回顾来增加医生的眼科知识。鼓励学者阅读课文，然后回答书后提出的问题。

学会仅提供以教育为目的的资料。这并不意味着它是所有医疗中唯一或最好的方法，也不可以取代医生的判断或为疾病的诊断提供具体建议。在使用前，包括超出资料范围的每种药物或治疗的所有适应证、禁忌证、副作用和替代药物，所有的信息和建议都应经过验证，并结合患者的病情和病史，还应注意生产商的包装说明书或其他独立的信息。本教程中提及的一些药物、器械和其他产品说明书仅供说明之用，并不表示认可。有的材料可能包括一些超出社区医疗标准的信息。这些应用未经 FDA 美国食品药品监督管理局批准，或者仅被批准应用于限定的研究环境。**FDA 声明内科医师有责任确定他或她想要使用的每科药物或设备的 FDA 规定应用状态，并在患者知情的情况下适当地按照法律使用它们。**对于因使用本手册的任何建议或信息而产生的所有索赔，学会声明免除因疏忽或其他原因造成的全部伤害和责任。

封面图片来自 BCSC 第 9 册《*葡萄膜炎与眼部炎症*》中的“结节病患者中大量的突变脂肪性角化物沉淀”。*（译者注：资料来源见前页原文。）*

Basic and Clinical Science Course

Louis B. Cantor, MD, Indianapolis, Indiana, *Senior Secretary for Clinical Education*
Christopher J. Rapuano, MD, Philadelphia, Pennsylvania, *Secretary for Lifelong Learning and Assessment*
Colin A. McCannel, MD, Los Angeles, California, *BCSC Course Chair*

Section 6

Faculty for the Major Revision

Robert W. Hered, MD, *Chair*, Maitland, Florida
Steven M. Archer, MD, Ann Arbor, Michigan
Rebecca Sands Braverman, MD, Aurora, Colorado
Arif O. Khan, MD, Abu Dhabi, United Arab Emirates
Katherine A. Lee, MD, PhD, Boise, Idaho
Gregg T. Lueder, MD, St Louis, Missouri
Mary A. O'Hara, MD, Sacramento, California
Kristina Tarczy-Hornoch, MD, DPhil, Seattle, Washington

The Academy wishes to acknowledge the *American Association for Pediatric Ophthalmology and Strabismus (AAPOS)* and the *American Academy of Pediatrics (AAP), Section on Ophthalmology*, for recommending faculty members to the BCSC Section 6 committee.

The Academy also wishes to acknowledge the following committees for review of this edition:

Committee on Aging: Aaron M. Miller, MD, MBA, Shenandoah, Texas

Vision Rehabilitation Committee: Terry L. Schwartz, MD, Cincinnati, Ohio

Practicing Ophthalmologists Advisory Committee for Education: Alice Bashinsky, MD, *Primary Reviewer*, Asheville, North Carolina; Edward K. Isbey III, MD, *Chair*, Asheville, North Carolina; David J. Browning, MD, PhD, Charlotte, North Carolina; Bradley D. Fouraker, MD, Tampa, Florida; Steven J. Grosser, MD, Golden Valley, Minnesota; Stephen R. Klapper, MD, Carmel, Indiana; James A. Savage, MD, Memphis, Tennessee; Michelle S. Ying, MD, Ladson, South Carolina

基础与临床科学教程

Louis B. Cantor，医学博士，印第安纳波利斯市，印第安纳州，*高级临床教育秘书*
Christopher J. Rapuano，医学博士，费城，宾夕法尼亚州，*终身学习与评估秘书*
Colin A. McCannel，医学博士，洛杉矶，加利福尼亚州，*BCSC 教程主席*

第 6 册

主要修订的教师

Robert W. Hered，医学博士，*大学教授*，梅特兰，佛罗里达州
Steven M. Archer，医学博士，安阿伯，密歇根州
Rebecca Sands Braverman，医学博士，奥罗拉，科罗拉多州
Arif O. Khan，医学博士，阿布扎比，阿拉伯联合酋长国
Katherine A. Lee，医学博士，哲学博士，博伊西，爱达荷州
Gregg T. Lueder，医学博士，圣路易斯，密苏里州
Mary A. O'Hara，医学博士，萨克拉曼多，加利福尼亚州
Kristina Tarczy-Hornoch，医学博士，哲学博士，西雅图，华盛顿

学会感谢*美国小儿眼科与斜视协会（AAPOS）*和*美国儿科学会（AAP）*，*眼科分会*推荐教师加入 BCSC 第 6 册的编委会。

学会致谢的评审委员会：

老龄化委员会：Aaron M. Miller，医学博士，MBA，谢南多厄，得克萨斯州

视觉康复委员会：Terry L. Schwartz，医学博士，辛辛那提，俄亥俄州

专业教育委员会：Alice Bashinsky，医学博士，*主审查员*，阿什维尔，北卡罗来纳州；Edward K. Isbey III，医学博士，*大学教授*，阿什维尔，北卡罗来纳州；David J. Browning，医学博士，哲学博士，夏洛特市，北卡罗来纳州；Bradley D. Fouraker，医学博士，坦帕市，佛罗里达州；Steven J. Grosser，医学博士，黄金谷，明尼苏达州；Stephen R. Klapper，医学博士，卡梅尔镇，印第安纳州；James A. Savage，医学博士，孟菲斯市，田纳西州；Michelle S. Ying，医学博士，莱德森，南卡罗来纳州。

European Board of Ophthalmology: Wagih Aclimandos, MB BCh, DO, FEBO, *EBO Chair*, London, United Kingdom; Peter J. Ringens, MD, PhD, *EBO Liaison*, Maastricht, Netherlands;Georges Caputo, MD, Paris, France; Rosario Gómez de Liaño, MD, Madrid, Spain; Peng T. Khaw, MD, PhD, London, United Kingdom; Birgit Lorenz, MD, PhD, Giessen, Germany; Francis L. Munier, MD, Lausanne, Switzerland; Seyhan B. Özkan, MD, Aydin, Turkey; Maria Papadopoulos, MBBS, London, United Kingdom; Nicoline E. Schalij- Delfos, MD, PhD, Leiden, Netherlands

The Academy also wishes to acknowledge the following committee for assistance in developing study questions and answers for this BCSC Section:

Self-Assessment Committee: Mitchell B. Strominger, MD, *Chair*, Boston, Massa chusetts; Deborah M. Costakos, MD, Milwaukee, Wisconsin; Theodore Curtis, MD, Mount Kisco, New York; Mark I. Salevitz, MD, Scottsdale, Arizona

Financial Disclosures

Academy staff members who contributed to the development of this product state that within the 12 months prior to their contributions to this CME activity and for the duration of development, they have had no financial interest in or other relationship with any entity discussed in this course that produces, markets, resells, or distributes ophthalmic health care goods or services consumed by or used in patients, or with any competing commercial product or service.

The authors and reviewers state that within the 12 months prior to their contributions to this CME activity and for the duration of development, they have had the following financial relationships:*

Dr Sands Braverman: Welch Allyn (C)

Dr Browning: Aerpio Therapeutics (S), Alcon Laboratories (S), Alimera Sciences (C), Genentech (S), Novartis Phar ma ceu ti cals (S), Ohr Phar ma ceu ti cals (S), Pfizer (S), Regeneron Phar maceu ticals (S), Zeiss (O)

Dr Fouraker: Addition Technology (C, L), Alcon Laboratories (C, L), KeraVision (C, L), OASIS Medical (C, L)

Dr Gómez de Liaño: Alcon Laboratories (C)

Dr Grosser: InjectSense (O), Ivantis (O)

Dr Hered: Moria Surgical (P)

Dr Isbey: Alcon Laboratories (S), Allscripts (C), Bausch + Lomb (S), Medflow (C), Oculos Clinical Research (S)

Dr Khaw: Isarna Therapeutics (C), Novartis (C), Santen (C)

Dr Lorenz: Bausch + Lomb (C), Bayer HealthCare Phar ma ceu ti cals (L), Clarity (L, S), Novartis Phar ma ceu ti cals (L, S), Spark Therapeutics (C)

Dr Miller: Alcon Laboratories (L), Credential Protection (O)

欧洲眼科学会：Wagih Aclimandos，MB BCh，DO，FEBO，*EBO 主席*，伦敦，英国；Peter J. Ringens，医学博士，哲学博士，*EBO 联络员*，马斯特里赫特，荷兰；Georges Caputo，医学博士，巴黎，法国；Rosario Gomez de Liano，医学博士，马德里，西班牙；Peng T. Khaw，医学博士，哲学博士，伦敦，英国；Birgit Lorenz，医学博士，哲学博士，吉森，德国；Francis L. Munier，医学博士，洛桑，瑞士；Seyhan B. Ozkan，医学博士，艾登省，土耳其；Maria Papadopoulos，MBBS，伦敦，英国；Nicoline E. Schalij-Delfos，医学博士，哲学博士，莱顿，荷兰。

学会还想感谢以下委员会的帮助，为 BCSC 教程提供学习的问题和答案：

自我评估委员会：Mitchell B. Strominger，医学博士，*主席*，波士顿，马萨诸塞州；Deborah M. Costakos，医学博士，密尔沃基，威斯康星州；Theodore Curtis，医学博士，芒特基斯科，纽约；Mark I. Salevitz，医学博士，斯科茨代尔，亚利桑那州。

财务信息

参与开发此产品的学会工作人员声明，在对发布此次 CME 活动 12 个月之前和开发该产品期间，他们与该教程中涉及的任何产品没有经济利益和其他关系，没有将其使用或应用于患者，包括产品的生产、市场出售、推广眼科医疗保健商品或服务中，没有与任何实体或金融机构产生关系，没有与任何产品或服务进行商业竞争。

作者和评审人员声明，在发布 CME 活动之前的 12 个月以及开发期间，他们拥有以下财务关系：*

Sands Braverman 博士：Welch Allyn (C)

Browning 博士：Aerpio Therapeutics (S), Alcon Laboratories (S), Alimera Sciences (C), Genentech (S), Novartis Pharmaceuticals (S), Ohr Pharmaceuticals (S), Pfizer (S), Regeneron Pharmaceuticals (S), Zeiss (O)

Fouraker 博士：Addition Technology (C, L), Alcon Laboratories (C, L), Kera Vision (C, L), OASIS Medical (C, L)

Gomez de Liano 博士：Alcon Laboratories (C)

Grosser 博士：InjectSense (O), Ivantis (O)

Hered 博士：Moria Surgical (P)

Isbey 博士：Alcon Laboratories (S), Allscripts (C), Bausch + Lomb (S), Medflow (C), Oculos Clinical Research (S)

Khaw 博士：Isarna Therapeutics (C), Novartis (C), Santen (C)

Lorenz 博士：Bausch + Lomb (C), Bayer HealthCare Pharmaceuticals (L), Clarity (L, S), Novartis Pharmaceuticals (L, S), Spark Therapeutics (C)

Miller 博士：Alcon Laboratories (L), Credential Protection (O)

Dr Schalij- Delfos: Novartis (C)

Dr Tarczy- Hornoch: Amgen (O), Mylan (O)

The other authors and reviewers state that within the 12 months prior to their contributions to this CME activity and for the duration of development, they have had no financial interest in or other relationship with any entity discussed in this course that produces, markets, resells, or distributes ophthalmic health care goods or services consumed by or used in patients, or with any competing commercial product or service.

*C = consultant fees, paid advisory boards, or fees for attending a meeting; L = lecture fees (honoraria), travel fees, or reimbursements when speaking at the invitation of a commercial sponsor; O = equity own-ership/stock options of publicly or privately traded firms (excluding mutual funds) with manufacturers of commercial ophthalmic products or commercial ophthalmic services; P = patents and/or royalties that might be viewed as creating a potential conflict of interest; S = grant support for the past year (all sources) and all sources used for a specific talk or manuscript with no time limitation

Recent Past Faculty

Daniel J. Karr, MD
Sylvia R. Kodsi, MD
Stephen P. Kraft, MD
Kanwal (Ken) Nischal, MD
Evelyn A. Paysse, MD

In addition, the Academy gratefully acknowledges the contributions of numerous past faculty and advisory committee members who have played an important role in the devel opment of previous editions of the Basic and Clinical Science Course.

American Academy of Ophthalmology Staff

Dale E. Fajardo, EdD, MBA, *Vice President, Education*
Beth Wilson, *Director, Continuing Professional Development*
Ann McGuire, *Acquisitions and Development Manager*
Stephanie Tanaka, *Publications Manager*
D. Jean Ray, *Production Manager*
Susan Malloy, *Acquisitions Editor and Program Manager*
Jasmine Chen, *Manager of E-Learning*
Beth Collins, *Medical Editor*
Eric Gerdes, *Interactive Designer*
Naomi Ruiz, *Publications Specialist*

Schalij–Delfos 博士：Novartis (C)

Tarczy–Hornoch 博士：Amgen (O), Mylan (O)

其他作者和审稿人声明：在发布 CME 活动之前 12 个月内及在此开发期间，他们与本教程中讨论的生产、营销、转售或所消费的眼科保健产品或服务的任何实体，或与任何竞争性商业产品或服务没有任何财务利益或其他关系。

*C= 顾问费，支付给顾问委员会或出席会议的费用；L= 应商业赞助商邀请发言时的演讲费（酬金）、差旅费或报销费用；O= 公开或私营贸易公司（不包括共同基金）与商业眼科产品制造商的股份 / 股票期权或商业眼科服务的费用；P= 可能被视为造成潜在利益冲突的专利和（或）版税；S= 过去 1 年（所有来源）的资助以及无时间限制的特定谈话或手稿的所有财务来源

近年卸任的教师

Daniel J. Karr，医学博士
Sylvia R. Kodsi，医学博士
Stephen P. Kraft，医学博士
Kanwal (Ken) Nischal，医学博士
Evelyn A. Paysse，医学博士

此外，学会衷心感谢以往的许多教师和咨询委员会成员，他们在“基础与临床科学教程”前几版的发展中发挥着重要的作用。

美国眼科学会工作人员

Dale E. Fajardo，EdD，工商管理硕士，*教育部副总裁*
Beth Wilson，*持续专业发展总监*
Ann McGuire，*采购和开发经理*
Stephanie Tanaka，*出版社经理*
D. Jean Ray，*生产部经理*
Susan Malloy，*采购编辑和项目经理*
Jasmine Chen，*电子学习经理*
Beth Collins，*医学编辑*
Eric Gerdes，*互动设计师*
Naomi Ruiz，*出版专家*

（翻译 // 审校 石一宁 杨嘉嵩）

CONTENTS

目录

General Introduction

The Basic and Clinical Science Course (BCSC) is designed to meet the needs of residents and practitioners for a comprehensive yet concise curriculum of the field of ophthalmology. The BCSC has developed from its original brief outline format, which relied heavily on outside readings, to a more convenient and educationally useful self-contained text. The Academy updates and revises the course annually, with the goals of integrating the basic science and clinical practice of ophthalmology and of keeping ophthalmologists current with new developments in the various subspecialties.

The BCSC incorporates the effort and expertise of more than 90 ophthalmologists, organized into 13 Section faculties, working with Academy editorial staff. In addition, the course continues to benefit from many lasting contributions made by the faculties of previous editions. Members of the Academy Practicing Ophthalmologists Advisory Committee for Education, Committee on Aging, and Vision Rehabilitation Committee review every volume before major revisions. Members of the European Board of Ophthalmology, organized into Section faculties, also review each volume before major revisions, focusing primarily on differences between American and European ophthalmology practice.

Organization of the Course

The Basic and Clinical Science Course comprises 13 volumes, incorporating fundamental ophthalmic knowledge, subspecialty areas, and special topics:

1 Update on General Medicine
2 Fundamentals and Principles of Ophthalmology
3 Clinical Optics
4 Ophthalmic Pathology and Intraocular Tumors
5 Neuro-Ophthalmology
6 Pediatric Ophthalmology and Strabismus
7 Oculofacial Plastic and Orbital Surgery
8 External Disease and Cornea
9 Uveitis and Ocular Inflammation
10 Glaucoma
11 Lens and Cataract
12 Retina and Vitreous
13 Refractive Surgery

In addition, a comprehensive Master Index allows the reader to easily locate subjects throughout the entire series.

References

Readers who wish to explore specific topics in greater detail may consult the references cited within each chapter and listed in the Basic Texts section at the back of the book. These references are intended to be selective rather than exhaustive, chosen by the BCSC faculty as being important, current, and readily available to residents and practitioners.

概述

“基础与临床科学教程”（BCSC）旨在满足住院医师和执业医师对眼科领域全面而简明课程设置的要求。BCSC 已经从最初的大纲格式（主要依赖于课外阅读）发展成为一种更方便、教育上更为有用的独立教材。学会每年对教程进行更新和修订，目标是将眼科基础科学与临床实践相结合，使眼科医生与各专科的新进展保持同步。

基础与临床科学教程（BCSC）凝聚了 13 个学科的 90 多名眼科医生的努力和专业知识，以及眼科学会编辑人员的共同努力工作。此外，本教程还得益于前几任学会人员所做的多年贡献，学会执业眼科医师教育咨询委员会、老龄委员会以及视力康复委员会都会在重大修订之前，审查每一册。欧洲眼科委员会也会组成分册编委会，审查每一册，然后进行重大修订，主要集中于美国和欧盟眼科实践之间的差异。

教程编制

“基础与临床科学教程”包括 13 册，包含基本的眼科知识、亚专业领域和专题：

1 医学最新进展
2 眼科学基础与原理
3 临床光学
4 眼病理学与眼内肿瘤
5 神经眼科学
6 小儿眼科与斜视
7 眼面部整形与眼眶手术
8 外眼疾病与角膜
9 葡萄膜炎与眼部炎症
10 青光眼
11 晶状体与白内障
12 视网膜与玻璃体
13 屈光手术

此外，一个全面的总索引便于读者在整个教程中寻找到主题。

参考文献

读者欲更详细地探讨特定主题，可参考书中每一章所引用的参考文献，以及书后的基础书籍一节列出的书籍。这些参考资料是有选择性的，并不详尽，由 BCSC 编委会选择重要的、最新进展的，并可以提供给住院医师和医生。

Multimedia

This edition of Section 6, *Pediatric Ophthalmology and Strabismus*, includes videos related to topics covered in the book. The videos were selected by members of the BCSC faculty to present important topics that are best delivered visually. This edition also includes an interactive feature, or "activity," developed by members of the BCSC faculty. Both the videos and the activity are available to readers of the print and electronic versions of Section 6 (www.aao .org/bcscvideo_section06) and (www.aao. org/bcscactivity_section06). Mobiledevice users can scan the QR codes below (a QR-code reader must already be installed on the device) to access the videos and activity.

Videos   Activity

Self-Assessment

Each volume of the BCSC is designed as an independent study activity for ophthalmology residents and practitioners. The learning objectives for this volume are given on page 7. The text, illustrations, and references provide the information necessary to achieve the objectives; the study questions allow readers to test their understanding of the material and their mastery of the objectives.

This Section of the BCSC has been approved by the American Board of Ophthalmology as a Maintenance of Certification (MOC) Part II self-assessment CME activity.

Conclusion

The Basic and Clinical Science Course has expanded greatly over the years, with the addition of much new text, numerous illustrations, and video content. Recent editions have sought to place greater emphasis on clinical applicability while maintaining a solid foundation in basic science. As with any educational program, it reflects the experience of its authors. As its faculties change and medicine progresses, new viewpoints emerge on controversial subjects and techniques. Not all alternate approaches can be included in this series; as with any educational endeavor, the learner should seek additional sources, including Academy Preferred Practice Pattern Guidelines.

The BCSC faculty and staff continually strive to improve the educational usefulness of the course; you, the reader, can contribute to this ongoing process. If you have any suggestions or questions about the series, please do not hesitate to contact the faculty or the editors.

The authors, editors, and reviewers hope that your study of the BCSC will be of lasting value and that each Section will serve as a practical resource for quality patient care.

多媒体

这一版的第 6 册，《*小儿眼科与斜视*》包括与书中主题相关的视频。这些视频由 BCSC 编委会挑选出来，用来展示最具视觉效果的重要主题。这个版本还包括一个由 BCSC 编委会开发的交互式功能或“活动”。读者可通过第 6 册的纸质版和电子版（www.aao.org/bcscvideosection06 和 www.aao.org/bcscactivitysection06）获取这些视频和活动。移动设备用户可扫描下面的二维码来访问视频和活动内容。

视频　　活动

自我评价

每册 BCSC 都是为眼科住院医师和执业医师设计的独立研究活动。本册的学习目标见第 7 页。教材、插图和参考文献提供了实现目标所需的信息，研究问题旨在让读者测试他们对教材的理解和对目标的掌握程度。

结论

近年来，“基础与临床科学教程”有了很大的扩展，具有大量的新内容、插图和视频内容。最新的版本试图在保持基础科学坚实基础的同时，更强调临床的适用性。与任何教育项目一样，它体现了作者的经验。随着学会的更换和医学的进步，对有争议的学科和技术产生了新的观点。不是所有的替代方法都可以包含在这个系列中；与任何教育努力一样，学习者应该寻求更多的资源，包括眼科学会的眼科临床指南 PPP。

BCSC 编委会不断努力提高教程的教育作用。作为读者，您可以为进行中的教程做一些贡献。如果您对该系列有任何疑问或不解，请立即与教师或编辑联系。

作者、编辑和评审者希望您的 BCSC 学习有持续的价值，并希望每个部分能够为患者高质量保健提供实用资源。

（李甸　译）

Objectives

Upon completion of BCSC Section 6, *Pediatric Ophthalmology and Strabismus*, the reader should be able to

- describe techniques for evaluating young children that provide the maximum information gain with the least trauma and frustration
- describe the anatomy and physiology of the extraocular muscles
- explain the classification and diagnosis of amblyopia
- describe the treatment options for amblyopia
- describe the commonly used tests for the diagnosis and measurement of strabismus
- classify the various esodeviations and exodeviations
- describe the management of each type of esodeviation and exodeviation
- describe various aspects of visual performance, including visual acuity, brightness sensitivity,
- summarize the steps for performing streak retinoscopy
- identify the steps for performing a manifest refraction using a phoropter or trial lenses
- describe the use of the Jackson cross cylinder
- identify pattern and vertical strabismus, as well as special forms of strabismus, and describe a treatment plan for each type
- list the most common lacrimal drainage system abnormalities found in children
- describe a management plan for the most common lacrimal drainage system abnormalities occurring in children
- list the most common diseases and malformations of the anterior segment occurring in children
- describe the diagnostic findings and treatment options for childhood glaucoma
- identify common types of childhood cataract and other lens disorders
- describe a diagnostic and management plan for childhood cataracts
- identify appropriate diagnostic tests for pediatric uveitis
- identify various vitreoretinal, optic disc, and metabolic diseases and disorders that occur in children
- describe the characteristic findings of accidental and nonaccidental ocular trauma in childhood
- list the characteristics of ocular tumors and phakomatoses occurring in children

目　标

完成 BCSC 第 6 册《*小儿眼科与斜视*》后，读者应能够掌握以下技能：

- 描述对于幼儿的创伤最小、干扰最少，且可获得最多信息的检测方法

- 描述眼外肌的解剖学和生理学
- 解释弱视的分类和诊断
- 描述弱视的治疗方案
- 描述斜视诊断和测量的常规检查方法
- 描述不同内斜视和外斜视的分型
- 描述每一类型内斜视和外斜视的处理方法
- 鉴别 pattern 斜视和垂直斜视及特殊类型斜视，并描述每一类型的治疗方案

- 描述不同类型儿童眼球震颤的特征，并解释其意义
- 斜视手术可能的并发症，以及手术并发症最小化的临床指南
- 描述儿童视力下降的诊断方法
- 列出儿童先天性和获得性眼部感染的各种原因，并描述每一类型感染的合理诊断和治疗方案
- 列出最常见的儿童泪道疾病
- 描述儿童泪道最常见疾病的治疗方案

- 列举儿童最常见的眼前节疾病和发育异常

- 描述儿童青光眼的诊断和治疗方案
- 鉴别儿童白内障的常见类型和其他晶状体疾病
- 描述儿童白内障的诊断及治疗计划
- 确定儿童葡萄膜炎的适当诊断方法
- 鉴别儿童的玻璃体视网膜、视盘以及代谢性疾病和异常

- 描述意外及非意外性儿童眼外伤的临床表现

- 列出儿童眼肿瘤及斑痣性错构瘤的特征

CHAPTER 1

The Pediatric Eye Examination

This chapter includes a related video, which can be accessed by scanning the QR code provided in the text or going to www.aao.org/bcscvideo_section06.

Children and their ophthalmic problems differ greatly from the patients and ocular conditions encountered in adult ophthalmology. Each developmental level in children requires a different approach for the examination, but with proper preparation and a positive attitude, the ophthalmologist can find the examination of pediatric patients to be both enjoyable and rewarding.

Examination of Children in the Outpatient Setting

An unworried child will allow a more pleasant and valuable examination. The atmosphere in the ophthalmology office or clinic, therefore, should be welcoming and positive. Preferably, a small room or section of the waiting area should be designated and designed for children. Parents and caregivers, as well as any adult patients, will be grateful for this separation. Also, because some children fear the white coat, many pediatric practitioners choose not to wear one.

A dedicated long pediatric examination lane with different types of distance fixation targets (including remotely activated videos and mechanical animals 6 meters from the examination chair) is optimal. Having several small toys readily available for near fixation is useful for the 1 toy, 1 look rule (Fig 1-1). Translucent, plastic finger puppets become silent accommodative near targets that can also provide a corneal light reflex if placed over a muscle light or penlight.

History and Examination: General Considerations and Strategies

For the pediatric history, it is important to obtain information about the pregnancy and neonatal period, with attention to maternal health and the patient's weight and gestational age at birth. The practitioner should ask whether the child has reached applicable developmental milestones, whether there are any neurologic problems, and whether there is a family history of strabismus or other childhood eye disorders.

The examination begins as the practitioner enters the room. An experienced practitioner may gather important information before formal examination begins. Visual behavior, abnormal head position, dysmorphic features, ability to ambulate, familial disorders (note parents and siblings), and family social dynamics can be effectively observed. A parent's smartphone may contain photos and videos that prove useful in establishing a diagnosis and a condition's progression over time.

第 1 章

小儿眼科检查

本章包含的相关视频，可通过扫描文本中提供的二维码或访问网页获得 www.aao.org/bcscvideo_section06。

儿童眼病与成人眼病有极大的不同。儿童在不同的发育阶段所需的检查不同，只要做好充分准备和具备积极的态度，眼科医生就会发现，给小患者检查是愉快而有成就感的。

门诊儿童检查

放松的孩子会更乐意接受检查而且其结果更有价值。因此，眼科诊所或门诊的氛围应该友好且活泼。最好为儿童指定和设计一个小房间或等候区，父母、护理人员以及成人患者都应该与之分隔。另外，有些孩子害怕白大衣，所以很多小儿科医生都不穿白大衣。

专用于儿童视力检查的通道应足够长，并且设计不同距离的视标（包括距检查椅 6m 距离的遥控视频和机械动物玩具）。准备几个小玩具，用于玩具尺检查近距离注视（图 1–1）。半透明的塑料手指木偶玩具可作为静态近距调节检查的视标，若套在笔灯或手电筒上，还可作为角膜映光检查的光源。

病史及检查：原则及策略

对于儿童病史，应注意询问妊娠期、新生儿期的相关信息，同时还应注意询问生产时产妇的健康情况、孩子的出生体重和胎龄等问题。医生还应询问孩子是否达到了相应生理发育期的指标，是否有神经系统问题，以及是否有斜视或其他儿童眼病的家族史。

医生一进入房间，检查就开始了。有经验的医生在正式检查前就已经收集到重要信息，可以有效地观察到孩子的视觉行为、异常头位、畸形、行走能力、家族的异常（注意父母和兄弟姐妹的情况）以及家庭的社会关系。家长的手机可能存有照片和视频，能为确诊和判断病情的进展提供有效的信息。

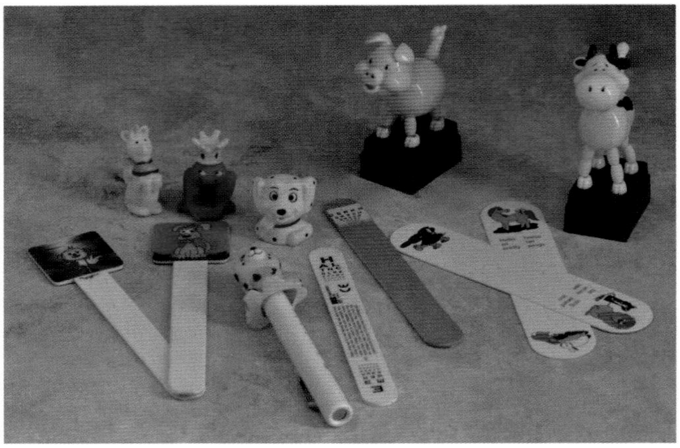

Figure 1-1 Small toys, pictures, and eye charts are used as accommodative near fixation targets. *(Courtesy of Robert W. Hered, MD.)*

The practitioner should sit at the child's eye level; note that some children are more contented sitting in a parent's lap. Introducing oneself to the child and family and establishing and maintaining eye contact with the child are important. Being relaxed, open, and playful during the examination helps create a "safe" environment. Gaining the child's confidence can lead to a faster and better examination, easier follow-up visits, and greater parental support.

cIt is helpful to first address a young child with easy questions. For example, children enjoy being regarded as "big" and correcting adults when they are wrong. The practitioner can tell a child, "You look so grown up," before grossly overestimating the patient's age or grade level and asking, "Is that right?" A simple joke can relax both child and parent.

Because cooperation may be fleeting, the examination elements that are most critical for diagnosis and management should be addressed early. If binocular fusion is in doubt, it should be checked first, before being disrupted by other tests, including those for visual acuity. When possible, the most threatening parts of the examination should be performed last.

A different vocabulary should be developed for working with children, such as "I want to show you something special" instead of "I need to examine you." Use "magic sunglasses" for the stereo glasses, "special flashlight" for the retinoscope, "funny hat" for the indirect ophthalmoscope, and "magnifying glass" for the indirect lens.

While checking vision, the practitioner can make the child feel successful by initially presenting objects that can be readily discerned and then saying, "That's too easy—let's try this one." Confrontation visual field testing can be performed as a counting-fingers game. Children might be coaxed into a slit-lamp examination if told they can "drive the motorcycle" by grabbing the handles of the slit lamp. Pushing the "magic button" on the child's nose while a distance fixation target is surreptitiously activated distracts and disarms the patient and allows for a more deliberate examination.

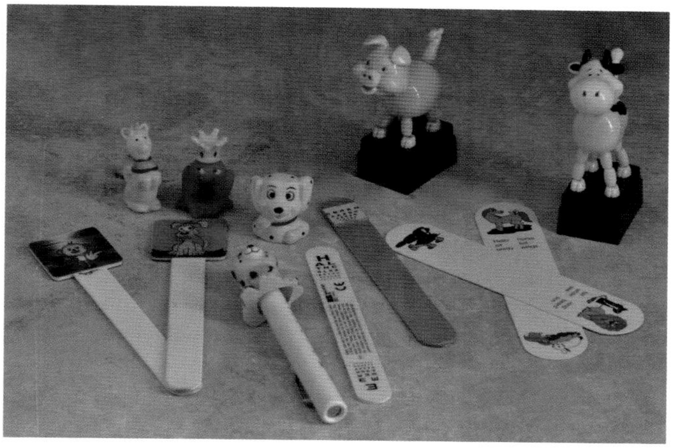

图 1–1　小玩具、图片和视力表被用作近距调节检查的视标。*（译者注：资料来源见前页原文。）*

医生和孩子的眼睛应该保持在同一水平高度，需要注意有些孩子喜欢坐在父母的腿上。医生向孩子和家长介绍自己、与孩子建立和保持眼神交流是很重要的。检查时放松、开放和嬉戏的氛围有助于创造一个“安全”的环境。获得孩子的信任可以使他们更快更好地接受检查，更容易进行随访，并得到其父母的充分支持。

最好先问孩子一些简单问题。例如，孩子们喜欢被视为“大人”，当成人错了的时候，孩子会指出错误。医生可以告诉孩子“你真懂事”，然后故意高估患儿的年龄或年级水平并问“是这样吗？”，一个简单的玩笑即可让孩子和父母都放松。

因为孩子能配合的时间可能很短暂，所以要抓紧完成对诊疗最关键的检查。如果考虑双眼融像功能有问题，应先进行相关的检查，因为其他检查（包括视力检查）可能会破坏融像而影响检查结果。如果可能的话，最难做的检查应该最后进行。

要对孩子使用不同的词汇，比如“我想给你看一些特别的东西”，而不是“我要给你做检查”，用“魔法太阳镜”替代立体镜、用“特殊手电筒”替代检眼镜、用“滑稽的帽子”替代间接检眼镜、用“放大镜”替代前置镜。

在检查视力的时候，医生可以先展示一些较易辨别的物体，让孩子有成就感，然后告诉他们：“那个太简单了，再试试这个。”面对面的视野检查可以做数手指游戏。如果告诉孩子“驾驶摩托车”来抓住裂隙灯的把手，他们可能会更愿意进行裂隙灯检查。当悄悄移动一个固定距离的视标时，按一下孩子的鼻子，告诉他上面有个“魔法按钮”，可以分散并缓和患儿的注意力，会使检查更仔细。

For examination of a difficult child, some combination of rest periods, persuasion, persistence, and rewards is usually successful. If a child is having a bad day, however, it is sometimes best to stop the examination and schedule another appointment. For the follow-up examination of an infant who was fussy during the first visit, ask the parent or other caregiver to bring the infant in hungry and then feed him or her during the examination. In infants and younger children, brief restraint may prevail. However, the practitioner must consider the physical and emotional consequences of restraining a child. Depending on the nature of the ocular problem, a sedated examination or an examination under anesthesia may be a better solution.

Examination: Specific Elements

The elements that constitute a complete pediatric ophthalmology examination parallel those that make up an adult examination but often require different techniques and devices. The following sections focus on these differences.

Visual Acuity Assessment

Visual acuity assessment requires different approaches depending on the age, developmental level, and cooperativeness of the child. In children, detection of amblyopia is of particular concern (see Chapter 6). Amblyopia is a developmental disorder of the central nervous system due to the abnormal processing of visual images, which leads to reduced visual acuity. Amblyopia is responsible for more cases of childhood-onset unilateral decreased vision than all other causes combined but is preventable or reversible with timely detection and intervention. Early detection of reduced vision from amblyopia is possible with the techniques described herein.

Ideally, accurate measurement of monocular distance visual acuity using a linear display of Sloan letters would be possible in all pediatric patients. Commonly, however, the child is preverbal, preliterate, or not fully cooperative. In these cases, clinical options include assessment of fixation behavior or testing with alternative eye charts designed for preliterate children.

In infants and toddlers, fixation behavior is observed to qualitatively assess visual acuity. Preferential looking and visual evoked potential testing may allow quantitative assessment of visual acuity in this young population (see the section "Alternative methods of visual acuity assessment in preverbal children"). *Fixation and following (tracking)* behavior is observed as the child's attention is directed to the examiner's face or to a small toy in the examiner's hand. Fixation preference is determined by observing how the patient responds to having one eye covered compared with the other eye covered. Children typically resist occlusion of the eye with better vision. Determining whether each eye can maintain fixation through smooth pursuit or a blink provides additional information; strong fixation preference for one eye indicates decreased vision in the nonpreferred eye.

给不配合的孩子检查时，休息、劝说、坚持和奖励都是有效的常用方法。如果一个孩子来检查时就不愉快，最好是停止检查，重新安排时间再来。对首次就诊时就烦躁不安的婴儿，后续复诊时，要让父母或护理人员在把孩子带来前使其保持饥饿状态，在检查过程中再给孩子喂食。对婴幼儿和低龄儿童做短暂的活动限制可能是有效的。但是，医生必须考虑到限制活动对患儿生理和心理上的影响。更好的处理方法是根据眼部问题的情况，进行镇静或麻醉后再做检查。

检查：具体检查项目

完整的儿童眼科检查的内容与成人检查的内容相同，但通常需要不同的技术和设备。以下各节重点介绍这些差异。

视力评估

视力评估需要根据儿童的年龄、发育水平以及合作程度采用不同的方法。对于儿童来说，弱视的检测尤为重要（见第 6 章）。弱视是由于视觉成像的异常加工而导致的中枢神经系统发育障碍，会造成视力下降。弱视主要导致的儿童期单侧视力下降，通过及时的检测和干预是可以预防或逆转的。使用本文所述的方法可以早期检测弱视所致的视力下降。

理想情况下，儿童的精确单眼远视力可以用线性排列的 Sloan 字母视标检测。然而，有时孩子可能不会说话、不认字，或不能配合。这种情况下，可通过评估患儿有无固视行为，或替换图形视标进行测试。

通过观察婴幼儿有无固视行为可以定性评估视力。优先注视和视觉诱发电位检查可以定量评估低龄儿童的视力（见“前言语期儿童视力检查替代方法”一节）。患儿注视医生的脸或手中的小玩具时，可以观察患儿的*固视和追随行为*。通过孩子对分别遮盖双眼的反应来确定其*固视偏好*。通常较好视力的眼被遮盖时，孩子会有抵抗行为。通过进一步观察眼球是否能连续追踪或瞬目，确定两眼是否都可以维持固视；如果固视偏好存在于一眼，则提示另一眼的有视力低下的情形。

Fixation behavior may be characterized by the CSM (Central, Steady, and Main-tained) method. *Central* refers to foveal fixation, tested monocularly. If the fixation target is viewed eccentrically, fixation is termed *uncentral* (UC). *Steady* refers to the absence of nystagmus and other motor disruptions of fixation (see Chapter 13). The S assessment is also performed monocularly. *Maintained* refers to fixation that is held after the opposite eye is uncovered. An eye that does not maintain fixation may be presumed to have lower visual acuity than the opposite eye. Maintained fixation is easier to identify in a patient with strabismus than in one without this defect. For children without strabismus or with a small angle of strabismic deviation, the *induced tropia test* may be useful (see Chapter 2 for strabismus terminology). First, the examiner directs the child's attention to a target. Then a 10–20 prism diopter base-down prism is placed in front of 1 eye, and the eyes are observed. The prism is then placed in front of the opposite eye. If the eyes move up, the child is fixating with the eye under the prism. If the child alternates fixation during the test, a strong preference is not present. If the child consistently fixates with the same eye, the opposite eye likely has decreased vision. The visual acuity of an eye that has eccentric fixation and nystagmoid movements when attempting fixation would be designated *uncentral, unsteady*, and *unmaintained* (UC, US, UM).

Monocular recognition testing—which involves identifying letters, numbers, or symbols (all termed *optotypes*) with each eye separately—is the preferred method of assessing visual acuity. Optotypes may be presented on a wall chart, computer monitor, or handheld card. The acuity test should be calibrated for the test distance used. Because of the potential for variable or inaccurate viewing distances when near vision is tested, measurement at distance is preferred.

In eye charts used for testing preliterate children, the optotypes may be symbols or letters for matching. Table 1-1 lists the expected recognition visual acuity, as measured by an ophthalmologist, for children at different ages; these visual acuity levels may differ from those used in primary care vision screening criteria. Copies of appropriate optotypes may be given to the parent before the test for at-home rehearsal to improve testability, as well as the speed and reliability of responses.

Various optotypes are available for recognition visual acuity testing in preliterate children. LEA symbols (Fig 1-2) and the HOTV test (Fig 1-3) are reliably calibrated and have high testability rates for preschool-aged children. For a shy child, testability may be improved by having the child point to match optotypes on a chart with those on a hand-held card rather than verbally identify them. Several symbol charts, such as Allen figures and the Light house chart, are not recommended by the World Health Organization and the National Academy of Sciences because the optotypes are considered confusing, cultur-ally biased, or nonstandardized. The Tumbling E chart is conceptually difficult for many preschool-aged children.

Table 1-1 Monocular HOTV Visual Acuity Test Results in Preschool Children

Age, y	Mean Visual Acuity	Threshold Visual Acuity[a]
2½	20/30	20/63
3	20/30	20/50
4	20/25	20/40
5	20/20	20/32

[a] Over 95% of children with normal vision are expected to achieve this level of visual acuity.

Information from Pan Y, Tarczy-Hornoch K, Cotter SA, et al; Multi-ethnic Pediatric Eye Disease Study Group. Visual acuity norms in preschool children: The Multi-ethnic Pediatric Eye Disease Study. *Optom Vis Sci.* 2009;86(6):607–612.

固视行为可以用 CSM（中心的、稳定的和持续的）方法来描述。*"中心的"*指黄斑中心凹的固视，单眼测量。如果是用中心凹以外的视网膜看固定视标，则称为*非中心注视*（UC）。*"稳定的"*是指没有眼球震颤和其他眼球运动障碍（见第 13 章）。"S 稳定性"的评估也是单眼进行的。*"持续的"*指的是另一眼去掉遮盖后被检眼仍固视。无固视眼的视力较对侧眼为差。有固视的斜视患者比没有固视的患者更易于诊断。对于没有斜视或小角度斜视的儿童，可用*诱导性斜视检测*（见第 2 章"斜视术语"）。首先，医生要使孩子的注意力集中在视标上。然后在 1 只眼前置一个 10 ~ 20° 底朝下棱镜进行观察。再将棱镜置于对侧眼前，如果被检查眼向上转动，说明置棱镜的眼是注视眼。如果患儿在检查过程中随放置棱镜的位置而改变注视，则说明患儿没有固视偏好。如果孩子始终用同 1 只眼固视，则对侧眼可能存在视力低下的情形。固视时表现为非中心注视和眼球震颤样运动，其视力为*非中心的、不稳定的和不持续的*（*UC，US，UM*）。

单眼识别检测，包括单眼识别字母、数字或符号（*均称为视标*），是评估视力的首选方法。视标可以显示在挂式视力表、计算机屏幕或手持卡上。根据检测距离计算视力。由于近视力检测时的距离变化或不准确，最好进行远距离测量。

给不识字的孩子查视力，视标可选用符号或字母。表 1–1 列出的是一位眼科医生测量的不同年龄儿童的预期视力，其视力水平可能与初级眼保健筛查标准中使用的标准不同。检测视力前，可提供适当的视标副本，让家长在家中给患儿做练习，以提高可测试性，以及检查速度和结果的可靠性。

可供不识字的孩子使用的视标有很多种类型。LEA 符号（图 1–2）和 HOTV 测试（图 1–3）经过可靠校准，在学龄前儿童中的可测试性较高。对于害羞的孩子，不需要说出，可以通过在手持卡片上指出与视力表匹配的视标，以此提高可测试性。世界卫生组织和国家科学院不推荐使用几种符号视力表，如 Allen 图和 Lighthouse 表，因为这些图表上的视标容易混淆，有文化偏见，或未标准化。翻转 E 表检查对于许多学龄前儿童来说是困难的。

表1–1　学龄前儿童单眼HOTV视力检查结果

年龄1岁	平均视力	阈值视力[a]
2.5	20/30	20/63
3	20/30	20/50
4	20/25	20/40
5	20/20	20/32

[a] 95%以上正常儿童的视力应该达到这个视力水平。

（译者注：资料来源见前页原文。）

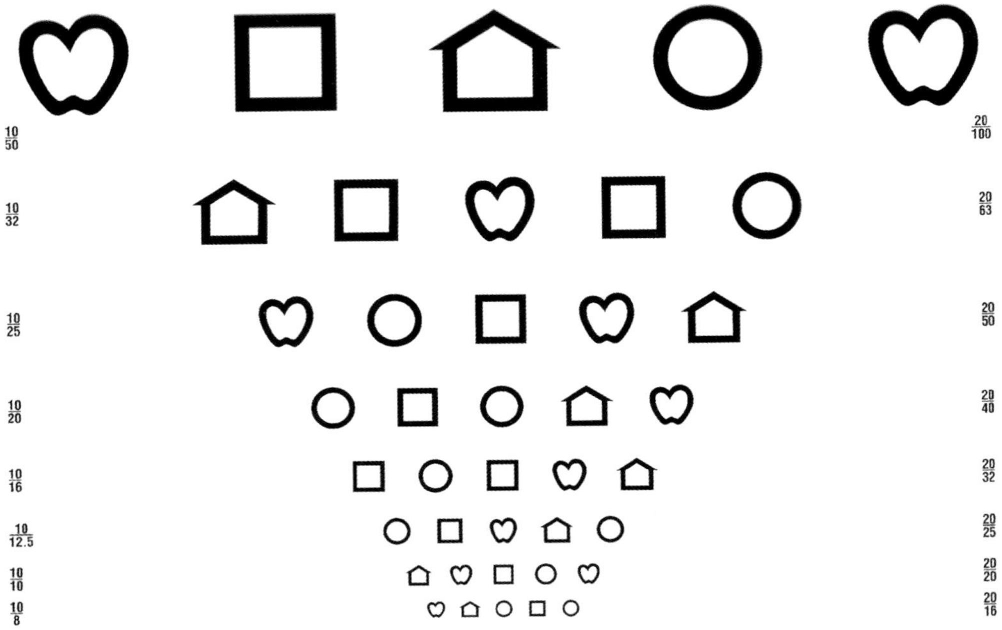

Figure 1-2 LogMAR (logarithm of the minimum angle of resolution) visual acuity chart with LEA symbols. *(Courtesy of the Good-Lite Company and Robert W. Hered, MD.)*

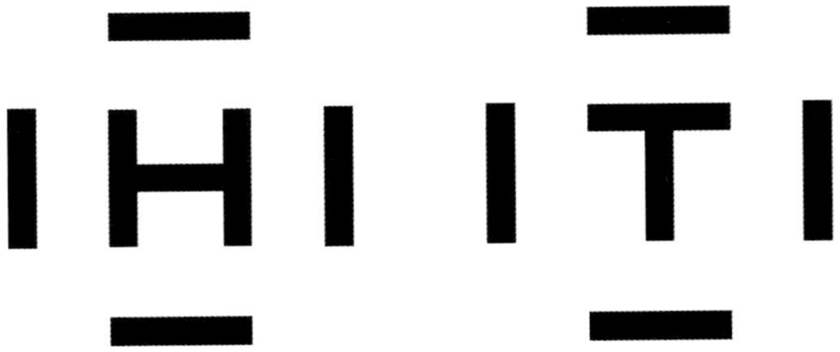

Figure 1-3 Crowded HOTV optotypes. *(Courtesy of the Good-Lite Company and Robert W. Hered, MD.)*

Because visual acuity may be overestimated when measured with isolated optotypes, particularly in amblyopia (see Chapter 6), a line of optotypes (linear acuity) or single optotypes surrounded by *contour interaction bars* ("crowding bars"; see Fig 1-3) should be used whenever possible. The optotypes should be spaced such that the distance between each optotype is no greater than the width of the optotypes on any given line. The design of the Bailey-Lovie and ETDRS (Early Treatment of Diabetic Retinopathy Study) charts incorporates appropriate linear-optotype spacing, a consistent number of optotypes on each line, and a logarithmic (logMAR) change in letter size from one line to the next (see Fig 1-2). See also BCSC Section 3, *Clinical Optics*, for further discussion of visual acuity charts.

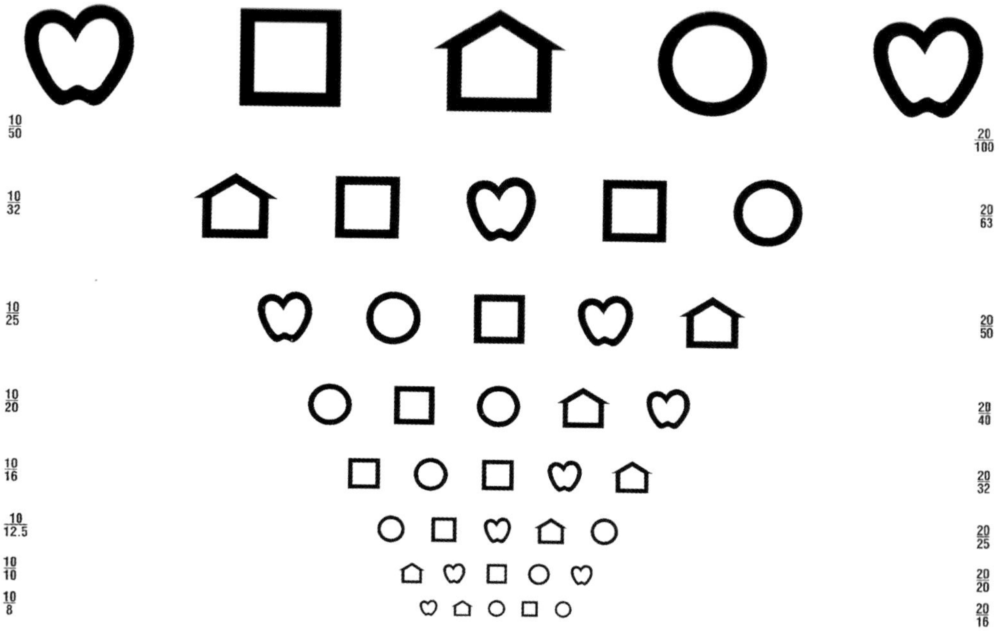

图 1–2　LogMAR（最小分辨角对数）视力表，带有 LEA 符号。*（译者注：资料来源见前页原文。）*

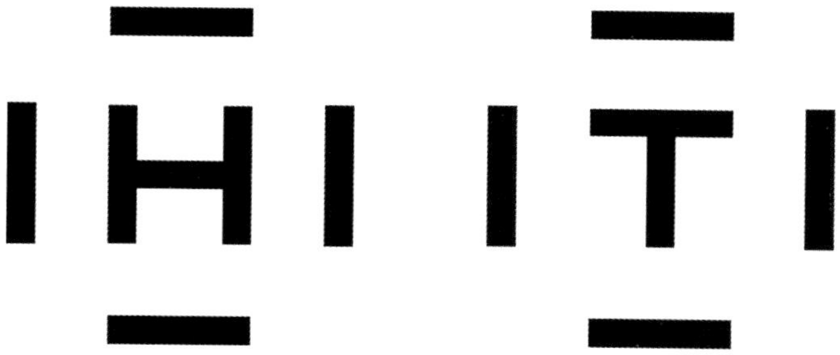

图 1–3　拥挤型 HOTV 视标。*（译者注：资料来源见前页原文。）*

用单独的视标测量视力时，特别是对弱视患者检查时（见第 6 章），可能会高估视力，因此检查应尽可能使用一行视标（线性排列视力）或由*环绕干扰条*（“拥挤条”）包围的单个视标（见图 1–3）。视标的间距应确保每个视标之间的距离不大于这一行上的视标宽度。Bailey–Lowie 视力表和 ETDRS（糖尿病视网膜病变早期治疗研究）视力表的设计包括适当的线性 – 视标间距、每行视标数相等，以及视标大小的上下行间呈对数变化（logMAR）（见图 1–2）。关于视力表的进一步讨论见 BCSC 第 3 册《*临床光学*》。

By convention, visual acuity is determined first for the right eye and then for the left. A patch or other occluder is used in front of the left eye as the acuity of the right eye is checked and vice versa. An adhesive patch is the most reliable occluder because it reduces the possibility that the child will "peek" around the occluder. Computerized visual acuity test systems allow for randomization of optotype presentation, preventing patients from memorizing optotypes and thus increasing test accuracy. Patients with nystagmus may show better binocular than monocular visual acuity. To assess monocular distance visual acuity in this situation, the fellow eye, rather than being occluded, should be fogged by using a translucent occluder or a lens +5.00 diopters (D) greater than the refractive error in that eye. Patients with poor vision may need to move closer to the chart until they can see the 20/400 line. In such cases, visual acuity is recorded as the distance in feet (numerator) over the size of the letter (denominator); for example, if the patient is able to read 20/400 optotypes at 5 ft, the acuity is recorded as 5/400. See the visual acuity conversion chart on the inside front cover of this book, which provides conversions of visual acuity measurements for the various methods in use.

The line with the smallest optotypes in which most of the optotypes are identified by the patient is recorded; if the patient misses a few optotypes on a line, a notation is made. For adults and children, visual acuity test results may vary depending on the chart used. The clinician should document the type of test performed, specifying the optotype and whether crowding was used, to facilitate comparison of measurements obtained at different times.

Age-appropriate optotypes are also used to determine uncorrected and corrected near visual acuity. Measuring near visual acuity in children with reduced vision is helpful for determining how they may function at school.

Alternative methods of visual acuity assessment in preverbal children

Two major methods are used to quantitate visual acuity in preverbal infants and toddlers: *preferential looking* (PL) and *visual evoked potential* (VEP).

Preferential looking tests In these tests, the child's response to a visual stimulus is observed to assess visual acuity. Teller Acuity Cards II (Stereo Optical, Inc, Chicago, IL), the LEA Grating Acuity Test (Good-Lite Company, Elgin, IL), and Patti Stripes Square Wave Grating Paddles (Precision Vision, Woodstock, IL) measure grating acuity, a form of resolution acuity, demonstrated by the subject's ability to detect patterns composed of uniformly spaced black and white stripes on a gray background. Grating acuity can be measured as early as infancy. Movement of the eyes toward the stripes indicates that the child can see them. Seeing narrower stripes denotes better vision (Fig 1-4, Video 1-1). The Cardiff Acuity Test, popular in Europe, uses vanishing optotypes for preferential looking.

Visual evoked potential Sweep visual evoked potential (VEP) can also be used to quantitatively assess visual acuity in preverbal patients. In this test, electrodes are placed over the occipital lobe to measure electrical signals produced in response to a visual stimulus. The child views a series of bar or grid patterns. If the stimulus is large enough for the child to discriminate, a visual impulse is recorded. Visual acuity is estimated based on the smallest stimulus width that produces a response.

根据惯例，检查视力时先查右眼，再查左眼。查右眼时，左眼用眼罩或遮挡板遮盖，反之亦然。黏性眼罩的遮盖最可靠，防止孩子从遮挡板周边空隙窥视。计算机视力检测系统可使视标随机化，防止患者背诵视标，提高检测的准确性。眼球震颤的双眼视力比单眼视力好。在这种情况下，为了准确评估单眼远视力，可使用半透明遮挡板或比检测眼屈光度大 +5.00D 的透镜做雾视。视力差的患者可能需要靠近视力表，直到能看到 20/400 的视标。这种情况下，视力记录为距离（分子，ft，1ft=0.3043m）除以字母大小（分母），如患者在 5ft（约 1.5m）处读取 20/400 大小的视标，则视力记录为 5/400。见本书封面内页的视力转换表，其中提供了各种视力测量方法的转换值。

记录患者能看到的最小一行视标；如果在该行患者有的几个视标不能识别出，则要进行记录。对于成人和儿童，视力检查的结果可随使用的视力表的不同而发生变化。临床医生应该记录使用的视力表类型，以及是否用了拥挤视标，以便对不同时间的测量结果进行比较。

适于不同年龄的视标也用于检测未矫正和矫正的近视力。对于伴有视力下降的儿童进行近视力的检测，有助于了解他们在学校时的视功能。

对于前言语期幼儿的视力评估方法

用于量化婴幼儿视力的方法主要有 2 种：*优先注视（PL）和视觉诱发电位（VEP）*。

优先注视检查　检测时，通过观察孩子对视觉刺激的反应来评估视力。Teller 视力表 II（Stereo Optical，Inc，Chicago，IL）、LEA 视力测试（Good-Lite Company，Elgin，IL）和 Patti 条纹板（Precision Vision，Woodstock，IL）可测量光栅视力，都是一种分辨率视力，表示受试者辨认灰色背景上的均匀黑白条纹图案的能力。婴儿期即可使用光栅视力测量。眼球向条纹的移动提示孩子能看见这些条纹。能看到的条纹越窄提示视力越好（图 1-4，视频 1-1）。在欧洲多用 Cardiff 视力测试，通过灰度逐渐减弱的视标来检查优先注视。

视觉诱发电位　扫式视觉诱发电位（VEP）也可用于定量评价前言语期幼儿的视力。检测时，将电极置于枕叶的部位，测量视觉刺激产生的电信号。患儿可看到一系列条形或网格状图案。如果刺激大到患儿足以辨别的程度，就可以记录到视觉冲动信号。根据产生反应的最小刺激宽度进行视力评估。

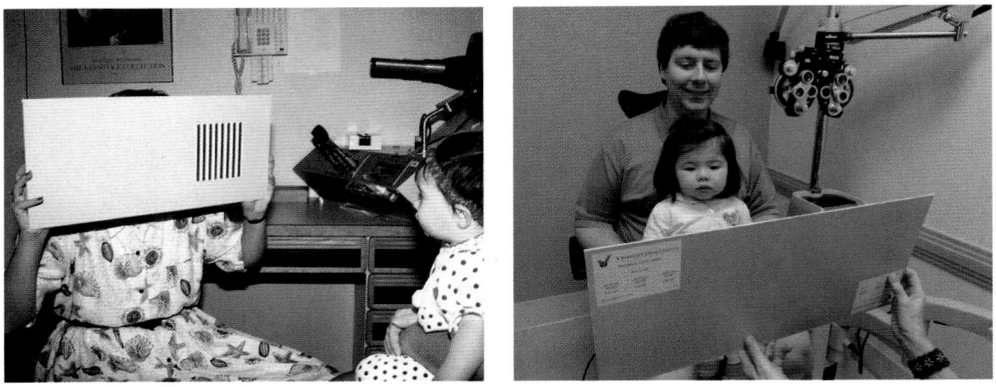

Figure 1-4 Teller Acuity Cards can be used to measure visual acuity in a preverbal child. If the pattern is visible to the child, the eyes gaze toward the grating; otherwise, the stripes blend into the gray background. *(Left image courtesy of John W. Simon, MD; right image courtesy of Lee R. Hunter, MD.)*

VIDEO 1-1 Teller Acuity Card.
Courtesy of Lee R. Hunter, MD.
Access all Section 6 videos at www.aao.org/bcscvideo_section06.

Red Reflex Examination and the Brückner Test

The Brückner test is performed in a semidark room using a direct ophthalmoscope to assess the red reflex from both eyes simultaneously at a distance of approximately 1 m. The clinician can quickly determine the clarity and symmetry of the 2 red reflexes and identify potentially amblyogenic conditions such as anisometropia, isoametropia, and ocular misalignment. A strabismic eye tends to give a brighter red reflex than does the fixating eye.

Dynamic Retinoscopy

Dynamic retinoscopy is a technique for measuring accommodation. For the test, the child is presented a distance fixation target, quickly followed by a near fixation target, while the retinoscopic reflex is observed. In a child with normal accommodation, the reflex will be neutralized at near focus. A poor accommodative response indicates a possible need for bifocal or reading glasses. Hypoaccommodation occurs much more frequently in children with Down syndrome or cerebral palsy than in the general pediatric population.

Visual Field Testing

Information about the visual fields can be obtained in very young patients, once visual fixation has developed (usually by 4 months of age). A peripheral target is presented while the child is fixating on an interesting central target. Movement of the eyes toward the peripheral target (an evoked saccade) confirms the field. Confrontation visual fields can be approximated in children old enough to identify fingers placed in each peripheral quadrant. School-aged children can often be evaluated with manual or automated perimetry.

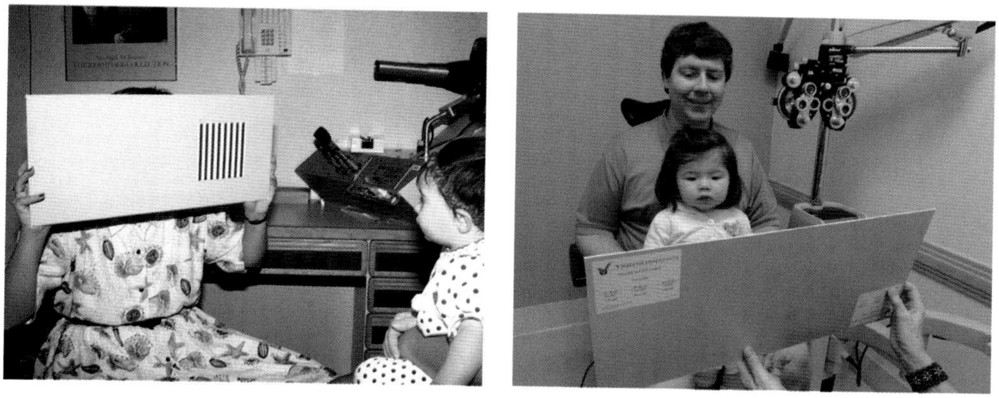

图 1–4　Teller 视力表用于测量前言语期幼儿的视力。如果孩子能看到图案，眼睛就会盯着光栅；否则，条纹就会融入灰色的背景中。*（译者注：资料来源见前页原文。）*

视频 1–1　Teller敏锐度卡。*（译者注：资料来源见前页原文。）*
大家可通过网站www.aao.org/bcscvideo_section06获得第6册的所有视频。

红光反射检查和 Brückner 试验

Brückner 检查在半暗室中进行，在 1m 远的距离、用直接检眼镜同时评估双眼的红光反射。医生可快速确定双眼红光反射的清晰度和对称性，判断是否存在弱视的病因，如屈光参差、屈光不正和斜视。斜视眼较注视眼的红光反射更明亮。

动态视网膜检影

动态视网膜检影是一种测量调节的技术。检测时，先给一个远距离的固定目标，紧接着给一个近距离的固定目标，其间观察视网膜检影的反射光。有正常调节能力的孩子，反射在近焦点处中和。如果调节反应差则提示需要双焦眼镜或阅读眼镜。Down 综合征或脑瘫儿童的调节不足发生率比一般儿童高。

视野检查

一旦固视形成（通常 4 个月大时），就可以进行视野检测。当孩子盯着一个有趣的中心目标时，再给一个周边的目标。当孩子的眼睛移向周边目标（诱发性扫视），可以确认其视野。当孩子的年龄增加到可以识别出每个周边象限的手指时，就可以进行面对面的视野检查。学龄儿童可以用手动或自动视野检查进行评估。

Pupil Testing

The pupillary light reflex is not reliably present until approximately 30 weeks' gestational age. Pupils are usually miotic in newborns and gradually increase in size until preadolescence. Accurate pupil testing in young children is complicated by the smaller pupil and difficulty controlling accommodation. Careful observation, remote or foot control of the room lights to allow continued observation during changes in room illumination, and use of appropriate distance fixation targets greatly facilitate pupil evaluation. Digital photography can also be useful for observing and documenting pupil size and symmetry.

Anterior Segment Examination

A successful anterior segment examination is usually possible in children but may require persistence and varied techniques. Children old enough to sit by themselves can usually be enticed to hold the "motorcycle handles" of the slit lamp long enough for a brief examination. A younger child may be positioned at the slit lamp while in a parent's lap. Children unable or unwilling to cooperate for standard slit-lamp examination may be examined with a portable slit lamp, surgical loupes, or a 20 D or 28 D handheld lens used with an indirect ophthalmoscope.

Intraocular Pressure Measurement

It is not always easy or possible to perform formal tonometry in children. Tonometry requires a relaxed patient. With a nonthreatening approach and experience, the practitioner may find that accurate testing is possible in children by using handheld devices such as the Icare tonometer (Icare Finland Oy, Helsinki, Finland) or Tono-Pen (Reichert Technologies, Depew, NY). The Tono-Pen or the Perkins Tonometer (Haag-Streit USA, Mason, OH) may be used to test infants when they are sleeping or feeding in the supine position.

Digital palpation, though not quantitative, can provide a gross assessment of intraocular pressure. Interpretation of the findings requires practice and involves correlation with formal tonometry results obtained in the same patient.

Cycloplegic Refraction

Because of the relationship between accommodation and ocular convergence, refraction with cycloplegic agents is a particularly important test in the evaluation of any patient who has issues relating to binocular vision and ocular motility.

Refraction technique

Refraction is generally performed after cycloplegia. The ophthalmologist's working distance and the child's visual axis are important considerations. To be accurate, retinoscopy must be performed on axis. The 2 main methods for refraction are loose lenses for infants and younger children and the phoropter for those old enough to sit in an examination chair.

瞳孔检查

30 孕周的胎儿才出现瞳孔光反射。新生儿的瞳孔常是缩小的，逐渐增大至青春前期。由于瞳孔小，调节控制困难，幼儿精确的瞳孔检查难度较大。仔细观察、遥控或脚控室内灯光，以便在室内照明变化时继续观察，并使用适当距离的固定视标，有助于瞳孔评估。还可以用数码照相来观察和记录瞳孔大小和对称性。

眼前节检查

只要有耐心并掌握一些技巧，就可以对儿童进行眼前节检查。引导自己能够坐立的孩子握住裂隙灯的“摩托车手柄”，进行简短的检查。更小的孩子可在裂隙灯面前坐在家长腿上。对于不能或不愿意配合标准裂隙灯检查的儿童，可使用便携式裂隙灯、手术放大镜或 20D/28 D 的手持透镜进行间接检眼镜检查。

眼压测量

对儿童进行常规眼压测量不容易，甚至是不可能的。眼压测量需要病人在放松的状态下进行。采用无伤害的方法，如 Icare 眼压计（Icare Finland Oy，Helsinki，Finland）或 Tono 笔（Reichert Technologies，Depew，NY）等手持设备，还要有丰富的经验，才可以对儿童进行准确眼压测量。Tono 笔或 Perkins 眼压计（Haag-Streit USA，Mason，OH）可在孩子处于仰卧体位、睡觉或喂养时测量。

手测眼压虽不能定量，但可以大致评估眼压水平。判断眼压需要有丰富的实践和经验，同时需要结合患者的常规眼压测量结果。

睫状肌麻痹验光

由于调节与集合的关联性，睫状肌麻痹验光是评价双眼视觉和眼球运动相关的问题重要检查。

验光技术

通常在睫状肌麻痹后进行验光。眼科医生的工作距离和孩子的视轴是重要因素。必须在视轴上进行检影验光才准确。验光方法主要有 2 种，对婴儿和幼儿用插片验光，而可以坐在检查椅上的儿童用综合验光仪验光。

Cycloplegic agents

Cyclopentolate hydrochloride (1%) is the preferred cycloplegic drug for routine use in children. Use of a weaker concentration of cyclopentolate (0.2% to 0.5%) is suggested in infants. *Tropicamide* (0.5% or 1%) is usually not potent enough for effective cycloplegia in children. Many ophthalmologists use a combination of cyclopentolate, tropicamide, and/or phenylephrine to achieve maximum pupil dilatation. *Atropine* (1%) drops or ointment is used by some ophthalmologists, particularly in young children with esotropia or dark irides, but this drug causes prolonged blurring and is more often associated with adverse effects (see the section "Adverse effects of cycloplegic agents"). Some ophthalmologists choose atropine to ensure complete cycloplegia in select cases of accommodative esotropia.

Table 1-2 gives the administration schedule and onset of action for commonly used cycloplegics. The duration of action varies greatly, and the pupillary effect occurs earlier and lasts longer than the cycloplegic effect; thus, a dilated pupil does not necessarily indicate complete cycloplegia. For patients with accommodative esodeviations, repeated cycloplegic examinations are essential when control of strabismus is precarious.

Eyedrops in children

Most young children are apprehensive about eyedrops. Fortunately, there are many approaches to administering eyedrops. If possible, to improve the child's cooperation for the remainder of the examination, someone other than the physician should instill the drops, which can be described to the child as being "like a splash of swimming pool water" that will "feel funny." Some practitioners administer a topical anesthetic drop first, while others use the cycloplegic drops alone; some use a compounded cycloplegic spray from an atomizer.

Adverse effects of cycloplegic agents

Adverse reactions to cycloplegic agents include allergic (or hypersensitivity) reaction with conjunctivitis, edematous eyelids, and dermatitis. These reactions are more common with atropine than with the other agents. Cycloplegic agents may also cause systemic symptoms, including fever, dry mouth, flushing, tachycardia, constipation, urinary retention, nausea, dizziness, and delirium. Treatment is discontinuation of the drug, with supportive measures as necessary. If the reaction is severe, physostigmine may be given. One drop of atropine, 1%, contains 0.5 mg of atropine. See also BCSC Section 2, *Fundamentals and Principles of Ophthalmology*, Part V: Ocular Pharmacology.

Table 1-2 Administration of Commonly Used Cycloplegic Agents

Medication	Administration Schedule	Onset of Action
Tropicamide	1 drop every 5 min × 2; wait 30 min	20–40 min
Cyclopentolate hydrochloride	1 drop every 5 min × 2; wait 30 min	30–60 min
Atropine sulfate	1 drop, wait 90 min Alternatively, 1–3 drops per day × 1–4 days; then 1 drop morning of appointment	45–120 min

睫状肌麻痹剂

盐酸环喷托酯滴眼液（1%）是首选的儿童常规睫状肌麻痹剂。建议婴儿使用低浓度的盐酸环喷托酯滴眼液（0.2% ~ 0.5%）。*托吡卡胺*（0.5% 或 1%）对儿童的睫状肌麻痹作用通常不足。许多眼科医生联合使用盐酸环喷托酯、托吡卡胺和（或）苯肾上腺素使瞳孔充分扩大。*阿托品*（1%）滴眼液或眼膏特别用于患有内斜视或虹膜色素多的幼儿，但会致长时间视物模糊，并常伴有副作用（见“睫状肌麻痹剂的副作用”一节）。一些眼科医生使用阿托品使调节性内斜视患者的睫状肌完全麻痹。

表 1–2 给出了常用睫状肌麻痹剂的用药时间表和起效时间。睫状肌麻痹的作用时间变化很大，瞳孔扩大效应比睫状肌麻痹效应出现得早且持续时间长。因此，瞳孔扩大并不意味着睫状肌完全麻痹。当调节性内斜视不稳定时，反复睫状肌麻痹检查非常必要。

儿童眼药水

大多数儿童害怕滴眼药水。但幸运的是，滴眼药的方法有很多种。为了提高孩子以后的配合度，医生尽量不要给孩子滴眼药，其他人可以把眼药水形容为“像游泳池里的水花一样”，会“感觉很有趣”。可以先滴 1 滴表面麻醉剂，或直接滴睫状肌麻痹剂，还可以使用喷雾器的复合睫状肌麻痹剂。

睫状肌麻痹剂的副作用

睫状肌麻痹剂的副作用包括结膜过敏（或超敏反应）、眼睑水肿和皮炎。这些副作用在阿托品的使用中更常见。睫状肌麻痹剂也可引起全身症状，包括发热、口干、潮红、心动过速、便秘、尿潴留、恶心、头晕和谵妄。治疗方法是停止用药，必要时采取支持治疗。如果反应严重，可给予毒扁豆碱治疗。一滴 1% 的阿托品滴眼液含有 0.5mg 阿托品。见 BCSC 第 2 册《*眼科学基础与原理*》的第 V 部分“眼科药理学”。

表1–2　常用睫状肌麻痹剂的使用

药品	用药方法	起效时间
托吡卡胺	5min 1滴 × 2次，等待30min	20~40min
盐酸环喷托酯	5min 1滴 × 2次，等待30min	30~60min
硫酸阿托品	1滴，等待90min 或者，每天1 ~ 3滴，连续滴1 ~ 4d； 预约门诊当天的早上滴1滴	45~120min

Fundus Examination

The fundus examination is typically the final component of a complete pediatric ophthalmology examination. Though often challenging to obtain in young children, an adequate view of the fundus is important for identifying pathology. After mydriasis is achieved, infants and small children can be examined with the indirect ophthalmoscope, often more easily by using decreased illumination. Examination may require restraint of some infants, particularly those being screened for retinopathy of prematurity (in these cases, a topical anesthetic, eyelid speculum, and scleral depression are necessary for a complete retinal evaluation). For many young children, the practitioner can obtain sufficient views by using diversionary targets such as illuminated toys and cartoons.

眼底检查

眼底检查通常是儿童眼科检查中的最后部分。虽然在幼儿中往往难以进行眼底检查，但充分的眼底检查对诊断疾病很重要。瞳孔扩大后，用间接检眼镜检查婴幼儿，减低光亮度会使操作更容易。检查可能需要固定婴儿的体位，尤其是筛查早产儿视网膜病变时（这时需要表麻、开睑器和巩膜顶压器对视网膜进行完整的评估）。医生可以使用发光的玩具和卡通动物等来分散幼儿的注意力。

（翻译 唐志萍 梅颖 // 审校 石一宁 布娟 // 章节审校 石广礼）

PART I

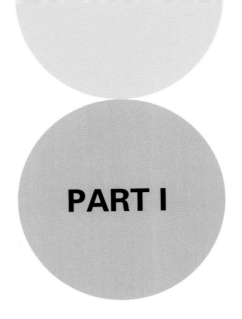

Strabismus

第一部分

斜视

CHAPTER 2

Strabismus Terminology

Definitions

The term *strabismus* is derived from the Greek word *strabismos*—"to squint, to look obliquely or askance"—and means ocular misalignment. This misalignment may be caused by abnormalities in binocular vision or by anomalies of neuromuscular control of ocular motility. Many terms are used in discussions of strabismus. Familiarity with this terminology can aid the reader in understanding these disorders; misuse of these terms could cause confusion. Unfortunately, some terms still in use are not correct physiologically.

Orthophoria is the ideal condition of perfect ocular alignment. In practice, orthophoria is seldom encountered, as a small heterophoria can be found in most people. Some ophthalmologists therefore prefer *orthotropia* to mean correct direction or position of the eyes under binocular conditions. Both terms are commonly used to describe eyes without manifest strabismus. *Heterophoria* is an ocular deviation kept latent by the fusional mechanism (latent strabismus). *Heterotropia* is a deviation that is present when both eyes are open and used for viewing (manifest strabismus). It is sometimes helpful to identify the deviating eye, particularly when vertical deviations or restrictive or paretic strabismus is being measured, or when amblyopia is present in a preverbal child.

Prefixes and Suffixes

A detailed nomenclature has evolved to describe the various types of ocular deviations. In this vocabulary, the prefix used indicates the relative position of the visual axes of the 2 eyes, or the direction of deviation.

Prefixes

Eso- The eye is rotated so that it is deviated nasally. Because the visual axes align at a point closer than the fixation target, this state is also known as *convergent strabismus*, one type of horizontal strabismus.

Exo- The eye is rotated so that it is deviated temporally. Because the visual axes are diverging from the fixation target, this state is also known as *divergent strabismus*, another form of horizontal strabismus.

Hyper- The eye is rotated so that it is deviated superiorly. This describes one type of *vertical strabismus.*

Hypo- The eye is rotated so that it is deviated inferiorly. This describes another type of *vertical strabismus.*

第 2 章

斜视术语

定义

*斜视*一词来源于希腊语 *strabismos*——“斜着看，歪着看”，意思是指眼位不正。这种眼位不正可能是由双眼视觉异常或眼运动的神经肌肉控制异常引起的。在讨论斜视时使用了许多术语。熟悉这些术语有助于读者理解这些疾病，误用术语会造成混淆。遗憾的是一些正在使用的术语在生理学意义上还是不够准确的。

*正位眼*是完美眼位的理想状态。但实际上，正位眼很少，绝大多数人都存在少量的斜视。因此，一些眼科医生更喜欢将*正位眼*理解为双眼视条件下眼睛注视方向和位置正常。这 2 个术语通常都用来描述没有显斜视的情况。*隐斜视*是指因融合机制的存在而不表现出来的隐性眼位偏斜（隐性斜视）。*斜视*是指使用双眼时眼位偏斜（显性斜视）。有时候确定斜视眼是有帮助的，特别是在垂直性斜视、限制性斜视或麻痹性斜视的检测中，或是对前言语期的幼儿弱视检测。

前缀和后缀

各种类型斜视已有详细的命名法来描述。在该词汇表中，使用的前缀表示两眼视轴的相对位置或偏斜方向。

前缀

Eso- 眼球向鼻侧偏斜。由于视轴交叉点比注视视标距离眼睛更近，这种状态也被称为*会聚性斜视*，是一种水平斜视。

Exo- 眼球向颞侧偏斜。由于视轴较注视视标更发散，这种状态也被称为*发散性斜视*，是另一种水平斜视。

Hyper- 眼球向上偏斜。是一种*垂直斜视*。

Hypo- 眼球向下偏斜。是一种*垂直斜视*。

Incyclo- The eye is rotated so that the superior pole of the vertical meridian is rotated nasally. This state is known as *intorsion*.

Excyclo- The eye is rotated so that the superior pole of the vertical meridian is rotated temporally. This state is known as *extorsion*.

Suffixes

-phoria A latent deviation (eg, esophoria, exophoria, right hyperphoria); the deviation is controlled by the fusional mechanism so that the eyes remain aligned under binocular conditions.

-tropia A manifest deviation (eg, esotropia, exotropia, right hypertropia); the deviation exceeds the control of the fusional mechanism so that the eyes are misaligned under binocular conditions. Heterotropias can be constant or intermittent.

Strabismus Classification Terms

Several methods of classifying ocular alignment and motility disorders are used, as no classification is perfect or all-inclusive. Terms used in these classifications are presented herein.

Age at onset

Infantile A deviation documented at or before age 6 months, presumably related to a defect present at birth. The term congenital is sometimes used, although it may be less accurate because the deviation is usually not present at birth.

Acquired A deviation with onset after 6 months of age, following a period of presumably normal ocular alignment.

Fixation

Alternating Spontaneous alternation of fixation from one eye to the other.

Monocular Fixation with one eye only.

Variation of the deviation size with gaze position or fixating eye

Comitant (concomitant) The size of the deviation does not vary by more than a few prism diopters in different positions of gaze or with either eye used for fixation.

Incomitant (noncomitant) The deviation varies in size in different positions of gaze or with the eye used for fixation.

Miscellaneous terms

Consecutive A strabismus that is in the direction opposite that of a previous strabismus. For example, consecutive exotropia is an exotropia that follows an esotropia.

Dissociated strabismus complex Consists of dissociated vertical deviation, dissociated horizontal deviation, and dissociated torsional deviation. The number of components varies, with some patients having all 3 and others having only 1. Dissociated vertical deviation is the most prevalent of the 3 components. The complex can be bilateral or unilateral; if it is bilateral, the degree of control of the deviation can vary between the eyes.

Incyclo-　眼球垂直径的上极向鼻侧旋转，称为*内旋*。

Excyclo-　眼球垂直径的上极向颞侧旋转，称为*外旋*。

后缀

-phoria　隐斜视，是隐性偏斜（如内隐斜、外隐斜、右上隐斜）。这种偏斜是在融合的可控范围内，因此在双眼视条件下可保持正位眼。

-tropia　斜视，是显性偏斜（如内斜视、外斜视、右上斜视）。这种偏斜超过了融合范围，因此在双眼视条件下眼位也偏斜。这种偏斜既可以是持续性的，也可以是间歇性的。

斜视分类术语

眼位和运动障碍的分类有几种，但均不够全面。下面介绍分类的术语。

发病年龄

婴儿的　在出生6个月或6个月之前发生的眼位偏斜，可能与出生时的缺陷有关。使用“先天性”一词并不准确，因为这种偏斜在出生时还不存在。

获得性的　出生 6 个月以后发生的眼位偏斜，此前眼位多正常。

注视

交替性的　从一眼到另一眼的自发性交替注视。

单眼的　只用一眼注视。

偏斜度随注视位置或注视眼而变化

共同性的（伴随性的）　在不同的注视眼位或用任一眼注视时，偏斜度不超过几个棱镜度的变化。

非共同性的（非伴随性的）　偏斜度随注视眼位和注视眼的不同而不同。

其他术语

连续性的　发生了与之前斜视方向相反的斜视。例如，连续性外斜视是内斜视之后发生的外斜视。

复合性分离性斜视　由分离性垂直斜视、分离性水平斜视和分离性旋转斜视组成。每个患者联合不同的种类，有的同时具有 3 种情况，有的仅有 1 种情况。其中分离性垂直斜视最常见。这种复合性斜视呈单眼或双眼；如果是双眼，两眼的斜视程度可不同。

Overelevation in adduction and overdepression in adduction These motility anomalies—frequently also called inferior oblique overaction and superior oblique overaction, respectively—can be caused by overaction of the oblique muscles, as well as by other mechanisms (see Chapter 11).

Underelevation in adduction and underdepression in adduction These motility anomalies—frequently also called inferior oblique underaction and superior oblique underaction, respectively—can be caused by underaction of the oblique muscles, as well as by other mechanisms (see Chapter 11).

Abbreviations for Types of Strabismus

Addition of the prime symbol (') to any of the following indicates that measurement of ocular alignment is made at near fixation (eg, E' indicates esophoria at near).

0 = 0 Orthophoria (orthotropia).

E, X, RH, LH Esophoria, exophoria, right hyperphoria, left hyperphoria at distance fixation, respectively.

ET, XT, RHT, LHT Constant esotropia, exotropia, right hypertropia, left hypertropia at distance fixation, respectively.

E(T), X(T), RH(T), LH(T) Intermittent esotropia, exotropia, right hypertropia, left hypertropia at distance fixation, respectively. The addition of parentheses around the T indicates an intermittent tropia.

RHoT, LHoT Right hypotropia, left hypotropia at distance fixation, respectively.

OEAd or IOOA Overelevation in adduction or inferior oblique overaction, respectively.

ODAd or SOOA Overdepression in adduction or superior oblique overaction, respectively.

UDAd or SOUA Underdepression in adduction or superior oblique underaction, respectively.

UEAd or IOUA Underelevation in adduction or inferior oblique underaction, respectively.

DSC Dissociated strabismus complex.

DHD, DTD, DVD Dissociated horizontal deviation, dissociated torsional deviation, dissociated vertical deviation, respectively.

内转时眼球上转过度或下转过度　是内转时的运动异常，分别称为下斜肌功能亢进和上斜肌功能亢进，是由斜肌过度收缩，以及其他机制引起的（见第 11 章）。

内转时上转不足或下转不足　在内转和内转不足的情况下，这些运动异常通常被分别称作下斜肌功能不足和上斜肌功能不足，是由斜肌收缩不足，以及其他机制引起的（见第 11 章）。

斜视类型缩写

下列情况中附加上撇符号（′）表示固定视近时所测眼位（例如，E′ 表示视近时内隐斜）。

0 = 0　正位。

E, X, RH, LH　依次为固定视远时的内隐斜、外隐斜、右上隐斜、左上隐斜。

ET, XT, RHT, LHT　依次为固定视远时的恒定性内斜视、外斜视、右上斜视、左上斜视。

E(T), X(T), RH(T), LH(T)　依次为固定视远时的间歇性内斜视、外斜视、右上斜视、左上斜视。T 表示间歇性。

RHoT, LHoT　为固定视远时的右下斜视、左下斜视。

OEAd 或 IOOA　为内转时眼球上转过度或下斜肌功能亢进。

ODAd 或 SOOA　为内转时眼球下转过度或上斜肌功能亢进。

UDAd 或 SOUA　为内转时眼球下转不足或上斜肌功能不足。

UEAd 或 IOUA　为内转时眼球上转不足或下斜肌功能不足。

DSC　为复合性分离性斜视。

DHD, DTD, DVD　为分离性水平斜视、分离性旋转斜视、分离性垂直斜视。

（翻译 梅颖 // 审校 石一宁 布娟 // 章节审校 石广礼）

CHAPTER 3

Anatomy of the Extraocular Muscles

This chapter includes a related activity, which can be accessed by scanning the QR code provided in the text or going to www.aao.org/bcscactivity_section06.

Origin, Course, Insertion, and Innervation of the Extraocular Muscles

There are 7 extraocular muscles (EOMs) in the human eye: the 4 rectus muscles (lateral, medial, superior, and inferior), the 2 oblique muscles, and the levator palpebrae superioris muscle. Figure 3-1 shows an anterior view of the EOMs and their relationships to one another. Cranial nerve (CN) VI (abducens) innervates the lateral rectus muscle; CN IV (trochlear), the superior oblique muscle; and CN III (oculomotor), the levator palpebrae, superior rectus, medial rectus, inferior rectus, and inferior oblique muscles. Cranial nerve III has an upper and a lower division: the upper division supplies the levator palpebrae and superior rectus muscles, and the lower division supplies the medial rectus, inferior rectus, and inferior oblique muscles. The parasympathetic innervation of the sphincter pupillae and ciliary muscle travels with the branch of the lower division of CN III that supplies the inferior oblique muscle. BCSC Section 5, *Neuro-Ophthalmology*, discusses the ocular motor nerves in more detail, and Section 2, *Fundamentals and Principles of Ophthalmology*, extensively illustrates the anatomical structures mentioned in this chapter.

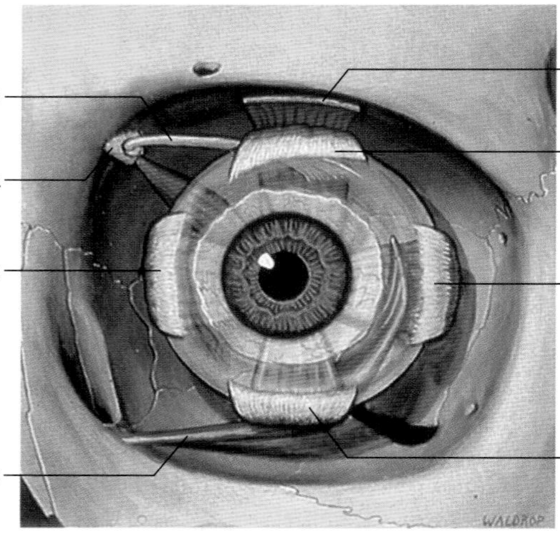

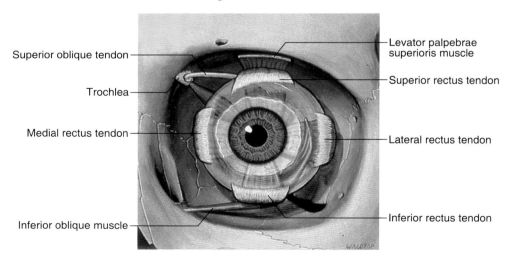

Figure 3-1 Extraocular muscles, frontal composite view, left eye. *(Reproduced with permission from Dutton JJ. Atlas of Clinical and Surgical Orbital Anatomy. Philadelphia: Saunders; 1994:23.)*

第 3 章

眼外肌解剖

本章相关内容，可扫描二维码访问，或访问网站 www.aao.org/bcscactivity_section06。

眼外肌的起点、经行、止点和神经支配

人眼有 7 条眼外肌（EOMs）：其中有 4 条直肌（外、内、上、下），2 条斜肌，以及提上睑肌。图 3–1 是眼外肌的前视图，显示了眼外肌 EOMs 及其相互关系。颅脑神经（CN）VI（外展神经）支配外直肌，颅脑神经 IV（滑车神经）支配上斜肌，颅脑神经 III（动眼神经）支配提上睑肌、上直肌、内直肌、下直肌和下斜肌。颅脑神经 III 分上下 2 支，上支支配提上睑肌和上直肌，下支支配内直肌、下直肌和下斜肌。支配瞳孔括约肌和睫状肌的副交感神经与支配下斜肌的颅脑神经 III 的下支一起并行。在 BCSC 第 5 册《*神经眼科学*》里，将更详细地讨论眼球运动神经，在第 2 册《*眼科学基础与原理*》中，将详细阐述本章提到的解剖结构。

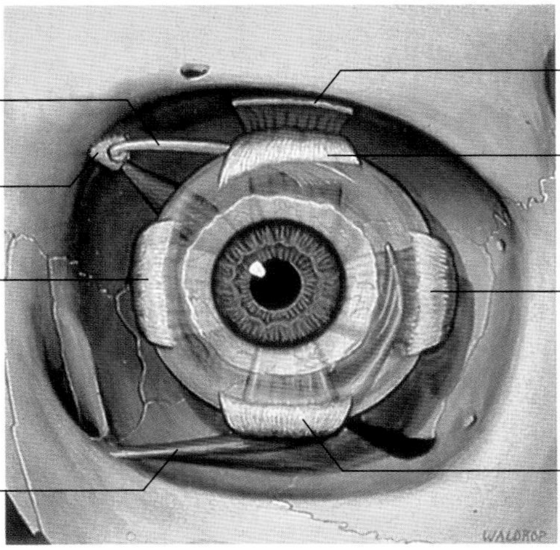

图 3–1 眼外肌，左眼正面图。*（译者注：资料来源见前页原文。）*

Table 3-1 summarizes the characteristics of the EOMs. The EOMs and their relationships to one another can be explored in Activity 3-1.

ACTIVITY 3-1 Extraocular muscles.
Activity developed by Mary A. O'Hara, MD.
Access the activity at *www.aao.org/bcscactivity_section06.*

Horizontal Rectus Muscles

The horizontal rectus muscles are the medial and lateral rectus muscles. Both arise from the annulus of Zinn. The *medial rectus muscle* courses along the medial orbital wall. The *lateral rectus muscle* courses along the lateral orbital wall.

Vertical Rectus Muscles

The vertical rectus muscles are the superior and inferior rectus muscles. The *superior rectus muscle* originates from the annulus of Zinn and courses anteriorly, upward over the eyeball, and laterally, forming an angle of 23° with the visual axis or the midplane of the eye in primary position (Fig 3-2; see also Chapter 4, Fig 4-3). The *inferior rectus muscle* also arises from the annulus of Zinn, and it then courses anteriorly, downward, and laterally along the floor of the orbit, forming an angle of 23° with the visual axis or midplane of the eye in primary position (see Chapter 4, Fig 4-4).

Oblique Muscles

The *superior oblique muscle* originates from the orbital apex, above the annulus of Zinn, and passes anteriorly and upward along the superomedial wall of the orbit. The muscle becomes tendinous before passing through the trochlea, a cartilaginous saddle attached to the frontal bone in the superior nasal orbit. The combination of the trochlea and the superior oblique tendon is known as the *tendon–trochlea complex.* The function of the trochlea is to redirect the tendon inferiorly, posteriorly, and laterally, with the tendon forming an angle of 51° with the visual axis or midplane of the eye in primary position (see Chapter 4, Fig 4-5). The tendon penetrates the Tenon capsule 2 mm nasally and 5 mm posteriorly to the nasal insertion of the superior rectus muscle. Passing under the superior rectus muscle, the tendon inserts posterior to the equator in the superotemporal quadrant of the eyeball, almost or entirely laterally to the midvertical plane or center of rotation.

The *inferior oblique muscle* originates from the periosteum of the maxillary bone, just posterior to the orbital rim and lateral to the orifice of the lacrimal fossa. It courses laterally, superiorly, and posteriorly, going inferior to the inferior rectus muscle and inserting under the lateral rectus muscle in the posterolateral portion of the globe, in the area of the macula. The inferior oblique muscle forms an angle of 51° with the visual axis or midplane of the eye in primary position (see Chapter 4, Fig 4-6). A stiff neurofibrovascular bundle containing the nerve to the inferior oblique runs anteriorly, along the lateral border of the inferior rectus muscle, to the myoneural junction. Most inferior oblique muscles have a single belly, but approximately 10% have 2 bellies; in rare cases, there are 3.

表 3–1 总结了眼外肌的特点。眼外肌及其相互关系将在示教 3–1 演示。

示教3-1　眼外肌。（*译者注：资料来源见前页原文。*）
大家可以通过网站 *www.aao.org/bcscactivity_section06*获得该演示活动视频。

水平直肌

水平直肌包括内直肌和外直肌，均起源于 Zinn 环。*内直肌*沿内侧眶骨壁经行。*外直肌*沿外侧眶骨壁经行。

垂直直肌

垂直直肌包括上直肌和下直肌。*上直肌*起源于 Zinn 环，向前、向上越过眼球经行。侧面观，与视轴或第一眼位的中间平面成 23° 角（图 3–2；另见第 4 章，图 4–3）。*下直肌*也起源于 Zinn 环，沿眶底向前、向下、向外经行，与视轴或第一眼位的中间平面成 23° 角（见第 4 章，图 4–4）。

斜肌

*上斜肌*起源于 Zinn 环上方的眶尖，沿内上眶壁向前、向上经行。肌肉在通过滑车（一个附着在眼眶鼻上方额骨上的软骨鞍）前变为肌腱。滑车和上斜肌肌腱的复合体称为*肌腱 – 滑车复合体*。滑车的功能是改变肌腱向下、向后、向外经行，使上斜肌肌腱与视轴或第一眼位的中间平面成 51° 角（见第 4 章，图 4–5）。上斜肌肌腱在 Tenon 囊鼻侧 2 mm 处、上直肌鼻侧止点后 5mm 处穿过，经上直肌下方，止于眼球颞上赤道部的后面，位于垂直中平面或眼球转动中心的颞侧。

*下斜肌*源于上颌骨骨膜、眶缘后、泪浅窝口外侧。向外、上、后经行，经下直肌下方，止于眼球后外侧黄斑区。下斜肌与视轴或第一眼位中间平面成角 51° （见第 4 章，图 4–6）。包含支配下斜肌神经的神经纤维血管束沿下直肌外侧，向前形成肌肉神经接点。下斜肌多为单肌腹，约 10% 为双肌腹，偶有 3 肌腹。

Table 3-1 Extraocular Muscles

Muscle	Approx. Length of Active Muscle, mm	Origin	Anatomical Insertion and Distance From Limbus, mm	Direction of Pull	Length of Tendon, mm	Arc of Contact, mm	Innervation
Medial rectus (MR)	40	Annulus of Zinn	Up to 5.5 mm from medial limbus	90°	4.5	7.0	Lower CN III
Lateral rectus (LR)	40	Annulus of Zinn	Up to 6.9 mm from lateral limbus	90°	7.0	12.0	CN VI
Superior rectus (SR)	40	Annulus of Zinn	Up to 7.7 mm from superior limbus	23°	6.0	6.5	Upper CN III
Inferior rectus (IR)	40	Annulus of Zinn	Up to 6.5 mm from inferior limbus	23°	7.0	6.5	Lower CN III
Superior oblique (SO)	32	Orbital apex, above annulus of Zinn (functional origin at the trochlea)	Posterior to equator in superotemporal quadrant	51°	26.0	7–8	CN IV
Inferior oblique (IO)	37	Behind inferior orbital rim, lateral to lacrimal fossa	Lateral to area of macula	51°	1.0	15.0	Lower CN III
Levator palpebrae superioris (LPS)	40	Orbital apex, above annulus of Zinn	Septa of pretarsal orbicularis and anterior surface of tarsus	—	14–20	—	Upper CN III

CN = cranial nerve.
See also Figures 4-2 through 4-6 in Chapter 4.

表 3-1　眼外肌

眼肌	肌长/mm	起点	附着点距角膜缘距离/mm	牵拉角/（°）	腱长/mm	接触弧/mm	支配神经
内直肌（MR）	40	Zinn环	鼻侧角膜缘后5.5mm	90	4.5	7.0	动眼神经下支
外直肌（LR）	40	Zinn环	颞侧角膜缘后6.9mm	90	7.0	12.0	外展神经
上直肌（SR）	40	Zinn环	上方角膜缘后7.7mm	23	6.0	6.5	动眼神经上支
下直肌（IR）	40	Zinn环	下方角膜缘后6.5mm	23	7.0	6.5	动眼神经下支
上斜肌（SO）	32	眶尖，Zinn环上方（功能起点在滑车处）	颞上象限赤道后方	51	26.0	7～8	滑车神经
下斜肌（IO）	37	下方眶缘后面，泪浅窝外侧	黄斑区外侧	51	1.0	15.0	动眼神经下支
提上睑肌（LPS）	40	眶尖，Zinn环上方	睑板前轮匝肌眶隔和睑板前表面	—	14～20	—	动眼神经上支

CN = 颅脑神经。
见第4章的图 4-2～4-6。

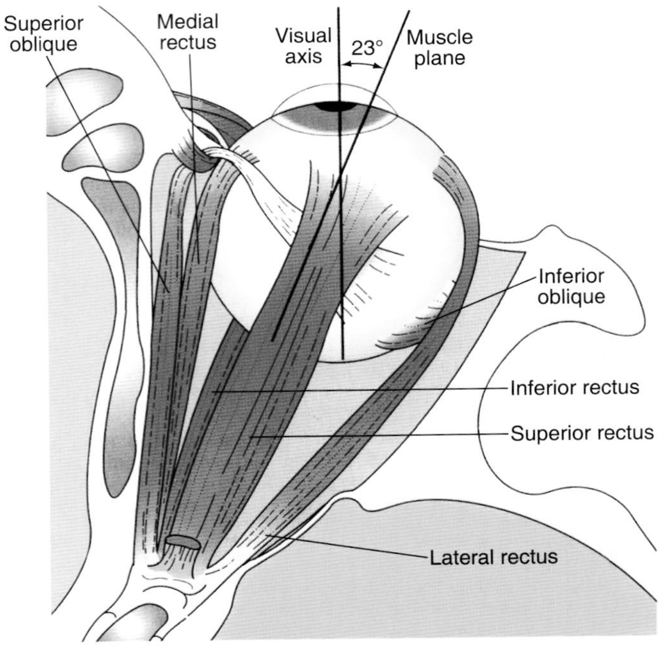

Figure 3-2 The extrinsic muscles of the right eyeball in primary position, seen from above. Note that only the origin and insertion of the inferior oblique muscle are visible in this view. *(Modified with permission from Yanoff M, Duker J, eds. Ophthalmology. 2nd ed. London: Mosby; 2004:549.)*

Levator Palpebrae Superioris Muscle

The levator palpebrae superioris muscle arises at the orbital apex from the lesser wing of the sphenoid bone, just superior to the annulus of Zinn. At its origin, the muscle blends with the superior rectus muscle inferiorly and with the superior oblique muscle medially. The levator palpebrae superioris passes anteriorly, lying just above the superior rectus muscle; the fascial sheaths of these 2 muscles are connected. The levator palpebrae superioris muscle becomes an aponeurosis in the region of the superior fornix. This muscle has both a cutaneous and a tarsal insertion. BCSC Section 7, *Oculofacial Plastic and Orbital Surgery*, discusses this muscle in detail.

Relationship of the Rectus Muscle Insertions

Starting at the medial rectus and proceeding to the inferior rectus, lateral rectus, and superior rectus muscles, the rectus muscle tendons insert progressively farther from the limbus. Drawing a continuous curve through these insertions yields a spiral, known as the *spiral of Tillaux* (Fig 3-3). The temporal side of each vertical rectus muscle insertion is farther from the limbus (ie, more posterior) than is the nasal side.

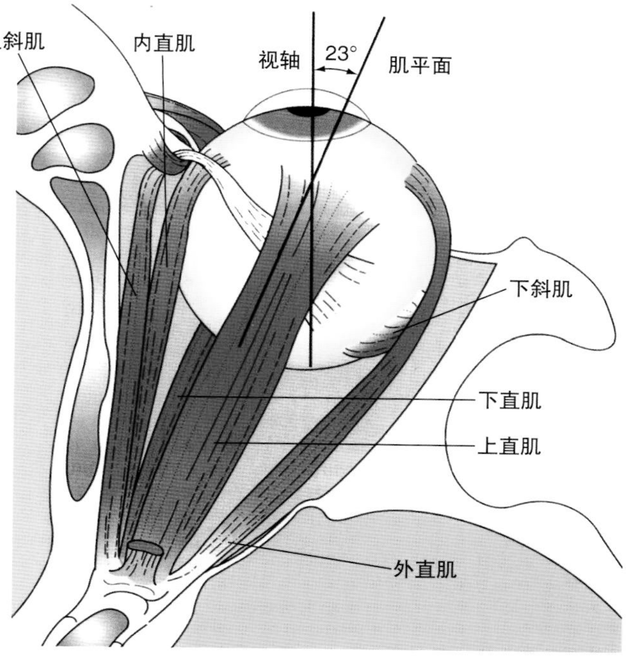

图 3–2　第一眼位时右眼眼外肌外观。该图中下斜肌仅见起点和附着点。*（译者注：资料来源见前页原文。）*

提上睑肌

提上睑肌起源于眶尖蝶骨小翼、Zinn 环上方。提上睑肌的起点于上直肌下方、上斜肌内侧与其混合，沿上直肌上方向前，2 条肌肉的筋膜相互连接，在上穹窿部形成腱膜。该肌肉在皮肤和睑板 2 处附着。在 BCSC 第 7 册《*眼面部整形与眼眶手术*》中会详细讨论该肌肉。

直肌附着点间的关系

4 条直肌附着点，以内直肌、下直肌、外直肌、上直肌的顺序，依次远离角膜缘，沿止点画 1 条连线就形成 1 个特殊的螺旋，称为 *Tillaux 螺旋*（图 3–3）。上下直肌的颞侧附着点比鼻侧附着点更远离角膜缘（或更偏后）。

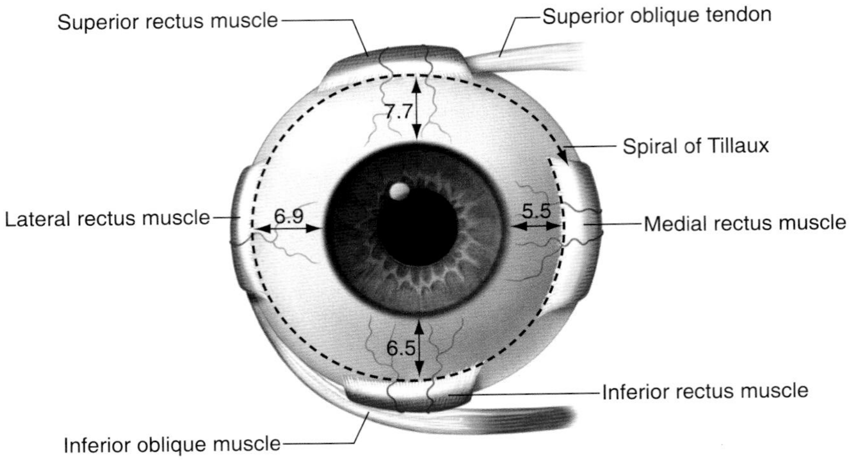

Figure 3-3 Spiral of Tillaux, right eye. Note: The insertion distances, given in millimeters, are maximum values. Insertion distances vary among individuals. *(Illustration by Christine Gralapp.)*

Blood Supply of the ExtraocularMuscles

Arterial System

The muscular branches of the ophthalmic artery provide the most important blood supply to the EOMs. The *lateral muscular branch* supplies the lateral rectus, superior rectus, superior oblique, and levator palpebrae superioris muscles; the *medial muscular branch*, the larger of the 2, supplies the inferior rectus, medial rectus, and inferior oblique muscles.

The lateral rectus muscle is partially supplied by the *lacrimal artery;* the *infraorbital artery* partially supplies the inferior oblique and inferior rectus muscles. The muscular branches give rise to the *anterior ciliary arteries* accompanying the rectus muscles; each rectus muscle has 1–4 anterior ciliary arteries. These pass to the episclera of the globe and then supply blood to the anterior segment. The commonly held notion that the lateral rectus has fewer ciliary vessels than the other rectus muscles has been challenged by anatomical work showing that the number of ciliary vessels is similar for the lateral rectus and the other rectus muscles and that these vessels may, in fact, contribute substantially to the blood supply of the anterior segment.

Johnson MS, Christiansen SP, Rath PP, et al. Anterior ciliary circulation from the horizontal rectus muscles. *Strabismus.* 2009; 17(1): 45–48.

Venous System

The venous system parallels the arterial system, emptying into the *superior* and *inferior orbital veins.* Generally, 4 or more *vortex veins* are located posterior to the equator; these are often found near the nasal and temporal margins of the superior rectus and inferior rectus muscles. Although the number and position of the vortex veins vary, the location of 2 of them in the orbit is consistent: the inferotemporal quadrant, just posterior to the inferior oblique muscle; and the superotemporal quadrant, just posterior to the superior oblique tendon.

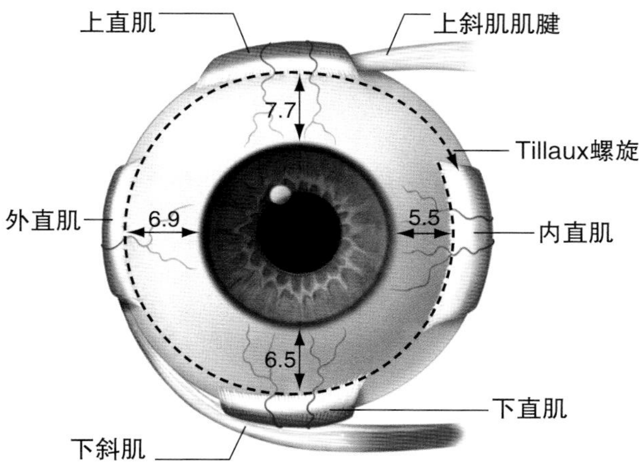

图 3–3　Tillaux 螺旋，右眼。注：附着点距离以 mm 为单位，此处标注的为最大值，该距离因人而异。*（译者注：资料来源见前页原文。）*

眼外肌的血液供应

动脉系统

眼动脉的肌支为眼外肌提供最重要的血液供应。*外侧肌支*负责供应外直肌、上直肌、上斜肌和提上睑肌，较大的 2 支*内侧肌支*负责供应下直肌、内直肌和下斜肌。

外直肌还有*泪腺动脉*参与供应；下斜肌和下直肌也有*眶下动脉*参与供应。眼动脉肌支形成*睫状前动脉*，与直肌伴行；每条直肌有 1~ 4 条睫状前动脉。这些睫状前动脉穿过表层巩膜为眼前节提供血液供应。以往普遍认为供应外直肌的睫状动脉分支数量少于其他直肌，现在有解剖学证据表明，所有直肌具有相同数量的睫状血管，并且对眼前节的血液供应非常重要。

Johnson MS, Christiansen SP, Rath PP, et al. Anterior ciliary circulation from the horizontal rectus muscles. *Strabismus*. 2009; 17(1): 45–48.

静脉系统

静脉系统与动脉系统伴行，注入*眶上*和*眶下静脉*。通常，赤道部后方有 4 条或 4 条以上的*涡静脉*分布，这些静脉常靠近上直肌和下直肌的鼻侧缘和颞侧缘。尽管涡静脉的数量和位置变异较大，但其中眼眶内有 2 条涡静脉的位置是固定不变的：在下斜肌后的颞下象限处，以及上斜肌肌腱后的颞上象限处。

Structure of the Extraocular Muscles

The important functional characteristics of muscle fibers are contraction speed and fatigue resistance. The eye muscles participate in motor acts that are among the fastest (saccadic eye movements) in the human body and among the most sustained (gaze fixation and vergence movements). Like skeletal muscle, EOM is voluntary striated muscle. However, EOM differs from typical skeletal muscle developmentally, biochemically, structurally, and functionally. In the EOMs, the ratio of nerve fibers to muscle fibers is very high (1:3–1:5) up to 10 times higher than the ratio of nerve axons to muscle fibers in skeletal muscle. This high ratio may enable accurate eye movements that are controlled by an array of systems ranging from the primitive vestibular-ocular reflex to highly evolved vergence movements.

The EOMs exhibit a distinct 2-layer organization: an outer *orbital layer*, which acts only on connective tissue pulleys (see the section The Pulley System, later in the chapter), and an inner *global layer*, whose tendon inserts on the sclera to move the globe (Fig 3-4). The muscle fibers of the orbital and global layers can be either singly or multiply innervated.

Singly innervated fibers are fast-twitch generating and resistant to fatigue. In the orbital layer, approximately 80% of the fibers are singly innervated. In the global layer, about 90% of the fibers are singly innervated. They can be subdivided into 3 groups (red, intermediate, and white), based on mitochondrial content. The red fibers are the most fatigue resistant; the white fibers, the least. The orbital singly innervated fibers are considered the major contributor to sustained EOM force in primary and deviated positions. Of all muscle fiber types, this type is the most affected by denervation from damage to the motor nerves or the end plates, as occurs after botulinum toxin injection.

The function of the multiply innervated fibers of the orbital and global layers is not clear. These fibers are not seen in elevator palpebrae superioris. They are thought to be involved in the finer control of fixation and in smooth and finely graded eye movements, particularly vergence control.

These novel properties of eye muscles lead to differential responses to local anesthetics and pharmaceuticals such as botulinum toxin and calcium channel blockers, as well as to disease processes such as myasthenia gravis and muscular dystrophy.

Finally, there is evidence for compartmentalization of rectus muscle innervation. For example, studies in primates and humans have shown distinct superior and inferior zones within the horizontal rectus muscles. The clinical significance of these observations is being investigated.

da Silva Costa RM, Kung J, Poukens V, Yoo L, Tychsen L, Demer JL. Intramuscular innervation of primate extraocular muscles: unique compartmentalization in horizontal recti. *Inv Ophthalmol Vis Sci.* 2011;52(5):2830–2836.

DemerJL.Compartmentalization of extraocular muscle function.*Eye(Lond).*2015;29(2):157–162.

眼外肌结构

肌纤维具有收缩速度和抗疲劳 2 个重要功能性特征。眼外肌参与人体最快速的运动（扫视运动）以及最持久的运动（注视和聚散运动）。与骨骼肌一样，眼外肌是自主横纹肌，然而从发育学、生物化学、结构以及功能方面看，眼外肌均不同于典型的骨骼肌。眼外肌中神经纤维与肌纤维的比例很高（1：3~1：5），高于骨骼肌中神经轴突与肌纤维比例的 10 倍。这种高比例受到从原始的前庭眼反射到高度进化的聚散运动等一系列系统的控制，使眼球运动精准。

眼外肌呈现清晰的双层结构：外侧的*眶层*，主要作用于结缔组织滑车（见章节后面的“滑车系统”部分），内侧的*球层*，其肌腱附着于巩膜上，使眼球转动。眶层和球层的肌纤维受到单一神经或多重神经支配。

单一神经支配的肌纤维能够快速收缩以及抗疲劳。在眶层，有大约 80% 的肌纤维是由单一神经支配的。在球层，有大约 90% 的肌纤维是由单一神经支配的。根据线粒体的含量，这些肌纤维分为 3 种（红纤维，中间色纤维，白纤维）。红纤维的抗疲劳能力最强，白纤维最差。无论在第一眼位还是偏斜位，受眶层单一神经支配的肌纤维都是眼外肌持续运动的主要纤维。在所有的肌纤维类型中，该类型的肌纤维最易受到运动神经或终板损害后的去神经支配影响，如发生在肉毒杆菌注射后。

由眶层和球层的多重神经支配的肌纤维的功能尚不明确。提上睑肌不存在多重神经支配的肌纤维。该类型纤维被认为参与了注视的精细控制，以及平滑的和精细分级的眼球运动，特别是对聚散运动的控制。

眼外肌的这些特点导致眼睛对局麻药和肉毒素、钙通道阻滞剂等的药物，以及对疾病发展，如重症肌无力和肌肉萎缩症，产生不同的反应。

最后，有证据显示，直肌的神经支配具有区域性。如对灵长类动物和人类的研究表明，水平直肌内有明显的上下区，其临床意义还在研究中。

da Silva Costa RM, Kung J, Poukens V, Yoo L, Tychsen L, Demer JL. Intramuscular innervation of primate extraocular muscles: unique compartmentalization in horizontal recti. *Inv Ophthalmol Vis Sci.* 2011;52(5):2830–2836.

DemerJL.Compartmentalization of extraocular muscle function.*Eye(Lond)*.2015;29(2):157–162.

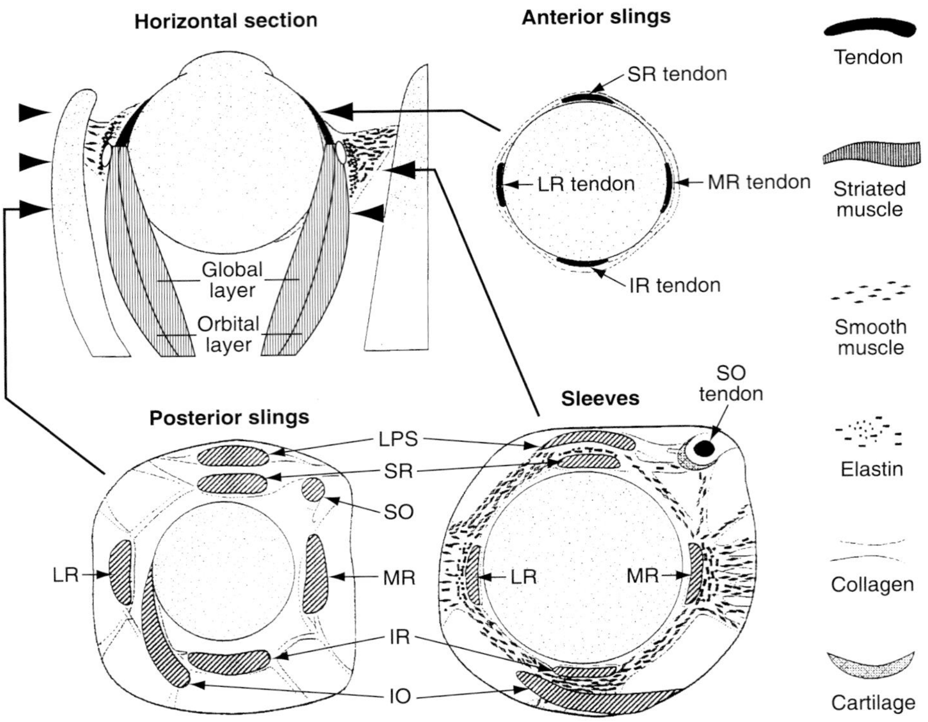

Figure3-4 Structure of orbital connective tissues. IO, inferior oblique; IR, inferior rectus; LPS, levator palpebrae superioris; LR, lateral rectus; MR, medial rectus; SO, superior oblique; SR, superior rectus. The 3 coronal views are represented at the levels indicated by arrows in horizontal section. *(Modified with permission from Demer JL, Miller JM, Poukens V. Surgical implications of the rectus extraocular muscle pulleys. J Pediatr Ophthalmol Strabismus. 1996;33(4):208–218.)*

Orbital and Fascial Relationships

Within the orbit, a complex musculofibroelastic structure suspends the globe, supports the EOMs, and compartmentalizes the fat pads (Fig 3-5). In recent years, the interconnectedness of the orbital tissues, as well as the extent and complexity of these connections, has come to light. The intense fibrous connections existing throughout the orbit can be illustrated clinically by the consequences of tissue entrapment in blowout fractures and of fibrosis of delicate fibrous septa after retrobulbar hemorrhage. The nature of these relationships remains under investigation.

Adipose Tissue

The eye is supported and cushioned within the orbit by a large amount of fatty tissue. External to the muscle cone, fatty tissue comes forward with the rectus muscles, stopping about 10 mm from the limbus. Fatty tissue is also present inside the muscle cone, kept away from the sclera by the Tenon capsule (see Fig 3-5).

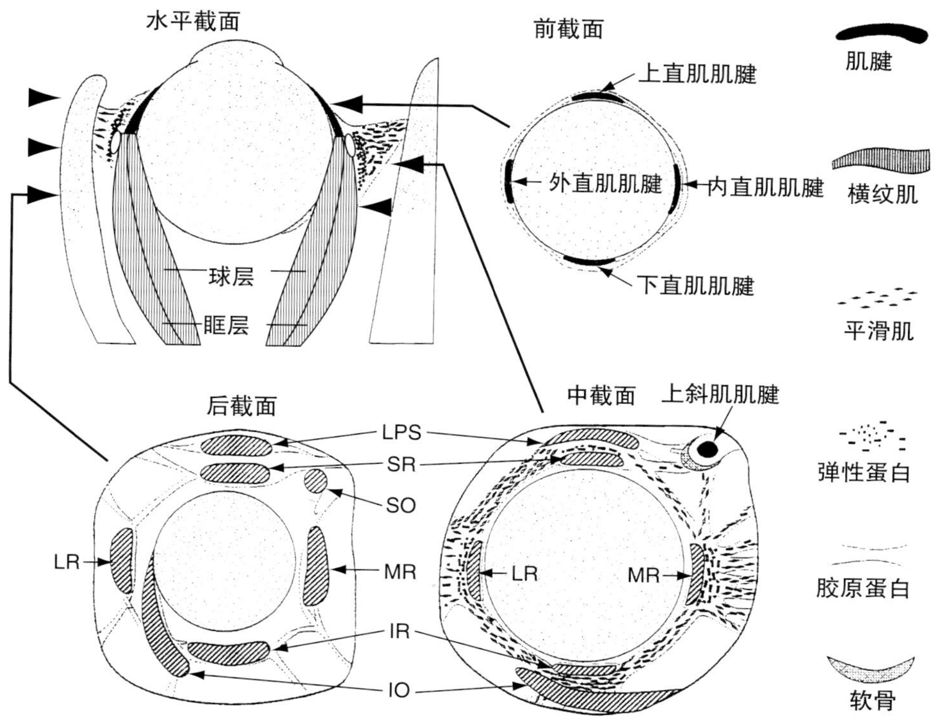

图 3-4　眼眶结缔组织结构。IO，下斜肌；IR，下直肌；LPS，提上睑肌；LR，外直肌；MR，内直肌；SO，上斜肌；SR，上直肌。3 个冠状面分别对应箭头所指的水平区域。*（译者注：资料来源见前页原文。）*

眼眶和筋膜关系

复杂的肌纤维弹性结构将眼球悬挂在眼眶内，支撑着眼外肌，并将脂肪垫分开（图 3-5）。近年来，对眼眶内组织的相互联系以及连接的范围和复杂性已研究得越来越清楚。爆裂性骨折后的组织嵌顿以及球后出血后纤维薄板的纤维化的临床结果进一步阐释了遍布眼眶的纤维组织连接的作用。这些连接的相互关系的本质仍在研究中。

脂肪组织

眼眶内大量的脂肪组织支撑着眼球，并起到缓冲作用。在肌圆锥外，脂肪组织与直肌一起前行，在距离角膜缘 10mm 处终止。脂肪组织也分布于肌圆锥内，使巩膜与 Tenon 囊分隔（见图 3-5）。

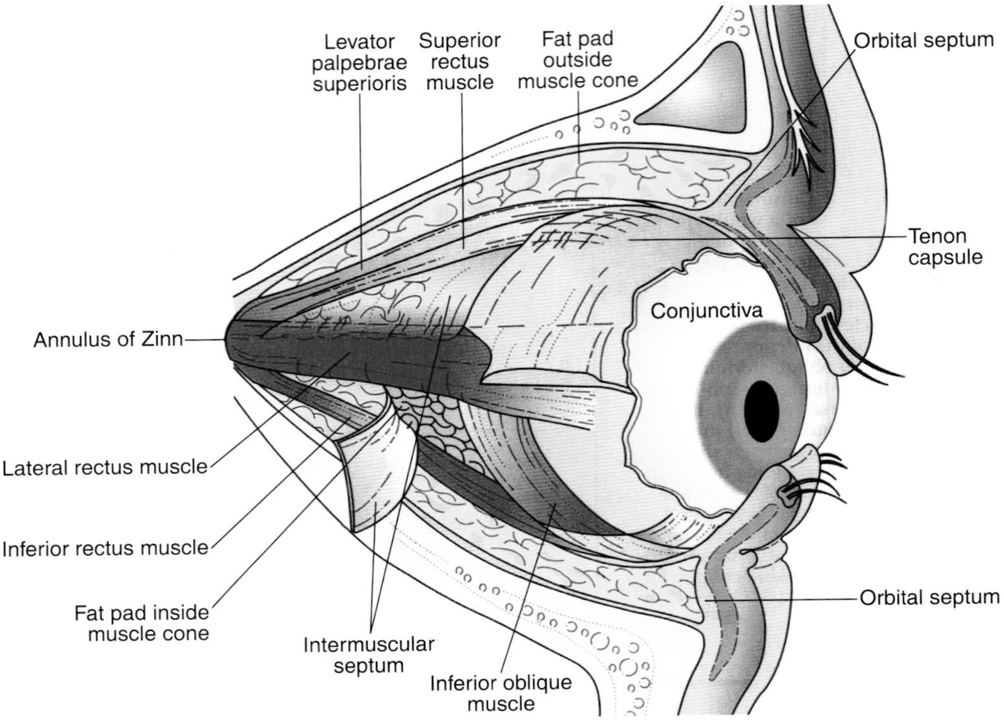

Figure 3-5 The muscle cone contains 1 fat pad and is surrounded by another; these 2 fat pads are separated by the rectus muscles and intermuscular septum. Note that the intermuscular septum does not extend all the way back to the apex of the orbit. *(Modified with permission from Yanoff M, Duker J, eds. Ophthalmology. 2nd ed. London: Mosby; 2004:553.)*

Muscle Cone

The muscle cone lies posterior to the equator. It consists of the EOMs, their sheaths, and the intermuscular septum (see Fig 3-5).

Muscle Capsule

Each rectus muscle has a surrounding fascial capsule that extends with the muscle from its origin to its insertion. These capsules are thin posteriorly, but near the equator they thicken as they pass through the sleeve of the Tenon capsule, continuing anteriorly with the muscles to their insertions. Anterior to the equator, between the undersurface of the muscle and the sclera, there is almost no fascia, only connective tissue footplates that connect the muscle to the globe. The smooth, avascular surface of the muscle capsule allows the muscles to slide easily over the globe.

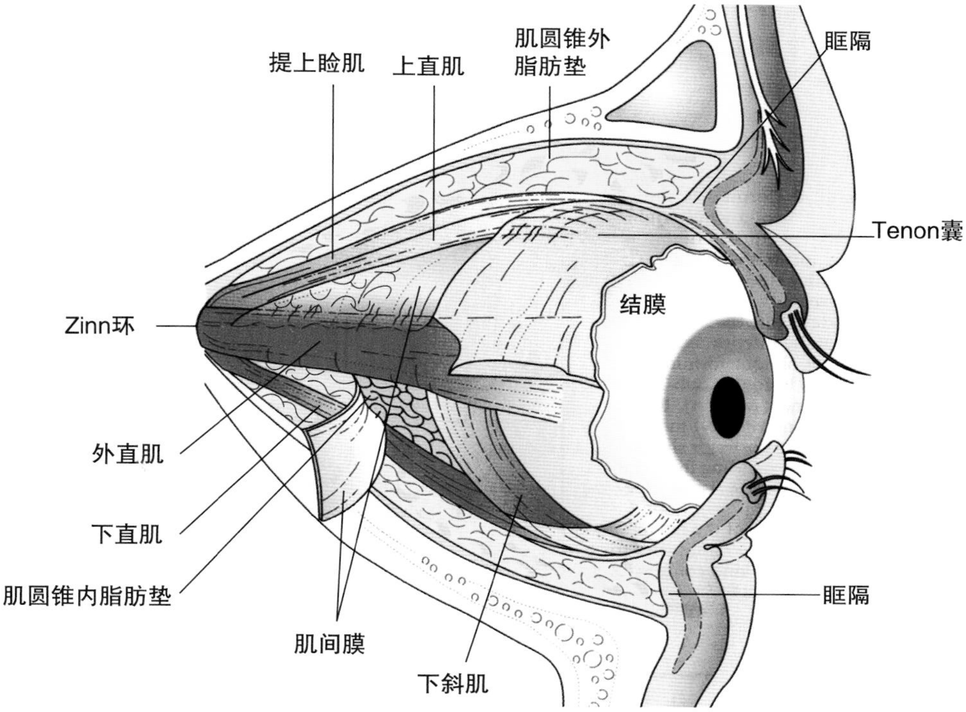

图 3–5　肌圆锥内包含 1 个脂肪垫，另 1 个脂肪垫包绕肌圆锥，2 块脂肪垫被直肌和肌间膈分开。注意：肌间膈没有延伸到眶尖的位置。*（译者注：资料来源见前页原文。）*

肌圆锥

肌圆锥位于赤道后，由眼外肌、肌鞘以及肌间膈组成（见图 3–5）。

肌鞘

每条直肌从起点到附着点均有纤维肌鞘包绕。眼球后部肌鞘薄，近赤道部的肌鞘增厚，其穿过 Tenon 囊，向前至附着点。在赤道部前方，肌肉下表面与巩膜之间几乎无筋膜，仅有结缔组织连接肌肉和眼球。肌鞘平滑的无血管表面使得肌肉能够轻松地在眼球上滑动。

The Tenon Capsule

The Tenon capsule (*fascia bulbi*) is the principal orbital fascia and forms the envelope within which the eyeball moves (Fig 3-6). The Tenon capsule fuses posteriorly with the optic nerve sheath and anteriorly with the intermuscular septum at a position 3 mm from the limbus. The posterior portion of the Tenon capsule is thin and flexible, enabling free movement of the optic nerve, ciliary nerves, and ciliary vessels as the globe rotates, while separating the orbital fat inside the muscle cone from the sclera. At and just posterior to the equator, the Tenon capsule is thick and tough, suspending the globe like a trampoline by means of connections to the periorbital tissues. The global layer of the 4 rectus muscles penetrates this thick fibroelastic tissue approximately 10mm posterior to their insertions. The oblique muscles penetrate the Tenon capsule anterior to the equator. The Tenon capsule continues forward over these 6 EOMs and separates them from the orbital fat and structures lying outside the muscle cone.

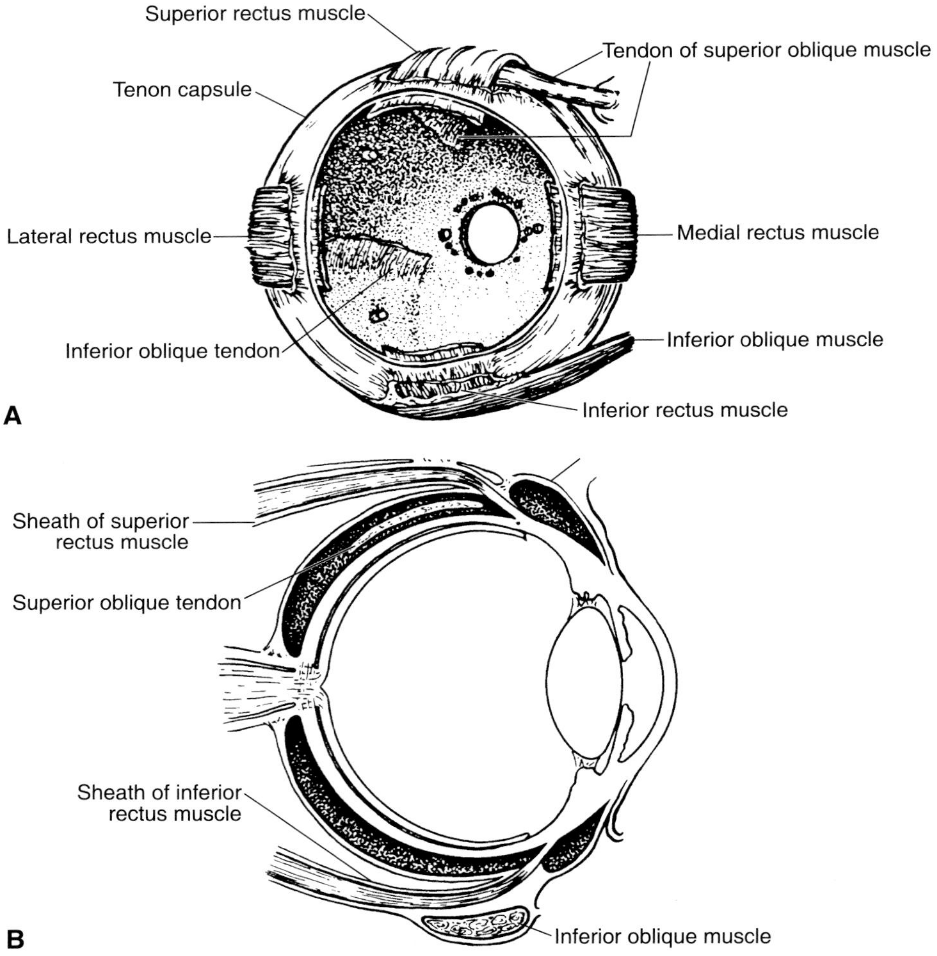

Figure 3-6 **A,** Anterior and posterior orifices of the Tenon capsule shown after enucleation of the globe. **B,** The Tenon space shown by injection with India ink. *(Modified with permission from von Noorden GK, Campos EC. Binocular Vision and Ocular Motility: Theory and Management of Strabismus. 6th ed. St Louis: Mosby; 2002:45.)*

Tenon 囊

Tenon 囊（*眼球筋膜*）是眼眶内主要的筋膜组织，包绕着在里面活动的眼球（图 3–6）。Tenon 囊向后与视神经鞘融为一体，向前在距离角膜缘 3mm 处与肌间膈融为一体。由于 Tenon 囊后部薄且柔韧，当眼球转动时，视神经、睫状神经和睫状血管可以自由运动，同时将肌圆锥内的脂肪与巩膜分隔开。在赤道部及偏后处，Tenon 囊变厚变硬，与眶周组织一起，将眼球像蹦床一样悬挂起来。4 条直肌的球层在距离它们附着点后大约 10mm 处穿过这厚层纤维弹性组织。斜肌在赤道前面穿过 Tenon 囊。Tenon 囊在 6 条眼外肌上继续前行，分隔眼外肌与肌圆锥外的眶周脂肪和其他组织。

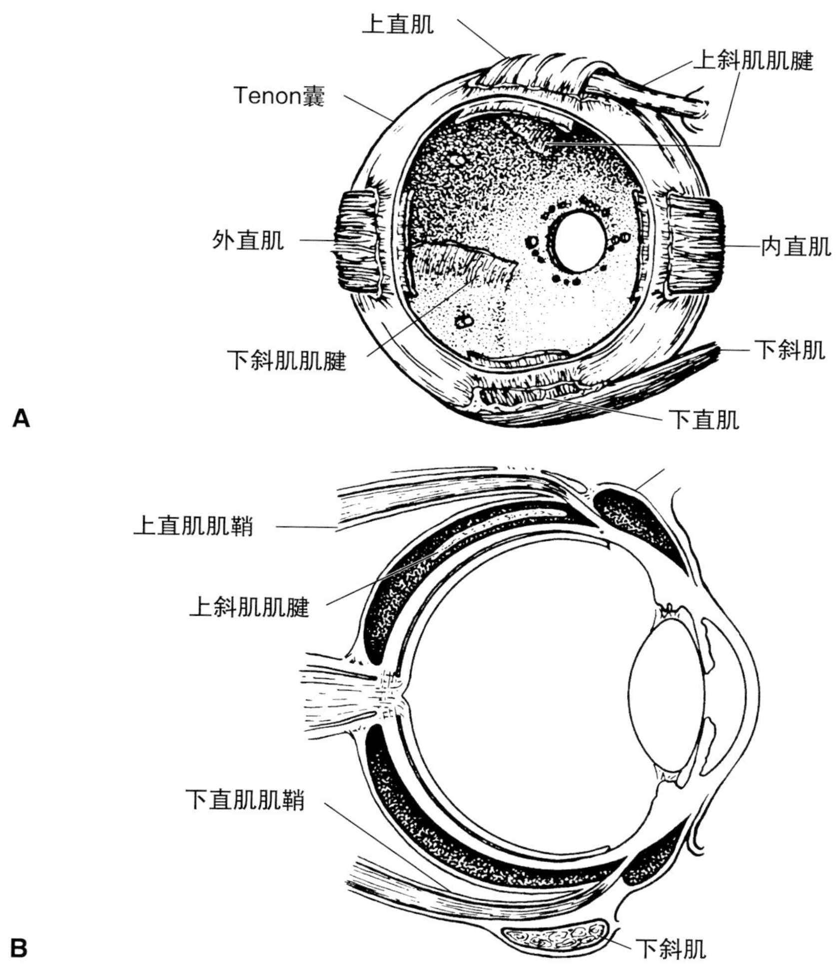

图 3–6　A. 眼球摘除后 Tenon 囊的前孔和后孔。**B.** 注入 India 墨后显示的 Tenon 囊空间。*（译者注：资料来源见前页原文。）*

The Pulley System

The 4 rectus muscles are surrounded by fibroelastic pulleys that maintain the position of the EOMs relative to the orbit. The pulleys consist of collagen, elastin, and smooth muscle, enabling them to contract and relax. Dynamic magnetic resonance imaging (MRI) studies show that, in some cases, the pulleys act mechanically as the rectus muscle origins. The pulleys may also serve to stabilize the muscle path, preventing sideslipping or movement perpendicular to the muscle axis (see Fig 3-4). Anteriorly, the pulleys merge with the *intermuscular septum*, which fuses with the conjunctiva 3 mm posterior to the limbus. The posterior section of the intermuscular septum separates the intraconal fat pads from the extraconal fat pads (see Fig 3-5). Numerous extensions from the EOM sheaths attach to the orbit and help support the globe.

The inferior oblique muscle originates inferonasally from the periosteum of the maxillary bone, near the orbital rim, adjacent to the anterior lacrimal crest, and it continues laterally, entering its connective tissue pulley inferior to the inferior rectus muscle, at the site where the inferior oblique muscle also penetrates the Tenon capsule. The inferior oblique pulley and inferior rectus pulley join to form the Lockwood ligament (see Fig 3-7). Attached to the conjoined inferior oblique and inferior rectus pulley complex is the dense neurofibrovascular bundle containing the inferior oblique motor nerve.

The *active pulley hypothesis* proposes that the pulley positions are shifted by the contraction of the orbital layer against the elasticity of the pulley suspension. This concept remains controversial: whether there is actual innervational control of the pulleys is still debated. However, high-resolution MRI scans have shown that the pulleys are located only a short distance from the globe center; therefore, small shifts in pulley position would confer large shifts in EOM pulling direction. Normal pulleys shift only slightly in the coronal plane, even during large eye movements. *Heterotopy (malpositioning)* of the rectus pulleys may cause some cases of incomitant strabismus and A or V patterns (see Chapter10), and these anomalies can mimic oblique muscle dysfunction by misdirecting the forces of the rectus muscles. Bony abnormalities, such as those seen with craniosynostosis, can also alter the direction of pull of rectus muscles by causing malpositioning of the pulleys.

The pulley model and its implications have been challenged by other high-resolution MRI studies, which show that during eye movements into eccentric fields, the posterior portions of rectus muscles shift. These findings are consistent with the more traditional model of eye muscle function, which is the "restrained shortest-path model."

Peragallo JH, Pineles SL, Demer JL. Recent advances clarifying the etiologies of strabismus. *J Neuroophthalmol.* 2015;35(2):185–193.

Anatomical Considerations for Ophthalmic Procedures

The nerves to the rectus muscles and the superior oblique muscle enter the muscles approximately one-third of the distance from the origin to the insertion (or trochlea, in the case of the superior oblique muscle). Damaging these nerves during anterior surgery is unlikely but not impossible. An instrument thrust more than 26 mm posterior to a rectus muscle's insertion may injure the nerve.

Cranial nerve IV is outside the muscle cone and is usually not affected by a retrobulbar block. However, any EOM could be reached by a retrobulbar needle and injured by injection of local anesthetic.

滑车系统

纤维弹性滑车包绕着 4 条直肌，维持眼外肌在眼眶内的相对位置。滑车由胶原蛋白、弹性蛋白和平滑肌组成，能够收缩和放松。动态磁共振成像（MRI）研究表明，有时滑车可作为直肌的力学起点。滑车还能稳定肌肉的运动路径，防止侧滑或垂直于肌肉轴的运动（见图 3–4）。滑车向前与*肌间膈*合并，而肌间膈在角膜缘后 3mm 处与结膜融合。肌间膈的后部将肌圆锥内、外的脂肪垫分开（见图 3–5）。眼外肌肌鞘广泛扩展连接到眼眶，支撑眼球。

下斜肌起源于鼻下方的上颌骨骨膜，接近眶缘，邻近前泪嵴，然后向外延伸，在下直肌下方融入结缔组织滑车，此处也是下斜肌穿过 Tenon 囊的位置。下斜肌滑车和下直肌滑车联合形成 Lockwood 韧带（见图 3–7）。致密的神经纤维血管束附着于下斜肌和下直肌的滑车复合体，其中含下斜肌的运动神经。

*功能性滑车假说*提出，随着眶层对抗滑车悬吊的弹性而产生的收缩，滑车的位置发生移动。对滑车是否存在神经支配的问题仍有争议。高分辨率的 MRI 扫描显示，滑车距离眼球中心很近，因此滑车位置微小的变化会使得眼外肌的牵拉方向发生很大的改变。在冠状面上，即使眼球大幅度地转动，正常的滑车位置改变也很小。直肌滑车的*异位*（*错位*）可能导致非共同性斜视和 A 征或 V 征（见第 10 章），这些异常通过改变直肌肌力，形成类似斜肌功能异常。骨性异常，如颅缝早闭，是由于滑车的错位改变了直肌的拉动方向。

高分辨率的 MRI 研究结果并不支持滑车模型及临床解释，研究表明当眼球转动到旁中心视野时，直肌的后部移位。这些结果与传统的眼肌功能模型（“限制性最短路径模型”）更吻合。

Peragallo JH, Pineles SL, Demer JL. Recent advances clarifying the etiologies of strabismus. *J Neuroophthalmol.* 2015;35(2):185–193.

眼科手术中的解剖问题

支配直肌和上斜肌的神经在起点到附着点的 1/3 处（在有的情况下是在上斜肌滑车处）进入肌肉。前路手术几乎不太可能损伤这些神经，但并非完全不可能。器械插入深度超过直肌附着点后 26 mm 处时，就可能损伤神经。

滑车神经位于肌圆锥外，通常不会受到球后阻滞麻醉的影响。而眼外肌可能被球后针头触及，并且受局麻药注射的损伤。

The nerve supplying the inferior oblique muscle enters the lateral portion of the muscle, where it crosses the inferior rectus muscle; surgery performed in this area can damage the nerve. Because parasympathetic fibers to the sphincter pupillae (for pupil constriction) and the ciliary muscle (for accommodation) accompany the nerve to the inferior oblique muscle, with a synapse in the ciliary ganglion, surgery in this area may also result in an enlarged pupil. In addition, an inferotemporal retrobulbar block can injure these nerves and the inferior oblique muscle.

An operation on the inferior oblique muscle requires careful inspection of the inferolateral quadrant to ensure that all bellies are identified. If, during a weakening or strengthening procedure, the presence of a second or third belly is not recognized, the action of the muscle may not be sufficiently altered, and additional surgery may be required.

The neurofibrovascular bundle along the lateral border of the inferior rectus muscle can become an ancillary insertion site for the inferior oblique muscle when the muscle is anteriorly or medially transposed. Anterior transposition of the inferior oblique creates an anti-elevation effect.

Maintaining the integrity of the muscle capsules during surgery reduces intraoperative bleeding and provides a smooth muscle surface with less risk of adhesion formation. If only the muscle capsule is sutured to the globe, the muscle can retract backward, causing a slipped muscle.

The surgeon can use the intermuscular septum (between the rectus muscles and especially the section between the rectus and oblique muscles) as a point of reference in locating a muscle that has been "lost" during surgery or as a result of trauma. Extensive dissections of the intermuscular septum are not necessary for rectus muscle recession surgery. However, during resection surgery, these connections should be severed to prevent unexpected consequences, such as the inferior oblique muscle being advanced with the lateral rectus muscle. Often, there are 2 frenula: one that connects the lateral rectus muscle to the underlying inferior oblique at its insertion and another that connects the superior rectus to the underlying superior oblique tendon. Usually, these must be disconnected during recessions and resections of either of these 2 rectus muscles.

The medial rectus is the only rectus muscle that does not have an oblique muscle running tangential to it. This makes surgery on the medial rectus less complicated but means that there is neither a point of reference if the surgeon becomes disoriented nor a point of attachment if the muscle is lost.

The inferior rectus muscle is distinctly bound to the lower eyelid by the fascial extension from its sheath. *Recession*, or weakening, of the inferior rectus muscle tends to widen the palpebral fissure and result in lower eyelid retraction. *Resection*, or strengthening, of the inferior rectus muscle tends to narrow the fissure by elevating the lower eyelid. Therefore, any alteration of the inferior rectus muscle maybe associated with achange in the palpebral fissure (Fig 3-7).

The superior rectus muscle is loosely bound to the levator palpebrae superioris muscle. The eyelid may be pulled downward after resection of the superior rectus muscle, thus narrowing the palpebral fissure. In contrast, the eyelid is not usually retracted upward with small or moderate recessions. In hypotropia, a pseudoptosis may be present because the upper eyelid tends to follow the superior rectus muscle (see Fig 3-7).

支配下斜肌的神经在下斜肌外侧进入肌肉，并与下直肌交叉。在这个区域的手术会损伤神经。因为支配瞳孔括约肌（瞳孔收缩）和睫状肌（调节）的副交感神经纤维，在睫状神经节交换神经元，也伴随着该神经到达下斜肌，因此在该区域的手术也可能导致瞳孔扩大。此外，颞下球后阻滞麻醉也会损伤这些神经和下斜肌。

对下斜肌进行手术需要仔细检查其外下象限，以确保找到所有的肌腹。如果在减弱和加强肌力的手术中，未找到第 2 或第 3 肌腹，则肌肉功能不能被有效地改变，可能需要再次手术。

当下斜肌向前或向内转位时，沿着下直肌外侧边缘走行的神经纤维血管束成为下斜肌的第 2 附着点。下斜肌的前移位抑制上转功能。

手术中，保持肌鞘的完整，可减少术中出血，提供平滑的肌肉表面，降低粘连形成的风险。如果仅将肌鞘缝合到眼球上，肌肉会向后缩回，造成肌肉滑脱。

医生可以利用肌间膈（在直肌之间，特别是直肌和斜肌之间），定位在手术中或是由于创伤而“丢失”的肌肉的参考点。直肌后徙术不需要广泛切断肌间膈。而在切除术时，应切断这些连接，以防止产生意外后果，如下斜肌被外直肌牵拉向前。通常，有 2 条系带：1 条连接外直肌和其下方的下斜肌附着点，另 1 条连接上直肌和其下方的上斜肌肌腱。后徙和切除 2 条直肌中的任意 1 条都必须切断相应的系带连接。

内直肌是唯一一条没有与斜肌相切的直肌。这使得内直肌上的手术相对简单，但也意味着如果医生辨不清方向时没有参考点，或者是肌肉丢失时没有附着点。

通过肌鞘的筋膜延伸，下直肌与下眼睑相连接。*后徙*或减弱下直肌肌力，会使睑裂开大，导致下眼睑退缩。*切除*或加强下直肌肌力，使下眼睑抬高，导致睑裂缩小。因此，任何下直肌的改变都可能造成睑裂的变化（图 3–7）。

上直肌与提上睑肌之间的黏附松弛。上直肌切除术后，上眼睑可能被向下牵拉，导致睑裂缩小。而少量上直肌后徙术后，上眼睑并不会退缩。下斜视可表现出假性上睑下垂，是由于上眼睑易受到上直肌的影响（图 3–7）。

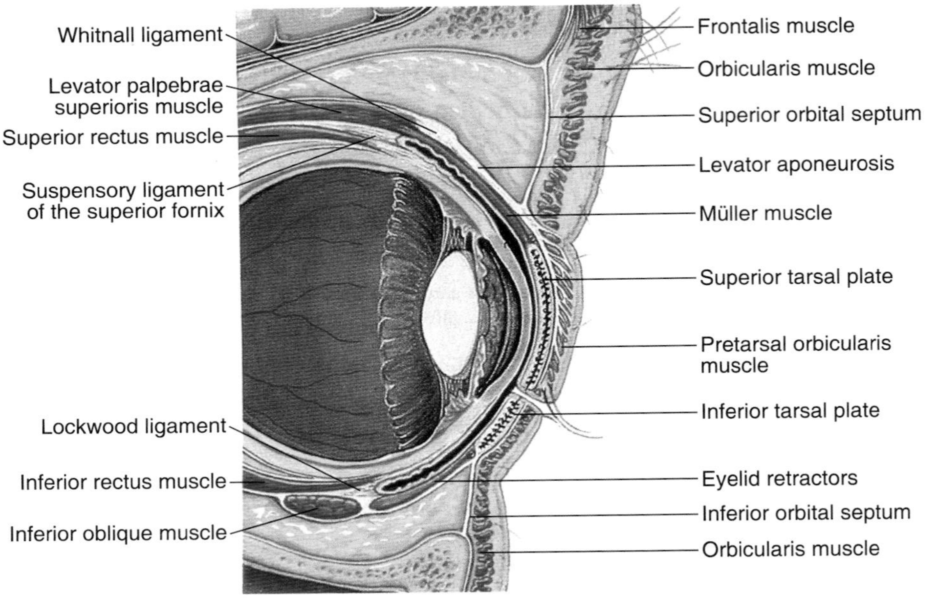

Figure 3-7 Attachments of the upper and lower eyelids to the vertical rectus muscles. *(Modified with permission from Buckley EG, Freedman S, Shields MB, eds. Atlas of Ophthalmic Surgery, Vol III: Strabismus and Glaucoma. St Louis: Mosby-Year Book; 1995:15.)*

The blood supply to the EOMs provides almost all of the temporal half of the anterior segment circulation and most of the nasal half of the anterior segment circulation, which also receives some blood from the long posterior ciliary artery. Therefore, simultaneous surgery on 3 rectus muscles may induce anterior segment ischemia, particularly in older or vasculopathic patients.

Whenever muscle surgery is performed, special care must be taken to avoid penetration of the Tenon capsule 10 mm or more posterior to the limbus. If the integrity of the Tenon capsule is violated posterior to this point, fatty tissue may prolapse through the capsule and form a restrictive adhesion to sclera, muscle, intermuscular septum, or conjunctiva, limiting ocular motility.

When surgery is performed near the vortex veins, accidental severing of a vein is possible. The procedures that present the greatest risk of damaging a vortex vein are recession or resection of the inferior rectus or superior rectus muscle, weakening of the inferior oblique muscle, and exposure of the superior oblique muscle tendon. Hemostasis can be achieved with cautery or with an absorbable hemostatic sponge.

The sclera is thinnest just posterior to the 4 rectus muscle insertions, an area that is the site of most eye muscle surgery, especially recession procedures. Thus, scleral perforation is always a risk during eye muscle surgery. See Chapter 14 for further discussion of EOM surgery.

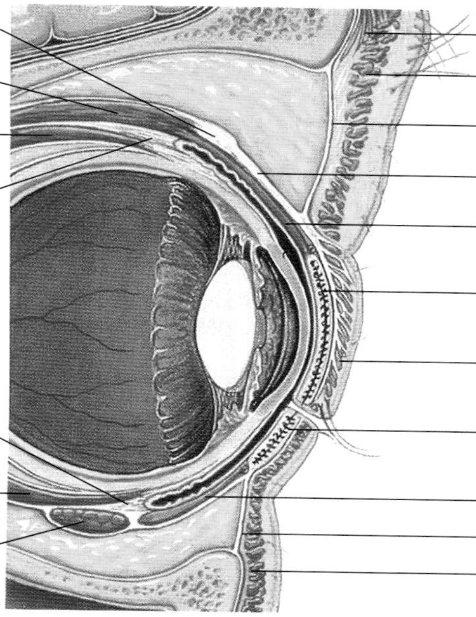

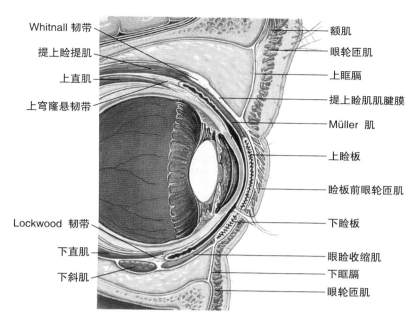

图 3–7　相对于垂直直肌上下眼睑的附属组织。*（译者注：资料来源见前页原文。）*

眼前节颞侧和大部分鼻侧的血液循环由眼外肌的血液供应，还接受睫状后长动脉的血液供应。因此，3 条直肌同时手术可能引起眼前节缺血，特别是老年人或血管病变患者。

进行眼外肌手术时，必须特别注意避免穿过角膜缘后 10 mm 以后的 Tenon 囊。如果 Tenon 囊的完整性受到破坏，脂肪组织可能从 Tenon 囊脱垂，并与巩膜、肌肉、肌间膈或结膜形成限制性粘连，从而限制眼球的运动。

手术部位靠近涡静脉时，有可能意外切断血管。上下直肌的后徙或切除术、下斜肌的减弱以及上斜肌肌腱的暴露最容易损坏涡静脉。

可通过烧灼或用可吸收止血海绵止血。4 条直肌附着点后面的巩膜最薄，此处是大多数眼外肌手术的部位，尤其是后徙术。因此，巩膜穿孔是眼外肌手术过程中始终存在的风险。有关眼外肌手术的进一步讨论，请参见第 14 章。

（翻译　梅颖　刘凤阳 // 审校　石一宁　布娟 // 章节审校　石广礼）

CHAPTER 4

Motor Physiology

Basic Principles and Terms

Ocular Rotations

While there are several coordinate systems that are useful for mathematical modeling of rotations of the eye, ocular rotations are clinically considered as *horizontal rotations* about a vertical axis, corresponding to medial and lateral gaze; vertical rotations about a horizontal axis, corresponding to upward and downward gaze; and *torsional rotations* about the line of sight. If a change in gaze position is broken down into a series of separate rotations about the horizontal and vertical axes, the final torsion of the eye for a given gaze direction could theoretically vary, depending on the sequence in which the rotations are applied. In practice, the final torsion of the eye is always the same for a given gaze direction, regardless of the sequence by which it arrives there *(Donder's law). Listing's law* specifies this relationship by stipulating that the orientation in a given gaze position is equivalent to that which would result from a single rotation around an axis lying in *Listing's plane.*

Positions of Gaze

- *Primary position* is the position of the eyes when they are fixating straight ahead.
- *Secondary diagnostic positions* are straight up, straight down, right gaze, and left gaze.
- *Tertiary diagnostic positions* are the 4 oblique positions of gaze: up and right, up and left, down and right, down and left, as well as the right and left head-tilt positions.
- *Cardinal positions,* which correspond to the primary fields of action of the extraocular muscles (EOMs) (see the section "Field of action"), are up and right, up and left, right, left, down and right, down and left (Fig 4-1).

See Chapter 7 for additional discussion of the positions of gaze.

Extraocular Muscle Action

The width of the insertion of each EOM serves to stabilize the eye and mitigate changes in action that would otherwise occur in different eye positions. For example, when the eye looks upward, the insertion of the medial rectus muscle also shifts upward. But this also tightens the inferior fibers and slackens the superior fibers, in effect shifting the net vector from the muscle downward toward its original position. See also Activity 3-1 in Chapter 3.

第 4 章

运动生理学

基本原则和术语

眼球转动

建立眼睛转动的数学模式时，使用坐标系非常有用。在临床上，眼睛转动可分为：沿垂直轴的水平转动，对应于向内、向外注视；沿水平轴的*垂直转动*，对应于向上、向下注视；以及沿视轴的*旋转转动*。如果注视位置的改变被分解成一系列沿水平和垂直轴的单独转动，从理论上看，对于给定注视方向的眼睛，其最后的转动方式可以是不同的，这取决于转动分解步骤的实施顺序。而在临床上，对于给定的注视方向，不论眼睛到达此状态的步骤顺序如何，其最终的旋转方式总是相同的（*Donder 法则*）。*Listing 法则*规定：给定注视位置的眼球运动相当于在 Listing 平面上的沿一轴进行的单次眼球转动。

注视位置

- *第一眼位*是眼睛注视正前方时所处的位置。
- 第二*诊断眼位*是眼睛注视正上方、正下方、右侧和左侧时所处的位置。
- *第三诊断眼位*是眼睛注视 4 个斜向位置（右上、左上、右下、左下），以及头向右和向左倾斜。
- *基本眼位*，对应于眼外肌（EOM）的主要功能视野（见“功能视野”一节），右上、左上、右、左、右下、左下（图 4–1）。

注视位置的其他相关内容参见第 7 章。

眼外肌功能

每条眼外肌的附着宽度有助于稳定并减少眼球运动时在不同位置上可能发生的变化。例如，当眼睛向上看时，内直肌的附着处也向上移动，但同时也会收紧下方的肌纤维，松弛上方的肌纤维，从而使净矢向量从肌肉向下指向原始位置。另见第 3 章的演示活动 3–1。

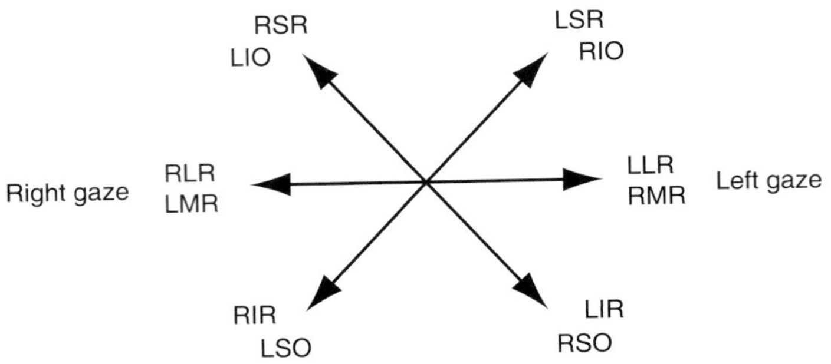

Figure 4-1 The 6 cardinal positions, which correspond to the primary fields of action of the extraocular muscles. RSR, right superior rectus; LIO, left inferior oblique; LSR, left superior rectus; RIO, right inferior oblique; RLR, right lateral rectus; LMR, left medial rectus; LLR, left lateral rectus; RMR, right medial rectus; RIR, right inferior rectus; LSO, left superior oblique; LIR, left inferior rectus; RSO, right superior oblique.

Muscle pulleys

Regardless of eye position or whether the insertion points have been moved surgically, the rectus muscles are still constrained to pass through the same openings in the Tenon capsule as they course from the orbital apex to the eye. The orbital connective tissue sheaths surrounding these openings have been described as muscle pulleys and have a specialized structure, including smooth muscle, that may provide active modulation of muscle action. See Chapter 3 for further discussion of muscle pulleys.

Arc of contact

In primary position, each muscle wraps around the globe for several millimeters before reaching its insertion on the sclera. The length of muscle in contact with the globe is called the *arc of contact* (see Chapter 3, Table 3-1, which gives the arc of contact for the EOMs). The point where the muscle first contacts the globe is the effective insertion of the muscle. As the muscle contracts and the eye rotates toward the muscle, the effective insertion moves forward on the globe, toward the scleral insertion point, as the arc of contact decreases. The muscle remains tangential to the globe at its effective insertion, maintaining the same torque through much of the eye movement.

Eye Movements

Motor Units

An individual motor nerve fiber and its several muscle fibers constitute a motor unit. The electrical activity of motor units can be recorded by *electromyography (EMG)*. An electromyogram is a useful research tool in the investigation of normal and abnormal innervation of eye muscles. A portable EMG device connected to an insulated needle is often used during injection of botulinum toxin into eye muscles to help the surgeon localize the appropriate muscle within the orbit, especially when the muscle has been operated on previously.

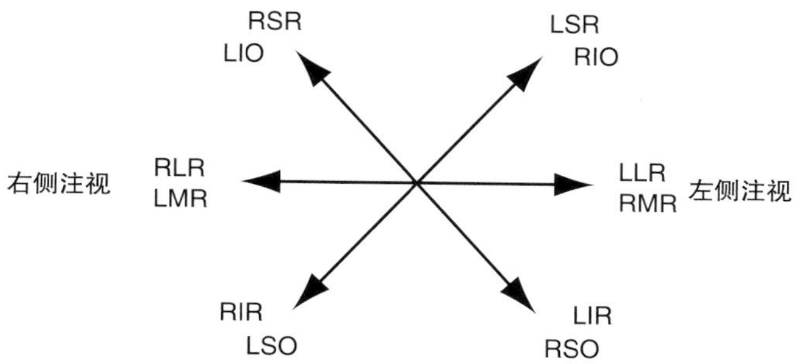

图 4–1　与眼外肌主要功能视野相对应的 6 个基本眼位。RSR，右上直肌；LIO，左下斜肌；ISR，左上直肌；RIO，右下斜肌；RLR，右外直肌；IMR，左内直肌；LLR，左外直肌；RMR，右内直肌；RIR，右下直肌；ISO，左上斜肌；LIR，左下直肌；RSO，右上斜肌。

肌肉滑车

无论眼睛的位置如何或肌肉附着点是否通过手术移动，直肌依然被限制在 Tenon 囊内相同的开口内，因为直肌是从眶尖走行至眼球的。围绕这些开口的眼眶结缔组织鞘被称为肌肉滑车，含有平滑肌等特殊的结构，可能能够主动调节肌肉功能。关于肌肉滑车的进一步讨论见第 3 章。

接触弧

第一眼位时，在插入巩膜前，每一条肌肉与眼球包绕数毫米。与眼球接触的肌肉长度称为*接触弧*（见第 3 章的表 3–1，其中给出了眼外肌的接触弧）。肌肉最先接触眼球处，即是肌肉的有效附着处。当肌肉收缩、眼球向肌肉转动时，有效附着处在眼球表面向前移动，随着接触弧的减少，眼球向巩膜插入点移动。肌肉在有效附着处与眼球相切，在大部分眼球运动中保持相同的扭矩。

眼球运动

运动单位

单个运动神经纤维及其支配的数条肌纤维构成一个运动单元。运动单元的电活动可以通过*肌电描记术（EMG）*记录。肌电图是研究眼肌正常和异常神经支配的有用工具。在给眼肌注射肉毒素的过程中，使用连接绝缘针的便携式肌电仪，可帮助手术医生在眼眶内定位相应的肌肉，特别是已行手术的肌肉。

Recruitment during fixation or following movement

Recruitment is the orderly increase in the number of activated motor units, thus increasing the strength of muscle contraction. For example, as the eye moves farther into abduction, more and more lateral rectus motor units are activated and brought into play by the brain to help pull the eye temporally. In addition, as the eye fixates farther into abduction, the firing frequency of each motor unit increases until it reaches a peak (several hundred per second, for some motor units).

Monocular Eye Movements

Ductions

Ductions are monocular rotations of the eye. *Adduction* is movement of the eye nasally; *abduction* is movement of the eye temporally. *Elevation* (*supraduction or sursumduction*) is an upward rotation of the eye; *depression* (*infraduction or deorsumduction*) is a down-ward rotation of the eye. *Intorsion* (*incycloduction*) is defined as a nasal rotation of the superior pole of the vertical meridian. *Extorsion* (*excycloduction*) is a temporal rotation of the superior pole of the vertical meridian.

The following are important terms relating to the muscles used in monocular eye movements:

- *agonist*: the primary muscle moving the eye in a given direction
- *synergist*: the muscle in the same eye as the agonist that acts with the agonist to produce a given movement (eg, the inferior oblique muscle is a synergist with the agonist superior rectus muscle for elevation of the eye)
- *antagonist*: the muscle in the same eye as the agonist that acts in the direction opposite to that of the agonist (eg, the medial rectus and lateral rectus muscles are antagonists)

Sherrington's law of reciprocal innervation states that increased innervation of a given EOM is accompanied by a reciprocal decrease in innervation of its antagonist. For example, as the right eye abducts, innervation of the right lateral rectus muscle increases and innervation of the right medial rectus muscle decreases.

Field of action

Field of action refers to the gaze position (one of the cardinal positions) in which the effect of the EOM is most readily observed. For the lateral rectus muscle, the direction of rotation and the position of gaze are both abduction; for the medial rectus muscle, they are both adduction. However, the direction of rotation and the gaze position are not the same for the vertical muscles. For example, the inferior oblique muscle, acting alone, is an abductor and elevator, pulling the eye up and out—but its elevating action is best observed in adduction. Similarly, the superior oblique muscle, acting alone, is an abductor and depressor, pulling the eye down and out—but its depressing action is best observed in adduction.

The clinical significance of fields of action is that a deviation (strabismus) that increases with gaze in some directions may result from weakness of the muscle normally pulling the eye in that direction, from restriction of its action by its antagonist muscle, or from a combination of these 2 factors.

固视和跟随运动中的启动

*启动*是指有序地增加运动单元的数量，从而增加肌肉收缩的强度。例如，随着眼球逐渐外转，越来越多的外直肌运动单元被激活，大脑发挥作用，帮助牵拉眼球向颞侧转动。另外，当眼睛进一步向外注视时，每个运动单元的放电频率增加，直到达到峰值（某些运动单元每秒可放电数百次）。

单眼运动

转动

转动是指单眼转动。*内转*是指眼球向鼻侧转动，*外转*是指眼球向颞侧转动。*上转*是眼球向上转动，*下转*是指眼球向下转动。*内旋*是指眼球垂直于径线的上极向鼻侧转动。*外旋*是指垂直于径线的上极向颞侧转动。

以下是单眼运动中与肌肉有关的重要术语：

- *主动肌*：在特定方向上转动眼球的主要肌肉。
- *协同肌*：在同一眼，协助主动肌一起产生特定运动的肌肉（如眼球上转时，下斜肌是上直肌的协同肌）。
- *拮抗肌*：在同一眼，作用方向与主动肌相反的肌肉（如内直肌和外直肌是拮抗肌）。

*神经交互支配的 Sherrington 法则*指出：增加某条眼外肌的神经支配，将伴随着其拮抗肌的神经支配减少。例如，右眼外转时，右眼外直肌的神经支配增加，而右眼内直肌的神经支配减少。

功能视野

*功能视野*是指眼外肌最主要的注视位置（基本眼位之一）。对于外直肌来说，其转动方向和注视位置均为外转，内直肌均为内转。而对于垂直肌肉来说，转动方向和注视位置是不同的。例如，单独作用时，下斜肌产生外转和上转，拉动眼球向上和向外，但其上转作用的最好观察位置是在内转时。同样地，上斜肌单独作用时产生外转和下转，拉动眼球向下和向外，但其下转作用的最好观察位置是在内转时。功能视野的临床意义在于，斜视角度在某些注视位置上增加，可能是由于正常情况下将眼球拉向该方向的肌肉力量弱，或是拮抗肌限制了它的作用，又或是二者的联合作用。

Primary, secondary, and tertiary actions

With the eye in primary position, the medial and lateral rectus muscles move the eye only horizontally and therefore have a primary horizontal action. Anatomical studies have shown compartmentalization of the innervation to the horizontal rectus muscles in some patients; this may explain the finding of small vertical actions of these muscles in these cases (see Chapter 3). The vertical rectus muscles have a direction of pull that is mostly vertical as their primary action, but in primary position, the angle of pull from origin to insertion is inclined 23° to the visual axis (or midplane of the eye), giving rise to a torsional effect as well. Intorsion is the secondary action of the superior rectus, and extorsion is the secondary action of the inferior rectus; because the net positions of the insertions are medial to the center of rotation of the eye, adduction is the tertiary action of both muscles. Because the oblique muscles are inclined 51° to the visual axis, torsion is their primary action, vertical rotation (depression/elevation) is their secondary action, and abduction is their tertiary action. The levator palpebrae superioris is also an EOM, and its sole action is elevation of the upper eyelid. See Table 4-1 for a summary of the EOM actions.

Changing muscle action with different gaze positions

The gaze position can alter the effect of EOM contractions on the rotation of the eye. In each of the cardinal positions, each of the 6 oculorotatory EOMs has different effects on the eye's rotation, based on the relationship between the visual axis of the eye and the orientation of the muscle plane to the visual axis. In each cardinal position, the angle between the visual axis and the direction of pull of the muscle being tested is minimized, thus maximizing the horizontal effect of the medial or lateral rectus or the vertical effect of the superior rectus, inferior rectus, superior oblique, or inferior oblique. By having the patient move the eyes to the 6 cardinal positions, the clinician can isolate and evaluate the ability of each of the 6 oculorotatory EOMs to move the eye. See also the section Binocular Eye Movements.

Table 4-1 Action of the Extraocular Muscles Referenced to Primary Position

Muscle[a]	Primary	Secondary	Tertiary
Medial rectus	Adduction	—	—
Lateral rectus	Abduction	—	—
Inferior rectus	Depression	Extorsion	Adduction
Superior rectus	Elevation	Intorsion	Adduction
Inferior oblique	Extorsion	Elevation	Abduction
Superior oblique	Intorsion	Depression	Abduction
Levator palpebrae superioris	Elevation of upper eyelid	—	—

[a] The superior muscles are intortors; the inferior muscles, extortors. The vertical rectus muscles are adductors; the oblique muscles, abductors.

With the eye in primary position, the horizontal rectus muscles share a common horizontal plane that contains the visual axis (Fig 4-2). The clinician can assess the relative strength of the horizontal rectus muscles by observing the horizontal excursion of the eye as it moves medially from primary position to test the medial rectus and laterally to test the lateral rectus. The actions of the vertical rectus and oblique muscles are more complex.

第一作用、第二作用和第三作用

当眼球处于第一眼位时，内、外直肌只能水平转动眼球，因此第一作用是水平的。解剖研究表明，某些患者的水平直肌的神经支配区域化，这也许可以解释这些病例中发现的水平肌肉的微小垂直运动（见第 3 章）。垂直直肌的第一作用是在垂直方向牵拉，但在第一眼位时，从肌肉起始端到附着端的走行方向与视轴（或眼球的中间平面）成 23° 角，这也会产生旋转作用。内旋是上直肌的第二作用，外旋是下直肌的第二作用；由于肌肉附着点位于眼球转动中心的内侧，内转是 2 条肌肉的第三作用。由于斜肌与视轴成 51° 角，因此其第一作用是旋转，垂直转动（下转 / 上转）是第二作用，外转是第三作用。提上睑肌也是一种眼外肌，其唯一的作用是抬高上睑。眼外肌的作用总结见表 4–1。

不同注视位置的肌肉作用变化

注视位置可以改变眼外肌收缩对眼球转动的影响。在每个基本眼位上，根据视轴和肌肉平面到视轴夹角之间的关系，6 条眼外肌中的每一条都对眼球的转动有不同的作用。在每个基本眼位上，使视轴与被拉肌肉方向之间的夹角最小，则使内直肌或外直肌的水平效应最大化，或使上直肌、下直肌、上斜肌或下斜肌的垂直效应最大化。通过让患者转动眼球至 6 个基本眼位，临床医生可以分离并评估 6 条眼外肌中每一条转动眼球的能力。另见“双眼运动”一节。

表 4 – 1　第一眼位时眼外肌的作用

肌肉[a]	第一作用	第二作用	第三作用
内直肌	内转	—	—
外直肌	外转	—	—
下直肌	下转	外旋	内转
上直肌	上转	内旋	内转
下斜肌	外旋	上转	外转
上斜肌	内旋	下转	外转
提上睑肌	抬高上睑	—	—

[a] 上方肌肉均为内旋肌，下方肌肉均为外旋肌，垂直直肌均为内转肌，斜肌均为外转肌。

当眼球处于第一眼位时，水平直肌共享一个包含视轴的水平面（图 4–2）。临床医生可以通过观察眼球从第一眼位向内侧转动（评估内直肌）和向外侧转动（评估外直肌）时的水平偏移量来评估水平直肌的相对强度。垂直直肌和斜肌的作用则更加复杂。

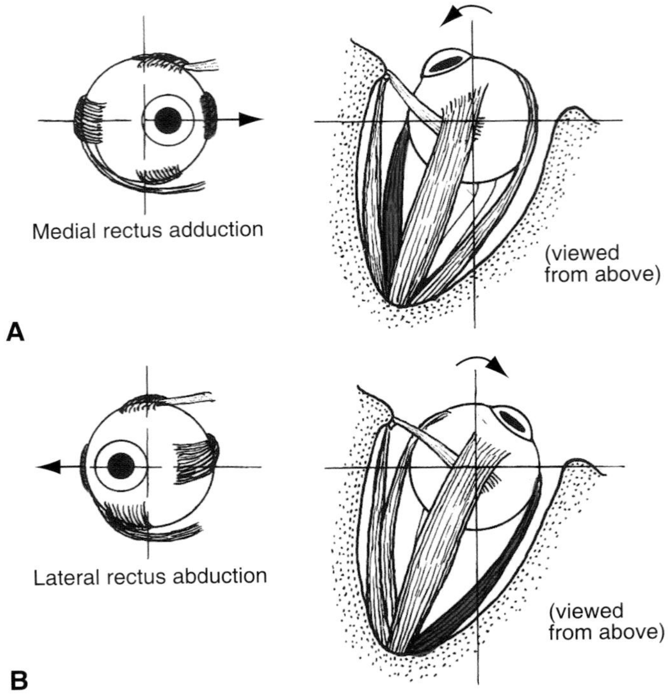

Figure4-2 The right horizontal rectus muscles. **A,** Right medial rectus muscle. **B,** Right lateral rectus muscle. *(Modified with permission from von Noorden GK. Atlas of Strabismus. 4th ed. St Louis: Mosby;1983:3.)*

With insertions anterior to the center of rotation of the globe and, in primary position, the 23° angle between the muscle planes and the visual axis (Figs 4-3, 4-4), the superior and inferior rectus muscles have 3 actions: primary vertical, secondary torsion, and tertiary adduction. The relative vertical strength of the vertical rectus muscles can be most readily observed by aligning the visual axis parallel to the muscle plane axis—that is, when the eye is rotated 23° into abduction. In this position, the superior rectus becomes a pure elevator and the inferior rectus a pure depressor. To minimize the vertical action of these muscles, the visual axis should be perpendicular to the muscle axis at a position of 67° of adduction. In this position, the superior rectus action would be pure intorsion, and the inferior rectus action would be pure extorsion. Because the globe cannot adduct this far, the vertical rectus muscles maintain significant elevating and depressing action even in maximal voluntary adduction.

With insertions posterior to the center of rotation of the globe and, in primary position, the 51° angle between the muscle planes and the visual axis (Figs 4-5, 4-6), the superior and inferior oblique muscles have 3 actions: primary torsion, secondary vertical, and tertiary abduction. In 51° adduction, the muscle plane is aligned with the visual axis, and the vertical action of the oblique muscle can be most readily observed. When the eye abducts 39°, the visual axis becomes perpendicular to the muscle plane, and the muscle action is mainly torsion.

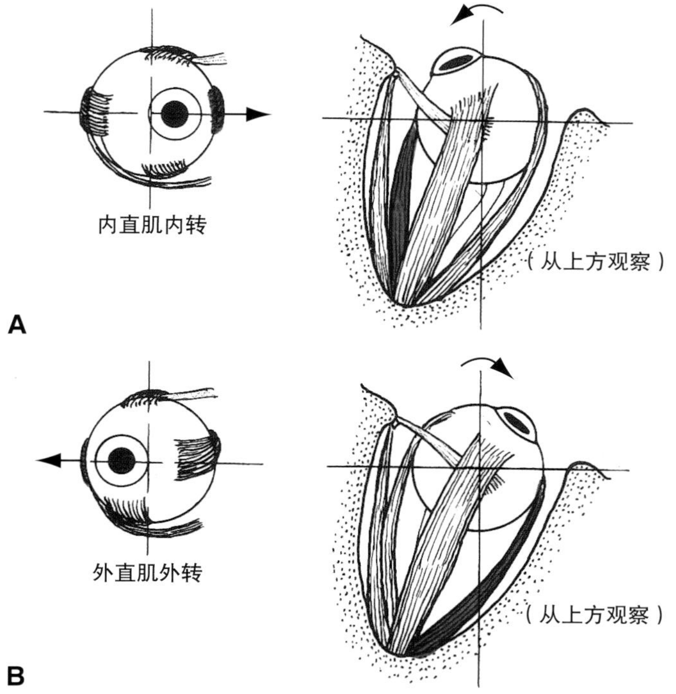

图 4–2　右眼水平直肌。**A.** 右眼内直肌。**B.** 右眼外直肌。*（译者注：资料来源见前页原文。）*

在第一眼位时，上直肌、下直肌的肌肉附着点位于眼球转动中心之前，肌肉平面与视轴之间存在 23° 夹角（图 4–3，图 4–4），上直肌和下直肌有 3 个作用：第一垂直转动、第二旋转和第三内转。当肌平面与视轴平行时，上、下直肌的垂直作用最易于观察，即眼球外转 23° 。在这个眼位时，上直肌呈单纯的上转肌，下直肌呈单纯的下转肌。尽量减少肌肉的垂直运动时，视轴应垂直于肌肉轴，眼球内转 67° 。在这个眼位上，上直肌的作用呈单纯的内旋，下直肌的作用呈单纯的外旋。由于眼球不能进行这么大角度的内转，垂直直肌即使在眼球进行最大限度的自主内转时，仍呈显著的上转和下转作用。

在第一眼位时，上斜肌、下斜肌的肌肉附着点位于眼球转动中心之后，肌肉平面和视轴之间存在 51° 夹角（图 4–5，图 4–6），上斜肌和下斜肌有 3 个作用：第一旋转、第二垂直转动和第三外转。在眼球内转 51° 时，肌肉平面与视轴平行时，最易于观察到斜肌的垂直作用。眼球外转 39° 时，视轴垂直于肌平面，肌肉作用以旋转为主。

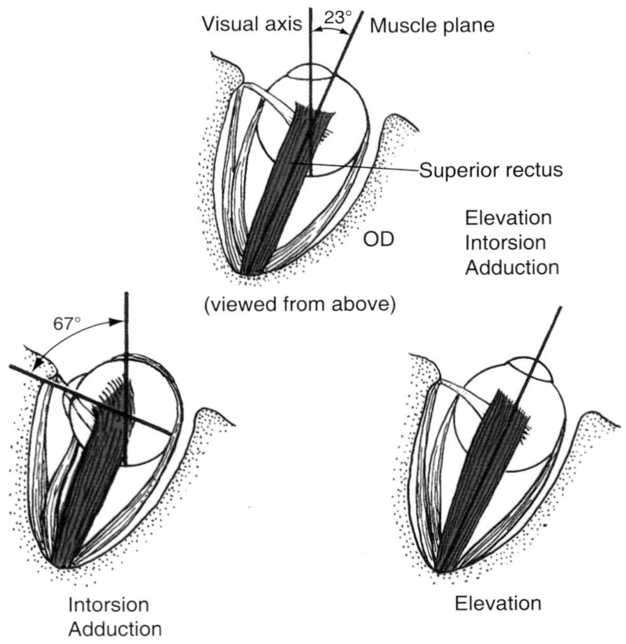

Figure4-3 The right superior rectus muscle, viewed from above. *(Modified with permission from von Noorden GK. Atlas of Strabismus. 4th ed. St Louis: Mosby; 1983:3.)*

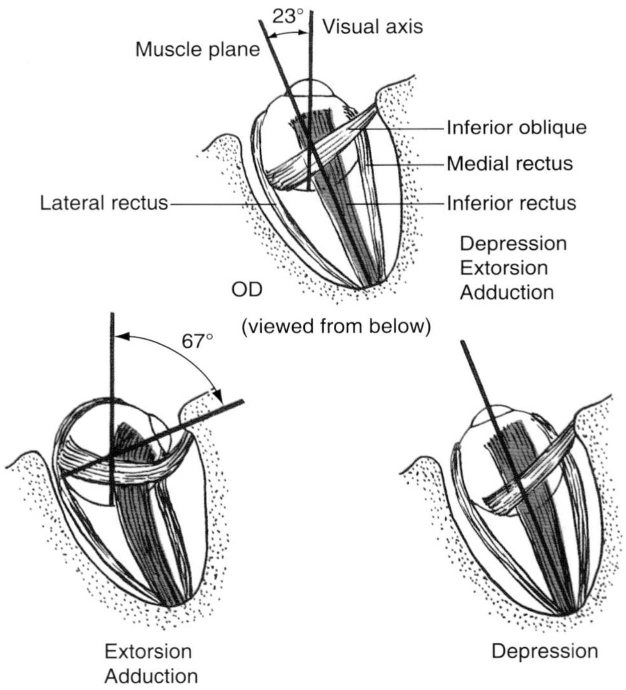

Figure 4-4 The right inferior rectus muscle, viewed from below. *(Modified with permission from von Noorden GK. Atlas of Strabismus. 4th ed. St Louis: Mosby;1983:5.)*

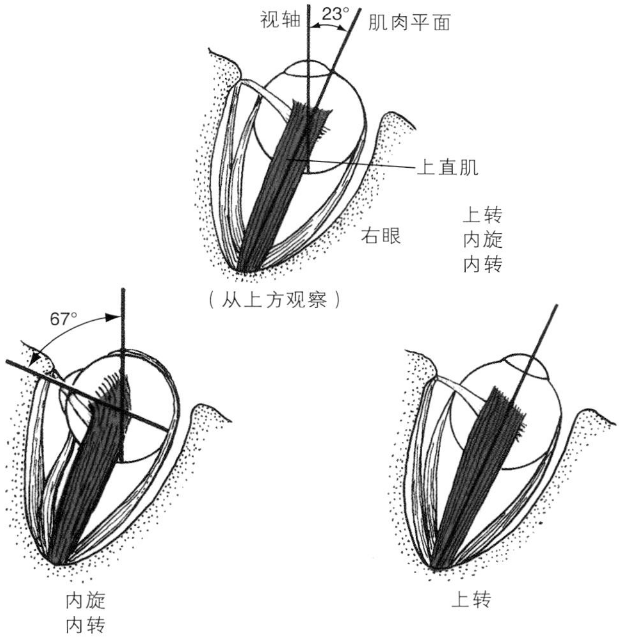

图 4–3　右眼上直肌，从上方观察。*（译者注：资料来源见前页原文。）*

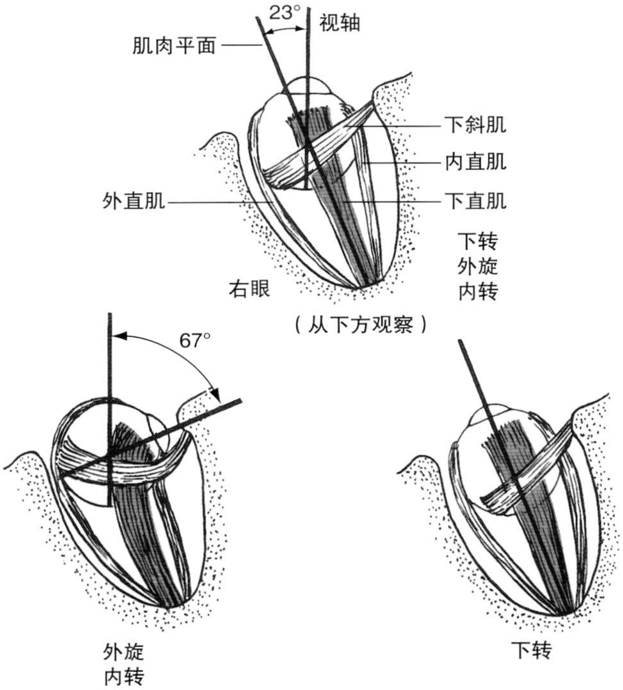

图 4–4　右眼下直肌，从下方观察。*（译者注：资料来源见前页原文。）*

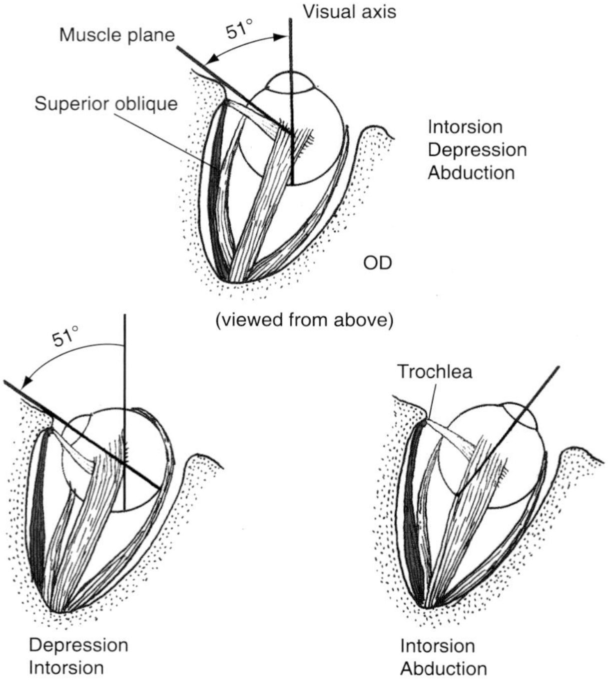

Figure 4-5 The right superior oblique muscle, viewed from above. *(Modified with permission from von Noorden GK. Atlas of Strabismus. 4th ed. St Louis: Mosby; 1983:7.)*

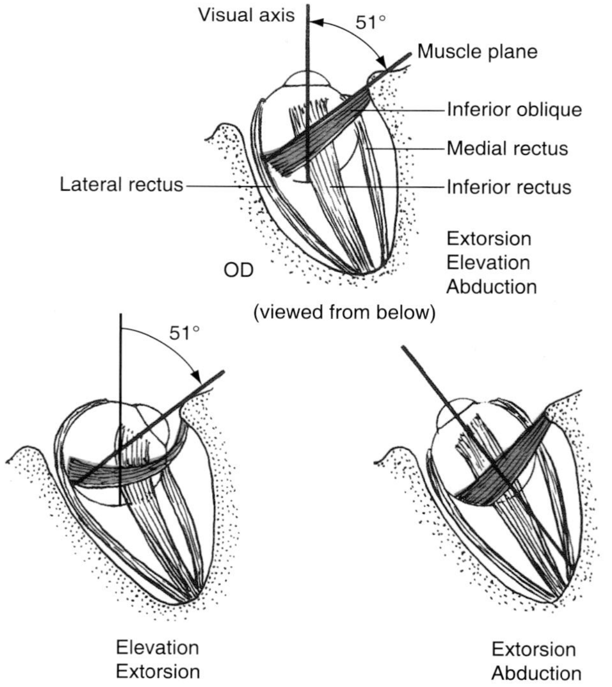

Figure 4-6 The right inferior oblique muscle, viewed from below. *(Modified with permission fromvon Noorden GK. Atlas of Strabismus. 4th ed. St Louis: Mosby;1983:9.)*

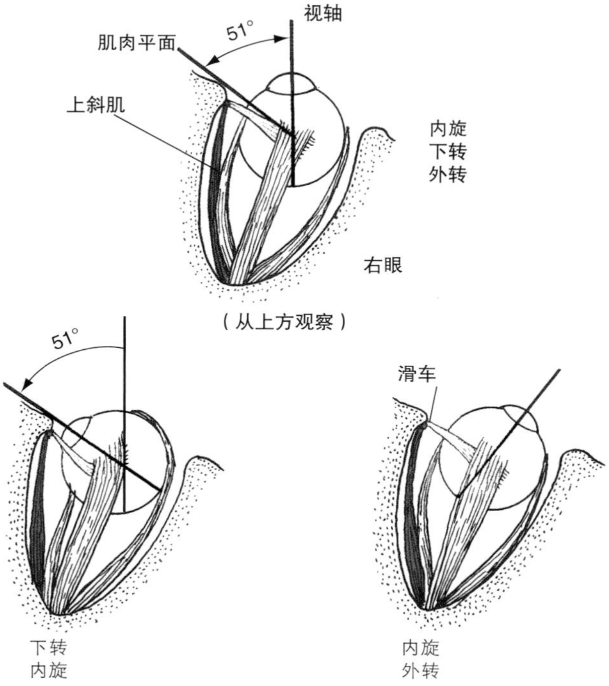

图 4–5　右眼上斜肌，从上方观察。*（译者注：资料来源见前页原文。）*

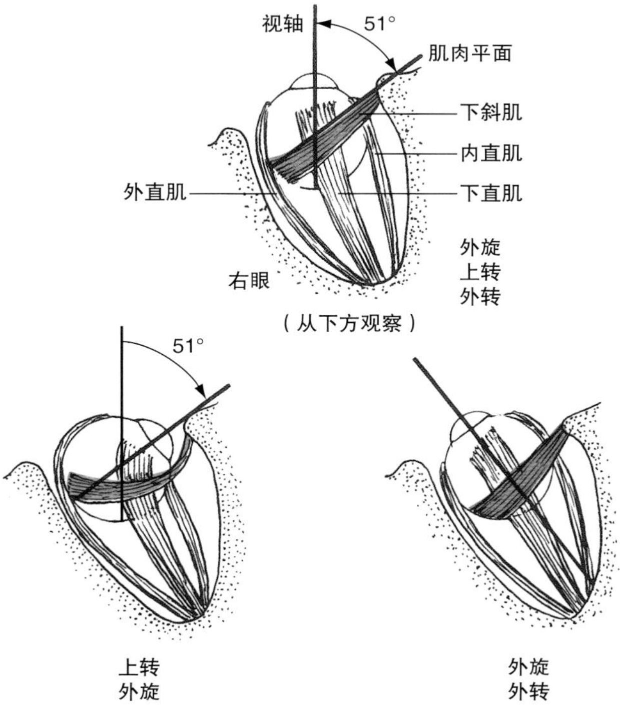

图 4–6　右眼下斜肌，从下方观察。*（译者注：资料来源见前页原文。）*

Binocular Eye Movements

When binocular eye movements are conjugate and the eyes move in the same direction, such movements are called *versions*. When the eye movements are dysconjugate and the eyes move in opposite directions, such movements are known as *vergences*.

Versions

Right gaze (*dextroversion*) is movement of both eyes to the patient's right. Left gaze (*levoversion*) is movement of both eyes to the patient's left. *Elevation*, or *upgaze* (*sursumversion*), is an upward rotation of both eyes. *Depression*, or *downgaze* (*deorsumversion*), is a downward rotation of both eyes. Dextrocycloversion is rotation of the superior pole of the vertical meridian of both eyes to the patient's right. Similarly, *levocycloversion* is movement of both eyes so that the superior pole of the vertical meridian rotates to the patient's left.

The term *yoke muscles* is used to describe 2 muscles (1 in each eye) that are the prime movers of their respective eyes into a given position of gaze. For example, when the eyes move into right gaze, the right lateral rectus muscle and the left medial rectus muscle are simultaneously innervated and contracted. These muscles are said to be "yoked" together. Each EOM in one eye has a yoke muscle in the other eye. See Figure 4-1, which shows the 6 cardinal positions of gaze and the yoke muscles whose primary actions are in those fields of gaze.

Hering's law of motor correspondence states that when the eyes move into a gaze direction, there is a simultaneous and equal increase in innervation to the yoke muscles for that direction. Hering's law has important clinical implications when the practitioner is evaluating a paralytic or restrictive strabismus. Because the amount of innervation supplied to both eyes is always determined by the fixating eye, the angle of deviation varies according to which eye is fixating. When the sound eye is fixating (prism over the affected eye when the prism alternate cover test is performed), the amount of misalignment is called the *primary deviation*. When the affected eye is fixating (prism over the sound eye when the prism alternate cover test is performed), the amount of misalignment is called the *secondary deviation*. The secondary deviation is larger than the primary deviation because of the increased innervation necessary to move the affected eye to the position of fixation. This extra innervation is shared by the yoke muscle in the sound eye, which causes excessive action of that muscle and a larger angle of deviation.

Vergences

Convergence is movement of both eyes nasally relative to a given starting position; *divergence* is movement of both eyes temporally relative to a given starting position. The medial rectus muscles are yoke muscles for convergence, and the lateral rectus muscles are yoked for divergence. With *vertical vergence* movements, one eye moves upward, and the other moves downward. *Incyclovergence* is a rotation of both eyes such that the superior pole of the vertical meridian is rotated nasally; *excyclovergence* is a rotation of both eyes such that the superior pole of the vertical meridian rotates temporally. Vergence movements are described in the following sections; see Table 4-2 for a classification of these movements.

Accommodative convergence of the visual axes Part of the near reflex (also called *near synkinesis, near triad*), which consists of accommodation, convergence, and miosis. A certain amount of accommodative convergence (AC) occurs with each diopter of accommodation (A), giving the *accommodative convergence/accommodation (AC/A) ratio.*

双眼运动

当双眼运动共轭且眼球朝着同一方向运动时，这种运动被称为*同向运动*。当眼球运动是非共轭，而且眼球向相反方向运动时，这种运动被称为*异向运动*。

同向运动

右侧注视是指双眼向患者的右侧转动。左侧注视是指双眼向患者的左侧转动。*上方注视*是指双眼向上转。*下方注视*是指双眼向下转。右侧旋转是双眼眼球的垂直径线上极向患者的右侧转动。类似地，*左眼旋转*是双眼眼球的垂直径线上极向患者的左侧转动。

“*配偶肌*”一词用于描述 2 条肌肉（每眼 1 条）的关系，是在指定注视位置上各眼的主要作用。例如，当眼球向右注视时，右眼的外直肌和左眼内直肌同时获得神经冲动并收缩。这 2 条肌肉“配偶”在一起。每一眼上的每条眼外肌都在对侧眼上有 1 条的配偶肌。如图 4–1 中显示出在这些注视区中的 6 个基本注视眼位及第一作用的配偶肌。

*运动对应关系的 Hering 法则*指出：当眼球转向某个方向注视时，配偶肌会获得朝这个方向上同步且等量增加的神经冲动。当医生评估麻痹性或限制性斜视时，Hering 法则具有重要的临床意义。由于双眼所获得的神经冲动总是由固视眼决定的，因此斜视角随固视眼的不同而变化。当健眼固视时（将棱镜置于患眼前，进行棱镜交替遮盖试验），测得的斜视度称为*第一斜视角*。当患眼固视时（将棱镜置于健眼前，进行棱镜交替遮盖试验），测得的斜视度称为*第二斜视角*。由于患眼移动到固视位置需要更多的神经冲动量，故第二斜视角大于第一斜视角。健眼的配偶肌接受了额外增加的神经冲动，从而导致该肌肉的过度作用并产生出更大的斜视角。

异向运动

*集合*是指相对于起始位置，双眼向鼻侧运动；*散开*是指相对于起始位置，双眼向颞侧运动。内直肌是用于集合的 1 对配偶肌，外直肌是用于散开的 1 对配偶肌。*垂直异向运动*是指一眼向上转，另一眼向下转。*内旋异向运动*则是指双眼内旋，使双眼在垂直径线的上极均向鼻侧旋转；*外旋异向运动*是双眼外旋，使双眼球垂直径线的上极均向颞侧旋转。异向运动在下一节描述，见表 4–2 运动分类。

视轴的调节性集合　是近反射（也称为近联动或者*近反射三联动*）的一部分，近反射包括调节、集合和瞳孔缩小。每一屈光度的调节（A）诱发一定量的调节性集合（AC），即*调节性集合 / 调节（AC/A）比*。

Abnormalities of this ratio are common and are important causes of strabismus (see Chapter 8). With an abnormally high AC/A ratio, the excess convergence tends to produce esotropia during near fixation that is greater than esotropia at distance. An abnormally low AC/A ratio tends to make the eyes less esotropic, or even exotropic, when the patient looks at near targets. Techniques for measuring this ratio are discussed in Chapter 7 under Convergence.

Fusional convergence A movement to converge and position the eyes so that similar retinal images project on corresponding retinal areas. Fusional convergence is activated when a target in the midline is seen with bitemporal retinal image disparity. See also Chapter 5.

Proximal (instrument) convergence An induced convergence movement caused by a psychological awareness that the object of fixation is near. This movement is particularly apparent when a person looks through an instrument such as a binocular microscope.

Table 4-2 Classification of Vergence Movements

Convergence	Divergence	Vertical Vergence	Cyclovergence
Accommodative convergence of the visual axes Fusional convergence Proximal (instrument) convergence Tonic convergence Voluntary convergence	Fusional divergence	Fusional vertical vergence	Fusional excyclovergence Fusional incyclovergence

Tonic convergence The constant innervational tone to the EOMs when a person is awake and alert. Because of the anatomical shape of the bony orbits and the position of the rectus muscle origins, the position of the eyes during complete muscle paralysis is divergent. Therefore, convergence tone is normally necessary in the awake state for the eyes to be aligned. For example, an esotropic patient under general anesthesia may become less esotropic or even exotropic with suspension of tonic convergence.

Voluntary convergence A conscious application of the near reflex.

Fusional divergence A movement to diverge and position the eyes so that similar retinal images project on corresponding retinal areas. Fusional divergence is activated when a target in the midline is seen with binasal retinal image disparity. See also Chapter 5.

Fusional vertical vergence A superior movement of one eye and inferior movement of the other to reduce vertical disparity so that similar retinal images project on corresponding retinal areas.

Fusional cyclovergence Intorsion of both eyes (incyclovergence) or extorsion of both eyes (excyclovergence) to reduce torsional disparity so that similar retinal images project on corresponding retinal areas. While it can be enhanced by special training, cyclovergence is normally very limited, and fusion of torsional disparity is mostly accomplished by sensory adaptation.

该比值的异常很常见，也是斜视的重要原因（见第 8 章）。当 AC/A 比值异常高时，视近时的过度集合产生的内斜视大于看远时。当 AC/A 比值异常低时，视近时内斜减少，甚至呈外斜。该比值的测量技术在第 7 章“集合”一节中讨论。

融像性集合　是指眼球集合并定位的运动，以使相似的视网膜图像投射到对应的视网膜区域。当伴有双颞侧视网膜图像视差的目标呈现在中线上时，融像性集合即被激活。另见第 5 章。

近感知性（器械性）集合　一种由心理意识到附近有固定物体而诱发的集合运动。当人通过双目显微镜这样的仪器观察时，这种运动特别明显。

表 4－2　异向运动分类

集合	散开	垂直异向运动	旋转异向运动
视轴的调节性集合	融像性散开	融像性垂直异向运动	融像性外旋异向运动
融像性集合			融像性内旋异向运动
近感知性 (器械性)集合			
张力性集合			
自主性集合			

张力性集合　指当人清醒和警觉时，眼外肌具有持续的神经冲动张力。由于骨性眼眶的解剖形状和直肌起源的位置，眼外肌完全麻痹时眼位是散开的。因此，在清醒状态下，张力性集合是正常情况下眼睛正位所必需的。例如，全身麻醉下的内斜视患者由于张力性集合消失，内斜视可能会减少，甚至变成外斜视。

自主性集合　指有意识的近反射。

融像性散开　指眼睛散开并定位的运动，以使相似的视网膜图像投射到对应的视网膜区域。当伴有双鼻侧视网膜视差的目标呈现在中线上时，融像性散开即被激活。另见第 5 章。

融合性垂直异向运动　指一眼向上运动，另一眼向下运动，以减小垂直视差，从而使相似的视网膜图像投影到对应的视网膜区域。

融合性旋转异向运动　指双眼内旋（内旋异向运动）或双眼外旋（外旋异向运动），以减小旋转视差，使相似的视网膜图像投射到对应的视网膜区域。虽然它可以通过特殊的训练来得到加强，但旋转异向运动很有限的，旋转视差的融合主要是通过感觉适应来完成的。

Supranuclear Control Systems for Eye Movement

Eye movements are directed and coordinated by several supranuclear systems. The *saccadic system* generates fast (up to 400°–500° per second) eye movements, such as eye movements of refixation. This system functions to place the image of an object of interest on the fovea or to shift gaze from one object to another. Saccadic movements require a sudden strong pulse of force from the EOMs to move the eye rapidly against the viscosity produced by the fatty tissue and the fascia in which the globe lies.

The *smooth-pursuit* system generates following, or pursuit, eye movements that maintain the image of a moving object on the fovea. Pursuit latency is shorter than saccade latency, but the maximum peak velocity of these slow pursuit movements is limited to 30°–60° per second. The involuntary *optokinetic system* utilizes smooth pursuit to track a moving object and then introduces a compensatory saccade to refixate. Tests of this system, performed with an optokinetic stimulus, are often used to detect visual responses in an infant or child with apparent vision loss, such as with ocular motor apraxia (see Chapter 12). The *vergence system* controls dysconjugate eye movement, as in convergence or divergence. Supranuclear control of vergence eye movements is not yet fully understood. There are also systems that integrate eye movements with body movements in order to stabilize the image on the retinas. The most clinically important of these systems is the vestibular-ocular system. Vestibular-ocular reflex responses are driven by the labyrinth, which involves the semicircular canals and otoliths (utricle and saccule) of the inner ears. The cervical, or neck, receptors also provide input for this reflex control. See BCSC Section 5, *Neuro-Ophthalmology*, for in-depth discussion of these systems.

眼球运动的核上控制系统

眼球运动由多个核上系统控制和协调。*扫视系统*产生快速（高达 400 ~ 500°/s）的眼球运动，如眼球再固视的运动。该系统的功能是将感兴趣的物体图像放置在黄斑中心凹处，或者将目光从一个物体转移到另一个物体上。扫视运动需要眼外肌产生一个骤然强大的脉冲力，以对抗眼球周围的脂肪和筋膜组织产生的黏性，使眼球快速运动。

*平滑追随系统*产生跟随或追随运动，以保持运动物体的图像处于黄斑中心凹。追随潜伏期比扫视潜伏期短，但这些缓慢的追随运动的最大速度峰值为 30 ~ 60° /s。非自主*眼动系统*利用平滑追随来跟踪运动的物体，然后引入补偿性的扫视来重新固视。用眼动刺激对该系统进行的检测，通常用于检测视力明显丧失的婴儿或儿童的视觉反应，如眼球运动失用症（见第 12 章）。*异向运动系统*控制着眼球的非共轭运动，如集合或散开。目前还不清楚眼球异向运动的核上控制。另外还有一些系统将眼球运动和身体运动相结合，以保证在视网膜上的图像稳定，临床上最重要的系统是*前庭 – 眼系统*。前庭 – 眼反射反应由耳迷路控制，包括内耳的半规管和耳石（椭圆囊和球囊）。颈部受体也为反射控制提供输入信号。有关这些系统的深入讨论，见 BCSC 第 5 册《*神经眼科学*》。

（翻译 汪晓倩 // 审校 石一宁 布娟 // 章节审校 石广礼）

CHAPTER 5

Sensory Physiology and Pathology

The Physiology of Normal Binocular Vision

If an area of the retina is stimulated by any means—externally by light or internally by mechanical pressure or electrical processes—the resulting sensation is always one of light, and the light is subjectively localized as coming from a specific visual direction in space. The imaginary line connecting the fixation point and the fovea is termed the *visual axis*, and normally, with central fixation, it is subjectively localized straight ahead.

Retinal Correspondence

If the stimulated areas of the retinas in the 2 eyes, or retinal locations, share a common subjective visual direction—that is, if stimulation of these 2 points results in the subjective sensation that the stimulating target or targets lie in the same direction—these retinal locations are said to be *corresponding*. When the image of an object in space falls on corresponding points, it is perceived as a single object. On the other hand, stimulation of *noncorresponding* or *disparate* retinal points results in the sensation of 2 visual directions for the same target, or diplopia.

With *normal retinal correspondence*, the foveae of the 2 eyes are corresponding points. Retinal areas in each eye that are essentially equidistant to the right or left and above or below the fovea are also corresponding points. The locus of points in space that stimulate corresponding points in each retina is known as the *horopter*. With symmetric convergence, the geometric relationship between corresponding points—for example, a point 1° nasal to the fovea in 1 eye would correspond to a point 1° temporal to the fovea in the other eye—gives a circle that passes through the nodal point of each eye and the point of fixation. This theoretical horopter is known as the *Vieth-Müller circle*. When the horopter is determined experimentally, the locus of points that are seen singly falls not on a circle but on a curve called the *empirical horopter* (Fig 5-1).

The horopter exists in both the horizontal and vertical planes. Although it might seem that the horopter would be a surface in space, the horizontal separation of the eyes causes points in the oblique quadrants to be vertically disparate. For symmetric convergence, the 3-dimensional horopter of points having both horizontal and vertical correspondence consists of a curved horizontal line and a sloped vertical line that intersect at the fixation point. Each fixation point has a unique horopter centered on that point.

第 5 章

感觉生理学与病理学

正常双眼视觉生理学

无论视网膜某区域受到任何方式的刺激，如外界光线、内部机械压力或电信号，其最终的感觉总是一种光，并且被主观定位为源于空间特定的视觉方向。将注视点与中心凹连接起来的假想线被称为*视轴*，通常在中心注视时，视轴被主观定位于正前方。

视网膜对应

如果双眼视网膜受刺激区域或视网膜定位有一个共同的视觉方向，也就是说，如果这 2 点刺激导致主观感觉刺激的目标位于同一方向，那么这些视网膜定位被认为是*对应的*。当空间一物体的像落在相对应的点上，它被认为是单一物体。而刺激*非对应的或不同的*视网膜点，会感觉同一目标的 2 个视觉方向，即为复视。

*正常视网膜对应*时，双眼中心凹为对应点。与中心凹上下左右基本等距的视网膜区域也是视网膜对应点。刺激每个视网膜对应点的空间区域被称为*双眼视界*。在对称性集合时，对应点之间的几何关系，经过每眼的结点和注视点，形成一个圆，例如，一眼鼻侧到中心凹的 1° 点对应于另一眼中心凹颞侧的 1° 点。理论上的双眼视界被称为 *Vieth–Müller* 圆。当实验确定了双眼视界时，看到单一点的对应点区域不是在一个圆上，而是在一条曲线上，称为*理想双眼视界*(图 5–1)。

双眼视界包括水平平面及垂直平面。虽然双眼视界可能是空间中的表面，但眼的水平分离导致斜象限中的点呈垂直分离。对称性集合时，具有水平及垂直对应点的三维双眼视界由相交于注视点的 1 条弯曲的水平线和倾斜的垂直线组成。每个注视点都具有以此点为中心的独立双眼视界。

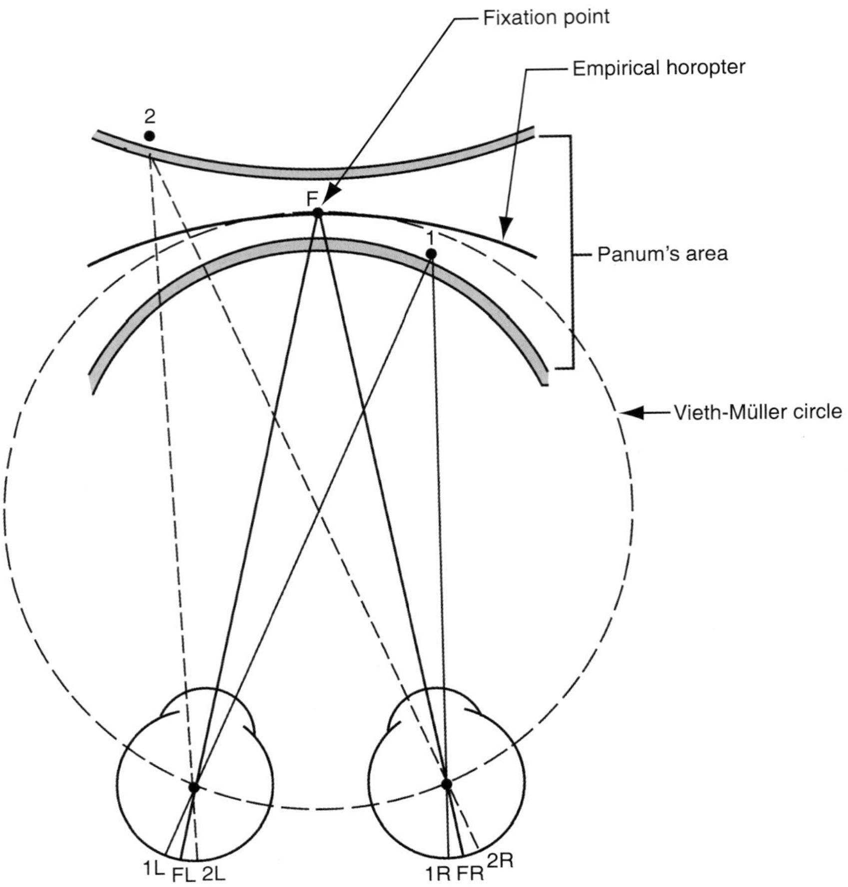

Figure 5-1 Empirical horopter. F = fixation point; FL and FR = left and right foveae, respectively. Point 1, falling within Panum's area, is seen singly and stereoscopically. Point 2 falls outside Panum's area and is therefore seen doubly.

If the horopter includes all points in space that stimulate corresponding retinal points, double vision would be expected when the target does not lie on the horopter. However, the visual system can combine slightly disparate points within a limited area surrounding the horopter, called *Panum's area of single binocular vision* (see Fig 5-1). Objects within Panum's area do not result in diplopia. Objects outside Panum's area stimulate widely disparate retinal points, resulting in physiologic diplopia. If an object is distal to Panum's area, uncrossed physiologic diplopia will result; if an object is proximal to Panum's area, crossed physiologic diplopia will result.

Fusion

Fusion is the cortical unification of 2 images of an object, 1 from each eye, into a single percept. For retinal images to be fused, they must be similar in size and shape. For fusion of macular images (*central fusion*) to occur, there can be very little dissimilarity between the images in each eye, because of the small receptive fields in the area near the fovea; otherwise, diplopia results. More image dissimilarity is tolerated in the periphery (peripheral fusion), where the receptive fields are larger. Fusion has been artificially subdivided into sensory fusion, motor fusion, and stereopsis.

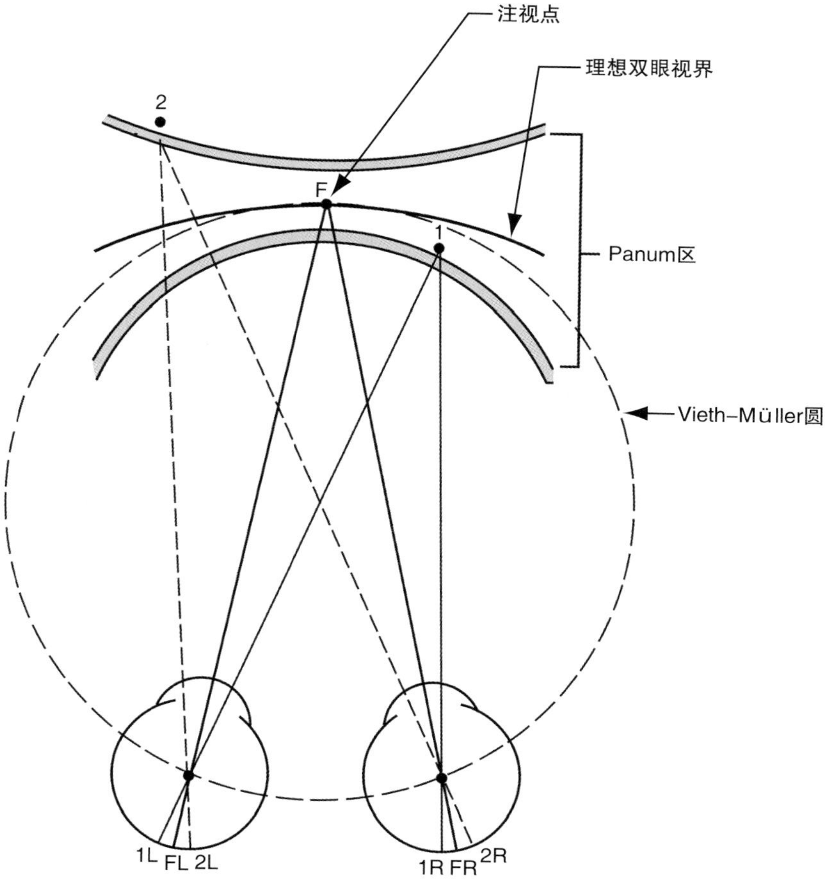

图 5–1　理想双眼视界。F 为注视点；FL 和 FR 为左眼及右眼的黄斑中心凹。点 1，落于 Panum 区内，单一、立体。点 2，落于 Panum 区外，所以看成 2 个。

如果双眼视界包括空间刺激的所有对应视网膜点，那么当目标不在双眼视界上时，将出现复视。然而，在双眼视界周围限定的范围内，视觉系统可以包容轻微的分离点，被称为 *Panum 区内双眼单视*（见图 5–1）。在 Panum 区内的物体不会出现复视。在 Panum 区外的物体广泛刺激不同的视网膜点，导致生理性复视。如果一个物体位于 Panum 区远端，会出现非交叉性生理复视；如果一个物体位于 Panum 区近端，则会出现交叉性生理复视。

融合

*融合*是皮质将一个物体在双眼的单个图像合成为单一感知。视网膜图像融合时，其大小和形状须相似。黄斑图像融合（*中心融合*）时，由于中心凹附近区域的感受野很小，双眼图像之间几乎无差异，否则会导致复视。周边区域耐受更大的图像差异（周围融合），因为其感受野较大。融合分为感觉融合、运动融合和立体视觉。

Sensory fusion

Sensory fusion is based on the innate, orderly topographic relationship between the retinas and the visual cortex, whereby images falling on corresponding (or nearly corresponding) retinal points in the 2 eyes are combined to form a single visual percept.

Motor fusion

Motor fusion is a vergence movement that allows similar retinal images to be maintained on corresponding retinal areas despite natural conditions (eg, heterophorias) or artificial causes that induce disparities. For example, when a progressive base-out prism is introduced before both eyes while a target is viewed, the retinal images move temporally over both retinas if the eyes remain in fixed position. However, because of a response called *fusional convergence* (see Chapter 4), the eyes instead converge, repositioning so that similar retinal images are projected on corresponding retinal areas. Measurement of fusional vergence amplitudes is discussed in Chapter 7.

Stereopsis

Stereopsis occurs when horizontal retinal disparity between the 2 eyes produces a subjective ordering of images of objects in depth, or 3 dimensions. It is the highest form of binocular cooperation and adds a unique quality to vision. The region of points with binocular disparities that result in stereopsis is slightly wider than Panum's area, so stereopsis is not simply a by-product of combining the disparate images from a point into a single visual percept. The brain interprets nasal disparity between 2 similar retinal images of an object in the midline as indicating that the object is farther away from the fixation point, and temporal disparity as indicating that the object is nearer. Binasal or bitemporal images are not a requirement for stereopsis; objects not in the midline in front of or behind the horopter also elicit stereopsis, even though their images fall on the nasal retina in 1 eye and the temporal retina in the other.

Stereopsis and depth perception (*bathopsis*) are not synonymous. Monocular cues—which include object overlap, relative object size, highlights and shadows, motion parallax, and perspective—also contribute to depth perception. Monocular patients can have excellent depth perception using these cues. Stereopsis is a *binocular* sensation of relative depth caused by horizontal disparity of retinal images.

Selected Aspects of the Neurophysiology of Vision

The decussation of the optic nerves at the chiasm is essential for the development of binocular vision and stereopsis. With decussation, visual information from corresponding retinal areas in each eye runs through the lateral geniculate body (lateral geniculate nucleus) and optic tracts to the visual cortex, where the information from both eyes is commingled and modified by the integration of various inputs. See BCSC Section 5, *Neuro-Ophthalmology*, Chapter 1, for further discussion.

感觉融合

感觉融合是指基于视网膜与视皮质之间内在的、有序的形态相关关系，图像落于双眼视网膜对应点（或接近对应点）上，合成单一视觉感知。

运动融合

运动融合是一种聚散运动，尽管自然条件（如隐斜视）或人工因素导致出现视差，仍可在视网膜对应区维持相似的视网膜图像。如当观察目标时，在双眼前放置逐步增加的底向外诱导三棱镜，如果眼睛的注视点不变，双眼视网膜图像会向颞侧位移。然而，由于融像性*集合反应*（见第 4 章），双眼反而集合，重新定位，从而将类似的视网膜图像投射到视网膜对应区域。有关融像性集合度的测量见第 7 章。

立体视觉

当双眼水平视差导致物体深度或三维图像的主观排序时，即产生立体视觉。它是双眼成像的最高级的形式，给视觉增加了其独特性。产生立体视觉的双眼视差区域比 Panum 区稍宽，因而立体视觉并不是将一点的差异图像组合成单一视觉感知的副产品。大脑将中线上物体在视网膜上的类似图像之间的鼻侧差异解释为物体离注视点较远，而将颞侧差异解释为物体离注视点较近。双鼻侧或双颞侧的图像并不是立体视觉的必要条件；物体不在双眼视界之前或之后的中线上，也会形成立体视觉，即使 1 只眼的图像落在鼻侧视网膜，另 1 只眼的图像落在颞侧视网膜。

立体视觉和深度感知觉（*视深*）是不同的。单眼线索，包括物体叠加、相对物体大小、增亮与阴影、运动视差及透视，也有助于深度感知觉。单眼患者用线索也可以获得良好的深度感知觉。立体视觉是由视网膜图像的水平视差引起的*双眼*相对深度感觉。

视觉神经生理学节选

视神经交叉对于双眼视觉及立体视觉的发育至关重要。通过视交叉，来源于每只眼视网膜对应区域的视觉信息穿过外侧膝状体（外侧膝状体核）及视神经束到达视皮层，来源于双眼的信息在这里经过整合，进行混合及修正。进一步讨论见 BCSC 第 5 册《*神经眼科学*》的第 1 章。

Visual Development

In the human retina, most of the ganglion cells are generated between 8 and 15 weeks' gestation, reaching a plateau of 2.2–2.5 million by week 18. After week 30, the retinal ganglion cell (RGC) population decreases dramatically during a period of rapid cell death (a process termed *apoptosis*) that lasts 6–8 weeks. Thereafter, RGC death continues at a low rate into the first few postnatal months. The RGC population is reduced to a final count of approximately 1.0–1.5 million. The loss of about 1 million RGC axons may serve to refine the topography and specificity of the retinogeniculate projection by eliminating inappropriate connections.

The continued development of visual function after birth is accompanied by major anatomical changes, which occur at all levels of the central visual pathways. The fovea is still covered by multiple cell layers and is sparsely packed with cones, which, in addition to neural immaturity, contributes to the estimated visual acuity of 20/400 in the newborn. During the first years of life, the photoreceptors redistribute within the retina, and foveal cone density increases fivefold to achieve the configuration found in the mature retina. In newborns, the white matter of the visual pathways is not fully myelinated. Myelin sheaths enlarge rapidly in the first 2 years after birth and then more slowly through the first decade of life. At birth, the neurons of the lateral geniculate body are only 60% of their average adult size. Their volume gradually increases until age 2 years. Refinement of synaptic connections in the striate cortex continues for many years after birth. The density of synapses declines by 40% over several years, attaining final adult levels at approximately age 10 years.

See BCSC Section 2, *Fundamentals and Principles of Ophthalmology*, for further discussion of ocular development.

Effects of Abnormal Visual Experience on the Retinogeniculocortical Pathway

Abnormal visual experience resulting from visual deprivation, anisometropia, or strabismus can powerfully affect retinogeniculocortical development. In studies of baby macaque monkeys, single-eyelid suturing usually produces axial myopia but no other significant anatomical changes in the eye. The lateral geniculate laminae that receive input from the deprived eye experience minor shrinkage, but these cells respond rapidly to visual stimulation, suggesting that a defect in the lateral geniculate body is not likely to account for amblyopia. In the striate cortex, monocular visual deprivation causes the regions of the visual cortex driven predominantly by the closed eye (ocular dominance columns) to radically narrow (Fig 5-2). This occurs because the 2 eyes compete for synaptic contacts in the cortex. As a result, the deprived eye loses many of the connections already formed at birth with postsynaptic cortical targets. The open eye profits by the sprouting of terminal arbors beyond their usual boundaries to occupy territory relinquished by the deprived eye (Fig 5-3). However, the benefit derived from invading the cortical territory of the deprived eye is unclear because visual acuity does not improve beyond normal. Positron emission tomography has shown that cortical blood flow and glucose metabolism are lower during stimulation of the amblyopic eye compared with the normal eye, suggesting the visual cortex as the primary site of amblyopia. Monocular deprivation also devastates binocularity because few cells can be driven by both eyes.

视觉发育

大多数人的视网膜神经节细胞在胚胎 8 ~ 15 周之间产生，18 周时细胞高达 220 万 ~ 250 万。30 周后，在细胞快速死亡（这个过程被称为*凋亡*）期，视网膜神经节细胞（RGC）的数量急剧减少，持续 6 ~ 8 周。此后，至出生后的最初几个月里，RGC 仍有少量死亡。RGC 的数量最终减少到大约 100 万 ~ 150 万。约 100 万个 RGC 轴突的丢失有助于消除不适当的连接，以改善视网膜膝状体的投射形态和特异性。

出生后视觉功能的持续发育伴随着解剖变化，这些变化发生在中央视觉通路的各个层面上。中心凹仍被多层细胞覆盖，视锥细胞稀疏堆积，其神经分化不成熟，估计新生儿的视力为 20/400。在出生后几年，光感受器在视网膜内重新分布，中心凹的视锥细胞密度增加 5 倍，达到成熟视网膜结构。在新生儿中，视觉通路的白质没有完全髓鞘化。髓鞘在出生后的前 2 年迅速扩张，之后至出生后前 10 年缓慢扩张。出生时，外侧膝状体的神经元仅为成人平均大小的 60%。它们的容量逐渐增大，直到 2 岁。在出生后的纹状体皮质中突触连接的精细化持续多年。突触的密度在几年内下降 40%，在大约 10 岁时最终达到成人水平。

关于视觉发育的更多讨论可见 BCSC 第 2 册《*眼科学基础与原理*》。

异常视觉经验对视网膜膝状体皮质通路的影响

由视觉剥夺、屈光参差或斜视引起的异常视觉经验会严重影响视网膜膝状体皮质的发育。在对幼猕猴的研究中，单眼睑缝合通常会导致轴性近视，但眼睛没有其他明显的解剖变化。接受被视觉剥夺的眼睛输入信息的外侧膝状体轻微收缩，但这些细胞对视觉刺激反应迅速，这表明外侧膝状体的缺陷不太可能导致弱视。在纹状体皮质中，主要通过闭合眼（主导眼）的单眼视觉剥离，导致视皮质区完全变窄（图 5–2）。这是由于双眼在视皮质的突触竞争。结果，被剥夺眼丧失了许多生后就与突触后皮质目标产生的连接。开放的眼在超出常规边界处，伸出终末树轴，占据被剥夺眼丧失的领域（图 5–3）。然而，尚不清楚侵占被剥夺眼丧失领域的益处，因为对视力并未有超过正常水平的提高。正电子放射断层扫描显示，与正常眼相比，弱视眼受刺激时皮质的血流和糖代谢较低，提示视皮层是弱视的主要部位。单眼剥夺也会破坏双眼视觉，因为很少有细胞受双眼支配。

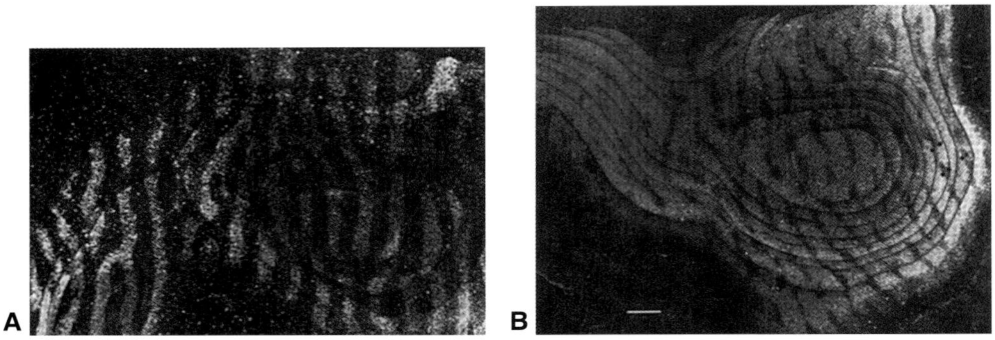

Figure 5-2 Change in ocular dominance columns in macaque visual cortex after monocular deprivation. Radioactive proline was injected into the normal eye and transported to the visual cortex to reveal the projections of that eye. In these sections, cut parallel to the cortical surface, white areas show labeled terminals. **A,** Normal monkey. There is roughly equal spacing of the stripes, which represent the injected eye (*bright*) and noninjected eye (*dark*). **B,** Monkey that had 1 eye sutured closed from birth for 18 months. The bright stripes (open, injected eye) are widened and the dark ones (closed eye) are greatly narrowed, showing the devastating physical effect of deprivation amblyopia. (Scale bar = 1 mm.) *(Reproduced with permission from Kaufman PL, Alm A. Adler's Physiology of the Eye. 10th ed. St Louis: Mosby; 2002:699. Originally from Hubel DH, Wiesel TN, LeVay S. Plasticity of ocular dominance columns in monkey striate cortex. Philos Trans R Soc Lond B Biol Sci. 1977;278(961):377–409.)*

There is a critical period in which visual development in the macaque is vulnerable to the effects of eyelid suturing. This period corresponds to the stage in which wiring of the striate cortex is still vulnerable to the effects of visual deprivation. During the critical period, the deleterious effects of suturing the right eyelid, for example, are correctable by reversal—that is, opening the sutured right eye and closing the left eye. After this reversal, the ocular dominance columns of the initially closed right eye appear practically normal, indicating that anatomical recovery of the initially shrunken columns was induced by opening the right eye and closing the left eye. However, when the right eye is sewn closed beyond the critical period, the columns of the right eye do not re-expand if the right eye is opened and the left eye closed.

Eyelid suturing in the baby macaque is a good model for visual deprivation amblyopia. In children, this condition can be caused by any dense opacity of the ocular media or occlusion by the eyelid. Visual deprivation can rapidly cause profound amblyopia.

There are other causes of amblyopia in children. Optical defocus resulting from anisometropia causes the cortical neurons driven by the defocused eye to be less sensitive (particularly to higher spatial frequencies, because they are most affected by blur) and to send out a weaker signal. This results in reduced binocular activity. The critical period for anisometropic amblyopia occurs later than that for strabismic amblyopia, and a prolonged period of unilateral blur is necessary before anisometropic amblyopia develops. Meridional (astigmatic) amblyopia does not develop during the first year of life and may not develop until age 3 years.

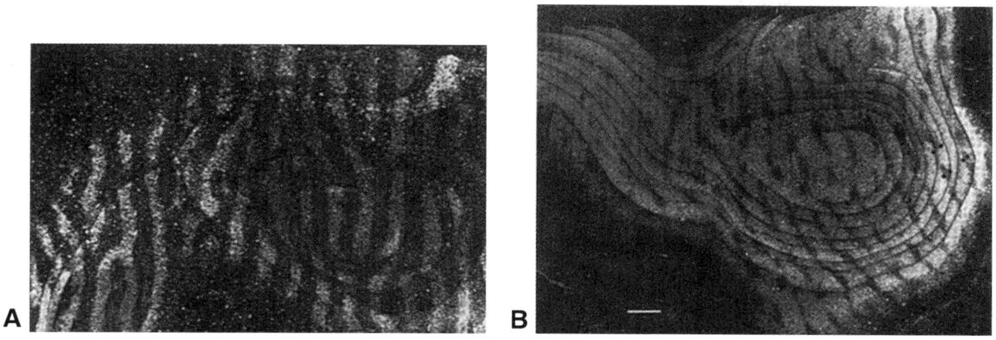

图 5–2　单眼剥夺后猕猴视皮质中优势眼柱的改变。放射性的脯氨酸被注射到正常的眼睛中，然后被输送到视觉皮层，显示眼的投射。在这部分，平行于皮质表面切割，白色区域显示标记的终端。**A.** 正常猴．条纹结构间距大致相等，代表被注射眼（*明亮*）和未被注射的眼（*黑暗*）。**B.** 从出生至 18 个月单眼被缝合的猕猴。明条纹（开放，被注射眼）变宽，暗条纹（闭合的眼睛）变狭窄，显示剥夺性弱视的生理破坏效应。（刻度尺 为 1mm。）（*译者注：资料来源见前页原文。*）

在视觉发育的关键时期，猕猴的视觉发育很容易受到眼睑缝合的影响。这个时期与纹状皮质连接发育相对应，仍然容易受到视觉剥夺的影响。例如，在这个关键时期，右眼睑缝合的损害，可以通过反转来纠正，即打开缝合的右眼并闭合左眼。在这一逆转之后，最初闭合的右眼的眼部优势柱看起来几乎正常，这表明通过打开右眼和闭合左眼可使优势柱最初的萎缩在解剖上恢复。但是，当右眼缝合超过关键时期，如果打开右眼，闭合左眼，则右眼的优势柱不会再扩大。

幼猕猴眼睑缝合是一种很好的剥夺性弱视模型。在儿童中，这种情况可能是由眼屈光介质的致密混浊或闭合眼睑引起的。视觉剥夺可迅速导致严重弱视。

儿童弱视还有其他原因。屈光参差引起的光学离焦使得皮质神经元的敏感度降低（尤其是高空间频率，易受模糊的影响），发出较弱的信号，导致双眼视觉活动减少。屈光参差性弱视的关键期比斜视性弱视出现得晚，在较长的单眼视觉模糊期后，才形成屈光参差性弱视。径线（散光性）弱视在出生后的第 1 年不会发生，直到 3 岁才有可能发生。

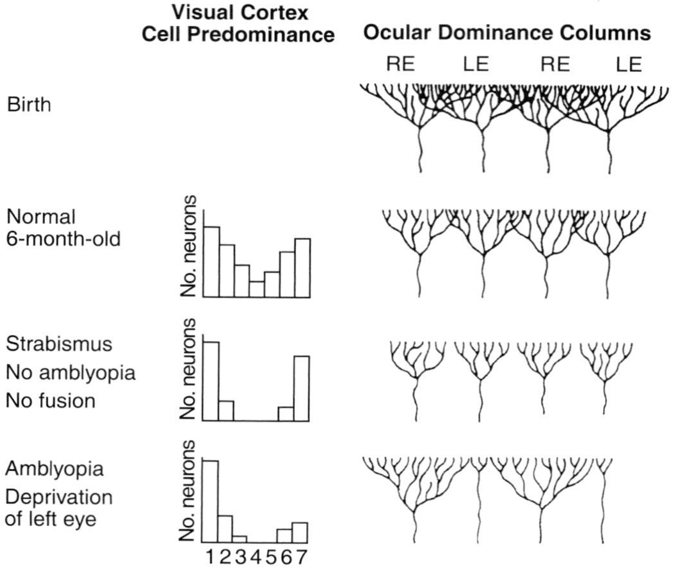

Figure 5-3 Anatomical and physiologic maturation of ocular dominance columns of the primary visual cortex in normal and deprived monkeys. *Birth*: Broad overlap of afferents from the lateral geniculate nucleus, hence little dominance by right eye (RE) versus left eye (LE). *Normal 6-month-old*: Regression of overlapping afferents from both eyes with distinct areas of monocular dominance. The bar graph shows the classic U-shaped distribution obtained by single cell recordings from the visual cortex. About half the cells are driven predominantly by the right eye and the other half by the left eye. A small number are driven equally by the 2 eyes. 1 = driven only by right eye; 2–6 = driven binocularly; 7 = driven only by left eye. *Strabismus*: Effect of artificial eye misalignment in the neonatal period on ocular dominance. The monkey alternated fixation (no amblyopia) and lacked fusion. Lack of binocularity is evident as exaggerated segregation into dominance columns. The bar graph shows the results of single-cell recordings obtained from this animal after age 1 year. Almost all neurons are driven exclusively by the right or left eye, with little binocular activity. *Amblyopia*: Effect of suturing the left eyelid shut shortly after birth. Dominance columns of the normal right eye are much wider than those of the deprivationally amblyopic left eye. The bar graph shows markedly skewed ocular dominance and little binocular activity. *(Modified with permission from Tychsen L. Binocular vision. In: Hart WM, ed.Adler's Physiology of the Eye: Clinical Application. 9th ed. St Louis: Mosby; 1992:810.)*

Strabismus can be artificially created in monkeys by the sectioning of an extraocular muscle. Alternating fixation develops in some monkeys after this procedure; they maintain normal acuity in each eye. Examination of the striate cortex reveals cells with normal receptive fields and an equal number of cells responsive to stimulation of either eye. However, the cortex is bereft of binocular cells (see Fig 5-3). After 1 extraocular muscle is cut, some monkeys do not alternately fixate; instead, they constantly fixate with the same eye, and amblyopia develops in the deviating eye. An important factor in the development of strabismic amblyopia is interocular suppression due to uncorrelated images in the 2 eyes. Strabismus prevents synchronous attainment of correlated images from the 2 foveae, resulting in abnormal input to the striate cortex. Another factor is the optical defocus of the deviated eye. The dominant eye is focused on the object of regard, while the deviated eye is oriented in a different direction; for the deviated eye, the object may be too near or too far to be in focus. Either mechanism can cause asynchrony or inhibition of 1 set of signals in the striate cortex. The critical period for development of strabismic amblyopia begins at approximately 4 months of age, during the time of ocular dominance segregation and sensitivity to binocular correlation.

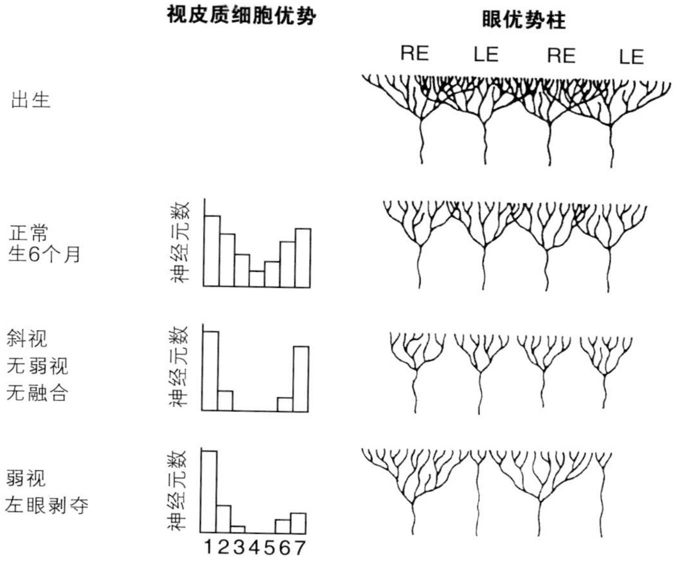

图 5–3　正常与视觉剥夺猴子的初级视皮层眼部优势柱的解剖和生理成熟度。*出生*：来自外侧膝状体神经核的传入神经广泛叠加，因此与左眼相比，右眼的优势较小。*正常 6 月龄*：双眼叠加传入神经回退，单眼优势区明显。条形图显示了由视觉皮质层单细胞记录获得的经典 U 形分布。大约一半的细胞主要由右眼驱动，另一半由左眼驱动。一小部分由双眼驱动。1 为仅由右眼驱动，2 ~ 6 为双眼驱动，7 为仅由左眼驱动。*斜视*：新生儿期人为眼位分离对眼部优势的影响。猴子交替注视（没有弱视），缺乏融合。当分离扩大，单眼优势，明显双眼视觉丧失。条形图显示了该动物 1 岁后获得的单细胞记录结果。几乎所有的神经元都是由右眼或左眼单独驱动的，几乎没有双眼活动。*弱视*：出生后立即缝合左眼睑的结果。正常右眼的优势柱比剥夺性弱视左眼的优势柱宽得多。柱状图显示明显的偏斜优势眼，几乎没有双眼活动。*（译者注：资料来源见前页原文。）*

猴子中，可以通过人为地切除 1 条眼外肌造成斜视。之后，一些猴子变成交替注视，保持每眼视力正常。纹状皮质检查显示，猴子具有正常接收野的细胞和对每只眼刺激都有相同数量的反应细胞。然而，大脑皮层缺少双眼细胞（见图 5–3）。1 条眼外肌切断后，有些猴子不交替注视，而是仅用一眼注视，致斜视眼形成弱视。导致斜视性弱视发生的一个重要因素是双眼不相关的图像导致双眼间的抑制。斜视阻止从 2 个中心凹同步获得相关的图像，从而导致纹状体皮质的异常输入。另一个因素是斜视眼的光学离焦。主导眼聚焦于注视对象，而斜视眼则指向不同的方向；对于斜视眼而言，物体可能太近或太远而无法对焦。任何一种机制都可能导致纹状体皮层一组信号的不同步或抑制。斜视性弱视发育的关键时期开始于约 4 月龄，此期间是眼部优势分离和双眼关联的敏感期。

Abnormal sensory input alone is sufficient to alter the normal anatomy of the visual cortex. Other areas of the cerebral cortex may also depend on sensory stimulation to form the proper anatomical circuits necessary for normal adult visual function, underscoring the importance of providing children with a stimulating sensory environment.

Abnormalities of Binocular Vision

When a manifest deviation of the eyes occurs, the corresponding retinal elements of the eyes are no longer directed at the same object. This places the patient at risk for 2 distinct visual phenomena: visual confusion and diplopia.

Visual Confusion

Visual confusion is the perception of a common visual direction for 2 separate objects. The 2 foveal areas are physiologically incapable of simultaneous perception of dissimilar objects. The closest foveal equivalent is *retinalrivalry*, wherein there is rapid alternation of the 2 perceived images (Fig 5-4). Confusion may be a phenomenon of extrafoveal retinal areas only. Clinically significant visual confusion is rare.

Diplopia

Double vision, or *diplopia*, usually results from an acquired misalignment of the visual axes that causes an image to fall simultaneously on the fovea of one eye and on a nonfoveal point in the other eye. As stated earlier, the object that falls on these disparate retinal points must be outside Panum's area to appear double. The same object is perceived as having 2 locations in subjective space, and the foveal image is always clearer than the nonfoveal image of the nonfixating eye. The perception of diplopia depends on the age at onset, its duration, and the patient's subjective awareness of it. The younger the child, the greater the ability to suppress, or inhibit, the nonfoveal image. Adults with acquired strabismus commonly present to the ophthalmologist because of diplopia.

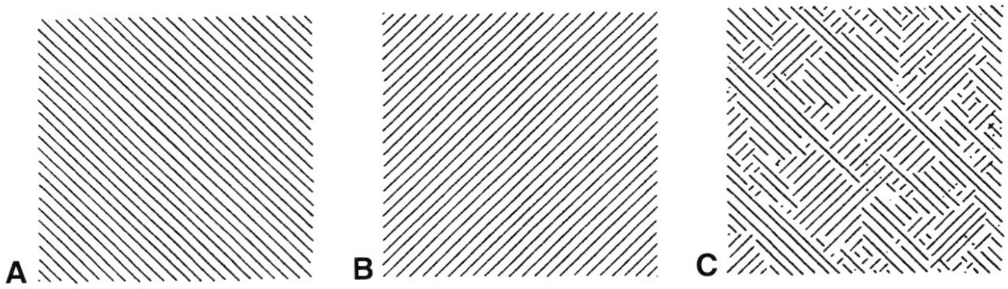

Figure 5-4 Rivalry pattern. **A,** Pattern seen by the left eye. **B,** Pattern seen by the right eye. **C,** Pattern seen with binocular vision. *(Reproduced with permission from von Noorden GK, Campos EC. Binocular Vision and Ocular Motility: Theory and Management of Strabismus. 6th ed. St Louis: Mosby; 2002:12.)*

The loss of normal binocular fusion in an individual unable to suppress disparate retinal images results in intractable diplopia, referred to as central fusion disruption (horror fusionis). This condition is typically seen in adults or visually mature children and can occur in a number of clinical settings, including prolonged visual deprivation due to monocular occlusion or a mature cataract, traumatic brain injury, or long-standing strabismus. Management is challenging.

仅仅是异常的感觉输入就可以改变视觉皮层的正常解剖结构。与中枢皮层一样，其他区域也依赖感觉刺激，以形成正常成人视觉功能所必需的解剖回路，提示为儿童提供刺激性感觉环境的重要性。

双眼视觉异常

当眼球明显分离时，对应的视网膜不再是同一物体。患者将面临 2 种不同的视觉现象：视觉混淆和复视。

视觉混淆

视觉混淆是对 2 个不同物体的共同视觉方向的感知觉。2 个中心凹区在生理上不能同时感知不同的物体。很接近的对等中心凹间存在视网膜竞争，其中 2 个感知图像快速交替（图 5–4）。混淆只是视网膜中心凹外区域的现象。临床上明显的视觉混淆很少见。

复视

重影，或称复视，通常是由于获得的视轴错位导致图像同时落在一眼的中心凹和另一眼的中心凹外。如前所述，落在这些不同视网膜点上的物体必须位于 Panum 区之外，才能出现双影。同一物体在主观空间有 2 个位置，中心凹图像总是比非注视眼的非中心凹图像清晰。复视的感觉取决于发病年龄、持续时间和患者对复视的主观意识。孩子越小，抑制或阻止非中心凹图像的能力就越强。成人的获得性斜视常是因为复视看眼科而被确诊。

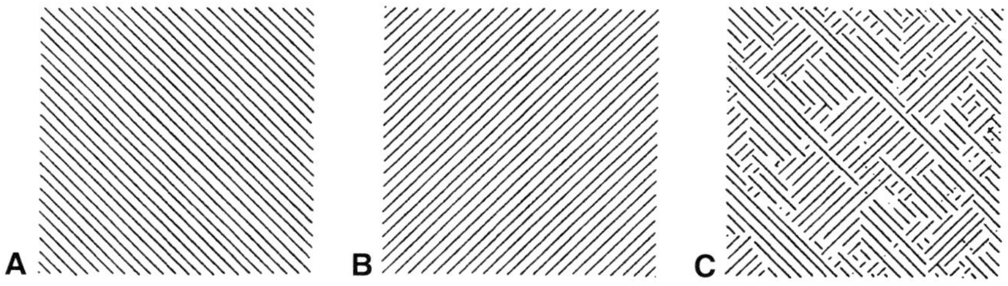

图 5–4　竞争模式。**A.** 左眼看到的图案。**B.** 右眼看到的图案。**C.** 用双眼视觉看到的图案。（*译者注：资料来源见前页原文。*）

无法抑制不同视网膜图像时，正常双眼融合的丧失导致顽固性复视，称为中心融合破坏（视像融合不能）。这种情况通常见于成人或视力成熟的儿童，可见于许多临床情况中，如单眼遮蔽或成熟白内障、创伤性脑损伤或长期斜视等导致的长期视觉剥夺。治疗有一定的难度。

El-Sahn MF, Granet DB, Marvasti A, Roa A, Kinori M. Strabismus in adults older than 60 years. *J Pediatr Ophthalmol Strabismus.* 2016;53(6):365–368.

Sensory Adaptationsin Strabismus

To avoid visual confusion and diplopia, the visual system uses the mechanisms of suppression and anomalous retinal correspondence (Fig 5-5). Pathologic suppression and anomalous retinal correspondence develop only in the immature visual system.

Suppression

Suppression is the alteration of visual sensation that occurs when an eye's retinal image is inhibited or prevented from reaching consciousness during binocular visual activity. Physiologic suppression is the mechanism that prevents physiologic diplopia (diplopia elicited by objects outside Panum's area) from reaching consciousness. Pathologic suppression may develop because of strabismic misalignment of the visual axes or other conditions resulting in discordant images in each eye, such as cataract or anisometropia. Such suppression can be regarded as an adaptation within the immature visual system to avoid diplopia. If a patient with strabismus and normal retinal correspondence (NRC) does not have diplopia, suppression is present, provided the sensory pathways are intact. In less obvious situations, several simple tests are available for clinical diagnosis of suppression (see Chapter 7).

The following classification of suppression may be useful for the clinician:

- *Central versus peripheral. Central suppression* is the mechanism that keeps the foveal image of the deviating eye from reaching consciousness, thereby preventing visual confusion. Peripheral suppression, another mechanism, eliminates diplopia by preventing awareness of the image that falls on the peripheral retina in the deviating eye, which corresponds to the image falling on the fovea of the fixating eye. This form of suppression is clearly pathologic, developing as a cortical adaptation only within an immature visual system. When strabismus develops after visual maturation/in adults, peripheral suppression does not develop and the patient is thus unable to eliminate the peripheral second image without closing or occluding the deviating eye.
- *Nonalternating versus alternating.* If suppression always causes the image from the dominant eye to be predominant over the image from the deviating eye, the suppression is nonalternating. This may lead to amblyopia. If the process switches between the 2 eyes, the suppression is described as *alternating.*
- *Facultative versus constant.* Suppression may be considered *facultative* if it is present only when the eyes are deviated and is absent in all other states. Patients with intermittent exotropia, for instance, often experience suppression when the eyes are divergent but may experience high-grade stereopsis when the eyes are straight. In contrast, *constant suppression* denotes suppression that is always present, whether the eyes are deviated or aligned. The suppression scotoma in the deviating eye may be either *relative* (permitting some visual sensation) or *absolute* (permitting no perception of light).

El-Sahn MF, Granet DB, Marvasti A, Roa A, Kinori M. Strabismus in adults older than 60 years. *J Pediatr Ophthalmol Strabismus*. 2016;53(6):365–368.

斜视的感觉适应

为了避免视觉混淆和复视，视觉系统采用抑制和异常视网膜对应的机制(图 5–5)。病理性抑制及异常视网膜对应仅发生在不成熟的视觉系统中。

抑制

抑制是指视觉感觉的改变，在双眼视觉活动中，一眼视网膜图像被抑制或被阻止进入知觉。生理性抑制是指阻止生理性复视（Panum 区外物体引发的复视）到达知觉的机制。病理性抑制可能是由于斜视性视轴错位或其他情况导致每只眼的图像不一致，如白内障或屈光参差。这种抑制是一种对不成熟视觉系统的适应，以避免复视。伴有正常视网膜对应的斜视患者没有复视，如果感觉通路完整，则会出现抑制。在不严重的情况下，可用简单方法对抑制进行临床诊断（见第 7 章）。

下面的抑制分类对医生有帮助：

- *中心与周围*。*中心抑制*是通过使斜视眼的中心凹图像不被感知，以防止视觉混淆的机制。周围性抑制是另外一种机制，阻止对落于斜视眼的周围视网膜图像的反应，其对应的注视眼视网膜图像落于中心凹，从而消除复视。这种抑制显然是病理性的，仅在不成熟的视觉系统中发展为皮质性适应。当视觉发育成熟后或成人出现斜视时，不能形成周围抑制，如果不闭合或遮挡斜视眼，那么患者就无法消除周围的第 2 幅图像。

- *非交替性与交替性*。如果抑制总是使注视眼的图像优于斜视眼的图像，则抑制是非交替性的。这可能导致弱视。如果这个过程在双眼间切换，则抑制为交替性的。

- *临时性与恒定性*。如果抑制仅在眼偏斜时出现，而在其他状态下均不出现，则认为是临时性的。如间歇性外斜视的患者，当眼偏斜时，常出现抑制，而当眼正位时，则出现高度立体视。相反，恒定性抑制时，无论是眼偏斜还是正位，始终存在抑制。斜视眼内的抑制暗点可能是相对的（有一些视觉感知），也可能是绝对的（对光无感知）。

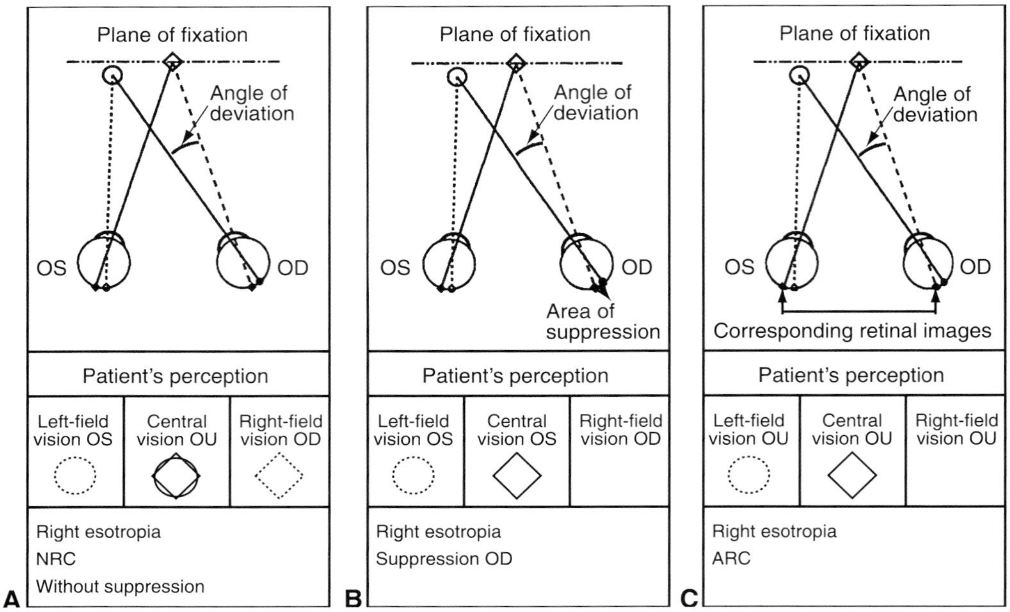

Figure 5-5 Retinal correspondence and suppression in strabismus. **A,** A patient with right esotropia with normal retinal correspondence (NRC) and without suppression would have diplopia and visual confusion, which is the perception of a common visual direction for 2 separate objects (represented by the superimposition of the images of the fixated diamond and the circle, which is imaged on the fovea of the deviating eye). **B,** The elimination of diplopia and confusion by suppression of the retinal image of the deviating/esotropic right eye. **C,** The elimination of diplopia and confusion by anomalous retinal correspondence (ARC), an adaptation of visual directions in the deviated right eye. *(Adapted with permission from Kaufman PL, Alm A. Adler's Physiology of the Eye. 10th ed. St Louis: Mosby; 2003:490.)*

Management of suppression

Therapy for suppression often includes the following:

- proper refractive correction
- amblyopia therapy using occlusion or pharmacologic treatment
- alignment of the visual axes, to permit simultaneous stimulation of corresponding retinal elements by the same object

Antisuppression orthoptic exercises may result in intractable diplopia and are not typically recommended.

Anomalous Retinal Correspondence

Anomalous retinal correspondence (ARC) is a condition wherein the fovea of the fixating eye has acquired an anomalous common visual direction with a peripheral retinal element in the deviating eye. ARC is an adaptation that restores some degree of binocular cooperation despite manifest strabismus. Anomalous binocular vision is a functional state that is superior to total suppression. In the development of ARC, normal sensory development is replaced only gradually and not completely. The more long-standing the deviation, the more deeply rooted the ARC may become. The period during which ARC may develop probably extends through the first decade of life.

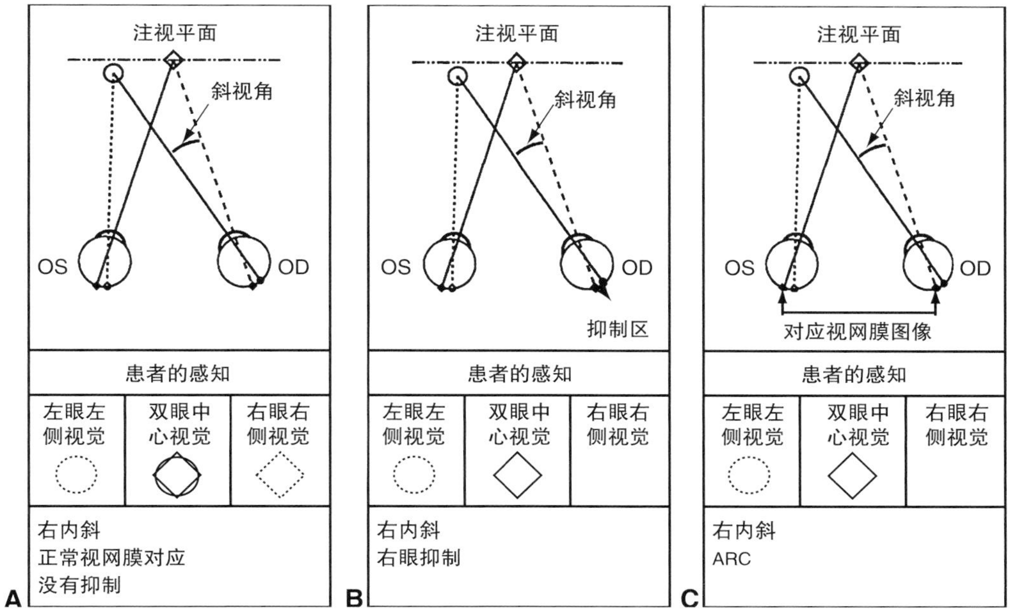

图 5–5　斜视的视网膜对应及抑制。**A.** 一个右眼内斜视患者，有正常的视网膜对应（NRC）、没有抑制，将出现复视及视觉混淆，这是一种对 2 个不同物体在共同视觉方向的感知（由注视的菱形和圆形的图像叠加而成，该图像在斜视眼的中心凹处）。**B.** 通过抑制斜视 / 内斜视右眼的视网膜图像，消除复视 / 视觉混淆。**C.** 通过异常视网膜对应（ARC）消除复视 / 视觉混淆，斜位右眼的视觉方向适应。*（译者注：资料来源见前页原文。）*

抑制的治疗

抑制治疗通常包括：

- 适当的屈光矫正。
- 弱视治疗，遮盖或药物。
- 调整视轴，使同一物体同时刺激对应的视网膜区域。

脱抑制的矫正训练可能会造成顽固性复视，通常不推荐。

异常视网膜对应

*异常视网膜对应（ARC）*是指注视眼的中心凹与斜视眼中的周边视网膜获得异常的共同视觉方向。ARC 是一种适应，尽管有明显的斜视，但仍能恢复一定程度的双眼视觉。异常双眼视觉是一种超出完全抑制的功能状态。在 ARC 的发展过程中，正常的感觉发育只是逐渐地，而不是完全地被取代。偏斜持续的时间越长，ARC 就可能越根深蒂固。ARC 的发展期可能到 10 岁前。

Paradoxical diplopia can occur when ARC persists after strabismus surgery. For example, when esotropic patients with proper or nearly proper ocular alignment after surgery report symptoms of a crossed diplopic localization of foveal or parafoveal stimuli, they are experiencing paradoxical diplopia (Fig 5-6). Paradoxical diplopia is typically a fleeting postoperative phenomenon, seldom lasting longer than a few days or weeks, but in rare cases it can persist much longer.

Testing for anomalous retinal correspondence

Testing for ARC is performed to determine how affected patients use their eyes in everyday life and to seek any vestiges of normal correspondence. As discussed earlier, ARC is a sensory adaptation to abnormal ocular alignment. Because the depth of the sensory rearrangement can vary widely, an individual can test positive for both NRC and ARC. Tests that closely simulate everyday use of the eyes are more likely to give evidence of ARC. The more dissociative the test, the more likely it is to produce an NRC response, unless the ARC is deeply rooted. Some of the more common tests (discussed at length in Chapter 7), in order of most to least dissociative, are the afterimage test, the Worth 4-dot test, the red-glass test (dissociation increases with the density of the red filter), amblyoscope testing, and testing with Bagolini striated lenses. If an anomalous localization response occurs in the more dissociative tests, the depth of ARC is greater.

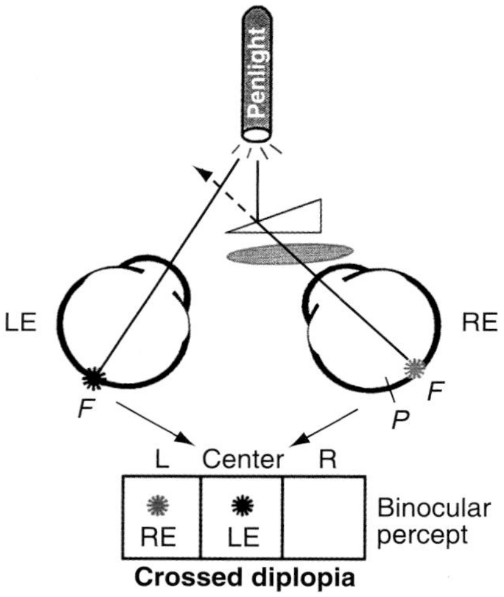

Figure 5–6 Paradoxical diplopia. Diagram of esotropia and ARC, wherein the deviation is being neutralized with a base-out prism. A red glass and base-out prism are placed over the right eye. The prism neutralizes the deviation by moving the retinal image of the penlight temporally, off the pseudofovea (P) to the true fovea (F). Because the pseudofovea is the center of orientation, the image is perceived to fall on the temporal retina and is projected to the opposite field, thus resulting in crossed diplopia. *(Modified with permission from Wright KW, Spiegel PH. Pediatric Ophthalmology and Strabismus. St Louis: Mosby; 1999:219.)*

Note that ARC is a binocular phenomenon, tested for and documented in both eyes simultaneously. It is not necessarily related to eccentric fixation (see Chapter 6), which is a monocular phenomenon found in testing 1 eye alone. Because some tests for ARC depend on separate stimulation of each fovea, the presence of eccentric fixation can significantly affect the test results (see also Chapter 7).

Monofixation Syndrome

The term monofixation syndrome is used to describe a particular presentation of a sensory state in strabismus. The essential feature of this syndrome is the presence of peripheral fusion with the absence of bifoveal fusion due to a central scotoma. The term microtropia was introduced separately to describe small-angle strabismus with a constellation of findings that largely overlap those of monofixation syndrome.

斜视手术后 ARC 持续存在时，会出现*矛盾性复视*。例如，当内斜视患者手术后获得正常或几乎正常的视轴，出现中心凹或旁中心凹刺激的交叉复视症状，即矛盾性复视（图 5-6）。矛性盾复视是术后的暂时现象，仅持续几天或几周，在极少数情况下可持续较长的时间。

异常视网膜对应的检测

异常视网膜对应的检测是为了确定受影响的患者在日常生活中如何用眼，并寻找正常对应的痕迹。如前所述，ARC 是对异常眼位的感觉适应。因为感觉重组的深度变异很大，可以同时检测正常视网膜对应和异常视网膜对应。检测与日常生活越相似，就越可能查出 ARC。检测与日常生活越偏离，越容易诱导 NRC，除非异常视网膜对应较为顽固。为了尽量使偏离最少，还有更常见的检测（见第 7 章中详细讨论），包括后像试验、Worth 4 点试验、红玻璃试验（随着红色滤光片密度的增加，偏离增加）、弱视仪试验，以及 Bagolini 线状镜试验。如果偏离较明显的试验出现异常定位反应，则异常视网膜对应的深度越大。

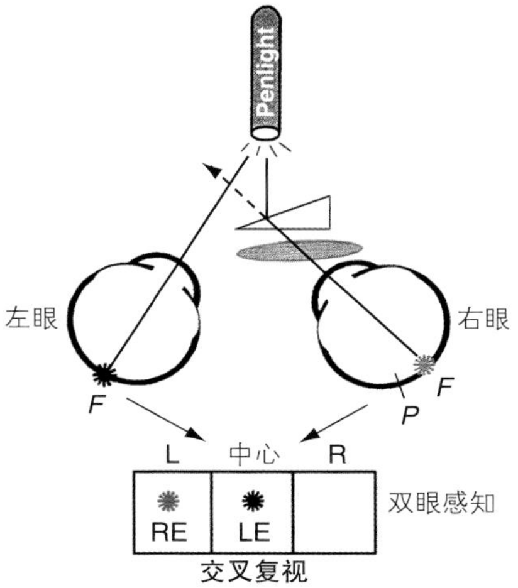

图 5-6　矛盾性复视。内斜视和异常视网膜对应图解，其中偏斜用底向外棱镜中和。在右眼前放置红玻片和底向外棱镜。棱镜通过将视网膜图像由假中心凹（P）暂时移到真中心凹（F）上来中和偏离。由于伪中心凹是定向的中心，图像被视为落在颞侧视网膜上，投射到相反的区域，从而导致交叉的复视。*（译者注：资料来源见前页原文。）*

应注意，ARC 是一种双眼现象，双眼要同时进行检查和记录。它并不一定与非中心注视相关（见第 6 章），非中心注视是一种单眼现象，单独检查一眼时发现。由于一些 ARC 的检查需分别刺激每眼的中心凹，检查结果会受非中心注视的影响（见第 7 章）。

单眼注视综合征

单眼注视综合征用于描述斜视中感觉状态的一种特殊表现。该综合征的基本特征是周边融像的存在，而因中心盲点导致双眼中心凹融像缺失。微斜视单独用于描述小角度的斜视，与单眼注视综合征的相关表现很相似。

A patient with monofixation syndrome may have no manifest deviation but usually has a small (≤8 prism diopters [Δ]) heterotropia; the heterotropia is most commonly an esotropia but is sometimes an exotropia or hypertropia. Stereoacuity is present but reduced. Amblyopia is a common finding.

Monofixation syndrome is a favorable outcome of infantile strabismus surgery and is present in a substantial minority of patients with intermittent exotropia. It can also be a primary condition that causes unilaterally decreased vision when no obvious strabismus is present. Monofixation syndrome can result from anisometropia or macular lesions as well.

Diagnosis

To diagnose monofixation syndrome, the clinician must demonstrate the absence of bimacular fusion by documenting a macular scotoma in the nonfixating eye under binocular conditions and the presence of peripheral binocular vision (peripheral fusion).

Vectographic projections of Snellen letters can be used to document the facultative scotoma of monofixation syndrome. Snellen letters are viewed through polarized analyzers or goggles equipped with liquid-crystal shutters so that some letters are seen with only the right eye, some with only the left eye, and some with both eyes. Patients with monofixation syndrome omit letters that are imaged only in the nonfixating eye. Various other tests for central suppression are more commonly used (see Chapter 7).

Testing stereoacuity is an important part of the monofixation syndrome evaluation. Any amount of gross stereopsis confirms the presence of peripheral fusion. Most patients with monofixation syndrome demonstrate stereopsis of 200–3000 seconds of arc. However, because some patients with this syndrome have no demonstrable stereopsis, other tests for peripheral fusion, such as the Worth 4-dot test and testing with Bagolini lenses, must be used in conjunction with stereoacuity measurement. Fine stereopsis (better than 67 seconds of arc) is present only in patients with bifoveal fixation.

Management

If associated amblyopia is clinically significant, occlusion therapy is indicated. Monofixation may decompensate to a larger heterotropia in adulthood, resulting in diplopia. Strabismus surgery may be required to restore fusion.

Ing MR, Roberts KM, Lin A, Chen JJ. The stability of the monofixation syndrome. *Am J Ophthalmol.* 2014;157(1):248–253.

单眼注视综合征的病人没有明显的斜视，常有小角度的斜视（≤ 8Δ）；最常见的是内斜，也有外斜或上斜。存在立体视觉，但偏低。常见弱视。

单眼注视综合征是婴儿斜视手术的较好结果，也存在于少数间歇性外斜中，也会引起没有明显斜视的单眼视力下降。单眼注视综合征也可由屈光参差或黄斑损伤引起。

诊断

诊断单眼注视综合征，必须在双眼条件下进行，存在非注视眼的黄斑盲点以及存在周边双眼视觉（周边融像），而没有双眼黄斑融像。

Snellen 字母的矢量投影可以记录单眼注视综合征的条件性盲点。通过偏振镜或有液晶快门的护目镜装置观察 Snellen 字母，一些字母只能被右眼看到，一些只能被左眼看到，还有一些能被双眼看到。单眼注视综合征的病人会遗漏仅成像于非注视眼的字母。可以使用其他各种检测中心抑制的检查方法（见第 7 章）。

立体视的检查是单眼注视综合征评估的重要部分。任何程度的总立体视证明周边融像的存在。大部分单眼注视综合征有 200 ~ 3000 弧秒的立体视。但是，因为有一些单眼注视综合征病人没有立体视，因此，在做其他周边融像的检查，如 Worth-4 点和 Bagolini 线状镜检查时，必须与立体视检查结合使用。精细立体视（小于67弧秒）仅存在于双眼黄斑中心凹注视的病人。

治疗

如果伴有严重的弱视，需要进行遮盖疗法。单眼注视在成年人呈大角度斜视，并导致复视。需要进行斜视手术重建融合。

Ing MR, Roberts KM, Lin A, Chen JJ. The stability of the monofixation syndrome. *Am J Ophthalmol.* 2014;157(1):248–253.

（翻译 张乐 刘念 // 审校 石一宁 布娟 // 章节审校 石广礼）

CHAPTER 6

Amblyopia

Amblyopia is a unilateral or, less commonly, bilateral reduction of best-corrected visual acuity (also referred to as *corrected distance visual acuity*) that cannot be attributed directly to the effect of any structural abnormality of the eye or visual pathways. Amblyopia signifies a failure of normal neural development in the immature visual system (see Chapter 5) and is caused by abnormal visual experience early in life resulting from one or a combination of the following:

- strabismus
- refractive error: anisometropia or bilateral high refractive error (isoametropia)
- visual deprivation in 1 or both eyes

Epidemiology

Amblyopia is responsible for more cases of childhood-onset unilateral decreased vision than all other causes combined, with a prevalence of 2%–4% in North America. It is also the most common cause of unilateral visual impairment in adults younger than 60 years.Amblyopia prevalence is increased in the setting of prematurity, developmental delay, or family history of amblyopia.

Pathophysiology

In early postnatal development, there are critical periods of cortical development during which neural circuits display a heightened sensitivity to environmental stimuli and are dependent on natural sensory experience for proper formation (see also Chapter 5). During these periods, the developing visual system is vulnerable to abnormal input due to visual deprivation, strabismus, or significant blur resulting from anisometropia or isoametropia. Conversely, the visual system's plasticity early in development allows the greatest opportunity for amblyopia reversal. The window of opportunity for treatment depends on the type of amblyopia (see the next section, Classification). For example, the critical period for reversal of visual deprivation amblyopia (eg, due to infantile cataracts) is shorter than that for reversal of infantile strabismic or anisometropic amblyopia.

第 6 章

弱视

弱视是单侧或较少见的双侧最佳矫正视力（*也称为矫正远视力*）的下降，没有任何直接的眼球或视路结构异常。弱视是指不成熟的视觉系统中神经未能正常发育（见第 5 章），并伴有以下一种或多种幼年早期的异常视觉经验：

- 斜视
- 屈光不正：屈光参差或双侧高度屈光不正（双眼屈光不正）
- 一眼或双眼的形觉剥夺

流行病学

弱视是儿童期发生的单侧视力下降的主要原因，高于其他所有原因之和，在北美发病率为 2% ~ 4%。也是 60 岁以下成年人中单侧视觉障碍最常见的原因。在早产儿、发育迟缓或有弱视家族史中，弱视的发病率较高。

病理生理学

出生后的早期发育中有皮质发育的关键期，在此期间，神经回路对环境刺激表现出高度的敏感性，正常的发育依赖于自然感知经验（见第 5 章）。此时，发育中的视觉系统容易受到异常传入的影响，如形觉剥夺、斜视或因屈光参差、双眼屈光不正引起的明显视觉模糊。相反，视觉系统在发育早期的可塑性为弱视的逆转提供了最大的可能。治疗的窗口期取决于弱视的类型(见下一节“分类”)。例如，视觉剥夺性弱视逆转的关键期(如婴儿白内障)比婴儿斜视或屈光参差性弱视的关键期短。

Amblyopic visual deficits result primarily from visual cortical changes. With abnormal visual experience early in life, cells of the primary visual cortex can lose their ability to respond to stimulation of 1 or both eyes, and the cells that remain responsive show significant functional deficiencies, including abnormally large receptive fields. Visual cortex deficiencies may account for the crowding phenomenon, in which optotypes are easier to recognize when isolated than when surrounded by similar forms (see Chapter 1). Abnormalities are also found in neurons within the lateral geniculate body, but the retina in amblyopia is essentially normal. Amblyopia is primarily a defect of central vision; the peripheral visual field is usually normal.

Classification

Strabismic Amblyopia

Strabismic amblyopia results from competitive or inhibitory interaction between neurons carrying nonfusible input from the 2 eyes. Constant, nonalternating heterotropias are the most likely deviations to cause amblyopia. The visual cortex becomes dominated by input from the fixating eye, with reduced responsiveness to input from the nonfixating eye. In young children with strabismus, suppression develops rapidly. This visual adaptation serves to avoid diplopia and visual confusion (see Chapter 5), but in a child who does not alternate fixation, constant suppression of input from the same eye can lead to amblyopia.

Several features distinguish strabismic amblyopia from other types of amblyopia. *Grating acuity* (see Chapter 1), the ability to resolve uniformly spaced stripes, is often reduced less than recognition acuity. Measurements obtained with Teller Acuity Cards II (Stereo Optical, Inc, Chicago, IL) and the LEA Grating Acuity Test (Good-Lite Company, Elgin, IL) may overestimate recognition visual acuity. Visual acuity measured through a neutral density filter declines less sharply for patients with strabismic amblyopia than for those with ocular disease (*neutral density filter effect*).

Eccentric fixation is the consistent use of a nonfoveal region of the retina during monocular viewing. Minor degrees of eccentric fixation, detectable only with special tests such as visuoscopy, are present in many patients with strabismic amblyopia. Clinically evident eccentric fixation results in a decentered position of the corneal light reflex when the amblyopic eye is fixating monocularly and implies visual acuity of 20/200 or worse, as well as a poorer prognosis. It should not be confused with an abnormal angle kappa (see Chapter 7).

Refractive Amblyopia

Refractive amblyopia results from consistent retinal defocus in 1 or both eyes. Anisometropia causes unilateral amblyopia; isoametropia causes bilateral amblyopia.

弱视的视觉功能低下主要是由视觉皮质的改变引起的。由于生命早期异常的视觉体验，主要的视皮质细胞丧失了对一眼或双眼刺激做出反应的能力，而保持反应的细胞表现出明显的功能低下，包括异常增大的感受野。视觉皮层功能低下可能导致拥挤现象，在这种现象中，单个视标比被相似形状包围时更容易识别 (见第 1 章)。在外侧膝状体的神经元也出现异常，但弱视的视网膜本质上是正常的。弱视主要是中心视力低下，周围视野正常。

分类

斜视性弱视

斜视性弱视是由神经元传入双眼不融合信号，造成神经元间相互竞争或抑制。恒定的、非交替性斜视最易引起弱视。视觉皮质由注视眼的输入占主导地位，对来自非注视眼的输入的反应性降低。患有斜视的儿童中，抑制迅速形成。这种视觉适应有助于避免复视和视觉混淆 (见第 5 章)，但对于不交替注视的儿童，同一眼的持续抑制会导致弱视。

斜视性弱视有几个特征，可区别于其他类型弱视。*条栅视力*（见第 1 章），指分辨均匀间隔条纹的能力，往往比认知视力下降得少。用 Teller 视力卡 II (Stereo Optical, Inc, Chicago, IL) 和 LEA 条栅视力测试 (Good–Lite Company, Elgin, IL)，可能高估认知视力。斜视性弱视患者通过中性密度滤光片测得的视力下降幅度小于其他眼部疾病的患者 (*中性密度滤光效果*)。

*非中心注视*是单眼注视时，始终用视网膜的非中心凹区域。斜视性弱视的许多小度数的非中心注视，只能用特殊的检查发现，例如视觉镜。临床上明显的非中心注视，在弱视眼单眼注视时，角膜光反射是偏中心的，提示为 20/200 或更差，预后也更差。不要与异常 kappa 角相混淆 (见第 7 章)。

屈光不正性弱视

屈光不正性弱视是由于单眼或双眼视网膜持续离焦所致。屈光参差引起单眼弱视；双眼屈光不正引起双眼弱视。

Anisometropic amblyopia

In anisometropic amblyopia, dissimilar refractive errors in the 2 eyes cause 1 retinal image to be chronically defocused. Considered more prevalent than strabismic amblyopia in some recent US studies, this condition is thought to result partly from the direct effect of image blur and partly from interocular competition or inhibition similar (but not identical) to that responsible for strabismic amblyopia. Levels of anisometropia that commonly lead to amblyopia are greater than 1.50 diopters (D) of anisohyperopia, 2.00 D of anisoastigmatism, and 3.00 D of anisomyopia. Higher levels are associated with greater risk. The eyes of a child with anisometropic amblyopia usually appear normal to the family and primary care physician, which may delay detection and treatment.

McKean-Cowdin R, Cotter SA, Tarczy-Hornoch K, et al; Multi-ethnic Pediatric Eye Disease Study Group. Prevalence of amblyopia or strabismus in Asian and non-Hispanic white preschool children: Multi-ethnic Pediatric Eye Disease Study. *Ophthalmology*. 2013;120(10): 2117–2124.

Multi-ethnic Pediatric Eye Disease Study Group. Prevalence of amblyopia and strabismus in African American and Hispanic children ages 6 to 72 months: The Multi-ethnic Pediatric Eye Disease Study. *Ophthalmology*. 2008;115(7):1229–1236.e1.

Isoametropic amblyopia

Isoametropic amblyopia (bilateral ametropic amblyopia) is bilaterally decreased visual acuity resulting from chronically defocused retinal images, which are due to similarly large uncorrected refractive errors in both eyes. Hyperopia exceeding 4.00–5.00 D and myopia exceeding 5.00–6.00 D are risk factors. Bilateral high astigmatism may cause loss of resolving ability specific to the chronically blurred meridians (*meridional amblyopia*). Most ophthalmologists recommend correction for eyes with more than 2.00–3.00 D of cylinder.

Visual Deprivation Amblyopia

The least common form of amblyopia, but the most severe and difficult to treat, is visual deprivation amblyopia (also known as *stimulus deprivation amblyopia, deprivation amblyopia, visual stimulus deprivation amblyopia, and form-vision deprivation amblyopia*), which is due to an eye abnormality that obstructs the visual axis or otherwise interferes with central vision. The most common cause is congenital or early-acquired cataract; other causes include blepharoptosis, periocular lesions obstructing the visual axis, corneal opacities, and vitreous hemorrhage. Visual deprivation amblyopia develops faster, and is deeper, than strabismic or anisometropic amblyopia. Unilateral visual deprivation tends to cause vision deficits in the affected eye that are more severe than the bilateral amblyopic deficits produced by bilateral deprivation of the same degree because interocular competition adds to the direct impact of image degradation (see Chapter 5). Even in bilateral cases, visual acuity can be 20/200 or worse if not treated early.

In children younger than 6 years, dense cataracts occupying the central 3 mm or more of the lens can cause severe visual deprivation amblyopia. Similar lens opacities acquired after age 6 years are generally less harmful. Small anterior polar cataracts, around which retinoscopy can be readily performed, and lamellar cataracts, through which a reasonably good view of the fundus can be obtained, may cause mild to moderate amblyopia or have no effect on visual development. Unilateral anterior polar cataracts, however, are associated with anisometropia and subtle optical distortion of the surrounding clear portion of the lens, which may cause anisometropic and/or mild visual deprivation amblyopia.

屈光参差性弱视

在屈光参差性弱视中，双眼不同程度的屈光不正导致长时间的一眼视网膜像离焦。美国最近的研究认为，这种情况比斜视性弱视更普遍，一部分是由于像模糊的直接作用造成，另一部分由于双眼间的竞争或抑制造成，类似于(但并不相同)斜视性弱视的原因。远视性屈光参差超过 1.50D、散光性屈光参差超过 2.00D 以及近视性屈光参差超过 3.00D 的屈光参差常常会导致弱视。屈光参差越大，弱视风险越大。屈光参差性弱视儿童的眼睛，通常在家人和初级保健医生看来是正常的，这样可能会延误诊断和治疗。

McKean-Cowdin R, Cotter SA, Tarczy-Hornoch K, et al; Multi-ethnic Pediatric Eye Disease Study Group. Prevalence of amblyopia or strabismus in Asian and non-Hispanic white preschool children: Multi-ethnic Pediatric Eye Disease Study. *Ophthalmology*. 2013;120(10): 2117–2124.

Multi-ethnic Pediatric Eye Disease Study Group. Prevalence of amblyopia and strabismus in African American and Hispanic children ages 6 to 72 months: The Multi-ethnic Pediatric Eye Disease Study. *Ophthalmology*. 2008;115(7):1229–1236.e1.

双眼屈光不正性弱视

屈光不正性弱视(双眼屈光不正性弱视)是长期的视网膜像离焦导致的双眼视力下降，双眼视力下降是由于双眼屈光度接近的高度屈光不正未予以矫正。远视超过 4.00 ~ 5.00D 和近视超过 5.00 ~ 6.00D 为危险因素。双眼高度散光可引起长期的特殊径线性模糊(*径线性弱视*)，从而丧失分辨能力。大多数眼科医生建议对于超过 2.00 ~ 3.00D 的柱镜进行矫正。

视觉剥夺性弱视

最少见的，但也是最严重和最难以治疗的弱视类型是视觉剥夺性弱视(也称为*刺激剥夺性弱视*，*剥夺性弱视*，*视觉刺激剥夺性弱视*，*和形态视觉剥夺性弱视*)，这是由于眼部异常，遮挡视轴或干扰了中心视力。最常见的原因是先天性或早期获得性白内障；其他原因包括上睑下垂、遮挡视轴的眼周病变、角膜混浊和玻璃体出血。视觉剥夺性弱视比斜视性或屈光参差性弱视发展更快、更严重。单眼视觉剥夺容易导致受累眼的视力低下，较同等程度的双眼剥夺引起的双眼弱视更严重，因为两眼间的竞争直接影响图像质量的下降(见第 5 章)。即便是双眼弱视，如果不及早治疗，视力可为 20/200 或者更差。

在 6 岁以下的儿童中，位于晶状体中心 3mm 或以上的密集白内障可导致严重的视觉剥夺性弱视。6 岁以后类似的获得性晶状体混浊危害较小。小的前极部白内障或层状的白内障，其周围可以进行视网膜检影，可进行较好眼底观察，可能导致轻度至中度的弱视，或对视觉发育没有影响。而单眼前极部白内障，伴有屈光参差和晶状体透明部分周围的微小光学畸变，可引起屈光参差和（或）轻度视觉剥夺性弱视。

Reverse amblyopia (occlusion amblyopia) is a form of visual deprivation amblyopia that can develop in the initially dominant eye if it is patched excessively during treatment of amblyopia in the other eye. See the section "Reverse amblyopia and new strabismus" for further discussion.

Detection and Screening

Amblyopia is preventable or reversible with timely detection and intervention. Risk factors for amblyopia include strabismus, anisometropia, isoametropia, and visual deprivation (eg, from ocular media opacities). Regular childhood screening through primary care or community-based programs facilitates early detection of amblyopia and amblyopia risk factors. Screening techniques include direct visual acuity measurement and testing for risk factors. Corneal light reflex tests and cover testing detect strabismus; the Brückner test (see Chapter 7) can reveal media opacities, strabismus, anisometropia, and isoametropia. Instrument-based vision screening is effective in preschool-aged and younger children: portable autorefractors identify refractive errors, while photoscreening devices detect strabismus, refractive errors, and abnormal red reflexes.

Donahue SP, Baker CN; Committee on Practice and Ambulatory Medicine, Section on Ophthalmology, American Academy of Pediatrics; American Association of Certified Orthoptists; American Association for Pediatric Ophthalmology and Strabismus; American Academy of Ophthalmology. Procedures for the evaluation of the visual system by pediatricians. *Pediatrics*. 2016;137(1):e20153597. doi: 10.1542/peds.2015-3597.

Evaluation

Amblyopia is diagnosed when a patient has a condition known to cause amblyopia and has decreased best-corrected visual acuity that cannot be explained by other diseases of the eye or visual pathways. Vision characteristics alone cannot differentiate amblyopia from other forms of vision loss. The crowding phenomenon, for example, is typical of amblyopia but not pathognomonic or uniformly demonstrable. Subtle afferent pupillary defects may occur in severe amblyopia, but only rarely. Amblyopia sometimes coexists with vision loss that is directly caused by an uncorrectable structural abnormality of the eye such as optic nerve hypoplasia or coloboma. If amblyopia is suspected in such a case, it is appropriate to undertake a trial of amblyopia treatment. Improvement in vision confirms that amblyopia was indeed present.

Multiple assessments of visual acuity are sometimes required to determine the presence and severity of amblyopia. (Assessment of visual acuity is discussed in Chapter 1.) In some cases, the clinician may assume that amblyopia is present and initiate treatment before decreased vision can be demonstrated. For example, if a clinician does not have access to a grating acuity test such as Teller Acuity Cards II, occlusion therapy may be started in a preverbal child in the presence of a high degree of anisometropia or shortly after surgery for a unilateral cataract.

反转性弱视(遮盖性弱视)是一种视觉剥夺性弱视，因为弱视眼过度遮盖，使最初的优势眼发生弱视。有关进一步讨论，见“反转性弱视和新斜视”一节。

发现与筛查

只要及时发现和干预，弱视是可预防的或可逆的。弱视的危险因素包括斜视、屈光参差、双眼屈光不正和视觉剥夺(如屈光间质混浊)。通过初级保健或社区为基础的项目，对儿童进行定期筛查，有助于早期发现弱视和弱视的危险因素。筛查技术包括直接视力检查和危险因素检测。角膜光反射法和遮盖试验检查斜视；Brückner 检查(见第 7 章)发现间质混浊、斜视、屈光参差和双眼屈光不正。仪器为基础的视觉筛查对于学龄前和幼儿是有效的：便携式自动验光仪确定屈光不正，照相筛查设备发现斜视、屈光不正和异常红光反射。

Donahue SP, Baker CN; Committee on Practice and Ambulatory Medicine, Section on Ophthalmology, American Academy of Pediatrics; American Association of Certified Orthoptists; American Association for Pediatric Ophthalmology and Strabismus; American Academy of Ophthalmology. Procedures for the evaluation of the visual system by pediatricians. *Pediatrics*. 2016;137(1):e20153597. doi: 10.1542/peds.2015-3597.

评估

当病人有引起弱视的条件，且其他眼或视路疾病不能解释最佳矫正视力下降原因时，即可诊断弱视。单独的视力低下并不能用于鉴别弱势与其他原因的视力低下。例如，拥挤现象是弱视的典型表现，但并不是弱势独有的或均有的表现。严重弱视可存在轻度传入性瞳孔阻滞，但极少见。有时弱视与眼部结构异常引起的视力丧失同时存在，如视神经发育不良或缺损。在怀疑弱视存在时，可进行试验性弱视治疗，有视力的改善则证明弱视确实存在。

有时需要多种的视力评估来确定弱视的存在和严重程度。(第 1 章中讨论了视力的评估。)有时临床医生认为已经存在弱视，并在未证明视力低下前就开始治疗。例如，医生没有进行条栅视力测试，如 Teller 视力卡 II，就开始对不会讲话的孩子进行遮盖疗法，而他们可能有高度屈光参差，或刚刚行单眼白内障手术。

When determining the severity of amblyopia in a young patient, the clinician should remember that both false-positive and false-negative errors may occur with fixation preference testing; a strabismic child may show a strong fixation preference despite having equal visual acuity, whereas an anisometropic child may alternate fixation despite having significant amblyopia. In addition, the young child's brief attention span frequently results in grating or recognition acuity measurements that fall short of the true limits of acuity; these measurements can mimic those of bilateral amblyopia or mask or falsely suggest a significant interocular difference. Finally, because test-retest variability can be up to a full line of letters in children, it is important for the clinician to evaluate trends when assessing response to treatment.

Treatment

Treatment of amblyopia involves the following steps:

1. Eliminate (if needed) any obstruction of the visual axis, such as a cataract.
2. Correct any significant refractive error.
3. Promote use of the amblyopic eye.

Cataract Removal

Cataracts capable of producing dense amblyopia require timely surgery. Removal of unilateral, visually significant congenital lens opacities within the first 6 weeks of life is necessary for optimal recovery of vision. In young children, significant cataracts with uncertain time of onset also deserve prompt and aggressive treatment if recent development is at least a possibility. For bilateral, dense congenital cataracts, surgery is recommended within the first 10 weeks of life. However, small partial cataracts may sometimes be managed nonsurgically; pharmacologic pupillary dilation may permit good vision despite a central opacity (see also the section Visual Deprivation Amblyopia, earlier in the chapter). Childhood cataract is discussed further in Chapter 23.

Refractive Correction

Refractive correction plays a key role in the treatment of all types of amblyopia, not just refractive amblyopia. Anisometropic, isoametropic, and even strabismic amblyopia may improve or resolve with refractive correction alone. Many ophthalmologists thus initiate amblyopia treatment with refractive correction, adding occlusion or pharmacologic or optical treatment later if necessary (see the following sections). Refractive correction for aphakia following cataract surgery in childhood is initiated promptly to avoid prolonging visual deprivation. For patients with high refractive error that is amblyogenic who will not or cannot wear glasses or contact lenses, refractive surgery may be an alternative in select cases.

在确定儿童弱视的严重程度时，临床医生应记住在进行固视偏好检查时，可能发生假阳性和假阴性的错误。斜视儿童在视力相同的情况下，也可能表现出强烈的固视偏好，而屈光参差的儿童尽管有明显的弱视，也出现交替性注视。此外，幼儿的短暂注意持续时间常导致条栅或认知视力测量低于真实的视力，使测量结果呈双眼弱视，掩盖或错误给出双眼间明显差异的假象。最后，因为儿童在测试－复测时可能一整行字母都在变化，所以临床医生在评估治疗反应时评估趋势是很重要的。

治疗

弱视的治疗包括以下步骤：

1. 消除（如果需要）视轴上的遮盖，如白内障。
2. 矫正明显的屈光不正。
3. 加强弱视眼的使用。

白内障摘除

能够产生重度弱视的白内障需要及时手术。单眼的明显可见的先天性晶状体混浊，需在出生后 6 周内摘除，以恢复最佳视力。如果幼儿明显的白内障，其发病时间不明、但近期有可能发展，也应及时和积极的治疗。对于双眼严重的先天性白内障，应在出生后 10 周内手术。然而，小范围的白内障有时可以非手术治疗，尽管有中心混浊（见本章“视觉剥夺性弱视”一节），药物的瞳孔扩大可以获得较好的视力。儿童白内障在第 23 章中进一步讨论。

屈光矫正

屈光矫正在各种类型弱视的治疗中起着至关重要的作用，而不仅仅是屈光不正性弱视。屈光参差性、屈光不正性及斜视性弱视，均可能仅通过矫正屈光不正而得到改善或治愈。因此，眼科医生从屈光不正矫正开始弱视治疗，如有必要，再加上遮盖、药物或光学治疗（见下一节）。儿童白内障手术后无晶体眼的屈光矫正应立即开始，以避免拖延形觉剥夺的时间。在特定情况下，对于有高度屈光不正，不想戴或不能戴框架眼镜或接触镜的患者，屈光手术可作为另一种选择。

In general, refractive correction in amblyopia should be based on the cycloplegic refraction. Often, full hyperopic correction is necessary to treat coexisting accommodative esotropia (see Chapter 8). Furthermore, because an amblyopic eye tends to have an impaired ability to control accommodation, it cannot reliably compensate for uncorrected hyperopia as would a child's normal eye. Thus, children with unilateral or bilateral amblyopia may need full or nearly full correction of their hyperopia during amblyopia treatment even if they do not have accommodative esotropia. Also, by ensuring clear distance vision in the fellow eye even under cycloplegia, full hyperopic correction may reduce the risk of reverse amblyopia, which can result from pharmacologic treatment with atropine (see the section "Reverse amblyopia and new strabismus"). Sometimes, however, symmetric reductions in plus-lens power help foster acceptance of glasses.

Writing Committee for the Pediatric Eye Disease Investigator Group; Cotter SA, Foster NC,Holmes JM, et al. Optical treatment of strabismic and combined strabismic-anisometropic amblyopia. *Ophthalmology.* 2012;119(1):150–158.

Occlusion Therapy

Occlusion therapy (patching) is commonly used to treat unilateral amblyopia. The sound eye is covered, obligating the child to use the amblyopic eye. Adhesive patches are usually employed, but spectacle-mounted occluders or opaque contact lenses are alternatives if skin irritation or inadequate adhesion is a problem. With spectacle-mounted occluders, close supervision is necessary to ensure that the patient does not peek around the occluder.

Full-time occlusion, defined as occlusion during all waking hours, can cause reverse amblyopia and strabismus (see the section Complications and Challenges of Therapy). For severe amblyopia, *part-time occlusion* of 6 hours per day achieves results similar to those obtained with prescribed full-time occlusion. The relative duration of patch-on and patch-off intervals should reflect the degree of amblyopia. For severe deficits (visual acuity of 20/125–20/400), 6 hours per day is preferred. For moderate deficits (visual acuity of 20/100 or better), 2 hours of daily patching may be effective. It is not necessary for the patient to engage in specific activities (eg, near work) while patched.

Follow-up timing depends on patient age and treatment intensity. Part-time treatment permits less frequent follow-up; reexamination 2–3 months after initiating treatment is typical. Subsequent visits can be at longer intervals, based on early response.

The desired endpoint of therapy for unilateral amblyopia is free alternation of fixation and/or linear recognition acuity that differs by no more than 1 line between the 2 eyes. The time required to complete treatment depends on amblyopia severity, treatment intensity, and patient adherence and age. More severe amblyopia and older children require more intensive or longer treatment. Occlusion during infancy may reverse substantial strabismic amblyopia in less than 1 month. In contrast, an older child who wears a patch only after school and on weekends may require several months to overcome a moderate deficit.

Adherence to occlusion therapy for amblyopia declines with increasing age. However, studies in older children and teenagers with strabismic or anisometropic amblyopia show that treatment can still be beneficial beyond the first decade of life. This is especially true in children who have not previously undergone treatment.

一般来说，弱视的屈光矫正应以睫状肌麻痹验光结果为基础。同时存在的调节性内斜视，需要对远视全部矫正 (见第 8 章)。此外，由于弱视眼调节功能障碍的患儿，不能像正常儿童眼准确地代偿未矫正的远视，所以，单眼或双眼弱视的儿童，即使没有调节性内斜视，在弱视治疗过程中可能需要远视全部矫正或接近全部矫正。而且，通过确保另一眼在睫状肌麻痹状态下远距离视力清晰，远视全部矫正可减少阿托品药物治疗的反转性弱视的风险 (见“反转性弱视和新斜视”一节)。然而，有时远视镜度数的对称性降低有助于加快儿童接受眼镜。

Writing Committee for the Pediatric Eye Disease Investigator Group; Cotter SA, Foster NC,Holmes JM, et al. Optical treatment of strabismic and combined strabismic-anisometropic amblyopia. *Ophthalmology*. 2012;119(1):150–158.

遮盖疗法

遮盖疗法 (眼罩) 是治疗单眼弱视的常用方法。遮盖健眼，迫使孩子使用弱视眼。通常使用黏性眼贴，如果出现皮肤刺激或黏附不牢时，可选用眼镜加盖眼罩或不透光的接触镜。而眼镜加盖眼罩必须严密监视，以确保孩子没有通过眼罩周围进行偷看。

全时间遮盖，定义为在所有清醒状态下的遮盖，可导致反转性弱视和斜视 (见“治疗的并发症和挑战”一节)。对于重度弱视，每天 6h 的*部分时间遮盖*与全时间遮盖的效果相似。遮盖和去遮盖间隔时间取决于弱视的程度。严重的视力低下 (视力为 20/125 ~ 20/400)，建议每天 6h。中度视力低下 (视力 20/100 或更好)，每天 2h 的遮盖即奏效。遮盖时，患儿不需要特定的活动 (如近距离工作)。

随访的时间取决于患者的年龄和治疗强度。部分时间遮盖治疗的随访频率较低，治疗后 2 ~ 3 个月复查。根据前一次的治疗反应，后续的复查间隔的时间可以更长。

单眼弱视治疗的理想终点是自由的交替固视和 (或) 两眼之间的单行认知视力差异不超过 1 行。完成治疗所需的时间取决于弱视的严重程度、治疗强度、患者的依从性和年龄。弱视越严重和儿童年龄越大，需要治疗的强度越大，治疗的时间越长。婴儿期的遮盖可能在 1 个月内重度的斜视性弱视好转。相比之下，大龄儿童只在放学后和周末才戴眼罩，所以中度弱视可能需要几个月的治疗。

随着年龄的增长，弱视遮盖疗法的依从性下降。然而，对伴有斜视或屈光参差性弱视的大龄儿童和青少年的研究表明，对 10 岁以上儿童治疗仍然有效。这对于以前没有接受过治疗的儿童更是如此。

Pharmacologic or Optical Treatment

Alternatives to occlusion therapy involve pharmacologic and/or optical degradation of the better eye's vision such that it becomes temporarily inferior to the amblyopic eye's vision, promoting use of the amblyopic eye. For patients with orthotropia or small-angle strabismus, an advantage of these treatments over occlusion therapy is that they allow a degree of binocularity, which is particularly beneficial in children with latent nystagmus.

Pharmacologic treatment of moderate amblyopia (visual acuity of 20/100 or better) is as effective as patching and may also be successful in more severe amblyopia (visual acuity of 20/125–20/400), particularly in younger children. A cycloplegic agent (usually atropine sulfate solution, 1%) is administered to the better-seeing eye so that it is unable to accommodate. Vision in the better eye is thus blurred at near and, if hyperopia is undercorrected, also for distance viewing. Atropine may be administered daily, but weekend administration is as effective for milder amblyopia. Regular follow-up is important to monitor for reverse amblyopia (see the section Complications and Challenges of Therapy).

Pharmacologic treatment is difficult for the child to thwart. It may not work well for myopic patients, however, because clear near vision persists in the dominant eye despite cycloplegia if the distance correction is not worn. In some children, attempts to accommodate with the dominant eye in the face of cycloplegia can increase accommodative convergence, worsening any underlying esotropia during treatment. Parents and caregivers should be counseled regarding the adverse effects of atropine, including light sensitivity, and potential systemic toxicity, the symptoms of which include fever, tachycardia, delirium, and dry mouth and skin (see Chapter 1).

Optical treatment involves the prescription of excessive plus lenses (fogging) or diffusing filters for the sound eye. This form of treatment avoids potential pharmacologic adverse effects and may be able to induce greater blur than cycloplegic agents. If the child wears glasses, a translucent filter, such as Scotch Magic Tape (3M, St Paul, MN) or a Bangerter foil (Ryser Optik AG, St Gallen, Switzerland), can be applied to the spectacle lens. Optical treatment may be more acceptable than occlusion therapy to many children and their parents, but patients must be closely monitored to ensure proper use (no peeking) of spectacle-borne devices.

Binocular Treatment

Binocular amblyopia treatments have recently shown some promise in amblyopic children with orthotropia or small-angle strabismus. In these treatments, the child engages in active or passive visual tasks that require simultaneous perception and are performed on an electronic device under dichoptic viewing conditions. The relative salience of amblyopic and fellow eye input can be adjusted over the course of treatment.

Birch EE, Li SL, Jost RM, et al. Binocular iPad treatment for amblyopia in preschool children. *J AAPOS.* 2015;19(1):6–11.

Holmes JM, Manh VM, Lazar EL, et al; for the Pediatric Eye Disease Investigator Group. Effect of a binocular iPad game vs part-time patching in children aged 5 to 12 years with amblyopia: a randomized clinical trial. *JAMA Ophthalmol.* 2016;134(12):1391–1400.

药物或光学治疗

遮盖疗法的替代方案包括对视力较好眼的药物和（或）光学压抑，使其视力暂时低于弱视眼，加强弱视眼的使用。正位或小角度斜视患者，这些治疗方法优于遮盖治疗，因为这样可以获得一定程度的双眼视，特别是对隐性眼球震颤的儿童有益。

药物治疗对中度弱视（视力 20/100 或更好），与遮盖治疗的疗效一样，对更严重的弱视（视力 20/125 ~ 20/400)，尤其是幼儿也有效。睫状肌麻痹剂 (1% 硫酸阿托品溶液）用于视力较好的眼，使其无法调节。较好眼看近时是模糊的，如果远视矫正不足，看远时也是模糊的。阿托品可以每日使用，但仅周末使用对轻度弱视同样有效。定期随访对监控反转性弱视很重要（见“治疗的并发症和挑战”一节）。

儿童很难抗拒药物治疗。而对近视患者并不奏效，因为尽管睫状肌麻痹了，如果不戴视远用矫正眼镜，优势眼的近距离视力仍然清晰。即使睫状肌麻痹，有时通过使用优势眼调节，增加调节性集合，使内斜视增加。应告知家长和看护者阿托品的副作用，包括畏光、潜在的全身毒性，其症状包括发烧、心动过速、谵妄 / 极度兴奋、口干和皮肤干燥（见第 1 章）。

光学治疗包括健眼前过量正镜（雾视）或加弥散滤片。这种方法避免了潜在的药物副作用，可产生较睫状肌麻痹剂更模糊的效果。眼镜镜片上可以加半透明滤光片，如 Scotch Magic Tape（3M,St Paul, MN）或 Bangerter 箔（Ryser Optik AG, St Gallen, Switzerland）。对于许多儿童和他们的父母来说，光学疗法可能比遮盖疗法更容易接受，但须严密监视，以确保适当使用（没有偷看）。

双眼治疗

在正位或小角度斜视的弱视儿童中，双眼弱视治疗取得了一些效果。治疗中，儿童参与需要同时感知的主动或被动视觉任务，通过电子设备，在双眼分视注视条件下完成。在治疗过程中，可对弱视眼和另一眼进行相对突显输入的调整。

Birch EE, Li SL, Jost RM, et al. Binocular iPad treatment for amblyopia in preschool children. *J AAPOS.* 2015;19(1):6–11.

Holmes JM, Manh VM, Lazar EL, et al; for the Pediatric Eye Disease Investigator Group. Effect of a binocular iPad game vs part-time patching in children aged 5 to 12 years with amblyopia: a randomized clinical trial. *JAMA Ophthalmol.* 2016;134(12):1391–1400.

Complications and Challenges of Therapy

Reverse amblyopia and new strabismus

Both occlusion therapy and pharmacologic treatment carry a risk of overtreatment, which can result in reverse amblyopia in the sound eye. Strabismus can also develop or worsen with amblyopia treatment (although strabismus can also improve with amblyopia treatment).

Full-time occlusion carries the greatest risk of reverse amblyopia and thus requires close monitoring. Consequently, most ophthalmologists do not use full-time occlusion in younger children. Children with binocular fusion, especially, may benefit from time spent viewing binocularly. The family of a strabismic child should be instructed to watch for a reversal of fixation preference with full-time occlusion and to report its occurrence promptly. Usually, iatrogenic reverse amblyopia can be treated successfully by judicious patching of the formerly worse-seeing, now better-seeing, eye. Sometimes, simply stopping treatment leads to equalization of vision.

During pharmacologic treatment, the risk of reverse amblyopia is greatest if daily treatment is coupled with undercorrection of hyperopic refractive error in the sound eye undergoing cycloplegia (see the section Refractive Correction, earlier in the chapter).

Poor adherence

Lack of adherence to the therapeutic regimen is a common problem that can prolong the treatment period or lead to outright failure. If difficulties derive from a particular treatment method, the clinician should seek a suitable alternative. Adhesive and cloth patches may not be covered by medical insurance in the United States; if treatment cost is a burden, pharmacologic treatment may facilitate adherence. If the skin becomes irritated from patch adhesives, switching to a different brand or applying skin lotion after patching may help. A barrier application of tincture of benzoin can protect the skin from contact with adhesive and help when patches do not adhere because of perspiration; however, it can make patch removal more traumatic.

Families who seem to lack sufficient motivation should be counseled concerning the importance of the therapy and the need for consistency in carrying it out. They can be reassured that once an appropriate routine is established, the daily effort required is likely to diminish, especially if the amblyopia improves. For an older child, it can also be helpful for the physician to explain and emphasize the importance of treatment adherence directly to the child in an age-appropriate manner. Further, it is important for the family to understand that amblyopia treatment is performed primarily to improve vision rather than ocular alignment (even though ocular alignment may sometimes improve) and, conversely, that improving ocular alignment (with surgery or glasses) does not obviate the need for treatment of associated amblyopia.

Adherence to a patching regimen in older children can be improved by creating goals and offering rewards or by linking patching to play activities (eg, decorating the patch or patching while the child plays a video game). For infants and toddlers, adherence to a patching regimen depends greatly on parental engagement and commitment. Arm splints and mittens are sometimes used as a last resort.

治疗的并发症和挑战

反转性弱视和新斜视

遮盖疗法和药物疗法都有过度治疗的风险，可能导致健眼的反转性弱视。斜视也会随弱视的治疗而发展或加重(虽然斜视也随弱视的治疗而改善)。

全时间遮盖承载着反转性弱视的最大风险，因此需要密切的监测。因此，大多数眼科医生不在幼儿中使用全时间遮盖。尤其是儿童有双眼融合，双眼注视更有益。在斜视儿童的家庭中观察全时间遮盖治疗时，出现固视偏好的反转这种现象时，应及时告知医生。通过遮盖原视力差眼而现在视力较好眼，医源性反转性弱视可以治愈。有时，仅仅停止治疗就会达到视力平衡。

在药物疗法中，如果健眼的睫状肌麻痹，并伴有远视矫正不足，出现反转性弱视的风险最大(见本章前面“屈光矫正”一节)。

依从性不良

缺乏对治疗方案的依从性是一个常见的问题，使治疗时间延长，或导致彻底的失败。如果困难是某种治疗方法，医生应寻找合适的替代方法。粘黏性眼贴和布质眼罩可能不包含在美国医疗保险范围内，如果是治疗费用负担问题，药物疗法可增加依从性。如果因使用黏性眼贴而皮肤过敏，可更换另一种不同的品牌，或在使用眼贴后涂抹护肤乳。苯偶氮酊隔层可保护皮肤不接触黏剂，并解决出汗而不黏的问题；但摘掉眼贴时可能有损伤。

对于缺乏足够动力的家庭，应告知治疗的重要性和坚持治疗的必要性。使他们确信，一旦建立了适当的治疗方案，特别是当弱视有所改善时，每天所花费的时间会逐步减少。对于大龄儿童，以适合其年龄的方式直接向儿童解释，并强调治疗依从性的重要性。此外，重要的是让家庭明白弱视治疗是为了改善视力，而不是改善眼位(即使眼位有时可能会改善)，相反，改善眼位的治疗(通过手术或眼镜)并不能取消对合并的弱视的治疗。

通过制定目标和提供奖励，或将遮盖与游戏活动联系起来(如孩子玩视频游戏时，戴眼罩或遮眼)，能提高大龄儿童对遮盖治疗的依从性。对于婴幼儿和初学走路的幼童，遮盖治疗的依从性很大程度上取决于父母。手臂夹板和手套有时是最后的手段。

Unresponsiveness

Sometimes even conscientious application of an appropriate therapeutic program fails to improve vision at all or beyond a certain level. Complete or partial unresponsiveness to treatment occasionally affects younger children but more often occurs in patients older than 5 years. When there is a significant deviation from the expected treatment response despite good adherence, reexamination may reveal subtle optic nerve or retinal anomalies. Neuroimaging may be considered if an occult compressive optic neuropathy is suspected.

In a prognostically unfavorable situation, decisions about treatment should take into account the patient's and parents' wishes. Amblyopia is not always fully correctable, even in younger children. Primary therapy may reasonably be terminated if there is a lack of demonstrable progress over 3–6 months despite good treatment adherence. Progress or lack thereof may be harder to quantify in preverbal children, however, so longer treatment is appropriate in this setting.

Recurrence

When amblyopia treatment is discontinued after complete or partial improvement of vision, up to one-third of patients show some degree of recurrence. Reducing the occlusion regimen (to 1–2 hours per day) or the frequency of pharmacologic treatment for a few months before cessation is associated with a decreased incidence of recurrence, although no randomized trial has compared tapered and nontapered cessation. If recurrence occurs, vision can usually be improved again with resumption of therapy. In a study of children who were between 7 and 12 years of age when treated for amblyopia, the vision improvements that occurred seemed to be mostly sustained after cessation of treatment other than spectacles. Younger patients may require periodic monitoring until vision is stable with spectacle treatment alone (eg, until age 8–10 years). With stable vision, 12-month examination intervals are acceptable.

Hertle RW, Scheiman MM, Beck RW, et al; Pediatric Eye Disease Investigator Group.Stability of visual acuity improvement following discontinuation of amblyopia treatment in children aged 7 to 12 years. *Arch Ophthalmol.* 2007;125(5):655–659.

无反应性

有时即使认真执行恰当的治疗方案，也会出现视力完全没有提高或没有超越一个特定的水平的情况。对治疗完全或部分无反应偶发于幼儿，更多发生在大于 5 岁的患者。当治疗反应与预期有明显偏差时，尽管依从性良好，也应重新检查，可能发现细微的视神经或视网膜病变。如果怀疑有隐匿性压迫性视神经病变，可以考虑神经影像学检查。

弱视预后不佳时，综合考虑患者和父母的意愿来决定是否治疗。即使是年幼患者，弱视并非都能完全治愈。如果在 3 ~ 6 个月内，尽管患者的治疗依从性好，如无明显好转，也需要考虑终止治疗。对于前语言期儿童，难以量化是否好转，可能需要更长时间的治疗。

复发

当弱视治疗使得视力完全或部分提高后中止弱视治疗，会有高达三分之一的患者表现出一定程度的弱视复发。尚没有对减量弱视治疗后终止治疗和直接终止治疗比较的随机试验研究。有研究显示在终止治疗前，减少遮盖治疗方案（每天 1 ~ 2h）或药物治疗的频率与复发率降低有一定关系。如果弱视复发，通常再次治疗可改善视力。一项研究发现，停止对 7 ~ 12 岁儿童的弱视治疗后，视力的改善仍在持续，而不需要眼镜矫正。年幼的患者可能需要一段时间的定期检查，一直到只通过眼镜矫正来稳定视力的状态（直到 8 ~ 10 岁）。如果视力保持稳定，可每年进行一次复诊。

Hertle RW, Scheiman MM, Beck RW, et al; Pediatric Eye Disease Investigator Group.Stability of visual acuity improvement following discontinuation of amblyopia treatment in children aged 7 to 12 years. *Arch Ophthalmol*. 2007;125(5):655–659.

（翻译 刘念 杨嘉嵩 // 审校 石一宁 钱学翰 // 章节审校 石广礼）

CHAPTER 7

Diagnostic Evaluation of Strabismus and Torticollis

This chapter includes related videos, which can be accessed by scanning the QR codes provided in the text or going to www.aao.org/bcscvideo_section06.

Obtaining a History in Cases of Strabismus or Torticollis

Both strabismus and torticollis are common presenting complaints to the pediatric ophthalmologist. Torticollis is an abnormal head position (AHP), such as a head turn or tilt.Although torticollis can be caused by a wide variety of ocular and nonocular conditions(discussed later in the chapter) and is not always associated with strabismus, it is a commonpresenting sign of strabismus. Thus, there is broad overlap in the diagnostic assessment of strabismus and torticollis.

Key questions for the clinician to ask when obtaining a strabismus or torticollis history include the following:

- At what age did the deviation or AHP appear? (Reviewing old photographs may be helpful.)
- Did onset coincide with trauma or illness?
- Is the deviation or AHP constant or intermittent?
- Is it present for distance or near vision or both?
- Is it present only when the patient is inattentive or fatigued?
- Is it associated with double vision or eyestrain?
- If a deviation is noted, is it present in all positions of gaze?
- If a deviation is noted, is it unilateral or alternating?
- Does the patient close 1 eye (squint)?
- Is there a history of other ocular disease or ocular surgery?

The clinician should review previous treatment, including amblyopia therapy, spectacle correction, and eye muscle surgery. The initial assessment should also include observation of the patient's habitual head position, head movement, and attentiveness. See Chapter 1 for a general discussion of examination of children.

第 7 章

斜视和斜颈的诊断和评价

本章所包含的相关视频，可通过扫描文中的二维码观看或访问网站观看 www.aao.org/bcscvideo_section06。

病史采集

斜视和斜颈是小儿眼科医生常见的疾病。斜颈是一种异常的头位，如头部转动或倾斜。虽然斜颈可以由多种眼部和非眼部疾病引起（在本章后面讨论），并不完全与斜视有关，但它是斜视的常见表现。因此，斜视和斜颈的诊断和评估多有重叠。

医师在采集斜视或斜颈病史时，需要提及的关键问题包括：

- 什么年龄出现斜视或异常头位？（看旧照片有所帮助。）
- 发病是否与外伤或疾病同时发生？
- 斜视或异常头位是持续性的还是间歇性的？
- 是看远或看近时出现，还是看远看近时都出现？
- 是否仅在患者注意力不集中时或疲劳时才出现？
- 是否与复视或视疲劳有关？
- 如果发现斜视，是否在所有注视方位都出现？
- 如果发现斜视，是单眼的还是交替的？
- 患者是否闭一眼（眯眼）？
- 是否有其他眼部疾病或眼部手术史？

医师应回顾此前的治疗，包括弱视治疗、眼镜矫正和眼肌手术。初步检查还应包括观察患者的习惯性头位、头部运动和注意力等。关于儿童检查的讨论见第 1 章。

Assessment of Ocular Alignment

Diagnostic Positions of Gaze

The *diagnostic positions of gaze* are a core set of 9 different gaze positions used in the comprehensive assessment of ocular alignment. They consist of

- *primary position:* The eyes fixate straight ahead on an object at infinity, which, for practical purposes, is considered to be 6 m, or 20 ft. For this position, the head should be straight.
- *6 cardinal positions:* Two muscles (1 in each eye) are the prime movers of their respective eyes into each of these positions of gaze (see Chapter 4).
- *straight up and straight down:* These do not isolate any single muscle, because the actions of both oblique and vertical rectus muscles affect elevation and depression from primary position; see Chapter 4.

For patients with vertical strabismus, the diagnostic positions of gaze also include forced head tilt toward the right shoulder and the left shoulder (see the section The 3-Step Test, later in this chapter). Near fixation (usually 33 cm in the primary position) and reading position (depending on the patient's symptoms) complete the list of clinically important test positions.

Tests for measuring ocular alignment can be grouped into 3 basic types: cover tests, corneal light reflex tests, and subjective tests.

Cover Tests

Foveal fixation in each eye, patient attention and cooperation, and the ability to make eye movements are all necessary for cover testing. If the patient is unable to maintain constant fixation on an accommodative target, cover tests should not be used. There are 3 main types of cover tests: cover-uncover, alternate cover, and simultaneous prism and cover. All can be performed at distance or near fixation.

The monocular *cover-uncover* test is the most important test for detecting manifest strabismus and for distinguishing a heterophoria from a heterotropia (Fig 7-1; Video 7-1). As the target is viewed, one eye is covered and the opposite eye observed for any movement, which would indicate a heterotropia. The occluder is then removed. If there is no movement of the noncovered eye when the occluder is introduced, movement of the *covered eye* in one direction with application of the occluder and then in the opposite direction (a fusional movement) with removal of the occluder would indicate a heterophoria. If the patient has a heterophoria, the eyes will be straight before and after the cover-uncover test; the deviation appears during the test because of interruption of binocular vision. A patient with a heterotropia, however, starts with a deviated eye and, after testing, ends with the same eye or—in the case of an *alternating heterotropia*—the opposite eye deviated. In patients with intermittent heterotropia, the eyes may be straight before testing but become dissociated after occlusion.

VIDEO 7-1 The cover-uncover test
Animation developed by Steven M. Archer, MD, and Kristina Tarczy-Hornoch, MD, DPhil.
Access all Section 6 videos at www.aao.org/bcscvideo_section06.

眼位的评估

诊断眼位

*注视诊断眼位*是指以 9 个不同注视方位为核心，评估双眼眼位的基本检查。包括以有下几种眼位

- *第一眼位：*眼直视前方无限远处的物体，实际上为 6m 或 20ft。在该眼位，头部应该垂直。
- *6 个基本眼位：*2 条肌肉（在每眼中有 1 条肌肉）起主要作用，将眼球转动所到各自的注视位置（见第 4 章）。
- *正上和正下：*这 2 种眼位不是由单独的一条眼肌完成的，因为从第一眼位上转或下转需要斜肌和垂直直肌的共同作用，见第 4 章。

对于垂直斜视患者，诊断眼位还包括使头部向右肩和左肩倾斜时的眼位（参见本章后面的“3 步测试法”一节）。视近（为第一眼位时的 33cm 处）和阅读眼位（取决于患者的症状）等都为临床重要的检测眼位。

评估眼位的检测分为 3 种基本类型：遮盖试验、角膜光反射试验和主观试验。

遮盖试验

遮盖试验的必要条件是，每眼均为中心凹固视，患者需集中注意力和并配合检查，以及能进行眼球运动。如果患者无法在调节视标上保持固视，则不宜进行遮盖试验。主要有 3 种类型的遮盖试验：遮盖 - 去遮盖、交替遮盖和棱镜下的遮盖试验。这几类试验都可以在远处或近处的固视点进行。

单眼的遮盖 - 去遮盖试验是检测显性斜视、鉴别隐性斜视与显性斜视的最重要的测试（图 7-1；视频 7-1）。注视目标时，遮盖一眼，另一眼有移动，提示有斜视。然后移开遮挡板。如果在遮盖一眼时，未遮盖的眼没有动，而遮盖眼在一个方向移动，再移开遮挡板，向相反方向移动（融像运动），提示隐性斜视。如果有隐性斜视，在遮盖 - 去遮盖试验前后，双眼都保持正位，而在测试过程中会出现的偏斜是因为双眼视觉的中断所致。而斜视患者，开始测试时斜视眼的眼位偏斜，测试结束时可能同一眼偏斜，或另一眼偏斜，即*交替性斜视*。间歇性斜视患者在测试前眼位可能是正位的，但在遮盖后会发生偏斜。

视频 7-1　遮盖–去遮盖试验。*（译者注：资料来源见前页原文。）*
大家可通过网站www.aao.org/bcscvideo_section06获得第6册的所有视频。

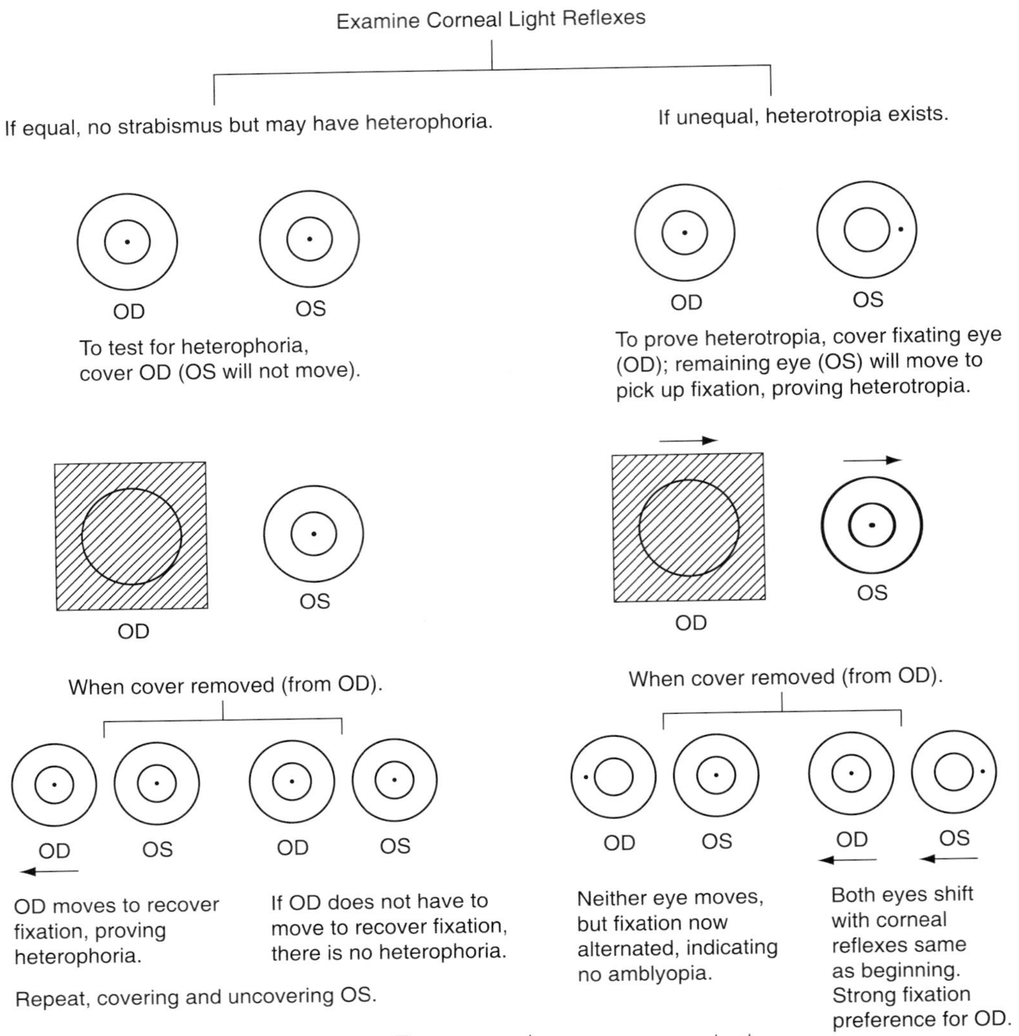

Figure 7-1 The monocular cover-uncover test.

The *alternate cover test* (Fig 7-2A; Video 7-2) detects both latent (heterophoria) and manifest (heterotropia) deviations. As the patient views the target, the examiner moves the occluder from one eye to the other, observing the direction of movement of each eye when it is uncovered. Because this test disrupts binocular fusion, dissociating the eyes, it does not distinguish between latent and manifest components. Testing should be performed at both distance and near fixation.

VIDEO 7-2 The alternate cover test.
Animation developed by Steven M. Archer, MD, and Kristina Tarczy-Hornoch, MD, DPhil.

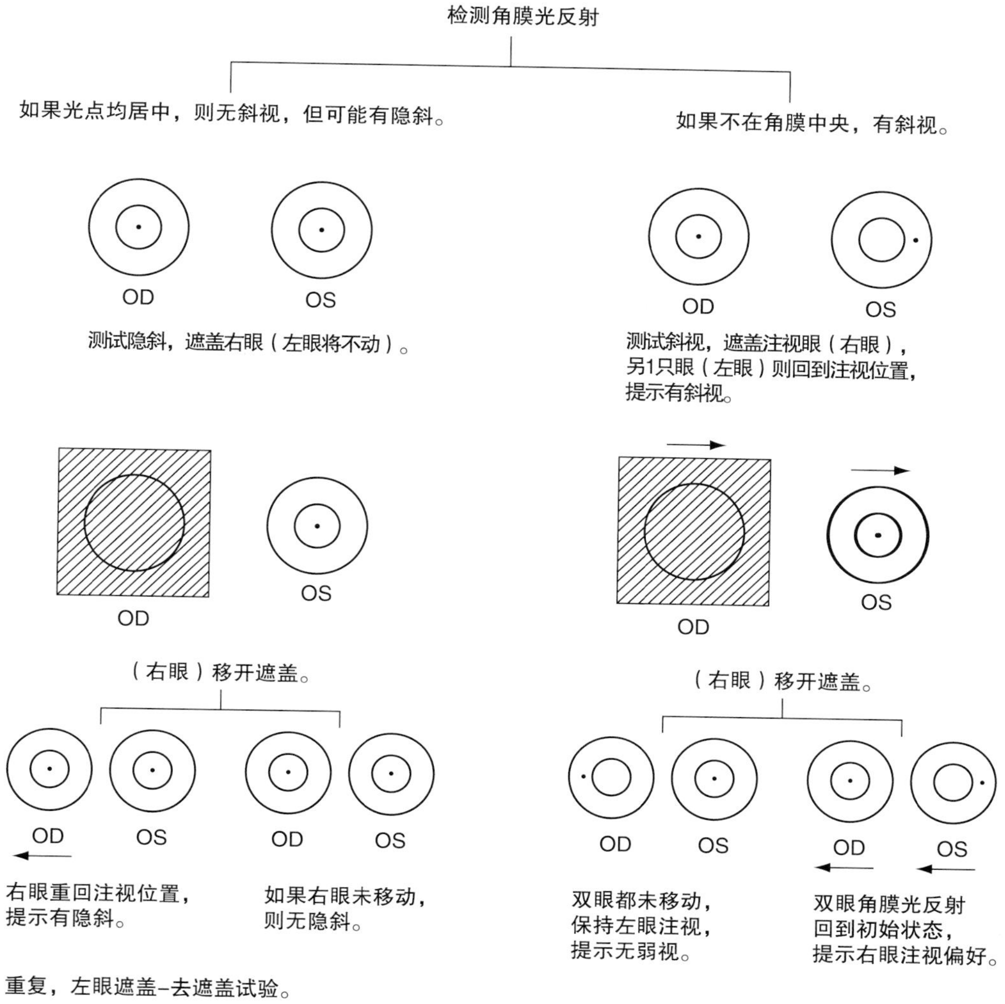
检测角膜光反射
如果光点均居中，则无斜视，但可能有隐斜。
如果不在角膜中央，有斜视。
OD
OS
OD
OS
测试隐斜，遮盖右眼（左眼将不动）。
测试斜视，遮盖注视眼（右眼），
另1只眼（左眼）则回到注视位置，
提示有斜视。
OD
OS
OD
OS
（右眼）移开遮盖。
（右眼）移开遮盖。
OD
OS
OD
OS
OD
OS
OD
OS
右眼重回注视位置，
提示有隐斜。
如果右眼未移动，
则无隐斜。
双眼都未移动，
保持左眼注视，
提示无弱视。
双眼角膜光反射
回到初始状态，
提示右眼注视偏好。
重复，左眼遮盖–去遮盖试验。

图 7–1　单眼的遮盖 – 去遮盖试验。

交替遮盖试验（图 7–2A；视频 7–2）检测潜在的（隐性斜视）和明显的偏斜（斜视）。当患者注视视标时，检查者将遮挡板从一眼移动到另一眼，观察移开遮盖时每眼的移动方向。因为该测试破坏了双眼融像，使眼分离，无法区别隐性和显性斜视。对远、近固视时都需要进行测试。

视频 7–2　交替遮盖试验。*（译者注：资料来源见前页原文。）*

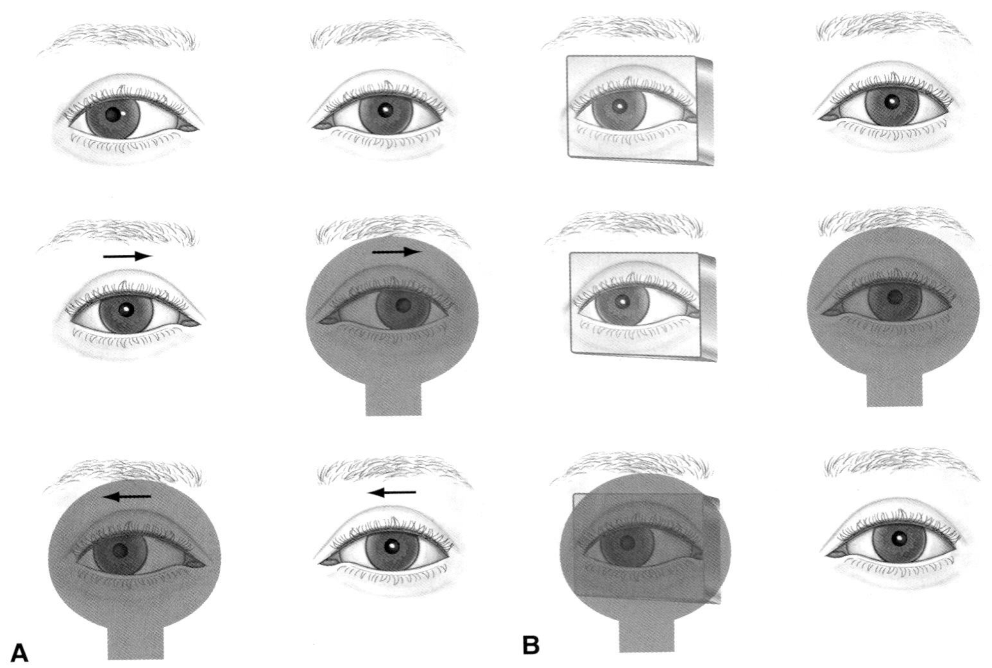

Figure 7-2 **A,**The alternate cover test. Top: Exotropia, left eye fixating. Middle and bottom: Both eyes move each time the cover alternates from one eye to the other. **B,**The prism alter-nate cover test. Top: The exotropia is neutralized with a prism of the correct power. Middle and bottom: The eyes do not move as the cover alternates from one eye to the other. *(Illustration developed by Steven M. Archer, MD; original illustration by Mark Miller.)*

In the *prism alternate cover test,* prisms of varying amount are held over one eye or both eyes during alternate cover testing; the amount of prism that neutralizes the deviation, such that eye movement is no longer seen as the occluder is moved from one eye to the other, represents the magnitude of the deviation (Fig 7-2B; Video 7-3). It may be necessary to use both horizontal and vertical prisms. This test measures the total deviation (heterotropia plus heterophoria).

VIDEO 7-3 The prism alternate cover test.
Animation developed by Steven M. Archer, MD, and Kristina Tarczy-Hornoch, MD, DPhil.

Two horizontal or 2 vertical prisms should not be stacked; such stacking can induce significant measurement errors. Deviations larger than the largest-available single prism are best measured by placing 1 prism in front of each eye, although this is not perfectly additive either. A horizontal prism and a vertical prism may be stacked over the same eye, however. Plastic prisms should always be held with the back surface (closest to the patient) in the patient's frontal plane. If the head is tilted, the prisms must be tilted accordingly. With incomitant (paretic or restrictive) strabismus, the primary and secondary deviations are measured by holding the prism over the paretic or restricted eye and the sound eye, respectively.

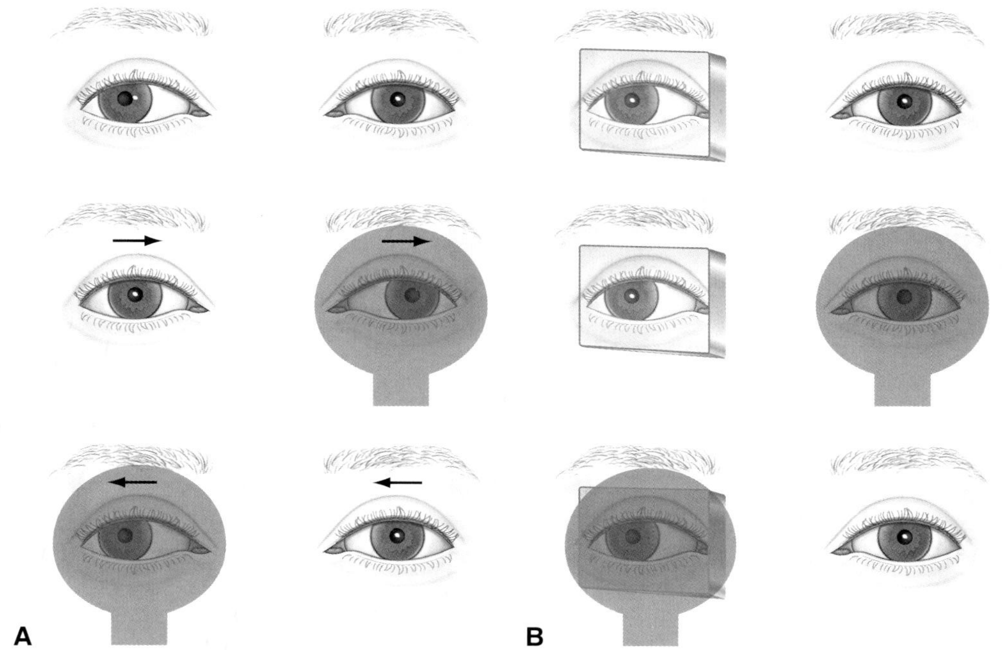

图 7–2　**A.** 交替遮盖试验。上图：外斜，左眼固视。中图和下图：每次遮挡板从 1 只眼换到另 1 只眼时，双眼都会移动。**B.** 棱镜辅助的交替遮盖试验。上图：一定度数的棱镜中和外斜。中图和下图：当遮挡板从一眼移到另一眼时，眼不会移动。*（译者注：资料来源见前页原文。）*

棱镜下的交替遮盖试验中，在交替遮盖时，在一眼或双眼前放置不同度数的棱镜；中和偏斜的棱镜度为斜视度数，即遮挡板在双眼间移动时，没有眼位的移动（图 7–2B；视频 7–3）。可能需要同时使用水平棱镜和垂直棱镜。该测试方法测量的是总偏斜度（斜视 + 隐斜）。

视频 7–3　棱镜下的交替遮盖试验。*（译者注：资料来源见前页原文。）*

2 个水平或 2 个垂直的棱镜不能叠加起来使用，这样叠加可能导致明显的测量错误。超过最大单个棱镜度数的斜视最好在每眼前放置一个棱镜来测量，尽管这也不是最好相加方法。而水平棱镜和垂直棱镜可以在同一眼前叠加放置。塑料棱镜的背面应始终放在患者额平面（尽量接近患者）。如果患者头部倾斜，棱镜必须相应倾斜。对于非共同性斜视（麻痹性或限制性斜视），通过将棱镜分别放置在麻痹或限制眼和健眼上，对第一眼位和第二眼位进行测量。

The *simultaneous prism and cover test* (Video 7-4) measures the manifest deviation during binocular viewing (only the heterotropia). The test is performed by placing a prism in front of the deviating eye and covering the fixating eye at the same time. The test is epeated using increasing prism powers until the deviated eye no longer shifts. This test has special application in monofixation syndrome. Under binocular conditions, patients with this syndrome often use peripheral fusion to exert some control over their deviation. The heterotropia alone is smaller than the total deviation (heterotropia plus heterophoria) measured by the prism alternate cover test. The simultaneous prism and cover test provides the best indication of the size of the deviation under real-life conditions.

VIDEO 7-4 The simultaneous prism and cover test.
Animation developed by Steven M. Archer, MD, and Kristina Tarczy-Hornoch, MD, DPhil.

Thompson JT, Guyton DL. Ophthalmic prisms. Measurement errors and how to minimize them. *Ophthalmology.* 1983;90(3):204–210.

Corneal Light Reflex and Red Reflex Tests

Corneal light reflex tests assess eye alignment using the location of the first Purkinje image, the image formed from reflection of a fixation light by the anterior corneal surface, which acts as a curved mirror. The Hirschberg and Krimsky tests are the main tests of this type. Though not as accurate as cover tests, they are useful for uncooperative patients and those with poor or eccentric fixation, in whom cover testing is not possible.

The *Hirschberg test* is based on the correlation between the decentration of the corneal light reflection and the ocular deviation. The ratio is about 22 prism diopters (Δ) per millimeter of decentration but can vary between 12Δ and 27Δ from one individual to the next. With an uncooperative child, it is not always possible to accurately measure the light reflex displacement, so gross estimates of the deviation are often used (although these are highly dependent on pupil size): 30Δ if the reflex is at the pupil margin, 60Δ if the reflex is in the middle of the iris, and 90Δ if the reflex is at the limbus (Fig 7-3).

The *Krimsky test* uses prisms to quantify the decentration of the corneal reflections from a handheld torch. This is done by holding a prism over either eye and adjusting the prism power until the corneal reflection is positioned symmetrically in each eye to approximate the near deviation (Fig 7-4; Video 7-5).

VIDEO 7-5 The Krimsky test.
Animation developed by Steven M. Archer, MD, and Kristina Tarczy-Hornoch, MD, DPhil.

棱镜下的遮盖试验（视频 7–4）测量在双眼注视时（仅有斜视）的显性偏斜。本实验是在斜视眼前面放置棱镜，同时遮盖固视眼来进行测试。不断增加棱镜的度数，反复测试，直到偏斜眼不再移动。该试验特别适用于单眼注视综合征。在双眼注视的情况下，这种综合征的患者常使用周边融像来控制眼的偏斜。单眼测量的斜视度数小于棱镜下的交替覆盖试验测量的总斜视度数（斜视加隐斜）。棱镜下的遮盖试验最适用于测量实际生活中的斜视度数。

视频 7–4　遮盖的同时进行棱镜试验。*（译者注：资料来源见前页原文。）*

Thompson JT, Guyton DL. Ophthalmic prisms. Measurement errors and how to minimize them. *Ophthalmology*. 1983;90(3):204–210.

角膜光反射和红光反射试验

角膜光反射试验是用第一 Purkinje 像的位置评估眼位，这是由固定光源照射角膜前表面（相当于曲面镜）反射后所形成的像。Hirschberg 试验和 Krimsky 试验为主要的测试方法。虽然不如遮盖试验准确，但对于不配合检查的患者和注视不佳或旁中心注视的患者有用，因为他们无法进行遮盖试验。

*Hirschberg 试验*基于角膜光反射点偏离角膜中心与眼偏斜之间的相关性。其偏中心比值为 22 棱镜度（Δ）/mm，但不同人的变化范围在 12 ~ 27 棱镜度（Δ）/mm。如果患儿不合作，就很难准确测量角膜光反射位置，常粗略估计偏斜的大小（高度依赖于瞳孔的大小）：如果反射光点位于瞳孔边缘，约 30Δ；如果反射光点位于虹膜中间，约为 60Δ；如果反射光点在角膜缘，约为 90Δ（图 7–3）。

*Krimsky 试验*是使用棱镜来量化手持手电筒的角膜光反射点的偏离程度。将棱镜放置在任一眼上，并调整棱镜的屈光度，直到角膜光反射点在双眼中对称，估算视近时的偏斜度数（图 7–4；视频 7–5）。

视频 7–5　Krimsky试验。*（译者注：资料来源见前页原文。）*

The *angle kappa*, the angle between the visual axis and the anatomical pupillary axis of the eye (Fig 7-5), can affect corneal light reflex measurements. The fovea is usually slightly temporal to the pupillary axis, making the corneal light reflection slightly nasal to the center of the cornea. This is termed *positive angle kappa*. A large positive angle kappa (eg, from temporal dragging of the macula in cicatricial retinopathy of prematurity) can simulate exotropia. If the position of the fovea is nasal to the pupillary axis, the corneal light reflection will be temporal to the center of the cornea. This *negative angle kappa* simulates esotropia. The angle kappa does not affect any of the cover tests.

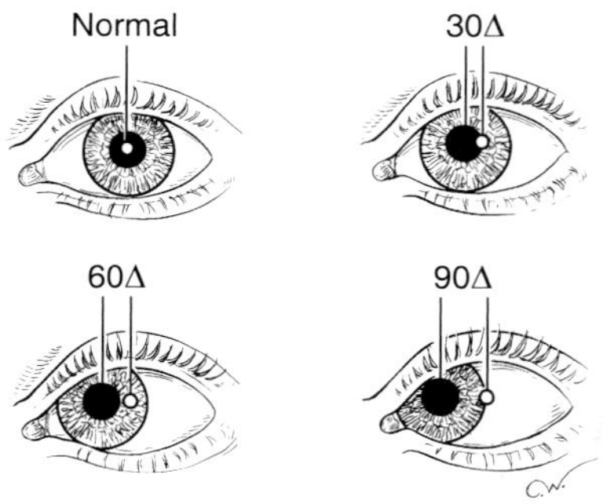

Figure 7-3 Hirschberg test, left eye. The extent to which the corneal light reflex is displaced from the center of an average-sized pupil provides an approximation of the angular size of the deviation (here, a left esotropia). Δ = prism diopter. *(Modified with permission from Simon JW, Calhoun JH. A Child's Eyes: A Guide to Pediatric Primary Care. Gaines-ville, FL: Triad Publishing Company; 1997:72.)*

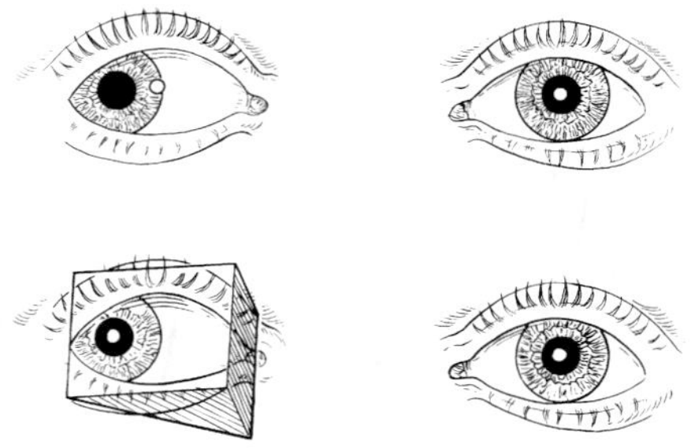

Figure 7-4 Krimsky test. The magnitude of the right exotropia is estimated by the power of the prism required to produce symmetric pu-pillary reflexes, as shown at bottom. *(Reprinted with permission from Simon JW, Calhoun JH. A Child's Eyes: A Guide to Pediatric Primary Care. Gainesville, FL: Triad Pub-lishing Company; 1997:72.)*

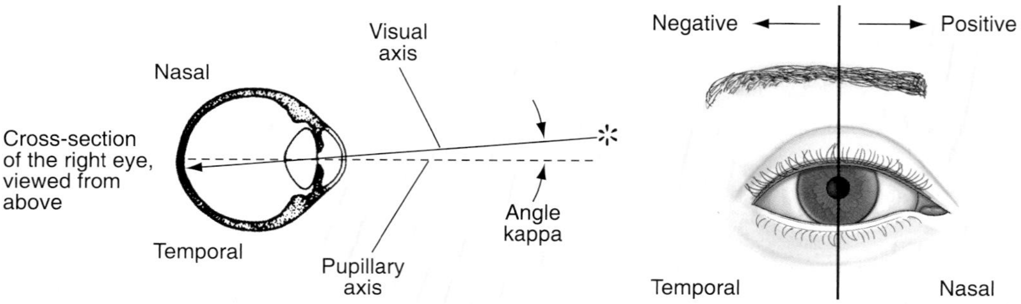

Figure 7-5 Angle kappa. A positive angle kappa (in which the corneal light reflex is nasally dis-placed; shown in cross-section for the right eye), if large enough, simulates exotropia, whereas a negative angle (in which the light reflex is temporally displaced) simulates esotropia. *(Modified with permission from Parks MM. Ocular Motility and Strabismus. Hagerstown, MD: Harper & Row; 1975.)*

In the *Brückner test*, the direct ophthalmoscope is used to obtain a red reflex simultaneously in both eyes. Foveation of the ophthalmoscope filament dims the red reflex. If strabismus is present, the deviated eye will have a lighter and brighter reflex than the fixating eye. Media opacities and refractive errors can also cause unequal red reflexes. Simultaneously, the positions of the corneal light reflexes can be assessed. This test is used mainly by primary care practitioners to screen for vision disorders.

*kappa 角*为眼的视轴和瞳孔轴之间的夹角（图 7–5），可以影响角膜光反射的测量。中央凹位于瞳孔轴偏颞侧，使角膜光反射点在角膜中心偏鼻侧。这被称为*正 kappa 角*。大角度的正 kappa 角（如早产儿视网膜病变视网膜的瘢痕将黄斑向颞侧牵拉）呈外斜状。如果中央凹的位置位于瞳孔轴鼻侧，角膜光反射点位于角膜中心的颞侧。这个*负 kappa 角*呈内斜状。kappa 角不受遮盖试验影响。

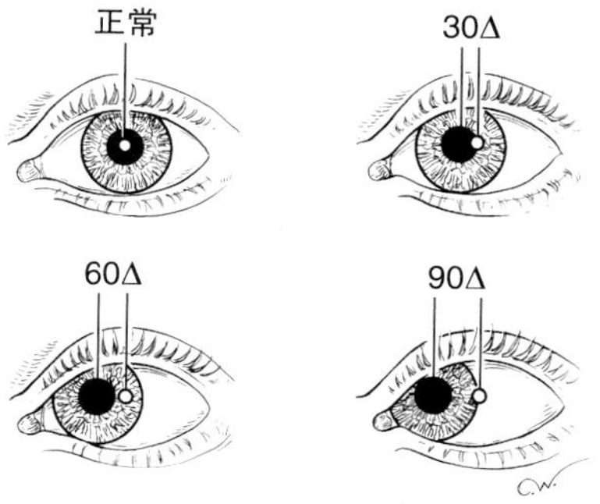

图 7–3　左眼的 Hirschberg 试验。根据角膜光反射点偏移平均瞳孔直径中心的程度估算斜视角度数（此为左眼内斜）。Δ= 棱镜屈光度*（译者注：资料来源见前页原文。）*

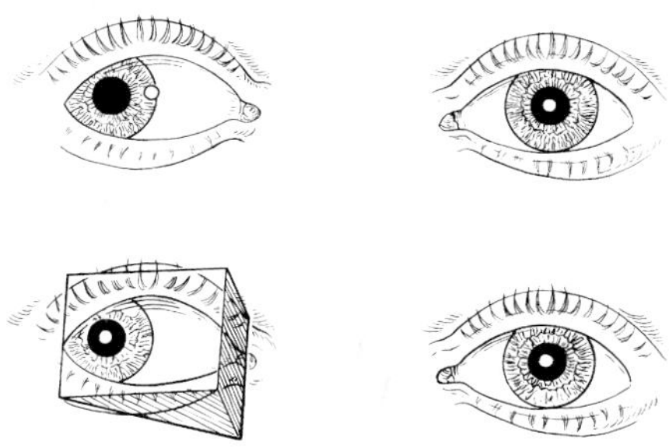

图 7–4　Krimsky 试验。将角膜光反射点调至对称正位瞳孔反射所需的棱镜度数，估算右眼外斜度数，如下图所示。*（译者注：资料来源见前页原文。）*

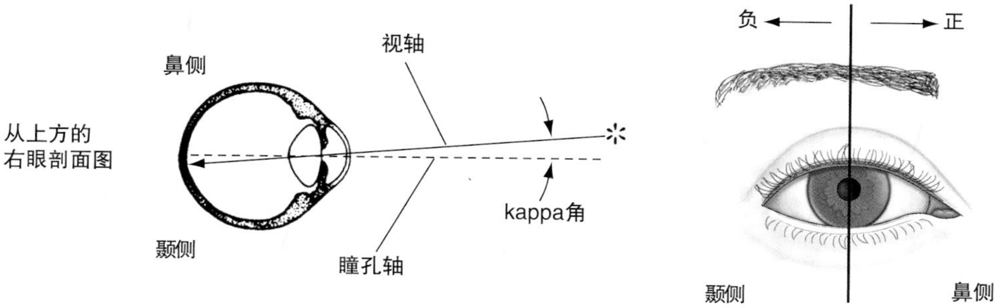

图 7–5　kappa 角。正 kappa 角（角膜光反射点在瞳孔中心的鼻侧；右眼的剖面图），如 kappa 角足够大，呈外斜状。负 kappa 角（角膜光反射点在瞳孔中心的颞侧），呈内斜状。*（译者注：资料来源见前页原文。）*

*Brückner 试验*是使用直接检眼镜同时照射双眼，观察双眼的红光反射。检眼镜灯丝落入中央凹使红色反射变暗。如果出现斜视，斜视眼的反射会比注视眼更明亮、红光反射也更强。间质混浊和屈光不正也会导致不均匀的红色反射。同时也可以评估角膜光反射点的位置。这项测试主要用于初级保健医生用来筛查视觉障碍。

Subjective Tests of Ocular Alignment

The *Maddox rod test assesses* ocular alignment using the patient's perception of the relative position of the images seen by each eye. For the eye viewing through the Maddox rod, a series of parallel cylinders convert a point source of light into a line image perpendicular to the cylinders. Like alternate cover testing, the test is dissociating and precludes fusion; thus, heterophorias and heterotropias cannot be differentiated. The test cannot assess alignment in patients with anomalous retinal correspondence (ARC) or suppression.

To test for horizontal deviations, the Maddox rod is held in front of 1 eye (eg, right eye) so that the cylinders are horizontal. The patient, fixating on a point source of light, sees a vertical line with the right eye and the point source of light with the left. Assuming normal retinal correspondence (NRC), in orthophoria, the point superimposes on the line; in esodeviations, the light is seen to the left of the line; and in exodeviations, the light is to the right of the line (see the section The Red-Glass (Diplopia) Test). The deviation is measured by finding the prism power that superimposes the point source on the line. Note, however, that unlike in cover testing with an accommodative target, accommodative convergence is not controlled by this technique. Vertical deviations can be assessed by orienting the cylinders vertically.

The *double Maddox rod test* (Fig 7-6) is used to measure cyclodeviations. Two Maddox rods are placed in a trial frame or phoropter and aligned vertically so that the patient sees 2 horizontal lines. A small vertical prism may be introduced to help separate the lines. The rod axes are rotated until the patient sees parallel lines. The angle of rotation indicates the magnitude and direction (intorsion or extorsion) of cyclodeviation. Traditionally, a red Maddox rod and a clear one were paired, but this was thought to bias the patient's localization of the cyclodeviation toward the eye with the red rod. Using the same color bilaterally avoids this bias. In congenital conditions such as congenital superior oblique palsy, the patient may not subjectively appreciate torsion or indicate any torsion with the double Maddox rod test. In these cases, seeing fundus torsion on indirect ophthalmoscopy can aid diagnosis.

The *Lancaster redgreen test* (and variations such as the Hess, Harms, and Lees screen tests) is useful for assessing ocular alignment in complicated incomitant strabismus in cooperative patients with NRC and no suppression (see Chapter 5), such as adults with acquired strabismus. Reversible redgreen goggles, redslit and greenslit projectors, and a grid projected or marked on a screen or wall are used in the test. With the red filter in front of the patient's right eye, the examiner projects a red slit onto the grid; the patient places the green slit so that it appears superimposed on the red slit. The relative positions of the streaks are recorded. The test is repeated for the 9 diagnostic positions of gaze, and the goggles are reversed to record deviations with the fellow eye fixating.

The *major amblyoscope* (Fig 7-7A) can be used to measure ocular alignment both objectively and subjectively. It may be particularly useful in adult strabismus, as it allows neutralization of torsional diplopia to assess fusional responses and can help characterize ARC. Separate, dissimilar targets are presented to each eye simultaneously, and the amblyoscope is adjusted until the patient sees the images superimposed. If the patient has NRC, the horizontal, vertical, and torsional deviations can be read directly from the calibrated scale of the amblyoscope (Fig 7-7B). See also the section Amblyoscope Testing, later in this chapter.

眼位的主观检查

*Maddox 杆试验是*利用患者对每眼接收到图像的相对位置来评估眼位。通过 Maddox 杆的一组平行的柱镜将一个点光源转换成垂直于柱镜的线条图像。与交替遮盖试验一样，该测试分离和阻止融像，因此不能区分隐斜和斜视。此测试不能评估视网膜异常对应（ARC）或有视觉抑制的眼位。

测量水平偏斜，将 Maddox 杆放在一眼（如右眼）的前面，柱镜处于水平位。病人注视点光源，右眼所见为垂直线条，左眼是点光源。假设在正视眼中，视网膜正常对应（NRC），光点叠加在垂直线上；光点在直线的左侧为内斜；光点在直线的右侧为外斜［见“红玻璃（复视）试验”一节］。通过加棱镜使光点叠加到垂直线上来测量偏斜的大小。然而，需注意的是与调节视标的遮盖试验不同，调节性集合不受此方法的限制。垂直偏斜可通过垂直放置柱镜来测量。

双 Maddox 杆试验（图 7–6）用于测量旋转斜视。2 个 Maddox 杆放置在一个试镜架或综合验光仪中，并垂直平行放置，患者看到 2 条水平线。放置一个小度数的垂直棱镜分离 2 条线。旋转 Maddox 杆轴位，直到患者看到平行的 2 条线。旋转的角度提示旋转偏斜的大小和方向（内旋或外旋）。传统使用 1 个红色 Maddox 杆和 1 个透明 Maddox 杆，但旋转偏斜会偏向红色 Maddox 杆的眼。双眼使用相同的颜色可以避免这种偏差。在先天性上斜肌麻痹等先天性疾病中，患者可能不会主观地意识到旋转，也不会通过双杆试验检测出旋转。用间接检眼镜检查有助于诊断眼底的旋转。

Lancaster 红 – 绿试验（包括 Hess、Harms 和 Lees 屏试验等）可用于评估复杂非共同性斜视的眼位，患者需配合良好、具有视网膜正常对应及无视觉抑制（见第 5 章），如成人的获得性斜视。测试中使用翻转的红绿镜、红裂隙和绿裂隙投影器以及投影或显示在屏幕或墙上的网格。当红色滤光片放置在患者右眼前，检查者将一条红色裂隙光投射到网格上；患者将绿色裂隙重合在红色裂隙上，使其看起来叠加在红色裂隙光带上。记录条纹的相对位置。重复测试 9 个注视诊断眼位。翻转红绿镜，另一眼注视，依此法记录偏斜程度。

大型弱视仪（图 7–7A）可测量客观和主观眼位，特别适用于成人的斜视，因为通过中和旋转复视，评估融像反应，还可以描述视网膜异常对应 ARC 的性质。将不同的分离视标同时放置在双眼前，调整弱视仪，直到患者看到叠加的图像。如果患者有正常视网膜对应 NRC，水平、垂直和旋转偏斜可直接从弱视仪的刻度上读取（图 7–7B）。另见本章后的“弱视仪试验”一节。

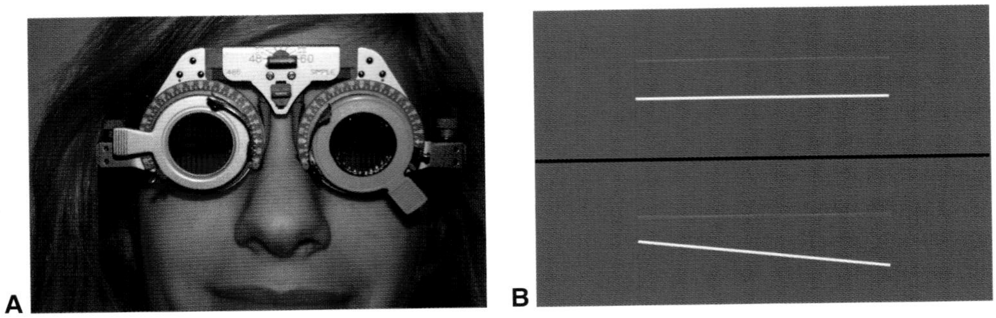

Figure7-6 Double Maddox rod test. **A,** The cylinders are aligned vertically, such that a patient with normal binocular vision sees 2 superimposed horizontal lines. **B,** Top: View seen by a pa-tient with a small left hypertropia and no torsion. Bottom: View seen by a patient with a small left hypertropia and extorsion. *(Part A courtesy of Scott Olitsky, MD; part B courtesy of Steven M. Archer, MD.)*

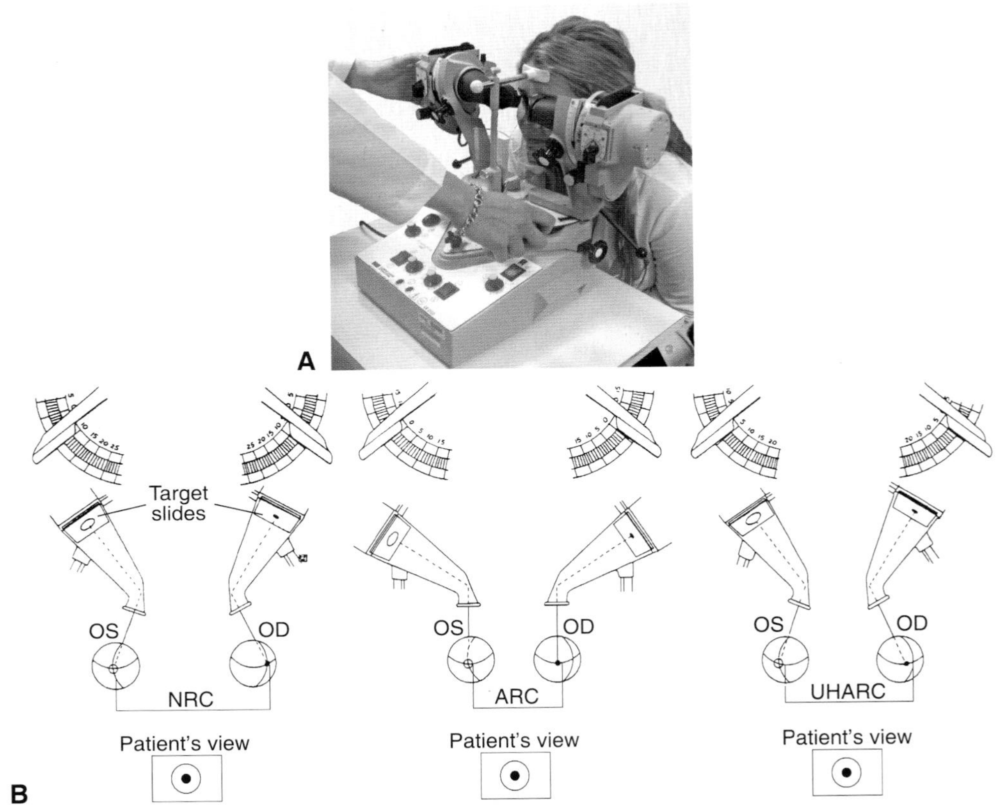

Figure 7-7 **A,** The major amblyoscope. Targets can be placed in each arm of the device to be presented separately to each eye. The arms can then be moved to compensate for ocular misalignment. **B,** Testing with a major amblyoscope for retinal correspondence in a patient with 20Δ of esotropia. NRC = normal retinal correspondence, with a fused percept when the angle of strabismus is fully compensated, presenting targets to the fovea of each eye; ARC = anomalous retinal correspondence (harmonious), with a fused percept in the absence of any compensation for the angle of strabismus, with one eye viewing the target foveally and the other extrafoveally; UHARC = unharmonious anomalous retinal correspondence, with a fused percept when the angle of strabismus is partially compensated. *(Part A courtesy of Steven M. Archer, MD; part B modified with permission from von Noorden GK, Campos EC. Binocular Vision and Ocular Motility: Theory and Management of Strabismus. 6th ed. St Louis: Mosby; 2002:229.)*

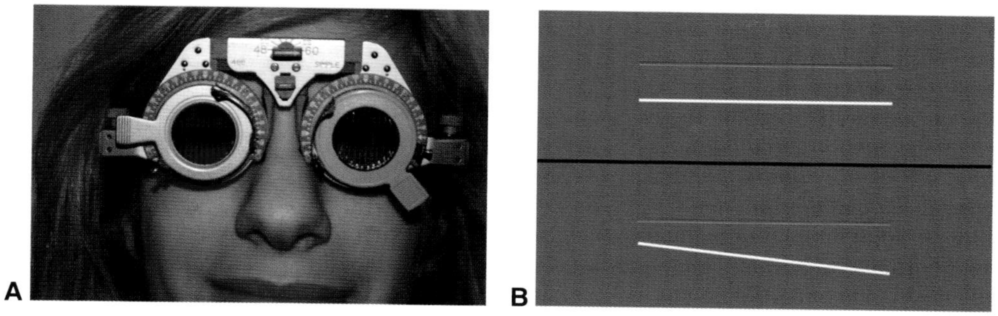

图 7-6　双 Maddox 杆试验。**A.** 柱镜垂直放置，双眼视正常的患者会看到 2 条重合的水平线条。**B.** 上图为左眼轻微上斜的患者所见，没有旋转。下图为左眼轻微上斜并外旋的患者所见。*（译者注：资料来源见前页原文。）*

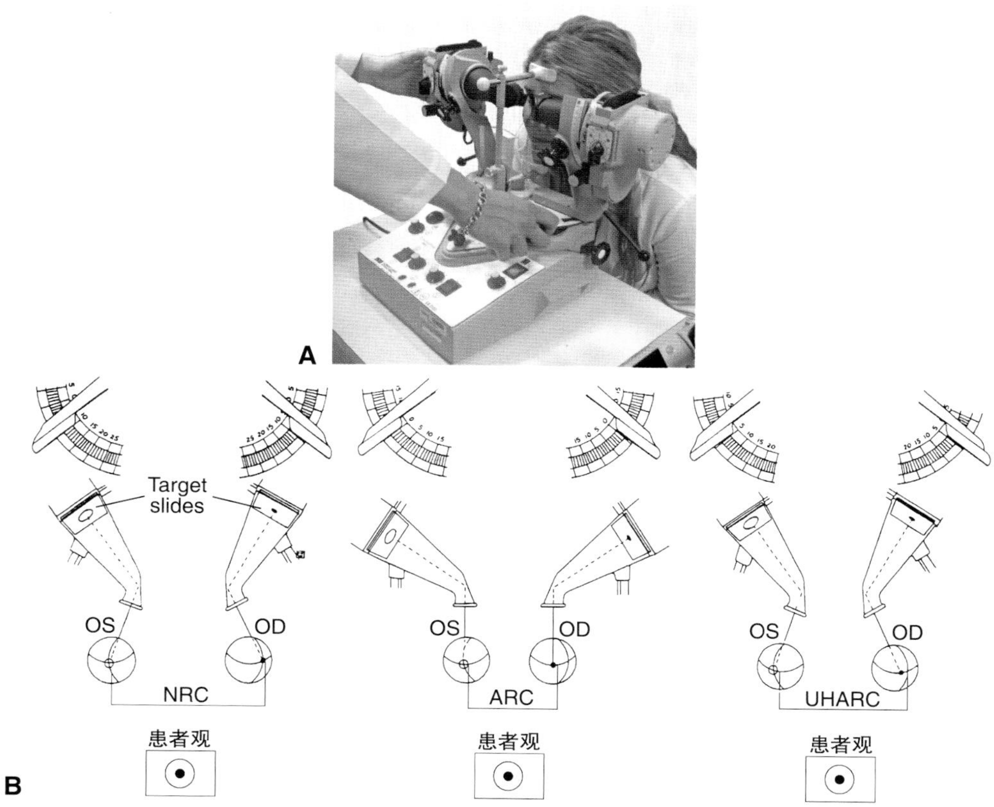

图 7-7　**A.** 弱视仪。视标放置在设备的 2 个镜筒中，分别对应一眼。然后可以通过移动镜筒来补偿眼位的偏斜。**B.** 用大型弱视仪检查 20Δ 内斜视的视网膜对应性。NRC= 正常视网膜对应，当斜视完全补偿时有融像知觉，视标落在每眼的中央凹；ARC= 异常视网膜对应（协调），在没有任何斜视补偿的情况下有融像知觉，视标落在一眼中央凹、另一眼中央凹外。UHARC= 不协调的异常视网膜对应，当斜视部分补偿时，具有融像知觉。*（译者注：资料来源见前页原文。）*

Assessment of Eye Movements

Ocular Rotations

Generally, versions are tested first; both eyes' movements into the 9 diagnostic positions of gaze are assessed. Limitations of movement and asymmetric excursion of the 2 eyes (such as "overaction") are noted. Spinning the child or the doll's head maneuver may be used to elicit vestibular-stimulated eye movements. If versions are not full, the examiner should test duction movements for each eye separately (Video 7-6). BCSC Section 5, *Neuro-Ophthalmology,* also discusses testing of the ocular motility system.

VIDEO 7-6 Versions and ductions.

Convergence

To determine the *near point of convergence,* the patient fixates on an object in the midsagittal plane, and the object, positioned initially at 40 cm, is moved toward the patient until 1 eye loses fixation and turns out. The distance from the object to the patient is then measured, giving the *near point of convergence,* which is normally 8–10 cm or less. The eye that maintains fixation is considered the dominant eye. This test does not distinguish between fusional convergence and accommodative convergence.

Accommodative convergence/accommodation ratio

The *accommodative convergence/accommodation (AC/A) ratio* is defined as the amount of convergence (in prism diopters) per unit change in accommodation (in diopters). There are 2 methods of clinical measurement (see also BCSC Section 3, *Clinical Optics*):

1. The *gradient method* derives the AC/A ratio by stimulating a change in accommodation using lenses, and dividing the resulting change in deviation (in prism diopters) by the change in lens power. An accommodative target must be used, and the working distance (typically 33 cm or 6 m) is held constant. Plus or minus lenses (eg, +1.00, +2.00, +3.00, −1.00, −2.00, −3.00) are used to vary the accommodative requirement (plus lenses at distance can be used only with uncorrected hyperopia). This method measures the *stimulus AC/A ratio,* which may differ from the *response AC/A ratio.* The latter can be determined only by simultaneously measuring the refractive state of the eyes to quantify the change in accommodation actually produced.
2. In the *heterophoria method,* the measurements of the distance and near deviations are used, along with the interpupillary distance, to calculate the AC/A ratio. Comparing distance and near deviations gives a rough clinical estimate. In accommodative esotropia, a near deviation exceeding distance deviation by 10Δ or more is considered to represent a high AC/A ratio. Note, however, that in intermittent exotropia, the near deviation may be smaller than the distance deviation despite a normal AC/A ratio, because of *tenacious proximal fusion* (see Chapter 9).

眼球运动评估

眼球转动

一般来说，首先检查双眼同向运动；在 9 个诊断眼位评估双眼眼球运动情况。观察是否存在双眼运动受限以及不协调（如“功能亢进”）。转动婴幼儿头部，可能诱导前庭眼刺激性眼球运动。如果双眼同向运动异常，检查者需要进行单眼转动试验（视频 7–6）。BCSC 第 5 册《*神经眼科学*》，也讨论了眼球运动系统的检查。

视频 7–6　双眼同向运动和单眼转动运动。

集合

测量*集合近点*时，患者需注视前方双眼中线矢状面上 40cm 的视标，检查者将视标沿双眼中线逐渐移向患者，直至一眼因不能维持注视而外转时终止，记录此时视标到患者的距离，称为*集合近点*，其正常值是 8~10cm 或更少。此时，维持注视的眼称为主导眼。此检查不能区分融像性集合和调节性集合。

调节性集合 / 调节比

调节性集合 / 调节比（*AC/A*）指每单位的调节（屈光度 D）引起的集合改变（棱镜度 Δ）。有 2 种方法测量（见 BCSC 第 3 册《*临床光学*》）：

1. *梯度法*：在双眼前加球镜刺激调节改变，记录相应斜视角（棱镜度 Δ），从而计算 AC/A。试验必须使用调节视标，并将其固定于工作距离（一般 33cm 或 6m）。用正球镜或负球镜（如：+1.00，+2.00，+3.00，−1.00，−2.00，−3.00）来相应减少调节或增加调节（视标固定于远处时，只有未矫正的远视眼才可使用正透镜）。此方法用于测量*刺激性 AC/A*，而*刺激性 AC/A* 与*反应性 AC/A* 存在差异。后者中真正产生的调节反应量只能通过检查双眼屈光状态获得。

2. *隐斜法*：分别测量看远和看近的斜视角，结合瞳距来计算 AC/A。将看远和看近的斜视角进行比较，只能给出粗略的临床估计。在调节性内斜视中，当看近内斜角超出看远内斜角 10Δ 或以上时，则认为是高 AC/A。不管怎样，请注意，间歇性外斜视患者的 AC/A 值即使正常，也可能有看近偏斜角小于看远偏斜角，因为*看近产生顽固性近感知集合*（见第 9 章）。

Fusional Vergence

Vergences are movements of the 2 eyes in opposite directions (see Chapter 4). Fusional vergences are motor responses that eliminate horizontal, vertical, and, to a limited degree, torsional image disparity.

- *Fusional convergence* eliminates bitemporal retinal image disparity and controls an exophoria.
- *Fusional divergence* eliminates binasal retinal image disparity and controls an esophoria.
- *Vertical fusional vergence* controls a hyperphoria or hypophoria.
- *Torsional fusional vergence* is cyclovergence that controls an incyclophoria or excyclophoria.

Fusional vergence can be measured using an amblyoscope, rotary prism, or bar prism; the prism power is gradually increased until diplopia occurs. Accommodation must be controlled during fusional vergence testing. Normal fusional vergence amplitudes are listed in Table 7-1. Fusional vergence can be altered by the following:

- *Compensatory mechanisms:* As a deviation evolves, a larger-than-normal fusional vergence develops. Large fusional vergences are common in compensated, longstanding vertical deviations and exodeviations.
- *Change in vision:* An improvement in vision may facilitate the fusional vergence mechanism and change a symptomatic intermittent deviation to an asymptomatic heterophoria.
- *State of awareness:* Fatigue, illness, or drug or alcohol ingestion may decrease the fusional vergence mechanism, converting a heterophoria to a heterotropia.
- *Orthoptics:* Orthoptic exercises may increase the magnitude of the fusional vergence mechanism (mainly fusional convergence). This treatment works best for near fusional convergence, particularly in convergence insufficiency.
- *Optical stimulation of fusional vergence:* In controlled accommodative esotropia, reducing the strength of the hyperopic or bifocal correction induces an esophoria that stimulates compensatory fusional divergence. In convergence insufficiency, baseout prism stimulates fusional convergence. Similarly, the power of prisms used to control diplopia may be decreased gradually to stimulate compensatory fusional vergence.

Table 7-1 Average Normal Fusional Vergence Amplitudes in Prism Diopters (Δ)

Testing Distance	Convergence	Divergence	Vertical
6 m	14	6	2.5
25 cm	38	16	2.6

Forced Duction, Active Force Generation, and Saccadic Velocity

- In the *forced duction test*, the eye is moved into various positions with the use of forceps to detect resistance to passive movement. This is usually done intraoperatively but can be done in clinic with topical anesthesia in cooperative patients.

融像性聚散

聚散是指双眼异向运动（见第 4 章）。聚散运动用以消除水平斜、垂直斜以及在一定程度上减少旋转斜所致的双眼视差。

- *融像性集合*消除双眼颞侧视网膜上的视差，控制外隐斜。
- *融像性散开*消除双眼鼻侧视网膜上的视差，控制内隐斜。
- *垂直融像功能*控制上隐斜和下隐斜。
- *旋转融像功能*控制内旋隐斜和外旋隐斜。

融像性聚散可用弱视仪、旋转棱镜或条状棱镜测量；逐渐增加棱镜度数至患者出现重影。检查过程中必须控制调节。正常融像性聚散范围见表 7–1。融像性聚散可能因以下情况而改变：

- *补偿机制*：随着斜视度进展，患者逐渐形成高于正常人的融像性聚散能力。常见于可代偿性长久的垂直斜视和外斜视。

- *视力变化*：视力改善可提高融像性聚散能力，使得有症状的间歇性斜视变为无症状的隐性斜视。
- *检查时状态*：疲劳、疾病、药物、酒精等可能降低融像性聚散的能力，使得隐斜变为显斜。

- *正视矫正*：正视矫正训练可增加融像性聚散的能力（主要是融像性集合）。此训练适于提高近正融像性集合范围，特别是集合不足时。

- *融像性聚散的光学刺激*：对于控制性调节性内斜视，降低远视度数或使用双焦镜会引起内隐斜，继而刺激补偿性融像性散开。当集合不足时，眼前加底向外棱镜，刺激融像性集合。同样，为了刺激补偿性融像性聚散，应逐渐降低用于控制复视的棱镜度数。

表7–1　融像性聚散范围的正常均值（棱镜度Δ）

检查距离	集合	散开	垂直
6 m	14	6	2.5
25 cm	38	16	2.6

被动牵拉试验、主动收缩试验、扫视速度

- *强迫转动试验 / 被动牵拉试验*中，用有齿镊依次向各个方向牵拉眼球，评估眼外肌被动运动的抵抗力。常用于术中检查，也可应用于门诊表面麻醉后配合的患者。

- In the *active force generation test,* the awake patient is asked to move a topically anesthetized eye while the examiner grasps it with forceps. If the muscle tested is paretic, the examiner feels less-than-normal tension.
- *Saccadic velocity* can be measured with instruments that track and record eye movement (eg, using magnetic search coils or video-based eye tracking). This measurement is useful for distinguishing paresis from restriction. For paretic muscles, saccadic velocity is low throughout the movement, whereas for restricted muscles, the velocity is initially normal but drops rapidly when the eye reaches the limit of its excursion. Clinical observation of saccadic velocity is qualitative: slow, *"floating" saccades indicate muscle paresis.*

See also BCSC Section 5, *Neuro-Ophthalmology.*

The 3-Step Test

There are 8 cyclovertical extraocular muscles (4 in each eye): the 2 *depressors* of each eye are the *inferior rectus (IR)* and *superior oblique (SO) muscles;* the 2 *elevators* of each eye are the *superior rectus (SR)* and *inferior oblique* (IO) *muscles.* Cyclovertical (especially superior oblique) muscle weakness often causes vertical deviations. The 3-*step test* (also called the *Parks-Bielschowsky 3-step test*) is an algorithm that helps identify a weak cyclovertical muscle. However, it is not always diagnostic, and results can be misleading, especially in patients with 1 of the following: more than 1 paretic muscle, previous strabismus surgery, skew deviation, or restrictions or dissociated vertical deviation (see Chapter 11). The 3-step test is performed as follows (Fig 7-8; see also Chapter 11, Fig 11-4):

- *Step 1:* Determine which eye is higher using the cover-uncover test (see Fig 7-1). Step 1 narrows the number of possible underacting muscles from 8 to 4. In the example shown in Figure 7-8, the right eye is higher than the left eye. This indicates weakness in 1 of the 2 depressors of the right eye (RIR, RSO) or 1 of the 2 elevators of the left eye (LIO, LSR). Draw an oval around these 2 muscle groups (see Fig 7-8A).
- *Step 2*: Determine whether the vertical deviation is greater in right gaze or in left gaze. In the example, the deviation is larger in left gaze. This implicates 1 of the 4 vertically acting muscles used in left gaze. Draw an oval around these (see Fig 7-8B). At the end of step 2, the 2 remaining possible muscles (1 in each eye) are either both intortors or both extortors and are either both superior or both inferior muscles (1 rectus and 1 oblique). In the example shown in Figure 7-8B, the increased left-gaze deviation eliminates 2 inferior muscles and implicates 2 superior muscles.
- *Step 3:* Known as the *Bielschowsky head tilt test,* the final step involves tilting the head toward the right shoulder and the left one during distance fixation. Head tilt to the right stimulates intorsion of the right eye (RSR, RSO) and extorsion of the left eye (LIR, LIO). Head tilt to the left stimulates extorsion of the right eye (RIR, RIO) and intorsion of the left eye (LSR, LSO). Normally, the 2 intortors and the 2 extortors of each eye have *opposite* vertical actions that cancel one another. If 1 intortor or 1 extortor is weak, the vertical action of the other ipsilateral torting muscle becomes manifest during the torsional response to head tilt.

- *主动收缩力激发试验 / 主动收缩试验*中，患者清醒状态下，表面麻醉后，检查者用有齿颞夹住结膜，嘱患者转动眼球。存在眼外肌麻痹时，检查者通过镊子可以感受到眼外肌力量的减弱。
- *扫视速度*可以用仪器追踪和记录眼球运动进行测量（例如：磁力搜索线圈或者视频眼追踪仪）。此方法可区分麻痹性斜视与限制性斜视。麻痹的肌肉使整个眼球运动过程中扫视速度降低，而限制性肌肉在扫视最初时的速度正常，当眼球到达其极限时，扫视速度突然下降。临床的扫视速度观察属于定性的：缓慢的、*“不固定”的扫视运动提示眼肌麻痹*。

见 BCSC 第 5 册《*神经眼科学*》。

3 步法试验

双眼共有 8 条垂直作用的眼外肌（每眼 4 条）：每眼的 2 条*下转肌*是*下直肌（IR）*和*上斜肌（SO）*，2 条*上转肌*是*上直肌（SR）*和*下斜肌（IO）*。垂直肌减弱（特别是上斜肌）常引起垂直斜视。*3 步法试验*（也称 *Parks–Bielschowsky 3 步法试验*）是鉴别垂直肌麻痹的操作步骤。但并不能够全部做出诊断，此方法也存在误判，特别当患者有以下情况时：存在 1 条以上的麻痹肌、曾行斜视矫正手术、反向偏斜，限制性或分离性垂直斜视（见第 11 章）。3 步法试验步骤如下（图 7–8；见第 11 章，图 11–4）：

- *第 1 步：*通过遮盖 – 去遮盖试验找到高位眼（见图 7–1）。第 1 步可以排除 8 条参与肌肉中的 4 条，如图 7–8，右眼比左眼高，因此麻痹肌为右眼下转肌之一（RIR,RSO）或左眼上转肌之一（LIO,LSR）。用椭圆形标出这 2 组眼外肌（见图 7–8A）。

- *第 2 步：*嘱患者双眼水平转动，明确向右转动还是向左转动时垂直分离更大。本例中：向左转动时垂直分离更大。提示向左注视时，4 条垂直肌中有 1 条参与。用椭圆形标出（见图 7–8B）。第 2 步后，剩下的这 2 条可能的垂直肌（每眼 1 条）或内旋肌，或外旋肌，或上方肌或下方肌（1 条直肌和 1 条斜肌）。如图 7–8B，向左转动垂直分离更大，提示可能的 2 条麻痹肌为上方眼外肌。

- *第 3 步：Bielschowsky 歪头试验*，嘱患者注视远处视标，头向右肩和左肩倾斜。向右侧歪头，诱发右眼内旋（RSR,RSO）和左眼外旋（LIR,LIO）。向左侧歪头，诱发右眼外旋（RIR,RIO）和左眼内旋（LSR,LSO）。正常情况下，每眼有 2 条内旋眼外肌和 2 条外旋眼外肌，它们在垂直方向上作用力*相反*、且相互抵消。如果 1 条内旋肌或外旋肌作用力不足，在歪头试验中，其另一条同侧旋转肌的垂直作用会更明显。

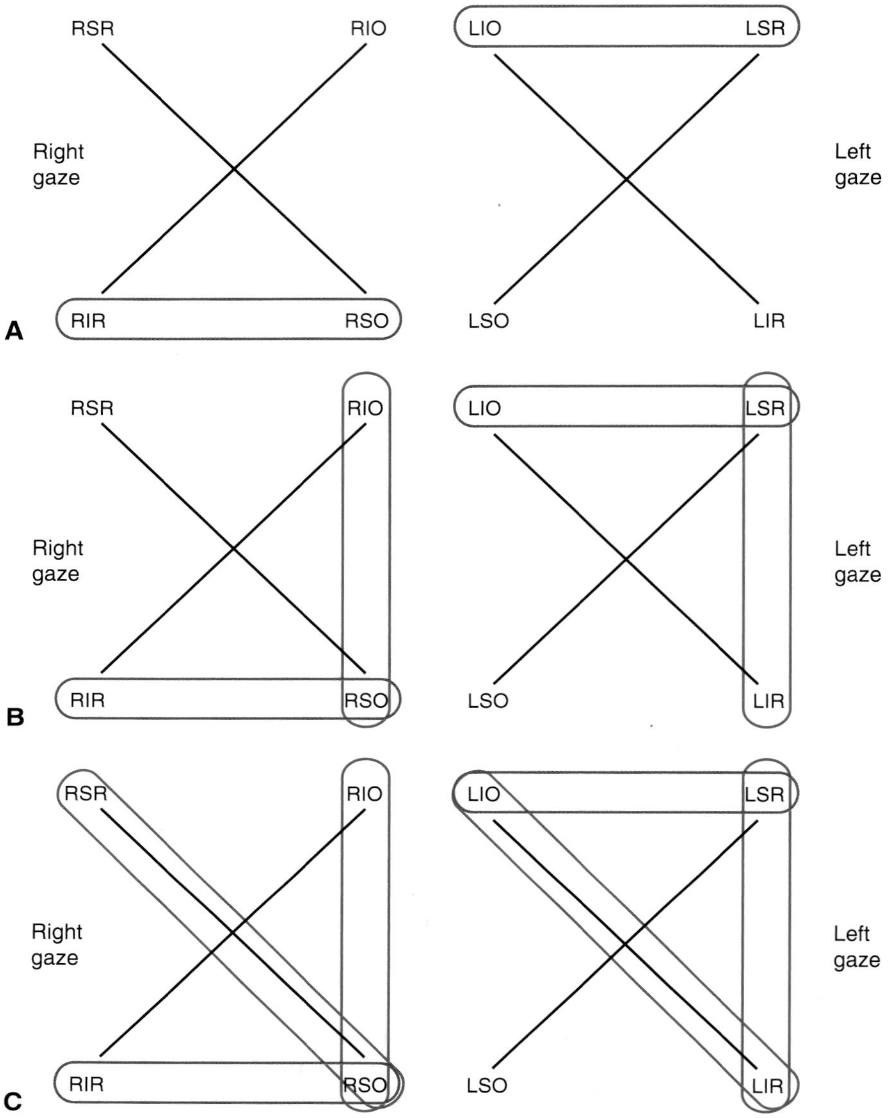

Figure 7-8 The 3-step test. The cyclovertical muscles are represented in their fields of action.**A,** Step 1: Right eye higher than left suggests weakness in 1 of the 2 depressors of the right eye (RIR or RSO) or in 1 of the 2 elevators of the left eye (LIO or LSR). **B,** Step 2: If the deviation furthermore worsens on left gaze, this implicates either the RSO or the LSR. Note that at the end of step 2, 1 depressor and 1 elevator of opposite eyes will be identified as the possible weak muscle. **C,** Step 3: If the right eye is furthermore higher in right head tilt than left head tilt, there is weakness of the RSO: right head tilt induces intorsion of the right eye, which depends on activation of both the RSO (a depressor) and the RSR (an elevator), and extorsion of the left eye, from activation of both the LIO (an elevator) and the LIR (a depressor). This rules out the LSR (which was still a candidate at the end of Step 2), and identifies the RSO as the weak muscle. LIO = left inferior oblique; LIR = left inferior rectus; LSR = left superior rectus; RIR = right inferior rectus; RSO = right superior oblique; RSR = right superior rectus.

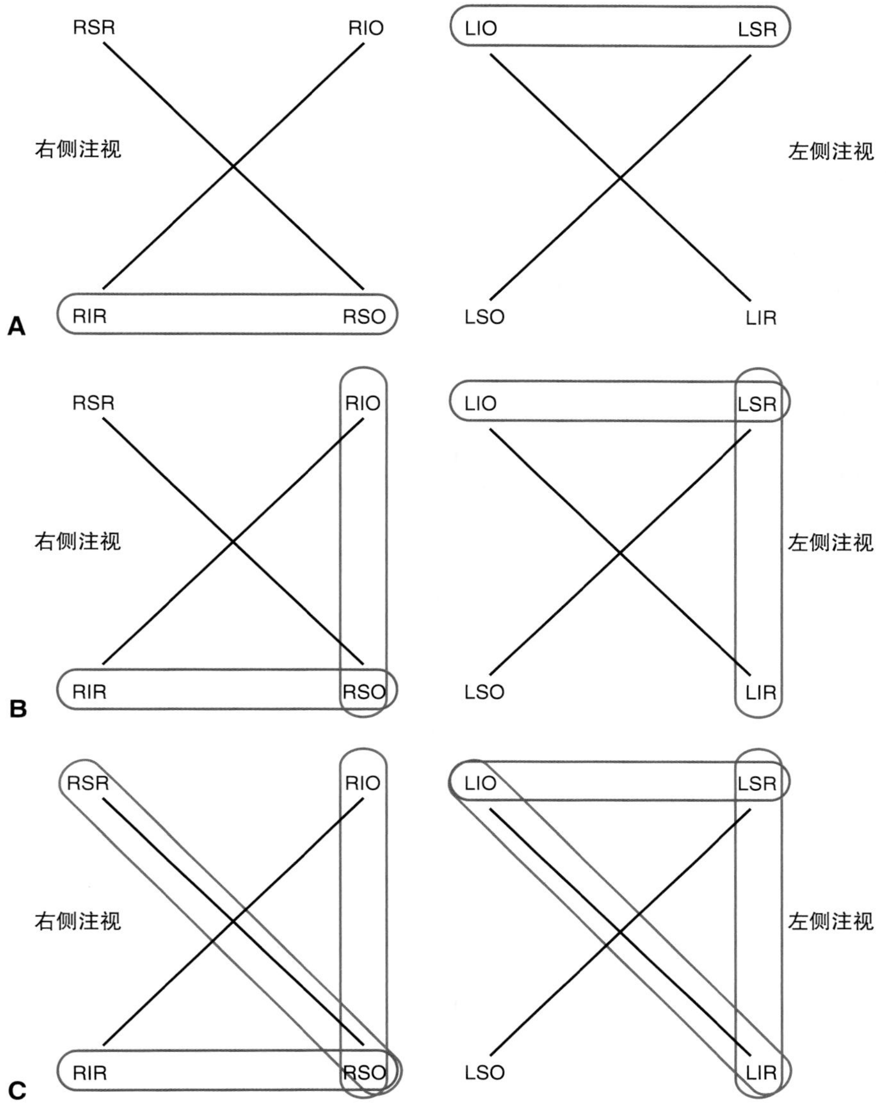

图 7–8　A. 3 步法试验。在各自诊断眼位标出 8 条垂直肌。A, 第 1 步：右眼比左眼高，证明右眼下转肌（RIR 或 RSO）中的 1 条麻痹，或者左眼上转肌中（LIO 或 LSR）的 1 条麻痹。**B.** 第 2 步：双眼向左转动，垂直分离更明显，可能的麻痹肌为 RSO 或 LSR。注意，进行第 2 步后，我们将判断麻痹肌为某一眼的上转肌或对侧眼的下转肌。**C.** 第 3 步：右侧歪头时右眼眼位更高，麻痹肌为 RSO：右侧歪头时右眼内旋，RSO（下转肌）和 RSR（上转肌）同时发挥内旋作用，左眼外旋，LIO（上转肌）和 LIR（下转肌）同时发挥内旋作用，排除 LSR（第 2 步后判断可能麻痹肌为 LSR 和 RSO 中的一个），判断麻痹肌为 RSO。LIO= 左眼下斜肌 ;LIR= 左眼下直肌 ;LSR= 左眼上直肌 ; RIR = 右眼下直肌 ; RSO = 右眼上斜肌 ; RSR = 右眼上直肌。

Tests of Sensory Adaptation and Binocular Function

Sensory binocularity involves the use of both eyes together to form a unified perception. Ideally, testing of this function is performed before binocularity or ocular alignment is disrupted by occlusion. The sensory response to strabismus is diplopia, suppression, or ARC (see Chapter 5). While a variety of sensory tests demonstrate these adaptations, the Worth 4-dot and stereopsis tests are the ones most commonly used in clinical practice. Sensory tests must be performed in conjunction with cover tests to determine whether a fusion response is due to normal alignment or ARC. Also, the clinician should remember that no sensory test can perfectly replicate habitual viewing conditions; the more dissociative the test, the greater the risk that it does not reflect habitual binocular function.

The Red-Glass (Diplopia) Test

In a strabismic patient, placing a red glass or filter before the fixating eye while the patient views a white light stimulates the fovea of the fixating eye and an extrafoveal area of the fellow eye. If the patient sees only 1 light (either red or white), suppression is present (Fig 7-9A). A 5Δ or 10Δ base-up prism placed in front of the deviated eye can move the image out of the suppression scotoma, causing the patient to experience diplopia. With NRC, the white light will be localized below and to one side of the red light (Fig 7-9B). Incorrect localization of the white light, for example, directly below the red light, indicates ARC (Fig 7-9C).

In the absence of suppression, the following results are possible:

- An esotropic patient without harmonious ARC experiences homonymous or *uncrossed* diplopia (see Chapter 5) (with the red glass over the *left* eye, the red light is perceived to the *left* of the white light—the *same* side as the red lens; Fig 7-9D). A patient with exotropia has *heteronymous* or *crossed* diplopia (with the red glass over the left eye, the red light is perceived to the *right* of the white light—the side *opposite* that of the red lens; Fig 7-9E). If the degree of separation between the 2images is consistent with the magnitude of the deviation measured by cover testing, the patient has NRC.
- If the patient sees the 2 lights superimposed so that they appear pinkish despite a measurable deviation, there is *harmonious* ARC.
- If the patient sees 2 lights (with uncrossed diplopia in esotropia and with crossed diplopia in exotropia) but the image separation is less than expected based on the measured deviation, there is *unharmonious* ARC. Some investigators consider this to be a testing artifact.

In the example shown in Figure 7-8C, the right hypertropia increases when the head is tilted to the right. This suggests that the vertical action of the right superior rectus muscle is unopposed, causing the right eye to move upward as it attempts to intort to maintain fixation; this indicates that the right superior oblique muscle is the weak muscle. (See also Chapter 11, Fig 11-3.)

感觉适应和同时视觉试验

感觉性同时视觉是指双眼同时形成一致的感知。理想状态下，需在同时视觉之前或通过遮盖打破双眼正位的条件下进行。对斜视的感觉性反应是复视、抑制或异常视网膜对应 ARC（见第 5 章）。尽管各种感觉试验都适合，但 Worth 4 点和立体视试验仍是临床上最常用的方法。感觉试验需结合遮盖试验，以确定融像反应是正常眼位，或是异常视网膜对应 ARC。医生应了解没有任何感觉试验能完全重复体现患者习惯性视觉状态，分离试验越多，其结果越不能反映习惯性同时视觉。

红玻璃（复视）试验

嘱患者双眼注视白灯，在斜视患者注视眼眼前放置红玻片或滤过片，从而刺激注视眼黄斑中心凹和对侧眼旁黄斑区。如果患者只看到 1 个灯（红灯或白灯），提示存在抑制（图 7-9A）。将 5Δ 或 10Δ 底朝上棱镜放置于偏斜眼前，棱镜使物体的成像离开抑制暗点，引发复视。对于正常视网膜对应患者，白灯位于红灯下方某一侧（图 7-9B）。如果白灯位置不正确，如白灯位于红灯正下方，提示存在异常视网膜对应（图 7-9C）。

如果不存在抑制，则可能有以下几种结果：

- 内斜视患者，没有协调异常视网膜对应 ARC，有同侧或*非交叉性*复视（见第 5 章）（红玻璃片置于*左*眼前，感知到红灯在白灯*左侧*，即与红玻璃片置放方位*相同*；图 7-9D）。外斜视患者，则存在*异侧或交叉性复视*（红玻璃片置于*左*眼前，感知到红灯在白灯*右侧*，即与红玻璃片置放方位*相反*；图 7-9E）。遮盖试验测量偏斜度，如果所感知的 2 个灯间距与其一致，则正常视网膜对应 NRC。

- 如果患者看到 2 个灯相重叠而呈现粉色，此时尽管有偏斜角存在，仍为*协调*异常视网膜对应 ARC。
- 如果患者看到 2 个灯（内斜视为非交叉复视，外斜视为交叉复视），但是 2 个灯间距小于所测偏斜角，为*不协调*异常视网膜对应 ARC。一些研究认为这种方法人为偏差较大。

图 7-8C 所示，右侧歪头时右眼上斜更明显。因为没有拮抗肌对抗右眼上直肌的垂直作用，导致内旋注视时右眼上转，为保持双眼单视，右眼上直肌发挥内旋作用，但这同时也使眼球上转，提示右眼上斜肌为麻痹肌（见第 11 章，图 11-3）。

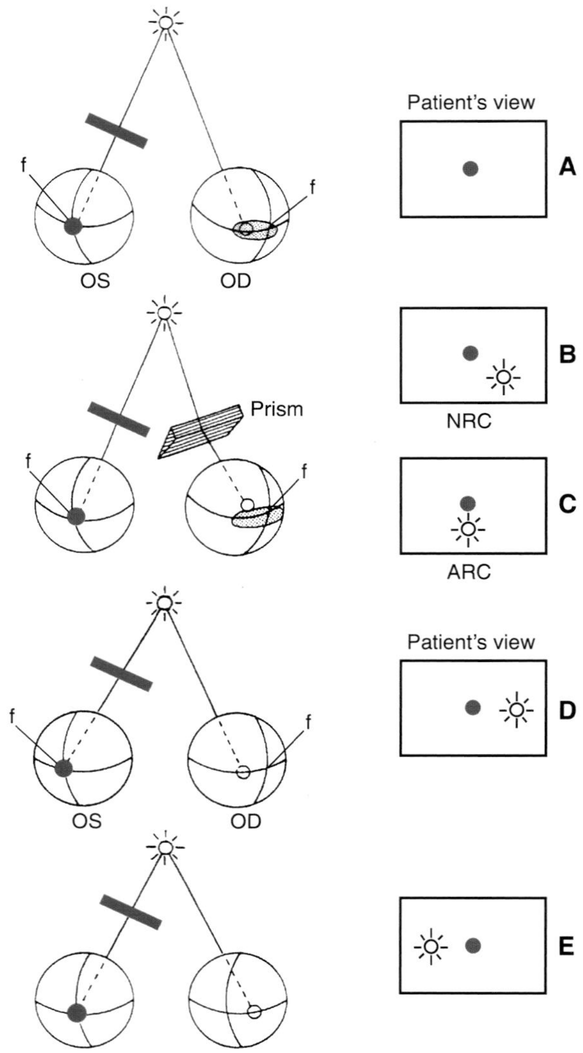

Figure 7-9 Red-glass test findings in diplopia, suppression, and ARC. *(see text for explanation; see also Chapter 5, Fig 5-5). (Modified with permission from von Noorden GK, Campos EC. Binocular Vision and Ocular Motility: Theory and Management of Strabismus. 6th ed. St Louis: Mosby; 2002:223.)*

Bagolini Lenses

Bagolini lenses have many narrow, parallel striations that, like Maddox rods, cause a point source of light to appear as a streak perpendicular to the striations. The lenses are usually placed with the striations at an angle of 135° (patient's view) for the right eye and at an angle of 45° for the left eye, and the patient fixates on a distant light. Orthotropic patients will see 2 line segments crossing at their centers, forming an "X." Figure 7-10 illustrates a range of possible subjective results. For a patient with monofixation syndrome and a central scotoma, 1 of the lines will be perceived as having a gap, corresponding to the scotoma.

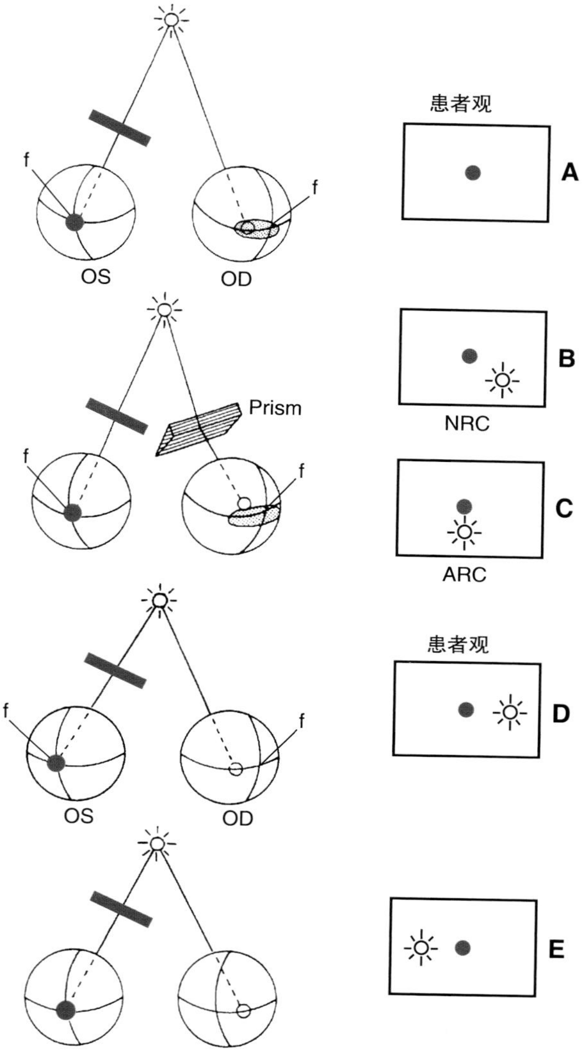

图 7–9　红玻璃试验检查复视、抑制和异常视网膜对应（图解见正文；也见第 5 章，图 5–5）。*（译者注：资料来源见前页原文。）*

Bagolini 镜

Bagolini 镜有许多细窄且相互平行的条纹，像 Maddox 杆，使光源变成 1 条光带，与条纹方向垂直。Bagolini 镜的条纹在右眼置于 135°（患者视角），左眼置于 45°，嘱患者注视远处点光源。正位眼患者将看到 2 条光线，在中点垂直交叉，呈“X”形。图 7–10 示意了可能的主观结果。如果患有单眼注视综合征和中心抑制暗点，将看到 1 条光线有中断，中断处与视网膜抑制区相对应。

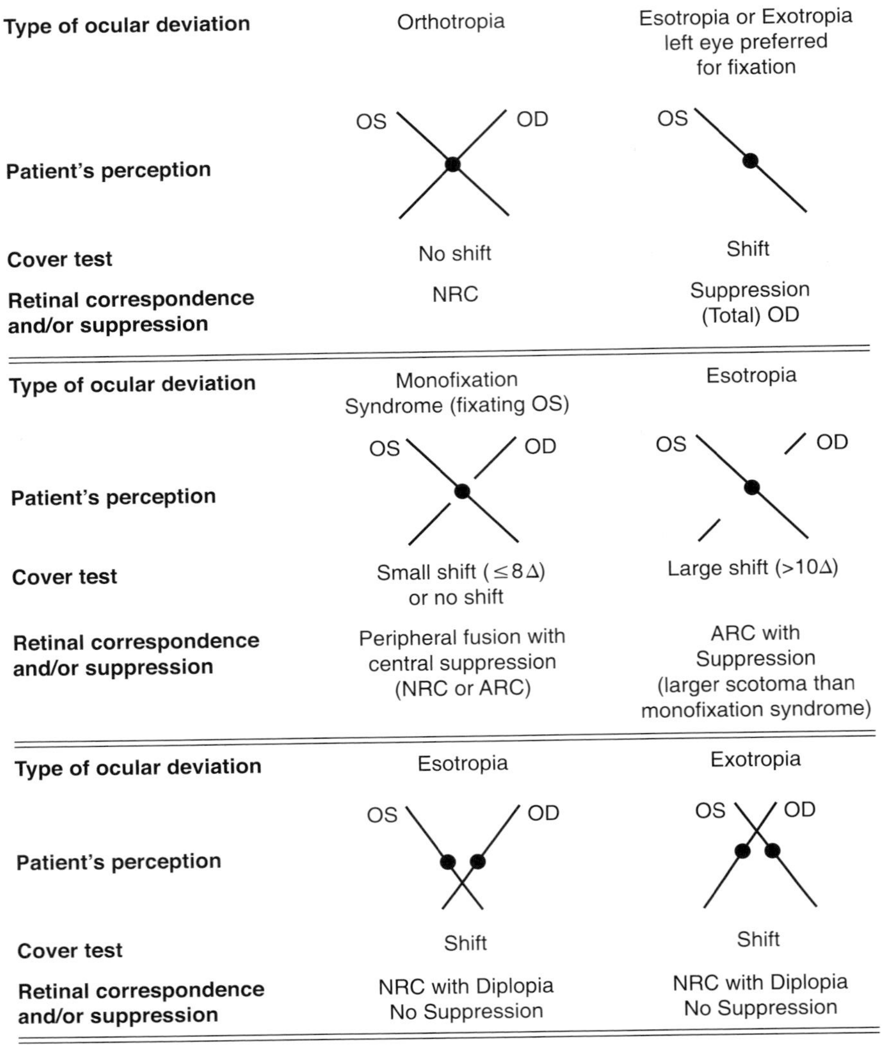

Figure 7-10 Bagolini striated lens test for retinal correspondence and suppression. For these figures, the Bagolini lens striations are oriented at 135° in front of the right eye (patient's view) and at 45° in front of the left eye, such that the patient sees a line segment at an angle of 45° with the right eye and a line segment at an angle of 135° with the left eye. The perception of the oblique lines seen by each eye under binocular conditions is shown. Examples of the types of strabismus in which these responses are commonly found are given.

Like Maddox rods, parallel Bagolini lenses can also assess torsion, but unlike Maddox rods, which are more dissociating, Bagolini lenses permit close-to-normal viewing and fusion and therefore reveal only manifest torsion; they also allow simultaneous cover testing.

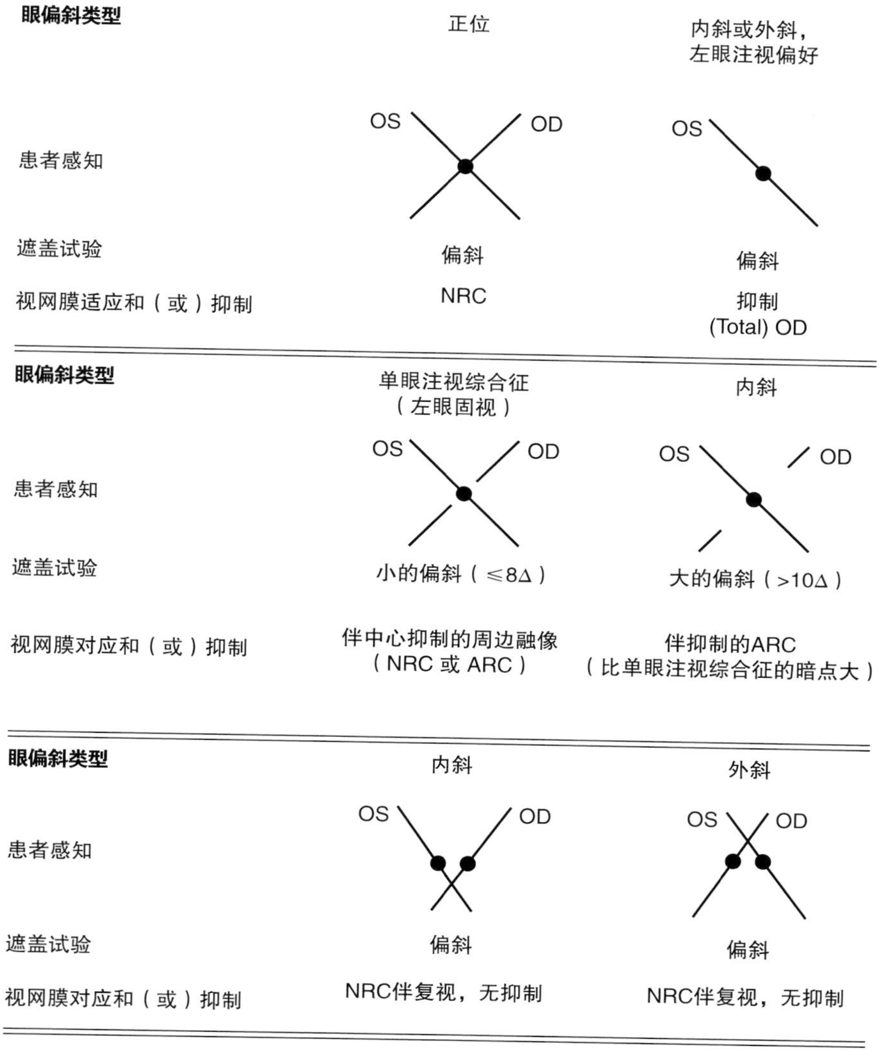

图 7-10　Bagolini 镜用于检查视网膜对应和抑制。如图，Bagolini 镜条纹分别位于右眼 135°（患者视角）和左眼 45°，从而患者右眼所见为 45° 的斜向光线，左眼所见为 135° 的斜向光线。图中展示了同时视条件下每一眼所感知的斜向光线。表格以不同斜视类型为例，展示相应双眼所见光线情况。NRC- 正常视网膜对应，ARC- 异常视网膜对应。

平行 Bagolini 镜与 Maddox 杆一样，能评估旋转。而与 Maddox 杆的像分离更大的情况不一样的是，Bagolini 镜只能允许接近正常的观察和融像，因此只能发现显性旋转；这 2 项检查需要与遮盖试验同时进行。

The 4Δ Base-Out Prism Test

The 4Δ base-out prism test can identify a small facultative scotoma in a patient with monofixation syndrome and no manifest deviation (see Chapter 5). A 4Δ base-out prism is placed before 1 eye during binocular viewing, while motor responses are observed (Fig 7-11); the test is then repeated with the prism over the other eye. Patients with bifixation usually show a version movement toward the apex of the prism, followed by a fusional convergence movement in which the eye with the prism maintains fixation while the fellow eye moves nasally to restore fusion. A similar response occurs regardless of which eye has the prism. In patients with monofixation, typically no movement is seen when the prism is placed before the nonfixating eye. When the prism is placed before the fixating eye, a refixation version movement occurs, but without any subsequent fusional convergence.

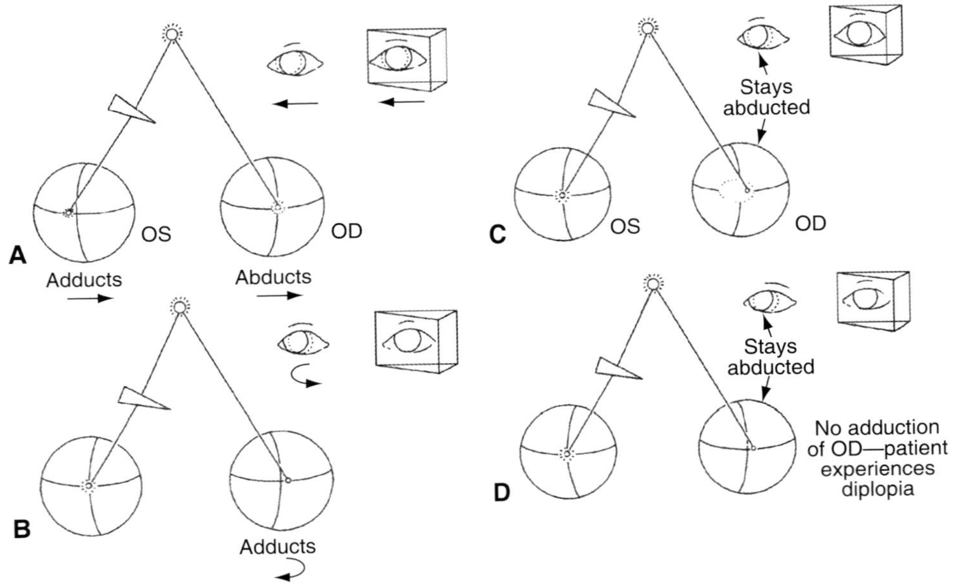

Figure 7-11 The 4Δ base-out prism test. **A,** When a prism is placed over the left eye, dextroversion occurs during refixation of that eye, indicating absence of foveal suppression in the left eye. If a suppression scotoma is present in the left eye, neither eye will move when the prism is placed before the left eye. **B,** Slow fusional adduction movement of the right eye is then observed, indicating absence of foveal suppression in the right eye. **C,** In a second patient, the absence of any such adduction movement (the right eye stays abducted after the dextrover-sion) suggests foveal suppression in the right eye. The patient does not experience diplopia. **D,** Weak fusion can also cause absence or delay of adduction movement, but in this case the patient experiences diplopia. *(Modified with permission from von Noorden GK, Campos EC. Binocular Vision and Ocular Motility: Theory and Management of Strabismus. 6th ed. St Louis: Mosby; 2002:220.)*

The 4Δ base-out prism test is the least reliable method of documenting a central suppression scotoma. Patients with bifixation may recognize diplopia when the prism is placed before an eye but make no convergence movement to correct for it. Patients with monofixation may switch fixation each time the prism is placed and show no version movement, regardless of which eye is tested.

4Δ 底朝外棱镜试验

4Δ 底朝外棱镜试验可检测出无明显偏斜的单眼注视综合征患者的微小条件性盲点（见第 5 章）。患者双眼注视一目标时，将 4Δ 底朝外棱镜置放于一眼前，观察眼球运动反应（图 7–11）；将棱镜置放于另一眼，重复一次。患者存在双注视时，双眼向棱镜尖端做同向运动，继而做融像性集合运动，即指放置棱镜的眼保持注视，对侧眼向鼻侧运动以恢复融像。无论棱镜放于哪只眼前，都有这样的现象。当患者为单眼注视时，棱镜放于非注视眼前时则无此典型眼球运动；而棱镜放于注视眼眼前时，注视眼向棱镜尖端做重新注视运动，但随后并没有融像性集合运动。

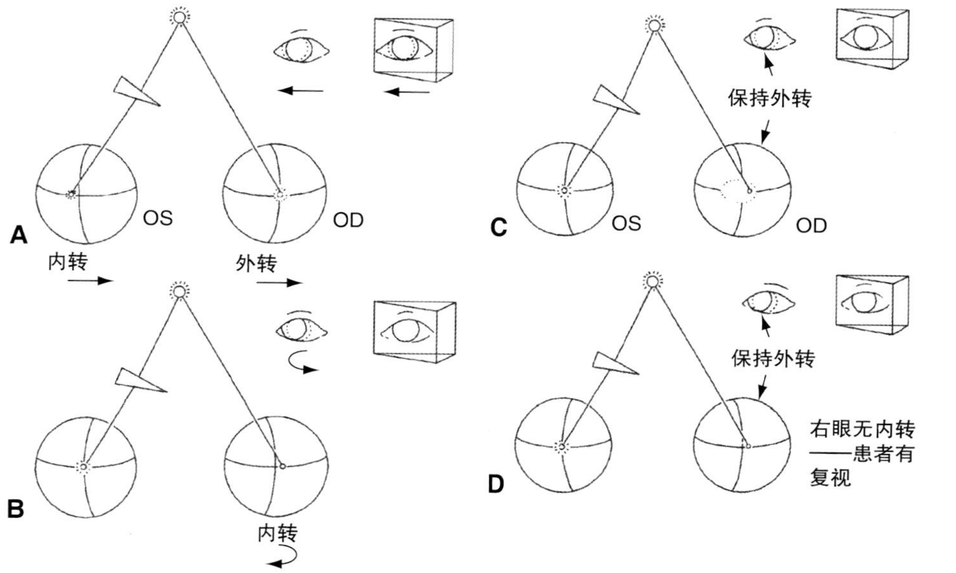

图 7–11　4Δ 底朝外棱镜试验。**A.** 棱镜置放于左眼，左眼向右转、再注视，提示左眼无黄斑中心凹抑制。如果左眼存在抑制盲点时，双眼此时都不会转动。**B.** 继而观察到右眼融像性内转，提示右眼中心凹抑制。**C.** 第 2 位患者无内转的眼球运动（右转后，右眼保持此外转位）表明右眼黄斑中心凹抑制。但患者无复视。**D.** 融像弱时，融像性集合运动也可能没有或延迟，但本例中，患者有复视。*（译者注：资料来源见前页原文。）*

4Δ 底朝外棱镜试验是检查中心抑制暗点的最不可靠的方法。原因在于，当棱镜加于任何一眼时，双注视时可能出现复视，但不发生融像性集合运动，而在眼前放置棱镜测试时出现交替的单注视，不表现出同向运动。

The Afterimage Test

This test involves stimulating the macula of each eye so as to produce a different linear afterimage in each eye, 1 horizontal and 1 vertical, by having each eye fixate on a linear light filament separately. The test can also be performed by covering a camera flash with black paper and exposing only a narrow slit; the center of the slit is covered with black tape to serve as a fixation point, as well as to protect the fovea from exposure. Because suppression scotomata extend along the horizontal retinal meridian and may obscure most of a horizontal afterimage, the vertical afterimage is induced in the deviating eye and the horizontal afterimage in the fixating eye. The patient is then asked to draw the relative positions of the perceived afterimages. Possible perceptions are shown in Figure 7-12. In patients with eccentric fixation (see Chapter 6), the afterimage is extrafoveal, and the test cannot be interpreted.

Amblyoscope Testing

Although its use has declined, the major amblyoscope (discussed earlier; see Fig 7-7) was for decades a mainstay in the assessment and treatment of strabismus. The amblyoscope can measure horizontal, vertical, and torsional deviations and can be particularly helpful in adult strabismus. Because it can neutralize torsion, this instrument is useful for distinguishing between central fusion disruption (see Chapter 5) and inability to fuse because of a large cyclodeviation. The amblyoscope can also assess fusion ability, suppression, retinal correspondence, fusional amplitudes, and stereopsis. In addition, it may be used in exercises designed to overcome suppression and increase fusional amplitudes.

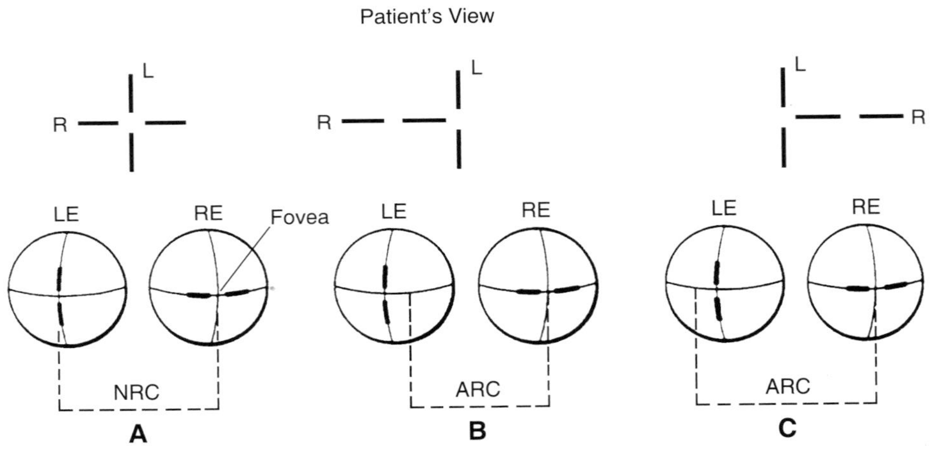

Figure 7-12 Afterimage test. **A,** Normal retinal correspondence. **B,** ARC in a case of esotropia. **C,** ARC in a case of exotropia. *(Modified with permission from von Noorden GK, Campos EC. Binocular Vision and Ocular Motility: Theory and Management of Strabismus. 6th ed. St Louis: Mosby; 2002:227.)*

后像试验

双眼分别注视线状灯丝，刺激黄斑，每眼形成 1 条线状后像，1 条水平线和 1 条垂直线。也可使用照相机闪光灯来实现，用黑纸遮住相机闪光灯，仅留出一条线形窄缝；并在窄缝中段用黑胶带覆盖，用来做注视点，同时也可保护黄斑中心凹，从而避免强光照射，因为抑制盲点沿着水平视网膜径线延伸，进而可掩盖绝大部分水平后像，因此偏斜眼形成垂直后像，注视眼形成水平后像。最后嘱患者画出所感知后像的相对位置关系。图 7–12 示几种可能的情况。对于旁中心注视（见第 6 章），后像位于黄斑中心凹旁，检测结果不能解释。

弱视仪检查

尽管大型弱视仪已经很少使用（见图 7–7），但它在斜视的评估和治疗中仍起着重要作用。弱视仪可以测量水平偏斜、垂直偏斜和旋转偏斜，特别是用于成人斜视。因为它能中和旋转斜视，而用于鉴别中心融像破坏（见第 5 章）和大度数旋转斜视的融像障碍。它也能评估融像能力、抑制、视网膜对应、融像范围和立体视觉。此外，也可以用于训练，以消除抑制、提高融像范围。

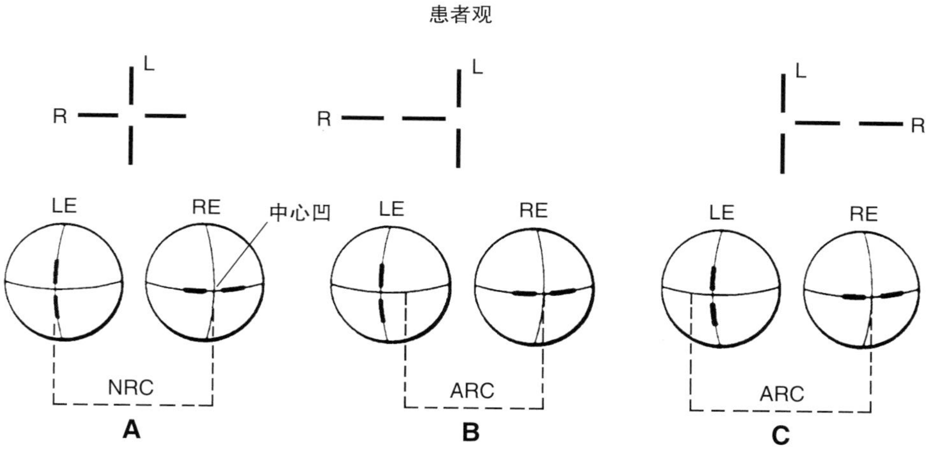

图 7–12　后像试验。**A.** 正常视网膜对应。**B.** 内斜视的异常视网膜对应。**C.** 外斜视的异常视网膜对应。*（译者注：资料来源见前页原文。）*

The Worth 4-Dot Test

The Worth 4-dot test (Fig 7-13) is often considered a test of sensory fusion; however, it does not evaluate sensory fusion directly as there is no fusible feature in the test. Its best use is to identify a suppression scotoma. The test uses red-green glasses and a target consisting of 4 illuminated dots: 1 red, 2 green, and 1 white. By convention, the red lens is placed in front of the right eye and the green lens in front of the left. The red lens blocks the green light, and the green lens blocks the red light, so the red and green dots are each seen by only 1 eye. The white dot is the only feature seen by both eyes, but it is seen in color rivalry in a patient with fusion. The *polarized Worth 4-dot test* uses polarized glasses rather than red and green ones. The stimulus lights can be presented in a wall-mounted display or with a Worth 4-dot flashlight. The test should be administered in good ambient light so that peripheral features in the room can stimulate motor fusion. The patient reports the number of dots seen:

- Seeing 2 dots indicates a suppression scotoma in the left eye.
- Seeing 3 dots indicates a suppression scotoma in the right eye.
- Seeing 4 dots indicates that if there is a suppression scotoma, it must subtend a smaller visual angle than the test target. The perception of 4 dots indicates some degree of sensory fusion, either NRC (if there is no manifest strabismus, or small-angle strabismus consistent with monofixation and peripheral fusion; see below) or harmonious ARC (if there is larger-angle manifest strabismus).
- Seeing 5 dots indicates diplopia, usually from larger-angle manifest strabismus without suppression or ARC.

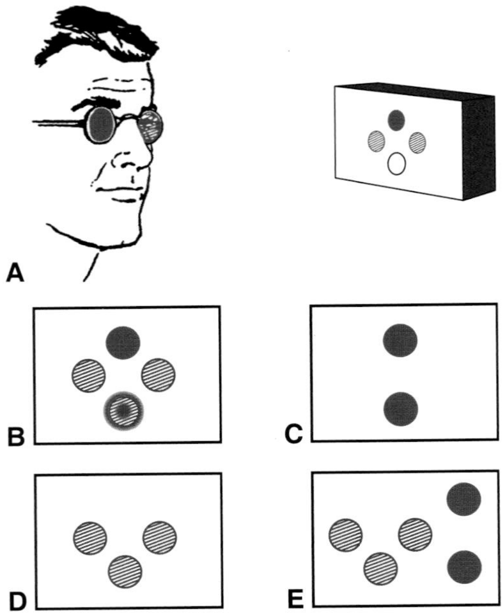

Figure 7-13 Worth 4-dot test. **A,** Looking through a pair of red-green glasses, the pa-tient views 4 illuminated dots (1 red, 2 green, 1 white) at 6 m (projected, or mounted in a box) and at 33 cm (on a Worth 4-dot flashlight). The possible responses are given in parts B through E. **B,** Patient sees all 4 dots: periph-eral fusion with orthophoria or strabismus with ARC. The dot in the 6 o'clock position is seen in color rivalry or, depending on ocular dominance, as predominantly red or predom-inantly green. **C,** Patient sees 2 red dots: sup-pression in left eye. **D,** Patient sees 3 green dots: suppression in right eye. **E,** Patient sees 5 dots: uncrossed diplopia with esotro-pia if the red dots appear to the right of the green dots, as in this figure; crossed diplopia with exotropia if the red dots appear to the left. (Modified with permission from von Noorden GK, Campos EC. Binocular Vision and Ocular Motility: Theory and Management of Strabismus. 6th ed. St Louis: Mosby; 2002:221.)

Worth 4 点试验

Worth 4 点试验是一种感觉融像功能测试；但不能直接评估感觉融像，因为试验中没有可融像功能。它最大的用处是可以检测抑制暗点。试验需要使用红绿眼镜和注视目标，其包括 4 个亮点：1 个红色、2 个绿色和 1 个白色。通常红色镜片置放于右眼眼前，绿色镜片置放于左眼眼前。红色镜片阻挡绿色光线，绿色镜片阻挡红色光线，所以一眼只看到 1 种，红色或绿色亮点。白点可双眼同时看到，但有融像时，其白色竞争为有色的。偏振 Worth 4 点试验使用偏振眼镜，而不是红绿眼镜。刺激光可安装在壁挂显示器上，或使用 Worth 4 点灯。此项试验须有良好的背景照明，这样周围物体可以刺激运动融像。患者可能看到的点数有：

- 看到 2 个点提示左眼抑制盲点。
- 看到 3 个点提示右眼抑制盲点。
- 看到 4 个点提示可能存在抑制盲点，抑制盲点比测试目标的视角小。4 个点的感知提示存在一定程度的感觉融像，或是正常视网膜对应（患者没有明显斜视或小度数斜视，此斜视与单眼注视和周围融像相一致；如下所示），或是协调异常视网膜对应（患者存在大度数显性斜视）。
- 看到 5 个点提示复视，患者存在大度数显性斜视，且没有抑制或异常视网膜对应。

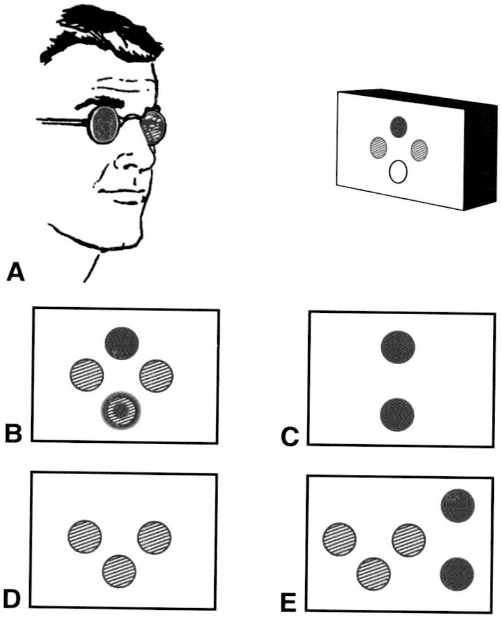

图 7–13 Worth 4 点试验。**A.** 患者戴红绿眼镜，注视 6m 远（投影或装在盒子上）和 33cm 远（Worth 4 点灯）的 4 个亮点（1 红、2 绿、1 白）。患者双眼看到的结果如 B ~ E 所示。**B.** 看到 4 个点：正位眼且存在周围融像，或斜视伴存在异常视网膜对应。6:00 钟位的点颜色呈竞争性变化，或由主导眼而定，呈现红色或绿色。**C.** 看到 2 个红点：左眼抑制。**D.** 看到 3 个绿点：右眼抑制。**E.** 看到 5 个点：内斜视为非交叉复视，即红点位于绿点右侧；外斜视为交叉复视，即红点位于绿点左侧。*（译者注：资料来源见前页原文。）*

In monofixation syndrome (see Chapter 5), the Worth 4-dot test can demonstrate both the presence of peripheral fusion and the absence of bifixation. The standard Worth 4-dot flashlight projects onto a central retinal area of 1° or less when viewed at 3 m (10 ft), well within the 1°–4° scotoma characteristic of monofixation syndrome, so patients with monofixation syndrome report seeing 2 or 3 lights, depending on fixation preference. As the Worth 4-dot flashlight is brought closer to the patient, the dots project onto more peripheral retina outside the central monofixation scotoma and a fusion response (4 lights) is obtained. This usually occurs between 0.67 and 1 m (2–3 ft).

Stereoacuity Tests

Stereopsis occurs when the 2 retinal images of an object in front of or behind the plane of fixation—which have small disparities due to the horizontal separation of the eyes—are cortically integrated, resulting in a perception of relative depth. Both *contour stereopsis* and *randomdot stereopsis tests* present horizontally displaced copies of the same stimulus to each eye separately (usually by having the patient wear polarized or red-green glasses). Contour stereopsis tests present horizontally displaced figures (one to each eye) that are recognizable to each eye individually. For contour stereoscopic figures with larger disparities, monocular cues in the form of decentration of the image seen by 1 eye are present, which could enable some patients to falsely pass. *Random-dot stereopsis tests* avoid such artifacts by embedding the stereoscopic figure in a background of similarly random dots; the dots in the area of the figure but not those in the background are shifted between the eyes, such that there is a stereoscopic percept, but neither eye alone can perceive the figure.

In the *Titmus* test, contour stereopsis is tested at near using polarized glasses. The ability to detect elevation of the fly's wings above the plane of the card indicates gross stereopsis (3000 seconds of arc). Finer levels of stereoacuity can also be demonstrated using stereoscopic images employing less horizontal disparity; at each level, the patient must identify the one stereoscopically presented figure out of a group of otherwise similar figures.

Clinically useful randomdot near stereopsis tests include the *Randot test*, which requires polarized glasses and measures stereoacuity down to 20 seconds of arc; the *TNO test*, which requires red-green glasses and measures stereoacuity down to 15 seconds of arc; the *Random-Dot E test*, a forced-choice test also requiring polarized glasses and employed mainly in pediatric vision-screening programs; and the *Lang stereopsis tests,* which do not require glasses to produce a random-dot stereoscopic effect and therefore may be useful in children who are not willing to put on glasses for testing.

Stereopsis can also be measured at distance using a chart projector with a vectographic slide, the Smart System PC-Plus (M&S Technologies, Inc.; Niles, IL), or the Frisby Davis Distance Stereotest (Stereotest Ltd, Sheffield, United Kingdom). Distance stereoacuity tests may be helpful in monitoring control of intermittent exotropia.

Assessment of the Field of Single Binocular Vision

The field of single binocular vision may be tested using a Goldmann perimeter. This assessment is useful for following recovery of a paretic muscle or measuring the outcome of surgery to alleviate diplopia. A small, white test object is followed by both eyes in the cardinal positions throughout the visual field. When the patient indicates that the test object is seen double, the point is plotted. The field of binocular vision normally measures about 45°–50° from the fixation point except where it is blocked by the nose (Fig 7-14). Weighted templates reflecting the greater importance of single binocular vision in primary and reading positions can be used to quantify the findings.

Worth 4 点试验可以检测到单眼注视综合征（见第 5 章）的周围融像的存在和双注视的缺失。手电筒 Worth 4 点试验投射到 1° 范围的视网膜中心，在 3m（10ft）处注视，正好落在单眼注视综合征的 1°~ 4° 盲点，由于注视偏好不同，单眼注视综合征患者可看到 2 个或 3 个点。再将 Worth 4 点灯移近，光点投射到中心单注视盲点的周围视网膜，在 0.67~1 m（2~3ft）处看到 4 个灯的融像反应。

立体视觉试验

由于双眼的水平分离导致小视差，双眼的 2 个视网膜图像位于注视平面之前或之后，通过皮质整合，形成相对深度感知，从而产生立体视觉。*轮廓立体视觉*和*随机点立体视觉试验*，分别给每眼相同且微小水平移位的刺激（戴偏振或红绿眼镜）。轮廓立体视觉试验呈现水平移位的图形（每眼 1 个），每眼可以单独识别。具有较大视差的轮廓立体图，存在单眼偏中心图像的线索，使患者假性通过试验。*随机点立体视觉试验*避免了这种伪像，将立体图形嵌入类似随机点的背景中；图形区内的点与背景中的点不同，并在双眼间交替，从而形成立体感知，但是仅单眼不能感知该图形。

在 *Titmus* 试验中，是通过在近处使用偏振镜来测试。轮廓立体视觉试验，在近处使用偏振镜。通过检测卡片平面上方的苍蝇翅膀的高度表示总立体视觉（3000 弧秒弧）。可用较少水平视差的立体图像检测更精细的立体视觉；在每个级别，患者需从一组类似的图形中识别出一个立体图形。

临床上的随机点近立体视觉试验包括 *Randot 试验*，需偏振镜，测量至 20 弧秒弧的立体视觉；*TNO 试验*，需红绿镜，测量至 15 弧秒度立体视觉；*随机点 E 试验*，是 1 种强迫选择测试，需偏振镜，主要用于小儿视力筛查项目；*Lang 立体视觉试验*，不需眼镜产生随机点立体效果，可用于不愿戴眼镜的儿童测试。

也可以进行远距离立体视觉测量，用带有矢量幻灯片的图表投影仪，如 Smart System PC-Plus（M&S Technologies，Inc.; Niles，IL），或 Frisby Davis Distance Stereotest（Stereotest Ltd，Sheffield，United Kingdom）。远距离立体视觉试验有助于监测间歇性外斜视的控制。

双眼单视的视野评估

使用 Goldmann 视野计测试双眼单视的视野范围。该评估可用于检测麻痹性斜视康复或斜视手术后复视的缓解。在基本眼位的视野范围，双眼追随的白色小视标。当患者看到 2 个视标时，标记该点。双眼视野距注视点约 45° ~ 50° ，除非被鼻子遮挡（图 7-14）。给出的模板反映出第一眼位和阅读眼位双眼单视的重要性，其可用于量化检测结果。

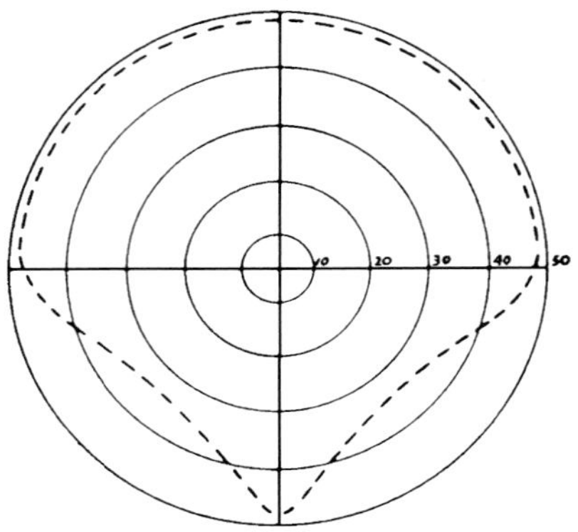

Figure 7-14 The normal field of single binocular vision.

Sullivan TJ, Kraft SP, Burack C, O'Reilly C. A functional scoring method for the field of binocular single vision. *Ophthalmology*. 1992;99(4):575–581.

The Prism Adaptation Test

In the prism adaptation test, binocular function is tested with prisms to align the visual axes to help predict whether fusion may be restored with surgical or prismatic alignment, especially in adults. This test is distinct from the use of prolonged prism adaptation to unmask a larger angle of deviation in acquired esotropia, as described in Chapter 8.

Torticollis: Differential Diagnosis and Evaluation

Torticollis is an abnormal head position (AHP): head turn, chin-up or chin-down, tilt, or any combination of these. Ocular torticollis, as opposed to nonocular torticollis, results from strabismus or other eye conditions; see Table 7-2 for the differential diagnosis of both ocular and nonocular torticollis.

Early diagnosis and correction of ocular conditions resulting in torticollis is impor-tant because prolonged AHP (primarily head tilt) in children can cause facial asymmetry or secondary musculoskeletal changes. Note, however, that facial asymmetry coexisting with head tilt is not always caused by the head tilt. For example, unicoronal craniosynostosis can result in strabismus with ocular torticollis and also directly cause facial asymmetry in dependent of the torticollis.

Ocular Torticollis

Sometimes an AHP and associated ocular abnormality simply have a shared underlying cause (eg, ocular tilt reaction), but more often, the AHP compensates for the ocular condition.

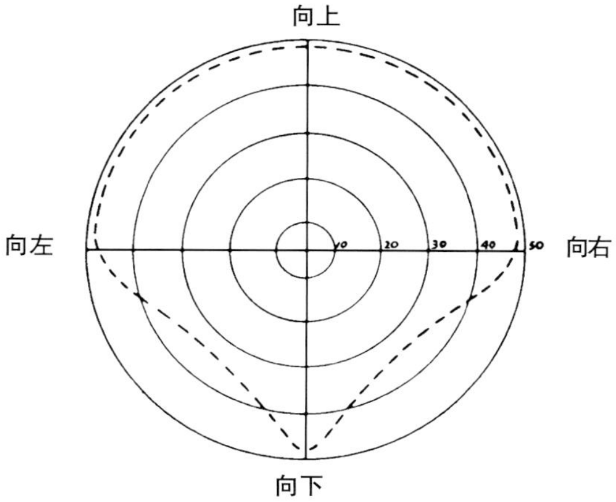

图 7–14　双眼单视的正常视野。

Sullivan TJ, Kraft SP, Burack C, O'Reilly C. A functional scoring method for the field of binocular single vision. *Ophthalmology*. 1992;99(4):575–581.

棱镜耐受试验

在棱镜耐受试验中，用保持视轴正位的棱镜测试双眼功能，以预测融像是否通过手术或棱镜矫正来恢复，特别是在成人。该测试与使用延长的棱镜耐受性试验不同，后者目的在于诱发大角度偏斜的获得性内斜视，见第 8 章所述。

斜颈的鉴别诊断和评估

斜颈是一种异常头位（AHP）：包括头部转动、下颌上抬或内收、倾斜或这些症状的组合。与非眼性斜颈相反，眼性斜颈是由斜视或其他眼部疾病引起的；有关眼性和非眼性斜颈的鉴别诊断见表 7–2。

早期诊断和矫正导致斜颈的眼部疾病非常重要，因为儿童长期异常头位 AHP（主要是头部倾斜）可导致面部发育不对称，或继发性肌肉骨骼改变。需注意，与头部倾斜共存的面部不对称并不一定是由头部倾斜引起的。例如，单角颅结节病可导致斜视伴斜颈，并且还直接导致面部不对称性。

眼性斜颈

有时异常头位与伴合并的眼部异常是共同的原因（如眼倾斜反应），但更常见的是异常头位补偿眼部异常。

Table 7-2 Differential Diagnosis of Torticollis

Ocular Torticollis	Nonocular Torticollis
Nystagmus	Congenital muscular torticollis
Infantile nystagmus syndrome (congenital motor or sensory nystagmus; null point)	Skeletal abnormalities
Fusion maldevelopment nystagmus syndrome (manifest latent nystagmus; less in adduction)	Congenital abnormalities (eg, Klippel-Feil syndrome)
Periodic alternating nystagmus (alternating null point)	Traumatic abnormalities
Spasmus nutans	Neurologic conditions
Acquired adult jerk nystagmus	Syringomyelia
A- or V-pattern esotropia or exotropia	Dystonia
Paretic strabismus	Posterior fossa lesions
Superior oblique palsy	Deafness in one ear
Duane retraction syndrome	Sandifer syndrome
Sixth nerve palsy	Psychogenic disease
Third nerve palsy	
Inferior oblique palsy	
Restrictive strabismus	
Brown syndrome	
Thyroid eye disease	
Orbital fracture	
Congenital fibrosis of extraocular muscles	
Supranuclear disorders	
Monocular elevation deficiency	
Dorsal midbrain syndrome	
Gaze palsy	
Dissociated vertical deviation	
Ocular tilt reaction	
Monocular blindness (with fusion maldevelopment nystagmus syndrome, or for centration of remaining field)	
Homonymous hemianopia	
Ptosis	
Refractive error	

Incomitant strabismus (eg, superior oblique palsy, Duane retraction syndrome, Brown syndrome, blowout fractures, thyroid eye disease) can cause an AHP that improves binocularity. Chin-up positioning in unilateral ptosis likewise enables binocularity. In rare cases, patients with superior oblique palsy show paradoxical head tilt to the wrong side, possibly to increase the separation between diplopic images when fusion is not possible.

In infantile nystagmus syndrome (congenital motor or sensory nystagmus) with a null point away from primary position, an AHP improves vision. In fusion maldevelopment nystagmus syndrome (manifest latent nystagmus), vision improves with an AHP that brings the fixating eye into adduction. With bilateral duction deficits (eg, congenital fibrosis of extraocular muscles) or bilateral ptosis, an AHP may be needed for foveation. Refractive errors may also cause an AHP.

Finally, monocular individuals and patients with homonymous hemianopia may have a variable head turn toward their blind side, perhaps to better center the total field of view accessible with saccadic eye movements.

表7-2　斜颈的鉴别诊断

眼性斜颈	非眼性斜颈
眼球震颤	先天性肌性斜颈
婴儿眼球震颤综合征（先天运动或知觉性眼球震颤，中和区）	骨骼异常
融像不良性眼球震颤综合征（表现为隐性眼球震颤，内转时摆动性较少）	先天性畸形（如Klippel-Feil综合征）
周期性交替性眼球震颤（交替性中和区）	创伤性畸形
点头状痉挛	神经系统的条件
获得性成人冲动性眼球震颤	脊髓空洞症
A型或V型内斜视或外斜视	肌张力障碍
麻痹性斜视	后窝病变
上斜肌麻痹	单耳耳聋
Duane眼球后退综合征	Sandifer综合征
第Ⅵ颅神经麻痹	心理疾病
第Ⅲ颅神经麻痹	
下斜肌麻痹	
限制性斜视	
Brown综合征	
甲状腺眼病	
眼眶骨骨折	
先天性眼外肌纤维化	
核上疾病	
单眼上转不足	
中脑背正中综合征	
凝视麻痹	
垂直分离性斜视	
眼倾斜反应	
单眼失明（伴融像不良性眼球震颤综合征，或残留中心视野）	
同侧偏盲	
上睑下垂	
屈光不正	

非共同性斜视（如上斜肌麻痹、Duane后退综合征、Brown综合征、爆裂性骨折、甲状腺眼病）可引起异常头位AHP，从而改善双眼视觉。通过下颌抬起，单眼上睑下垂可以获得双眼视觉。在极少数情况下，上斜肌麻痹的患者表现为矛盾性头部倾斜到相反一侧，可能是由于不能融像时，为增加了复视图像之间的分离。

在婴儿眼球震颤综合征（先天性运动或感觉性眼球震颤）中，第一眼位远离中和区，异常头位可改善视力。融像不良性眼球震颤综合征（表现为隐性眼球震颤）的异常头位使眼球内转，以改善视力。双侧转动缺陷（如先天性眼外肌纤维化）或双侧上睑下垂可能需要异常头位实现中心凹注视。屈光不正也会引发异常头位。

最后，独眼和同侧偏盲的患者可能会转向盲侧，也许是为了使扫视运动进入到视野中心。

Diagnostic evaluation of ocular torticollis

To identify ocular causes of an AHP, motility testing should be done, with particular attention to gaze positions opposite those favored. Nystagmus is usually obvious, but subtle nystagmus may be visible only during slit-lamp or fundus examination. Fundus examination may reveal extorsion suggestive of superior oblique palsy, or conjugate torsion (extorsion in one eye and intorsion in the other), as seen in the ocular tilt reaction. If placing the patient in the supine position eliminates the head tilt, a musculoskeletal etiology is unlikely. If monocular occlusion eliminates the AHP, the torticollis probably serves binocular fusion.

眼性斜颈的诊断

为了鉴别异常头位的眼部原因，应进行运动性试验，特别注意与偏好相反的注视位置。眼球震颤通常很明显，但细小的眼球震颤只有在裂隙灯或眼底检查时才发现。眼底检查可发现黄斑外转，提示上斜肌麻痹，或共轭旋转（一眼黄斑外旋和另一眼黄斑内旋），与双眼倾斜反应相同。如果患者取仰卧位可消除头部倾斜，则不太可能是肌肉骨骼病因。如果遮挡一眼，异常头位消失，则可能是为了双眼融像而发生斜颈。

（翻译 杨嘉嵩 龚慧 谭薇 // 审校 石一宁 钱学翰 // 章节审校 石广礼）

CHAPTER 8

Esodeviations

An *esodeviation* is a latent or manifest convergent misalignment of the visual axes. Esodeviations are the most common type of childhood strabismus, accounting for more than 50% of ocular deviations in the pediatric population. In adults, esodeviations and exodeviations are equally prevalent.

Repka MX, Yu F, Coleman A. Strabismus among aged fee-for-service Medicare beneficiaries. *J AAPOS.* 2012;16(6):495–500.

Epidemiology

Esodeviations occur with equal frequency in males and females and are more common in African Americans and white ethnic groups than in Asian ethnic groups in the United States. Risk factors for the development of esotropia include anisometropia, hyperopia, neurodevelopmental impairment, prematurity, low birth weight, craniofacial or chromosomal abnormalities, maternal smoking during pregnancy, and family history of strabismus. The prevalence of esotropia increases with age (higher prevalence at 48–72 months compared with 6–11 months), moderate anisometropia, and moderate hyperopia. In some families, a mendelian inheritance pattern has been observed. Amblyopia develops in approximately 50% of children who have esotropia.

Esodeviations can result from innervational, anatomical, mechanical, refractive, or accommodative factors. There are several major types of esodeviations, and they can be classified as comitant or incomitant (Table 8-1).

Cotter SA, Varma R, Tarczy-Hornoch K, et al; Joint Writing Committee for the Multi-Ethnic Pediatric Eye Disease Study and the Baltimore Pediatric Eye Disease Study Groups. Risk factors associated with childhood strabismus. *Ophthalmology*. 2011;118(11):2251–2261.

Pseudoesotropia

Pseudoesotropia refers to the appearance of esotropia when the visual axes are in fact aligned. The appearance may be caused by a flat and broad nasal bridge, prominent epicanthal folds, a narrow interpupillary distance, or a negative angle kappa (see Chapter 7). Less than the expected amount of sclera is seen nasally, creating the impression that the eye is deviated inward (Fig 8-1). This is especially noticeable when the child gazes to either side. Because no real deviation exists, results of both corneal light reflex testing and cover testing are normal.

第 8 章

内斜视

内斜视是视轴隐性或显性集合异常，是最常见的儿童斜视类型，占儿童斜视的 50% 以上。而成人的内斜视和外斜视发病率则一样。

Repka MX, Yu F, Coleman A. Strabismus among aged fee-for-service Medicare beneficiaries. *J AAPOS.* 2012;16(6):495–500.

流行病学

男性和女性的内斜视发病率相同，在美国，非洲裔和白人内斜视患者比亚裔更常见。内斜视的危险因素包括屈光参差、远视、神经发育障碍、早产而、低出生体重、颅面或染色体异常、妊娠期母亲吸烟和斜视家族史。内斜视的发病率随着年龄的增长（48 ~ 72 个月的发病率高于 6 ~ 11 个月）、中度屈光参差和中度远视而增加。一些家庭呈现 Mendel 遗传模式。大约 50% 的内斜视儿童患有弱视。

神经、解剖、机械、屈光或调节因素可能导致内斜视。有几种主要类型的内斜，可分为共同性或非共同性（表 8–1）。

Cotter SA, Varma R, Tarczy-Hornoch K, et al; Joint Writing Committee for the Multi-Ethnic Pediatric Eye Disease Study and the Baltimore Pediatric Eye Disease Study Groups. Risk factors associated with childhood strabismus. *Ophthalmology.* 2011;118(11):2251–2261.

假性内斜视

*假性内斜视*是指外观呈内斜视，而视轴正位。这种现象可能是由扁平而宽的鼻梁、明显的内眦赘皮、窄瞳孔间距或负 kappa 角的外观所致（见第 7 章）。所见的鼻侧的巩膜减少，造成眼睛向内偏斜的印象（图 8–1）。当孩子向任一侧注视时，特别明显。由于不存在眼位异常，因此角膜光反射试验和遮盖试验均正常。

Table 8-1 Major Types of Esodeviation

Comitant Esotropia
Infantile (congenital) esotropia
Ciancia syndrome
Accommodative esotropia
Refractive (normal AC/A ratio)
Nonrefractive (high AC/A ratio)
Partially accommodative
Acquired nonaccommodative esotropia
Basic
Cyclic
Sensory (deprivation)
Divergence insufficiency
Primary (age-related distance esotropia)
Secondary
Spasm of the near reflex
Consecutive esotropia
Spontaneous
Postsurgical
Nystagmus and esotropia
Fusion maldevelopment nystagmus syndrome
Nystagmus blockage syndrome
Incomitant Esotropia
Sixth nerve palsy
Medial rectus muscle restriction following excessive resection
Slipped or lost lateral rectus muscle following surgery
Thyroid eye disease
Medial orbital wall fracture with entrapment
Congenital fibrosis of the extraocular muscles
Esotropia associated with high myopia
Duane retraction syndrome
Möbius syndrome

AC/A = accommodative convergence/accommodation.

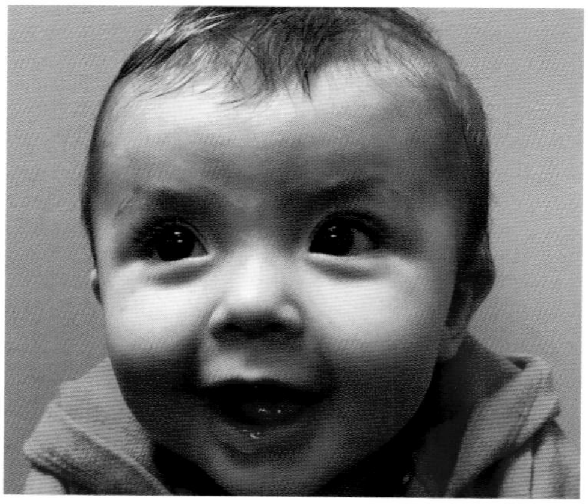

Figure 8–1 Infant girl with pseudoesotropia. The child is looking to right gaze, and the broad epicanthal folds create the appearance of a left esotropia. *(Courtesy of Katherine A. Lee, MD, PhD.)*

Infantile (Congenital) Esotropia

Infantile esotropia is defined as an esotropia that is present by 6 months of age. Some ophthalmologists refer to this disorder as *congenital esotropia,* although the deviation is usually not manifest at birth.

表8-1　主要类型的内斜视

共同性内斜视

婴儿（先天性）内斜视
　Ciancia综合征
调节性内斜视
　屈光性内斜视（正常AC/ A比）
　非屈光性内斜视（高AC / A比）
　部分调节性内斜视
获得性非调节性内斜视
　基本型内斜视
　周期性内斜视
　感知性内斜视（剥夺性）
　分散不足
　　原发性（年龄相关的视近内斜视）
　　继发性
　近反射痉挛
　连续内斜视
　　自发性
　　手术后
眼球震颤与内斜视
　融合发育不良性眼球震颤综合征
　眼球震颤阻滞综合征

非共同性内斜视

Ⅵ颅经麻痹
内直肌过度切除后的运动受限
手术后外直肌滑脱或丢失
甲状腺眼病
眶内壁骨折伴内陷
先天性眼外肌纤维化
内斜视伴有高度近视
Duane后退综合征
Möbius 综合征

AC/A =调节性集合/调节。

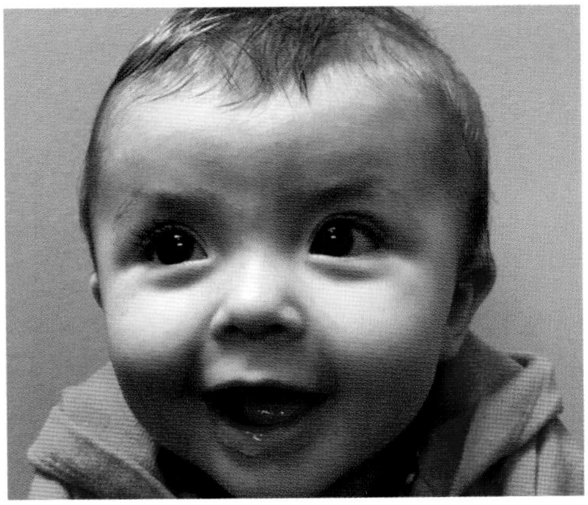

Figure 8–1　女婴假性内斜视。患儿向右侧注视时，宽内眦赘皮造成左眼内斜视的假象。*（译者注：资料来源见前页原文。）*

婴儿（先天性）内斜视

*婴儿内斜视*指 6 个月内的内斜视。一些眼科医生称其为*先天性内斜视*，尽管这种斜视不发生在出生时。

Variable, transient, intermittent strabismus is commonly noted in the first 2–3 months of life. Also, it is common to see both intermittent esotropia and exotropia in the same infant (termed *ocular instability of infancy*). This condition should resolve by 3 months of age but sometimes persists, especially in premature infants. If an esotropia is present after age 2 months, is constant, and measures 30 prism diopters (Δ) or more, it is unlikely to resolve and will probably require surgical intervention.

Patients with infantile esotropia often have a family history of esotropia or other strabismus, but well-defined genetic patterns are unusual. Infantile esotropia occurs more frequently in children born prematurely and in up to 30% of children with neurologic and developmental problems, including cerebral palsy and hydrocephalus. Infantile esotropia has been associated with an increased risk of development of mental illness by early adulthood (2.6 times higher in patients with infantile esotropia than in controls).

Olson JH, Louwagie CR, Diehl NN, Mohney BG. Congenital esotropia and the risk of mental illness by early adulthood. *Ophthalmology*. 2012;119(1):145–149.

Pathogenesis

The cause of infantile esotropia remains unknown. The debate regarding its etiology has focused on the implications of 2 conflicting theories. The Worth "sensory" concept proposes that infantile esotropia results from a congenital deficit in a "fusion center" in the brain. According to this theory, the goal of restoring binocularity is futile. In contrast, the Chavasse theory proposes that the primary problem in infantile esotropia is one of motor development, which is potentially curable if ocular alignment is achieved in infancy. Several authors have reported favorable sensory results in infants operated on between 6 months and 2 years of age, and these encouraging results have become the basis for the practice of early surgery for infantile esotropia.

Clinical Features and Evaluation

The eyes may have equal vision, in which case alternate fixation or cross-fixation will be present. Cross-fixation, the use of the adducted eye for fixation of objects in the contralateral visual field, is associated with large-angle esotropias (Fig 8-2). Amblyopia is, however, commonly associated with infantile esotropia, and when it is present, a fixation preference can be observed.

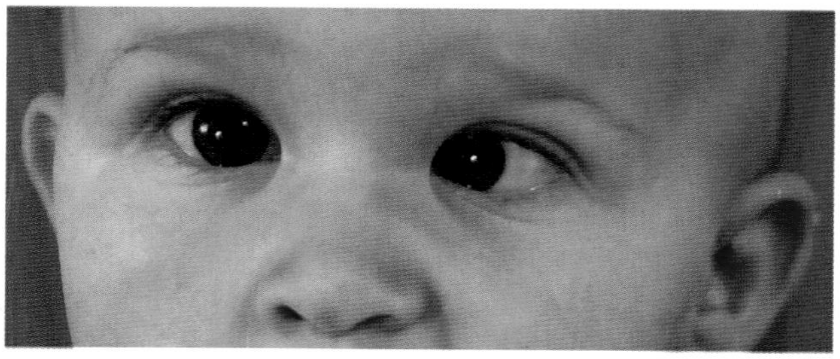

Figure 8-2 Infant boy with left esotropia. Cross-fixation of the right eye from the adducted position. *(Courtesy of Katherine A. Lee, MD, PhD.)*

在婴儿出生后 2 ~ 3 个月常会见到不稳定的、一过性的、间歇性的斜视。还在同一婴儿中见到间歇性内斜和外斜同时存在（称为*婴儿期的眼不稳定性*）。这种情况在 3 个月左右消失，但有时会持续存在，特别是早产儿。如果在 2 个月之后存在恒定的内斜视，≥ 30Δ 棱镜度，则不太可能恢复，需手术干预。

婴儿型内斜视的患者常有内斜视或其他斜视的家族史，但没有一定的遗传模式。婴儿型内斜视常见于早产儿，伴神经系统和发育问题的儿童可高达 30%，包括脑瘫和脑积水。婴儿内斜视与成年早期患精神疾病的风险增加有关（婴儿内斜视患者比对照组高 2.6 倍）。

Olson JH, Louwagie CR, Diehl NN, Mohney BG. Congenital esotropia and the risk of mental illness by early adulthood. *Ophthalmology*. 2012;119(1):145–149.

病因

婴儿型内斜视的原因尚不清楚。病因学有 2 个相互矛盾的理论。Worth 提出“感知”的概念，婴儿型内斜视是由大脑皮质的“融合中心”先天性缺陷引起的。根据这一理论，恢复双眼视是不可能的。相反，Chavasse 的理论认为，婴儿型内斜视的问题是运动发育异常，如果在婴儿期达到眼位正位，斜视是可以治愈的。有文献报道，6 月龄到 2 岁的患儿实施手术，可恢复良好感知，这是婴儿型内斜视进行早期手术的根据。

临床特征和评估

双眼视力相等，可存在交替注视或交叉注视。交叉注视，即用内斜视眼注视对侧眼视野的物体，这与大角度内斜视有关（图 8–2）。弱视常伴有婴儿型内斜视，且出现注视偏好。

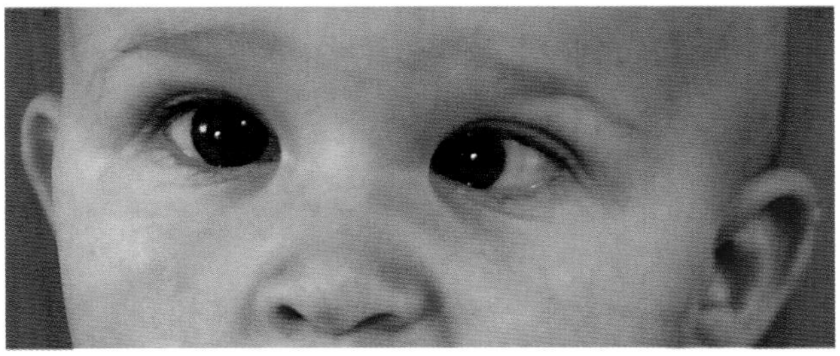

图 8–2　男婴左眼内斜视。右眼自内转位交叉注视。*（译者注：资料来源见前页原文。）*

Versions and ductions are often normal initially. The deviation is comitant and characteristically larger than 30Δ. Overelevation in adduction and dissociated strabismus complex develop in more than 50% of patients, usually after 1–2 years of age. There may be an apparent abduction deficit because of cross-fixation; children with equal vision in both eyes have no need to abduct either eye on side gaze. If amblyopia is present, the better-seeing eye will fixate in all fields of gaze, making the amblyopic eye appear to have an abduction deficit. The infant's ability to abduct each eye can be demonstrated with the doll's head maneuver or by observation after patching either of the patient's eyes. The clinician can also hold the infant and spin in a circle, which stimulates the vestibular-ocular reflex and helps demonstrate full abduction.

Asymmetry of monocular horizontal smooth pursuit is normal in infants up to age 6 months, with the nasal-to-temporal direction less well developed than the temporalto-nasal. Patients with infantile esotropia, however, have persistent smooth-pursuit asymmetry throughout their lives. Fusion maldevelopment nystagmus syndrome (also known as *latent* and *manifest latent nystagmus*) is also a commonly associated motility anomaly. Cycloplegic refraction characteristically reveals low hyperopia (+1.00 to +2.00 diopters [D]). Hyperopia greater than 2.00 D should prompt consideration of spectacle correction; reduction of the strabismic angle with glasses indicates the presence of an accommodative component.

A severe form of infantile esotropia, referred to as *Ciancia syndrome*, consists of largeangle esotropia (>50Δ), abducting nystagmus, and mild abduction deficits. Children with this syndrome uniformly use cross-fixation.

Management

Significant hyperopic refractive error should be corrected by prescribing the full cycloplegic refraction. A small-angle esotropia that is variable in degree or intermittent may be more likely to respond to hyperopic correction than would a large-angle or constant esotropia.

Ocular alignment is rarely achieved without surgery in early-onset esotropia. Previously, it was thought that concurrent amblyopia should be fully treated before surgery. However, it has recently been shown that successful postoperative alignment is as likely to occur in patients with mild to moderate amblyopia at the time of surgery as it is in those whose amblyopia has been fully treated preoperatively. When ocular alignment is achieved earlier, there may be the added benefits of better fusion, stereopsis, and long-term stability.

The goal of surgical treatment of infantile esotropia is to reduce the deviation to orthotropia or as close to it as possible. In the presence of normal vision, this ideally results in the development of some degree of sensory fusion. Alignment within 8Δ–10Δ of orthotropia frequently results in the development of the monofixation syndrome, characterized by peripheral fusion, central suppression, and favorable appearance (see Chapter 5). This small-angle strabismus generally represents a stable, functional surgical outcome even though bifoveal fusion is not achieved; it is therefore considered a successful surgical result. In addition, the child's psychological and motor development may improve and accelerate after the eyes are straightened.

最初，眼球同向运动和转动是正常的。斜视是共同性的，斜视度数多大于 30Δ。50% 以上患者在 1 ~ 2 岁后发生内转高位和复合性分离性斜视。由于交叉注视，可呈现外展功能缺陷；还由于双眼视力相同，侧视时眼睛不需要外转。如果有弱视，所有注视视野均使用视力较好眼，弱视眼呈现外展功能缺陷。婴儿的眼外转能力可以通过洋娃娃头手法或遮盖任一眼后进行观察。还可以抱婴儿旋转一圈，刺激前庭 – 眼反射，有助于显示完全外展功能。

水平追随运动的不对称性在 6 月龄以下婴儿中是正常的，鼻侧 – 颞侧方向运动的发育不如颞侧 – 鼻侧方向运动的发育。而水平追随不对称性在婴儿型内斜视的患者持续终生。融合发育不良性眼球震颤综合征（也称为*隐性和显性 – 隐性眼球震颤*）也是一种常伴发的运动异常。睫状肌麻痹验光呈低度远视（+1.00 ~ +2.00D）。大于 2.00 D 的远视应立即行眼镜矫正；若戴镜减小了斜视度，提示存在调节因素。

一种严重的婴儿型内斜视，称为 Ciancia 综合征，其症状有大角度内斜视（> 50Δ）、外转位眼球震颤和轻度外展功能缺陷。同样，患有该综合征的儿童使用交替注视。

治疗

应完全睫状肌麻痹的远视屈光矫正。与大角度或恒定性斜视相比较，变化的或间歇性小角度内斜视对远视矫正有效。

没有手术的早发内斜视很少获得眼正位。以前认为伴有弱视时，手术前应先进行充分的弱视治疗。而最近研究表明，轻中度弱视的患者经过手术治疗后同样可获得眼正位，与充分治疗弱视后再手术矫正的结果一样。越早获得眼正位，越有益于融合、立体视觉和长期稳定性。

婴儿型内斜视手术治疗的目标是减少内斜视度数，尽可能接近正位。在视力正常的情况下，此目标促进一定程度的感觉融合发展。8Δ ~ 10Δ 的小度数斜视的正眼位常常发展为单视注视综合征，其特征为周围融合、中心抑制和正常外观（见第 5 章）。这种小度数斜视常表示实施了稳定的功能性手术，即便没有实现双眼中心凹融合，也可以认为手术成功。此外，眼睛正位后，儿童心理和运动发育可能会得到改善和加速。

Most ophthalmologists in North America agree that surgery should be undertaken early. The belief is that the eyes should be aligned by 2 years of age, preferably earlier, to optimize binocular cooperation. Surgery can be performed in healthy children as early as age 4 months. The Congenital Esotropia Observational Study showed that when patients present with constant esotropia of at least 40Δ after 10 weeks of age, the deviations are unlikely to resolve spontaneously. Smaller angles can be monitored, as they may improve spontaneously. A prospective, multicenter European study (ELISSS) comparing early (age 6–24 months) versus delayed (age 32–60 months) strabismus surgery showed a small improvement in gross binocularity in the early-surgery group; however, a higher number of procedures were performed in the early-surgery group.

Various surgical approaches have been suggested for infantile esotropia. The most commonly performed initial procedure is recession of both medial rectus muscles. Recession of a medial rectus muscle combined with resection of the ipsilateral lateral rectus muscle is also effective. Two-muscle surgery spares the other horizontal rectus muscles for subsequent surgery should it be necessary, which is not uncommon. For infants with large deviations (typically >60Δ), some surgeons operate on 3 or even 4 horizontal rectus muscles at the time of the initial surgery, or they add botulinum toxin injection to the medial rectus muscle recession. Significant inferior oblique muscle overaction can be treated at the time of the initial surgery. Chapter 14 discusses surgical procedures in detail.

Injection of botulinum toxin to the medial rectus muscles has also been used as primary treatment of infantile esotropia. In a recent study, botulinum toxin injection was associated with a substantially higher reoperation rate than was strabismus surgery, and children treated with botulinum toxin were found to have a higher rate of postoperative abnormal binocularity. Botulinum toxin may be most useful for smaller deviations.

Leffler CT, Vaziri K, Schwartz SG, et al. Rates of reoperation and abnormal binocularity following strabismus surgery in children. *Am J Ophthalmol.* 2016;162:159–166.e9.

Pediatric Eye Disease Investigator Group. The clinical spectrum of early-onset esotropia: experience of the Congenital Esotropia Observational Study. *Am J Ophthalmol.* 2002; 133(1):102–108.

Simonsz HJ, Kolling GH, Unnebrink K. Final report of the early vs. late infantile strabismus surgery study (ELISSS), a controlled, prospective, multicenter study. *Strabismus.* 2005; 13(4):169–199.

Accommodative Esotropia

Accommodative esotropia is defined as a convergent deviation of the eyes associated with activation of the accommodative reflex. All accommodative esodeviations are acquired and can be characterized as follows:

- onset typically between 6 months and 7 years of age, averaging 2½ years of age (can be as early as age 4 months)
- usually intermittent at onset, becoming constant
- comitant
- often hereditary
- sometimes precipitated by trauma or illness
- frequently associated with amblyopia
- possibly occurring with diplopia (especially with onset at an older age), which usually disappears with development of a facultative suppression scotoma in the deviating eye

大多数北美眼科医生都认为应该尽早进行手术，应该在 2 岁之前或更早，使眼恢复正位，以使双眼协调达到最佳状态。健康儿童可以在 4 月龄进行手术。“先天性内斜视观察研究项目”显示，当患者在 10 周后出现持续性达 40Δ 的内斜视时，斜视不可能自愈。较小度数的内斜可以监测，可能自愈。一项前瞻性多中心的欧洲研究（ELISSS），比较了早期（6 ~ 24 月龄）与迟发（32 ~ 60 月龄）斜视的手术效果，结果显示早期手术组的双眼视功能有小的改善，而早期手术组需要进行更多次手术。

多种手术方法可用于婴儿型内斜视。最常用的手术是双眼内直肌后徙。双眼内直肌后徙联合同侧外直肌缩短也有效。双肌肉手术可以节约其他水平直肌，其在后续手术中可能用到，临床经常出现这种情况。对于斜视度数较大（通常 > 60Δ）的婴儿，一些医生在初次手术时，对 3 条、甚至 4 条水平直肌进行手术，或将肉毒杆菌毒素注射到后徙的内直肌。在初次手术时，可以同时治疗下斜肌亢进。第 14 章详细讨论手术步骤。

将肉毒杆菌毒素注射到内直肌已被用于婴儿型内斜视初次治疗。最近研究表明，与斜视手术相比，肉毒杆菌毒素注射伴有显著增高的再次手术率，并且用肉毒杆菌毒素治疗的儿童的术后异常双眼视功能更高。肉毒杆菌毒素对较小度数斜视最有效。

Leffler CT, Vaziri K, Schwartz SG, et al. Rates of reoperation and abnormal binocularity following strabismus surgery in children. *Am J Ophthalmol.* 2016;162:159–166.e9.

Pediatric Eye Disease Investigator Group. The clinical spectrum of early-onset esotropia: experience of the Congenital Esotropia Observational Study. *Am J Ophthalmol.* 2002; 133(1):102–108.

Simonsz HJ, Kolling GH, Unnebrink K. Final report of the early vs. late infantile strabismus surgery study (ELISSS), a controlled, prospective, multicenter study. *Strabismus.* 2005; 13(4):169–199.

调节性内斜视

*调节性内斜*视指伴调节反射激活的眼集合性偏斜。所有调节性内斜视都是获得性的，其特征如下：

- 发病年龄在 6 月龄 ~ 7 岁，平均年龄为 2.5 岁（最早可发生在 4 月龄）。
- 发病早期常呈间歇性，逐步呈恒定性。
- 共同性。
- 常有遗传性。
- 有时有创伤或疾病引起。
- 常伴有弱视。
- 可能发生复视（特别是较大年龄发病的患者），通常随偏斜眼的条件性抑制盲点形成而消失。

Types of accommodative esotropia are listed in Table 8-1 and discussed in the following sections.

Pathogenesis and Types of Accommodative Esotropia

Refractive accommodative esotropia

The mechanism of refractive accommodative esotropia involves 3 factors: uncorrected hyperopia, accommodative convergence, and insufficient fusional divergence. Because of uncorrected hyperopia, the patient must accommodate to focus the retinal image. Accommodation is accompanied by the other components of the near reflex, namely convergence and miosis. If the patient's fusional divergence mechanism is insufficient to compensate for the increased convergence tonus, esotropia results. The angle of esotropia is approximately the same at distance and near fixation and is generally between 20Δ and 30Δ. Patients with refractive accommodative esotropia have an average of +4.00 D of hyperopia.

High AC/A ratio accommodative esotropia

Patients with a *high accommodative convergence/accommodation (AC/A) ratio* (see Chapter 7) have an excessive convergence response for the amount of accommodation required to focus while wearing their full cycloplegic correction. In this form of esotropia, the deviation is present only at near or is much larger at near.

The refractive error in high AC/A ratio accommodative esotropia (also called *nonrefractive accommodative esotropia*) averages +2.25 D. However, this esotropia can occur in patients with a normal level of hyperopia or high hyperopia, with emmetropia, or even with myopia.

Partially accommodative esotropia

Patients with partially accommodative esotropia show reduction in the angle of esotropia when wearing glasses but have a residual esotropia despite provision of the full hyperopic correction. This is more likely to occur if there is a long delay in refractive correction. In some cases, partially accommodative esotropia results from decompensation of a pure refractive accommodative esotropia; in other instances, an initial nonaccommodative esotropia subsequently develops an accommodative component.

Evaluation

The 2 eyes can have equal vision, or amblyopia can be present. Versions and ductions may be normal, or overelevation in adduction or dissociated strabismus complex (discussed in Chapter 11) may be present. The examiner should measure the deviation using an accommodative target at distance and at near. Alternate cover testing at the initial examination typically reveals an intermittent comitant esotropia that is larger at near than at distance.

调节性内斜视的类型列于表 8-1 中，并随后讨论。

调节性内斜视的发病机制和类型

屈光性调节性内斜视

*屈光性调节性内斜视*的发病机制涉及 3 个因素：未矫正的远视、调节性集合和融合性散开不足。由于未矫正远视，患者需调节物像，以聚焦到视网膜上。调节伴随其他近反射，即集合和瞳孔缩小。如果患者的融合性散开功能不能补偿增加的集合张力，则会产生内斜视。在视近和视远时的内斜视度数大致相同，通常在 20Δ ～ 30Δ 之间。屈光性调节性内斜视的远视平均为 +4.00D。

高 AC/A 比的调节性内斜视

*高调节性集合 / 调节比（AC/A）*的患者（见第 7 章）即使在睫状肌完全麻痹下进行屈光矫正，仍对于聚焦所需的调节量产生过度的集合反应。这种内斜视仅在视近时出现，或视近时增大。

高 AC/A 比的调节性内斜视（也称为*非屈光性调节性内斜视*）的屈光度数平均为 +2.25D。而这种内斜视可发生在正常远视状态或高度远视，正视眼，甚至近视眼。

部分调节性内斜视

部分调节性内斜视患者，戴镜时斜视度数减小，但尽管进行了完全远视屈光矫正，仍有残余内斜视。如果长期没有进行屈光矫正，这种情况更容易发生。有时部分调节性内斜视只因为单纯的屈光性调节性内斜视代偿不全所致。还有由初发的非调节性内斜视发展成为调节性内斜。

评估

双眼视力相等或有弱视。同向运动和单眼转动正常，或内转高位或复合性分离斜视（第 11 章讨论）。分别在远距离及近距离使用调节视标测量斜视度。最初的交替遮盖试验呈间歇性共同性内斜视，视近斜视度大于视远。

Management

Refractive accommodative esotropia

Treatment of refractive accommodative esotropia consists of correction of the full amount of hyperopia, as determined under cycloplegia. If binocular fusion is maintained, the refractive correction can later be decreased to 1.00–2.00 D less than the full cycloplegic refraction. Amblyopia, if present, may respond to spectacle correction alone, but treatment with occlusion or atropine may be necessary if the amblyopia persists after a period of spectacle wear (see Chapter 6).

Parents must understand not only that full-time wear of the glasses is important but also that the refractive correction can only help control the strabismus, not "cure" it. Once full-time wear has begun, the esotropia may increase when the child is not wearing glasses, because the child makes a strong accommodative effort to produce an image that is as clear as the one experienced with refractive correction. Discussing these issues with the parents at the time the prescription is given is helpful.

Strabismus surgery may be required when a patient with presumed refractive accommodative esotropia does not achieve an ocular alignment within the fusion range (up to 8Δ–10Δ) with correction (partially accommodative esotropia). Before proceeding with surgery, the ophthalmologist should recheck the cycloplegic refraction to rule out latent uncorrected hyperopia.

High AC/A ratio accommodative esotropia

A high AC/A ratio can be managed optically or surgically; it can also be observed.

- *Bifocals.* Plus lenses for hyperopia reduce accommodation and therefore accommodative convergence. Bifocal glasses further reduce or eliminate the need to accommodate for near fixation. If bifocals are used, the initial prescription should be for flat-top style bifocals (see the chapter on refraction in BCSC Section 3, *Clinical Optics*) with the lowest plus power needed (up to +3.00 D) to achieve ocular alignment at near fixation. To increase the likelihood that the child will use the bifocal segment, it should be set high enough that the top of the bifocal segment bisects the pupil. Progressive bifocal lenses have been used successfully in older children who know how to use bifocal glasses. An ideal response to bifocal glasses is restoration of normal binocular function (fusion and stereopsis) at both distance and near fixation. An acceptable response is fusion at distance and less than 10Δ of residual esotropia at near with bifocals (signifying the potential for fusion). While some children improve spontaneously with time, others need to be slowly weaned from bifocal glasses. The process of reducing the bifocal power in 0.50–1.00 D steps can be started at about age 7 or 8 years and should be completed by age 10–12 years. If a child cannot be weaned from bifocals, surgery may be considered.
- *Surgery.* Surgical management of high AC/A ratio accommodative esotropia is controversial. Some ophthalmologists advocate surgery (medial rectus muscle recessions with or without posterior or pulley fixation) to normalize the AC/A ratio, which may allow discontinuation of bifocals. The risk of overcorrection at distance is low (<10%). Some ophthalmologists use prism adaptation, which entails using prisms preoperatively to neutralize a deviation for a certain length of time. The prism neutralization can then be used to predict the outcome of surgery and determine the maximum deviation.

治疗

屈光性调节性内斜视

屈光性调节性内斜视的治疗包括在睫状肌麻痹下完全远视矫正。如果双眼融合存在，屈光矫正以后可较睫状肌麻痹下的屈光度降低 1.00 ~ 2.00D。如果存在弱视，单独配镜矫正可能有效果；但如果配镜一段时间后弱视仍存在，则需遮盖治疗或阿托品治疗 (见第 6 章)。

父母不仅要懂得全天候戴镜的重要性，还要懂得屈光矫正只能帮助控制斜视，而不能“治愈”。一开始全天候戴镜，当患儿取下眼镜时内斜视会增加，因为孩子为了能得到与戴镜矫正时一样清晰的图像，会更努力地调节。医生开配镜处方时就与父母讨论这些问题是很有帮助的。

在融合范围内（至 8 ~ 10Δ）进行了屈光矫正 (部分调节性内斜视)，屈光性调节性内斜仍不能获得眼正位，则需斜视手术治疗。在进行手术前，眼科医生应再次进行睫状肌麻痹性验光，排除隐性未矫正的远视。

高 AC/A 比值的调节性内斜视

高 AC/A 比值可进行视光矫正或手术治疗，也可以观察。

- *双焦眼镜*。正附加眼镜可减少调节，因此调节性集合也减少。双焦眼镜可进一步减少或消除近注视的调节。如果使用双焦眼镜，初始处方应该用平顶双光眼镜（见 BCSC 第 3 册《*临床光学*》，验光一章），用最低的正附加度数（加至 + 3.00 D）达到视近时眼球正位。为了使儿童可以使用双焦镜，应将双焦段顶部设置足够高，以平分瞳孔。渐进式双焦镜可以于用年长儿童，他们知道如何使用双焦镜。双焦镜理想的效果是分别在视近和视远时，正常双眼功能（融合和立体视觉）都恢复。可接受的双光镜效果是在视远时有融合，但在视近时残余小于 10Δ 内斜视（提示潜在的融合）。有些儿童随着时间自发改善，其他的可逐渐摘掉双焦镜。从 7 ~ 8 岁开始减少双焦镜的度数，每次减少 0.50 ~ 1.00D，10 ~ 12 岁完成。如果儿童不能脱离双光镜，应考虑手术。

- *手术*。手术治疗高 AC/A 比的调节性内斜视是有争议的。一些眼科医生提倡通过手术 (内直肌后徙术，伴有或不伴有后固定或滑车固定) 使 AC/A 比值恢复正常，这样可以摘掉双光镜。视远时过矫的风险较低 (< 10%)。一些眼科医生使用棱镜耐受正，手术前需要使用一段时间棱镜来中和偏斜。棱镜中和可以用于预测手术，并确定最大偏差度。

- *Observation*. Many patients show a decrease in the near deviation with time, and binocular vision at both distance and near fixation ultimately develops. Some ophthalmologists observe the near deviation as long as the distance alignment allows for the development of peripheral fusion.

For the long-term management of both refractive and high AC/A ratio accommodative esotropia, it is important to remember that hyperopia usually increases until age 5–7 years before it starts to decrease. Therefore, if the esotropia with correction increases, the cycloplegic refraction should be repeated and the full correction prescribed.

If glasses correct all or nearly all the esotropia and if some degree of sensory binocular cooperation or fusion is present, the clinician may begin to reduce the hyperopic correction to create a small esophoria, which is thought to stimulate fusional divergence. An increase in the fusional divergence, combined with the Natural decrease of both the hyperopia and the high AC/A ratio, may enable the patient to eventually maintain straight eyes without bifocals or glasses altogether.

Partially accommodative esotropia

Treatment of partially accommodative esotropia consists of strabismus surgery for the deviation that persists while the patient wears the full hyperopic correction. It is important that the patient and parents understand *before* surgery that its purpose is to produce straight eyes with spectacle wear—not to enable the child to discontinue wearing glasses altogether. In older patients, refractive surgery may be considered to both reduce the hyperopic refractive error and improve the ocular alignment.

Acquired Nonaccommodative Esotropia

Several types of comitant esotropia not associated with activation of the accommodative reflex may develop in later infancy (>6 months), childhood, or even adulthood. The causes of these acquired nonaccommodative esotropias are varied.

Basic Acquired Nonaccommodative Esotropia

Basic acquired nonaccommodative esotropia is a comitant esotropia that develops after age 6 months and is not associated with an accommodative component. As in infantile esotropia, the amount of hyperopia is not significant, and the angle of deviation is similar when measured at distance and near. Acquired esotropia may be acute in onset. In such cases, the patient immediately becomes aware of the deviation and may have diplopia. A careful evaluation is important to rule out an accommodative or paretic component. Temporary but prolonged disruption of binocular vision—such as may result from a hyphema, preseptal cellulitis, mechanical ptosis, or prolonged patching for amblyopia—is a known precipitating cause of acquired nonaccommodative esotropia. In patients with acquired nonaccommodative esotropia, fusion is thought to be tenuous, so this temporary disruption of binocular vision upsets the balance, resulting in esotropia. Because the onset of nonaccommodative esotropia in an older child may be a sign of an underlying neurologic disorder, neuroimaging and neurologic evaluation may be indicated, especially when other symptoms or signs of neurologic abnormality are present, such as lateral incomitance, deviation greater at distance than near, abnormal head position, or concomitant headache.

- *观察*。很多病人的视近斜视度随时间变化而降低，并且最终视远和视近的双眼视发育正常。一些医生观察到，当视远眼位形成周围融合时，就会出现视近的偏斜。

从长远看屈光性和高 AC/A 比的调节性内斜视的治疗，需要记住，远视一直增加到 5 ~ 7 岁，之后开始减少。因此，如果屈光矫正时内斜视继续增加，应进行反复睫状肌麻痹验光，并给完全矫正处方。

如果眼镜矫正了全部内斜视，而且存在一定程度的感知双眼协调或融合，医生应开始减少远视的矫正度数，并形成一个小内斜，以刺激融合性散开。融合散开的增加，伴随远视和高 AC/A 比的降低，可能最终会使患者在摘掉双光镜或眼镜后而保持正位。

部分调节性内斜视

部分调节性内斜视的治疗包括斜视手术，针对那些全天候配戴远视完全矫正而仍存在斜视的患者。非常有必要让*患者*及其家长在手术*前*知道，其目的是让眼正位，而并不是摘掉眼镜。在年龄稍大的患者中，屈光手术可减少远视，并改善眼正位。

获得性非调节性内斜视

不伴随调节反射激活的几类共同性内斜视，可以在婴儿期（>6 月龄）、儿童期，甚至成年期发生。这些获得性非调节性内斜视的原因有多种。

基本型获得性非调节性内斜视

基本型获得性非调节性内斜视是一种共同性内斜视，发生于出生 6 个月后，不伴有调节成分。幼儿型内斜视的远视度数高，视远和视近的斜视度一样。获得性内斜视是急性发病，这样会立即发现眼位偏斜和复视。仔细的评估是非常重要的，需排除调节性或麻痹性斜视。临时但会长时间破坏双眼视的情况有以下几种——前房积血、膈前眶蜂窝织炎、机械性上睑下垂或长时间遮盖治疗弱视，以上为导致获得性非调节性内斜视的原因。获得性非调节性内斜视的融合很弱，所以暂时打破双眼视觉会干扰这种平衡，导致内斜视。因为年长孩子出现非调节性内斜视提示神经系统疾病，特别是存在的其他神经系统异常的症状或体征，如侧向非共同性、视远斜视度大于视近、异常头位或伴随头痛，应该继续进行神经影像学和神经系统评估。

Many patients with acquired nonaccommodative esotropia have a history of normal binocular vision; thus, the prognosis for restoration of single binocular vision with prisms and/or surgery is good. Therapy consists of amblyopia treatment, if necessary, and surgical correction or botulinum toxin injection as soon as possible after the onset of the deviation. The Prism Adaptation Study showed a smaller undercorrection rate (approximately 10% less) when the amount of surgery was based on the prism-adapted angle.

Jacobs SM, Green-Simms A, Diehl NN, Mohney BG. Long-term follow-up of acquired nonaccommodative esotropia in a population-based cohort. *Ophthalmology*. 2011;118(6): 1170–1174.

Repka MX, Connett JE, Scott WE. The one-year surgical outcome after prism adaptation for the management of acquired esotropia. *Ophthalmology*. 1996;103(6):922–928.

Cyclic Esotropia

Cyclic esotropia is a rare form of strabismus; other forms of cyclic strabismus occur but are even rarer. Onset of cyclic esotropia is typically during the preschool years. The esotropia is comitant and intermittent, usually occurring every other day (48-hour cycle). Variable intervals and 24-hour cycles have also been documented.

Fusion and binocular vision are usually absent or defective on the strabismic day, with marked improvement or normalization on the orthotropic day. Occlusion therapy may convert the cyclic deviation into a constant one.

Surgical treatment of cyclic esotropia is usually effective. The amount of surgery is based on the maximum angle of deviation present when the eyes are esotropic.

Sensory Esotropia

Monocular vision loss (due to cataract, corneal clouding, optic nerve or retinal disorders, or various other entities) may cause sensory (deprivation) esotropia. Conditions preventing clear and focused retinal images and symmetric visual stimulation must be identified and remedied promptly, if possible, to prevent irreversible amblyopia. If surgery or botulinum toxin injection is indicated for strabismus, it is generally performed only on the eye with a significant vision deficit.

Divergence Insufficiency

In divergence insufficiency, the characteristic finding is an esodeviation that is greater at distance than at near. The deviation is horizontally comitant, and fusional divergence is reduced. There are 2 forms of divergence insufficiency: a primary, isolated form; and a secondary form that is rare and associated with neurologic abnormalities, including pontine tumors, increased intracranial pressure, or severe head trauma. In these secondary cases, the divergence insufficiency is probably due to a mild sixth nerve paresis. Patients with secondary divergence insufficiency require neuroimaging to rule out treatable intracranial lesions.

许多获得性非调节性内斜视患者既往双眼视觉正常，因此，棱镜和（或）手术治疗后可以较好地恢复双眼单视功能，预后较好。治疗包括弱视治疗，必要时斜视一旦发生后尽快进行手术矫正或肉毒杆菌毒素注射。棱镜耐受研究项目（Prism Adaptation Study）显示，当手术量是基于棱镜耐受调整的，矫正不足率较小 (低于 10%)。

Jacobs SM, Green-Simms A, Diehl NN, Mohney BG. Long-term follow-up of acquired nonaccommodative esotropia in a population-based cohort. *Ophthalmology*. 2011;118(6): 1170–1174.

Repka MX, Connett JE, Scott WE. The one-year surgical outcome after prism adaptation for the management of acquired esotropia. *Ophthalmology*. 1996;103(6):922–928.

周期性内斜视

周期性内斜视是一种罕见的斜视类型，还有其他周期性斜视，但更为罕见。周期性内斜视常发生在学龄前。内斜视是共同性和间歇性的，常隔日发生 (48h 为 1 个周期)。也有变化的间歇周期和 24h 周期。

在斜视日，融合和双眼视觉功能缺失或功能不全，而在眼正位日，功能明显改善或正常。遮盖治疗会将周期性内斜视转成恒定性。

手术治疗周期性内斜视有效。手术的设计量是基于内斜视日的最大偏离度数。

感觉性内斜视

单眼视力丧失 (由于白内障、角膜混浊、视神经或视网膜疾病或其他眼部疾病) 可引起感觉性 (剥夺性) 内斜视。当存在妨碍形成清晰的和聚焦的视网膜像、对称的视觉刺激时，需及时诊断和及时治疗，以防止形成不可逆的弱视。只有存在明显的视觉损害时，才考虑实施手术或注射肉毒杆菌毒素。

散开不足

散开不足的临床特点是视远的内偏斜角大于视近的内偏斜角。眼位偏斜为水平的共同性，融合性散开减少。有 2 种散开不足：原发性的、孤立的形式和继发性的形式，后一种较为罕见，与神经系统异常相关，包括脑桥肿瘤、颅内高压及严重的头部外伤。继发性病例中，散开不足可能是由于第Ⅵ对脑神经轻度麻痹引起。继发性散开不足需进行神经影像检查，以排除可治疗的颅内病变。

Primary divergence insufficiency is an increasingly diagnosed type of adult strabismus. More recently termed *age-related distance esotropia*, the entity is a slowly progressing, benign condition that occurs predominantly in patients older than 50 years. Affected individuals report a gradual onset of horizontal diplopia that is present at distance but not at near. Imaging may demonstrate thinning, elongation, and rupture of the connective tissue between the lateral and superior rectus muscles and sagging and elongation of the lateral rectus muscles. Management consists of base-out prisms, botulinum toxin injection of the medial rectus muscles, and strabismus surgery. In patients with agerelated distance esotropia, reestablishment of binocular fusion generally occurs following treatment.

Chaudhuri Z, Demer JL. Sagging eye syndrome: connective tissue involution as a cause of horizontal and vertical strabismus in older patients. *JAMA Ophthalmol.* 2013;131(5): 619–625.

Spasm of the Near Reflex

Spasm of the near reflex (also known as *ciliary spasm or convergence spasm*) is a spectrum of abnormalities of the near response. The etiology is generally thought to be functional, related to psychological factors such as stress and anxiety. In rare cases, it can be associated with organic disease. Patients present with varying combinations of excessive convergence, increased accommodation, and miosis. Patients may present with acute esotropia alternating with orthotropia. Substitution of a convergence movement for a gaze movement with horizontal versions is characteristic. Monocular abduction is normal despite marked limitation of abduction on version testing. Pseudomyopia may occur.

Treatment consists of cycloplegic agents such as atropine or homatropine, hyperopic correction, and bifocal glasses. Counseling to address underlying psychological issues may be helpful. If the spasm cannot be broken, botulinum toxin injection of the medial rectus muscles and strabismus surgery may be considered with caution.

Kaczmarek BB, Dawson E, Lee JP. Convergence spasm treated with botulinum toxin. *Strabismus.* 2009;17(1):49–51.

Consecutive Esotropia

Consecutive esotropia refers to an esotropia that follows a history of exotropia. It can arise spontaneously, or it can develop after surgery for exotropia. Spontaneous consecutive esotropia is rare and almost always occurs in the setting of neurologic disorders or with very poor vision in 1 eye. Postsurgical consecutive esotropia, on the other hand, is not uncommon. Fortunately, it often resolves over time without treatment. In fact, an initial small overcorrection is desirable after surgery for exotropia, as it is associated with an improved long-term success rate. Treatment options for consecutive esotropia include base-out prisms, hyperopic correction, alternating occlusion, botulinum toxin injection, and strabismus surgery. In postsurgical consecutive esotropia, unless the deviation is very large or a slipped or "lost" muscle is suspected, surgery or botulinum toxin injection may be postponed for several months after onset because of the possibility of spontaneous improvement.

成人斜视中诊断出原发性散开不足的病例在增加。近来，称为*年龄相关性视远内斜眼*，这是一种进展缓慢的良性疾病，主要发生在50岁以上。患者逐渐出现水平复视，发生在视远时，而不是在视近时。影像检查显示外直肌和上直肌之间的筋膜组织变薄、拉长和撕裂，以及外直肌松弛和拉长。治疗包括底朝外棱镜、内直肌肉毒杆菌毒素注射和斜视手术。一般在治疗后，年龄相关性视远内斜视的双眼融合可以恢复。

Chaudhuri Z, Demer JL. Sagging eye syndrome: connective tissue involution as a cause of horizontal and vertical strabismus in older patients. *JAMA Ophthalmol.* 2013;131(5): 619–625.

近反射痉挛

近反射痉挛（也称为*睫状体痉挛或集合性痉挛*）是一系列的视近反应异常。病因是功能性的，多与压力和焦虑等心理因素有关，偶与器质性疾病相关。患者存在过度集合、调节增强和瞳孔缩小。患者可能会出现急性内斜视，与眼正位交替。用集合运动替代凝视运动、伴有水平异向运动为其特征。尽管在异向试验中外转明显受限，但单眼外转是正常的。可有假性近视。

治疗包括睫状肌麻痹剂药物（如阿托品或后马托品）、远视的屈光矫正和双焦镜。咨询有助于解决潜在心理问题。如果痉挛不能缓解，可考虑在内直肌注射肉毒杆菌毒素和进行斜视手术，但需慎重。

Kaczmarek BB, Dawson E, Lee JP. Convergence spasm treated with botulinum toxin. *Strabismus.* 2009;17(1):49–51.

连续性内斜视

*连续性内斜视*是指外斜视病史后发生的内斜视。它可以是自发性的，也可以发生于外斜视手术后。自发性连续性内斜视罕见，总是伴有神经系统病变，或单眼低视力极差。术后的连续性内斜视并不少见，常不需治疗即可自愈。外斜视手术可以小度数过矫，因为远期治疗效果较好。连续性内斜视的治疗方案包括底朝外棱镜、远视的屈光矫正、交替遮盖、肉毒杆菌毒素注射和斜视手术。除非偏斜度非常大，或肌肉滑落或“丢失”，术后的连续性内斜视应在病发几个月后再考虑进行手术或肉毒杆菌毒素注射，因为患者有可能自发改善。

A slipped or lost lateral rectus muscle (discussed in Chapter 14) produces various amounts of esotropia and incomitance, depending on the amount of slippage, and should be suspected in consecutive esotropia following lateral rectus recession surgery if a significant abduction deficit is present. However, if the ipsilateral medial rectus muscle was resected at the time of the lateral rectus recession, the consecutive esotropia could be due to a tight medial rectus muscle. Forced duction testing helps differentiate between these 2 causes. In cases of a slipped or lost lateral rectus muscle, surgical exploration is required. (See Chapter 14, Fig 14-1, and the accompanying discussion.)

Nystagmus and Esotropia

Several types of nystagmus are associated with esotropia. *Fusion maldevelopment nystagmus syndrome* (also known as *latent and manifest latent nystagmus*) is a common feature of infantile esotropia. Ciancia syndrome (discussed earlier in this chapter) is a severe form of infantile esotropia associated with an abducting nystagmus. *Nystagmus blockage syndrome* occurs in children with congenital motor nystagmus, who use convergence to "damp," or decrease the amplitude or frequency of, their nystagmus, resulting in esotropia. See also Chapter 13.

Incomitant Esotropia

There are several positional, restrictive, and innervational abnormalities of the extraocular muscles that may result in incomitant esotropia (see Table 8-1).

Sixth Nerve Palsy

Weakness of the lateral rectus muscle due to palsy of the abducens nerve results in incomitant esotropia. Sixth cranial nerve palsy occurring in the neonatal period is rare and usually transient. Most cases of suspected congenital sixth nerve palsy are actually infantile esotropia with cross-fixation. Congenital sixth nerve palsy may be difficult to differentiate from esotropic Duane retraction syndrome, which is more common in young infants (see Chapter 12), as the unique retraction feature of this syndrome may not yet be evident. A distinguishing characteristic is that for an equal amount of abduction deficit, the deviation in primary position is usually much larger in sixth nerve palsy than it is in esotropic Duane retraction syndrome.

Pathogenesis

Congenital sixth nerve palsy is usually benign and transient and may be caused by the increased intracranial pressure associated with the birth process. Sixth nerve palsy in older children is associated with intracranial lesions in approximately one-third of cases, which may have additional neurologic findings. Other cases may be related to infectious or immunologic processes involving cranial nerve VI. The most common cause of isolated, transient sixth nerve palsy in a child is thought to be a virus; in an adult, a microvascular occlusive event.

滑落或丢失的外直肌（第 14 章中讨论）产生不同程度的非共同性内斜视，取决于滑落的程度。外直肌后徙术后出现明显的外展不足，应考虑连续性内斜视。如果外直肌后徙时切除同侧内直肌，连续性内斜视可能是由于内直肌缝线过紧所致。被动牵拉试验有助于区分这 2 个原因。如果外直肌滑脱，需手术探查。（见第 14 章，图 14–1，及其讨论。）

眼球震颤和内斜视

几种类型的眼球震颤伴有内斜视。*融合发育不良性眼球震颤综合征*（也称为*隐性*和*显性 – 隐性眼球震颤*）是一种常见的幼儿型内斜视。Ciancia 综合征（见本章讨论）是一种严重的幼儿型内斜视，伴有外展性眼球震颤。*眼球震颤阻滞综合征*是发生在先天性运动性眼球震颤的儿童身上，即使用集合“抑制”或减少眼球震颤的振幅或频率，导致内斜视。见第 13 章。

非共同性内斜视

眼外肌的位置异常、限制和神经支配异常可导致非共同性内斜视（见表 8–1）。

第Ⅵ颅神经麻痹

外展神经麻痹引起的外直肌无力可表现为非共同性内斜视。第Ⅵ颅神经麻痹罕见在新生儿期，是暂时性的。大多数疑似先天性第Ⅵ颅神经麻痹实际上是婴儿型内斜视的交叉注视。先天性第Ⅵ神经麻痹与内斜视性 Duane 后退综合征很难鉴别，后者更常见于婴幼儿（见第 12 章），而综合征特有的后退现象可能尚不明显。一个突出的特征是，因为存在外展不足的程度一样，第Ⅵ颅神经麻痹的第一眼位斜视角大于内斜视性 Duane 眼球后退综合征中第一眼位的斜视度。

发病机制

先天性第 VI 颅神经麻痹是良性和暂时性的，可能是出生过程中颅内压升高导致的。年长婴儿第 VI 颅神经麻痹中，约 1/3 伴有颅内病变，有其他神经症状。其他可能与累及第 VI 颅神经的感染或免疫有关。在儿童群体中，孤立的一过性第 VI 颅神经麻痹的最常见原因是病毒引起，在成年人中，微血管闭塞是最常见原因。

Clinical features and evaluation

Older children and adults may report diplopia. Often there is a compensatory head turn toward the side of the para lyzed lateral rectus muscle, adopted to place the eyes in a position where they are best aligned. If a child presents soon after onset of the deviation, vision in the eyes is usually equal. The esotropia increases in gaze toward the side of the paralyzed lateral rectus muscle, and versions show limited or no abduction of the affected eye (Fig 8-3). Results of the saccadic velocity test show slowing of the affected lateral rectus muscle, and active force generation tests document weakness of that muscle.

A careful history should be taken, including antecedent infections, head trauma, and hydrocephalus, as well as hypertension and diabetes mellitus in adults. In light of the high prevalence of associated intracranial lesions in children with sixth nerve palsy, neurologic evaluation and magnetic resonance imaging of the head and orbit are usually indicated, even in the absence of other focal neurologic findings.

Management

Patching may be necessary to prevent or treat amblyopia if the child is not using a compensatory head posture or if the child is very young. Press-on prisms are sometimes used to correct diplopia in primary position. Correction of a significant hyperopic refractive error may help prevent the development of an associated accommodative esotropia. Botulinumtoxin injection of the ipsilateral medial rectus muscle is sometimes employed to temporarily decrease the esotropia. If the deviation does not resolve after 6 months of treatment, surgery may be indicated. Options include horizontal rectus muscle surgery if abduction is at least partially preserved or vertical rectus muscle transposition surgery if abduction is absent (see Chapter 14).

See BCSC Section 5, *Neuro-Ophthalmology*, for further discussion of sixth nerve palsy.

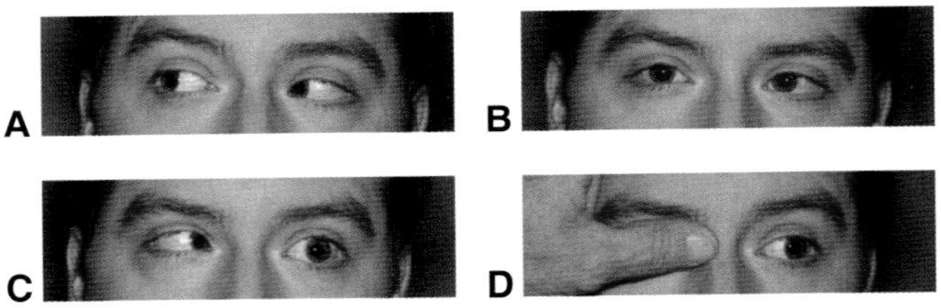

Figure 8-3 Sixth nerve palsy, left eye. **A,** Right gaze. **B,** Esotropia in primary position. **C,** Limited abduction, left eye. **D,** Abduction is still incomplete, but there is further abduction when the left eye is fixating, a finding that is important in the plan for surgical correction. *(Courtesy of Edward L. Raab, MD.)*

Other Forms of Incomitant Esotropia

Medial rectus muscle restriction may result from thyroid eye disease, orbital myositis, medial orbital wall fracture with medial rectus entrapment, excessive medial rectus muscle resection, or congenital fibrosis of the extraocular muscles. Duane retraction syndrome and Möbius syndrome begin as paralytic disorders, and secondary restriction of the medial rectus may develop later. In patients with high myopia, esotropia may develop because of prolapse of the posterior globe between displaced lateral and superior rectus muscles.

For further discussion of these special forms of strabismus, see Chapter 12 in this volume and BCSC Section 5, *Neuro-Ophthalmology.*

临床特征和评价

大龄儿童和成年人可有复视。通常有一个代偿性的头转向麻痹的外直肌一侧，最大限度保持正眼位。如果出现斜视后立即代偿头位，视力常是相等的。当朝向麻痹性外直肌一侧注视时，内斜视增加，同向运动受限或麻痹眼不能外展 (图 8–3)。扫视速度试验显示受累外直肌速度变缓和主动收缩试验记录肌肉力量的减弱。

认真采集病史，包括以前的感染、头部创伤、脑积水以及成人高血压和糖尿病等病史。因为儿童相关的颅内病变伴有较高的第 VI 颅神经麻痹发病率，即使没有局灶性神经病灶，也需要进行颅脑和眼眶的神经系统评估和磁共振成像检查。

治疗

如果孩子没有代偿头位或年龄太小，需遮盖预防弱视或治疗弱视。压贴棱镜可用于矫正第一眼位的复视。远视的屈光矫正有助于防止相关调节性内斜视的发展。肉毒杆菌毒素注射同侧内直肌以暂时减少内斜视。如果 6 个月后斜视没有改善，可考虑手术治疗。若外展功能部分保留，行水平直肌手术；若外展功能丧失，则须行垂直直肌转位手术 (见第 14 章)。

见 BCSC 第 5 册《*神经眼科学*》，有关第Ⅵ颅神经麻痹的讨论。

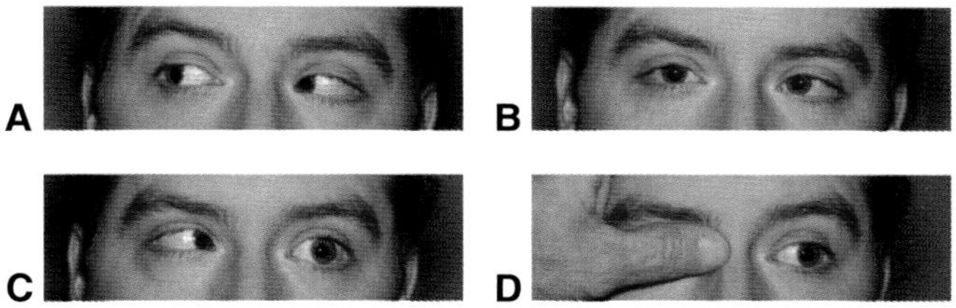

图 8–3　第Ⅵ颅神经麻痹，左眼。**A.** 右注视。**B.** 第一眼位内斜。**C.** 外展受限，左眼。**D.** 外展不足，但左眼注视时可进一步外展，在计划实施手术矫正时，这一体征非常重要。*（译者注：资料来源见前页原文。）*

其他形式的非共同性内斜视

*内直肌限制*的病因有甲状腺眼病、眶肌炎、眶内壁骨折伴内直肌嵌顿、过度内直肌切除以及先天性眼外肌纤维化。Duane 后退综合征和 Möbius 综合征开始呈麻痹性，随后呈现继发性内直肌受限。高度近视会发展为内斜视，因为在移位的外直肌和上直肌之间，后部眼球向前脱出。

有关特殊类型的斜视进一步讨论，见本册第 12 章和 BCSC 第 5 册《*神经眼科学*》。

（翻译 谭薇 杨乐 // 审校 石一宁 丁娟 // 章节审校 石广礼）

CHAPTER 9

Exodeviations

An exodeviation is a manifest (exotropia) or latent (exophoria) divergent strabismus. Risk factors for exotropia include maternal substance abuse and smoking during pregnancy, premature birth, perinatal morbidity, genetic anomalies, family history of strabismus, and uncorrected refractive errors.

Pseudoexotropia

The term *pseudoexotropia* refers to an appearance of exodeviation when in fact the eyes are properly aligned. Pseudoexotropia is much less common than pseudoesotropia (see Chapter 8 for discussion of pseudoesotropia) and may occur when there is a wide interpupillary distance or a positive angle kappa with or without other ocular abnormalities (see the discussions of angle kappa in Chapter 7 of this volume and in BCSC Section 3, *Clinical Optics*).

Exophoria

Exophoria is an exodeviation controlled by fusion under normal binocular viewing conditions. An exophoria is detected when binocular vision is interrupted, as during an alternate cover test or monocular visual acuity testing. Exophoria is relatively common, and patients are usually asymptomatic, although with prolonged near work, they may experience asthenopia. Decompensation of an exophoria to an exotropia may occur when the patient is ill or under the influence of sedatives or alcohol. Treatment is recommended when an exophoria becomes symptomatic.

Intermittent Exotropia

Intermittent exotropia is the most common type of manifest exodeviation.

Clinical Characteristics

The onset of intermittent exotropia is usually before age 5 years, and the exotropia typically continues into adulthood. The exodeviation becomes manifest during times of visual inattention, fatigue, stress, or illness. Parents of affected children often report that the exotropia occurs late in the day or when the child is daydreaming or tired. Exposure to bright light often causes exodeviation and a reflex closure of 1 eye (which is why strabismus is sometimes referred to as a "squint").

第 9 章

外斜视

外斜视是显性（外斜）或隐性（隐性外斜）散开性斜视。外斜视的危险因素包括孕期母亲药物滥用/吸毒和吸烟、早产、围产期患病、基因异常、斜视家族史以及未矫正的屈光不正。

假性外斜视

*假性外斜视*指外观呈外斜状，而眼位正位。假性外斜视较假性内斜视少见（见第 8 章的假性内斜视），有较宽的瞳距，或正 kappa 角，可伴有或不伴有其他眼部异常（见第 7 章 kappa 角，和 BCSC 第 3 册《*临床光学*》）。

隐性外斜视

隐性外斜视是在正常双眼视觉条件下，受融合控制的外偏斜。当双眼视觉中断时，可检测到隐性外斜视，如交替遮盖试验或单眼视力测试时。隐性外斜视较常见，常无症状，但近距离工作时间过长，可能出现视疲劳。当人在生病时，或在镇静剂、酒精的作用下，隐性外斜视的失代偿则成为外斜视。

间歇性外斜视

间歇性外斜视是最常见的一类显性外斜视。

临床特点

间歇性外斜视在 5 岁前发病，持续到成年。当注意力不集中、疲劳、压力或生病时，外斜视显现。患儿的父母会发现孩子在下午，或发呆，或疲劳时候出现外斜。在强光下常会引起外斜，并反射性地闭合一眼（这是为什么斜视有时被称为“眯眼”）。

Exodeviations are usually larger when the patient views distant targets, and they may be difficult to elicit at near. Because most parental interactions with young children occur at near, parents of a child with intermittent exotropia may not notice it initially. Intermittent exotropia can be associated with small hypertropias, A and V patterns (see Chapter 10), and overelevation and underelevation in adduction (see Chapter 11).

Left untreated, intermittent exotropia may remain stable, resolve, or progress, sometimes to constant exotropia. Because of suppression, children younger than 10 years with intermittent exotropia rarely report diplopia. They retain normal retinal correspondence and good binocular function when orthotropic. Amblyopia may occur if the strabismus is poorly controlled or becomes constant. Adults with poorly controlled intermittent or constant exotropia often experience significant psychological stress, anxiety, and depression because of their strabismus. Adults with strabismus often report reduced quality of life, obtain lower levels of education, and may have limited career choices and advancement opportunities.

Evaluation

The clinical evaluation begins with a history, including the age at onset of the strabismus, frequency and duration of misalignment, circumstances under which the deviation is manifest, and whether the exotropia is becoming more frequent with time. The clinician should determine whether symptoms such as diplopia, asthenopia, or difficulty with interpersonal interactions secondary to ocular misalignment are present.

Exodeviation control may be categorized as follows:

- *Good control*: Exotropia manifests only after cover testing, and the patient resumes fusion rapidly without blinking or refixating.
- *Fair control*: Exotropia manifests after fusion is disrupted by cover testing, and the patient resumes fusion only after blinking or refixating.
- *Poor control*: Exotropia manifests spontaneously and may remain manifest for an extended time.

Some ophthalmologists use the Newcastle Control Score for Intermittent Exotropia to quantitatively grade the control exhibited by patients with this deviation.

Because visual acuity and alignment tests are dissociating and may adversely affect assessment of strabismus control, they should be performed after sensory tests for stereopsis and fusion. Prism and alternate cover testing should be used to evaluate the exodeviation at fixation distances of 6 m and 33 cm. A far-distance measurement at 30 m or greater (eg, at the end of a long hallway or out a window) may uncover a latent deviation or elicit an even larger one. The deviation at near fixation is often smaller than the deviation at distance fixation. This difference is usually due to tenacious proximal fusion, a slow-to-dissipate fusion mechanism at near. The difference may sometimes be due to a high accommodative convergence/accommodation (AC/A) ratio, but a high AC/A ratio occurs much less commonly in exotropia than in esotropia (see Chapter 7, which discusses measurement of AC/A ratios). The exodeviation is termed *basic intermittent exotropia* when the size of the deviation at distance fixation is within 10 prism diopters (Δ) of the deviation size at near fixation. Some children have a larger deviation at near than at distance; this is distinct from convergence insufficiency (discussed later in the chapter).

外斜视在视远时更明显，而视近时很少引起。因为父母与孩子的交流多在近距离，间歇性外斜患儿的父母在最初可能并没有发现。间歇性外斜视可伴有小度数上斜，A 和 V 征 (见第 10 章)，以及内转高位和低位 (见第 11 章)。

如果不治疗，间歇性外斜视可能维持稳定、自愈或发展，一些转为恒定性外斜视。因为存在抑制，10 岁以下的间歇性外斜视很少有复视。他们保持正常视网膜对应，当眼正位时，可保持良好的双眼视功能。如果间歇性斜视控制不佳，或发展为恒定性，则形成弱视。控制不好的间歇性外斜视，或恒定性外斜视的成人，常有很大的心理压力、焦虑和抑郁。有报告称成人斜视会降低生活质量，获得的教育水平较低，并有可能限制职业的选择和发展的机会。

评估

临床评估从病史着手，包括斜视的发病年龄、频率和偏斜的持续时间，出现斜视的环境，外斜视显现是否随着时间的推移变得更加频繁。医师需确定是否伴有复视、视疲劳，或因眼位偏斜造成人际交流障碍。

外斜视控制可分为如下几类：

- *控制力良好*：外斜视只有在遮盖试验时才显现，病人不需要眨眼或重新注视，即可迅速恢复融合。
- *控制力一般*：遮盖试验打破融合后，外斜视显现，但需眨眼或重新注视，才可恢复融合。
- *控制力差*：外斜视自然显现，并可长时间持续。

一些眼科医生采用“间歇性外斜视 Newcastle 控制评分法”量化分级病人对偏斜的控制程度。

因为视力和眼位试验可能分离，对评估斜视控制产生负面影响，需要在进行立体视觉和融合功能的感觉试验后再进行视力和眼位的试验。分别注视 6m 和 33cm 处，进行棱镜和交替遮盖试验，评估外偏斜度。在 30m 或更远的距离检查 (如长走廊的尽头或窗外) 可能会发现隐性斜视或诱发更大度数的斜视。视近时的偏斜度通常小于视远时的。这种差异是由于顽固性近端融合，即视近时延缓分离的融合机制，也可能是高的调节性集合 / 调节 (AC/A) 比，但外斜视的高 AC/A 比的发生率比内斜视的低 (见第 7 章“AC/A 比测量”)。*基本型间歇性外斜视*是指视远时的偏斜与视近时差异在 10Δ 以内。一些儿童视近时的偏斜比视远时偏斜更大，这是与集合不足的区别（本章稍后讨论）。

When the exodeviation at distance is larger than the deviation at near fixation by 10Δ or more, the near exodeviation should be remeasured after 1 eye is occluded for 30–60 minutes (the patch test). The patch test eliminates the effects of tenacious proximal fusion, helping distinguish between pseudodivergence excess and true divergence excess. A patient with pseudodivergence excess has similar distance and near measurements after the patch test. A patient with true divergence excess continues to have a significantly larger exodeviation at distance. Many patients with true divergence excess also have a high AC/A ratio. For these patients, the AC/A ratio can be determined by measuring the near deviation with and without +3.00 diopter (D) lenses (while the patient wears corrective lenses, if necessary), after the patch test is completed. The measurements are then compared. Alternatively, the distance deviation can be measured with and without −2.00 D lenses to determine the AC/A ratio.

American Academy of Ophthalmology Pediatric Ophthalmology/Strabismus Panel. Preferred Practice Pattern Guidelines. *Esotropia and Exotropia*. San Francisco, CA: American Academy of Ophthalmology; 2012. For the latest guidelines, go to www.aao. org/ppp.

Treatment

All patients with exodeviations should be monitored as some will require treatment. Opinions vary widely regarding the timing of surgery and the use of nonsurgical treatments. Patients who have well-controlled, asymptomatic intermittent exotropia and good binocular fusion can be observed. Untreated strabismus often results in poor self-esteem in adults and children. Adults with strabismus report a wide range of difficulties with social interactions, which improve significantly after surgery.

Nonsurgical management

Correction of refractive errors Corrective lenses should be prescribed for significant refractive errors. Correction of even mild myopia may improve control of the exodeviation. Mild-to-moderate degrees of hyperopia are not routinely corrected in children with intermittent exotropia because refractive correction may worsen the deviation. Children with marked hyperopia (>+4.00 D) may be unable to sustain accommodation, which results in a blurred retinal image and manifest exotropia. In these patients, correction of refractive errors with glasses or contacts may improve retinal image clarity and help control the exodeviation.

In some cases, overcorrection of myopia by 2.00–4.00 D can stimulate accommodative convergence to help control the exodeviation. It can be effective as a temporizing measure to promote fusion and delay surgery in children with an immature visual system. This therapy may cause asthenopia in school-aged children, however. For patients whose initial overcorrection results in control, the prescription can be gradually tapered and surgery may be avoided.

Occlusion therapy Occlusion therapy (patching) for amblyopia may improve exotropic deviations. For patients without amblyopia, part-time patching of the dominant (nondeviating) eye or alternate patching (alternating which eye is patched each day) in the absence of a strong ocular preference can improve control of small-to moderate-sized deviations, particularly in young children. The improvement is often temporary, however, and many patients eventually require surgery.

Prisms Although they can be used to promote fusion in intermittent exotropia, base-in prisms are seldom chosen for long-term management because they can cause a reduction in fusional vergence amplitudes.

与视近的偏斜相比，视远时的偏斜大 10Δ 或更多时，遮盖一眼 30 ~ 60min（遮盖试验）后，重新测量视近偏斜度。遮盖试验消除了顽固性近端融合的影响，以帮助鉴别假性散开过度和真性散开过度。伴假性散开过度的患者在遮盖试验后，视远和视近的偏斜试验值相同。伴真性散开过度的患者在遮盖试验后，视远时持续有更大的外斜视。伴真性散开过度的患者也伴高 AC/A 比，确定这类 AC/A 比时，需在遮盖试验后、通过加和减 +3.00D（必要时戴矫正镜），检测视近时的偏斜量，比较测量结果；或者视远时，通过加和减 –2.00D，检测偏斜量，确定 AC/A 比。

American Academy of Ophthalmology Pediatric Ophthalmology/Strabismus Panel. Preferred Practice Pattern Guidelines. *Esotropia and Exotropia*. San Francisco, CA: American Academy of Ophthalmology; 2012. For the latest guidelines, go to www.aao. org/ppp.

治疗

所有外斜视都应随访，因为一些患者需进行治疗。关于手术时机和非手术治疗方法的意见分歧很大。控制良好的、无症状的间歇性外斜视和双眼融合良好的患者可以观察。未治疗的成人及儿童斜视患者常有自卑心理。有报告称成人斜视患者存在较大的社交障碍，手术后有明显改善。

非手术治疗

屈光不正的矫正　明显的屈光不正需要矫正。轻度近视的矫正可以改善外斜视的控制。儿童轻度 ~ 中度远视伴间歇性外斜视不用矫正，因为屈光矫正可能使偏斜加重。伴有明显远视（>+4.00D）的儿童可能不能保持调节，会产生模糊的视网膜像和显性外斜视。可配戴框架眼镜或接触镜矫正屈光不正，以改善视网膜像的清晰度和帮助控制外斜视。

有时近视过矫 2.00 ~ 4.00D 可刺激调节性集合，以帮助控制外斜视。对视觉系统发育尚未成熟的儿童，是一种有效的促进融合、延迟手术的暂时措施。但这种治疗方法可能引起学龄儿童的视疲劳。对于最初采取过矫方法进行控制的患者，可逐渐降低处方度数，且可能避免手术。

遮盖治疗　针对弱视患者的遮盖治疗（遮盖）可改善外偏斜。在没有弱视、没有明显的注视偏好的情况下，部分时间遮盖优势（未偏斜）眼或交替遮盖（每日交替遮盖一眼）可以改善小到中度偏斜，特别是幼儿。但偏斜的改善常是暂时的，许多患者最终需要手术。

棱镜　尽管棱镜可以促进间歇性外斜视的融合，但不应长期使用基底朝内棱镜，因为会降低融像性聚散幅度。

Surgical treatment

Factors influencing the decision to proceed with surgery include strabismus that is frequently manifest, poorly controlled, worsening (especially at near), symptomatic; poor self-image; and difficulty with personal or professional relationships. Strabismus surgery in adults is reconstructive, not cosmetic, and may alleviate anxiety and depression in some patients.

Surgical treatment of exotropia typically consists of bilateral lateral rectus muscle recession or unilateral lateral rectus muscle recession combined with medial rectus muscle resection. Large (>**50**Δ) deviations may require surgery on 3 or 4 muscles; for small deviations, single-muscle recession is sometimes performed. The optimal age for surgery and the choice of procedure are debatable. Caution is advised when surgery is considered for patients with true divergence excess exotropia, as they are at risk for postoperative diplopia and esotropia at near.

Adams GG, McBain H, MacKenzie K, Hancox J, Ezra DG, Newman SP. Is strabismus the only problem? Psychological issues surrounding strabismus surgery. *J AAPOS.* 2016;20(5):383–386.

Joyce KE, Beyer F, Thomson RG, Clarke MP. A systematic review of the effectiveness of treatments in altering the Natural history of intermittent exotropia. *Br J Ophthalmol.* 2015;99(4):440–450.

Postoperative alignment A small-angle esotropia in the immediate postoperative period tends to resolve and is desirable because of its association with a reduced risk of recurrent exotropia. Patients may experience diplopia while esotropic, and they should be advised of this possibility preoperatively. An esodeviation that persists beyond 3–4 weeks or that develops 1–2 months after surgery (*postsurgical esotropia*) may need further treatment, such as hyperopic correction, base-out prisms, patching to prevent amblyopia, or additional surgery. Bifocal glasses can be used for a high AC/A ratio and should be discussed preoperatively with patients who have true divergence excess. Unless deficient ductions suggest a slipped or "lost" muscle, a delay of a few months is recommended before reoperation for postsurgical esotropia, as spontaneous improvement may occur.

Because of the possibility of persistent consecutive esodeviations, some ophthalmologists prefer to delay surgery in young children who have good preoperative visual acuity and stereopsis. Others, however, consider surgical delay a risk factor for recurrence of strabismus. Long-term follow-up studies of the effectiveness of surgical treatment of intermittent exotropia show high recurrence rates. Patients may require multiple surgeries to maintain ocular alignment long term.

Convergence Insufficiency

Convergence insufficiency (CI) is an exodeviation that is greater at near fixation than at distance fixation. It is characterized by poor fusional convergence amplitudes and a remote near point of convergence (normal fusional vergence amplitudes are given in Chapter 7, Table 7-1). This sometimes results in symptoms of asthenopia, blurred near vision, and diplopia during near work, usually in older children or adults. Convergence insufficiency is a common complication of Parkinson disease. Rarely, accommodative spasms occur when accommodation and convergence are stimulated in an effort to overcome the CI.

手术治疗

手术治疗的决定因素包括常常呈显性的、控制差的、逐渐加重（特别在视近时）、有症状的斜视，自我形象不佳，存在个人或职业交流困难。成人的斜视手术目的功能重建，而非美容性的，而且可减轻患者的焦虑和抑郁。

外斜视手术有双眼外直肌后徙术，或单眼侧外直肌后徙联合内直肌切除术。大角度（>50Δ）的外斜视需在 3 ~ 4 条肌肉上实施手术；小角度外斜视有时仅需单一肌肉后徙术。手术的最佳年龄和术式的选择是有争议的。患者有真性散开过度外斜视时，手术应慎重考虑，因为存在术后视近时出现复视和内斜的风险。

Adams GG, McBain H, MacKenzie K, Hancox J, Ezra DG, Newman SP. Is strabismus the only problem? Psychological issues surrounding strabismus surgery. J AAPOS. 2016;20(5):383–386.

Joyce KE, Beyer F, Thomson RG, Clarke MP. A systematic review of the effectiveness of treatments in altering the Natural history of intermittent exotropia. Br J Ophthalmol. 2015;99(4):440–450.

术后眼正位　术后小角度内斜视可逐渐恢复，且是一种理想状态，因为它可减少外斜视复发。出现内斜视时有复视，所以应在术前告知其可能性。在手术后持续 3 ~ 4 周以上或继续发展 1~2 个月的内斜视（手术后内斜视），需要进一步治疗，如矫正远视、基底朝外棱镜、遮盖以避免弱视，抑或再次手术。高 AC/A 比患者可以戴双焦镜，并且伴真性散开过度的患者应在术前告知。手术后内斜视需再次手术时，建议推迟数月，因为可能出现自发性的改善，除非发生肌肉滑落或“丢失”导致的外展功能不足。

因为可能存在连续性内斜视，对术前有良好视力和立体视的幼儿，可推迟手术。然而，有人认为推迟手术是斜视复发的危险因素。通过长期随访研究手术疗效，提示间歇性外斜视的复发率高。患者需要多次手术来维持长期正眼位。

集合不足

集合不足（CI）是视近时眼偏斜大于视远的一种外斜视，其特征为融像性集合幅度低下和集合近点移远（正常融像性聚散幅度见第 7 章，表 7–1）。有时表现为视疲劳、近视力模糊以及近距离工作时复视，常见于青少年或成人。集合不足是 Parkinson 病的常见并发症。罕见有调节痉挛，是因为努力克服集合不足，而刺激调节与集合。

Treatment of symptomatic CI typically involves orthoptic exercises. Base-out prisms can be used to stimulate and strengthen fusional convergence amplitudes. Stereograms, "pencil push-ups," and computer-based or office-based convergence training programs are all viable options. If these exercises fail, base-in prism reading glasses may alleviate symptoms. Surgical treatment, usually medial rectus muscle resection, may be indicated in patients whose problems persist despite medical therapy.

Constant Exotropia

Constant exotropia is encountered most often in older patients with sensory exotropia or in patients with a history of long-standing intermittent exotropia, which has decompensated. Constant exotropia also occurs in persons with infantile or consecutive exotropia. A patient with an exotropia that is constant can have basic, pseudodivergence excess, or true divergence excess exotropia—the same forms seen in intermittent exotropia.

Surgical treatment is the same as that for intermittent exotropia, discussed earlier in the chapter.

Some patients with constant exotropia have an enlarged field of peripheral vision because they have large areas of nonoverlapping visual fields. These patients may notice a field constriction when the eyes are straightened.

Infantile Exotropia

Infantile exotropia is much less common than infantile esotropia. Constant infantile exotropia is apparent before age 6 months as a large-angle deviation (Fig 9-1). The risk of amblyopia is higher in constant exotropia than in intermittent exotropia. Although infants with constant exotropia may be otherwise healthy, the risk of associated neurologic impairment or craniofacial disorders is increased in these patients. A careful developmental history is thus important, and referral for neurologic assessment should be considered if there are indications of developmental delay. Patients with constant infantile exotropia are operated on early in life, and outcomes are similar to those for infantile esotropia (see Chapter 8). Early surgery can lead to monofixation with gross binocular vision, but restoration of normal binocular function is rare. Dissociated vertical deviations and overelevation in adduction may develop (see Chapter 11).

Sensory Exotropia

Esotropia or exotropia may develop as a result of any condition that severely reduces vision or the visual field in 1 eye. It is not known why some individuals become esotropic and others exotropic after unilateral vision loss. In addition, although both sensory esotropia and sensory exotropia occur in infants and young children, the latter predominates in older children and adults. If the vision in the exotropic eye can be improved, peripheral fusion may be reestablished after surgical realignment, provided the sensory exotropia has not been present for an extended period. Loss of fusional abilities, known as central fusion disruption, can lead to constant and permanent diplopia despite anatomical realignment when adult-onset sensory exotropia has been present for several years before vision rehabilitation.

治疗集合不足需要做正视训练。基底朝外棱镜可用于刺激和提高融像性集合幅度。还可以选择立体图、“铅笔移近移远法”，以及基于计算机的或办公室的集合训练程序。训练不成功时，可以戴基底朝内棱镜阅读以减轻症状。对于仍不能解决问题的患者可手术治疗，多用内直肌切除术。

恒定性外斜视

在成人中，恒定性外斜视多为感觉性外斜视，或由长期间歇性外斜视的失代偿演变而来。恒定性外斜视也发生于婴儿或连续性外斜视。恒定性外斜视分为基本型、假性散开过度或真性散开过度性外斜视——与间歇性外斜视相同。

手术治疗与间歇性外斜视一样，已在前面进行讨论。

有的恒定性外斜视的患者有很大的周边视野，因为非重叠视野范围很大。可能在直视时感到视野变窄。

婴儿型外斜视

婴儿型外斜视比婴儿型内斜视少见。恒定性婴儿型外斜视是指 6 月龄前出现的大角度偏斜（图 9-1）。恒定性外斜视导致弱视的风险高于间歇性外斜视。虽然伴恒定性外斜视的婴儿在其他方面健康，但合并神经系统损害或颅面部疾病的风险增加。因此详细的发育史很重要，如果发现发育迟缓，应转诊，进行神经系统评估。恒定性婴儿型外斜视应尽早进行手术，且效果与婴儿型内斜视相同（见第 8 章）。早期手术可形成双眼单视，但很难恢复正常双眼视功能。可能出现垂直分离性偏斜和内转高位（见第 11 章）。

感觉性外斜视

内斜视或外斜视可能发展为严重视力减退或仅有一眼视野。尚不清楚在单眼视力丧失后，为何一些患者变为内斜视，另一些变为外斜视。尽管感觉性内斜视和感觉性外斜视都发生于婴幼儿中，但后者以青少年和成人为主。假如感觉性外斜视存在时间不长，外斜视眼视力可以改善，则周围融合可能在手术复位后重建。融合功能丧失，即*中心融合破坏*，可导致解剖结构复位正眼位后，仍存在恒定性永久性复视，成人在视力恢复之前，已经存在多年的感觉性外斜视。

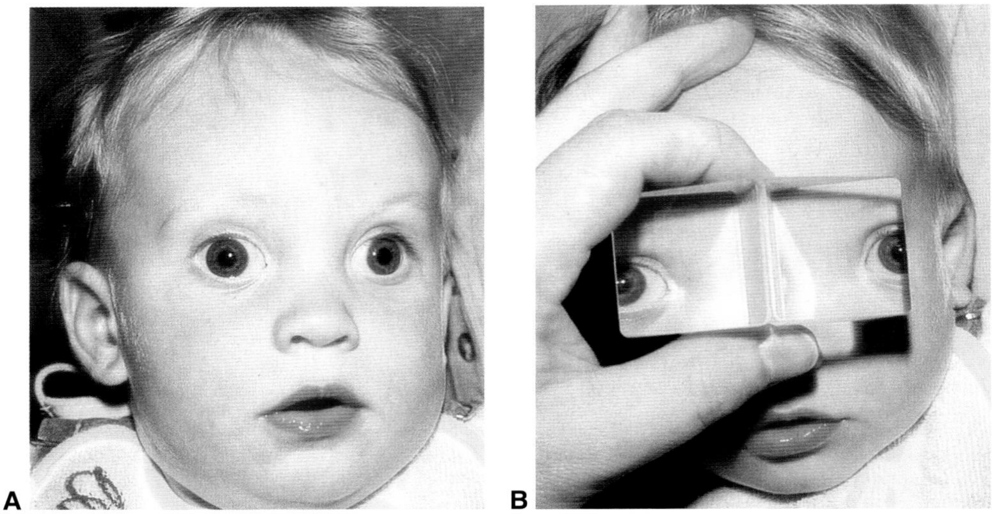

Figure 9-1 Infantile exotropia. **A,** This 10-month-old infant with infantile exotropia also shows developmental delay. **B,** Krimsky test. Two base-in prisms are used to measure the large exotropia. *(Reproduced from Wilson ME. Exotropia. Focal Points: Clinical Modules for Ophthalmologists. San Francisco: American Academy of Ophthalmology; 1995, module 11.)*

Consecutive Exotropia

Exotropia that occurs after a period of esotropia is called *consecutive exotropia*. Rarely, exotropia may develop spontaneously in a patient who was previously esotropic and never underwent strabismus surgery. Much more commonly, consecutive exotropia develops after previous surgery for esotropia (*postsurgical exotropia*), usually within a few months or years after the initial surgery. However, in some patients who had surgery for infantile esotropia, consecutive exotropia may not develop until adulthood. Consecutive exotropia may be intermittent or constant.

Other Forms of Exotropia

Exotropic Duane Retraction Syndrome

The most widely used classification of Duane retraction syndrome defines 3 types. Patients with type 2 can present with exotropia, usually accompanied by deficient adduction and a head turn away from the affected side. See Chapter 12 for further discussion.

Neuromuscular Abnormalities

A constant exotropia may result from third nerve palsy, internuclear ophthalmoplegia, or myasthenia gravis. These conditions are discussed in Chapter 12 of this volume and in BCSC Section 5, *Neuro-Ophthalmology.*

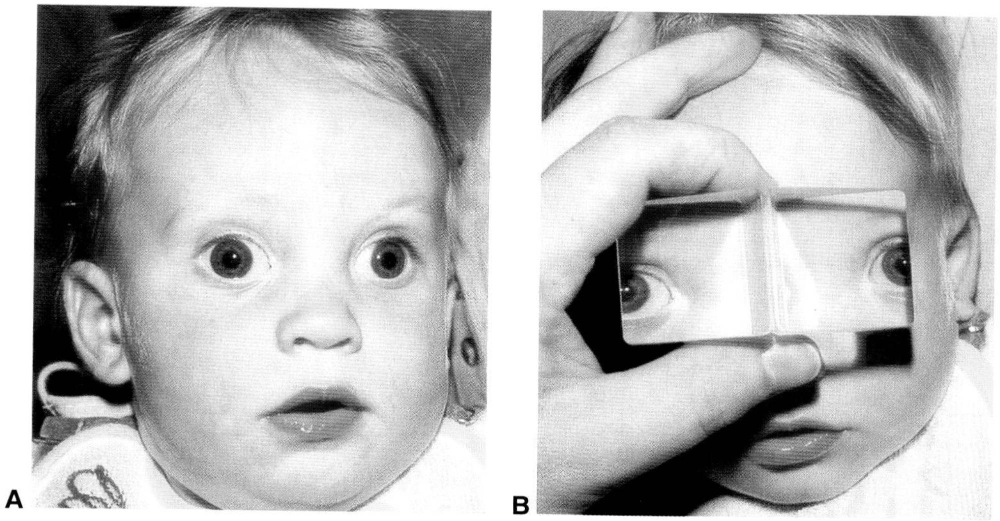

图 9–1　婴儿型外斜视。**A.** 这个 10 月龄的患儿患婴儿型外斜视，伴发育迟缓。**B.** Krimsky 试验。用 2 个基底朝内棱镜测量大度数外斜视。*（译者注：资料来源见前页原文。）*

连续性外斜视

内斜视一段时期后发生的外斜视称为*连续性外斜视*。既往有内斜视但未行斜视手术也可能自发成为外斜视的现象较为罕见。连续性外斜视多见于曾行内斜视手术的（*手术后外斜视*）患者，通常在首次手术后数月或数年。而曾行婴儿型内斜视手术的患者，其连续性外斜至成年才出现。连续性外斜视可为间歇性或恒定性。

其他形式的外斜视

外斜视型 Duane 后退综合征

Duane 后退综合征分 3 型。2 型患者有外斜视，常伴有内转不足，头偏离受累眼。进一步讨论见第 12 章。

神经肌肉异常

第Ⅲ颅神经麻痹、核间眼肌麻痹或重症肌无力可导致恒定性外斜视。见本册第 12 章和 BCSC 第 5 册《*神经眼科学*》。

Dissociated Horizontal Deviation

Dissociated strabismus complex may include vertical, horizontal, and/or torsional components (see Chapter 2 and Chapter 11). It may be associated with infantile esotropia. When a dissociated abduction movement is predominant, the condition is called *dissociated horizontal deviation (DHD)*. Though not a true exotropia, DHD can be confused with a constant or intermittent exotropia. Dissociated vertical deviation and latent nystagmus often coexist with DHD (Fig 9-2). In rare cases, patients may manifest both DHD and intermittent esotropia. DHD must be differentiated from anisohyperopia associated with intermittent exotropia, in which the exotropic deviation is present during fixation with the normal eye but is masked during fixation with the hyperopic eye because of accommodative convergence. Treatment of DHD usually consists of unilateral or bilateral lateral rectus recession in addition to any necessary oblique or vertical muscle surgery.

Convergence Paralysis

Convergence paralysis is distinct from convergence insufficiency and usually secondary to an intracranial lesion, most commonly in association with dorsal midbrain syndrome (see BCSC Section 5, *Neuro-Ophthalmology*). It is characterized by normal adduction and accommodation, with exotropia and diplopia present at attempted near fixation only. Apparent convergence paralysis due to malingering or lack of effort can be distinguished from true convergence paralysis by the absence of pupillary constriction with attempted near fixation.

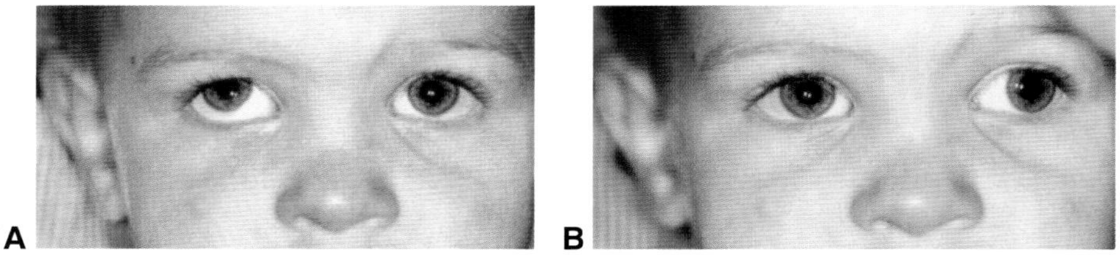

Figure 9-2 Dissociated strabismus complex. **A,** When the patient fixates with the left eye, a prominent vertical deviation is observed in the right eye. **B,** However, when the patient fixates with the right eye, a prominent horizontal deviation is noted in the left eye. *(Reproduced from Wilson ME. Exotropia. Focal Points: Clinical Modules for Ophthalmologists. San Francisco: American Academy of Ophthalmology; 1995, module 11.)*

Treatment of convergence paralysis is difficult and often limited to use of base-in prisms at near to alleviate the diplopia. Plus lenses may be required if accommodation is limited. Monocular occlusion is indicated if diplopia cannot be otherwise treated.

分离性水平斜视

分离性斜视综合征包括垂直、水平、和（或）旋转（见第 2 章和第 11 章）。可伴婴儿型内斜视。当分离性外转 / 外展运动明显时，称为*分离性水平斜视*（DHD）。虽然不是真性外斜视，但 DHD 可与恒定性或间歇性外斜视混淆。分离性垂直斜视和隐性眼球震颤常与 DHD 同时存在（图 9–2）。罕见病例中，患者可能同时表现为 DHD 和间歇性内斜视。DHD 必须与异向性远视 / 远视性参差相关的间歇性外斜视相鉴别，在调节性集合作用下，表现为正常眼注视时产生外斜视，但远视眼注视时外斜视不显示。DHD 的治疗包括单眼或双眼外直肌后徙术，必要时行斜肌或垂直肌手术。

集合麻痹

集合麻痹不同于集合不足，常继发于颅内病变，最常见于背侧中脑综合征（见 BCSC 第 5 册《*神经眼科学*》）。特征为内收和调节正常、仅视近时出现外斜视和复视。但诈病或不努力而产生集合不足，可以通过努力视近时没有瞳孔收缩体征，与真性集合麻痹相鉴别。

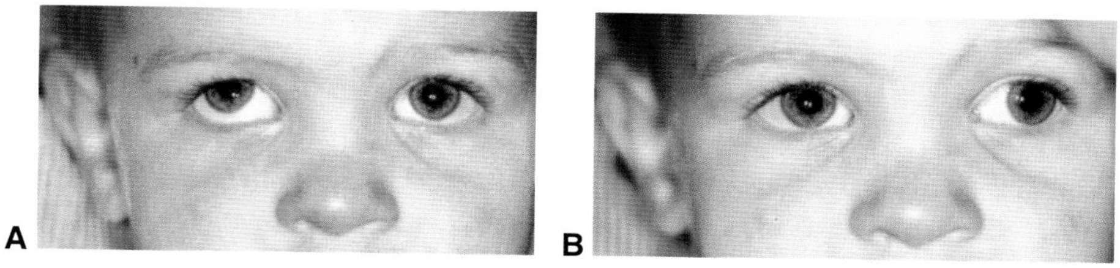

图 9–2　分离性斜视综合征。**A.** 患者左眼注视，可见右眼有明显的垂直偏斜。**B.** 然而，患者用右眼注视时，可见左眼明显的水平偏斜。*（译者注：资料来源见前页原文。）*

集合麻痹的治疗困难，可以有限地使用基底朝内棱镜，缓解视近时的复视。调节不足时可能需使用正镜。如复视无法治疗，可行单眼遮盖。

（翻译　杨乐　刘建 // 审校　石一宁　丁娟 // 章节审校　石广礼）

CHAPTER 10

Pattern Strabismus

Pattern strabismus is a horizontal deviation in which there is a difference in the magnitude of deviation between upgaze and downgaze. The term *V pattern* describes a horizontal deviation that is more divergent (less convergent) in upgaze than in downgaze, while the term *A pattern* describes a horizontal deviation that is more divergent (less convergent) in downgaze than in upgaze. An A or V pattern is found in 15%–25% of horizontal strabismus cases. Less common variations of pattern strabismus include Y, X, and λ (lambda) patterns.

Etiology

The following conditions are associated with various types of pattern strabismus or considered causes of these patterns.

- *Oblique muscle dysfunction*. Apparent inferior oblique muscle overaction (overelevation in adduction [OEAd]; see Chapter 11) is associated with V patterns (Fig 10-1), and apparent superior oblique muscle overaction (overdepression in adduction [ODAd]) with A patterns (Fig 10-2). These associations may be due to the tertiary abducting action of these muscles in upgaze and downgaze, respectively; however, oblique dysfunction is frequently associated with ocular torsion that can also contribute to A or V patterns (see below).
- *Orbital pulley system abnormalities.* Abnormalities (heterotopia) of the orbital pulley system (see Chapter 3) have been described as a cause of simulated oblique muscle overactions and of altered rectus muscle pathways and functions that can result in A or V patterns. These pulley effects may help explain the observation that patients with upward-or downward-slanting palpebral fissures (Fig 10-3) may show A or V patterns because of an underlying variation in orbital configuration, which is reflected in the orientation of the fissures. Similarly, patients with craniofacial anomalies (see Chapter 18) may have a V-pattern strabismus with marked elevation of the adducting eye as a manifestation of rotation of the orbits, pulley system, and muscle pathways.
- *Ocular torsion.* While not as consequential as pulley dystopia, ocular torsion displaces the anterior path of the vertical rectus muscles. Extorsion displaces the superior rectus muscle temporally and the inferior rectus muscle nasally, which tends to produce a V pattern. Intorsion displaces the superior rectus nasally and the inferior rectus temporally, which tends to produce an A pattern.

第 10 章

A–V 型斜视

*A–V 型斜视*是一种在向上注视和向下注视时偏斜有明显差异的水平斜视。*V 型*为一种向上注视比向下注视时散开更多（集合更少）的水平斜视，同时 *A 型*为一种向下注视比向上注视时散开更多（集合更少）的水平斜视。水平斜视中有 15% ~ 25% 是 A 型或 V 型。少见的 A–V 型斜视包括 Y，X，λ（lambda）型。

病因学

以下情况可能伴随不同类型的 A–V 型斜视，或是其原因。

- *斜肌功能障碍*。明显的下斜肌功能亢进（内转时眼球上转过度，*OEAd*，见第 11 章）导致 V 型（图 10–1），而明显的上斜肌功能亢进（内转时眼球下转过度，*ODAd*）导致 A 型（图 10–2）。这可能分别与向上注视与向下注视时这些肌肉的第三功能外转作用有关；然而，斜肌功能异常与其旋转功能有关，也导致 A 或 V 型的眼球（见下文）。

- *眶滑车系统异常*。异常。眶滑车系统异常（隐斜视）（见第 3 章）是假性斜肌功能亢进和直肌走行路线改变的原因，可以导致 A 或 V 型。滑车效应可解释睑裂向上或向下 – 倾斜的患者（图 10–3）多表现出 A 或 V 型的，可能因为眶结构的改变反映在睑裂的位置上。同样的，伴颅面畸形的患者（见第 18 章）可有内转高位的 V 型斜视，提示存在眶、滑车系统和肌肉经行的旋转。

- *眼球旋转*。与滑车异位的结果不同，眼球旋转是垂直直肌前段异位。外旋是上直肌向颞侧异位，和下直肌向鼻侧异位，从而导致 V 型斜视。内旋是上直肌向鼻侧异位和下直肌向颞侧异位，从而导致 A 型斜视。

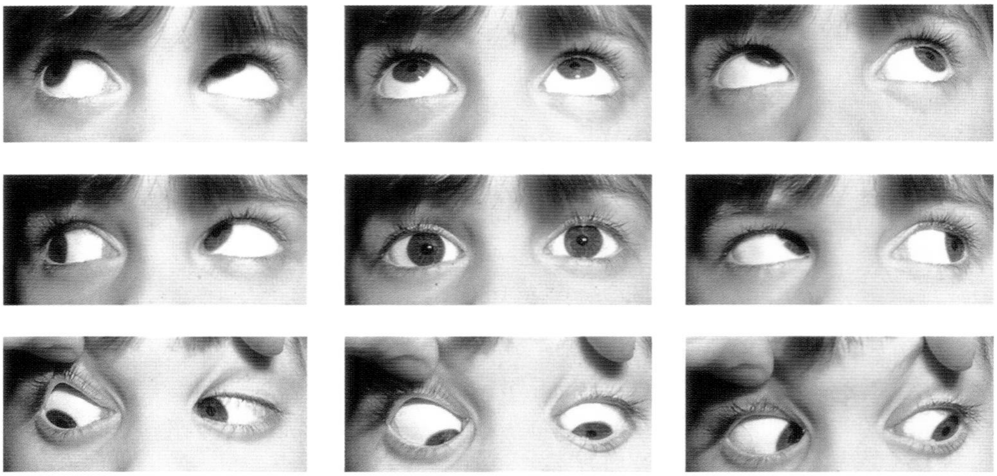

Figure 10-1 V pattern with exotropia in upgaze and esotropia in downgaze. Note overelevation in adduction and limitation of depression in adduction.

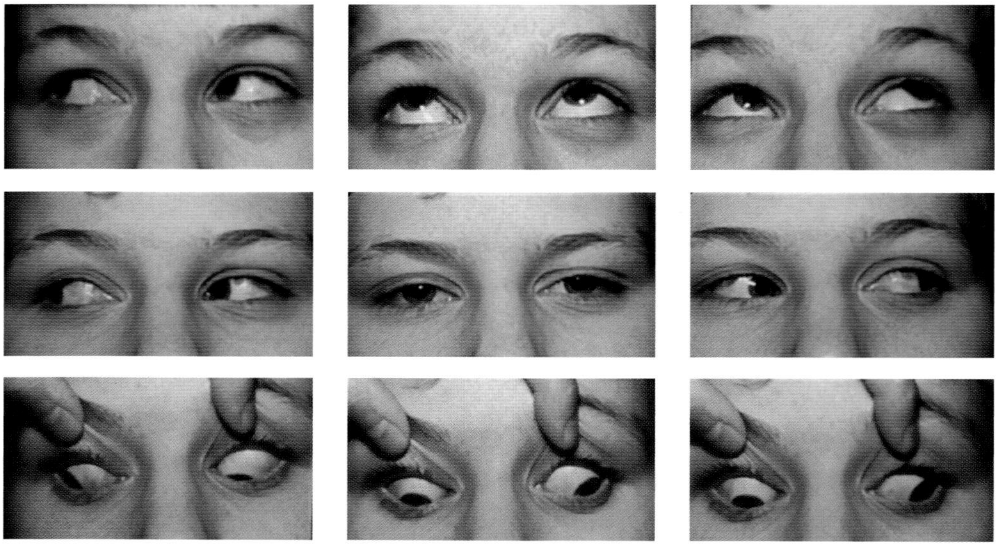

Figure 10-2 A-pattern exotropia with overdepression and underelevation in adduction. *(Modified with permission from Levin A, Wilson T, eds. The Hospital for Sick Children's Atlas of Pediatric Ophthalmology and Strabismus. Philadelphia: Lippincott Williams & Wilkins; 2007:11.)*

Figure 10-3 Palpebral fissures that slant downward temporally, sometimes associated with a V-pattern horizontal deviation. *(Courtesy of Edward L. Raab, MD.)*

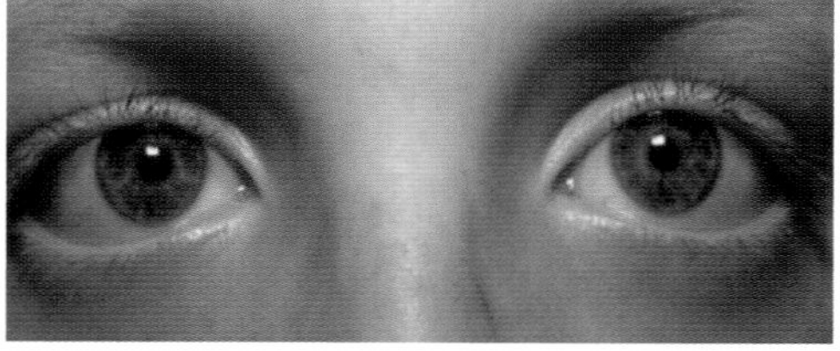

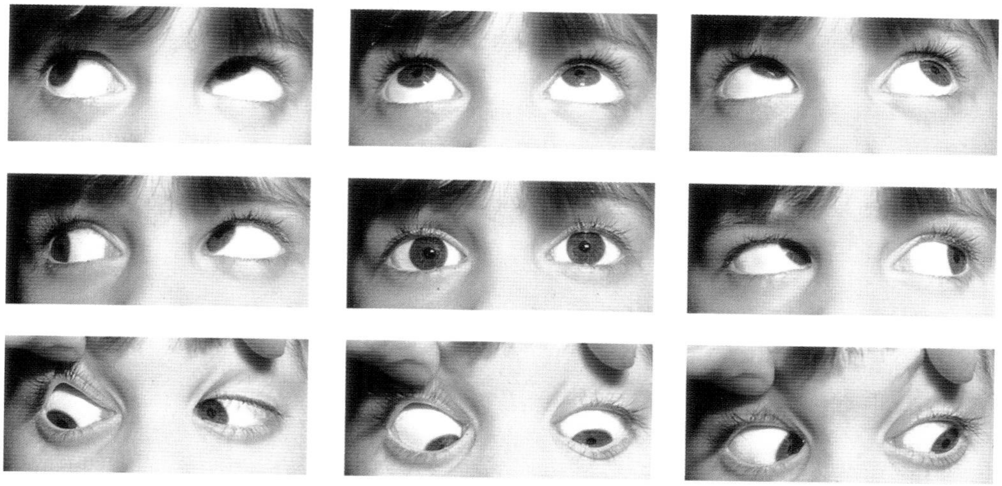

图 10–1　向上注视的外斜视伴 V 型和向下注视的内斜视伴 V 型。注意内转时眼球上转过度和内转时眼球下转受限。

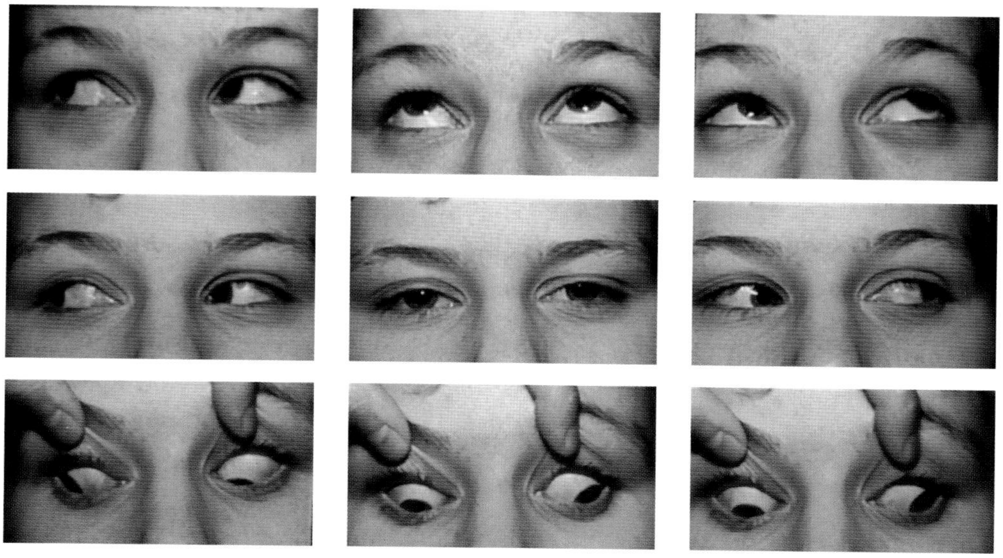

图 10–2　A 型外斜视伴内转时眼球下转过度和内转时眼球上转不足。*（译者注：资料来源见前页原文。）*

图 10–3　向颞下侧倾斜的睑裂，伴 V 型水平斜视。*（译者注：资料来源见前页原文。）*

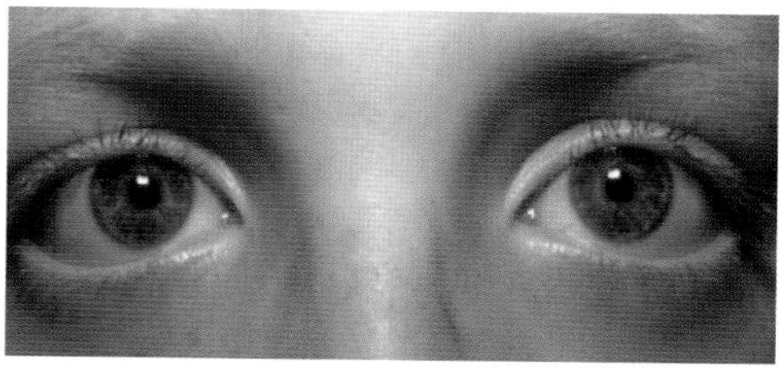

- *Restricted horizontal rectus muscles.* Contracture of the lateral rectus muscles in large-angle exotropia may result in an X pattern, with globe slippage in adduction.
- *Anomalous innervation.* Sometimes seen in isolation and sometimes associated with other congenital cranial dysinnervation disorders (see Chapter 12), this most commonly produces a Y pattern.
- *Selective innervation of superior or inferior compartments of the horizontal rectus muscles.* This is a possible contributing factor to A and V patterns and is under investigation (see Chapter 3).

Clinical Features and Identification of Pattern Strabismus

The presence of A and V patterns is determined by measuring alignment while the patient fixates on an accommodative target at distance, with fusion prevented with the prism alternate cover test, in primary position and in straight upgaze and downgaze, approximately 25° from the primary position. Proper refractive correction is necessary during measurement because an uncompensated accommodative component can induce exaggerated convergence in downgaze. The examiner should look specifically for apparent oblique muscle overaction (OEAd or ODAd) because of its frequent association with pattern strabismus.

An A pattern is considered clinically significant when the difference in measurement between upgaze and downgaze is at least 10 prism diopters (Δ). For a V pattern, this difference must be at least 15Δ because there is normally some physiologic convergence in downgaze.

V Pattern

The most common type of pattern strabismus, V pattern occurs most frequently in patients with infantile esotropia. The pattern is usually not present when the esotropia first develops but becomes apparent during the first year of life or later. V patterns may also occur in patients with superior oblique palsies, particularly if they are bilateral, and in patients with craniofacial malformations.

A Pattern

A pattern is the second most common type of pattern strabismus and occurs most frequently in patients with exotropia and in persons with spina bifida.

Y Pattern

Patients with Y patterns (pseudo-overaction of the inferior oblique muscle) have normal ocular alignment in primary position and downgaze, but the eyes diverge in upgaze. These patients appear to have overacting inferior oblique muscles, but the deviation is thought to be due to anomalous innervation of the lateral rectus muscles in upgaze. Clinical characteristics that help identify this form of strabismus include the following: the overelevation is not seen when the eyes are moved directly horizontally, but it becomes manifest when the eyes are directed horizontally and slightly into upgaze; there is no fundus torsion; there is no difference in vertical deviation with head tilts; and there is no superior oblique muscle underaction.

- *受限的水平直肌*。大角度外斜视的外直肌挛缩可能导致 X 型，并伴内收时眼球下降。
- *神经支配异常*。独立存在或与先天性颅骨神经支配异常有关（见第 12 章），其最容易导致 Y 型。
- *水平直肌上转或下转功能的选择性神经支配*。这可能是导致 A 和 V 型的一个因素，目前正在研究（见第 3 章）。

A–V 型斜视的临床特征及鉴别

让患者注视远距离的调节性视标，棱镜交替遮盖试验打破融合，测量在第一眼位以及自第一眼位垂直向上注视、垂直向下注视 25°，来确定 A 和 V 型眼位。测量时需要屈光矫正，因为未代偿的调节成分导致在向下注视时的过度收敛。应特别注意明显的斜肌功能亢进（OEAd 或 ODAd），因为它常与 A–V 型斜视有关。

在向上注视和向下注视时的差别至少 10Δ 时，A 型有临床意义，对于 V 型，差别至少需 15Δ，因为向下注视时存在正常的生理性收敛。

V 型

V 型是最常见的 A–V 型斜视类型，婴儿型内斜视多见。刚发生内斜视时并不出现 V 型，但在 1 岁或之后变得明显。V 型可能出现在上斜肌麻痹的患者，特别是双侧的，以及伴颅面畸形的患者。

A 型

A 型占 A–V 型斜视类型的第二位，多见于外斜视及伴脊柱裂的患者。

Y 型

伴 Y 型的患者（假性下斜肌功能亢进）在第一眼位和向下注视时眼正位，但向上注视时散开。这些患者表现出下斜肌功能亢进，但其眼位偏斜可能是向上注视时的外直肌异常神经支配所致。鉴别这种形式斜视的临床特征有：无眼水平转动时的过度上转，但当眼水平运动并轻微向上注视时，过度上转变得明显；没有眼底旋转；与伴头倾斜时的垂直偏斜没有差异；没有上斜肌功能不足。

Kushner BJ. Pseudo inferior oblique overaction associated with Y and V patterns. *Ophthalmology.* 1991;98(10):1500–1505.

X Pattern

In X-pattern strabismus, an exodeviation is present in primary position and increases in both upgaze and downgaze. This pattern is usually associated with overelevation and overdepression in adduction when the eye moves slightly above or below direct side gaze. X patterns are most commonly seen in patients with large-angle exotropia.

λ Pattern

This rare pattern is a variant of A-pattern exotropia. In λ-pattern strabismus, the horizontal deviation is the same in primary position and upgaze but increases in downgaze. The λ pattern is usually associated with ODAd.

Management

Clinically significant patterns (see the section Clinical Features and Identification of Pattern Strabismus) are typically treated surgically, in combination with **correction of** the underlying horizontal deviation.

Surgical Correction of Pattern Deviations: General Principles

The following are strategies for surgical correction of pattern deviations. See Chapter 14 for further discussion of some of the procedures and concepts mentioned here.

- For pattern strabismus associated with apparent overaction of the oblique muscles (OEAd, ODAd), weakening of the oblique muscles is performed.
- For patients with no apparent overaction of the oblique muscles or a pattern inconsistent with oblique dysfunction, vertical transposition of the horizontal muscles is performed. The muscles are transposed from one-half to a full tendon width. The medial rectus muscles are always moved toward the "apex" of the pattern (ie, upward in A patterns and downward in V patterns). The lateral rectus muscles are moved toward the open end (ie, upward in V patterns and downward in A patterns). A useful mnemonic is MALE: medial rectus muscle to the apex, lateral rectus muscle to the empty space. These rules apply whether the horizontal rectus muscles are weakened or tightened (Fig 10-4).

  If transposition of horizontal rectus muscles is used to treat pattern strabismus when there is associated ocular torsion, it will exacerbate the torsion (extorsion with V pattern and intorsion with A pattern), which itself can contribute to the pattern. Conversely, when rectus muscle transposition is used to treat torsion, it will make any associated pattern strabismus worse.

Kushner BJ. Pseudo inferior oblique overaction associated with Y and V patterns. *Ophthalmology*. 1991;98(10):1500–1505.

X 型

X– 型斜视中，外斜视出现在第一眼位，并在向上注视和向下注视时斜视都增加。当轻微向上或向下垂直注视时，X– 型斜视多伴随内转时眼球上转过度和下转过度。X 型最常见于大角度外斜视的患者。

λ 型

这种罕见的类型是 A– 型外斜的变异。在 λ 型斜视中，水平偏斜在第一眼位和向上注视时一致，但向下注视时加重。多伴有内转时眼球下转过度（ODAd）。

治疗

临床上明显的 A–V 型（见 A–V 型斜视的临床特征及鉴别一节）通常手术治疗，并联合水平斜视的矫正。

A–V 型斜视的手术矫正：总原则

以下是手术矫正 A–V 型斜视的策略。第 14 章将进一步讨论有关步骤和概念。

- A–V 型斜视伴有明显的斜肌功能亢进（内转时眼球*上转过度*，内转时眼球*下转过度*），可行斜肌功能减弱。
- 对于无明显斜肌功能亢进，或不符合斜肌功能异常的患者，可行水平直肌垂直移位。肌肉移位 1/2 ~ 1 个肌腱宽度。内直肌移至“顶点”（如 A 型上移，V 型下移）。外直肌移至开口端（如 V 型上移与 A 型下移）。符号 MALE 便于记忆：内直肌到顶点，外直肌到开口端。这些法则用于水平直肌是被减弱还是被加强（图 10–4）。

若使用水平直肌移位术治疗伴旋转的 A–V 型斜视时，则会使眼球旋转加重（V 型外旋和 A 型内旋），旋转本身参与 A–V 型斜视。相反，若使用直肌移位术治疗旋转，则会加重 A–V 型斜视。

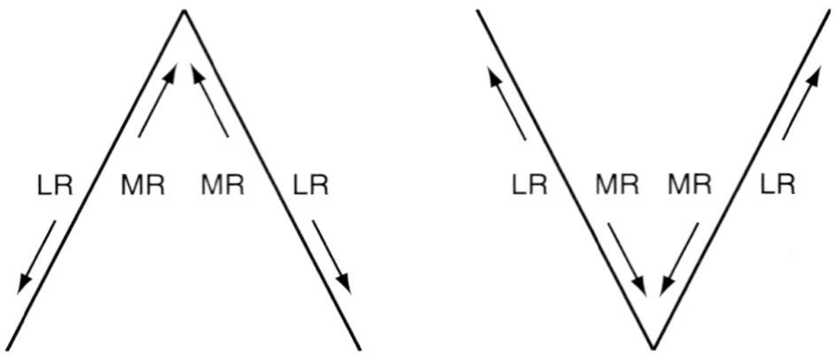

Figure 10-4 Direction of displacement of medial rectus (MR) and lateral rectus (LR) muscles in procedures to treat A-pattern *(left)* and V-pattern *(right)* deviations. *(Reprinted with permission from von Noorden GK, Campos EC. Binocular Vision and Ocular Motility: Theory and Management of Strabismus. 6th ed. St Louis: Mosby; 2002:388.)*

- When horizontal rectus muscle recession-resection surgery is the preferred choice because of other pertinent factors (eg, prior surgery, unimprovable vision in 1 eye), displacement of the rectus muscle insertions should be in mutually opposite directions, according to the rules stated previously. Unlike what occurs when both horizontal rectus muscles of an eye are moved in the same direction, this displacement has little, if any, vertical effect in the primary position. This procedure should be used with caution in patients with binocular fusion as it can produce symptomatic torsion.
- Some surgeons adjust the amount of horizontal surgery because of the potential effect of oblique muscle weakening on the horizontal deviation, particularly for superior oblique muscle surgery, but this is controversial. Some believe that bilateral superior oblique weakening causes a change of 10Δ–15Δ toward convergence in primary position and suggest modifying the amount of horizontal surgery to compensate for this expected change. For inferior oblique muscle weakening procedures, the amount of horizontal rectus muscle surgery does not need to be altered, because the inferior oblique muscle weakening does not substantially change primary position alignment.
- Surgery on the vertical rectus muscles (eg, temporal displacement of the superior rectus muscles for A-pattern esotropia or temporal displacement of the inferior rectus muscles for V-pattern esotropia) is rarely used because transposition of the horizontal rectus muscles that are being operated on for the underlying esotropia or exotropia is usually sufficient.

Surgical Treatment of Specific Patterns

Table 10-1 summarizes the surgical treatment of pattern strabismus (see also Chapter 14).

V pattern

For V-pattern esotropia or exotropia associated with OEAd, weakening of the inferior oblique muscles is performed. For patients who also have dissociated vertical deviation (DVD; see Chapter 11), anterior transposition of the inferior oblique muscle may improve both the V pattern and the DVD. Because patients with V-pattern infantile esotropia who are younger than 2 years are at risk of developing DVD, anterior transposition of the inferior oblique may be considered preemptively for this group.

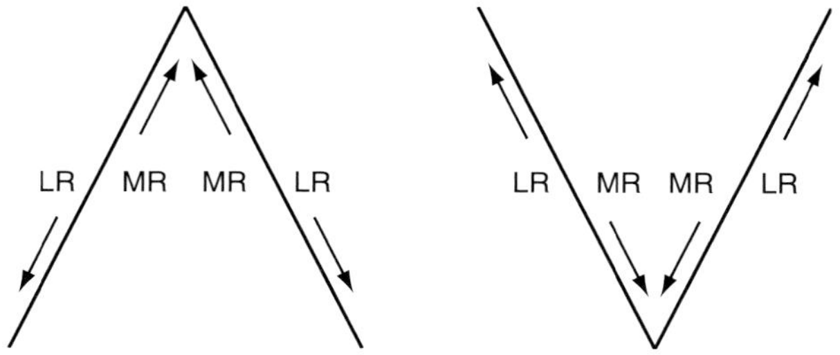

图 10–4　手术治疗 A– 型斜视 *（左）* 和 V– 型斜视 *（右）* 时，内直肌（MR）和外肌直（LR）的移位方向。*（译者注：资料来源见前页原文。）*

- 由于其他相关因素 (如手术前，一眼视力无法改善)，首选水平直肌的后徙 – 切除术时，根据前面的规则，直肌止点的移位方向应该是相反的。与一眼中的 2 条水平直肌向同一方向运动的情况不同，这种位移在第一眼位几乎没有垂直效应。对于双眼融合患者，这种手术应慎用，因为会产生症状性旋转。

- 由于斜肌减弱手术，特别是上斜肌减弱手术，对水平偏斜的潜在影响，一些医生会调整水平肌肉手术的量，但这一方法存在争议。有人认为双侧上斜肌的减弱术会引起第一眼位集合时 10 ~ 15Δ 的改变，建议改变水平肌肉移位的量来补偿这一预期的变化。进行下斜肌减弱手术时，水平肌肉手术的量不需要改变，因为下斜肌减弱对第一眼位的斜视角无大的影响。

- 很少采用垂直直肌手术 (如 A– 型内斜视的上直肌向颞侧位移，或 V– 型内斜视的下直肌向颞侧位移)，因为水平直肌的移位足以矫正潜在的内斜视或外斜视。

特殊 A–V 型斜视的手术治疗

表 10–1 总结了 AV 型斜视的手术治疗 (见第 14 章)。

V 型斜视

伴有内转时眼球上转过度 OEAd 的 V– 型内斜视或外斜视，行下斜肌减弱术。伴分离性垂直斜视 (DVD; 见第 11 章)，行下斜肌的前移位可以同时改善包括 V 型斜视和 DVD。由于小于 2 岁的 V– 型婴儿型内斜视可能发展成 DVD，所以可优先考虑下斜肌的前移位。

Table 10-1 Surgical Treatment of Pattern Strabismus

Type of Pattern	Most Common Clinical Association	Treatment: With OEAd or ODAd	Treatment: Without OEAd or ODAd	Treatment: Other
V Pattern	Infantile esotropia	Weakening of inferior oblique muscles	Vertical transposition of horizontal rectus muscles	If DVD present, anterior transposition of inferior oblique muscles
A Pattern	Exotropia	Weakening of superior oblique muscles	Vertical transposition of horizontal rectus muscles	
Y Pattern	Pseudo-inferior oblique overaction			Superior transposition of lateral rectus muscles
X Pattern	Large-angle exotropia (pseudo-overaction due to contracture of lateral rectus muscles)			Recession of lateral rectus muscles
λ Pattern	Variant of A-pattern exotropia	Weakening of superior oblique muscles		

DVD = dissociated vertical deviation; ODAd = overdepression in adduction; OEAd = overelevation in adduction.

For patients with V-pattern esotropia or exotropia not associated with OEAd, appropriate vertical transposition of the horizontal rectus muscles is performed (see Fig 10-4).

A pattern

For A-pattern exotropia or esotropia associated with ODAd, weakening of the superior oblique muscles is performed. Tenotomy of the posterior 7/8 of the insertions is an effective method for treating up to 20Δ of A pattern, without a significant effect on torsion. Lengthening of the oblique tendon by recession, insertion of a spacer, or a split-tendon lengthening procedure may also be used to weaken the superior oblique muscles. Bilateral superior oblique tenotomy is a very powerful procedure that may correct up to 40Δ–50Δ of A pattern. There is a risk of induced torsion with this procedure, which may be symptomatic for patients with binocular fusion.

For patients with A-pattern exotropia or esotropia not associated with ODAd, appropriate vertical transposition of the horizontal rectus muscles is performed (see Fig 10-4).

Y pattern

Because Y patterns are not due to overaction of the inferior oblique muscles, weakening these muscles is not an effective treatment. Superior transposition of the lateral rectus muscles can improve this pattern but does not eliminate it.

X pattern

表10-1　AV征手术治疗

		治疗方法		
斜视	伴随的最常见临床症状	伴随OEAd或ODAd	无OEAd或ODAd	其他
V 型	婴儿型内斜视	下斜肌减弱术	水平直肌的垂直移位	如伴有DVD, 下斜肌前移位
A型	外斜	上斜肌减弱术	水平直肌的垂直移位	
Y型	假性下斜肌亢进			外直肌上移位
X型	大角度外斜(外直肌挛缩造成的假性斜视)			外直肌后徙术
λ型	A型外斜视的变异	上斜肌减弱术		

DVD =分离性垂直斜视；ODAd = 内转时眼球下转过度；OEAd = 内转时眼球上转过度。

不伴有内转时眼球上转过度 OEAd 的 V– 型内斜视或外斜视，需要进行适当的水平直肌垂直移位 (见图 10–4)。

A 型斜视

伴有内转时眼球下转过度 ODAd 的 A– 型外斜视或内斜视，行上斜肌减弱术。止点处的后 7/8 肌腱切断术，可有效治疗 20Δ 的 A 型斜视，而没有明显的旋转效应。通过后徙、植入物插入或肌腱分离延长术也可减弱上斜肌。双侧上斜肌腱切断术是一种非常有效的手术，可矫正多达 40 ～ 50Δ 的 A– 型斜视。这种手术对于双眼融合患者有诱发症状性旋转的风险。

不伴有内转时眼球下转过度 ODAd 的 A– 型外斜视或内斜视，行水平直肌适当的垂直移位 (见图 10–4)。

Y 型

由于 Y 型不是下斜肌亢进所致，减弱下斜肌无效。外直肌上移位可以改善 Y 型斜视，但不能完全消除。

X patterns are usually due to pseudo-overaction of the oblique muscles, which is caused by contracture of the lateral rectus muscles in large-angle exotropia. Recession of the lateral rectus muscles alone usually improves the pattern.

λ *pattern*

As stated earlier, these patterns are typically associated with ODAd. Appropriate superior oblique weakening procedures may be used in patients with this pattern.

X 型

X 型是斜肌的假性功能亢进造成的，大角度外斜视是外直肌挛缩引起的。单独外直肌后徙术即可改善。

λ 型

如前所述，这些类型斜视通常与内转时眼球下转过度 ODAd 有关。可采用上斜肌减弱术。

（翻译 刘建 芮莹 // 审校 石一宁 丁娟 // 章节审校 石广礼）

CHAPTER 11

Vertical Deviations

This chapter includes a related video, which can be accessed by scanning the QR code provided in the text or going to www.aao.org /bcscvideo section06.

A vertical deviation can be termed a hyperdeviation of the higher eye or a hypodeviation of the lower, fellow eye. By convention, vertical deviations are named according to the hypertropic eye. However, the term *hypotropia of the nonfixating* eye is used to describe the patient who has a strong fixation preference for the hypertropic eye.

Surgical treatment of these conditions is discussed in Chapter 14.

A Clinical Approach to Vertical Deviations

The evaluation and diagnosis of vertical deviations are complicated by the need to consider *dissociated vertical deviation (DVD).* In a patient with a completely comitant deviation, there is no movement of either eye on prism alternate cover testing with the same amount of prism used for either eye (prism placed base down over one eye or base up over the other). When there is an incomitant hyperdeviation due to restriction or cyclovertical muscle paresis, the amount of prism needed to neutralize the deviation may be different depending on which eye is fixating. This is the difference between a primary and secondary deviation according to Hering's law (see Chapter 4). Once the neutralizing prism for a given eye is found, however, neither eye moves when alternate cover testing is performed.

In some cases, the examiner encounters a more confusing situation that appears to violate Hering's law. For example, suppose the examiner finds the prism that neutralizes a patient's right hypertropia. That is, if the prism is held over an occluded right eye with the left eye fixating, there is no movement of the right eye when the occluder is moved to the left eye, and fixation switches to the right eye. However, when the occluder is moved back to the right eye, the left eye moves (either upward from a hypotropic position under cover or downward from a hypertropic position) as it resumes fixation. This inability to find a single prism that neutralizes the refixation movement for both eyes indicates the presence of DVD.

Some patients have both "true" hypertropia and DVD. In these patients, there is no way to quantify how much of the deviation is DVD and how much is true hypertropia, although several estimation methods have been advocated. Often, however, one is predominant and the other, smaller component can be ignored. For the sake of simplicity, this chapter does not discuss true hypertropia and DVD in combination but only as separate entities.

第 11 章

垂直斜视

本章包括一个相关视频，可以通过扫描文本中提供的二维码或访问网站查看 www.aao.org /bcscvideo section06.

垂直斜视可称为高眼位的上斜视或对侧低眼位的下斜视。根据习惯，垂直斜视以高眼位的眼命名。而*非注视眼的下斜视*是描述强烈注视偏好的上斜视患者。

第 14 章讨论手术治疗。

垂直斜视的临床治疗

垂直斜视的评估和诊断较为复杂，需要考虑*分离性垂直斜视（DVD）*。当完全共同性斜视时，任意一眼使用等量棱镜交替遮盖试验（基底朝下棱镜置于一眼，或基底朝上棱镜置于另一眼），没有眼位移动。当由于限制或旋转垂直肌麻痹而出现的非共同性斜视时，中和斜视所需的棱镜量可能会因注视眼的不同而不同。根据 Hering 法则，产生第 1 斜视角和第 2 斜视角的差异（见第 4 章）。但是，一旦找到一眼的中和棱镜度，交替遮盖试验时，双眼都不动。

有时检查者会遇到违反了 Hering 法则的情况。例如，检查者发现了中和右斜视的棱镜度。也就是说，如果将棱镜放在右眼上，遮盖右眼，用左眼注视；当遮盖左眼、用右眼注视时，右眼没有移动。而当遮盖移回右眼时，左眼在恢复注视时移动（从遮盖时的下斜视位置向上，或从上斜视位置向下）。出现这种无法找到单一棱镜，以中和双眼的再注视移动的现象，提示存在分离性垂直斜视 DVD。

有人同时存在“真性”上斜视和分离性垂直斜视 DVD。在这些患者中，虽然使用几种估计方法。但仍无法量化 DVD 度数和真性上斜视度数，常多以一种情况为主，另一种情况可以忽略。为了简单起见，本章不讨论真性上斜视联合 DVD，仅分别对单独概念进行讨论。

Vertical Deviations With Marked Horizontal Incomitance

Many vertical deviations are characterized by a hypertropia that is much greater on gaze to one side. They are often, but not exclusively, associated with oblique muscle abnormalities.

Overelevation and Overdepression in Adduction

There are several causes of overelevation in adduction (OEAd) and overdepression in adduction (ODAd) (Tables 11-1, 11-2). These include true overaction and underaction of the oblique muscles, as well as several conditions that can simulate oblique muscle overactions. These cases have also been termed *oblique muscle pseudo-overactions.*

In some patients, such as those with large-angle exotropia or thyroid eye disease, clinical examination of versions appears to show overaction of both the superior and the inferior oblique muscles. In such cases, elevation or depression of the vertical rectus muscle of the opposite, abducting eye is restricted in the lateral portion of the bony orbit. The clinical findings can be explained as an attempt by the vertical rectus muscle to overcome this restriction through extra innervation, which, according to Hering's law, is distributed to the yoke oblique muscle as well (see Chapter 4). Alternatively, overelevation may be due to slippage of a tight lateral rectus muscle as the eye adducts and rises above or below the midline (see Chapter 10).

Table 11-1 Causes of Overelevation in Adduction

Inferior oblique muscle overaction (primary or secondary)
Dissociated vertical deviation
Large-angle exotropia
Rectus muscle pulley heterotopia
Orbital dysmorphism (eg, craniofacial syndromes)
Duane retraction syndrome
Anti-elevation syndrome after contralateral inferior oblique muscle anterior transposition
Contralateral inferior rectus muscle restriction (eg, after orbital floor fracture, in thyroid eye disease)
Skew deviation

Table 11-2 Causes of Overdepression in Adduction

Superior oblique muscle overaction (primary or secondary)
Large-angle exotropia
Rectus muscle pulley heterotopia
Orbital dysmorphism (eg, craniofacial syndromes)
Duane retraction syndrome
Brown syndrome (rarely)
Contralateral superior rectus muscle contracture (eg, after muscle resection)
Skew deviation

垂直斜视伴有明显的水平非共同性

许多垂直斜视的特征是一侧注视时上斜视增加。常（但不完全）与斜肌异常有关。

内转时眼球上转过度和下转过度

内转时眼球上转过度（OEAd）和下转过度（ODAd）的原因有很多（表 11-1,11-2）。这些包括真正的斜肌功能亢进和功能低下，以及类似斜肌功能亢进。也称为*假性斜肌功能亢进*。

大角度外斜视或甲状腺眼病的患者，同向运动检查上斜肌和下斜肌均有亢进。这时存在对侧眼外转时，垂直直肌的上转或下转受限于外侧眶骨。根据 Hering 法则，临床表现可以解释为垂直直肌通过更多的神经冲动克服这一限制，这异常冲动也作用于配偶肌的斜肌（见第 4 章）。另外，上转过度也可能是由于内转并高于或低于中线时，缝合的外侧直肌滑脱（参见第 10 章）。

表11-1　内转时眼球上转过度的原因

下斜肌亢进(原发性或继发性)
分离性垂直斜视
大角度外斜视
直肌滑车异位
眼眶畸形(如颅面综合征)
Duane后退综合征
对侧下斜肌前移位后抗上转综合征
对侧下直肌受限(如眶底骨折后，甲状腺眼病)
反向偏斜

表11-2　内转时眼球过度下转的原因

上斜肌亢进(原发性或继发性)
大角度外斜视
直肌滑车异位
眼眶畸形(如颅面综合征)
Duane后退综合征
Brown综合征(少见)
对侧上直肌挛缩(如肌肉切除后)
反向偏斜

Malposition of the rectus muscle pulleys can lead to anomalous movements that can simulate oblique muscle overactions. This can be seen in craniofacial syndromes. For example, an inferiorly displaced lateral rectus muscle pulley can cause depression in abduction or, if this is the fixating eye, OEAd of the contralateral eye and a V-pattern deviation that simulate inferior oblique muscle overaction. Conversely, a superiorly displaced lateral rectus muscle can produce ODAd—simulating a superior oblique overaction—along with an A-pattern deviation. Lateral and medial malpositioning of vertical rectus muscles can also create pseudo-overactions of oblique muscles. The treatment implication is that apparent oblique dysfunction or A and V patterns associated with anomalous pulley positions respond poorly to oblique muscle surgery.

Other causes of OEAd and ODAd include the upshoots and downshoots of Duane retraction syndrome, superior or inferior rectus muscle restriction (causing extra innervation of contralateral oblique muscles), limitation of elevation in abduction after inferior oblique anterior transposition (anti-elevation syndrome), and rare cases of Brown syndrome.

Inferior oblique muscle overaction

Overaction of the inferior oblique muscle is one cause of OEAd. The overaction is termed *primary* when it is not associated with superior oblique muscle palsy. It is called *secondary* when it accompanies palsy of the superior oblique muscle or the contralateral superior rectus muscle. The eye is elevated in adduction, both on horizontal movement and in upgaze (Fig 11-1).

One explanation of primary overaction relates to vestibular factors governing postural tonus of the extraocular muscles. Some authors have questioned whether primary inferior oblique overaction truly exists, preferring to describe the movement merely as OEAd.

Clinical features Primary inferior oblique muscle overaction has been reported to develop between ages 1 and 6 years in up to two-thirds of patients with infantile strabismus (esotropia or exotropia). It also occurs, less frequently, in association with acquired esotropia or exotropia and, occasionally, in patients with no other strabismus. Bilateral overaction can be asymmetric, often in patients with poor vision in 1 eye, which leads to greater overaction in that eye.

With the eyes in lateral gaze, alternate cover testing shows that the higher (adducting) eye refixates with a downward movement and that the lower (abducting) eye refixates with an upward movement. When inferior oblique muscle overaction is bilateral, the higher and lower eyes reverse their direction of movement in the opposite lateral gaze. These features differentiate inferior oblique overaction from DVD, in which neither eye refixates with an upward movement, whether adducted, abducted, or in primary position. A V-pattern horizontal deviation (see Chapter 10) and extorsion are common with overacting inferior oblique muscles.

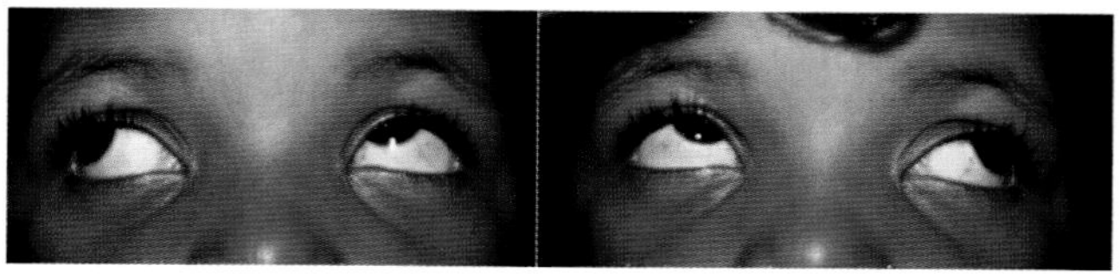

Figure 11-1 Bilateral inferior oblique muscle overaction. Overelevation in adduction, seen best in the upper fields of gaze. *(Courtesy of Edward L. Raab, MD.)*

直肌滑车的异位导致异常运动，类似斜肌功能亢进，也见于颅面综合征。例如，下移位的外侧直肌滑车可能导致外转时下转，或是注视眼，则对侧眼出现类似下斜肌功能亢进的内转时眼球上转过度（OEAd）和 V 型斜视。相反，上移位的外侧直肌可产生内转时眼球下转过度（ODAd）的类似上斜肌亢进，并伴有 A 型斜视。垂直直肌的外侧和内侧异位也会造成假性斜肌功能亢进。治疗结果提示，明显的斜肌功能障碍或与异常滑车位置相关的 A 型和 V 型，斜肌手术效果较差。

内转时眼球上转过度（OEAd）和内转时眼球下转过度（ODAd）的其他病因包括 Duane 后退综合征、上直肌或下直肌限制（引起对侧斜肌的额外神经冲动）、下斜肌前移位后外转上转受限（抗上转综合征）以及罕见的 Brown 综合征。

下斜肌功能亢进

下斜肌功能亢进是内转时眼球上转过度（OEAd）的病因之一。原发性功能亢进与上斜肌麻痹无关。继发性指伴随上斜肌麻痹或对侧上直肌麻痹。眼球水平运动和向上注视时，内转时眼球上转过度（图 11–1）。

一种解释是，原发性功能亢进与眼外肌体位性张力的前庭控制因素有关。有人怀疑原发性下斜肌功能亢进是否真实存在，故仅将肌肉运动描述为内转过度上转（OEAd）。

临床表现　原发性下斜肌功能亢进发生在 2/3 的 1 ~ 6 岁婴儿型斜视（内斜视或外斜视），也发生在获得性内斜视或外斜视患者，偶尔发生在没有斜视的患者。一眼视力较差时，双眼功能亢进不对称，视力较差导致其功能亢进。

当外侧注视时，交替遮盖试验显示，高位（内转状）眼再注视时眼向下运动，下位（外转状）眼再注视时眼向上运动。当双眼下斜肌功能亢进时，向对侧的外侧注视的高位眼和低位眼的运动方向相反。这些特征用于鉴别分离性垂直斜视 DVD，后者在内转、外转或第一眼位时，任意一眼的再注视都没有眼的向上运动。下斜肌亢进常伴有 AV 型水平斜视（见第 10 章）和外旋。

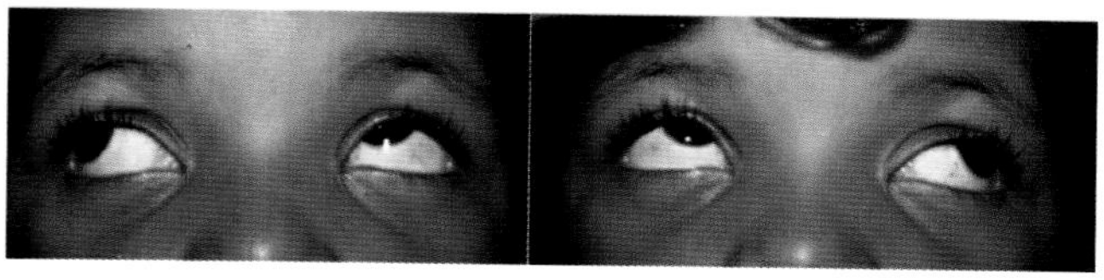

图 11–1　双侧下斜肌功能亢进。内转时眼球上转过度，注视上方时观察最明显。*（译者注：资料来源见前页原文。）*

Management For cases in which inferior oblique overaction produces a functional problem—V-pattern strabismus, hypertropia in primary position, or symptomatic hypertropia in side gaze—a procedure to weaken the inferior oblique muscle (recession, disinsertion, myectomy, or anterior transposition) is indicated. Some surgeons grade the weakening procedure according to the severity of the overaction. Weakening of the inferior oblique muscles generally has an insignificant effect on horizontal alignment in primary position.

Superior oblique muscle overaction

Superior oblique muscle overaction is one of several causes of ODAd.

Clinical features A vertical deviation in primary position often occurs with unilateral or asymmetric bilateral overaction of the superior oblique muscles. The lower eye has the overacting superior oblique muscle in unilateral overaction and the more prominently overacting superior oblique in bilateral cases. The overacting superior oblique muscle causes a hypotropia of the adducting eye, which is accentuated in the lower field of gaze (Fig 11-2). A horizontal deviation, most often exotropia, may be present and may lead to an A pattern (see Chapter 10). Intorsion is common with superior oblique muscle over action. Most cases of bilateral superior oblique overaction are primary overactions.

Management In a patient with clinically significant hypertropia or hypotropia or an A pattern, a procedure to weaken the superior oblique tendon (recession, tenotomy, tenectomy, or lengthening by insertion of a silicone spacer or nonabsorbable suture or by split-tendon lengthening) is appropriate. Significant intorsion will also be reduced with any of these procedures. Many surgeons are reluctant to perform superior oblique tendon weakening in patients with fusion because torsional or asymmetric vertical effects can cause diplopia. As with inferior oblique muscle overaction, the horizontal deviation can be corrected during the same operative session. Some surgeons, anticipating a convergent effect in primary position, alter the amount of horizontal rectus muscle surgery when simultaneously weakening the superior oblique muscles.

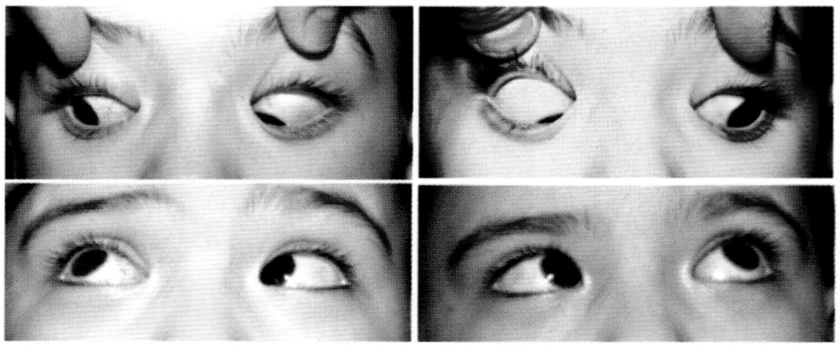

Figure 11-2 *Top row,* Bilateral superior oblique muscle overaction. Overdepression in adduction, seen best in the lower fields of gaze. *Bottom row,* Associated bilateral inferior oblique underaction. *(Courtesy of Edward L. Raab, MD.)*

治疗　对于下斜肌功能亢进导致功能性问题——V 型斜视、第一眼位上斜视或侧位注视时的症状性上斜视，应采用减弱下斜肌的方法（后徙术、断腱术、肌肉切除术或前转位术）。一些医生根据亢进的严重程度对减弱手术进行分级。下斜肌减弱术对第一眼位的水平眼位的作用不大。

上斜肌亢进

上斜肌功能亢进是引起内转时眼球下转过度（ODAd）的原因之一。

临床表现　由于单眼或不对称的双眼的上斜肌功能亢进，在第一眼位发生垂直性偏斜。单侧上斜肌亢进时，下位眼的上斜肌功能亢进，而双侧时，上斜肌功能亢进更明显。功能亢进的上斜肌导致内转眼的下斜视，向下注视时更明显（图 11–2）。伴有水平斜视，最常见外斜视，并导致 A 型斜视（见第 10 章）。上斜肌功能亢进常合并内旋。双眼上斜肌功能亢进多为原发性。

治疗　对于临床上明显的上斜视、下斜视或 A 型斜视，可采用上斜肌减弱术（后徙术、肌腱切开术、肌腱切除术、硅胶垫片植入、不可吸收缝线的肌腱延长或肌腱分离延长术）。这些方法也可以减少内旋。对融合患者，许多医生不行上斜肌腱减弱手术，因为旋转性或不对称性垂直效应可导致复视。与下斜肌功能亢进一样，在手术中，可同时矫正水平偏斜。一些外科医生先预测第一眼位的集合效应，在减弱上斜肌的同时，调整水平直肌的手术量。

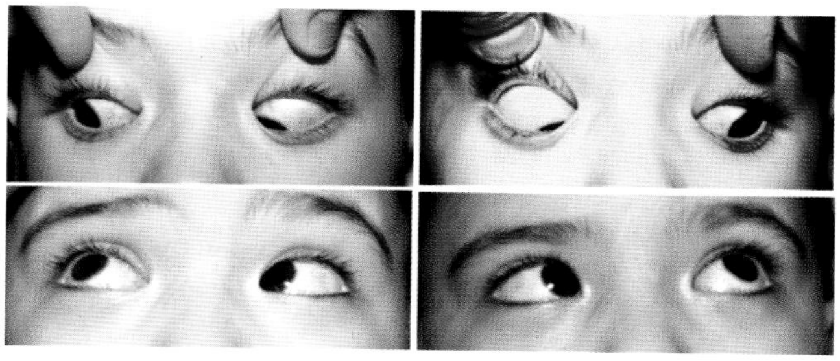

图 11–2　*上排*，双侧上斜肌功能亢进。内转时眼球下转过度，注视下方时最明显。*下排*，伴双眼下斜肌功能低下。*（译者注：资料来源见前页原文。）*

Superior Oblique Muscle Palsy

The most common paralysis of a single cyclovertical muscle is fourth nerve (trochlear) palsy, which involves the superior oblique muscle. The palsy can be congenital or acquired; if the latter, it is usually a result of closed head trauma or, less commonly, vascular problems of the central nervous system, diabetes mellitus, or a brain tumor. Direct trauma to the tendon or the trochlear area is an occasional cause of unilateral superior oblique muscle palsy. Results of one study showed that most patients with congenital superior oblique palsy had an absent ipsilateral trochlear nerve and varying degrees of superior oblique muscle hypoplasia.

The same clinical features (discussed in the next section) can be observed when there is a congenitally lax, attenuated, or even absent superior oblique tendon or an unusual course of the muscle, or when there are malpositioned orbital pulleys—although, strictly speaking, these are not paralytic entities. Superior oblique muscle underaction can also occur in several craniofacial abnormalities (see Chapter 18).

To differentiate congenital from acquired superior oblique muscle palsy, the clinician can examine childhood photographs of the patient for a preexisting compensatory head tilt, although manifestations of congenital palsy sometimes become apparent only later in life. The presence of a large vertical fusional amplitude supports a diagnosis of congenital superior oblique palsy, whereas associated neurologic disorders suggest an acquired condition. Facial asymmetry from long-standing head tilting indicates chronicity. Diagnostic evaluation, including neuroimaging, often fails to identify an etiology but may still be warranted for acquired superior oblique palsy without a history of trauma. Neurologic aspects of superior oblique muscle palsy are discussed in BCSC Section 5, *Neuro-Ophthalmology.*

Yang HK, Kim JH, Hwang JM. Congenital superior oblique palsy and trochlear nerve absence: a clinical and radiological study. *Ophthalmology*. 2012;119(1):170–177.

Clinical features, evaluation, and diagnosis

Either the normal or the affected eye can be preferred for fixation. Examination of versions usually reveals underaction of the involved superior oblique muscle and overaction of its antagonist inferior oblique muscle; however, the action of the superior oblique muscle can appear normal.

Unilateral superioroblique palsy In a unilateral palsy, the hyperdeviation is typically incomitant, especially in the acute stages. Over time, contracture of the ipsilateral superior rectus or contralateral inferior rectus muscle can lead to "spread of comitance," with the result that there is minimal difference in the magnitude of the hypertropia when the patient looks from one side to the other. If depression cannot be evaluated because of the eye's inability to adduct (eg, in third nerve palsy), superior oblique muscle function can be evaluated by observing whether the eye intorts, as judged by the movement of surface landmarks or examination of the fundus, when the patient attempts to look downward and inward from primary position. Weakness of the superior oblique muscle also results in extorsion of the eye. If the degree of extorsion is large enough, subjective incyclodiplopia, in which the patient describes the image as appearing to tilt inward, can occur.

上斜肌麻痹

最常见的单一旋转垂直肌麻痹是Ⅳ颅神经（滑车神经）麻痹，累及上斜肌。可是先天性的，或是后天的，后者常是闭合性头部外伤的结果，或（不太常见的）中枢神经系统的血管问题、糖尿病或脑瘤。偶见肌腱或滑车区的直接损伤导致的单眼上斜肌麻痹。一项研究显示，大多数先天性上斜肌麻痹伴有同侧滑车神经缺如和不同程度的上斜肌发育不全。

当存在先天性松弛、薄变、上斜肌腱缺如、肌肉径行异常或眶滑车异位，尽管严格地说，这些并不是麻痹，也可以观察到同样的临床特征（下一节讨论）。上斜肌功能低下也见于部分颅面畸形（见第 18 章）。

先天性和获得性上斜肌麻痹的鉴别，可以参考患者童年时期的照片，以确定先前是否存在代偿性头倾斜，尽管有时先天性麻痹只是在以后的生活中表现出来。大的垂直融合幅度支持先天性上斜肌麻痹的诊断，而伴随的神经功能障碍提示为获得性。长期头倾斜导致的面部不对称，说明其慢性过程。诊断评估，包括神经影像学，往往不能确定病因，但对于无外伤史的获得性上斜肌麻痹仍有必要。上斜肌麻痹的神经学方面的讨论见 BCSC 第 5 册《*神经眼科学*》。

Yang HK, Kim JH, Hwang JM. Congenital superior oblique palsy and trochlear nerve absence: a clinical and radiological study. *Ophthalmology*. 2012;119(1):170–177.

临床特征、评估和诊断

无论是正常眼还是受累眼都可以作为注视眼。同向运动检查常显示，累及的上斜肌功能不足，其拮抗肌下斜肌亢进；然而，上斜肌也可以表现为功能正常。

单眼上斜麻痹　单眼麻痹的上斜视呈非共同性，特别是急性期。随着时间的推移，同侧上直肌或对侧下直肌的挛缩会导致“共同性扩散”，当患者从一侧向另一侧注视时，上斜视幅度的差别很小。若眼球不能内转（如Ⅲ颅神经麻痹）而无法评估下转时，上斜肌功能可以通过观察眼球是否内旋，即当患者从第一眼位向下、向内看时，通过眼表标志的运动或眼底检查进行评估。上斜肌功能低下也导致眼外旋。如果外旋角度足够大，就会发生主观上的内旋性复视，患者主诉图像向内倾斜。

The diagnosis of unilateral superior oblique muscle palsy is further established by results of the 3-step test (also called the *Parks-Bielschowsky 3-step test*) (Fig 11-3; see also Chapter 7, Fig 7-8) and the double Maddox rod test to measure torsion. However, results of the 3-step test can be confounded in patients with DVD, entities involving restriction, additional paretic muscles, previous strabismus surgery, or skew deviation. Intorsion of the higher eye on fundus examination—instead of the expected extorsion—suggests skew deviation, especially when there are associated neurologic findings. In addition, if the patient is placed in a supine position, the vertical tropia is more likely to decrease with skew deviation than with superior oblique palsy. Some ophthalmologists document serial changes in the deviation by means of the Hess screen or the Lancaster red-green test or by plotting the field of single binocular vision. (See Chapter 7 for further discussion of some of the tests mentioned in this section.)

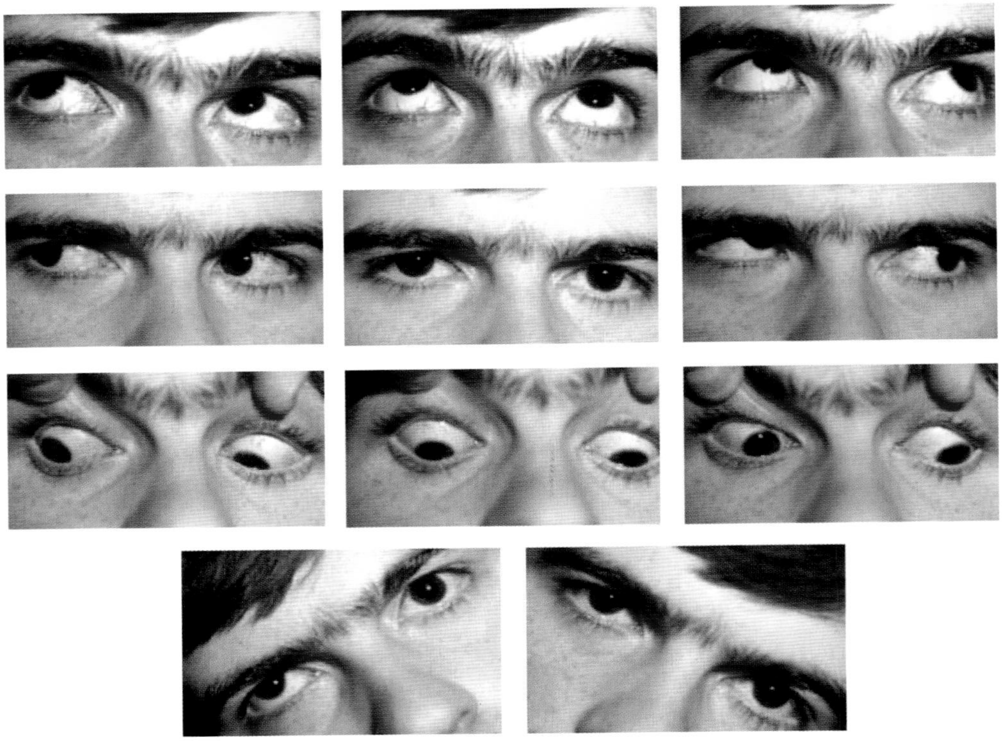

Figure 11-3 Right superior oblique palsy. There is a right hypertropia in primary position that increases in left gaze and with head tilt to the right. Note accompanying overaction of the right inferior oblique muscle. *(Courtesy of Edward L. Raab, MD.)*

INHIBITIONAL PALSY OF THE CONTRALATERAL ANTAGONIST Patients who fixate with the paretic eye can exhibit so-called *inhibitional palsy of the contralateral antagonist* (Fig 11-4). If a patient with right superior oblique palsy uses the right eye to fixate on an object that is located up and to the left, the innervation of the right inferior oblique muscle required to move the eye into this gaze position is reduced because the right inferior oblique muscle does not have to overcome the normal antagonistic effect of the right superior oblique muscle (Sherrington's law). According to Hering's law, less innervation is also received by the yoke muscle of the right inferior oblique muscle, which is the left superior rectus muscle. This decreased innervation can lead to the impression that the left superior rectus muscle is paretic.

单眼上斜肌麻痹可通过 3 步试验（也称 *Parks–Bielschowsky* 3 步试验）（图 11–3；见第 7 章，图 7–8）确诊，以及双 Maddox 杆试验测量转矩。当存在分离性垂直斜视 DVD、限制因素、其他肌肉麻痹、以前的斜视手术或反向偏斜时，3 步试验结果可能会混淆。进行眼底检查，见高位眼内旋，而不是外旋，提示存在反向偏斜，特别是伴有神经系统症状。此外，如果患者仰卧位，反向偏斜的垂直性斜视较上斜肌麻痹时减少。通过 Hess 屏试验、Lancaster 红绿试验或绘制双眼单视视野，医生可以记录偏斜的连续变化。（本节提到的试验见第 7 章。）

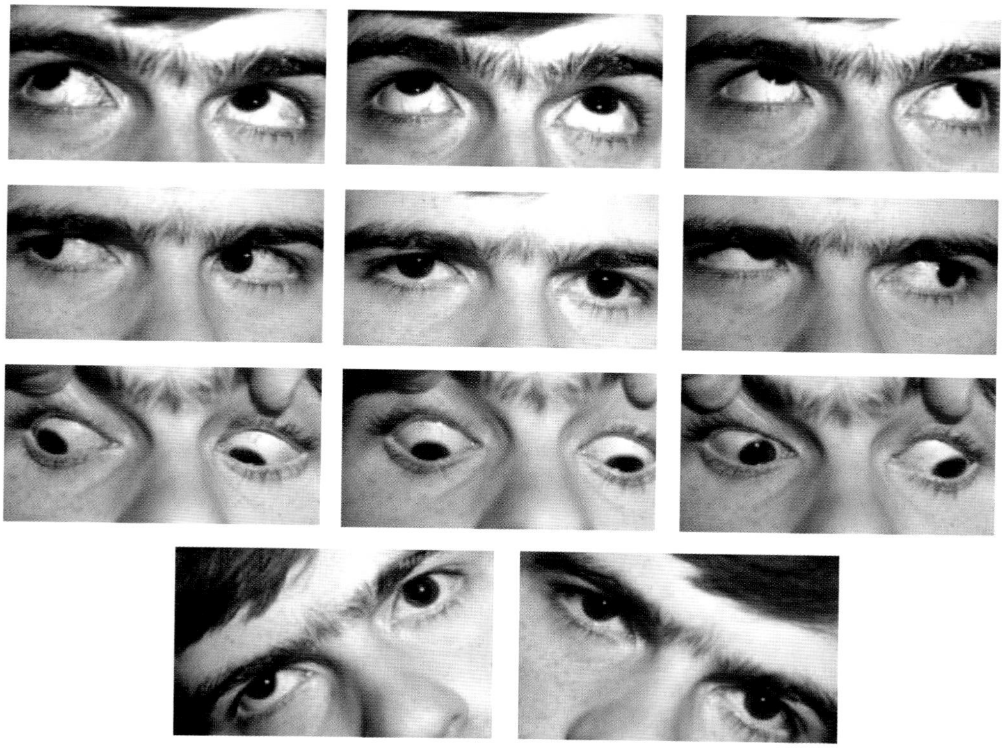

图 11–3　右上斜肌麻痹。第一眼位右上斜视，且左侧注视时增加、头向右倾斜。注意伴随右下斜肌功能亢进。*（译者注：资料来源见前页原文。）*

对侧拮抗肌的抑制性麻痹　用麻痹眼注视的患者可以表现出*对侧拮抗肌的抑制性麻痹*（图 11–4）。如果右上斜肌麻痹患者用右眼注视左上方物体，则朝这个注视位运动时需要的右下斜肌神经冲动减弱，因为右下斜肌不需要克服右上斜肌的正常拮抗性作用（Sherrington 定律）。根据 Hering 定律，右下斜肌的配偶肌，左眼上直肌接受的神经冲动也减弱，这种减弱的神经冲动导致左眼上直肌麻痹的假象。

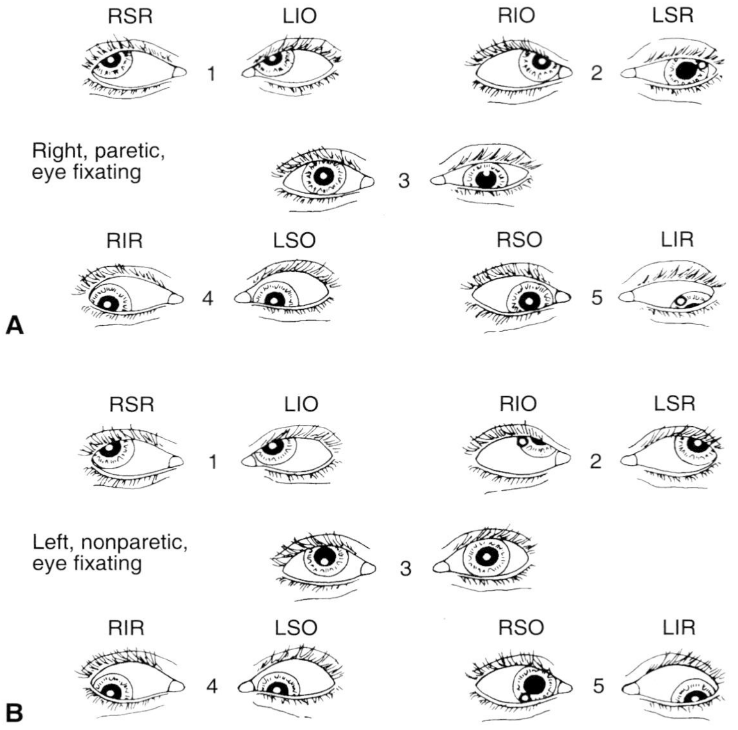

Figure 11-4 Palsy of right superior oblique muscle. **A**, With the palsied right eye fixating, little or no vertical difference appears between the 2 eyes in the right field of gaze (1 and 4). In primary position (3), a left hypotropia may be present because the right elevators require less innervation to stabilize the eye in primary position, and thus the left elevators will receive less-than-normal innervation. When gaze is up and left (2), the RIO needs less-than-normal innervation to elevate the right eye because its antagonist, the RSO, is palsied. Consequently, its yoke, the LSR, will be apparently underacting, and pseudoptosis with pseudopalsy of the LSR will be present. When gaze is toward the field of action of the palsied RSO muscle (5), maximum innervation is required to move the right eye down during adduction, and thus the yoke LIR will be overacting. **B**, With the unaffected left eye fixating, no vertical difference appears in the right field of gaze (1 and 4). In primary position (3), the right eye is elevated because of unopposed elevators. When gaze is up and left (2), the RIO shows marked overaction because its antagonist is palsied. The action of the LSR is normal. When gaze is down and left (5), normal innervation required by the fixating normal eye does not suffice to fully move the palsied eye into that field of gaze. (See also Chapter 7, Fig 7-8.) LIO = left inferior oblique; LIR = left inferior rectus; LSO = left superior oblique; LSR = left superior rectus; RIO = right inferior oblique; RIR = right inferior rectus; RSO = right superior oblique; RSR = right superior rectus. *(Reproduced with permission from von Noorden GK. Atlas of Strabismus. 4th ed. St Louis: Mosby; 1983:24–25.)*

Bilateral superior oblique palsy Bilateral superior oblique palsy occurs commonly after head trauma but is sometimes congenital. It can be differentiated from unilateral superior oblique muscle palsy by the following criteria:

- *Unilateral* cases usually show little if any V pattern and less than 10° of extorsion in downgaze. Subjective incyclodiplopia is uncommon. The Bielschowsky headtilt test (step 3 of the 3-step test) yields positive results for the involved side only. Abnormal head positions—usually a tilt toward the shoulder opposite the side of the weakness—are common. The oblique muscle dysfunction is confined to the involved eye.

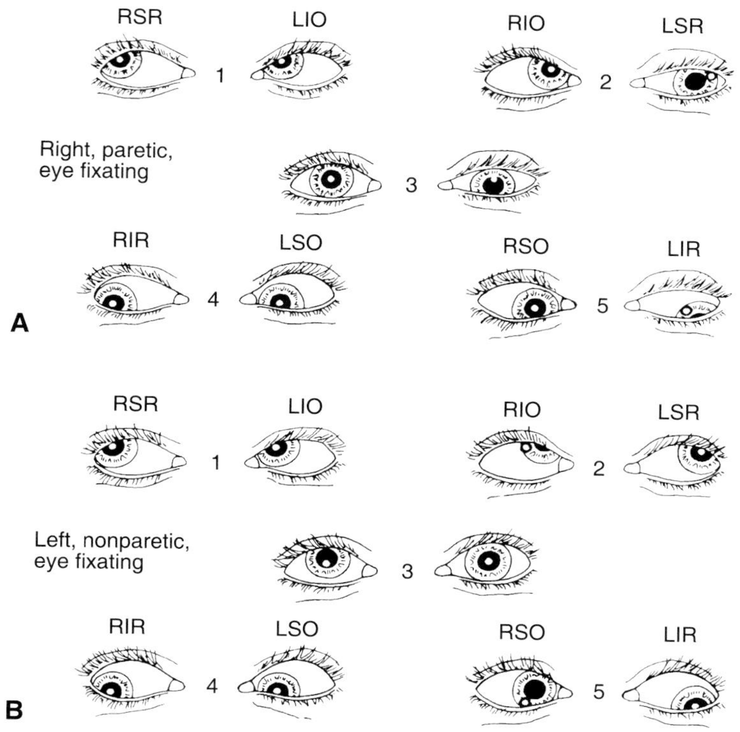

图 11-4　右眼上斜肌麻痹。**A.** 麻痹的右眼注视，在右侧注视野，双眼没有或有较小的垂直斜视度（1 和 4）；在第一眼位（3）可能存在左眼下斜视，因为右眼上转肌需要较小的神经冲动来维持第一眼位，因此左眼上转肌将得到少于正常的神经冲动；当向上方和左侧注视时（2），右眼下斜肌 RIO 需要少于正常的神经冲动来上转右眼，因为右眼下斜肌的拮抗剂右眼上斜肌 RSO 麻痹，继而其配偶肌左眼上直肌 LSR 明显功能低下，出现假性上睑下垂和左眼上直肌 LSR 假性麻痹；当向麻痹的右眼上斜肌 RSO 作用的方向注视时（5），需要最大的神经冲动来使右眼内转、下转，因而其配偶肌左眼下直肌 LIR 功能亢进。**B.** 用正常的左眼注视时，在右侧注视野（1 和 4），没有明显的垂直斜视；在第一眼位（3）由于上转肌没有对抗，右眼上转；当向上、向左侧注视时（2），因拮抗剂麻痹，右眼下斜肌 RIO 功能明显亢进；左眼上直肌 LSR 运动正常。当向下方和左侧注视时（5），正常左眼注视所需的正常神经冲动不能满足麻痹眼在这个方向的完全运动。（见第 7 章，图 7-8）LIO= 左眼下斜肌；LIR= 左眼下直肌；LSO= 左眼上斜肌；LSR= 左眼上直肌；RIO= 右眼下斜肌；RIR= 右眼下直肌；RSO= 右眼上斜肌；RSR= 右眼上直肌。*（译者注：资料来源见前页原文。）*

双眼上斜肌麻痹　双眼上斜肌麻痹常发生在头部创伤后，但有时是先天性的。根据以下标准可与单眼上斜肌麻痹鉴别：

- *单眼*病例中，向下注视时可有较小的 V 型和小于 10° 的外旋。主觉的内旋性复视不常见。Bielschowsky 歪头试验（3 步法中的第 3 步）仅受累侧呈阳性。异常头位较常见——头位通常是向功能减弱侧相反的肩部倾斜。上斜肌功能障碍仅限于受累眼。

- *Bilateral* cases usually show a V pattern. Extorsion is 10° or more in downgaze; more than 15° of extorsion in primary position is highly suggestive of bilateral involvement. Subjective incyclodiplopia is common in acquired bilateral cases. The Bielschowsky head-tilt test yields positive results on tilt to each side—that is, right head tilt produces a right hypertropia and left head tilt, a left hypertropia. There is bilateral oblique muscle dysfunction. Patients may exhibit a chin-down head position. Symmetric palsies may show little or no hypertropia in primary position.

MASKED BILATERAL SUPERIOR OBLIQUE PALSY Markedly asymmetric bilateral superior oblique palsy that initially appears to be unilateral is called *masked bilateral palsy.* Signs of masked bilateral palsy include bilateral objective fundus extorsion, esotropia in downgaze, and even the mildest degree of oblique muscle dysfunction on the presumably uninvolved side. Masked bilateral palsy is more common in patients with head trauma. Surgical overcorrection of unilateral superior oblique palsy can produce a pattern of hypertropia and 3-step-test findings similar to those of superior oblique palsy in the contralateral eye and should not be mistaken for masked bilateral palsy.

Management

For small, symptomatic deviations that lack a prominent torsional component—especially those that have become comitant—prisms that compensate for the hyperdeviation in primary position may be used to overcome diplopia. Abnormal head position, significant vertical deviation, diplopia, and asthenopia are indications for surgery. Common operative strategies are discussed in the following sections (see Chapter 14 for details of the procedures and for related videos).

Unilateral superior oblique muscle palsy There are many options for surgical treatment of a unilateral palsy. Any of the 4 cyclovertical muscles in each eye could potentially be operated on to correct the hypertropia. Some surgeons use a uniform approach and weaken the ipsilateral antagonist inferior oblique muscle. For other surgeons, the surgical plan is informed by superior oblique tendon laxity. Tendon laxity is assessed at the time of surgery by forced duction testing, in which the globe is pushed (translated) posteriorly into the orbit while it is simultaneously extorted, thus placing the superior oblique tendon on stretch (Video 11-1). If the tendon is lax, they perform a superior oblique tightening procedure; if it is not, they usually perform an inferior oblique weakening procedure. Other ophthalmologists use tendon laxity only as diagnostic confirmation of superior oblique palsy.

VIDEO 11-1 Oblique muscle forced duction testing.
Access all Section 6 videos at www.aao.org /bcscvideo_section06.

- *双眼*病例中，表现为 V 型。在向下注视时，外旋大于 10°；在第一眼位外旋超过 15° 时，高度提示双眼上斜肌受累。在获得性双眼病例中，主觉内旋性复视较常见。在向每侧倾斜时，Bielschowsky 歪头试验都是阳性，即向右侧头倾出现右上斜视，向左侧头倾出现左上斜视。这是因为双眼上斜肌功能障碍。患者常表现下颌内收位。对称性麻痹在第一眼位常没有上斜视。

隐性双眼上斜肌麻痹　明显非对称性双眼上斜肌麻痹最初表现为单眼麻痹，称为隐性双眼上斜肌麻痹。隐性双眼上斜肌麻痹的体征包括客观性双眼底外旋、向下注视时内斜视以及可能源于未受累眼的轻度上斜肌功能障碍。隐性双眼上斜肌麻痹常见于头部创伤。单眼上斜肌麻痹手术过矫能引起上斜视，3 步法试验结果类似于对侧眼上斜肌麻痹，这时不应误认为隐性双眼上斜肌麻痹。

治疗

小而无明显旋转的、有症状的斜视，特别是变成共同性，用棱镜补偿第一眼位上斜视、纠正复视。异常头位、明显的垂直斜视、复视和视疲劳都是手术的指征。常规手术方案随后章节讨论（见第 14 章手术操作和相关视频）。

单眼上斜肌麻痹　手术治疗单眼麻痹有许多方案。对每只眼的 4 条旋转垂直肌中的任何 1 条实施手术，都可以矫正上斜视。有的医生用均匀法，减弱同侧的拮抗肌下斜肌，其他医生则行上斜肌肌腱松弛。肌腱松弛是根据手术中被动牵拉试验进行评估，即眼球向后推入（转入）眼眶同时外旋，这样使上斜肌肌腱伸展（视频 11-1）。如果肌腱是松弛的，则实施上斜肌加强术；反之，则实施下斜肌减弱术。还有医生仅用肌腱松弛度来证实上斜肌麻痹的诊断。

视频11-1　斜肌被动牵拉试验。
*大家可以通过网站*www.aao.org/bcscvideo_section06获得第6册的所有视频。

Many surgeons take a tailored approach, reflecting the variety of hypertropia patterns that may occur with superior oblique palsy. For example, if underaction of an affected right superior oblique muscle is the most prominent feature, then the deviation will be greatest in down-left gaze. Another patient, by contrast, may predominantly exhibit overaction of the antagonist inferior oblique muscle, with the greatest deviation in up-left gaze. Because each of the 8 cyclovertical muscles has a somewhat different field of action, surgery involving some muscles will be more appropriate than others, depending on the field of gaze in which the deviation is largest (Table 11-3). In addition, some surgeons believe that superior oblique tightening is the most effective procedure for addressing a marked head tilt in children with congenital superior oblique palsy. Extorsion in unilateral superior oblique palsy rarely produces symptoms, but when it does, it can be corrected with a Harada-Ito procedure.

If the hyperdeviation is greater than 15 prism diopters (Δ) in primary position, surgery usually involves at least 2 muscles. Ipsilateral inferior oblique weakening and superior oblique tightening represent a particularly powerful combination but carry an increased risk of problematic iatrogenic Brown syndrome or overcorrection. In the unusually severe case with a vertical deviation greater than 35Δ in primary position, 3-muscle surgery is usually required.

Whatever the approach, it is important to avoid overcorrection of a long-standing unilateral superior oblique muscle palsy. Because there are often no sensory or motor adaptations tohypertropia in the opposite direction, disabling diplopia can result.

Bilateral superior oblique muscle palsy Surgical planning for treatment of bilateral superior oblique muscle palsy can be complex. If the paresis is asymmetric, hypertropia in primary position may be present and require many of the same considerations as hypertropia in unilateral palsy. In addition, there is often symptomatic extorsion or a V pattern that needs to be addressed.

If the palsies are symmetric (minimal hypertropia in primary position), both inferior oblique muscles can be weakened if they are overacting and hypertropia is present in side gaze. Bilateral superior oblique muscle tightening should be performed when hypertropia in side gaze is accompanied by V-pattern esotropia or symptomatic extorsion, especially in downgaze. If there is symptomatic extorsion but minimal hypertropia in side gaze, bilateral Harada-Ito procedures can be performed. Other, less commonly used approaches, such as bilateral inferior rectus muscle recessions, serve to add extra innervational drive on downgaze to help overcome the superior oblique deficits.

Table 11-3 Surgical Treatment of Unilateral Superior Oblique Palsy

	Difference in Hypertropia Between Right and Left Gaze	
Characteristic	**Large (>15Δ)**	**Moderate (<15Δ)**
Greater deviation in (contralateral) upgaze	Inferior oblique weakening	Inferior oblique weakening Ipsilateral superior rectus recession Contralateral superior rectus tightening (rarely)
Greater deviation in (contralateral) downgaze	Superior oblique tightening	Contralateral inferior rectus recession Ipsilateral superior rectus recession (if restricted)

Δ = prism diopters.

许多外科医生根据上斜肌麻痹所出现的各种上斜视变异，采取量身定制的方法。例如，如果以受累的右眼上斜肌功能不足为主，则在左下方注视时斜视度最大。相反，如果主要表现为拮抗剂下斜肌功能亢进，则在左上方注视时斜视度最大。因为 8 条旋转垂直肌的每一条肌肉都有不同的作用区域，因此手术累及的较为适合肌肉，取决于哪个注视方向的斜视度最大（表 11-3）。另外，有的医生认为，对于有明显头位倾斜的先天性上斜肌麻痹的儿童，上斜肌加强术是最有效的手术方式。单眼上斜肌麻痹的外旋少有症状，若有症状，则行 Harada-Ito 手术矫正。

第一眼位上斜视大于 15Δ 时，需对至少 2 条肌肉进行手术，同侧下斜肌减弱术和上斜肌加强术是一种非常强的手术组合，可造成医源性 Brown 综合征和过矫的风险。在第一眼位垂直斜视大于 35Δ 的严重病例中，则需对 3 条肌肉进行手术。

无论何种方法，避免过矫长期存在的单眼上斜肌麻痹是很重要的。因为在相反方向，对上斜视没有感知适应和运动适应，否则可能会产生融合无力性复视。

双眼上斜肌麻痹　双眼上斜肌麻痹的手术治疗方案比较复杂。如果在第一眼位表现为非对称性麻痹性上斜视，则与单眼上斜肌麻痹的手术方案相同，另外，还需解决有症状的外旋和 V 型。

如果上斜肌麻痹是对称性的（第一眼位有微小的上斜视），当向侧方注视时出现功能亢进和上斜视，需减弱双眼的下斜肌；当向侧方注视时，特别是向下注视时伴随 V 型内斜视或有症状的外旋，行双眼上斜肌加强术；如果有症状性的外旋，伴随侧方注视时微小的上斜视，行双眼 Harada-Ito 手术。较少使用的手术方法，如双眼下直肌后徙，通过增加向下注视的额外神经冲动，克服上斜肌功能不全。

表11-3　单眼上斜肌麻痹的手术治疗

特征	向右侧和左侧注视时上斜视的差异 大（>15△）	 中度（<15△）
在对侧上方注视时较大的斜视度	下斜肌减弱	下斜肌减弱 同侧上直肌后徙 对侧上直肌加强（罕见）
在对侧下方注视时较大的斜视度	上斜肌加强	对侧下直肌后徙 同侧上直肌后徙（如果有限制）

Δ=棱镜度。

Inferior Oblique Muscle Palsy

Whether inferior oblique muscle palsy (Fig 11-5) actually exists has been questioned. Most cases are considered to be congenital or posttraumatic.

Clinical features

Inferior oblique palsy is suspected when the patient has hypotropia and 3-step-test results consistent with this diagnosis. As with Brown syndrome, a prominent feature is deficient elevation when the eye is in adduction. The features that distinguish inferior oblique palsy from Brown syndrome are listed in Table 11-4.

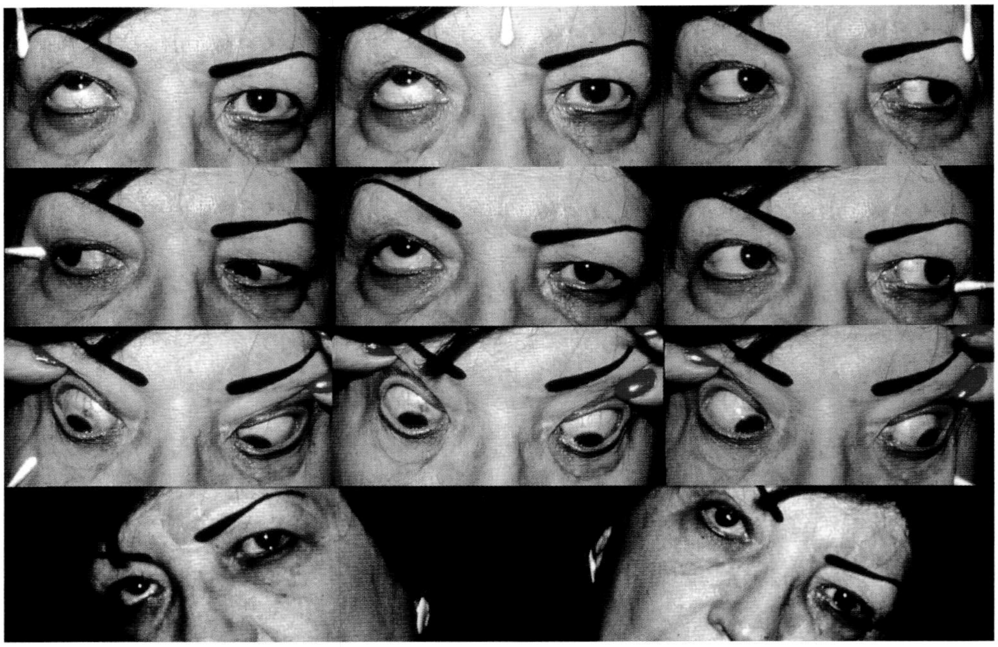

Figure 11-5 Left inferior oblique palsy. When the patient fixates with the paretic eye, there is a right hypertropia in primary position that is also most prominent in right gaze and with head tilt to the right—the 3-step test is consistent with this diagnosis. This patient had no abnormal neurologic findings. *(Courtesy of Steven M. Archer, MD.)*

Management

Indications for treatment of inferior oblique muscle palsy are abnormal head position, vertical deviation in primary position, and diplopia. Management consists of weakening either the ipsilateral superior oblique muscle or the contralateral superior rectus muscle.

Table 11-4 Comparison of Inferior Oblique Muscle Palsy and Brown Syndrome

Features	Inferior Oblique Muscle Palsy	Brown Syndrome
Forced duction test	Negative	Positive
Strabismus pattern	A pattern	None or V pattern
Superior oblique muscle overaction	Usually significant	None or minimal
Torsion	Intorsion	None
Head-tilt test	Positive	Negative

下斜肌麻痹

是否真正存在下斜肌麻痹一直受到质疑（图 11–5）。许多病例为先天性或创伤后性的。

临床特点

当患者有下斜视，且 3 步法试验与下斜肌麻痹诊断一致时，需考虑下斜肌麻痹。与 Brown 综合征一样，内转时出现明显的上转不足的特征。下斜肌麻痹和 Brown 综合征的鉴别见表 11–4。

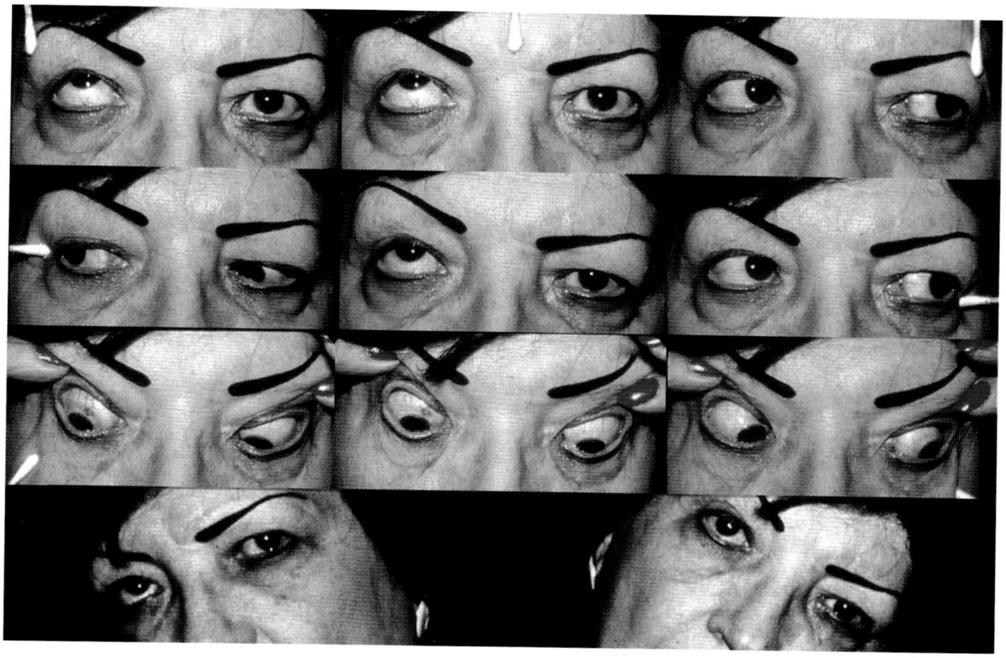

图 11–5　左眼下斜肌麻痹。当患者用麻痹眼注视时，第一眼位出现右眼上斜视，同时右眼上斜视在向右侧注视时和右侧头倾时也最明显，3 步法试验与此诊断一致。发现神经性系统异常。（译者注：资料来源见前页原文。）

治疗

治疗下斜肌麻痹的指征有异常头位、第一眼位垂直性斜视和复视。治疗方案包括同侧上斜肌减弱术或对侧上直肌减弱术。

表 11–4　下斜肌麻痹与Brown综合征的比较

特点	下斜肌麻痹	Brown综合征
被动牵拉试验	阴性	阳性
斜视型	A型	无或V型
上斜肌功能亢进	明显	无或较小
旋转	内旋	无
歪头试验	阳性	阴性

Skew Deviation

Skew deviation is an acquired vertical strabismus that can mimic superior or inferior oblique palsy. The deviation is due to peripheral or central asymmetric disruption of supranuclear input from the otolith organs. Intorsion of the hypertropic eye on fundus examination—rather than the expected extorsion in superior oblique palsy—suggests skew deviation, particularly when there are associated neurologic findings. In addition, if the patient is placed in a supine position, the vertical tropia is more likely to decrease with skew deviation than with superior oblique palsy. Similarly, if there is extorsion of the hypotropic eye on fundus examination—instead of the expected intorsion in inferior oblique palsy—then skew deviation is the likely diagnosis. See BCSC Section 5, *Neuro-Ophthalmology*, for additional discussion.

Other Conditions With Incomitant Vertical Deviations

Incomitant hypertropia may occur in several other conditions. These include innervational problems, such as third nerve palsy with aberrant regeneration and the upshoots and downshoots in Duane retraction syndrome, and mechanical disorders, such as Brown syndrome and thyroid eye disease or those due to orbital tumors and orbital implants (eg, tube shunts, scleral buckles). These topics are discussed elsewhere in this book and in other BCSC volumes.

Vertical Deviations With Horizontal Comitance

Most patients with vertical deviations demonstrate some lateral incomitance. However, in vertical deviations not associated with apparent oblique muscle dysfunction, the difference between the deviations in right gaze and left gaze is usually less than 10Δ.

Monocular Elevation Deficiency

Monocular elevation deficiency (previously termed *double-elevator palsy*) involves a limitation of upward gaze with a hypotropia that is similar in adduction and abduction. There are 3 forms of this motility pattern, each with a different cause: restriction of the inferior rectus muscle; deficient innervation of elevator muscles (paresis of 1 or both elevator muscles or a monocular supranuclear gaze disorder); a combination of restriction and elevator muscle deficit.

Clinical features

All 3 forms of monocular elevation deficiency are characterized by hypotropia of the involved eye with limited elevation, a chin-up head position with binocular fusion in downgaze, and ptosis or pseudoptosis (Fig 11-6). True ptosis is present in 50% of affected patients. These are features of third nerve palsy, as well. Therefore, if any other feature of third nerve palsy is present, that condition should be suspected rather than monocular elevation deficiency.

The clinical features of each form of monocular elevation deficiency are as follows:

反向偏斜

反向偏斜是一种类似上斜肌或下斜肌麻痹的获得性垂直性斜视，是由于发自耳石器官的、周边或中心非对称性的核上性神经传入中断所致。在眼底检查时，上斜视眼内旋，与上斜肌麻痹的外旋不同，特别是伴随相关的神经系统异常时，提示反向偏斜。另外，如果患者仰卧位，反向偏斜的垂直斜视度的减少较上斜肌麻痹明显。在眼底检查时，下斜视眼外旋，而不是下斜肌麻痹的内旋，可以诊断反向偏斜。进一步讨论见 BCSC 第 5 册《*神经眼科学*》。

其他非共同性垂直性斜视

非共同性上斜视可能出现在其他几种情况中。有神经支配问题，如在 Duane 后退综合征中的Ⅲ颅神经麻痹伴异常的再生、上射和下射；还有机械性异常，如 Brown 综合征、甲状腺眼病、眼眶肿瘤和眼眶植入物（如引流管和巩膜扣带）。这些问题在本套书的其他图书中讨论。

伴随水平共同性的垂直斜视

多数垂直斜视伴侧方的非共同性。但垂直性斜视不伴随明显的斜肌功能障碍时，在向右注视和向左注视两者间的斜视度差异小于 10Δ。

单眼上转不足

单眼上转不足（之前称为*双上转肌麻痹*）包括伴下斜视的向上注视时受限，在内转和外转时表现相似的下斜视。有 3 种运动类型，每种都有不同的病因：下直肌的限制、上转肌的支配神经缺陷（1 条或 2 条上转肌麻痹，或单眼核上性注视障碍）；联合限制和上转肌功能不足。

临床特点

3 种单眼上转不足是以受累眼的下斜视和有限的上转、下颌上抬伴向下注视时双眼融合以及上睑下垂或假性上睑下垂为特征（图 11-6）。真性上睑下垂占 50%。这也是Ⅲ颅神经麻痹的特征，因此，如果有Ⅲ颅神经麻痹的其他表现，则不考虑单眼上转不足。

每种类型的单眼上转不足的临床特点如下：

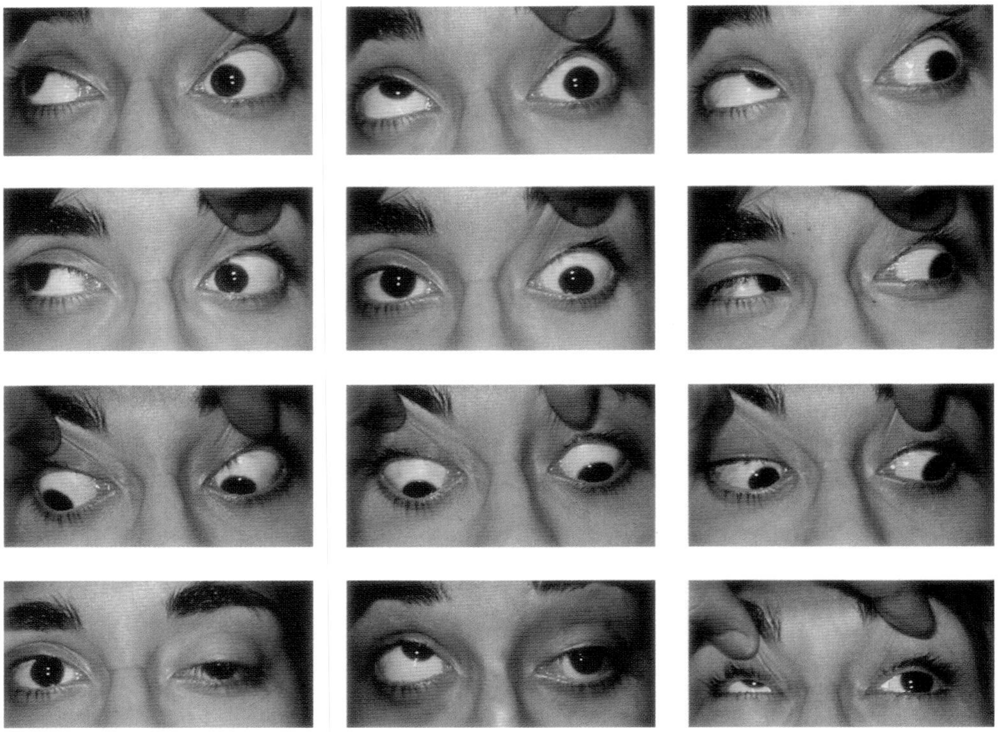

Figure 11-6 Monocular elevation deficiency of the left eye. *Top row,* No voluntary elevation of the left eye above horizontal. *Second row,* Hypotropia of the left eye across the horizontal fields of gaze. *Third row,* Depression of the left eye is unaffected. *Bottom row, left,* Ptosis (true and pseudo-) of the left upper eyelid during fixation with the right eye (in the top 3 rows, the left upper eyelid is elevated manually). *Bottom row, center,* Persistence of ptosis and marked secondary overelevation of the right eye during fixation with the left eye. *Bottom row, right,* Bell phenomenon, with the left eye elevating above the horizontal on forced eyelid closure.

- restriction
  - positive forced duction on elevation
  - normal force generation and saccadic velocity (no muscle paralysis)
  - often an extra or deeper lower eyelid fold on attempted upgaze
  - poor or absent Bell phenomenon
- elevator muscle innervational deficit
  - negative forced duction on elevation
  - reduced force generation and saccadic velocity
  - preservation of Bell phenomenon (indicating a supranuclear cause) in many cases
- combination of restriction and elevator muscle deficit
  - positive forced duction on elevation
  - reduced force generation and saccadic velocity

In support of this classification, studies using magnetic resonance imaging have shown either focal thickening of the inferior rectus muscle, supporting a restrictive etiology, or normal ocular motor nerves, suggesting a central unilateral disorder of upgaze.

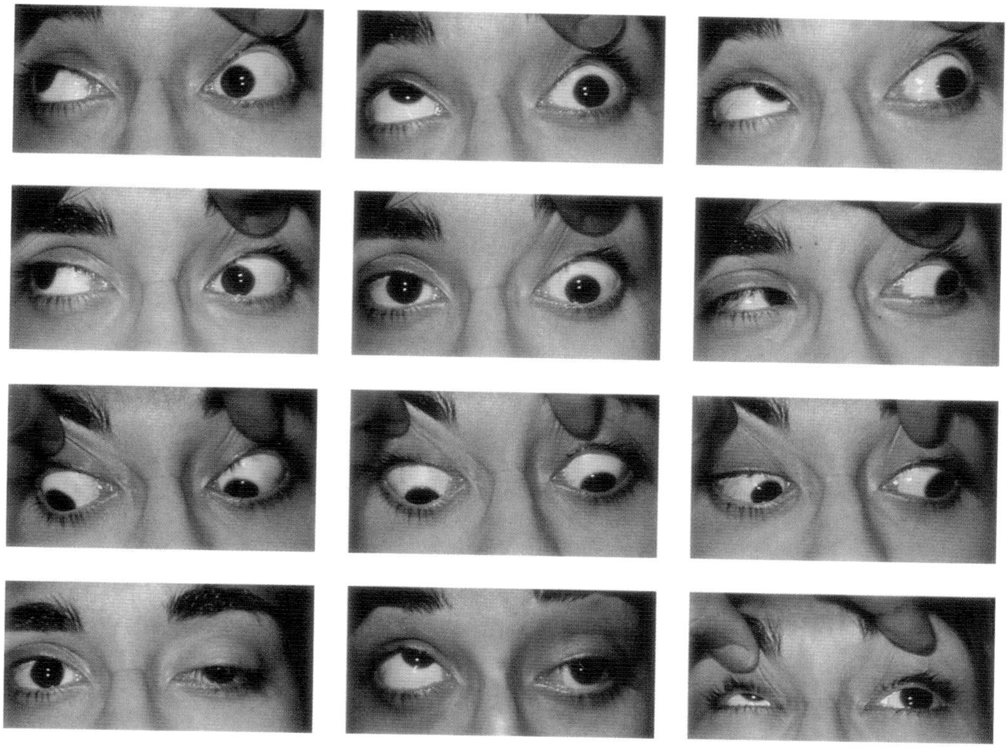

图 11-6　左眼单眼上转不足。*最上行*，水平线以上注视时，左眼没有自主上转。*第二行*，在水平注视野转动时，左眼下斜视。*第三行*，左眼下转时，未受累。*最后一行左图*，用右眼注视时（前 3 行图中，左眼上睑被人为抬起），左上眼睑上睑下垂（真性和假性）。*最后一行中间图*，用左眼注视时，持续性上睑下垂及右眼明显继发性睑过度上转。*最后一行右图*，Bell 现象，左眼被动性眼睑闭合时，左眼上转超过水平线。

- 受限
  - 上转时被动牵拉试验阳性；
  - 正常的肌肉力量激发和扫视速度（无肌肉麻痹）；
  - 努力向上注视时，产生额外的或更深的下睑皱褶；
  - Bell 现象差或缺如。
- 上转肌神经支配缺陷
  - 上转时，被动牵拉试验阴性；
  - 肌力激发和扫视速度减弱；
  - 许多病例中存在 Bell 现象（提示核上性病因）。
- 受限和上转肌功能不足并存
  - 上转时，被动牵拉试验阳性；
  - 肌力激发和扫视速度减弱。

磁共振成像（MRI）研究支持这种分类法，下直肌局限性增厚的影像支持限制性病因学；正常的眼球运动神经的影像提示中枢单侧向上注视障碍。

Kim JH, Hwang JM. Congenital monocular elevation deficiency. *Ophthalmology*. 2009;116(3): 580–584.

Management

Indications for treatment include a large vertical deviation in primary position, with or without ptosis, and an abnormal chin-up head position. If restriction originating inferiorly is present, the inferior rectus muscle should be recessed. If there is no restriction, the medial and lateral rectus muscles can be transposed toward the superior rectus muscle (*Knapp procedure*). Alternatively, the surgeon can recess the ipsilateral inferior rectus and either recess the contralateral superior rectus muscle or resect the ipsilateral superior rectus muscle. Ptosis surgery should be deferred until the vertical deviation has been corrected and the pseudoptosis component eliminated.

Orbital Floor Fractures

Clinical features and management of orbital floor fractures are discussed in Chapter 27 of this volume and in BCSC Section 7, *Oculofacial Plastic and Orbital Surgery*. The discussion in this chapter focuses on motility abnormalities in patients with these fractures.

Clinical features

Diplopia in the immediate postinjury stage is common and not necessarily an indication for urgent intervention. Indications and timing for surgical repair are discussed in Chapter 27 of this volume and in BCSC Section 7, *Oculofacial Plastic and Orbital Surgery*. Depending on the site of the bony trauma, muscles can be either restricted due to entrapment or paretic due to muscle contusion or nerve damage. "Flap tears" of the inferior rectus muscle have also been described by some authors as a cause of limitation of elevation, depression, or both. Paresis of a muscle may resolve over several months. If the fracture requires surgery, the range of eye movements may improve. By contrast, fibrosis after trauma may cause restriction to persist even after successful repair of the fracture.

Management

Treatment of strabismus is usually necessary when diplopia persists in primary position or downgaze or there is an associated compensatory head position. Some mild limitations of eye movements can be managed with prisms.

Planning of eye muscle surgery depends on the fields where diplopia is present and on the relative contributions of muscle restriction and paresis. Any flap tear discovered on exploration of the inferior rectus muscle should be repaired. For hypotropia in primary position (Fig 11-7), recession of the ipsilateral inferior rectus muscle can be effective, especially if the muscle is restricted on forced duction testing. Similarly, an incomitant esotropia (with diplopia on side gaze) due to restriction on the medial side may be improved by recession of the ipsilateral medial rectus muscle.

Initially, hypertropia due to weakness of the inferior rectus muscle without entrapment is managed with observation because the weakness may improve with time. If recovery is not complete within 6–12 months of the injury and there is at least a moderate degree of active force, resection of the affected muscle can be performed. If the hypertropia is large, the procedure can be combined with recession of the ipsilateral superior rectus muscle or recession of the contralateral inferior rectus muscle, with or without the addition of a posterior fixation suture (*fadenoperation*). Transposition of the ipsilateral medial and lateral rectus muscles to the inferior rectus muscle (*inverse Knapp procedure*) may be necessary for treatment of complete, chronic inferior rectus muscle palsy or when a crippling amount of recession has been necessary to relieve restriction.

Kim JH, Hwang JM. Congenital monocular elevation deficiency. *Ophthalmology*. 2009;116(3): 580–584.

治疗

治疗指征包括第一眼位较大的垂直性斜视，伴或不伴上睑下垂及异常的下颌上抬头位。如果源于下方的限制，需下直肌后徙术。如果没有限制，则内直肌和外直肌向上直肌转位（*Knapp 法*）。也可选择行同侧下直肌后徙术，联合对侧上直肌后徙术或同侧上直肌切除术。上睑下垂手术应推迟，在垂直斜视矫正和假性上睑下垂因素消除后考虑。

眶底骨折

眶底骨折临床特点和治疗的讨论见第 27 章和 BCSC 第 7 册《*眼面部整形与眼眶手术*》。本章集中讨论集中在骨折患者的眼球运动异常。

临床特征

复视常在伤后立即出现，但并不需要紧急处理。手术适应证和修复时机的讨论见第 27 章和 BCSC 第 7 册《*眼面部整形与眼眶手术*》。根据骨折的部位，可能因肌肉嵌顿而运动受到限制，或因肌肉挫伤或神经损伤导致麻痹。下直肌的“皮瓣样撕裂”也是上转、下转或同时运动受限的原因。肌肉麻痹可在数月后逐渐恢复。如果骨折手术，则眼球运动幅度可能改善。反而在成功修复骨折后，伤后肌肉纤维化将引起持续性的运动受限。

治疗

当第一眼位或向下注视时出现复视，或有相关的代偿头位时，需进行斜视手术。轻度眼球运动限制可用棱镜。

眼肌手术设计取决于哪个视野出现复视，以及相关的麻痹性或受限肌肉。探查发现的下直肌皮瓣样撕裂均需修复。对于第一眼位的下斜视（图 11-7），特别是被动牵拉试验时肌肉运动受限，同侧的下直肌后徙有效。同样，内侧受限导致的非共同性内斜视（伴侧视时复视），同侧内直肌后徙可改善。

起初无嵌顿的下直肌减弱导致的上斜视，只需观察，因为肌肉力量可能随时间而改善。如果在外伤后 6 ~ 12 月内未完全恢复，并且肌肉有中度主动收缩力，可行受累肌肉切除术。如果上斜视度数较大，则手术可联合同侧上直肌后徙和对侧下直肌后徙，伴或不伴后固定术（*Faden 术*）。同侧内直肌和外直肌向下直肌转位（*反向 Knapp 法*）可用于治疗完全性慢性的下直肌麻痹，或为解除限制需长量 / 致残量后徙。

Other Conditions With Comitant Vertical Deviations

Other conditions and disorders featuring a hypertropia that does not change markedly from right to left gaze include innervational problems, such as superior division (partial) palsy of the third cranial nerve; and mechanical disorders, such as thyroid eye disease, congenital fibrosis of the extraocular muscles, and orbital tumors. These topics are discussed elsewhere in this volume and in other BCSC Sections.

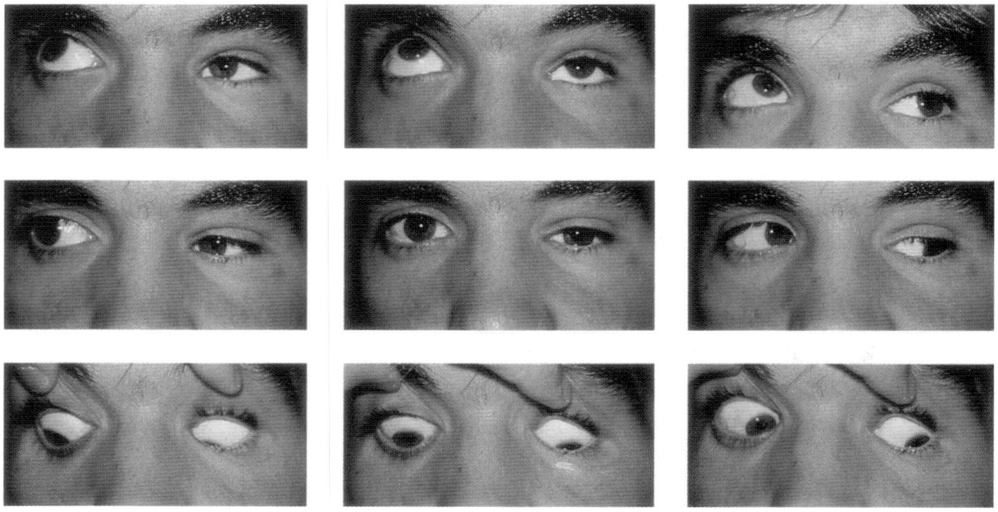

Figure 11-7 Old orbital floor fracture, left eye, with inferior rectus muscle entrapment. Note limitation of elevation of the left eye and pseudoptosis from enophthalmos. The eyelids are elevated manually in the bottom row.

Dissociated Vertical Deviation

Dissociated vertical deviation (DVD) is an innervational disorder found in more than 50% of patients with infantile strabismus (esotropia or exotropia). There are 2 explanations for the origin of DVD. One theory is that DVD is a vertical vergence movement to damp latent nystagmus, with the oblique muscles playing the principal role. An alternative theory suggests that deficient fusion allows the primitive dorsal light reflex, which is prominent in other species, to emerge.

Brodsky MC. Dissociated vertical divergence: a righting reflex gone wrong. *Arch Ophthalmol.* 1999;117(9):1216–1222.

Guyton DL. Ocular torsion reveals the mechanisms of cyclovertical strabismus: the Weisenfeld lecture. *Invest Ophthalmol Vis Sci.* 2008;49(3):847–857.

Clinical Features

Dissociated vertical deviation usually presents by age 2 years, whether or not any horizontal deviation has been surgically corrected. Either eye slowly drifts upward and outward, with simultaneous extorsion, when occluded or during periods of visual inattention (Fig 11-8). Some patients attempt to compensate by tilting the head, for reasons that still have not been conclusively identified.

伴随共同性垂直性斜视的其他异常

从右侧向左侧注视时上斜视无显著改变的其他异常，包括神经支配问题，如Ⅲ颅神经上支（部分）麻痹；机械性障碍，如甲状腺眼病、先天性眼外肌纤维化和眼眶肿瘤。这些在本书和 BCSC 其他分册讨论。

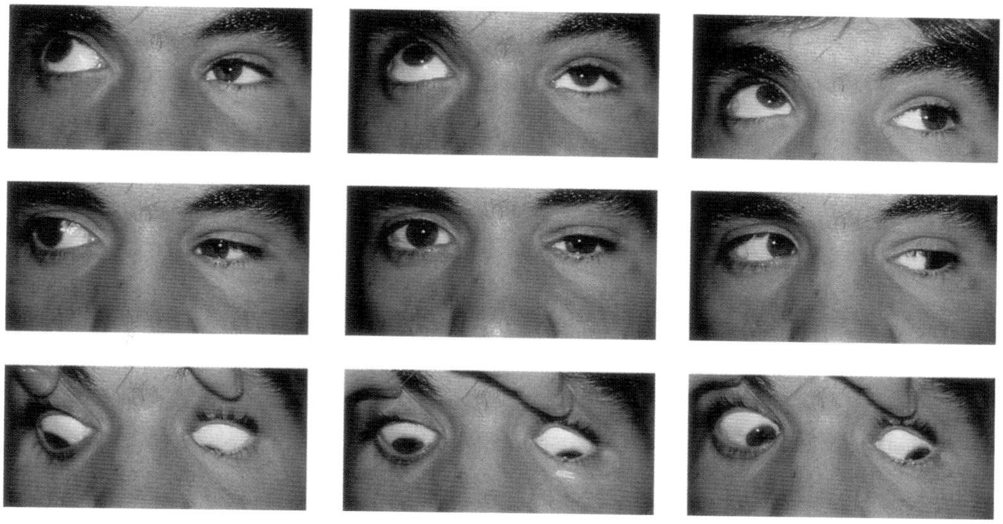

图 11–7　陈旧性眶底骨折，左眼，伴下直肌嵌顿。左眼上转限制及因眼球内陷导致的假性上睑下垂。最下面行是人为抬高眼睑。

分离性垂直斜视

分离性垂直斜视（DVD）是一种异常神经支配，见于 50% 的婴儿型斜视（内斜或外斜）。DVD 的病因有 2 种解释。一种理论认为，DVD 是一种抑制隐性眼球震颤的垂直性聚散运动，其中斜肌为主要作用。另一种理论认为，融像缺陷导致出现原始背侧光反射，后者在其他物种中比较明显。

Brodsky MC. Dissociated vertical divergence: a righting reflex gone wrong. *Arch Ophthalmol.* 1999;117(9):1216–1222.

Guyton DL. Ocular torsion reveals the mechanisms of cyclovertical strabismus: the Weisenfeld lecture. *Invest Ophthalmol Vis Sci.* 2008;49(3):847–857.

临床特点

无论之前是否行水平斜视矫正手术，分离性垂直斜视 DVD 常在 2 岁时出现，当遮盖或注意力不集中时，任意一眼出现缓慢的向上向外漂移，同时伴外旋（图 11–8）。有时患者通过歪头来代偿，其原因目前尚未确定。

DVD is usually the most prominent component of the *dissociated strabismus complex (DSC)*, but sometimes the principal dissociated movement is one of abduction *(dissociated horizontal deviation, DHD)*, and occasionally it is almost entirely a torsional movement *(dissociated torsional deviation, DTD)*. DVD is usually bilateral but is frequently asymmetric. It may occur spontaneously (manifest DVD) or only when 1 eye is occluded (latent DVD). An eye with latent DVD can give the appearance of inferior oblique overaction when it is occluded by the nose during adduction. In addition to DHD, latent nystagmus and horizontal strabismus are often associated with DVD. These entities are manifestations of deficient binocular vision.

Measurement of DVD is difficult and imprecise. In one method, a base-down prism is placed in front of the upwardly deviating eye while it is behind an occluder. The occluder is then switched to the fixating lower eye. The prism power is adjusted until the deviating eye shows no downward movement to refixate. These steps are then repeated for the other eye. Measurements obtained with this technique are confounded by any coexisting true hypertropia, but it does provide a rough estimate for surgical planning.

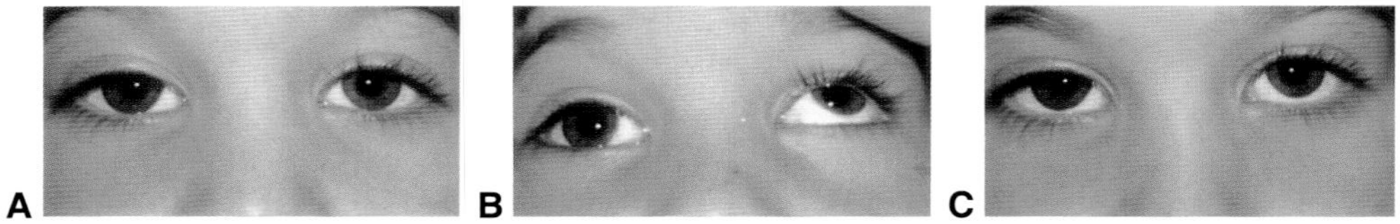

Figure 11-8 Dissociated vertical deviation, left eye. **A,** Straight eyes during binocular viewing conditions. **B,** Large left hyperdeviation immediately after the eye is covered and then uncovered. **C,** The left eye comes back down to primary position without a corresponding right hypotropia.

Management

Treatment of DVD is indicated if the deviation is noticeable (generally more than 6Δ–8Δ) and occurs frequently during the day. When DVD is unilateral or highly asymmetric, encouraging fixation by the eye with greater DVD by optically blurring the fellow eye is sometimes sufficient. Because DVD can mimic OEAd, distinguishing it from overaction of the inferior oblique muscles is important, as the surgical approaches to these 2 conditions are different in most cases.

Surgery on the vertical muscles often improves the condition but rarely eliminates it. Recessions of the superior rectus muscle, ranging from 6 to 10 mm according to the size of the hypertropia, can be effective. If there is residual DVD after superior rectus muscle recession, inferior rectus muscle resection or plication can be performed. Inferior oblique muscle anterior transposition is also effective in treating DVD, especially if it is accompanied by inferior oblique muscle overaction. Bilateral surgery is performed whenever both eyes can fixate; asymmetric surgery is an option if the DVD is asymmetric.

分离性垂直斜视 DVD 是最主要的*分离性斜视综合征（DSC）*表现，但有时分离性运动表现为外展性的（*分离性水平斜视，DHD*），偶尔表现为完全的旋转性运动（*分离性旋转斜视，DTD*）。DVD 常为双眼非对称性，为自发性出现（显性 DVD），或一眼遮盖时出现（隐性 DVD）。隐性 DVD 内转时被鼻子遮挡，呈现下斜肌功能亢进的外观。除了分离性水平斜视 DHD 以外，分离性垂直斜视 DVD 常伴随隐性眼球震颤和水平斜视。这是双眼视功能缺陷的表现。

分离性垂直斜视 DVD 的测量很难且不精准。检测方法之一，是将基底朝下的棱镜置于向上偏斜眼前，同时遮盖该眼；然后遮盖板移至注视的低位眼。调整棱镜度直至偏斜眼不再出现下转再注视的运动。然后，对另一眼进行同样检测。这种方法常与同时存在的真性上斜视混淆，但为手术提供了粗略的评估。

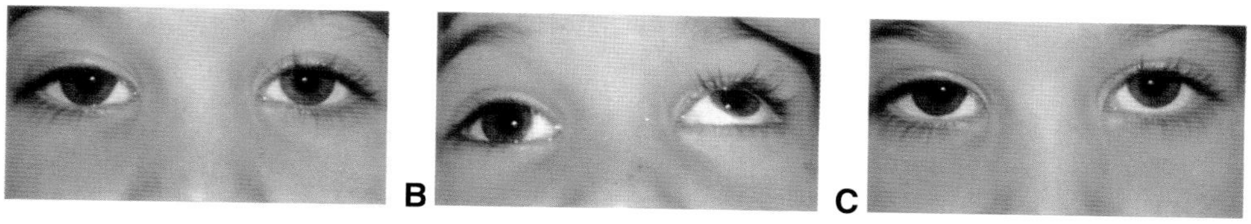
A B C

图 11–8　分离性垂直斜视，左眼。**A.** 双眼视时，眼正位。**B.** 当一眼遮盖和去遮盖后，立即出现较大的左眼上斜视。**C.** 左眼向下恢复到第一眼位，不伴相应的右眼下斜视。

治疗

分离性垂直斜视 DVD 的治疗指征为斜视度较显著（大于 6 ~ 8Δ），且常白天出现。当 DVD 呈单侧或明显非对称性，可以使用 DVD 明显的眼进行注视，而光学雾视对侧眼，有时即可矫正 DVD。DVD 的表现类似于内转过度上转 OEAd，与下斜肌功能亢进的鉴别非常重要，因为在多数病例中，这 2 种情况的手术方法是不同的。

垂直肌的手术常能改善 DVD，但很少能消除。根据上斜视的程度行上直肌后徙 6~10mm 即有效。如果在上直肌后徙后有残存的 DVD，可行下直肌切除或折叠术。下斜肌前转位在治疗伴下斜肌功能亢进的 DVD 是有效的。双眼均能注视时，可行双眼手术；如果 DVD 是非对称性，则可选择非对称性手术。

（翻译　芮莹　马玉红 // 审校　石一宁　丁娟 // 章节审校　石广礼）

CHAPTER 12

Special Motility Disorders

See BCSC Section 5, *Neuro-Ophthalmology*, for additional discussion of several entities covered in this chapter, and see Chapter 14 in this volume for discussion of some of the surgical procedures mentioned in this chapter.

Congenital Cranial Dysinnervation Disorders

Congenital cranial dysinnervation disorders (CCDDs) are a group of strabismus entities that have in common a developmental defect of one or more cranial nerves. There can be nuclear hypoplasia, nerve misdirection, and/or or absence of the nerves themselves. These anomalies lead to various patterns of abnormal innervation of the eye muscles that often result in secondary abnormal structural changes to the affected muscles, usually stiffening or contracture. Onset of the innervation anomalies can be as early as the first trimester in utero. Included in this group are Duane retraction syndrome, congenital fibrosis of the extraocular muscles, Möbius syndrome, and some cases of congenital fourth nerve palsy (see Chapter 11). In recent work, congenital Brown syndrome has been postulated to be a form of CCDD.

Gutowski NJ, Chilton JK. The congenital cranial dysinnervation disorders. *Arch Dis Child.* 2015;100(7):678–681.

Duane Retraction Syndrome

Duane retraction syndrome is a spectrum of ocular motility disorders characterized by anomalous co-contraction of the medial and lateral rectus muscles on actual or attempted adduction of the involved eye or eyes; this co-contraction causes the globe to retract. Horizontal eye movement can be limited to various degrees in both abduction and adduction. An upshoot or downshoot often occurs when the affected eye is innervated to adduct; vertical slippage of a tight lateral rectus muscle by 1–2 mm, which has been demonstrated by magnetic resonance imaging (MRI) studies, is the typical cause. Less commonly, anomalous vertical rectus muscle activity is responsible for upshoots and downshoots.

Although most affected patients have Duane retraction syndrome alone, many associated systemic defects have been noted, such as Goldenhar syndrome (hemifacial microsomia, ocular dermoids, ear anomalies, preauricular skin tags, and eyelid colobomas) and Wildervanck syndrome (sensorineural hearing loss and Klippel-Feil anomaly with fused cervical vertebrae). Studies of patients with Duane retraction syndrome related to prenatal thalidomide exposure show that the underlying defect in development occurs between the fourth and sixth weeks of gestation.

第 12 章

特殊运动障碍

本章所涉及问题的补充讨论，见 BCSC 第 5 册《*神经眼科学*》；有关手术操作见第 14 章。

先天性颅神经支配障碍

先天性颅神经支配障碍（CCDDs）是一组斜视性疾病，通常有一条或多条颅神经发育缺陷。可能存在核性发育不全、神经走形错位、和（或）神经本身的缺如。这些异常形成各种眼肌的异常神经支配的模式，导致受累肌肉的继发性结构改变，常为僵硬或挛缩。神经支配异常可早在宫内前 3 个月发生。这组疾病中包括 Duane 后退综合征、先天性眼外肌纤维化、Möbius 综合征以及一些先天性第Ⅳ颅神经麻痹（见第 11 章）。近年将先天性 Brown 综合征也列入 CCDD 的一种。

Gutowski NJ, Chilton JK. The congenital cranial dysinnervation disorders. *Arch Dis Child.* 2015;100(7):678–681.

Duane 后退综合征

Duane 后退综合征是一组眼球运动障碍，特点为眼内转时，受累眼或双眼内直肌和外直肌异常同时收缩；这种同时收缩引起眼球后退。眼球水平运动的内转和外转均有不同程度受限。当受累眼内转时，发生眼的上射和下射；磁共振成像（MRI）证实，收缩的外直肌垂直滑脱 1 ~ 2mm 为典型原因。垂直肌肉异常运动为上射和下射的少见原因。

尽管多数患者只患 Duane 后退综合征，但还伴有许多系统缺陷，如 Goldenahar 综合征（半侧面矮小症、眼部皮肤病、耳部异常、耳前皮肤附赘以及眼睑缺损）、Wildervanck 综合征（感觉神经性听力缺失和 Klippel–Feil 异常伴颈椎融合）。与产前使用反应停（镇静剂）有关的 Duane 后退综合征患者的研究显示，缺陷的形成在妊娠第 4 ~ 6 周之间。

Most cases of Duane retraction syndrome are sporadic, but approximately 5%–10% show autosomal dominant inheritance. Instances of links to more generalized disorders have been reported. Discordance in monozygotic twins raises the possibility that the intrauterine environment may play a role in the development of this syndrome. A higher prevalence in females is reported in most series, and there is a predilection for the left eye.

In most anatomical and imaging studies, the nucleus of the sixth cranial nerve is absent or hypoplastic and an aberrant branch of the third cranial nerve innervates the lateral rectus muscle. Results of electromyographic studies have been consistent with this finding. Although Duane retraction syndrome is considered an innervational anomaly, tight and broadly inserted medial rectus muscles and fibrotic lateral rectus muscles, with corresponding forced duction abnormalities, are often encountered during surgery.

Clinical features

The most widely used classification of Duane retraction syndrome defines 3 types, but they may represent differences only in the severity of horizontal rotation limitations. Type 1 refers to poor abduction, frequently with esotropia in primary position (Fig 12-1); type 2 refers to poor adduction and exotropia (Fig 12-2); and type 3 refers to poor abduction and adduction, with esotropia, exotropia, or no primary position deviation (Fig 12-3). Approximately 15% of cases are bilateral; the type may differ between the 2 eyes. The spectrum of dysinnervation among cases means that classification of patients based on these categories can be arbitrary in some situations, especially in deciding between type 1 and type 3. *Synergistic divergence* is a rare and bizarre motility disturbance that is often classified as a fourth type of Duane syndrome. There is usually exotropia, and when the affected eye looks in the direction that should result in adduction, it actually abducts even further—a finding colorfully described as "the ocular splits." Synergistic divergence can be unilateral or bilateral and can be due to biallelic *COL25A1* mutations.

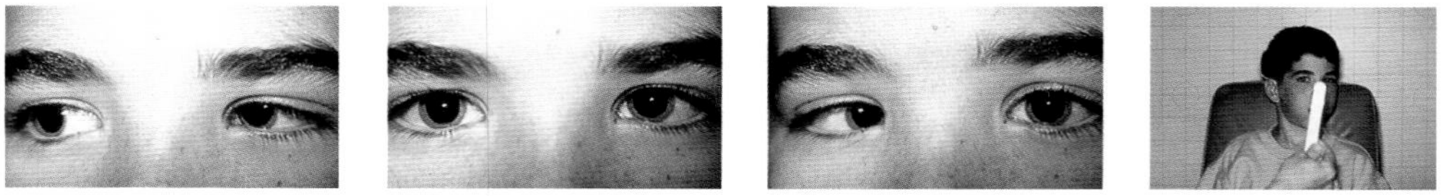

Figure 12-1 Type 1 Duane retraction syndrome with esotropia, left eye, showing limitation of abduction, almost full adduction, and retraction of the globe on adduction. *Far right,* Compensatory left head turn. *(Courtesy of Edward L. Raab, MD.)*

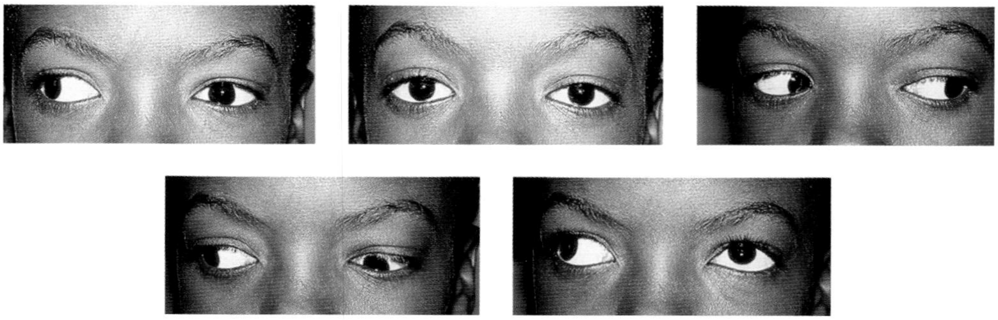

Figure 12-2 Type 2 Duane retraction syndrome, left eye. *Top row,* Full abduction and marked limitation of adduction. *Bottom row,* Variable upshoot and downshoot of the left eye with extreme right-gaze effort. The typical primary position exotropia is not present in this patient. *(Courtesy of Edward L. Raab, MD.)*

多数 Duane 后退综合征是散发的，但 5% ~ 10% 为常染色体显性遗传。已报告了与更广泛疾病有关的实例。单卵双胞胎的不一致增加了宫内环境对该综合征发展的作用。女性发病率较高，更常见于左眼。

解剖和影像研究提示，Ⅵ颅神经核缺如或发育不全，以及Ⅲ颅神经异常分支支配外直肌。肌电图研究的结果与其一致。尽管 Duane 后退综合征属神经支配异常，手术中常见紧张且宽附着的内直肌和纤维化的外直肌，并伴随相应的被动牵拉异常。

临床特征

Duane 后退综合征最常分为 3 型，但它们可能仅在水平转动受限的严重程度上存在差异。1 型指外转受限，第一眼位内斜视（图 12-1）；2 型指内转受限和外斜（图 12-2）；3 型指外转和内转均受限，伴有内斜、外斜或无第一眼位偏斜（图 12-3）。15% 为双眼发病，双眼的类型可能不同。这些病例的神经异常支配提示，这种分类有时过于武断，特别是对 1 型和 3 型的诊断。*协同开散*是一种罕见而复杂的运动障碍，常被分为 4 型 Duane 后退综合征，常有外斜视，当受累眼本应向内转方向时，实际呈现更多的外转——这一表现被生动地描述为“眼球分离”。协同开散可是单眼或双眼的，由于双等位基因 *COL25A1* 突变所致。

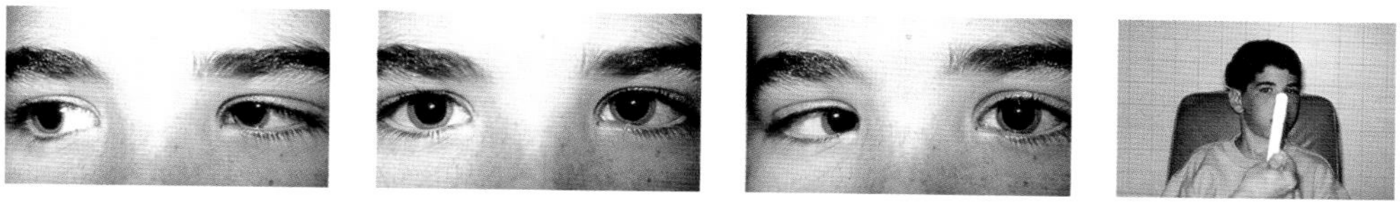

图 12–1　1 型 Duane 后退综合征伴内斜视，左眼外转受限，几乎是全部内转，眼球在内转时后退。*右眼看远处时，头左转代偿。*（*译者注：资料来源见前页原文。*）

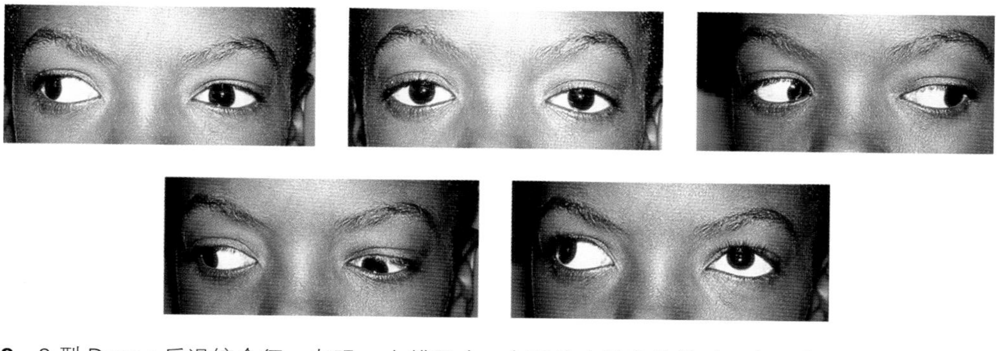

图 12–2　2 型 Duane 后退综合征，左眼。*上排图中*，右眼最大限度外转时，左眼内转受限。*下排图中*，最大程度右侧注视时，左眼不同程度上射和下射。典没有型的第一眼位外斜视。（*译者注：资料来源见前页原文。*）

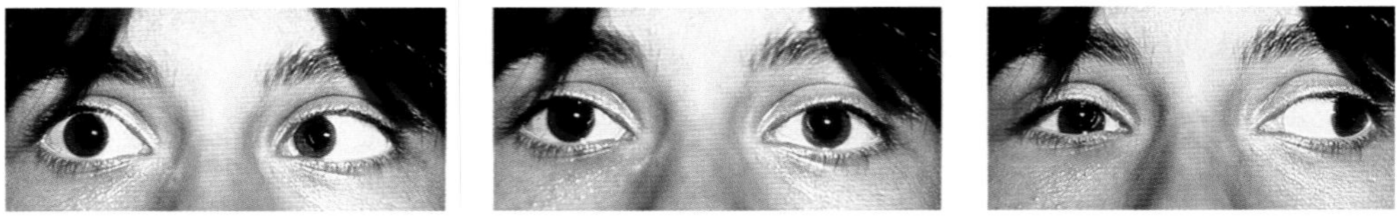

Figure 12-3 Type 3 Duane retraction syndrome, right eye. Severe limitation of abduction and adduction, with palpebral fissure narrowing even though adduction cannot be accomplished. There is no deviation in primary position. *(Courtesy of Edward L. Raab, MD.)*

Type 1 (with esotropia and limited abduction) is the most common form of Duane retraction syndrome, accounting for 50%–80% of cases in several series. Affected individuals or their caregivers often incorrectly believe that the normal eye is turning in excessively, not realizing that the involved eye is failing to abduct. Observation of globe retraction on adduction obviates the need for neurologic investigation for sixth nerve palsy, from which it must be differentiated; however, retraction can be difficult to appreciate in an infant. Another indicator that the condition is not sixth nerve palsy is the relatively small esotropia in primary position (usually <30 prism diopters [Δ]) in the setting of a severe abduction deficit. A further point of differentiation is that even in esotropic Duane retraction syndrome, a small-angle exotropia is sometimes present on gaze to the side opposite that of the affected eye, a finding that does not occur in lateral rectus muscle paralysis. Finally, examination at the slit lamp can help confirm the diagnosis in mild cases: if the vertical slit-lamp beam cast from the cornea onto the lower eyelid is disrupted by globe retraction when the eye adducts, Duane retraction syndrome is present.

Management

No surgical approach will normalize rotations. Surgery is reserved for cases with a primary position deviation, a head turn, marked globe retraction, or large upshoots or downshoots. Because Duane retraction syndrome is a spectrum of motility disorders, the surgical plan must be individualized for the patient. In many patients with this syndrome, the eyes are properly aligned in at least 1 position of gaze, allowing the development of binocular vision. The main goal of surgery is to centralize this field of single binocular vision to eliminate the need for a head turn. Expansion of the field of single binocular vision, while laudable, is more relevant in patients with sixth nerve palsy than in those with Duane syndrome, who rarely report diplopia in ipsilateral gaze.

For unilateral type 1 Duane retraction syndrome, recession of the medial rectus muscle on the involved side has been the procedure most often used to correct the primary position deviation and eliminate the head turn. Adding recession of the opposite medial rectus (bilateral surgery) has been advocated by some surgeons, but the rationale is unclear, as this does not increase innervation to the lateral rectus muscle (as it would in sixth nerve paresis) and any decrease in medial rectus innervation is offset by a decrease in anomalous innervation to the lateral rectus muscle of the involved eye. These operations do not usually improve abduction significantly. Primary position overcorrection can occur due to excessive medial rectus recession, and the resulting exotropia will worsen in the field of gaze in which the involved eye is adducted. Recession of the lateral rectus muscle of the uninvolved eye can offset this effect to some extent.

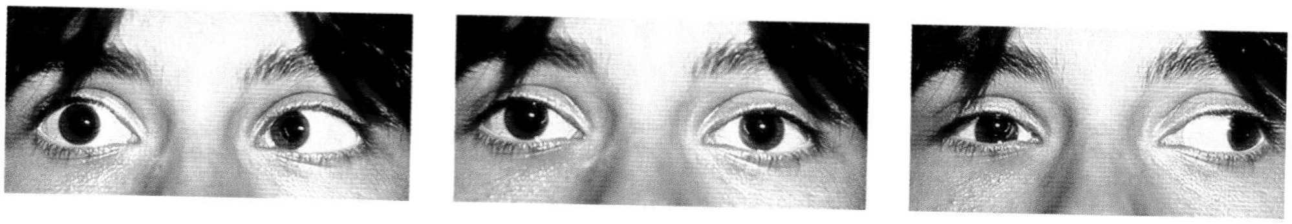

图 12-3　3 型 Duane 后退综合征，右眼。严重的外转和内转受限，内转不能时仍伴睑裂变窄。没有第一眼位偏斜。*（译者注：资料来源见前页原文。）*

1 型（伴内斜和外转受限）是最常见的 Duane 眼球后退综合征，占 50% ~ 80%。患者和护士常误认为其是正常眼内转过度，并没有意识到是受累眼不能外转。当观察到内转时眼球后退时，可排除对Ⅵ颅神经麻痹的神经系统检查，但是必须进行鉴别诊断。婴儿很难评估眼球后退。另一个排除Ⅵ颅神经麻痹的指征是第一眼位轻度内斜（<30 棱镜度［Δ］）伴重度外转不足。另一鉴别点是，即使是内斜型 Duane 后退综合征，向受累眼相反方向注视时，有时出现轻度外斜，这种情况在外直肌麻痹时不会出现。最后，裂隙灯检查可以帮助确诊疑似病例：如果垂直裂隙光束从角膜照射到下眼睑时，会因内转时的眼球后退而中断，即可确诊 Duane 后退综合征。

治疗

手术不能使眼球转动正常。第一眼位偏斜、头位转动、明显的眼球后退或较大的上射下射时考虑手术。由于 Duane 后退综合征是眼球运动异常，手术方案需个性化设计。许多患此综合征患者至少在一个注视位置时眼正位，双眼视觉得以发育。手术的主要目标是将这一双眼单视视野转变成中心视野，以消除头位转动。单眼双视范围的扩大虽很值得，但Ⅵ颅神经麻痹比 Duane 综合征患者更重要，因为 Duane 综合征少有同侧注视的复视。

单侧 1 型 Duane 后退综合征，多行受累眼的内直肌后徙术进行第一眼位偏斜矫正和消除头位转动。有些医生建议增加对侧眼内直肌后徙（双眼手术），但是基本原理尚不清楚，因为这不能增加外直肌的神经冲动（与Ⅵ颅神经麻痹一样），任何对内直肌神经冲动的减少，可抵消受累眼外直肌的异常神经冲动的减少。这些手术不能明显改善外转。由于过度内直肌后徙，可发生第一眼位过矫，并且在受累眼内转的注视范围内所产生的外斜视会严重。未受累眼的外直肌后徙可以在一定程度上抵消这种影响。

Because of concern that lateral rectus muscle resection will exacerbate globe retraction, most surgeons do not favor this approach. Occasionally, however, there are patients with minimal co-contraction in whom a small resection (<3–4 mm) can produce dramatic improvement in abduction. Partial or full lateral transposition of both vertical rectus muscles or the superior rectus alone, usually with medial rectus recession, with or without posterior scleral fixation (myopexy), has been shown to improve abduction in some patients.

The most commonly recommended surgery for type 2 Duane retraction syndrome is recession of the lateral rectus muscle on the involved side; resection of the medial rectus muscle is avoided. Some surgeons recess both lateral rectus muscles if a large-angle exotropia is present, but when a fixating unaffected eye is operated on, the effect of increased contralateral medial rectus innervation (and associated lateral rectus anomalous innervation) must be considered.

Patients with type 3 Duane retraction syndrome often have straight eyes near the primary position and do not require surgical treatment for their minimal head turn or horizontal strabismus. Globe retraction may be severe enough to warrant treatment and can be lessened by recession of both the medial and the lateral rectus muscles, which may also reduce any upshoot or downshoot in adduction. This is also an option for treating retraction in type 1 and type 2 Duane retraction syndrome. The lateral recession must be large to improve the retraction. Other procedures to address an upshoot or downshoot include splitting of the lateral rectus muscle in a Y configuration, retroequatorial fixation of the lateral rectus muscle and, more recently, deactivation of the lateral rectus muscle, such as by disinsertion and reattachment to the lateral periosteum of the orbit with a subsequent transposition procedure.

Rosenbaum AL. Costenbader Lecture. The efficacy of rectus muscle transposition surgery in esotropic Duane syndrome and VI nerve palsy. J *AAPOS*. 2004;8(5):409–419.

Congenital Fibrosis of the Extraocular Muscles

Congenital fibrosis of the extraocular muscles (CFEOM), or congenital fibrosis syndrome, is a group of rare congenital disorders in which EOM restriction is present and fibrous tissue replaces these muscles. Some forms have been noted to be inherited, usually as an autosomal dominant trait but occasionally in an autosomal recessive fashion. Cases of CFEOM involve developmental defects of cranial nerve nuclei and of the nerves themselves, resulting in dysinnervation and abnormal structure of the EOMs.

Heidary G, Engle EC, Hunter DG. Congenital fibrosis of the extraocular muscles. *Semin Ophthalmol.* 2008;23(1):3–8.

Clinical features

Depending upon the type of CFEOM, there may be various combinations of esotropia with limited abduction, exotropia with limited adduction, limited elevation with chin-up head position, and ptosis.

Strabismus fixus involves the horizontal rectus muscles, usually the medial rectus muscles, causing severe esotropia. The condition is usually sporadic and can be acquired late.

Vertical retraction syndrome affects the superior rectus muscle and causes inability to depress the eye.

由于外直肌切除术可能加剧眼球后退，多数手术医生不赞成这种方法。偶有患者有微量的共同收缩，少量切除（< 3 ~ 4 mm）即可明显改善外转。垂直直肌或上直肌的部分或完全外侧移位，同时伴有内直肌后徙、伴有或不伴有后巩膜固定（肌肉固定）已证明可改善一些患者的外转。

2 型 Duane 后退综合征最常推荐的手术是受累眼的外直肌后徙术，避免内直肌切除术。如果有大角度外斜视，一些医生行双侧外直肌后徙术，但对固视的未受累眼实施手术时，必须考虑增加的对侧眼内直肌神经冲动（和相关的外直肌异常神经支配）。

3 型 Duane 后退综合征患者在第一眼位正位，较小的头位转动或水平斜视不需要手术。严重的眼球后退需要治疗，内直肌和外直肌后徙术可以减轻眼球后退，也可以减少内转时的上射或下射。这也是治疗 1 型和 2 型 Duane 后退综合征的选择。外直肌后徙必须足够大，以改善眼球后退。其他改善上射或下射的方法包括外直肌 Y 字形劈开术、外直肌赤道后固定术及外直肌功能减弱术，如转位术后再行外直肌切断并外侧骨膜固定术。

Rosenbaum AL. Costenbader Lecture. The efficacy of rectus muscle transposition surgery in esotropic Duane syndrome and VI nerve palsy. J *AAPOS*. 2004;8(5):409–419.

先天性眼外肌纤维化

先天性眼外肌纤维化（CFEOM）或先天性纤维化综合征，是一组罕见的先天性疾病，表现为眼外肌受限和纤维组织替代眼外肌。有一些是遗传性的，为常染色体显性遗传，偶尔为常染色体隐性遗传。先天性眼外肌纤维化（CFEOM）是颅神经核和神经本身发育缺陷，导致眼外肌（EOMs）的神经支配异常和结构异常。

Heidary G, Engle EC, Hunter DG. Congenital fibrosis of the extraocular muscles. *Semin Ophthalmol.* 2008;23(1):3–8.

临床特征

根据先天性眼外肌纤维化（CFEOM）的类型，有多种不同组合，内斜视伴外转受限、外斜视伴内转受限、上转受限伴下颌抬高头位以及上睑下垂。

*固定性斜视*累及水平直肌，多为内直肌，引起严重的内斜视。常为散发，也可为迟发性。

*垂直性后退综合征*累及上直肌，导致无法使眼球下转。

Diagnosis of CFEOM depends on finding limited voluntary motion with restriction, which is usually severe and can be confirmed with forced duction testing. The congenital onset is important in distinguishing the syndrome from thyroid eye disease.

Management

Surgery for CFEOM is difficult and requires release of the restricted muscles (ie, weakening procedures). Fibrosis of the adjacent tissues may be present as well. A good surgical result aligns the eyes in primary position, but full ocular rotations cannot be restored and the outcome is unpredictable.

Sener EC, Taylan Sekeroglu H, Ural O, Oztürk BT, Sanaç AS. Strabismus surgery in congenital fibrosis of the extraocular muscles: a paradigm. *Ophthalmic Genet.* 2014;35(4):208–225.

Möbius Syndrome

Clinical features

Möbius syndrome (or "sequence"; see Chapter 15 discussion of sequence) is a rare condition characterized by the association of both sixth and seventh nerve palsies, the latter causing masklike facies. Patients may also manifest gaze palsies that can be attributed to abnormalities in the paramedian pontine reticular formation or the sixth cranial nerve nucleus. Many patients also have limb, chest, and tongue defects. Some geneticists believe that Möbius syndrome is one of a family of syndromes in which hypoplastic limb anomalies may be associated with orofacial and cranial nerve defects. Poland syndrome (absent pectoralis muscle) is another variant.

Patients with Möbius syndrome exhibit 1 of 3 patterns of ocular motility involvement, which are likely related to the severity and timing of the in utero insult:

- orthotropia in primary position with marked deficits in abduction and adduction (40% of cases) (Fig 12-4)
- esotropia with cross-fixation and sparing of convergence (50% of cases)
- large exotropia with absence of convergence (10% of cases)

Some patients appear to have palpebral fissure changes on adduction or vertical EOM involvement. Those with exotropia and vertical limitation may harbor *TUBB3* mutations.

Carta A, Mora P, Neri A, Favilla S, Sadun AA. Ophthalmologic and systemic features in Möbius syndrome: an Italian case series. *Ophthalmology.* 2011;118(8):1518–1523.

MacKinnon S, Oystreck DT, Andrews C, Chan WM, Hunter DG, Engle EC. Diagnostic distinctions and genetic analysis of patients diagnosed with moebius syndrome. *Ophthalmology.* 2014;121(7):1461–1468.

Management

Medial rectus muscle recession has been advocated for patients with large-angle esotropia, but caution should be exercised in the presence of a significant limitation of adduction. Some surgeons have endeavored to improve abduction by performing vertical rectus muscle transposition procedures after medial rectus muscle restriction has been relieved.

先天性眼外肌纤维化（CFEOM）的诊断依据是限制性自主运动，常很严重，并且通过被动牵拉试验证实。先天发病是甲状腺眼病的重要鉴别点。

治疗

先天性眼外肌纤维化（CFEOM）手术很困难，需要松解受限的肌肉（即减弱手术）。也可能存在邻近组织纤维化。较好的手术效果是使第一眼位正眼位，但无法恢复完全的眼球转动，而且无法预测手术效果。

Sener EC, Taylan Sekeroglu H, Ural O, Oztürk BT, Sanaç AS. Strabismus surgery in congenital fibrosis of the extraocular muscles: a paradigm. *Ophthalmic Genet*. 2014;35(4):208–225.

Möbius 综合征

临床特征

Möbius 综合征（或“序列”；见第 15 章序列的讨论）是一种罕见的疾病，其特征与Ⅵ和Ⅶ颅神经麻痹相关，后者导致面具脸。还可出现注视麻痹，这是因脑桥旁正中网状结构或Ⅵ颅神经核异常。许多患者还有肢体、胸和舌缺陷。一些遗传学家认为，Möbius 综合征是综合征家系之一，其中肢体发育不全的异常可能与口面神经和颅神经缺陷有关。Poland 综合征（胸大肌缺如）是另一种变异亚型。

Möbius 综合征表现出受累的 3 种眼球运动之一，可能与子宫内损害的严重程度和时间有关：

- 第一眼位眼正位视，伴明显的外转和内转缺陷（40%的病例）（图 12–4）。
- 内斜视，伴交叉注视和集合回避（50%的病例）。
- 大的外斜视，伴集合缺失（10%的病例）。

一些患者在内转时伴睑裂改变或垂直眼外肌受累。有外斜视和垂直运动受限的患者可能有 *TUBB3* 突变。

Carta A, Mora P, Neri A, Favilla S, Sadun AA. Ophthalmologic and systemic features in Möbius syndrome: an Italian case series. *Ophthalmology*. 2011;118(8):1518–1523.

MacKinnon S, Oystreck DT, Andrews C, Chan WM, Hunter DG, Engle EC. Diagnostic distinctions and genetic analysis of patients diagnosed with moebius syndrome. *Ophthalmology*. 2014;121(7):1461–1468.

治疗

对大角度内斜视患者建议行内直肌后徙术，但当存在显著的内转受限时，应慎重。一些手术医生为了尽量改善外转，在解除内直肌受限后，行垂直直肌转位术。

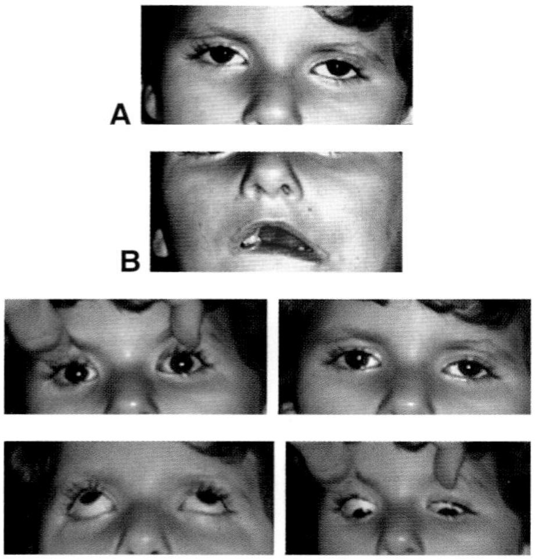

Figure 12-4 Möbius syndrome. **A,** Straight eyes in primary position. **B,** The patient cannot smile because of bilateral seventh nerve palsy. **C,** Bilaterally absent adduction and severely limited abduction. **D,** Vertical movements are not affected. *(Courtesy of Edward L. Raab, MD.)*

Miscellaneous Special Forms of Strabismus

Brown Syndrome

Although it is included in most lists of vertical deviations (see Chapter 11), Brown syndrome is best considered a special form of strabismus. The characteristic restriction of elevation in adduction was originally thought to be caused by shortening of the supposed sheath of the superior oblique tendon. It is now attributed to various abnormalities of the tendon–trochlea complex (see Chapter 3), and evidence indicates that structural problems within the orbit but remote from the superior oblique tendon, including instability of the lateral rectus pulley, can present an identical clinical picture (pseudo–Brown syndrome). Recent work suggests that congenital Brown syndrome may be a form of CCDD.

Most cases are congenital. Prominent causes of the acquired form include trauma in the region of the trochlea, iatrogenic causes such as scleral buckles and tube shunts, orbital tumors, and systemic inflammatory conditions such as rheumatoid arthritis. The latter often results in intermittent Brown syndrome, which may resolve spontaneously. Sinusitis can also lead to Brown syndrome; thus, patients with acute-onset presentation of Brown syndrome of undetermined cause should undergo imaging of the orbits and paranasal sinuses to investigate this possibility. The condition is bilateral in approximately 10% of cases. Resolution of congenital Brown syndrome has been thought to be unusual, but a report by Dawson and colleagues describes spontaneous improvement in 75% of cases, often after many years.

Dawson E, Barry J, Lee J. Spontaneous resolution in patients with congenital Brown syndrome. *J AAPOS.* 2009;13(2):116–118.

Clinical features

Well-recognized clinical features of Brown syndrome include deficient elevation in adduction that improves in abduction but often not completely (Fig 12-5). Several findings differentiate Brown syndrome from inferior oblique muscle paralysis (see Chapter 11, Table 11-4).

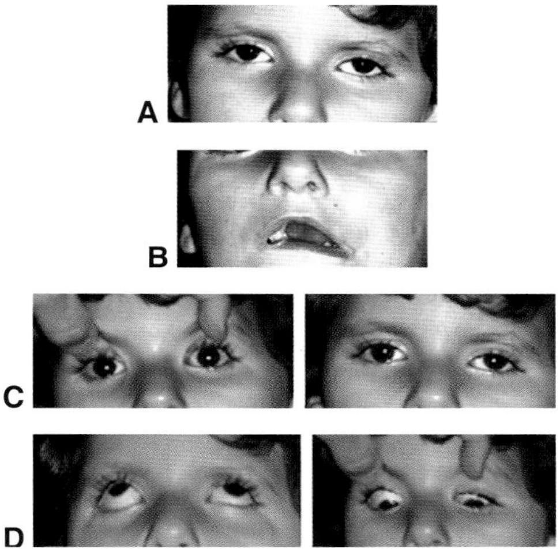

图 12-4　Möbius 综合征。**A.** 第一眼位正位。**B.** 因双侧Ⅶ颅神经麻痹，患者不能笑。**C.** 双眼不能内转和严重的外转受限。**D.** 垂直运动不受累。*（译者注：资料来源见前页原文。）*

斜视的其他特殊形式

Brown 综合征

虽然将 Brown 综合征归类于垂直分离（见第 11 章），但最好将其视为一种特殊形式的斜视。最初认为内转时上转的特征性受限是上斜肌腱缩短。现在认为是肌腱——滑车复合体异常（见第 3 章），并且有证据表明，是眶内、远离上斜肌腱的结构问题，包括外直肌滑车的不稳定性，表现出相似的临床表现（假性 Brown 综合征）。最近的研究表明，先天性 Brown 综合征可能是先天性颅神经支配异常（CCDD）眼病的一种形式。

大多数病例是先天性的。获得性的主要原因有滑车创伤、医源性原因（巩膜扣带和引流管）、眼眶肿瘤和全身性炎性病症（类风湿性关节炎）。后者常导致间歇性 Brown 综合征，可自愈。鼻窦炎也可导致 Brown 综合征，患者出现急性发作的、不明原因的 Brown 综合征时，应进行眼眶和鼻窦的影像检查，以排除这种可能性。大约 10% 的病例是双侧的。先天性 Brown 综合征的治疗方案与一般不同，但 Dawson 等发现，75% 的病例常在多年后自行改善。

Dawson E, Barry J, Lee J. Spontaneous resolution in patients with congenital Brown syndrome. *J AAPOS.* 2009;13(2):116–118.

临床特征

Brown 综合征的临床特征包括内转时上转不足，外转时会改善，但不完全（图 12–5）。一些症状可以将 Brown 综合征与下斜肌麻痹相鉴别（见第 11 章，表 11–4）。

An unequivocally positive forced duction test demonstrating restricted passive elevation in adduction is essential for the diagnosis. Retropulsion of the globe during this test stretches the superior oblique tendon and accentuates the restriction. In restrictions involving the inferior rectus muscle or its surrounding tissues, by contrast, the limitation of passive elevation is accentuated by forceps-induced proptosis of the eye rather than by retropulsion.

Attempts at elevation straight upward usually cause divergence (V pattern) due to lateral diversion of the globe as it meets resistance from the tight superior oblique tendon (see Fig 12-5). This finding is an important point of distinction from inferior oblique muscle paralysis, which is more likely to exhibit an A pattern. In adduction, the palpebral fissure widens and overdepression in adduction can be observed in severe cases of Brown syndrome (see Chapter 11, Table 11-2). This differs from overdepression in adduction in true superior oblique muscle overaction, which occurs less abruptly with increasing adduction. In mild Brown syndrome, no hypotropia is present in primary position. Severe cases of Brown syndrome with a primary position hypotropia are often accompanied by a chin-up head position or a head turn away from the side of the affected eye.

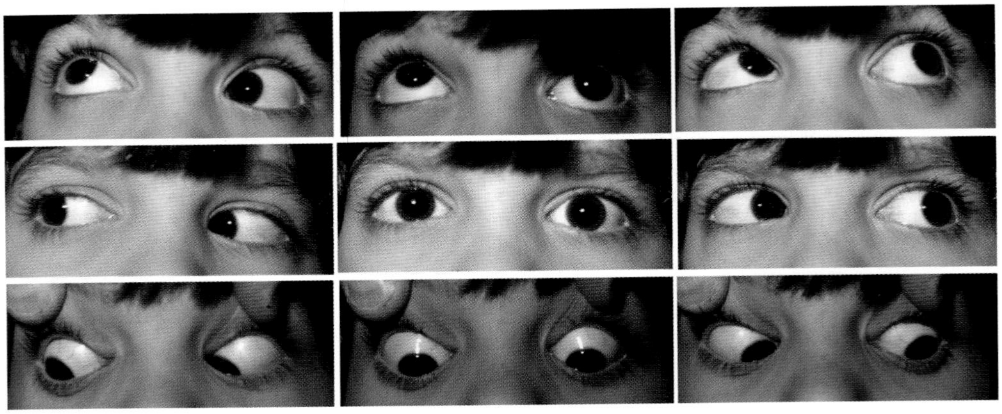

Figure 12-5 Brown syndrome, left eye. No elevation of the left eye when adducted; left eye is depressed instead. Elevation is also severely limited in straight-up gaze and moderately so even in up-and-left gaze. Note the characteristic divergence in straight-up gaze and lack of ipsilateral superior oblique overaction. *(Courtesy of Edward L. Raab, MD.)*

Management

Observation alone is appropriate for mild congenital Brown syndrome. When Brown syndrome is secondary to rheumatoid arthritis or other systemic inflammatory diseases, resolution may occur as systemic treatment brings the underlying disease into remission or when corticosteroids are injected near the trochlea.

Surgery is indicated for more severe congenital cases. Superior oblique tenotomy nasal to the superior rectus muscle is definitive treatment; however, iatrogenic superior oblique muscle paresis occurs in a significant minority of patients after this procedure. Careful handling of the intermuscular septum during surgery can reduce the incidence of this sequela. To reduce the consequences of superior oblique muscle palsy after tenotomy, some surgeons perform simultaneous ipsilateral inferior oblique muscle weakening. Other current options include insertion of an inert spacer or suture between the cut ends of the superior oblique tendon, and split-tendon lengthening of the tendon (see Chapter 14).

明确的被动牵拉试验阳性对诊断至关重要，提示内转时被动上转受限。在被动牵拉试验中，眼球的回退拉伸了上斜肌腱，并使限制加重。相反，下直肌或其周围组织的受限时，被动上转受限加重是因为镊子引起的眼球突出，而不是眼球回退。

当试图垂直向上转时，常会引起散开（V 型）（见图 12–5），这是由于有紧张的上斜肌腱的阻力，眼球向外侧散开。这是与下斜肌麻痹的鉴别要点，其通常表现为 A 型。重度的 Brown 综合征病例中，在内转时睑裂扩大，且内转过度下转（见第 11 章，表 11–2）。这不同于真正的上斜肌功能亢进的内转过度下转，后者内转时不会突然加重。轻度的 Brown 综合征中，第一眼位没有下斜视。重度的 Brown 综合征第一眼位有下斜视，常伴有下颌上抬头位或头位转向受累眼对侧。

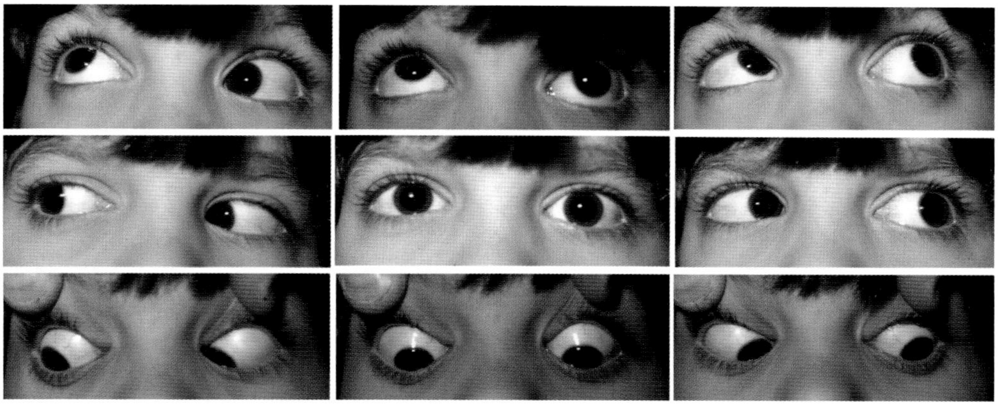

图 12–5　Brown 综合征，左眼。左眼内转时无上转；左眼反而下转。直视向上注视时上转严重受限，甚至在左右注视时也会中度受限。注意直视向上注视时，出现特征性散开，并缺乏同侧的上斜肌功能亢进。*（译者注：资料来源见前页原文。）*

治疗

轻度先天性 Brown 综合征仅需观察。继发于类风湿性关节炎或其他全身性炎性疾病时，因为全身治疗或在滑车附近注射皮质类固醇使病情缓解，Brown 综合征可能会自愈。

手术适用于严重的先天性病例。进行上直肌鼻侧的上斜肌切除术，但偶发生医源性上斜肌麻痹。术中小心处理肌间隔可减少这种后遗症的发生。为了减少上斜肌腱切断术后的上斜肌麻痹，一些医生同时行同侧下斜肌减弱术。目前其他选择包括在上斜肌腱的切开端之间植入隔离条或缝线，以及行肌腱延长的劈裂肌腱法（见第 14 章）。

Wright KW. Brown's syndrome: diagnosis and management. *Trans Am Ophthalmol Soc.* 1999; 97:1023–1109.

Third Nerve Palsy

In children, third nerve palsy can be congenital (more appropriately termed *dysinnervation*) or can be caused by conditions such as trauma, inflammation, or viral infection. It can also occur as a manifestation of ophthalmoplegic migraine, after vaccination, or (infrequently) as a result of a neoplastic lesion. In adults, the usual causes are intracranial aneurysm, microvascular infarction, inflammation, trauma, infection, or tumor. See BCSC Section 5, *Neuro-Ophthalmology*, for detailed discussion of the causes and manifestations of third nerve palsy. This section is concerned primarily with the Principles of treatment of the strabismus.

Clinical features

Complete paralysis results in limited adduction, elevation, and depression of the eye, causing exotropia and often hypotropia. These findings are expected because the remaining unopposed muscles are the lateral rectus (abductor) and the superior oblique (abductor and depressor), except when the cause of the paralysis involves the nerves supplying these muscles as well. Upper eyelid ptosis is usually present, often with pseudoptosis due to the depressed position of the involved eye (Fig 12-6).

The clinical findings and treatment may be complicated by misdirection (aberrant regeneration) of the damaged nerve, presenting as anomalous eyelid elevation, pupil constriction, or vertical excursion of the globe—any or all of which can occur upon attempted rotation into the field of action of the EOMs supplied by the injured nerve. A miotic pupil is sometimes noted in congenital cases, irrespective of whether there is aberrant regeneration. Affected adults report incapacitating diplopia unless the involved eye is occluded by ptosis or other means.

Management

Except in congenital cases, it is advisable to wait at least 6 months, possibly even up to 12 months, for spontaneous recovery before proceeding with surgical correction. Patients with at least partial recovery are much better candidates for good functional and cosmetic results. Because the visual system is still developing in pediatric patients, amblyopia is a common finding that must be treated aggressively.

In adults with previously good binocular vision, occlusion from associated ptosis may actually be beneficial by preventing incapacitating diplopia associated with a limited or absent field of single binocular vision; ptosis repair should not be done without prism adaptation testing to demonstrate that the patient can achieve satisfactory binocular vision with prism. The incidence of diplopia in patients younger than 8 years is low because of suppression (see Chapter 5).

Third nerve palsy presents difficult surgical challenges because multiple EOMs, including the levator muscle, are involved. Replacing all the lost rotational forces on the globe is impossible; therefore, the goal of surgery is adequate alignment for binocular function in primary position and in slight downgaze for reading.

Wright KW. Brown's syndrome: diagnosis and management. *Trans Am Ophthalmol Soc.* 1999; 97:1023–1109.

Ⅲ颅神经麻痹

儿童的Ⅲ颅神经麻痹可以是先天性的（称为*神经支配异常更适当*），或由创伤、炎症或病毒感染引起。Ⅲ颅神经麻痹也可出现在眼麻痹性偏头痛、接种疫苗后或肿瘤（不常见）。成人常见原因是颅内动脉瘤、微血管梗死、炎症、创伤、感染或肿瘤。Ⅲ颅神经麻痹病因和临床表现见 BCSC 第 5 册《*神经眼科学*》。本节主要讨论斜视的治疗原则。

临床特征

完全性麻痹会导致内转、上转和下转受限，引起外斜视和下斜视。这些是可预期的，因为留下的是无拮抗的外直肌（外转）和上斜肌（外转和下转），支配这些肌肉的神经也可能受累。也常见上睑下垂，由于受累眼下转，表现为假性上睑下垂（图 12–6）。

临床表现和治疗可因受损神经的异常走行（异常再生）而变得复杂，表现为异常眼睑上提、瞳孔收缩或眼球垂直偏斜——当眼球转向受损神经支配的眼外肌的视野时，可能出现这些表现。无论是否存在神经的异常再生，先天性病例中有时出现瞳孔缩小。除非有上睑下垂或用其他方式遮挡，成年患者会失代偿性复视。

治疗

除先天性病例外，建议进行手术矫正前，至少等待 6 ~ 12 个月，因为可能自愈。自行恢复不全的患者，术后也可能有较好功能恢复和美容效果。由于患儿的视觉系统仍在发育，弱视较为常见，必须积极治疗。

有良好双眼视觉的成人中，眼睑下垂的遮挡有益于防止失代偿性复视和伴随的双眼单视视野受限或缺失。上睑下垂手术前应进行棱镜适应试验，以检测患者用棱镜是否能获得满意的双眼视觉。小于 8 岁的患者，由于发生抑制，复视发生率较低（见第 5 章）。

Ⅲ颅神经麻痹手术较为困难，因为累及多条眼外肌（EOMs），包括上睑提肌。不可能恢复眼球上缺失的所有旋转力。因此，手术目的是第一眼位获得双眼视功能所需的适当正位，以及阅读时轻微向下注视的能力。

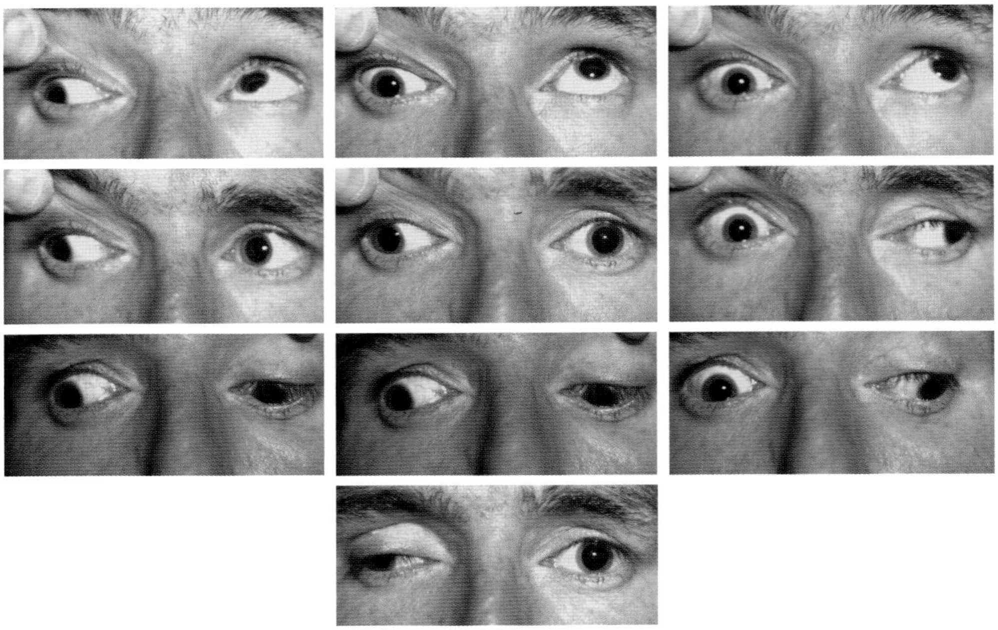

Figure 12-6 Third nerve palsy, right eye, with ptosis *(bottom photo)* and limited adduction, elevation, and depression (upper eyelid elevated manually in top 9 photos). *(Courtesy of Edward L. Raab, MD.)*

Selection of the surgical procedure is dictated by the number of involved muscles and their condition, as well as by the presence or absence of noticeable paradoxical rotations. In a case of incomplete paralysis, a large recession-resection of the horizontal rectus muscles to correct the exodeviation, with supraplacement of both to correct the hypotropia, is effective. Some surgeons perform a concurrent superior oblique tenotomy to reduce the hypotropia. For complete paralysis, one suggested approach is a large recession of the lateral rectus muscle, combined with either a large medial rectus resection or fixation of the globe to the nasal orbital periosteum. Disinsertion of the lateral rectus muscle and reattachment to the lateral orbital periosteum can maximize inactivation of the muscle. Splitting and transposition of the lateral rectus muscle to the nasal side of the globe has also been described. Transfer of the superior oblique tendon to the upper nasal quadrant of the globe has been used as well; however, anomalous eye movements can result from this procedure. Most surgeons reserve correction of ptosis for a subsequent procedure, which allows for more accurate positioning of the upper eyelid.

Fourth Nerve Palsy

Paralysis of cranial nerve IV (trochlear) is discussed in Chapter 11 and BCSC Section 5, *Neuro-Ophthalmology.*

Sixth Nerve Palsy

Paralysis of cranial nerve VI (abducens) is less common in children than in adults. This entity is discussed in Chapter 8. See BCSC Section 5, *Neuro-Ophthalmology*, for additional discussion.

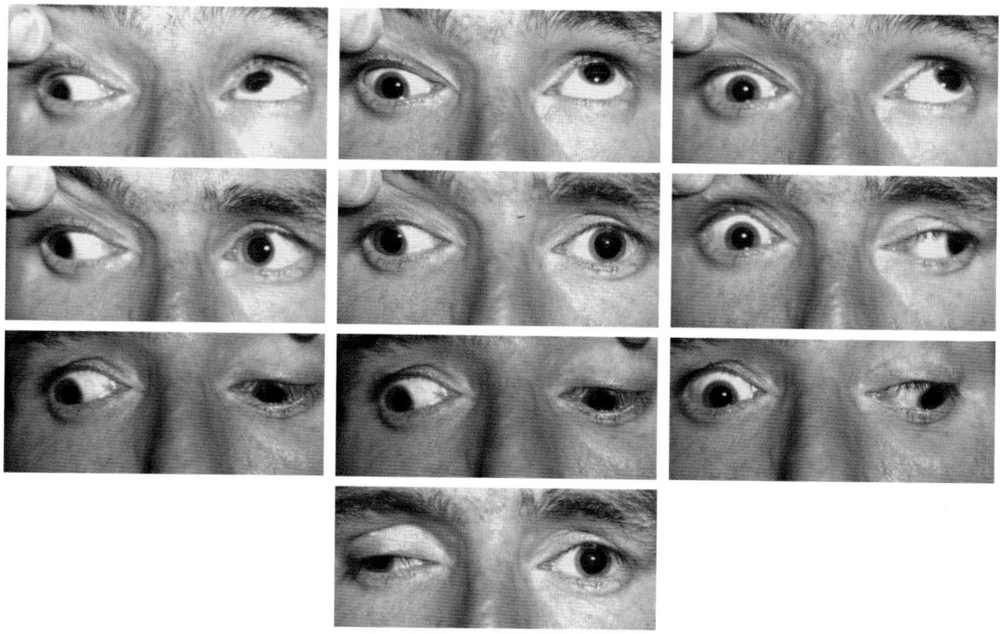

图 12-6　Ⅲ颅神经麻痹，右眼，上睑下垂（*底部照片*）和内转、上转和下转受限（前 9 张照片，用手上提上睑）。*（译者注：资料来源见前页原文。）*

手术的选择取决于受累的肌肉数量及其状况，以及是否存在明显的矛盾性旋转。在不完全麻痹时，对水平直肌进行较大后徙——切除以矫正外斜视、并且两者上移位可以矫正下斜视，都可奏效。一些手术医生同时行上斜肌肌腱切开术以减少下斜视。完全麻痹时，建议较大的外直肌后徙，同时较多内直肌切除术或将眼球固定到鼻侧眶骨膜。外直肌断腱术和眶外侧骨膜再固定术，可以使眼肌完全失去活动度。也有报道将外直肌劈裂和转位到眼球鼻侧。还有将上斜肌腱转位到眼球鼻上象限，但这个术式可导致异常眼球运动。大多数手术医生二次行上睑下垂矫正术，使上眼睑定位更准确。

Ⅳ颅神经麻痹

第 11 章和 BCSC 第 5 册《*神经眼科学*》讨论 Ⅳ 颅神经（滑车）麻痹。

Ⅵ颅神经麻痹

儿童的Ⅵ颅神经（外展）麻痹比成人少见，见第 8 章。进一步讨论见 BCSC 第 5 册《*神经眼科学*》。

Thyroid Eye Disease

Thyroid eye disease (TED) affects the eye and the orbit in various ways. Only motility disturbances are covered in this volume.

Edema, inflammation, and fibrosis of the EOMs due to lymphocytic infiltration occur in this disease. Not only do these pathologies restrict motility, but the massively enlarged muscles can cause compressive optic neuropathy. Detection of muscle enlargement by orbital imaging helps confirm the diagnosis.

The myopathy is not caused by thyroid dysfunction. Rather, both conditions probably result from a common autoimmune disease. Thyroid-stimulating immunoglobulins likely mediate TED and may be regarded as a functional biomarker for this condition. Some patients also have myasthenia gravis (another autoimmune disease, discussed later in this chapter), complicating the clinical findings. An association between severity of TED and smoking has recently become apparent; the hazard ratio for strabismus surgery is almost double in patients with thyroid disease who smoke.

Clinical features

The muscles affected in TED, in decreasing order of severity and frequency, are the inferior rectus, medial rectus, superior rectus, and lateral rectus. The condition is usually bilateral but is often asymmetric. Forced duction testing almost always shows restriction in one or more directions.

Most often, the patient presents with some degree of upper eyelid retraction, proptosis, hypotropia, and esotropia (Fig 12-7). TED is a common cause of acquired vertical deviation in adults, especially women, but rarely causes motility problems in children.

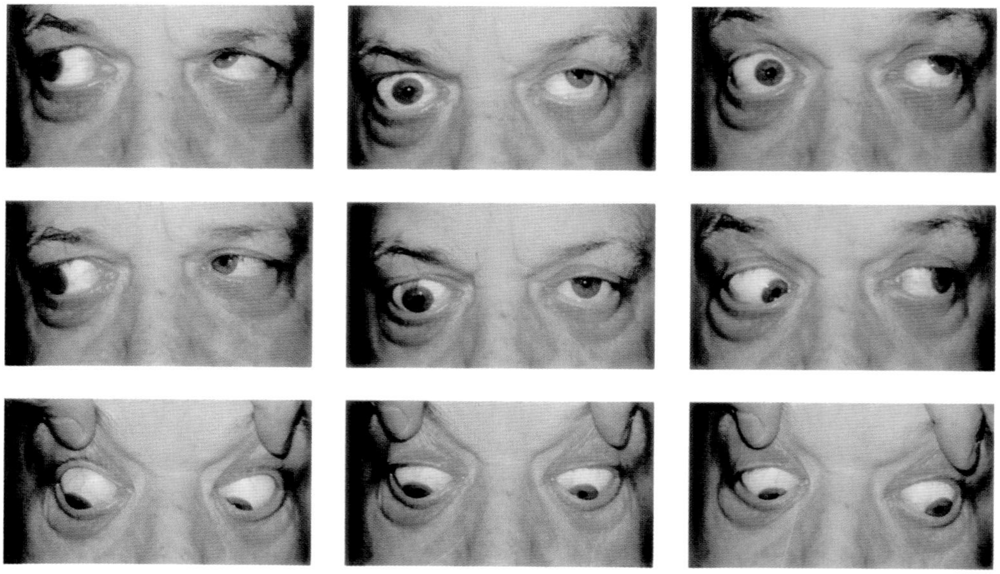

Figure 12-7 Thyroid eye disease. Note right upper eyelid retraction and restrictive right hypotropia with very limited elevation. Other rotations are not affected in this patient.

甲状腺眼病

甲状腺眼病（TED）影响眼球和眼眶的诸多方面。本节仅讨论运动障碍。

由于淋巴细胞浸润，引起眼外肌（EOMs）水肿、炎症和纤维化。这些病理改变不仅使眼球运动受限，明显增粗的肌肉还可引起压迫性视神经病变。眼眶影像检查见到眼肌增粗有助于确诊。

眼肌病不是由甲状腺功能障碍引起的。相反，这 2 种情况可能都是由一种常见的自身免疫性疾病引起的。甲状腺刺激免疫球蛋白可能介导甲状腺眼病（TED），并且可以视为是其功能性生物标志物。一些患者还同时患有重症肌无力（另一种自身免疫性疾病，本章后面会讨论），临床表现比较复杂。近年研究表明，甲状腺眼病（TED）的严重程度与吸烟明显相关，吸烟的甲状腺疾病患者的斜视手术风险增加 2 倍。

临床特征

甲状腺眼病（TED）受累眼肌的严重程度和发病率从高到低依次为：下直肌、内直肌、上直肌和外直肌。通常是双眼的，但不对称。被动牵拉试验在一个或多个方向运动受限。

在大多数情况下，患者会出现一定程度的上睑退缩、眼球突出、下斜视和内斜视（图 12–7）。甲状腺眼病是成人获得性垂直斜视的常见原因，特别是女性，但很少引起儿童的眼球运动障碍。

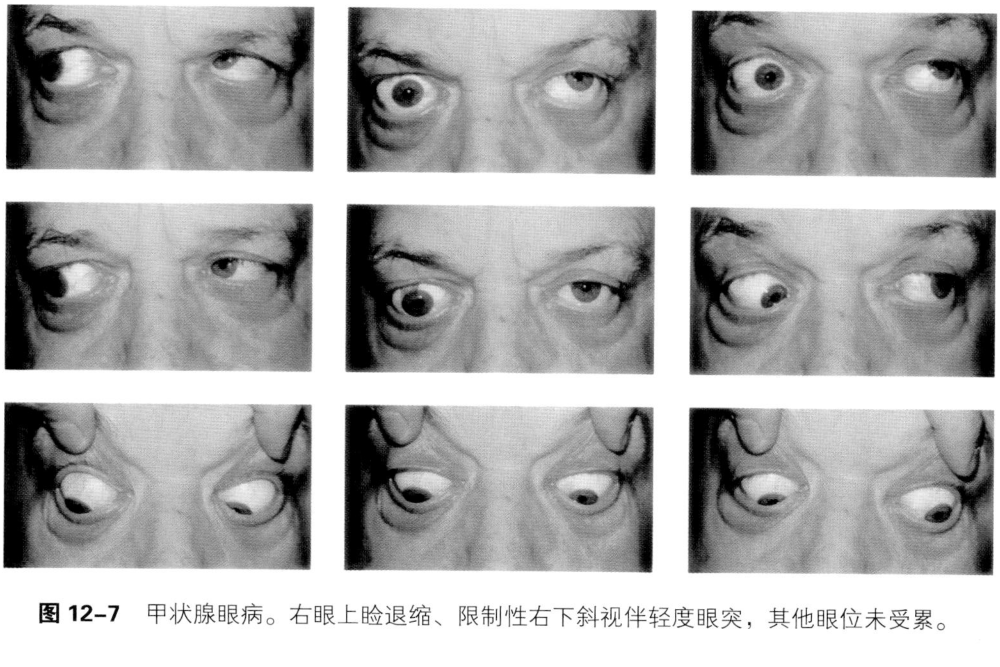

图 12–7　甲状腺眼病。右眼上睑退缩、限制性右下斜视伴轻度眼突，其他眼位未受累。

Management

Diplopia and abnormal head position are the principal indications for strabismus surgery. The operation may eliminate diplopia in primary gaze but rarely restores normal motility because of the restrictive myopathy, the need for large recessions in some cases to place the eye in primary position, and the ongoing underlying disease.

It is best to perform surgery after strabismus measurements and thyroid function tests have stabilized. In cases in which orbital decompression is necessary, strabismus surgery should be delayed until after that has been done. In the meantime, prisms may alleviate diplopia. Botulinum toxin may reduce the severity of fibrosis when injected into tight muscles in the acute phase. In studies of surgery performed before stability was achieved in patients with severe head positions, the results were favorable, but half the patients required further surgery.

Recession of the affected muscles is the preferred surgical treatment, addressing the tight muscles in 1 or both eyes. Resection procedures usually worsen restriction, but in carefully selected cases they may be helpful as part of the surgical plan. Slight initial undercorrection of hypotropia is desirable because late progressive overcorrection is common, especially with inferior rectus muscle recessions. Limited depression of the eyes after inferior rectus muscle recessions can interfere with patients' bifocal use.

Because proptosis and eyelid retraction can increase after EOM surgery, eyelid surgery is best delayed until after all EOM surgery has been completed.

Chronic Progressive External Ophthalmoplegia

Clinical features

Chronic progressive external ophthalmoplegia (CPEO) is a rare form of mitochondrial cytopathy that can affect various body systems. It usually begins in childhood with ptosis and slowly progresses to total paralysis of the eyelids and EOMs. CPEO may be sporadic or familial. Although a true pigmentary retinal dystrophy is rare, constricted visual fields and electrodiagnostic abnormalities can occur. The diagnosis of CPEO is confirmed when muscle biopsy results show ragged red fibers or when specific alterations of mitochondrial DNA are detected. *Kearns-Sayre syndrome* is characterized by retinal pigmentary changes, CPEO, and cardiomyopathy (especially heart block).

See BCSC Section 2, *Fundamentals and Principles of Ophthalmology*, Section 5, *Neuro-Ophthalmology*, and Section 12, *Retina and Vitreous*, for additional information on these and other mitochondrial disorders.

Management

It is important to ensure that the patient's cardiac status is evaluated, because lifethreatening arrhythmias can occur in Kearns-Sayre syndrome. Treatment options for the ocular motility disorder are limited; small surgical series report a high rate of long-term undercorrections. Cautious surgical elevation (suspension) of the upper eyelids can lessen a severe chin-up head position.

Myasthenia Gravis

Myasthenia gravis is a disorder in which antibodies directed against acetylcholine receptors cause muscle dysfunction. Onset in childhood is uncommon. A transient neonatal form, caused by the placental transfer of acetylcholine receptor antibodies of mothers with myasthenia gravis, exists but usually subsides rapidly. Another variant is not immune mediated and exhibits a familial predisposition.

治疗

复视和异常头位是斜视手术指征。手术可消除第一眼位的复视，但因为是限制性眼肌病，很少能恢复正常的眼球运动（有时还需要大量后徙以将眼球置于第一眼位），以及持续存在的原发病。

手术前最好测量斜视度，并待甲状腺功能稳定后再实行。需要行眶减压手术的病例，斜视手术应推迟，同时应用棱镜减轻复视症状。急性期，给紧张的肌肉注射肉毒杆菌毒素，可以减少纤维化的程度。研究显示，稳定期前行手术矫正明显头位的结果尚好，但是有一半的患者需要进一步的手术。

受累肌肉后徙术是首选的手术治疗，解除单眼或双眼紧张的肌肉。切除术常加重运动限制，但某些病例也可以作为手术一部分。下斜视初次手术可轻度欠矫，因为病情进展到后期，常见过矫，特别是下直肌切除术更常见，下直肌后徙的下转受限会影响患者双焦镜的使用。

因为眼外肌（EOM）手术会加重眼球突出及眼睑退缩，所以眼睑手术最好在眼外肌（EOM）手术后再实施。

慢性进行性眼外肌麻痹

临床表现

慢性进行性眼外肌麻痹（CPEO）是一种罕见的线粒体病，可累及多个系统。通常起病于儿童时期，表现为上睑下垂，之后缓慢进展到眼睑和眼外肌（EOMs）完全麻痹。慢性进行性眼外肌麻痹（CPEO）有散发性或家族性。虽然真性色素性视网膜变性很罕见，但可有视野缩小及电生理异常。肌肉活检显示破碎的红色纤维或线粒体 DNA 特殊改变可以确诊慢性进行性眼外肌麻痹（CPEO）。Kearns-Sayre 综合征的特征是视网膜色素病变、慢性进行性眼外肌麻痹（CPEO）和心肌病（尤其是传导阻滞）。

更多信息和其他线粒体疾病见 BCSC 第 2 册《*眼科学基础与原理*》、第 5 册《*神经眼科学*》和第 12 册《*视网膜与玻璃体*》。

治疗

Kearns-Sayre 综合征可能发生危及生命的心律失常，因此评估患者的心脏功能非常重要。眼球运动障碍的治疗方法有限，小样本的手术病例报道了远期的欠矫率比较高。谨慎施行上睑抬高术（悬吊术）可以减轻严重的下颌抬高头位。

重症肌无力

重症肌无力是乙酰胆碱受体的抗体导致肌肉功能障碍。童年期少见发病。母亲患重症肌无力时，经胎盘转移的乙酰胆碱受体抗体，可以引起新生儿的一过性重症肌无力，常迅速好转。还有一种重症肌无力不是免疫介导的，且有家族倾向。

The disease may be purely ocular. In its most severe form, it frequently occurs as part of a major systemic disorder that involves other skeletal muscles, especially in patients who have not received immunosuppressive therapy. Generalization to systemic myasthenia is less common in childhood-onset ocular myasthenia than in the adult-onset form.

See BCSC Section 5, *Neuro-Ophthalmology*, for an in-depth discussion of the diagnosis of myasthenia gravis, along with its ocular and systemic aspects. Additional information is available on the website of the Myasthenia Gravis Foundation of America (www.myasthenia.org).

Clinical features

The principal ocular manifestation of myasthenia gravis is weakening of the EOMs, including the levator muscle. Most cases (90%) exhibit both ptosis and limited ocular rotations (Fig 12-8). The ocular signs can resemble those of any unilateral or bilateral ophthalmoplegia, including internuclear ophthalmoplegia.

Table 12-1 compares the features of TED with those of CPEO and myasthenia gravis.

Ortiz S, Borchert M. Long-term outcomes of pediatric ocular myasthenia gravis. *Ophthalmology.* 2008;115(7):1245–1248.

Table 12-1 Differentiation of Conditions Producing Ptosis and Extraocular Muscle Involvement

	Thyroid Eye Disease	Chronic Progressive External Ophthalmoplegia	Myasthenia Gravis
Age	Rare in children	Any age	Any age
Muscle preferentially involved	Inferior rectus muscles, medial rectus muscles	Levator palpebrae, all ocular motor muscles	Levator palpebrae, any ocular motor muscle
Fatigability	No, unless coexistent with myasthenia gravis	No	Yes
Response to edrophonium	No, unless coexistent with myasthenia gravis	No	Yes
Other eye signs	External eye signs	Pigmentary retinopathy, optic neuropathy	No
Forced ductions	Restriction	Restriction if long-standing	Normal
Clinical course	May resolve or progress	Slowly progresses	Fluctuates; may involve generalized weakness
Eyelids	Retraction	Ptosis	Ptosis
Diplopia	Yes	No	Yes
Other signs and symptoms	Tachycardia, arrhythmia, tremor, weight loss, diarrhea, heat intolerance	Heart block, retinopathy (manifestations of Kearns-Sayre syndrome)	Dysphagia, jaw weakness, limb weakness, dyspnea

这种疾病可以只有眼部表现。严重时，作为全身系统性功能障碍的一部分，常累及其他骨骼肌，特别是在没有接受免疫抑制治疗的患者中。与成人相比，儿童患者发病形式少有系统性重症肌无力的患者，多为眼部肌无力。

BCSC 第 5 册《*神经眼科学*》深入讨论重症肌无力的诊断，以及眼部和系统性改变。更多信息见美国重症肌无力基金会网站（www.myasthenia.org）。

临床表现

重症肌无力的主要表现是眼外肌（EOM）肌力减弱，包括提上睑肌。大多数（90%）表现为上睑下垂和眼球运动受限（图 12-8）。眼部体征呈单眼或双眼的眼肌麻痹，包括核间性眼肌麻痹。

表 12-1 比较了甲状腺眼病（TED）、慢性进行性眼外肌麻痹（CPEO）和重症肌无力的临床特征。

Ortiz S, Borchert M. Long-term outcomes of pediatric ocular myasthenia gravis. *Ophthalmology*. 2008;115(7):1245–1248.

表12-1　累及上睑下垂及眼外肌运动异常疾病的鉴别

	甲状腺眼病	慢性进行性眼外肌麻痹	重症肌无力
年龄	儿童少见	任何年龄	任何年龄
受累肌肉	下直肌，内直肌	提上睑肌， 所有眼球运动肌肉	提上睑肌， 所有眼球运动肌肉
是否易疲劳	否，除非合并重症肌无力	没有	是
是否对腾喜龙有反应	否，除非合并重症肌无力	没有	是
其他眼部体征	外眼体征	视网膜色素 上皮层病变，视神经病变	否
被动牵拉试验	限制	长期可能受限	正常
病程	可缓解或进展	缓慢进展	波动，可伴有全身性无力
眼睑	退缩	上睑下垂	上睑下垂
复视	有	无	有
其他体征和症状	心动过速，心律失常，震颤，体重下降，腹泻，怕热	心脏阻滞，视网膜病变 （Kearns–Sayre综合征）	吞咽困难，咀嚼无力， 四肢无力，呼吸困难

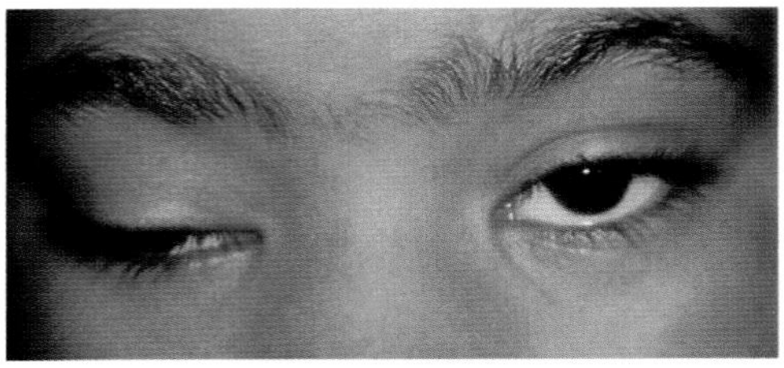

Figure 12-8 Myasthenia gravis. Bilateral ptosis (right more than left) with right hypotropia.

Management

A full discussion of treatment of the various forms of myasthenia gravis is beyond the scope of this chapter. In adults, the ocular manifestations are frequently resistant to the usual systemic myasthenia treatment. However, pediatric ocular myasthenia is often successfully managed with pyridostigmine alone. In adults and children in whom the ocular deviation has stabilized, standard eye muscle surgery can help restore binocular function in at least some gaze positions. Ptosis occasionally requires surgical repair.

Esotropia and Hypotropia Associated With High Myopia

In highly myopic patients, extremely increased axial length can cause the elongated globe to herniate between the superior and lateral rectus muscles. High-resolution MRI studies have shown stretching and dehiscence of the intermuscular septum between these 2 muscles. They have also demonstrated inferior slippage of the lateral rectus pulley and other supporting tissues, along with medial displacement of the superior rectus. These anomalies cause a progressively worsening hypotropia and esotropia. The medial rectus is often tight, exacerbating the severity of the esotropia.

Various surgical procedures have been devised to overcome the defect by stabilizing the position of the lateral rectus muscle. An effective option is a joining of the superior and lateral rectus muscles, usually with a nonabsorbable suture, to reposition the globe. Recession of the medial rectus muscle may also be necessary if the muscle is tight.

Yamaguchi M, Yokoyama T, Shiraki K. Surgical procedure for correcting globe dislocation in highly myopic strabismus. *Am J Ophthalmol.* 2010;149(2):341–346.

Internuclear Ophthalmoplegia

The anatomical and functional features of the *medial longitudinal fasciculus (MLF)* are discussed in BCSC Section 5, *Neuro-Ophthalmology*. The MLF integrates the nuclei of the cranial nerves governing ocular motility and has major connections with the vestibular nuclei. An intact MLF is essential for production of conjugate eye movements. Lesions of the MLF result in a typical pattern of dysconjugate movement called *internuclear ophthalmoplegia (INO)*. Abnormalities of this pathway are frequently seen in patients with demyelinating disease, but they may also occur in patients who have had cerebrovascular accidents or brain tumors.

Clinical features

On horizontal versions, the eye ipsilateral to the MLF lesion adducts slowly and incompletely or not at all, whereas the abducting eye exhibits a characteristic horizontal jerk nystagmus (see Chapter 13). Both eyes adduct normally on convergence. Skew deviation may be present, in addition to exotropia.

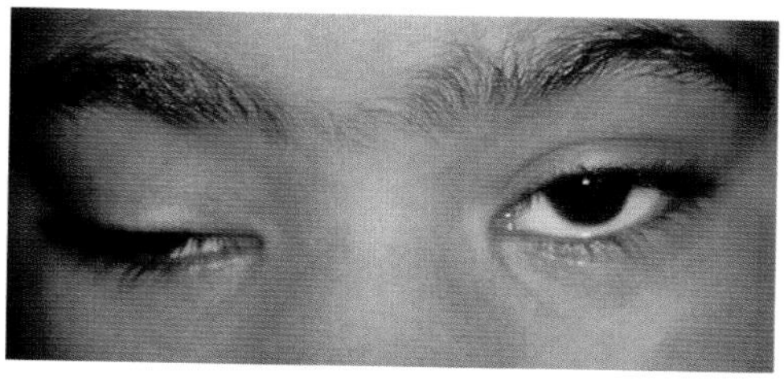

图 12–8　重症肌无力。双眼上睑下垂（右眼较左眼重）伴右眼下斜视。

治疗

关于各种类型重症肌无力的治疗超出本章的讨论范围。成人中，眼部表现常常对全身性肌无力治疗有耐受。而儿童眼部肌无力仅用溴吡斯的明即可奏效。当成人和儿童眼部情况稳定后，眼外肌手术可以重建注视眼位的双眼视功能。上睑下垂有时需手术。

与高度近视相关的内斜视和下斜视

在高度近视患者，极度增长眼轴导致扩大的眼球从上直肌和外直肌之间疝出。高分辨率 MRI 研究显示，这 2 条肌肉间的肌间隔拉伸和断裂。还表现出外直肌滑车和其他支持组织的下移，以及上直肌的内侧移位。这些异常导致下斜视和内斜视进行性加重。内直肌很紧张，加剧了内斜视的严重程度。

多种手术设计用于稳定外直肌的位置、治疗这些缺陷。有效的方式是上直肌和外直肌连接，恢复眼球位置，常用不可吸收缝线。如果内直肌紧张，也可以采用内侧直肌后徙术。

Yamaguchi M, Yokoyama T, Shiraki K. Surgical procedure for correcting globe dislocation in highly myopic strabismus. *Am J Ophthalmol*. 2010;149(2):341–346.

核间性眼肌麻痹

*内侧纵束（MLF）*的解剖学和功能特征见 BCSC 第 5 册《*神经眼科学*》的讨论。内侧纵束（MLF）整合了控制眼球运动的颅神经核，并与前庭核有重要联系。完整的内侧纵束（MLF）是产生眼共轭运动的基础。内侧纵束（MLF）的病变导致典型的共轭运动障碍，称为*核间眼肌麻痹（INO）*。这一通路的异常多见于脱髓鞘疾病，也可能发生在脑血管意外或脑肿瘤的患者。

临床表现

水平同向运动时，内侧纵束（MLF）病变的同侧眼内转缓慢，且不完全或不能内转，而外转时表现出特征性的水平冲动型眼球震颤（见第 13 章）。双眼集合时内转正常。除了有外斜视，还有反向偏斜。

Management

If exotropia persists, medial rectus muscle resection and unilateral or contralateral lateral rectus muscle recession (to limit exotropia in lateral gaze) can help eliminate diplopia, particularly in bilateral cases.

Ocular Motor Apraxia

Ocular motor apraxia, also known as *saccadic initiation failure*, is a rare supranuclear disorder of ocular motility, sometimes including strabismus. The congenital form may be familial, most commonly autosomal dominant.

This condition has been associated with premature birth and developmental delay. Bilateral lesions of the frontoparietal cortex, agenesis of the corpus callosum, hydrocephalus, and Joubert syndrome (abnormal eye movements, developmental delay, microcephaly, hypoplasia of the cerebellar vermis, and retinal dysplasia, among several anomalies) also have been associated with the condition, as have type 3 Gaucher disease and ataxia-telangiectasia. Several case reports have identified mass lesions of the cerebellum that compress the rostral part of the brainstem. Neurodevelopmental evaluation and imaging of the brain are advisable for assessment of children with ocular motor apraxia, especially if there is an associated vertical apraxia. The differential diagnosis of acquired ocular motor apraxia includes conditions that affect the generation of voluntary saccades, including metabolic and degenerative diseases such as Huntington chorea.

Clinical features

In ocular motor apraxia, normal voluntary horizontal saccades cannot be generated. Instead, changes in horizontal fixation are accomplished by a head thrust that overshoots the target, followed by a rotation of the head back in the opposite direction once fixation is established. The initial thrust serves to break fixation; an associated blink serves the same purpose. Vertical saccades and random eye movements are intact, but horizontal vestibular and optokinetic nystagmus are impaired. The head thrust may improve in late childhood. See also BCSC Section 5, *Neuro-Ophthalmology*.

Superior Oblique Myokymia

Superior oblique myokymia is a rare entity whose cause is poorly understood. Some evidence indicates that it is caused by ephaptic transmission between fourth cranial nerve fibers perhaps due, in some cases, to damage by vascular compression.

Clinical features

In superior oblique myokymia, there are abnormal torsional movements of the eye that cause diplopia and monocular oscillopsia. Usually, patients are otherwise neurologically normal. Recurrences may persist indefinitely.

治疗

如果外斜视持续存在，内直肌切除术和单眼或对侧眼外直肌后徙术（限制外侧方注视的外斜视）可以消除复视，特别是累及双眼。

眼球运动失用症

眼球运动失用症，也称为*眼跳起始失败*，是一种罕见的眼球运动性核上病变，有时伴斜视。先天性形式有家族性，最常见的是常染色体显性遗传。

这与早产和发育迟缓有关。前额叶皮质的双侧病变、胼胝体发育不全、脑积水和 Joubert 综合征（异常的眼球运动，发育迟缓，小头畸形，小脑蚓部发育不全和视网膜发育不良等几种异常）还伴随其他病情，如伴有 3 型 Gaucher 病和共济失调 – 毛细血管扩张症。有报告发现，小脑病灶压缩了脑干的腹侧部。神经发育评估和脑成像可用于评估儿童的眼球运动失用症，特别是存在相关的垂直失用症。获得性眼球运动失用症的鉴别诊断包括影响自主扫视产生的条件，包括代谢性和退行性疾病，如 Huntington 舞蹈病。

临床表现

在眼球运动失用症中，不能产生正常的自主水平扫视。通过甩头，即头部超过注视目标，建立水平固视；随后，当固视建立后，将头部回转向相反方向。最初的头部伸出及眨眼是为了打破固视。垂直扫视和随机眼球运动是完整的，但水平前庭性眼球震颤和视动性眼球震颤功能受损。大龄儿童的甩头会改善。见 BCSC 第 5 册《*神经眼科学*》。

上斜肌肌纤维颤搐

上斜肌肌纤维颤搐是一种罕见病变，其原因尚不清楚。一些证据表明是由于血管压迫造成Ⅳ颅神经纤维神经元间传递。

临床表现

上斜肌肌纤维颤搐时，眼球异常旋转运动，导致复视和单眼振动性幻视。通常，患者神经系统正常。复发可能会持续存在。

Management

Treatment is not necessary if the patient is not disturbed by the visual symptoms. Various systemic medications (such as carbamazepine, phenytoin, propranolol, baclofen, gabapentin) and topical timolol have produced inconsistent results but have been advocated as first-line treatment because some patients will benefit, at least in the short term. Effective surgical treatment requires that the superior oblique muscle be disconnected from the globe by generous tenectomy. Because this typically results in a superior oblique palsy, some surgeons perform simultaneous inferior oblique muscle weakening.

Williams PE, Purvin VA, Kawasaki A. Superior oblique myokymia: efficacy of medical treatment. *J AAPOS.* 2007;11(3):254–257.

Strabismus Associated With Other Ocular Surgery

Refractive surgery that produces monovision, facilitating visual clarity at distance and near without optical aids (performed mainly in adults of presbyopic age; see BCSC Section 13, *Refractive Surgery*), can result in dissimilar sensory input to the 2 eyes. The dissimilarity can impair motor fusion, particularly in patients with marginally controlled heterophorias.

Retinal distortion due to an epiretinal membrane or after retinal detachment repair can also distort the retinal image (metamorphopsia, micropsia, or macropsia) to impair motor or sensory fusion. The diplopia rarely improves with surgery for the epiretinal membrane; fogging the eye with a translucent filter or tape (Bangerter; Ryser Optik AG, St Gallen, Switzerland) is the main treatment option.

The *dragged-fovea diplopia syndrome* occurs when an epiretinal membrane displaces the fovea, placing foveal fusion in conflict with peripheral fusion. Prism and alternate cover testing shows a small heterotropia corresponding to the foveal displacement. But under binocular conditions, that prism eliminates the diplopia only briefly, until a fusion movement brings the peripheral retinae back into alignment. Treatment involves fogging the eye, sometimes in combination with a small amount of prism.

Surgery for retinal detachment can lead to restricted rotations and scarring from dissection of the EOMs and the application of devices (such as a scleral buckle) required to bring about reattachment (see BCSC Section 12, *Retina and Vitreous*). Surgical correction of the resultant strabismus is often difficult. Consultation with a retina surgeon is recommended if removal of a scleral buckle is contemplated.

Tube shunts are another potential source of scarring and interference with ocular rotations (see BCSC Section 10, *Glaucoma*). Treatment may require removal, relocation, or substitution of the device, which creates a dilemma if it has been functioning well.

The EOMs can be damaged from retrobulbar injections, either by direct injury to the muscles or from toxicity of the injected material. Because of the usual site of these injections, the vertical rectus muscles are the most vulnerable.

Injection of botulinum toxin into the eyelids can result in diffusion of this substance and a transient paralyzing effect on any of the EOMs.

Laceration or inadvertent excision of an entire section of the medial rectus muscle is one of several serious ocular and orbital complications of pterygium removal or endoscopic sinus surgery. Restoration of function can be an extremely difficult surgical challenge.

治疗

如果患者不受视觉症状的影响，则无须治疗。各种全身性药物（如卡马西平、苯妥英、普萘洛尔、巴氯芬、加巴喷丁）和噻吗洛尔眼液产生的效果不同，但一直视为一线用药，因为一些患者至少在短期内有效。有效的手术治疗是将上斜肌广泛肌腱切除术完全与眼球分离，这会导致上斜肌麻痹，有些医生同时行下斜肌减弱术。

Williams PE, Purvin VA, Kawasaki A. Superior oblique myokymia: efficacy of medical treatment. *J AAPOS.* 2007;11(3):254–257.

与其他眼科手术相关的斜视

屈光手术的单眼视设计，可以提供裸眼清晰的视远及视近（主要在老视患者，见 BCSC 第 13 册《*屈光手术*》），但会导致双眼视觉输入不同。这种差异可能损害运动融合功能，特别是处于隐斜视控制临界状态的患者。

视网膜前膜或视网膜脱离复位术后的视网膜扭曲导致视网膜成像变形（视物变形症、小视症或大视症），影响运动或感觉融合。视网膜前膜手术不能改善复视，主要的治疗方法是通过半透明滤片或贴膜（Bangerter; Ryser Optik AG, St Gallen, Switzerland）产生雾视。

当视网膜前膜使中心凹移位时，中心凹融合与周围融合发生冲突，产生*中心凹牵拉复视综合征*。棱镜和交替遮盖试验与中央凹位移对应的斜视。在双眼条件下，融合运动使周边视网膜回到正眼位前，棱镜可短暂地消除复视。治疗有雾视，有时联合少量的棱镜。

视网膜脱离手术中，切断眼外肌和其他视网膜复位的材料（如巩膜扣带）可能导致旋转受限和瘢痕（见 BCSC 第 12 册《*视网膜与玻璃体*》）。手术很难矫正其产生的斜视。如果考虑取出巩膜扣带，需要咨询视网膜手术医生。

青光眼阀也是潜在瘢痕形成的原因，并影响眼球旋转（见 BCSC 第 10 册《*青光眼*》）。需要移除、重新放置或用新的装置替代，但如果其功能尚好，会难以抉择。

球后注射会损伤眼外肌（EOMs），可能直接损伤肌肉，或有注射物的毒性影响。由于这些部位通常是垂直肌最易受累的部位。

眼睑注射肉毒素可导致药物扩散，对眼外肌（EOMs）产生一过性麻痹。

内直肌撕裂或意外切除是翼状胬肉切除或鼻窦内窥镜手术的严重并发症之一。功能重建极其困难。

Conjunctival scarring and symblepharon can also result in restrictive strabismus after pterygium surgery or other surgery or trauma involving the conjunctiva, particularly in the lateral canthal area. Treatment involves lysis or excision of the fibrotic band. The resulting defect can be managed with conjunctival recession, conjunctival transposition, or an amniotic membrane graft.

Kushner BJ, Kowal L. Diplopia after refractive surgery: occurrence and prevention. *Arch Ophthalmol.* 2003;121(3):315–321.

De Pool ME, Campbell JP, Broome SO, Guyton DL: The dragged-fovea diplopia syndrome. *Ophthalmology.* 2005;112(8):1455–1462.

结膜瘢痕和睑球粘连导致翼状胬肉手术、其他结膜手术或创伤后产生限制性斜视，特别是在外眦部。治疗包括溶解或切除纤维条索。通过结膜后退、结膜转位或羊膜移植弥补缺损区。

Kushner BJ, Kowal L. Diplopia after refractive surgery: occurrence and prevention. *Arch Ophthalmol.* 2003;121(3):315–321.

De Pool ME, Campbell JP, Broome SO, Guyton DL: The dragged-fovea diplopia syndrome. *Ophthalmology.* 2005;112(8):1455–1462.

（翻译 孙西宇 张哲 // 审校 石一宁 丁娟 // 章节审校 石广礼）

CHAPTER 13

Childhood Nystagmuss

This chapter includes related videos, which can be accessed by scanning the QR codes provided in the text or going to www.aao.org/bcscvideo _section06.

Nystagmus is an involuntary, rhythmic oscillation of the eyes. The prevalence of nystagmus in preschool children in the United States is estimated to be 0.35%. Nystagmus can be due to a motor defect that is compatible with relatively good vision, an ocular abnormality that impairs vision or fusion, or a neurologic abnormality. Distinguishing between these causes can be challenging. See BCSC Section 5, *Neuro-Ophthalmology*, for additional discussion of nystagmus.

General Features

The plane of nystagmus can be horizontal, vertical, or torsional, or a combination of these. The condition is often characterized as either *jerk nystagmus*, which has a slow and a fast component, or *pendular nystagmus*, in which the eyes oscillate with equal velocity in each direction. By convention, jerk nystagmus is described by the direction of its fastphase component; for example, a right jerk nystagmus consists of a slow movement to the left, followed by a fast movement (jerk) to the right. Nystagmus is conjugate (as opposed to dysconjugate) when its direction, frequency (number of oscillations per unit of time), and amplitude (magnitude of the eye movement) are the same in both eyes.

Nystagmus characteristics may change with gaze direction. Pendular nystagmus can become jerk nystagmus on side gaze. Jerk nystagmus can have a *null point or null zone* (gaze position in which the intensity [frequency × amplitude] is diminished and the vision improves), or it can decrease in intensity with gaze in the direction opposite that of the fast-phase component (analogous to Alexander's law for vestibular nystagmus). The abnormal head position that patients assume in order to reduce nystagmus can be the most prominent manifestation of their condition.

第 13 章

儿童眼球震颤

本章包括相关视频，可通过扫描文本中提供的 QR 码或访问网站 www.aao.org/bcscvideo_section06

眼球震颤是一种不自主、有节律摆动的眼球运动。美国学龄前儿童眼球震颤的发病率为0.35%。眼球震颤可以是一种运动缺陷伴有相对较好的视力或损害视力或融合功能的眼部异常或是神经异常。很难鉴别这些原因。有关眼球震颤的其他讨论见 BCSC 第 5 册《*神经眼科学*》。

一般特征

眼球震颤的方向可以是水平的、垂直的、旋转的或多种混合。通常表现分为冲动型眼球震颤——具有快相和慢相，以及钟摆型眼球震颤——2 个方向的摆动速度相同。按照惯例，快相方向为冲动型眼球震颤的方向，如右侧冲动型眼球震颤由向左侧的缓慢运动，然后向右侧的快速移动（冲动）。当双眼的眼球震颤的方向、频率（每单位时间的摆动次数）和幅度（眼球运动的幅度）一致时，眼球震颤是共轭的（与共轭失调相反）。

眼球震颤特征可能随注视方向而改变。钟摆型眼球震颤可在侧方注视时转变成冲动型眼球震颤。冲动型眼球震颤可以有*中和点或中和带*（眼球震颤强度 [频率 × 幅度] 消失、且视力提高的注视位置），或在快相相反方向的注视，眼球震颤强度降低（类似于前庭性眼球震颤的 Alexander 定律）。患者为减少眼球震颤而采取的异常头位是其突出的临床表现。

Nomenclature

The National Eye Institute (NEI) has reclassified eye movement abnormalities, including nystagmus. For abnormalities affected by changes in terminology, this chapter uses the terms recommended by the NEI-sponsored Committee for the Classification of Eye Movement Abnormalities and Strabismus (https://www.nei.nih.gov /sites /default /files /nei-pdfs /cemas.pdf), with traditional designations in parentheses.

Types of Childhood Nystagmus

Infantile Nystagmus Syndrome (Congenital Nystagmus)

Congenital motor nystagmus

Congenital motor nystagmus (CMN) is a binocular, conjugate nystagmus with several distinctive features (Table 13-1; Video 13-1). It is often recognized in the first few months of life. CMN is not indicative of central nervous system abnormalities. Patients typically have nearly normal visual function. The nystagmus is uniplanar (ie, the plane of the nystagmus remains the same in all positions of gaze) and is most often horizontal. When CMN has a jerk waveform, it shows an exponential increase in velocity during the slow phase (Fig 13-1). A null point may be present, with right jerk nystagmus to the right of the null point and left jerk to the left of the null point. If the null point is not in primary position, the patient may adopt an abnormal head position to improve vision by placing the eyes near the null point. This head position becomes more pronounced as the child approaches school age. Head bobbing or movement may be present initially but usually decreases with age. Nystagmus amplitude may diminish with age. Oscillopsia is rare.

VIDEO 13-1 Infantile nystagmus syndrome (congenital motor nystagmus).
Courtesy of Agnes M.F. Wong, MD, PhD.
Access all Section 6 videos at www.aao.org /bcscvideo _section06.

CMN worsens with fixation and may worsen with illness or fatigue. Convergence damps (reduces the intensity of) the nystagmus. Thus, near visual acuity is often better than distance acuity. Occasionally, children with CMN overconverge to damp the nystagmus *(nystagmus blockage syndrome)*, resulting in esotropia. Clinicians should take care not to confuse it with cases in which esotropia and nystagmus happen to coexist or cases of infantile strabismus with fusion maldevelopment nystagmus syndrome (latent nystagmus). Patients with nystagmus blockage syndrome characteristically present with an esotropia that "eats up prism" as the strabismic deviation increases upon attempted measurement, and with nystagmus that is least apparent when the deviation is largest.

Approximately two-thirds of CMN patients exhibit a paradoxical inversion of the optokinetic nystagmus (OKN) response, which is unique to CMN. Normally, when a patient with right jerk nystagmus views an optokinetic drum rotating to the patient's left (eliciting a "pursuit left, jerk right" response), the intensity of the right jerk nystagmus increases. However, patients with CMN exhibit a damped right jerk nystagmus or possibly even a left jerk nystagmus when viewing an optokinetic drum rotating to the left.

命名

美国国家眼科研究所（NEI）对眼球运动异常重新进行了分类，包括了眼球震颤。本章使用 NEI 支持的眼球运动异常及斜视委员会建议的命名 (https://www.nei.nih.gov/sites/default/files/nei-pdfs/cemas.pdf)，括号中附传统命名。

儿童眼球震颤的类型

婴儿眼球震颤综合征（先天性眼球震颤）

先天性运动性眼球震颤

*先天性运动性眼球震颤（CMN）*是一种双眼、共轭性眼球震颤，具有多种明显的特征（表 13-1; 视频 13-1），出生几个月即可发现。先天性运动性眼球震颤（CMN）并不表示中枢神经系统异常。患者的视觉功能正常。眼球震颤在同一平面（即不同注视位，眼球震颤平面相同），且是水平的。当先天性运动性眼球震颤（CMN）有冲动时，表示在慢相期呈指数增长（图 13-1）。如果存在中和点，在中和点右侧有一个向右冲动的眼球震颤，并在中和点左侧向左冲动。如果中和点不在第一眼位，则患者采用异常头位，将眼置于中和点附近，以改善视力。到入学年龄时，这个头位更加明显。最初可能存在头部摆动或移动，但随着年龄而减小。眼球震颤的幅度可能会随着年龄的增长而减少。振动性幻视很少见。

视频13-1　婴儿眼球震颤综合征（先天性运动性眼球震颤）。*（译者注：资料来源见前页原文。）*

大家可以通过网站www.aao.org/bcscvideo_section06获得第6册的所有视频。

先天性运动性眼球震颤（CMN）随固视而恶化，并因疾病或疲劳而恶化。集合使眼球震颤减轻（降低振幅）。因此，近视力优于远视力。有时，先天性运动性眼球震颤（CMN）的儿童过度集合，以抑制眼球震颤*（眼球震颤阻滞综合征）*，导致内斜视。临床医生应注意与内斜视合并眼球震颤或融合不良性眼球震颤综合征（隐形眼球震颤）的婴幼儿斜视鉴别。眼球震颤阻滞综合征的内斜视表现为特征性“吃掉棱镜（eats up prism）”现象，测量时斜视度会增加，当斜视度最大时眼球震颤最小。

先天性运动性眼球震颤（CMN）的 2/3 表现出反转的视动性眼球震颤（OKN）反应，这是先天性运动性眼球震颤（CMN）独有的。正常情况下，当右侧冲动性眼球震颤患者注视向左转动的视动鼓（引发一个“追踪左侧，冲动右侧”的反应），右侧冲动性眼球震颤强度增加。而当先天性运动性眼球震颤（CMN）患者注视向左旋转的视动鼓时，右侧冲动性眼球震颤减弱，或是左侧冲动性眼球震颤。

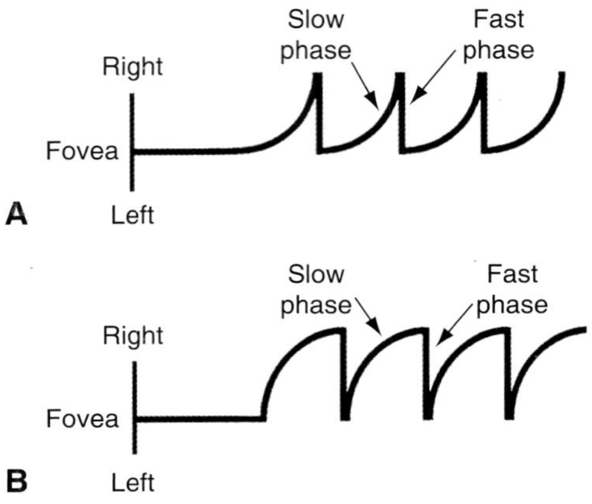

Figure 13-1 Left jerk nystagmus. **A**, Electronystagmographic evaluation of infantile nystagmus syndrome (congenital motor nystagmus) shows an exponential increase in velocity during the slow phase. **B**, An exponential decrease in velocity during the slow phase is the waveform characteristic of fusion maldevelopment nystagmus syndrome (latent nystagmus).

Table 13-1 Features of Congenital Motor Nystagmus

Conjugate
Horizontal
Uniplanar
Worsens with attempted fixation
Improves with convergence
Null point often present with abnormal head position
"Inverted" optokinetic nystagmus response in two-thirds of patients
Oscillopsia usually not present
Severe visual impairment uncommon

X-linked mutations in the FERM domain-containing-7 gene *(FRMD7)* underlie many cases of typical CMN.

Congenital sensory nystagmus

Congenital sensory nystagmus is secondary to an early-onset, bilateral abnormality of the pregeniculate afferent visual pathway. Inadequate retinal image formation interferes with the normal development of the fixation reflex. If the visual deficit is present at birth, the resulting nystagmus becomes apparent in the first 3 months of life. Its severity is somewhat correlated with the degree of vision loss. The waveform of sensory nystagmus can be pendular or jerk and cannot be distinguished from that of CMN.

Searching, slow, or wandering conjugate eye movements may also be observed. Searching nystagmus—defined as a roving or drifting, typically horizontal movement of the eyes without fixation—is usually seen in children whose visual acuity is worse than 20/200. Pendular nystagmus typically occurs in patients with visual acuity better than 20/200 in at least 1 eye. Jerk nystagmus is often associated with visual acuity between 20/60 and 20/100.

Table 13-2 lists some conditions that are associated with congenital sensory nystagmus.The abnormality may be obvious, as with cataracts; subtle, as with optic nerve hypoplasia or foveal hypoplasia; or not visible on examination, as with some retinal dystrophies.

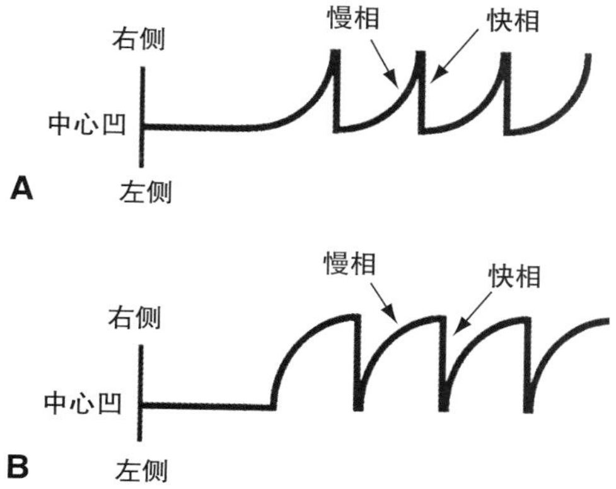

图 13–1　左冲动性眼球震颤。**A.** 眼球震颤电图评估婴儿眼球震颤综合征（先天性运动性眼球震颤）在慢相期呈指数增长。**B.** 在慢相期呈指数下降，这是融合发育不良性眼球震颤（隐性眼球震颤）的特征波形。

表13–1　先天性运动性眼球震颤特征

共轭性
水平性
同一平面的
固视时加重
集合时减轻
中和点伴异常头位
2/3表现为“反转的”视动性眼球震颤反应
震动性幻视：不常见
严重的视力障碍：不常见

含有 FERM 结构域的 –7 基因（*FRMD7*）中的 X 连锁突变是先天性运动性眼球震颤（CMN）不同类型的发病基础。

先天性感觉性眼球震颤

先天性感觉性眼球震颤继发于早发性双侧外侧膝状体前视觉传入通路异常。不良的视网膜成像影响了固视反射的正常发育。出生时存在视觉缺陷，可导致眼球震颤在出生后 3 个月内显现。其严重程度与视力丧失程度相关。感觉性眼球震颤的波形呈钟摆型或冲动型，不易与先天性运动性眼球震颤（CMN）鉴别。

还可观察到搜寻的、缓慢的、漂移的共轭眼运动。搜寻性眼球震颤——定义为漂移不定、没有固视的水平运动——常发生在视力低于 20/200 的儿童。钟摆型眼球震颤常发生在至少一眼视力高于 20/200 的患者。冲动型眼球震颤常发生在视力为 20/60 ~ 20/100 的患者。

表 13–2 列出了伴先天性感觉性眼球震颤的眼病。伴白内障的异常易于发现，视神经或黄斑中心凹发育不良的病灶微小，视网膜营养不良在检查时不易发现。

Central Vestibular Instability Nystagmus (Periodic Alternating Nystagmus)

Central vestibular instability nystagmus (periodic alternating nystagmus) is an unusual form of jerk nystagmus that can be congenital (as a form of CMN) or acquired (especially with Arnold-Chiari malformation). The nystagmus periodically changes direction owing to a shifting null point (Video 13-2). The cycle begins with a typical jerk nystagmus, which slowly damps; this leads to a 10-to 20-second period of no nystagmus, followed by jerk nystagmus in the opposite direction. The cycle repeats every few minutes. Some children adopt an alternating head turn to take advantage of the changing null point.

VIDEO 13-2 Central vestibular instability nystagmus (periodic alternating nystagmus).

Table 13-2 Ocular Conditions Associated With Congenital Sensory Nystagmus

Bilateral anterior segment abnormalities
Congenital cataract
Congenital glaucoma
Iridocorneal dysgenesis
Primary retinal abnormalities
Leber congenital amaurosis
Achromatopsia
Blue-cone monochromatism
Congenital stationary night blindness (X-linked and autosomal recessive)
Bilateral vitreoretinal abnormalities
Sequelae of severe retinopathy of prematurity
Coloboma involving macula
Familial exudative vitreoretinopathy
Norrie disease
Retinal dysplasia
Congenital retinoschisis
Retinoblastoma
Foveal hypoplasia
Albinism
Aniridia
Isolated foveal hypoplasia
Bilateral optic nerve disorders
Optic nerve hypoplasia
Optic nerve coloboma
Optic nerve atrophy
Bilateral congenital infectious chorioretinitis
Congenital toxoplasmosis involving macula
Congenital cytomegalovirus infection
Congenital rubella
Congenital lymphocytic choriomeningitis virus infection
Congenital syphilis
Generalized central nervous system disorder
Aicardi syndrome

中枢前庭不稳定眼球震颤（周期性交替性眼球震颤）

*中枢前庭不稳定性眼球震颤（周期性交替性眼球震颤）*是一种少见的冲动型眼球震颤，可以是先天性（作为先天性运动性眼球震颤 [CMN] 的一种）或获得性（特别是伴 Arnold-Chiari 畸形）。由于中和点移动，眼球震颤周期性地改变方向（视频 13-2）。循环始于冲动型眼球震颤，慢慢地被抑制，10 ~ 20s 没有眼球震颤，之后反方向冲动型眼球震颤。该循环每隔几分钟一次。有些儿童转头找到变换的中和点。

视频13-2　中枢前庭不稳定性眼球震颤（周期性交替性眼球震颤）。

表13-2　与先天性感觉眼球震颤相关的眼部疾病

双眼前节异常
先天性白内障
先天性青光眼
虹膜角膜发育异常
原发性视网膜异常
Leber先天性黑矇
色盲
蓝色锥体全色盲
先天性静止性夜盲症（X连锁及常染色体隐性遗传）
双眼玻璃体视网膜异常
严重的早产儿视网膜病变后遗症
累及黄斑的眼缺损
家族性渗出性玻璃体视网膜病变
Norrie病
视网膜发育不良
先天性视网膜劈裂
视网膜母细胞瘤
中心凹发育不全
白化病
无虹膜症
孤立性中心凹发育不全
双眼视神经病变
视神经发育不全
视神经缺损
视神经萎缩
双眼先天性感染性脉络膜视网膜炎
先天性弓形虫病累及黄斑
先天性巨细胞病毒感染
先天性风疹
先天性淋巴细胞性脉络丛脑膜炎病毒感染
先天性梅毒
广泛中枢神经系统病变
Aicardi综合征

Fusion Maldevelopment Nystagmus Syndrome (Latent Nystagmus)

Fusion maldevelopment nystagmus syndrome (FMNS) (latent nystagmus) is a conjugate, horizontal jerk nystagmus and a marker of fusion maldevelopment, which occurs as a result of infantile-onset strabismus or (less commonly) decreased vision in 1 eye. When either eye is occluded, a conjugate jerk nystagmus develops, with the direction of the fastphase component toward the uncovered eye. Left jerk nystagmus occurs upon covering the right eye, and right jerk nystagmus upon covering the left (Video 13-3). This is the only nystagmus that reverses direction depending on which eye is fixating. The nystagmus damps when the fixating eye is in adduction, so the preferred head turn also reverses direction with change of fixation (Fig 13-2). Amplitude, frequency, and velocity of the nystagmus can also vary depending on which eye is fixating.

VIDEO 13-3 Fusion maldevelopment nystagmus syndrome (latent nystagmus).
Courtesy of Robert W. Hered, MD.

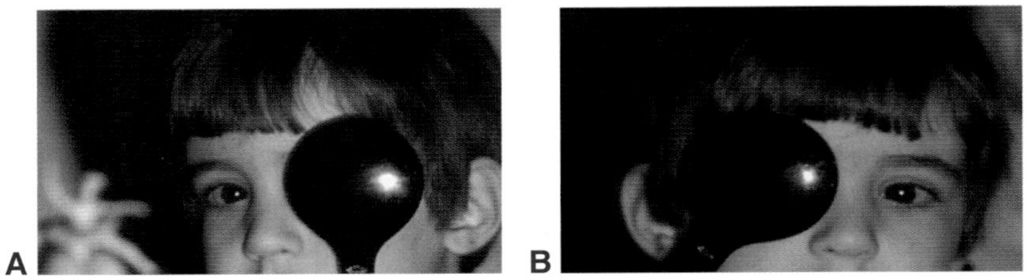

Figure 13-2 Fusion maldevelopment nystagmus syndrome (latent nystagmus). **A,** A right head turn occurs during fixation with the right eye. **B,** The head turn reverses direction during fixation with the left eye. The nystagmus damps with the fixating eye in adduction. *(Courtesy of Edward L. Raab, MD.)*

Fusion or binocular viewing damps FMNS, and disruption of fusion (eg, by occlusion) increases it. FMNS may manifest even when both eyes are open if only 1 eye is being used for viewing (eg, the other eye is suppressed or amblyopic); this is sometimes referred to as *manifest latent nystagmus.* Electronystagmographic evaluation of both fully latent and manifest forms of FMNS shows similar waveforms, with a slow phase of constant or exponentially decreasing velocity (see Fig 13-1B). FMNS is distinct from infantile nystagmus syndrome that has a latent component, worsening when 1 eye is covered. Like other hallmarks of infantile strabismus with which it is associated (dissociated vertical deviation and oblique muscle overaction), FMNS becomes more prominent with age.

Richards M, Wong A, Foeller P, Bradley D, Tychsen L. Duration of binocular decorrelation predicts the severity of latent (fusion maldevelopment) nystagmus in strabismic macaque monkeys. *Invest Ophthalmol Vis Sci.* 2008;49(5):1872–1878.

融合发育不良眼球震颤综合征（隐性眼球震颤）

*融合发育不良性眼球震颤综合征（FMNS）（隐性眼球震颤）*是共轭水平的冲动型眼球震颤，融合发育不良为其特征，是婴儿期一眼发生斜视或（不常见）视力低下的结果。当遮盖一眼时，共轭冲动型眼球震颤发生，快相的方向指向未遮盖眼。遮盖右眼时，发生左侧冲动型眼球震颤，而遮盖左眼时，发生右侧冲动型眼球震颤（视频 13–3）。这是唯一的随注视眼改变方向的眼球震颤。当眼球内转时，眼球震颤被抑制，因此头转动也会随固视改变而反转方向（图 13–2）。眼球震颤的振幅、频率和速度也随注视眼而变化。

视频13–3　融合发育不良性眼球震颤综合征（潜伏性眼球震颤）。
（译者注：资料来源见前页原文。）

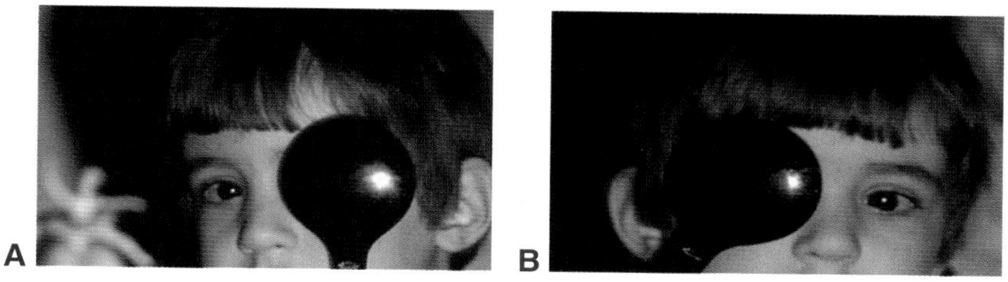

图 13–2　融合发育不良性眼球震颤综合征（潜伏性眼球震颤）。**A.** 右眼注视时，头转向右。**B.** 左眼注视时，头向反向转动。注视眼内转时，眼球震颤被抑制。*（译者注：资料来源见前页原文。）*

融合或双眼视觉抑制融合发育不良性眼球震颤综合征（FMNS），而打破融合（如遮盖）会加重。如果只用一眼观察（如压抑另一眼或另一眼为弱视），即使睁开双眼也出现融合发育不良性眼球震颤综合征（FMNS），这种现象有时称作“*显性 – 隐性眼球震颤*”。完全隐性和显性发育不良性眼球震颤综合征（FMNS）的眼球震颤电图显示相似波形，并伴有一个恒速或呈指数下降的慢相（见图 13–1B）。与婴幼儿眼球震颤综合征不同的是，融合发育不良性眼球震颤综合征（FMNS）呈隐性，遮盖一眼会加重。与婴儿型斜视的其他特征一样（分离垂直偏斜和斜肌功能亢进），融合发育不良性眼球震颤综合征（FMNS）随着年龄的增长而加重。

Richards M, Wong A, Foeller P, Bradley D, Tychsen L. Duration of binocular decorrelation predicts the severity of latent (fusion maldevelopment) nystagmus in strabismic macaque monkeys. *Invest Ophthalmol Vis Sci.* 2008;49(5):1872–1878.

Acquired Nystagmus

Spasmus nutans syndrome

Spasmus nutans syndrome (spasmus nutans) is an idiopathic acquired nystagmus that manifests during the first 2 years of life, presenting as a triad of generally small-amplitude, high-frequency ("shimmering"), dysconjugate nystagmus; head nodding; and torticollis. The nystagmus is binocular but often asymmetric, sometimes appearing to be monocular. The plane of the nystagmus can be horizontal, vertical, or torsional; the nystagmus can vary with gaze position, and it is occasionally intermittent. The head nodding and torticollis appear to be compensatory movements that maximize vision. The natural history of spasmus nutans syndrome is diminution of the abnormal head and eye movements by 3–4 years of age. Spasmus nutans syndrome is a benign disorder in most cases, but there is a high incidence of associated strabismus, amblyopia, and developmental delay.

Spasmus nutans–like nystagmus has been seen with chiasmal or suprachiasmal tumors and retinal dystrophies such as congenital stationary night blindness. Neuroradiologic investigation is warranted when there is any evidence of optic nerve dysfunction (eg, disc pallor, relative afferent pupillary defect) or any sign of neurologic abnormality. Because subtle optic disc pallor and relative afferent pupillary defects can be difficult to assess in children, some investigators prefer neuroimaging for all young children with nystagmus resembling spasmus nutans syndrome.

See-saw nystagmus

See-saw nystagmus is an unusual but dramatic type of dysconjugate nystagmus that has both vertical and torsional components. If the 2 eyes are envisioned as being placed on an imaginary see-saw, one at either end, they "roll down the plank" as one end of the see-saw rises, with the high eye intorting and the low eye extorting. As the direction of the see-saw changes, so does that of the eye movement. Thus, the eyes make alternating movements of elevation and intorsion, followed by depression and extorsion (Video 13-4).

VIDEO 13-4 See-saw nystagmus.
Courtesy of Agnes M.F. Wong, MD, PhD.

This type of nystagmus is often associated with rostral midbrain or suprasellar lesions, most often craniopharyngioma in children. Confrontation visual field testing may elicit a bitemporal defect. Neuroradiologic evaluation is necessary. A congenital form of see-saw nystagmus can be seen in disorders of decussation, such as Joubert syndrome.

Vertical nystagmus

Vertical nystagmus is uncommon. Congenital vertical nystagmus is sometimes seen in infants with inherited retinal dystrophies. Downbeat nystagmus (upward slow phase with downward fast phase) (Video 13-5), which often features a null point in upgaze, may occur as a congenital disorder associated with good vision and normal neurologic findings. More commonly, vertical nystagmus is acquired, secondary to structural abnormalities such as Arnold-Chiari malformations or use of medications such as codeine, lithium, anxiolytics, and anticonvulsants. Neurologic evaluation is usually indicated in patients with unexplained acquired vertical nystagmus.

获得性眼球震颤

点头状痉挛综合征

*点头状痉挛综合征（点头状痉挛）*是一种特发性获得性眼球震颤，在出生后头 2 年出现，表现为三联症：小幅度、高频率（“闪硕的”）、共轭失调性眼球震颤，点头和斜颈。眼球震颤多为双眼的，但不对称，有时为单眼的。眼球震颤平面呈水平的、垂直的或旋转的。眼球震颤随注视位置而变化，偶为间歇性。点头和斜颈是为获得最佳视力的补偿性运动。在 3 ~ 4 岁前，点头状痉挛综合征的头部和眼部异常运动会减少。点头状痉挛综合征多为良性，但斜视、弱视和发育迟缓等并发症的发病率较高。

类点头状痉挛眼球震颤中发现视交叉或视交叉上肿瘤，以及视网膜营养不良症，如先天性静止性夜盲。有视神经功能障碍（如视盘苍白、相对性瞳孔传入缺陷）或神经系统异常症状时，需行神经放射学检查。儿童的轻微视盘苍白和相对性瞳孔传入缺陷较难评估，故对幼儿患有类点头状痉挛综合征的眼球震颤，均行神经影像检测。

跷跷板式眼球震颤

*跷跷板式眼球震颤*是一种少见但特殊的共济失调性眼球震颤，既有垂直性，又有旋转性震颤。如果将双眼放在一个虚拟跷跷板上，两端各置一眼，随着跷跷板 1 端上升，而“从跷板上滚下”，同时高处眼睛内旋，低处眼睛外旋。随着跷跷板方向的改变，眼球运动方向也随之改变。因此，双眼先交替上转和内旋，再交替下转和外旋（视频 13–4）。

视频13–4　跷跷板式眼球震颤。*（译者注：资料来源见前页原文。）*

这种眼球震颤常伴有中脑腹侧部病变或鞍上病变，儿童最常见的是颅咽管瘤。面对面视野检测可查出双颞侧缺损。须行神经放射学检查。先天性跷跷板式眼球震颤可见于 Joubert 综合征等视交叉病变。

垂直性眼球震颤

垂直性眼球震颤并不常见。先天性垂直性眼球震颤偶见于婴儿遗传性视网膜营养不良症。下射性眼球震颤（向上慢相，向下快相）（视频 13–5）为先天性疾病，常表现为向上注视时中和点，其视力较好且神经系统功能正常。常见的垂直性眼球震颤是获得性的，继发于结构异常，如 Arnold–Chiari 畸形或使用药物（可待因、锂、抗焦虑药以及抗痉挛药等）。对于不明原因的后天性垂直性眼球震颤患者，应行神经系统功能评估。

VIDEO 13-5 Downbeat nystagmus.
Courtesy of Janet C. Rucker, MD.

Monocular nystagmus

Monocular nystagmus has been reported to occur in severely amblyopic or blind eyes *(Heimann-Bielschowsky phenomenon)*. The oscillations are pendular, chiefly vertical, slow, variable in amplitude, and irregular in frequency.

Nystagmus-Like Disorders

Induced Convergence-Retraction (Convergence-Retraction Nystagmus)

Induced convergence-retraction (convergence-retraction nystagmus) is not a true nystagmus; rather, the abnormal eye movements are saccades. In children and adults, induced convergence-retraction is part of the dorsal midbrain syndrome, which is associated with paralysis of upward gaze, eyelid retraction, and pupillary light–near dissociation. In children, it commonly occurs secondary to congenital aqueductal stenosis or a pinealoma. The phenomenon is best elicited by having the patient attempt an upgaze saccade (Video13-6) (eg, track a downward-rotating optokinetic drum). Co-contraction of all horizontal extraocular muscles occurs upon attempted upgaze, causing globe *retraction. Convergence* also occurs, because the medial rectus muscles overpower the lateral rectus muscles (voluntary convergence, however, may be impaired).

VIDEO 13-6 Induced convergence-retraction (convergence-retraction nystagmus).

Opsoclonus

Not a true nystagmus, opsoclonus consists of involuntary saccades that are rapid and multidirectional, often accompanied by somatic dyskinesias. Opsoclonus can occur intermittently and often presents as eye movements with very high frequency and large amplitude (Video 13-7). Causes of opsoclonus in children include acute postinfectious cerebellar ataxia, viral encephalitis, and paraneoplastic manifestations of neuroblastoma.

VIDEO 13-7 Opsoclonus.
Courtesy of Agnes M.F. Wong, MD, PhD.

视频13-5　下行性眼球震颤。*（译者注：资料来源见前页原文。）*

单眼球震颤

单眼球震颤发生于重度弱视或失明眼（*Heimann–Bielschowsky 现象，一种分离性眼球震颤*）。眼球震颤为钟摆型，呈垂直性、慢速、振幅变化和不规律的运动。

类眼球震颤疾病

诱导性集合 – 后退（集合 – 后退性眼球震颤）

*诱导性集合 – 后退（集合 – 后退性眼球震颤）*并不是真性眼球震颤，相反，异常眼球运动为扫视运动。在儿童与成人的诱导性集合 – 后退属于背侧中脑综合征的一部分，伴向上注视麻痹、眼睑后退以及瞳孔的光 – 近反射分离。儿童的诱导性集合 – 后退继发于先天性中脑导水管狭窄或松果体瘤。患者向上扫视时（视频 13–6）最容易引发这种现象（如跟踪向下旋转的视动鼓）。向上注视时，所有水平眼外肌同时收缩，引起眼球后退。也发生集合，因为内直肌力量强于外直肌（但已损害自主性集合）。

视频 13–6　诱导性集合–后退（集合–后退性眼球震颤）。

视性眼阵挛

非真性眼球震颤，视性眼阵挛有快速、多方向的不自主扫视，伴有躯体运动障碍。视性眼阵挛可能是间歇性的，常表现为眼球极高频的大幅度运动（视频 13–7）。儿童视性眼阵挛的病因包括急性感染后小脑性共济失调、病毒性脑炎和神经母细胞瘤的副肿瘤性表现。

视频 13–7　视性眼阵挛。*（译者注：资料来源见前页原文。）*

Evaluation

History

Family history may aid diagnosis and provide prognostic information. Although CMN is often sporadic, X-linked recessive, X-linked dominant, autosomal recessive, and autosomal dominant inheritance occur as well. X-linked mutations in *FRMD7* underlie many cases of typical CMN and central vestibular instability nystagmus. Congenital sensory nystagmus can be associated with other inherited ocular conditions (see Table 13-2).

The history should include questions about the pregnancy and birth, because factors such as intrauterine exposure to infection, maternal use of drugs or alcohol, prematurity, and other prenatal or perinatal events can affect development of the visual system and contribute to nystagmus.

For children older than 3 months, parental observations regarding head tilts, head movements, gaze preference, and viewing distances can aid in diagnosis.

Ocular Examination

Visual acuity

The level of visual function can help determine the cause of the nystagmus. Patients with nystagmus and nearly normal visual function usually have CMN, which is a benign entity. Markedly decreased visual acuity usually suggests either retinal or optic nerve abnormalities.

Because monocular occlusion can increase nystagmus intensity, particularly in FMNS (latent nystagmus), monocular acuity should be tested with at least one of the following: a fogging lens (+5.00 diopters [D] greater than the refractive error) or translucent occluder placed over the nontested eye, polarizing lenses with a polarized chart, or an occluder positioned several inches in front of the nontested eye. Binocular visual acuity is often better than monocular acuity and should be measured at distance and near, with any desired head position permitted, to assess the child's true functional vision. Near visual acuity is usually better than distance. Children with a distance acuity below 20/400 can sometimes read as well as the 20/40 to 20/60 level at near.

In preverbal children, the optokinetic drum can be used to estimate visual acuity. If vertical rotation of an optokinetic drum elicits a vertical nystagmus superimposed on the child's underlying nystagmus, the visual acuity is usually 20/400 or better. Preferential looking tests such as Teller Acuity Cards II (described in Chapter 1) can also be used; in patients with horizontal nystagmus, the responses can be more easily assessed with the cards held vertically.

Pupils

Pupil responses are normal in CMN. Sluggish or absent responses to light, or a relative afferent defect in asymmetric cases, indicates a bilateral anterior visual pathway abnormality such as optic nerve or retinal dysfunction. However, normal responses can be seen with some sensory abnormalities such as foveal hypoplasia and achromatopsia. The normal response to darkness is the immediate dilation of the pupil. If, instead of dilating, the pupils paradoxically constrict, optic nerve or retinal disease may be present.

Anterior segment

Examination of the anterior segment may reveal a direct cause of decreased vision (eg, congenital cataracts, corneal opacities) or clues to the cause of decreased vision (such as aniridia, or iris transillumination in albinism, both of which are associated with foveal hypoplasia).

评估

病史

家族病史可辅助诊断，并提供预后信息。虽然先天性运动性眼球震颤（CMN）常常散发，也有 X 连锁隐性遗传、X 连锁显性遗传、常染色体隐性遗传和常染色体显性遗传。*FRMD7* 的 X 染色体突变产生先天性运动性眼球震颤（CMN）和中央前庭不稳定性眼球震颤。先天性感觉性眼球震颤可能与其他遗传性眼部疾病有关（见表 13–2）。

病史应包括询问妊娠与生育情况，因为宫内感染、孕妇吸毒或酗酒、早产及其他产前或围产期异常等因素可影响视觉系统发育，造成眼球震颤。

父母对 3 个月以上儿童的头部倾斜、头部运动、注视偏好和注视距离的观察有助于诊断。

眼部检查

视力

视觉功能水平可有助于确定眼球震颤的原因。患有眼球震颤且视觉功能接近正常多有先天性运动性眼球震颤（CMN），是一种良性病变。视力显著下降通常提示存在视网膜或视神经异常。

由于单眼遮盖可增加眼球震颤强度，特别是在融合发育不良性眼球震颤综合征（FMNS）（潜伏性眼球震颤）中，应使用以下一种方法测试单眼视力：雾视透镜（大于验光屈光度 +5.00D）或半透明遮板遮盖非测试眼；使用偏光镜片及偏光表；或将遮板置于非测试眼前方几厘米处。双眼视力通常好于单眼视力，应测近视力和远视力，头部置于任何位置，以评估该儿童的真实功能性视力。近视力好于远视力。远视力低于 20/400 的儿童，近视力有时可以达到 20/40~20/60。

对于前语言期儿童，可用视动鼓评估视力。视动鼓垂直旋转导致在眼球震颤基础上叠加垂直性眼球震颤，则视力为 20/400 以上。也可用 Teller Acuity Cards II（见第 1 章的介绍）等选择性注视法，通过垂直手持卡片更容易评估水平眼球震颤患者的反应。

瞳孔

先天性运动性眼球震颤（CMN）的瞳孔反应正常。在非对称病例中，光反应迟缓或缺失或相对性传入缺陷提示，存在双侧前视觉通路异常，如视神经或视网膜功能障碍。然而，反应正常时可有感觉异常，如中央凹发育不良和全色盲。对黑暗的正常反应是瞳孔立即放大。如果瞳孔矛盾性收缩而不是放大，则存在视神经或视网膜病变。

眼前节

眼前节检查可发现视力下降的直接原因（如先天性白内障、角膜混浊），或视力下降的原因线索（如无虹膜或白化病虹膜透照，均与中央凹发育不良有关）。

Ocular motility

Nystagmus may be associated with strabismus for a variety of reasons. Early-onset strabismus may cause FMNS (latent nystagmus); convergence may be used to damp nystagmus; or poor vision may be the underlying cause of both nystagmus and strabismus.

Fundus

Optic nerve hypoplasia and foveal hypoplasia are common causes of congenital sensory nystagmus that may be diagnosed on fundus examination. A child with congenital sensory nystagmus from a retinal dystrophy may have vascular attenuation or optic disc pallor but may have a normal fundus; electroretinography may be required for diagnosis in patients with nystagmus and decreased vision but normal-appearing fundi (see Table 13-2, which lists primary retinal abnormalities that cause nystagmus).

Treatment

Prisms

The use of prisms can improve anomalous head positions by shifting perceived object location toward the null point. For a patient with a left head turn and a null point in right gaze, the prism before the right eye should be oriented base-in, and the prism before the left eye oriented base-out. This shifts the retinal images to the patient's left and perceived object location to the right; objects in front of the patient are now imaged on the fovea when the patient is in right gaze, reducing the amount of head turn required to use the null point gaze position.

In patients with binocular fusion, bilateral base-out prisms can improve vision by inducing convergence, which damps nystagmus (amounts are determined by trial and error).

Prisms can be used as the sole treatment of nystagmus or as a trial to predict surgical success. With powers ranging up to 40 prism diopters, Press-On (Fresnel) prisms (3M, St Paul, MN), inexpensive plastic pieces that can be cut and then applied to glasses, can be used for both purposes. **Ground-in prisms** cause less distortion and are preferred for patients who require only small amounts of prism.

Other nonsurgical treatment options for nystagmus are discussed in Chapter 9 of BCSC Section 5, *Neuro-Ophthalmology*.

Surgery

Extraocular muscle surgery for nystagmus may correct a stable anomalous head position by shifting the null point closer to the primary position; this is achieved with medial rectus recession in one eye and lateral rectus recession in the other *(Anderson procedure)* or a recess-resect procedure in both eyes *(Kestenbaum procedure)*. Surgery can similarly alleviate compensatory head positions in adults with acquired nystagmus. Bilateral medial rectus recession can treat esotropia resulting from nystagmus blockage syndrome (using larger-than-normal recessions for the amount of esotropia, sometimes in combination with posterior fixation sutures). Extraocular muscle surgery may also improve vision in nystagmus by increasing foveation time, as reported with recession or tenotomy of all 4 horizontal rectus muscles. See Chapter 14 for further discussion of surgical procedures mentioned in this chapter.

眼球运动

眼球震颤与斜视有关的原因很多。早发性斜视可能引起融合发育不良性眼球震颤综合征（FMNS）（潜伏性眼球震颤）；集合可抑制眼球震颤；或者视力低下引起眼球震颤和斜视。

眼底

视神经发育不全和中央凹发育不良先天性感觉缺陷型眼球震颤的常见原因，眼底检查即可诊断。视网膜营养不良症导致先天性感觉性眼球震颤儿童可能会血管变细、视神经盘苍白，但眼底正常。对于眼球震颤、视力下降、眼底正常的患者需视网膜电图进行诊断（见表 13–2，列出了引起眼球震颤的主要视网膜异常）。

治疗

棱镜

通过棱镜将感知物的位置移向零点位，改善头位异常。对于向左转头并伴有右眼注视零点位的患者，右眼前的棱镜基底向内，左眼前的棱镜基底向外。从而将视网膜图像移动到患者左侧，将感知物体移动到右侧；现在，当患者右眼注视时，患者面前的物体在中央凹上成像，减少了零点位注视所需要的转头量。

对于双眼融合的患者，双侧基底向外棱镜诱导集合、改善视力，抑制眼球震颤（反复测试，确定抑制量）。

棱镜可作为眼球震颤的治疗或预测手术的测试。压贴（Fresnel）棱镜（3M，St Paul，MN）的棱镜度可达 40 △，廉价的塑料镜片剪切后贴于眼镜，可满足以上 2 种用途。磨削棱镜用于棱镜度小的患者可减少畸变。

眼球震颤的其他非手术治疗见 BCSC 第 5 册《*神经眼科学*》第 9 章中讨论。

手术

眼球震颤眼外肌手术，是通过将零点位移近第一眼位，以矫正异常头位。通过一眼内直肌后徙术、另一眼外直肌切除术（*Anderson 手术*），或双眼后徙——切除术（*Kestenbaum 手术*）。同样地，成人的获得性眼球震颤也可通过手术减轻代偿头位。双眼内直肌后徙术可治疗眼球震颤阻滞综合征引起的内斜视（大于内斜视正常后徙量，有时联合后固定缝合术）。眼外肌手术增加中心凹时间，从而改善眼球震颤视力，如 4 个水平直肌的后徙术或腱切断术。本章所述手术的进一步讨论见第 14 章。

In a Kestenbaum or Anderson procedure, the eyes are rotated toward the direction of the head turn and away from the preferred gaze position, moving both eyes in the same direction. For patients with infantile nystagmus syndrome (congenital nystagmus), a left head turn, and null point in right gaze, the eyes are surgically rotated to the left by recessing the right lateral and left medial rectus muscles and resecting the right medial and left lateral rectus muscles. The right-gaze effort, which damps nystagmus, now brings the eyes from this leftward-rotated position to primary position, instead of from primary position into right gaze; in other words, the null point has been shifted toward the primary position (Fig 13-3).

Suggested amounts of recession and resection are listed in Table 13-3. The total amount of surgery for each eye (in millimeters) is equal in order to rotate each globe an equal amount. For head turns of 30°, 40% augmentation is recommended; for turns of 45°, 60% augmentation is used. Augmentation may restrict motility, but this is usually necessary to achieve a satisfactory result.

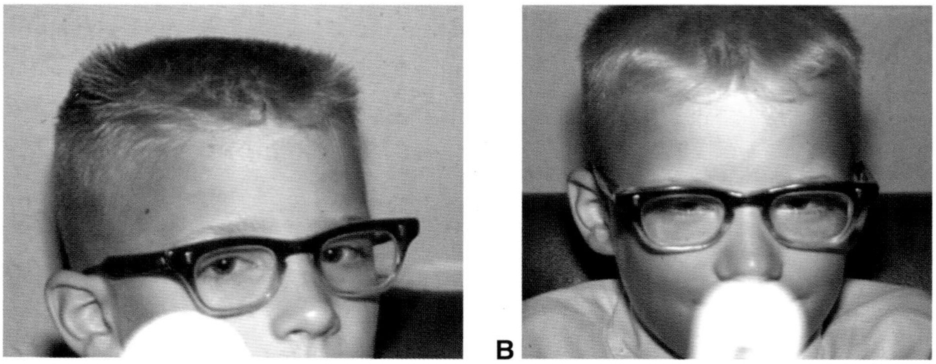

Figure 13-3 **A,** Infantile nystagmus syndrome with the null point in right gaze. **B,** Null point shifted by the Kestenbaum procedure, reducing the head turn. *(Courtesy of Edward L. Raab, MD.)*

Table 13-3 Amount of Recession and Resection for Kestenbaum Procedure, With Modifications[a]

Procedure	Kestenbaum, mm	40% Augmented, mm	60% Augmented, mm
Eye adducted in null point			
Recess medial rectus	5.0	7.0	8.0
Resect lateral rectus	8.0	11.0	12.5
Eye abducted in null point			
Recess lateral rectus	7.0	10.0	11.0
Resect medial rectus	6.0	8.5	9.5

[a] Amounts listed are for the original Kestenbaum procedure plus 2 modifications in which the amount of surgery is increased.

在 Kestenbaum 或 Anderson 手术中，双眼朝着转头方向旋转，并远离选择注视位，双眼朝相同方向移动。婴儿眼球震颤综合征（先天性眼球震颤），伴左转头和右侧注视零点位，通过后徙右眼外直肌和左眼内直肌，并切除右眼内直肌和左眼外直肌，将双眼手术旋转至左侧。将原来抑制眼球震颤的向右注视，转变为眼左转至第一眼位，而不是从第一眼位转为右眼注视。换句话说，将零点位向第一眼位移动（图 13–3）。

后徙术和切除术的量见表 13–3。每眼的手术总量（mm）相等，使双眼的旋转量相等。转头 30° 时，建议增强 40%，转头 45° 时，增强 60%。增强术可能限制运动，但结果满意。

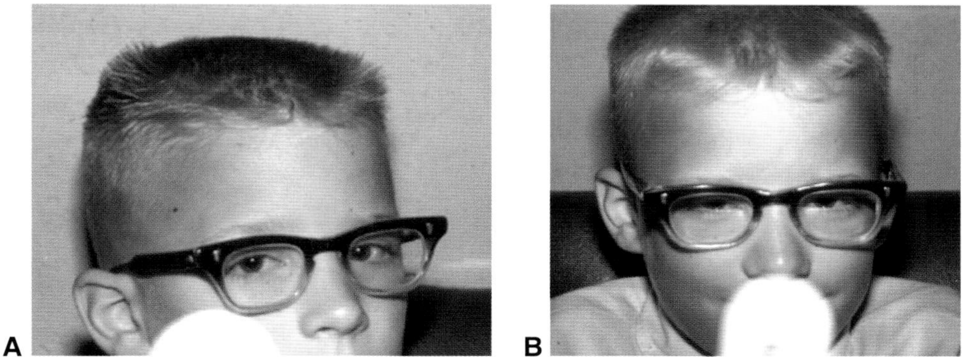

图 13–3　A. 婴儿眼球震颤综合征伴右侧注视零点位。**B.** 经 Kestenbaum 手术转移零点位，减少转头。*（译者注：资料来源见前页原文。）*

表13–3　Kestenbaum改良术的后徙和切除量[a]

手术	Kestenbaum/mm	增强40%/mm	增强60%/mm
眼内转为零点位			
后徙内直肌	5.0	7.0	8.0
切除外直肌	8.0	11.0	12.5
眼外转为零点位			
后徙外直肌	7.0	10.0	11.0
切除内直肌	6.0	8.5	9.5

[a]所列手术量为原Kestenbaum手术量加2项改良的增加手术量。

Similarly, chin-up or chin-down positions may be ameliorated by use of a vertical prism (apex toward the null point) or surgery on vertical rectus or oblique muscles, rotating the eyes away from the preferred gaze position. For a chin-up, eyes-down position, the inferior rectus muscles are recessed and the superior rectus muscles are resected, usually by 8–10 mm in each eye. Alternatively, combined weakening of a vertical rectus muscle and an oblique muscle in each eye can be used. For a chin-up position, the inferior rectus and superior oblique muscles are weakened; for a chin-down position, the superior rectus and inferior oblique muscles are weakened. Improvement of head tilt in nystagmus has been reported with torsional surgery involving the oblique muscles or transposition of the vertical rectus muscles.

For nystagmus patients with strabismus, surgery to shift the null point is performed on the dominant eye; surgery on the nondominant eye is then adjusted to account for the strabismus. For example, a patient who is right-eye dominant with a right head turn and null point in left gaze would undergo right medial rectus recession and right lateral rectus resection, as shown in Table 13-3. This would contribute to reducing the angle of an esodeviation or increasing the angle of an exodeviation. Surgery would then be performed on the nonpreferred eye to correct the residual or resultant deviation.

Other types of nystagmus surgery are less widely practiced. The goal of recession of all 4 horizontal rectus muscles to a position posterior to the equator (8-to 10-mm recessions of medial rectus muscles and 10-to 12-mm recessions of lateral rectus muscles) is to improve vision. Simple 4-muscle tenotomy, which involves disinserting and reattaching the horizontal rectus muscles without recession or resection, has produced similar results, improving recognition time and foveation time on electronystagmography, with modest improvements in visual acuity (approximately 1 line on average).

Hertle RW, Dell'Osso LF, FitzGibbon EJ, Thompson D, Yang D, Mellow SD. Horizontal rectus tenotomy in patients with congenital nystagmus: results in 10 adults. *Ophthalmology*. 2003; 110(11):2097–2105.

同样地，可通过使用垂直棱镜（尖向零点位）或垂直直肌或斜肌手术，改善下颌抬高或下颌内收，双眼旋转、远离选择注视眼位。下颌抬高、双眼向下位时，后徙下直肌、切除上直肌，每只眼 8 ~ 10mm。另外，同时行每只眼垂直肌和斜肌减弱术。下颌抬高时，减弱下直肌和上斜肌；下颌内收时，减弱上直肌和下斜肌。有报告称，斜肌旋转手术或垂直肌转位术可改善眼球震颤的头倾斜。

眼球震颤伴斜视时，主眼行移动零点位手术，然后非主眼行斜视手术。例如，患者右眼为主眼、伴头右转、左侧注视零点位，行右眼内直肌后徙术和右眼外直肌切除术，如表 13–3 所示。这将减少内斜视或增加外斜视度数。然后对非主眼行残余斜视矫正术。

其他眼球震颤手术较少使用。将 4 条水平直肌后徙至眼球赤道后位置（内直肌后徙 8 ~ 10mm，外直肌后徙 10 ~ 12mm）的目标是改善视力。单纯的 4 条肌腱断腱术，包括断腱和重新附着水平直肌，不行后徙术或切除术，得到的结果相似，眼球震颤电图显示改善了识别时间和中心凹时间，视力略有改善（平均提高约视力表的 1 行）。

Hertle RW, Dell'Osso LF, FitzGibbon EJ, Thompson D, Yang D, Mellow SD. Horizontal rectus tenotomy in patients with congenital nystagmus: results in 10 adults. *Ophthalmology*. 2003; 110(11):2097–2105.

（翻译 张哲 许志强 // 审校 石一宁 // 章节审校 石广礼）

CHAPTER 14

Surgery of the Extraocular Muscles

This chapter includes related videos, which can be accessed by scanning the QR codes provided in the text or going to www.aao.org /bcscvideo_section06.

While orthoptic exercises or prism glasses are sufficient for some patients with strabismus, many require surgery in order to correct their alignment. Most often, this is achieved with incisional surgery. Chemodenervation, covered at the end of this chapter, is an alternative for some patients.

Evaluation

The history and a detailed evaluation of ocular motility, as part of a complete ophthalmologic examination, provide the information necessary for the surgeon to plan optimal strabismus surgery. Evaluation, tailored to the type of case, may include sensory binocularity testing, forced duction testing, active force generation, and saccadic velocity measurement. Simulation of the target postoperative alignment with prisms or an amblyoscope may be used to assess the risk of diplopia and the potential for single binocular vision (see Chapter 7 for discussion of these tests). Preoperative discussions should address the expectations of the patient and family, as well as the risks and potential complications of strabismus surgery, especially if surgery on the only eye with good vision is considered.

Indications for Surgery

Surgery of the extraocular muscles (EOMs) is performed to improve visual function, appearance, patient well-being, or any combination of these. It may relieve asthenopia (a sense of ocular fatigue) in patients with heterophorias or intermittent heterotropias, or it may relieve the diplopia that often accompanies adult-onset strabismus. Alignment of the visual axes can establish or restore binocular fusion and stereopsis, especially if the preoperative deviation is intermittent or of recent onset. Correction of esotropia expands the binocular visual field. Some patients require an abnormal head position to relieve diplopia or to improve vision. For these patients, surgical treatment may not only increase the field of binocular vision but also shift it to a more useful, centered location.

Correction of strabismus should be considered reconstructive rather than merely cosmetic, as it has many functional and psychosocial benefits.

第 14 章

眼外肌手术

本章包含相关视频，可扫描文中的二维码或访问网站 www.aao.org/bcscvideo_section06。

虽然正视训练或棱镜已可矫正一部分斜视，但多数患者需通过手术矫正眼位正位。最常用的是手术方式，一些可使用化学去神经疗法，见本章最后部分。

评估

病史和眼球运动的评价作为完整眼科检查的一部分，为医师提供斜视手术所需的必要信息。根据类型进行评价，包括感觉性双眼视觉试验、被动牵拉试验、主动收缩试验以及扫视速度测量。采用棱镜或弱视镜（同视机）模拟术后眼位，以评估复视的风险和单双眼视觉的可能性（关于这些试验的讨论见第 7 章）。术前讨论重点是考虑患者和家属的期望，以及斜视手术的风险和潜在并发症，特别是对唯一视力良好的眼睛进行手术。

手术适应证

通过眼外肌（EOMs）手术改善视觉功能、外貌、患者生活以及所有相关的方方面面。可缓解隐斜视或间歇性隐斜视的视疲劳（眼的疲劳感），或缓解成年斜视伴有的复视。视轴正位可建立或恢复双眼视像融合和立体视觉，特别是术前斜视间歇性的，或近期发生的。内斜视矫正可扩大双眼视野。有些患者需要异常头位缓解复视或改善视力，手术治疗不仅可以提高双眼视野，还可以将其移动到更有用的中心位置。

斜视矫正更应注重功能重建，而不仅仅是美容性的，因为手术可改善患者的视觉功能和心理。

Gunton KB. Impact of strabismus surgery on health-related quality of life in adults. *Curr Opin Ophthalmol.* 2014;25(5):406–410.

Planning Considerations

Vision

When a child has amblyopia, some surgeons prefer to treat the amblyopia before strabismus surgery, whereas others believe that the prognosis for binocular vision is better if surgery is not delayed. If a patient has dense amblyopia or permanent vision loss due to other causes, surgery is usually performed only on the eye with poor vision.

General Considerations

Symmetric surgery

The amount of surgery is based on the size of the preoperative deviation. One commonly used surgical formula for medial rectus muscle recession or lateral rectus muscle resection for esodeviations is given in Table 14-1 (also see the section Rectus Muscle Tightening Procedures, later in this chapter). Surgical options for infants with large-angle esotropia (>60 prism diopters [Δ]) include combined recession-resection of 3 or 4 horizontal rectus muscles or bilateral medial rectus muscle recessions of 7.0 mm. Augmentation of the latter with botulinum toxin has been advocated.

A commonly used surgical formula for exodeviation is provided in Table 14-2. Some surgeons use bilateral lateral rectus muscle recessions of 9.0 mm or greater for deviations larger than 40Δ. Others prefer to limit lateral rectus recession to no more than 8.0 mm and add resection of 1 or both medial rectus muscles for larger-angle exotropias.

Lueder GT, Galli M, Tychsen L, Yildirim C, Pegado V. Long-term results of botulinum toxin–augmented medial rectus recessions for large-angle infantile esotropia. *Am J Ophthalmol.* 2012;153(3):560–563.

Table 14-1 Surgical Amounts for Esodeviation

Angle of Esotropia, Δ	Recession MR OU, mm	or	Resection LR OU, mm
15	3.0		4.0
20	3.5		5.0
25	4.0		6.0
30	4.5		7.0
35	5.0		8.0
40	5.5		9.0
50	6.0		9.0

LR = lateral rectus; MR = medial rectus; OU = both eyes *(oculi uterque).*

Table 14-2 Surgical Amounts for Exodeviation

Angle of Exotropia, Δ	Recession LR OU, mm	or	Resection MR OU, mm
15	4.0		3.0
20	5.0		4.0
25	6.0		5.0
30	7.0		6.0
40	8.0		7.0

LR = lateral rectus; MR = medial rectus; OU = both eyes *(oculi uterque).*

Gunton KB. Impact of strabismus surgery on health-related quality of life in adults. *Curr Opin Ophthalmol.* 2014;25(5):406–410.

手术设计的思考

视力

当儿童有弱视时，一些手术医生主张先治疗弱视，再行斜视手术，另一些认为立即手术对双眼视觉预后更好。如果因其他原因导致患者严重弱视或永久性失明，则通常仅对视力较差的那只眼实施手术。

总体思考

对称外科手术

手术量根据术前斜视度数确定。内斜视通常采用手术公式，行内直肌后徙术或眼外直肌切除术，见表 14–1（也可见本章的“直肌紧缩手术”）。婴儿的大度数内斜视（>60 Δ）的手术方案包括联合后徙——切除 3 或 4 条水平直肌或后徙双眼内直肌 7.0 mm，可用肉毒杆菌毒素辅助加强后者效果。

外斜视的常用手术公式见表 14–2。有些手术医生采用双眼外直肌后徙 9.0 mm 以上，矫正> 40 Δ 斜视。其他手术医生多采用外直肌后徙 8.0 mm，同时内直肌切除 1 或 2 条，矫正大度数外斜视。

Lueder GT, Galli M, Tychsen L, Yildirim C, Pegado V. Long-term results of botulinum toxin–augmented medial rectus recessions for large-angle infantile esotropia. *Am J Ophthalmol.* 2012;153(3):560–563.

表14–1　内斜视手术量

内斜视度/Δ	后徙术 MR OU/mm	或	切除术 LR OU/mm
15	3.0		4.0
20	3.5		5.0
25	4.0		6.0
30	4.5		7.0
35	5.0		8.0
40	5.5		9.0
50	6.0		9.0

LR=外直肌；MR=内直肌；OU=双眼 *(oculi uterque)*。

表14 – 2　外斜视手术量

外斜视度/Δ	后徙术 LR OU/mm	或	切除术 MR OU/mm
15	4.0		3.0
20	5.0		4.0
25	6.0		5.0
30	7.0		6.0
40	8.0		7.0

LR = 外直肌；MR = 内直肌；OU = 双眼 *(oculi uterque)*。

Monocular horizontal rectus recess-resect procedures

The values given in Tables 14-1 and 14-2 may also be used in unilateral recess-resect procedures, with the surgeon selecting the appropriate number of millimeters for each muscle. For example, for an esotropia measuring 30Δ, the surgeon would recess the medial rectus muscle by 4.5 mm and resect the lateral rectus muscle by 7.0 mm. For an exodeviation measuring 15Δ, the surgeon would recess the lateral rectus muscle by 4.0 mm and resect the antagonist medial rectus muscle by 3.0 mm. Unilateral surgery for exotropia beyond the given values (ie, >40Δ) is likely to result in a limited rotation; thus, a 3-or 4-muscle procedure is preferable if there is at least moderately good visionin each eye.

Incomitance

When the size of the deviation varies in different gaze positions, the surgical plan should be designed with a goal of making the postoperative alignment more comitant.

Vertical incomitance of horizontal deviations

The treatment of horizontal deviations that differ in magnitude in upgaze and downgaze—such as *A* or *V patterns*—is discussed in Chapter 10.

Horizontal incomitance

When the size of the esodeviation or exodeviation changes significantly between right and left gaze, paresis, paralysis, or restriction is suggested. In general, restrictions must be relieved for surgery to be effective, and the surgical amounts usually used to correct a misalignment of a given size may not be applicable.

When there is no restriction to account for an incomitant deviation, the deviation is treated as if it were caused by a weak muscle, whether from neurologic, traumatic, or other causes. If the weak muscle exhibits little or no force generation, transposition procedures are usually indicated. Otherwise, treatment consists of some combination of resection of the weak muscle (or advancement if it has been previously recessed) and weakening of its direct antagonist or yoke muscle.

In some cases, both restriction and weakness are present, particularly in long-standing paretic or paralytic strabismus, and a combination of treatment strategies is necessary. Forced duction and active force generation testing are helpful in these cases.

Distance–near incomitance

Treatment of horizontal distance–near incomitance has classically consisted of medial rectus muscle surgery for deviations greater at near and lateral rectus muscle surgery for deviations greater at distance. Evidence suggests that, regardless of which muscles are operated on, the improvement in distance–near incomitance is similar.

Archer SM. The effect of medial versus lateral rectus muscle surgery on distance-near incomitance. *J AAPOS.* 2009;13(1):20–26.

单眼水平直肌后徙 – 切除术式

表 14–1 和 14–2 中列出的数值也可用于单眼后徙——切除术，手术医生确定每条肌肉的量。如内斜视 30 Δ 时，内直肌后徙 4.5 mm、外直肌切除 7.0 mm。外斜视 15 Δ 时，外直肌后徙 4.0 mm、拮抗的内直肌切除 3.0 mm。单眼外斜视手术超过一定量（>40 Δ）时，可导致旋转受限，因此，如果每只眼均有良好视力，应选择在 3 或 4 条肌肉实施手术。

非共同性

当不同的注视位置的斜视度数发生变化时，手术设计应使术后眼位更具共同性。

水平斜视的垂直非共同性

向上注视和向下注视时的水平斜视度数不同的治疗方法——如 *A 型*或 *V 型*——见第 10 章的讨论。

水平非共同性

在右侧和左侧注视时，内斜视或外斜视的度数显著不同，提示存在部分麻痹、麻痹或运动受限。运动受限必须缓解限制因素，手术方可奏效，且不宜采用通常用于矫正一定度数的斜视手术量。

当非共同性斜视不存在限制性因素时，则多由肌力减弱引起，有神经性、创伤性或其他原因。如果牵拉试验肌力很弱或无肌力，提示采用转位术或肌力弱的肌肉切除术（如果之前已行后徙术，则为徙前术），联合其直接拮抗肌或配偶肌的减弱术。

有时限制因素和肌力减弱同时存在，特别是长期部分或完全麻痹性斜视，且需要联合治疗。在这些情况下，被动牵拉和主动收缩试验很有帮助。

远—近非共同性

水平远—近非共同性的治疗方法包括视近斜视度数较大时，实施内直肌手术，以及视远斜视度数较大时，实施外直肌手术。有证据表明，无论对哪条肌肉手术，远—近非共同性的改善都一样。

Archer SM. The effect of medial versus lateral rectus muscle surgery on distance-near incomitance. *J AAPOS.* 2009;13(1):20–26.

Cyclovertical Strabismus

In many patients with cyclovertical strabismus, the deviation differs between right and left gaze and, on the side of the greater deviation, often between upgaze and downgaze as well. In general, surgery should be performed on those muscles whose field of action corresponds to the greatest vertical deviation unless results of forced duction testing reveal contracture that requires a weakening procedure for a restricted muscle. For example, for a patient with a right hypertropia that is greatest down and to the patient's left, the surgeon should consider either tightening the right superior oblique muscle or weakening the left inferior rectus muscle. (Tightening and weakening of the oblique muscles are discussed later in this chapter.) If the right hypertropia is the same in left upgaze, straight left gaze, and left downgaze, then any of the 4 muscles whose greatest vertical action is in left gaze may be chosen for surgery. In this example, the left superior rectus muscle or right superior oblique muscle could be tightened, or the left inferior rectus muscle or right inferior oblique muscle could be weakened. Larger deviations may require surgery on more than 1 muscle.

Prior Surgery

In the surgical treatment of residual or recurrent strabismus after previous surgery, procedures on EOMs that have not undergone prior surgery are technically easier and somewhat more predictable than on those that have. Unfortunately, when previous surgery has resulted in muscle restriction or weakness with limited duction (due to excessive recession or slipped or "lost" muscle), reoperation on the involved muscle is usually necessary. If the restriction is a result of retinal detachment surgery, correction can usually be accomplished without removal of scleral explants. For an eye that has previously undergone glaucoma surgery such as trabeculectomy or implantation of a tube shunt, strabismus surgery should be planned to minimize the risk of disrupting the filtering bleb.

Surgical Techniques for the Extraocular Muscles and Tendons

Step-by-step descriptions of each surgical procedure are beyond the scope of this volume. See the Basic Texts section of this volume for a list of texts describing surgical technique.

Approaches to the Extraocular Muscles

Fornix incision

The fornix incision (Video 14-1) is made in either the superior or, more frequently, the inferior quadrant. The incision is located on bulbar conjunctiva, not actually in the fornix, 1–2 mm to the limbal side of the cul-de-sac, so that bleeding is minimized. The incision is made parallel to the fornix and is approximately 8–10 mm in length.

VIDEO 14-1 Fornix incision.
Access all Section 6 videos at www.aao.org /bcscvideo_section06.

旋转垂直斜视

许多旋转垂直斜视，右侧注视和左侧注视时的偏斜不同，且偏斜较大的一侧，向上和向下注视时的偏斜也不同。一般对最大垂直斜视的作用肌肉进行手术，除非被动牵拉试验提示有肌肉挛缩，需对受限肌肉行减弱术。如右眼上斜视的患者，向下和向左斜视度最大，应考虑行右上斜肌紧缩术或左下直肌减弱术。（本章将讨论斜肌的紧缩术和减弱术。）如果右眼上斜视时，在左上注视、左侧注视以及左下注视时相同，则可选择左侧注视时最大垂直作用所累及的 4 条肌肉中的任意 1 条肌肉进行手术，其中，可行左上直肌或右上斜肌紧缩术、左下直肌或右下斜肌减弱术。较大度数斜视需要对 1 条以上肌肉实行手术。

既往手术

对既往手术后的残余或复发性斜视进行手术时，应对未手术的眼外肌（EOM）进行手术，且比已手术的眼外肌（EOM）有较好的预测性。但是，当既往手术导致肌肉受限或肌力减弱、伴转动受限（由于过度后徙、肌肉滑脱或“丢失”）时，需再次对相关肌肉手术。如果肌肉受限是视网膜脱离手术所致，可以不取出巩膜植入物进行矫正。曾行青光眼手术，如小梁切除术或引流管植入术，斜视手术尽量少影响滤泡。

眼外肌和肌腱的手术

分步描述每个手术的分解操作步骤超出本章的范围。有关手术技巧的描述见本章列表的具体内容。

眼外肌的方法

穹窿切口

穹窿切口（视频 14–1）可在上象限进行，但更常在下象限进行。实际上切口不在穹窿，位于球结膜，距角膜缘 1 ~ 2 mm 的结膜囊，这样可尽量减少出血。切口与穹窿平行，长度为 8 ~ 10 mm。

视频 14–1　穹窿切口。

大家可以通过网站www.aao.org/bcscvideo_section06获得第6册的所有视频。

Bare sclera is exposed by incising the Tenon capsule deep to the conjunctival incision. Using this exposed bare sclera, the surgeon engages the muscle with a succession of muscle hooks. The conjunctival incision is pulled over the hook that has passed under the muscle. All 4 rectus muscles and both oblique muscles can be explored, if necessary, through inferotemporal and superonasal conjunctival incisions.

When properly placed, the 2-plane incision can be self-closing at the end of the operation by gentle massage of the tissues into the fornix, with the edges of the incision splinted by the overlying eyelid. Some surgeons prefer to close the incision with conjunctival sutures.

Limbal incision

The fused layer of conjunctiva and Tenon capsule is cleanly severed from the limbus. Some surgeons make the limbal incision (*peritomy)* 1–2 mm posterior to the limbus to spare limbal stem cells (Video 14-2). A short radial incision is made at each end of the peritomy so that the flap of conjunctiva and Tenon capsule can be retracted to expose the muscle for surgery. At the completion of the operation, the flap is reattached, without tension, close to its original position with a single suture at each corner. If the conjunctiva is restricted from prior surgery or shortened by a long-standing deviation, closure should involve recession of the anterior edge.

VIDEO 14-2 Limbal incision.

Rectus Muscle Weakening Procedures

Table 14-3 defines various rectus muscle weakening procedures and describes when each is used. The most common is simple recession (Video 14-3), for which typical amounts of surgery for esotropia and exotropia are given in Tables 14-1 and 14-2, respectively. Because the conventional technique for rectus muscle recession involves passing sutures within thin sclera with the attendant risk of perforation, some surgeons prefer *a hangback recession*, in which the recessed tendon is suspended by sutures that pass through the thicker stump of the original insertion. Although it is not known where the tendon reattaches to the sclera, empirical experience indicates that this method is usually reliable.

VIDEO 14-3 Recession of extraocular rectus muscle.
Courtesy of Scott A. Larson, MD, Ronald Price, MD, and George Beauchamp, MD.

Rectus Muscle Tightening Procedures

Although also referred to as strengthening procedures, muscle tightening procedures (defined in Table 14-4) do not actually give the muscles more strength. Rather, they produce a tightening effect that tends to offset the opposite action of the antagonist muscle. For this purpose, surgeons usually use the *resection* technique (Video 14-4); typical amounts of surgery for esotropia and exotropia are given in Tables 14-1 and 14-2, respectively. *Plication* of the muscle can be used as an alternative to produce a similar effect. A previously recessed rectus muscle can also be tightened by advancing its insertion toward the limbus.

向结膜切口深处切开 Tenon 囊，暴露巩膜。通过暴露的巩膜，医生用一连串肌肉拉钩找到肌肉。将肌肉下方的肌钩拉出结膜切口。通过颞下和鼻上结膜切口可以找到 4 条直肌和 2 条斜肌。

当切口位置得当时，手术结束时，轻轻按摩组织退回穹窿，切口的 2 个平面自动闭合，切口的边缘可被覆盖的眼睑夹合。有的手术医生用结膜缝线缝合切口。

角膜缘切口

将结膜和 Tenon 囊的融合层从角膜缘切开。一些手术医生在角膜缘后 1 ~ 2mm 行角膜缘切口（*球结膜环形切开术*），避开角膜缘干细胞（视频 14–2）。在球结膜环形切开的开口处做一个短的放射状切开，以便结膜瓣和 Tenon 囊回退，暴露肌肉。手术完成后，在没有张力的情况下，瓣在接近原位置复位，每个角缝合 1 针。如果因既往手术或长期偏斜，使结膜受限或缩短，则缝合时应将结膜前缘后徙。

视频 14–2　角膜缘切口。

直肌减弱术

表 14–3 定义了各种直肌减弱术，及每种方法的适应证。最常见的是单纯后徙术（视频 14–3），内斜视和外斜视的手术量分别见表 14–1 和 14–2。因为直肌后徙术的常规技术需在薄巩膜内穿过缝线，并伴有穿孔的风险，一些手术医生选用*悬吊后徙术*，即将后徙的肌腱缝合在肌肉原附着点较厚的残端。尽管不清楚肌腱重新附着巩膜的位置，但经验表明这种方法是可靠的。

视频 14-3　眼外直肌后徙术。*（译者注：资料来源见前页原文。）*

直肌紧缩术

虽然肌肉紧缩术（定义见表 14–4）也称为加强术，但实际上并未增加肌力，相反，它们产生了紧缩效果，可抵消拮抗肌的相反作用。为此，常用*切除术*（视频 14–4），内斜视和外斜视的手术量分别见表 14–1 和 14–2。肌肉*折叠术*是产生类似效果的替代术式。已行后徙术的直肌，也可将其附着点前移向角膜缘，实现紧缩。

Table 14-3 Weakening Procedures Used in Strabismus Surgery

Procedure	Indications
Myotomy: cutting across a muscle *Myectomy:* removal of a portion of muscle	Used by some surgeons to weaken the inferior oblique muscles
Marginal myotomy: cutting partway across a muscle, usually following a maximal recession	Used to weaken a rectus muscle further
Tenotomy: cutting across a tendon *Tenectomy:* removal of a portion of tendon	Both used routinely to weaken the superior oblique muscle; some surgeons interpose silicone spacers to control the weakening effect
Recession: removal and reattachment of a muscle (rectus or oblique) so that its insertion is closer to its origin	The standard weakening procedure for rectus muscles
Denervation and extirpation: ablation of the entire portion of the muscle, along with its nerve supply, within the Tenon capsule	Used only on severely or recurrently overacting inferior oblique muscles
Recession and anteriorization: movement of the muscle's insertion anterior to its original position	Used primarily on the inferior oblique muscle to reduce its elevating action; particularly useful with coexisting inferior oblique overaction and DVD
Posterior fixation suture (fadenoperation): attachment of a rectus muscle to the sclera 11–18 mm posterior to the insertion using a nonabsorbable suture; fixation to the muscle's pulley may be an alternative for medial rectus muscles	Used to weaken a muscle by decreasing its mechanical advantage; often used in conjunction with recession; sometimes used in high AC/A ratio accommodative esotropia and in incomitant strabismus

AC/A = accommodative convergence/accommodation; DVD = dissociated vertical deviation.

Table 14-4 Tightening Procedures Used in Strabismus Surgery

Procedure	Indication
Resection: removal of a segment of muscle followed by reattachment to the original insertion	The standard tightening procedure for rectus muscles
Advancement: movement of a previously recessed muscle toward its insertion	Used to correct a consecutive deviation
Tuck: folding and securing, reducing tendon length	Used on the superior oblique tendon
Plication: folding and securing to the sclera	Used on rectus muscles to impart a similar effect as resection

VIDEO 14-4 Resection of extraocular rectus muscle.

Courtesy of Scott A. Larson, MD, and Johanna Beebe, MD.

Rectus Muscle Surgery for Hypotropia and Hypertropia

For reasonably comitant vertical deviations, recession and resection of vertical rectus muscles are appropriate. Recessions are generally preferred as a first procedure. Approximately 3Δ of correction in primary position can be expected for every millimeter of vertical rectus muscle recession. For comitant vertical deviations less than 10Δ that accompany horizontal deviations, displacement of the reinsertions of the horizontal rectus muscles in the same direction, by approximately one-half the tendon width (up for hypotropia, down for hypertropia), performed during a recess-resect procedure, is often sufficient.

表14–3　斜视手术中的减弱术

手术	适应证
肌切开术：横截面切开肌肉 *肌切除术*：　切除一部分肌肉	一些手术医生用于下斜肌减弱
边缘肌切开术：中间部分横截面切开肌肉，常在最大限度的后徙术后	用于进一步减弱直肌
肌腱切断术：横截面切开肌腱 *肌腱切除术*：切除一部分肌腱	常规二者都用于上斜肌减弱；一些手术医生植入硅胶片，控制减弱效果
后徙术：切除并再附着肌肉（直肌或斜肌），使其附着位置更接近原始位置	直肌的标准减弱术
去神经和灭火术：在Tenon囊内消除整条肌肉及其神经供应	仅用于严重或复发性下斜肌功能亢进
后徙和前移术：　将肌肉附着点向前移至其原始位置	主要用于下斜肌的上转作用减弱；特别用于下斜肌亢进合并DVD
后固定缝线术（Faden术）：用不可吸收缝合线，将直肌固定于距原始附着点后11～18 mm处巩膜上；固定肌肉滑车上可替代内直肌	通过降低肌肉的机械力矩，来减弱肌力；经常与后徙术同用；有时用于高AC/A的调节性内斜视和非共同性斜视

AC/A = 调节性集合/调节；DVD = 分离性垂直偏斜。

表14–4　斜视手术中的紧缩术

手术	适应证
切除术：切除一段肌肉，然后将其复位到原始附着部位	直肌的标准紧缩术
前徙术：　将之前后徙的肌肉移至其原始附着部位	用于矫正连续性偏斜
卷折术：　折叠并固定、缩短肌腱长度	用于上斜肌腱
折叠术：　折叠并固定到巩膜	用于直肌，产生与切除相似的效果

视频 14-4　眼外直肌切除术。*（译者注：资料来源见前页原文。）*

下斜视和上斜视的直肌手术

有的共同性垂直斜视，适用于垂直直肌的后徙术和切除术。后徙术常为首选手术。垂直直肌后徙 1mm，可矫正第一眼位 3Δ。共同性垂直偏斜< 10Δ、伴水平偏斜时，在后徙——切除术同时，进行相同方向水平直肌移位即可，移位约 1/2 肌腱宽度（下斜视向上移位，上斜视向下移位）。

Adjustable Sutures

Some surgeons use adjustable sutures (Video 14-5) to avoid an immediately obvious poor result or to increase the likelihood of success with 1 operation, but this modification does not ensure long-term satisfactory alignment. The surgeon completes the operation using externalized sutures and slip knots that enable the position of the surgical muscle to be altered during the early postoperative period. This technique can be used in children; however, general anesthesia is usually required.

Another alternative, used mainly in adults, is performance of surgery with the patient awake. Anesthetic agents that might affect ocular motility are avoided, and the patient's dynamic ocular motility and ocular alignment are observed and adjusted at the time of surgery. This technique can be difficult in patients with significant scarring, individuals with thyroid eye disease, and children.

VIDEO 14-5 Adjustable sutures for extraocular rectus muscles.
Courtesy of Scott A. Larson, MD.

Oblique Muscle Weakening Procedures

Weakening the inferior oblique muscle

Table 14-3 lists muscle weakening procedures, including those involving the inferior oblique muscle. These procedures are most commonly used for treatment of overelevation in adduction when it is believed to be due to inferior oblique muscle overaction. In all these procedures, the surgeon must be sure that the entire inferior oblique muscle is weakened, because the distal portion and the insertion can be anomalously duplicated (Videos 14-6, 14-7).

VIDEO 14-6 Strabismus surgery: inferior oblique—partial and complete hooking.
Courtesy of John D. Ferris, FRCOphth, and Peter E. J. Davies, FRANZCO, MPH.

VIDEO 14-7 Inferior oblique weakening procedures.

In cases that show marked asymmetry of the overactions of the inferior oblique muscles and no superior oblique muscle paralysis, unilateral surgery only on the muscle with the more prominent overaction is often followed by a significant degree of overaction in the fellow eye. Therefore, some surgeons recommend bilateral inferior oblique muscle weakening for asymmetric cases. A symmetric result is the rule and overcorrections are rare; however, inferior oblique muscles that are not overacting at all—even when there is overaction in the fellow eye—should not be weakened.

Secondary overaction of the inferior oblique muscle occurs in many patients who have superior oblique muscle paralysis. A weakening of that inferior oblique muscle typically corrects up to 15Δ of vertical deviation in primary position. The amount of vertical correction is roughly proportional to the degree of preoperative overaction (see Chapter11). Frequently, a weakening procedure is performed on each inferior oblique muscle for V-pattern strabismus (see Chapter 10).

可调节缝线

一些手术医生使用可调节缝合线（视频 14–5），以避免手术后即刻出现的明显不理想结果，或增加 1 次性手术成功的可能性，但这种改良并不能确保满意的长期眼正位。在术后早期，手术医生使用外预留的缝线和滑结调整肌肉位置完成手术。这种技术可用于儿童，常需全身麻醉。

另一种替代方案是在患者清醒的情况下进行手术，主要用于成人。避免使用麻醉剂对眼球运动的影响，即在手术时观察患者的动态眼球运动和眼正位，并进行调整。这种技术在有明显疤痕、甲状腺眼病和儿童患者身上有一定难度。

视频 14–5　用于眼外直肌的可调节缝合线。*（译者注：资料来源见前页原文。）*

斜肌减弱术

下斜肌减弱术

表 14–3 列出了肌肉减弱术，包括涉及下斜肌的肌肉减弱术。当考虑内转过度上转是由下斜肌功能亢进所致时，最常用此手术。医生需确定整条下斜肌肌力减弱，因为肌肉远端和附着点可能发生异常重叠（视频 14–6、14–7）。

视频 14–6　斜视手术：下斜肌——部分和完整钩住。
（译者注：资料来源见前页原文。）

视频 14–7　下斜肌减弱术。

当下斜肌功能亢进呈现明显非共同性且无上斜肌麻痹时，若仅针对功能亢进较明显的肌肉行单眼手术，常伴随呈现对侧眼的显著功能亢进。因此，一些外科医生建议不对称性病例应行双眼下斜肌减弱术。对称是手术的最终目的，很少见过度矫正，即使对侧眼出现功能亢进，下斜肌完全没有功能亢进，就不应行减弱术。

继发性下斜肌功能亢进多患有上斜肌麻痹。下斜肌减弱术在第一眼位最多矫正垂直偏斜 15Δ。垂直矫正量与术前功能亢进的程度成正比（见第 11 章）。V 型斜视常行 2 条下斜肌减弱术（见第 10 章）。

Moving the insertion of the inferior oblique muscle anteriorly to a point adjacent to the lateral border of the inferior rectus muscle *(inferior oblique anterior transposition, inferior oblique anteriorization)* weakens the normal actions of the inferior oblique. Because the neurofibrovascular bundle along the lateral border of the inferior rectus muscle can then serve as the effective origin for the distal portion of the muscle, anteriorization also allows the inferior oblique muscle to actively oppose elevation of the eye; that is, this muscle becomes an anti-elevator (see Chapter 3). This procedure is effective for treatment of dissociated vertical deviation (DVD) and is especially useful when DVD and inferior oblique overaction coexist.

Weakening the superior oblique muscle

Procedures to weaken the superior oblique muscle include tenotomy (Video 14-8); tenectomy; split-tendon lengthening; placement of a spacer of silicone, fascia lata, or nonabsorbable suture between the cut edges of the tendon to functionally lengthen it; and recession. The purpose of spacers is to prevent an excessive gap between the cut edges, but they have the disadvantage of possible adhesion formation, which can alter motility. Unilateral weakening of a superior oblique muscle is not commonly performed except as treatment for Brown syndrome (see Chapter 12) or for isolated inferior oblique muscle weakness, which is rare. Unilateral superior oblique muscle weakening can affect not only vertical alignment but also torsion, potentially creating undesired extorsion. Many ophthalmologists favor a tenotomy of only the posterior 75%–80% of the tendon to preserve the torsional action, which is controlled by the most anterior tendon fibers.

VIDEO 14-8 Superior oblique muscle tenotomy.

Bilateral weakening of the superior oblique muscle can be performed for A-pattern deviations and can be expected to cause an eso-shift in downgaze and almost no change in upgaze. If this procedure is performed on patients with normal binocularity, it may cause vertical or torsional strabismus with subsequent diplopia, which must be considered and discussed with the patient preoperatively.

Oblique Muscle Tightening Procedures

Tightening the inferior oblique muscle

Inferior oblique muscle tightening is seldom performed. To be effective, advancement of the inferior oblique muscle requires reinsertion more posteriorly and superiorly, which is technically difficult and exposes the macula to possible injury.

Tightening the superior oblique muscle

Tightening the superior oblique tendon is discussed in Chapter 11. Tucking the superior oblique tendon enhances both its vertical and torsional effects (Video 14-9). The anterior half of the superior oblique tendon alone may be advanced temporally and somewhat anteriorly, in the *Fells modification of the Harada-Ito procedure*, to reduce extorsion in patients with superior oblique muscle paralysis (Video 14-10).

将下斜肌附着点前移至下直肌外缘（*下斜肌前转位术，下斜肌前部化*）可减弱下斜肌的正常功能。因为沿下直肌外侧的神经纤维血管束可以作为肌肉远端部分的有效供给，前部化使下斜肌主动对抗上转，即前部化肌肉成为对抗上转的肌肉（见第 3 章）。此术式可有效治疗分离性垂直斜视（DVD），当离性垂直斜视（DVD）和下斜肌功能亢进同时存在时，特别有用。

上斜肌减弱

上斜肌减弱手术包括肌腱切断术（视频 14–8），肌腱切除术，分裂肌腱延长，在肌腱的切口边缘置放硅胶植入条、阔筋膜或不可吸收缝合线等，达到功能性延长和后徙。隔离条的目的是防止切口边缘的间隙过大，但缺点是可能形成粘连，改变眼球的运动。除了用于治疗 Brown 综合征（见第 12 章）或罕见的孤立性下斜肌肌力减弱外，单眼上斜肌减弱术并不常采用。单眼上斜肌减弱术不仅影响垂直眼位，还影响旋转，产生外旋。许多眼科医生只切除肌腱后部的 75% ~ 80%，以保持旋转功能，因它旋转功能由前部肌腱纤维控制。

视频 14–8　上斜肌肌腱切断术。

双眼上斜肌减弱术可用于 A 型斜视，并会导致向下注视的内偏移，而向上注视无变化。如果患者双眼视觉正常，则术后的垂直性或旋转性斜视会产生复视，术前需考虑到这一点，并与患者讨论。

斜肌紧缩术

下斜肌紧缩术

下斜肌退缩术很少实施。为了达到手术效果，下斜肌的附着点需进一步向后和向上重新固定，技术上有一定难度，且暴露黄斑可能会产生损伤。

上斜肌收缩

第 11 章讨论了上斜肌肌腱紧缩。卷折上斜肌腱可以增强其垂直和旋转功能（视频 14–9）。*Fells 改良的 Harada–Ito 术*仅将上斜肌肌腱的前半部分向颞侧偏前移位，以减少上斜肌麻痹的外旋（视频 14–10）。

VIDEO 14-9 Superior oblique tucking.

VIDEO 14-10 Strabismus surgery: Fells modification of the Harada-Ito procedure.
Courtesy of John D. Ferris, FRCOphth, and Peter E. J. Davies, FRANZCO, MPH.

Stay Sutures

A stay (pull-over) suture is a temporary suture that is attached to the sclera at the limbus or under a rectus muscle insertion, brought out through the eyelids, and secured to periocular skin over a bolster to fix the eye in a selected position during postoperative healing. Some surgeons believe that this technique is particularly useful in cases with severely restricted ocular rotations. Its disadvantages are that patients experience some discomfort and that the limbal attachment of the stay suture tends to be lost before the desired interval of 10–14 days after placement.

Transposition Procedures

Transposition procedures involve redirection of the paths of the EOMs. In the treatment of sixth nerve palsy, Duane retraction syndrome, and monocular elevation deficiency, these procedures utilize 1 or both muscles adjacent to the abnormal muscle to provide a tonic force vector (Video 14-11). The effect of the transposition can be augmented by resecting the transposed muscles or by using offset posterior fixation sutures (*Foster modification*). Vertical deviations are a possible complication of vertical rectus muscle transposition surgery. Transposition of only the superior rectus muscle, combined with recession of the medial rectus muscle, can also be effective.

VIDEO 14-11 Strabismus surgery: lateral rectus and medial rectus inferior full-tendon transfers.
Courtesy of John D. Ferris, FRCOphth, and Peter E. J. Davies, FRANZCO, MPH.

Posterior Fixation

Posterior fixation is a procedure in which a rectus muscle is sutured to the sclera far posterior to its insertion. The result is weakening of the muscle in its field of action with little or no effect on the alignment in primary position. This procedure is particularly useful for treatment of incomitant strabismus. A similar effect may be achieved, at least for medial rectus muscles, by fixation to the muscle pulley.

视频 14-9　上斜肌卷折术。

视频 14-10　斜视手术：Fells改良的Harada–Ito术。*（译者注：资料来源见前页原文。）*

留置缝线

留置（牵拉）缝线是一种临时缝线，其附着在角膜缘或直肌附着点下的巩膜上，穿过眼睑引出，并用衬垫固定在眼周皮肤上，以便在术后愈合期间将眼球固定在指定眼位。一些手术医生认为，这对眼球旋转严重受限的病例特别有用，缺点是患者会感到不适，并且在留置所需的时间（即 10 ~ 14d）内，留置缝线的角膜缘附着点常会丢失。

转位术

转位术累及眼外肌（EOM）径行的重新定向。在Ⅵ颅神经麻痹、Duane 后退综合征和单眼上转不足的治疗中，手术利用与异常肌肉相邻的 1 或 2 条肌肉形成张力矢状力（视频 14-11）。转位肌肉的切除或抵消后固定缝合术（*Foster 改良术*），可以增强转位术效果。垂直斜视是垂直直肌转位手术的并发症。单纯上直肌转位术联合内直肌后徙术也是有效的。

视频 14–11　斜视手术：外直肌和内直肌下方全肌腱转位术。
（译者注：资料来源见前页原文。）

后固定术

后固定术是一种将直肌缝合到其附着点后的巩膜上的手术。手术结果是在其作用区域中的肌力减弱，对第一眼位几乎没有影响。特别适用于治疗非共同性斜视。至少固定内直肌滑车可产生类似效果。

Complications of Strabismus Surgery

Diplopia

Diplopia can occur after strabismus surgery, occasionally in older children but more often in adults. Surgery can move the fixated image out of a suppression scotoma. In the several months following surgery, various responses are possible:

- Fusion of the 2 images may occur.
- A new suppression scotoma may form, corresponding to the new angle of alignment. If the initial strabismus was acquired before age 10 years, the ability to suppress is generally well developed.
- Diplopia may persist.

Prolonged postoperative diplopia is uncommon. However, if strabismus was first acquired in adulthood, diplopia that was symptomatic before surgery is likely to persist unless comitant alignment and fusion are regained. Prisms that compensate for the deviation may be helpful during the preoperative evaluation to assess the fusion potential and the risk of bothersome postoperative diplopia.

A patient with unequal vision can often ignore the dimmer, more blurred image. Further treatment is indicated for patients whose symptomatic diplopia persists after surgery, especially if it is severe and present in the primary position. If vision in the eyes is equal or nearly so, temporary or permanent prisms should be tried to address any residual diplopia. If this approach fails, additional surgery or botulinum toxin injection may be considered. In some cases, intractable diplopia can be controlled only by occluding or blurring the less-preferred eye with a MIN lens (Fresnel, Bloomington, MN), Bangerter foil (Ryser, St Gallen, Switzerland), or Scotch Magic Tape (3M, St Paul, MN).

Unsatisfactory Alignment

Unsatisfactory postoperative alignment—overcorrection, undercorrection, or development of an entirely new strabismus problem—is perhaps better characterized as a disappointing outcome of strabismus surgery, rather than as a complication. Alignment in the immediate postoperative period, whether satisfactory or not, may not be permanent. Among the reasons for this unpredictability are poor fusion, poor vision, and contracture of scar tissue. Reoperations are often necessary.

Iatrogenic Brown Syndrome

Iatrogenic Brown syndrome can result from superior oblique muscle tightening procedures. Taking care to avoid excessive tightening of the tendon when these procedures are performed minimizes the risk of this complication. A tuck can sometimes be reversed if reoperation is undertaken soon after the original surgery. Observation is also an option, as superior oblique tucks tend to loosen with time (see Chapter 12).

Anti-Elevation Syndrome

Inferior oblique anteriorization can result in restricted elevation of the eye in abduction, known *as anti-elevation syndrome.* Reattaching the lateral corner of the muscle anterior to the spiral of Tillaux increases the risk of this syndrome; "bunching up" the insertion at the lateral border of the inferior rectus muscle may reduce the risk.

斜视手术的并发症

复视

复视可发生于斜视手术后，偶尔发生于年龄较大的儿童，更常见于成人。手术将固定像移出了抑制暗点。手术后的几个月内会产生各种反应：

- 出现 2 个像的融合。
- 形成新的抑制暗点，对应于新的眼正位角度。如果斜视发生在 10 岁前，会形成较好的抑制能力。
- 复视持续存在。

术后的长期复视不常见。而首次斜视发生在成年期，手术前已经存在的复视会持续，除非重新获得共同性眼正位和融合。术前用棱镜补偿偏斜，有助于对融合潜力和较麻烦的术后复视风险进行评估。

视力不等的患者常会忽略更暗淡、更模糊的图像。对于手术后持续存在的症状性复视，特别是症状严重且在第一眼位出现，则需要进一步治疗。如果两眼视力相等或接近，则使用临时性或永久性棱镜来解决残存复视。如果这种方法无效，需考虑进行手术或肉毒杆菌毒素注射。有时只能用 MIN 镜片（Fresnel, Bloomington, MN）、Bangerter 膜（Ryser, St Gallen, Switzerland）或 Scotch Magic 胶带（3M, St Paul, MN）遮挡或雾化非主眼，控制难治性复视。

不满意眼位

不能令人满意的术后眼位——过度矫正、矫正不足或出现新的斜视问题——都是令人失望的斜视手术结果，而不是并发症。无论是否满意，术后即刻眼位并不是永久性的。其中不可预测性的原因包括融合不良、视力不佳和瘢痕组织挛缩。通常需要再次手术。

医源性 Brown 综合征

医源性 Brown 综合征由上斜肌紧缩术引起。手术时，应避免肌腱过度紧缩，以最大限度地降低这种并发症的风险。如果在初始手术后很快行二次手术，折卷（tuck）尚可逆。也可进行观察，因为上斜肌折卷往往会随着时间的推移而松弛（见第 12 章）。

抗上转综合征

下斜肌前部化可导致外转时上转受限，称为*抗上转综合征*。将肌肉的侧角附着于 Tillaux 螺旋前会增加这种综合征的风险；将下直肌外侧边缘的附着点“缝合在一起”，以降低这种风险。

Lost and Slipped Muscles

A rectus muscle that sustains trauma or that slips out of the sutures or instruments while unattached to the globe during an operation can retract through the Tenon capsule and become inaccessible ("lost") posteriorly in the orbit. This consequence is most severe when it involves the medial rectus muscle, because that muscle is the most difficult to recover.

The surgeon should immediately attempt to find the lost muscle, if possible with the assistance of a surgeon experienced in this potentially complex surgery. Malleable retractors and a headlight are helpful. Minimal manipulation should be used to bring into view the anatomical site through which the muscle and its sheath normally penetrate the Tenon capsule where, it is hoped, the distal end of the muscle can be recognized and captured. If inspection does not reliably indicate that the muscle has been identified, sudden bradycardia when traction is exerted can be confirmatory. Recovery of the medial rectus muscle has been achieved by using a transnasal endoscopic approach through the ethmoid sinus or by performing a medial orbitotomy. Transposition surgery may be required if the lost muscle is not found, but anterior segment ischemia may be a risk. Where to reattach the recovered muscle depends on several factors in the particular case and is largely a matter of judgment.

A slipped muscle is the result of inadequate imbrication of the muscle during strabismus surgery, which allows it to recede posteriorly within its capsule postoperatively. Clinically, the patient manifests a weakness of that muscle immediately postoperatively, with limited rotations and possibly decreased saccades in its field of action (Fig 14-1). Surgery should be performed as soon as possible in order to secure the muscle before further retraction and contracture take place.

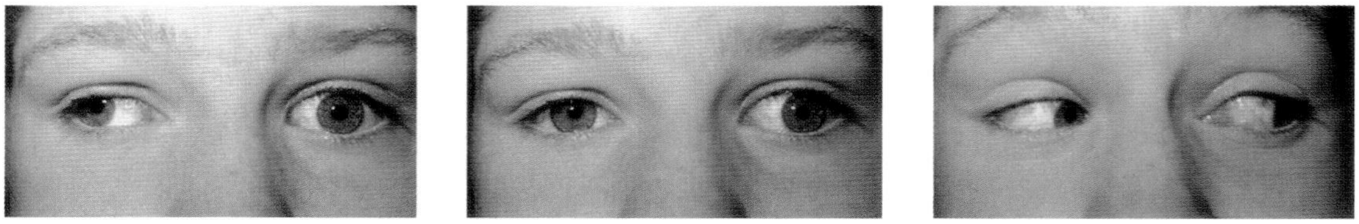

Figure 14-1 Slipped left medial rectus muscle. ***Left,*** Gaze right shows inability to adduct the left eye. ***Center,*** Exotropia in primary position. ***Right,*** Gaze left shows full abduction. Note that the left palpebral fissure is wider than the right, especially with attempted adduction.

In reoperations for strabismus with deficient rotations, slippage or a stretched scar should be suspected and the involved muscles explored. The pseudotendon must be excised to restore the function of the muscle.

Pulled-in-Two Syndrome

Dehiscence of a muscle during surgery has been termed *pulled-in-two syndrome (PITS).* The dehiscence usually occurs at the tendon–muscle junction, and the inferior rectus may be the most frequently affected muscle. Advanced age, various myopathies, previous surgery, trauma, or infiltrative disease may predispose a muscle to PITS by weakening its structural integrity. Treatment is recovery, when possible, using techniques similar to those used for lost muscles, and re-anastomosis of the muscle.

肌肉丢失和滑脱

直肌受到外伤或手术期间附着于眼球之前时，从缝合线或器械中滑脱，可能通过Tenon囊收缩，在眼眶后无法触及（“丢失”）。当累及内直肌时，后果是最严重，因为内直肌最难复位。

在这种复杂的情况下，应请经验丰富的医生帮助，立即寻找丢失的肌肉。可伸缩开睑器和头灯很有帮助。探查特定解剖部位时，即解剖上肌肉及其肌鞘穿透 Tenon 囊处，操作动作尽量小，找到肌肉的远端，并抓住肌肉。如果不能确认已经找到的肌肉，牵拉肌肉突然发生心动过缓即可确定。还可用鼻内窥镜穿过筛窦或行内侧眶切开术来使内直肌复位。如果无法找到丢失的肌肉，则需要转位术，但有前节缺血的风险。在特定情况下，肌肉的复位位置取决于的几个因素，主要取决于判断。

在斜视手术时，肌肉重叠不足导致了肌肉滑脱，术后肌肉在其囊内向后回缩。临床上，患者术后立即出现该肌肉作用范围内的功能不足，伴有旋转受限和扫视减少（图 14–1）。应尽快进行手术，以便在发生进一步收缩和挛缩之前保护肌肉。

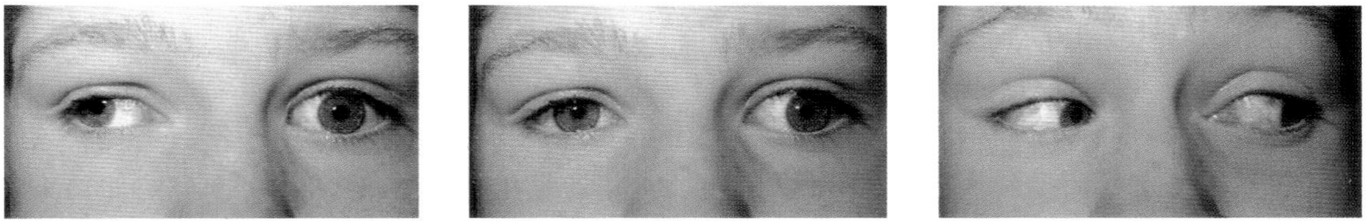

图 14–1　左眼内直肌滑脱。***左图：*** 右侧注视时，左眼无法内转。***中图：*** 第一眼位时，左眼呈外斜视。***右图：*** 左侧注视时，左眼完全外转。注意，特别是内转时，左侧睑裂比右侧宽。

对旋转不足的斜视再次手术时，应对相关的肌肉进行探查，排除肌肉滑脱或瘢痕。必须切除假性肌腱，以恢复肌肉的功能。

Pulled-in-Two 综合征

手术过程中，肌肉的分离被称为 *pulled-in-two 综合征（PITS）*。分离常发生在肌腱——肌肉结合处，下直肌是最常受累的肌肉。高龄、各种肌病、既往手术、创伤或浸润性疾病易发生 PITS，可能是肌肉结构的完整性的减弱。使用丢失肌肉和肌肉再吻合方法进行恢复。

Perforation of the Sclera

During reattachment of an EOM, a needle may penetrate the sclera and pass into the suprachoroidal space or perforate the choroid and retina. Perforation can lead to retinal detachment or endophthalmitis (see BCSC Section 9, *Uveitis and ocular Inflammation*); in most cases, it results in only a small chorioretinal scar, with no effect on vision. Most perforations are unrecognized unless specifically looked for by ophthalmoscopy. If vitreous escapes through the perforation site, many surgeons apply immediate local cryotherapy or laser therapy. Topical antibiotics are generally given during the immediate postoperative period, even when vitreous has not escaped. Ophthalmoscopy during the postoperative period is an appropriate precaution, with referral to a retina con sul tant if needed.

Postoperative Infections

Intraocular infection is uncommon following strabismus surgery. Mild conjunctivitis develops in some patients and may be caused by allergy to suture material or postoperative medications, as well as by infectious agents. Preseptal and orbital cellulitis with proptosis, eyelid swelling, chemosis, and fever are rare (Fig 14-2). These conditions usually develop 2–3 days after surgery and generally respond well to systemic antibiotics. Patients should be warned of the signs and symptoms of orbital cellulitis and endophthalmitis and instructed to seek emergency consultation if necessary.

Pyogenic Granuloma and Foreign-Body Granuloma

Pyogenic granuloma (lobular capillary hemangioma) consists of a lobular proliferation of capillaries with edema that typically develops at the conjunctival incision site (Fig 14-3). It is prone to ulceration or bleeding but usually resolves spontaneously. Persistent lesions may require surgical excision. In rare cases, suture can cause foreign-body granulomas and allergic reactions (Fig 14-4).

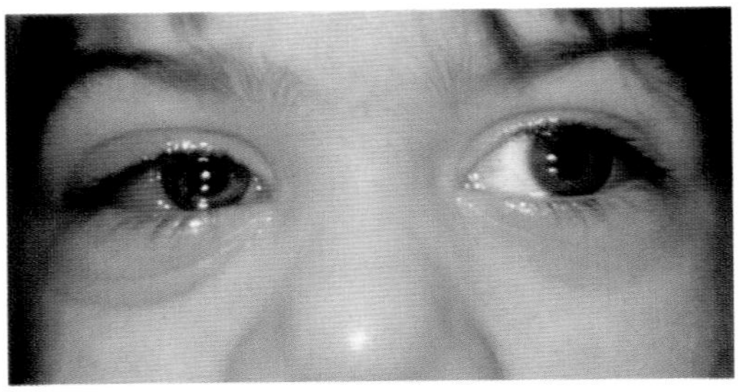

Figure 14-2 Orbital cellulitis, right eye, 2 days after bilateral recession of the lateral rectus muscles.

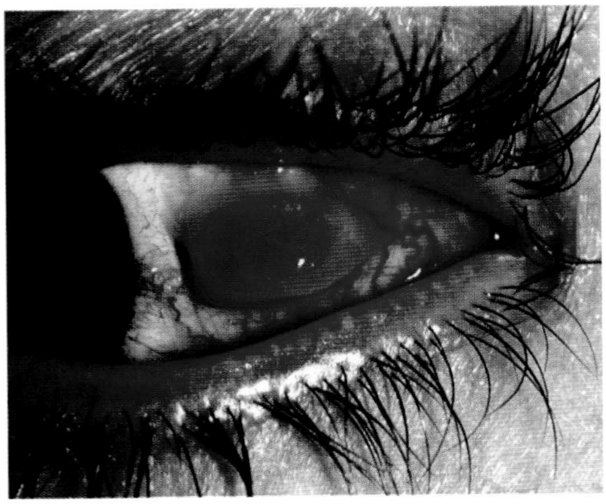

Figure 14-3 Postoperative pyogenic granuloma over the left lateral rectus muscle. *(From Espinoza GM, Lueder GT. Conjunctival pyogenic granulomas after strabismus surgery. Ophthalmology. 2005;112(7): 1283–1286.)*

巩膜穿孔

复位眼外肌（EOM）时，缝针可能穿透巩膜，进入脉络膜上腔，或穿透脉络膜和视网膜。穿孔可导致视网膜脱离或眼内炎（见 BCSC 第 9 册《*葡萄膜炎与眼部炎症*》）。大多数仅产生小的脉络膜视网膜疤痕，对视力没有影响。不使用眼底镜进行特别检查时，大多数穿孔不被识别。如果穿孔处玻璃体脱出，医生会立即采用局部冷冻或激光治疗。即使没有发生玻璃体脱出，术后亦应立即给予局部抗生素。术后眼底镜检查是一种适当的预防措施，如果需要，可请视网膜专家会诊。

术后感染

斜视手术后眼内感染并不常见。部分患者出现轻度结膜炎，可能由缝合材料或术后药物过敏以及感染引起。眶膈前和眶蜂窝织炎伴眼球突出、眼睑水肿、球结膜水肿和发热的情况很少见（图 14–2）多在手术后 2 ~ 3d 出现，全身性抗生素治疗有效。应告知患者眶蜂窝织炎和眼内炎的体征和症状，需急诊就诊。

化脓性肉芽肿和异物肉芽肿

化脓性肉芽肿（小叶性毛细血管瘤）包括通常在结膜切口部位形成的小叶性毛细血管增生伴水肿（图 14–3）。其容易形成溃疡或出血，但常自行消退。病变持续存在则需要手术切除。在极少数情况下，缝线产生异物肉芽肿，并引起过敏反应（图 14–4）。

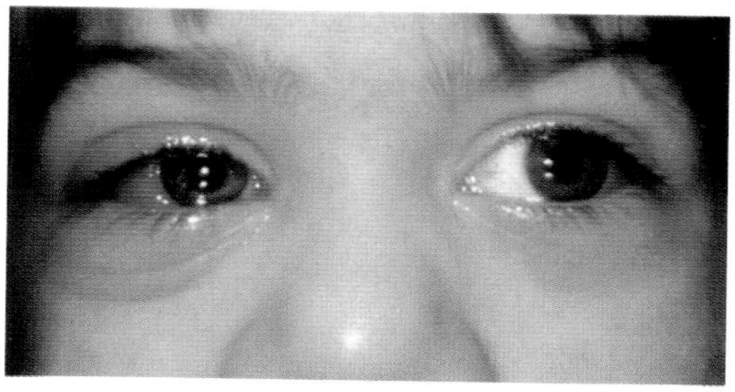

图 14–2　眶蜂窝织炎，右眼，双眼外直肌后徙术后 2 天。

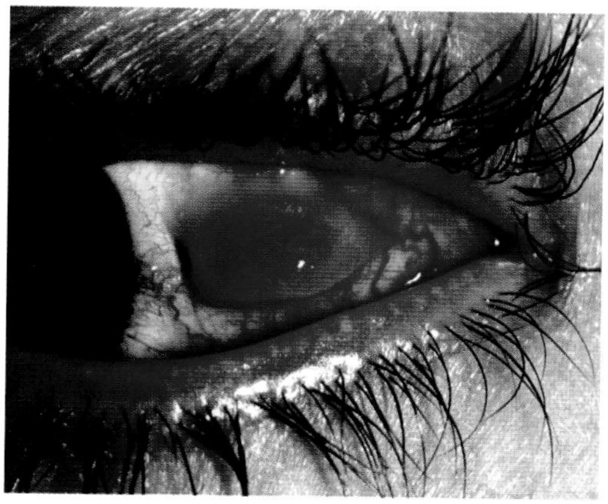

图 14–3　左眼外直肌术后化脓性肉芽肿。*（译者注：资料来源见前页原文。）*

Epithelial Cyst

A noninflamed, translucent subconjunctival mass may develop if conjunctival epithelium is buried during muscle reattachment or incision closure (Fig 14-5). Occasionally, the cyst resolves spontaneously. Topical steroids may be helpful; persistentcases may require surgical excision. In some cases, the cyst is incorporated into the muscle tendon, so careful exploration is mandatory to identify this complication.

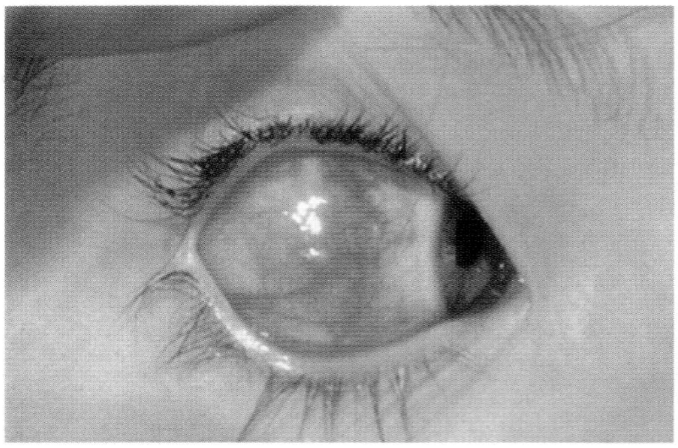

Figure 14-4 Allergic reaction to chromic gut suture. Allergic reactions are rare with modern synthetic suture material such as polyglactin.

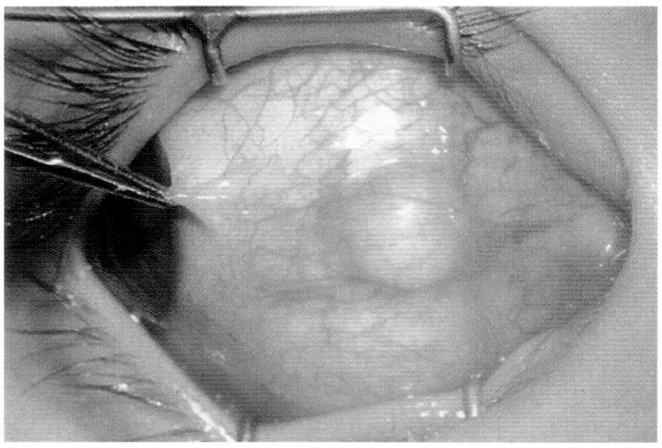

Figure 14-5 Postoperative epithelial cyst following right medial rectus muscle recession.

Conjunctival Scarring

Satisfaction from improved alignment may occasionally be overshadowed by unsightly scarring of the conjunctiva and the Tenon capsule. The tissues remain hyperemic and salmon pink instead of returning to their usual whiteness. This complication may occur as a result of the following:

- *Advancement of thickened Tenon capsule too close to the limbus.* In resection procedures, pulling the muscle forward may advance the Tenon capsule. The undesirable result is exaggerated in reoperations, when the Tenon capsule may be hypertrophied.
- *Advancement of the plica semilunaris.* During surgery on the medial rectus muscle using the limbal approach, the surgeon may mistake the plica semilunaris for a conjunctival edge and incorporate it into the closure. Though not strictly a conjunctival scar, the advanced plica, now pulled forward and hypertrophied, retains its fleshy color (Fig 14-6).

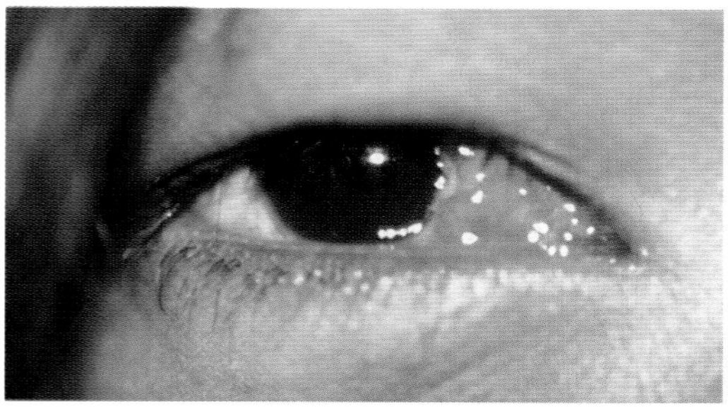

Figure 14-6 Hypertrophy involving the plica semilunaris. *(Courtesy of Scott Olitsky, MD.)*

Treatment options include conjunctivoplasty with resection of scarred conjunctiva and transposition of adjacent conjunctiva, resection of subconjunctival fibrous tissue, recession of scarred conjunctiva, and amniotic membrane grafting.

上皮囊肿

肌肉复位或切口闭合时，结膜上皮的包埋可出现非炎症性的、半透明的结膜下包块（图 14-5）。囊肿偶会自行消退。局部类固醇眼药有效；病情持续则需要手术切除。有时，囊肿与肌腱混合，必须仔细探查。

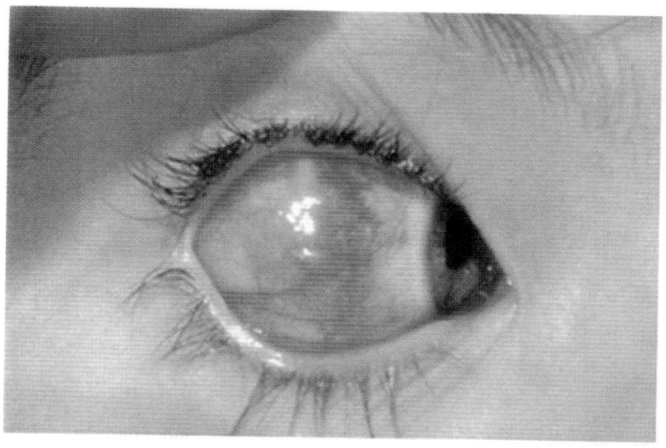

图 14-4　对铬肠缝线的过敏反应。现代合成缝合材料（如 polyglactin）很少发生过敏反应。

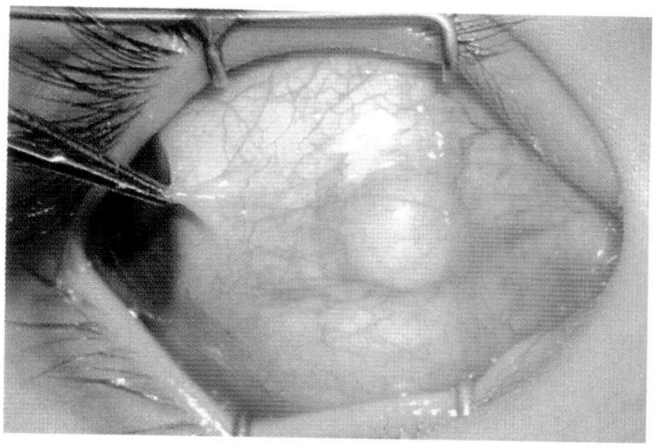

图 14-5　右眼内直肌后徙术后上皮囊肿。

结膜瘢痕

即使眼位恢复满意，但结膜和 Tenon 囊的疤痕仍令人不悦，组织呈充血的肉粉色，而不是正常的白色。其原因有：

- *增生厚的 Tenon 囊太靠近角膜缘*。切除术中，向前拉肌肉可将 Tenon 囊前移。当 Tenon 囊增生时，这种效果更为明显。

- *半月皱襞前移*。经角膜缘的内直肌手术时，手术医生误将半月皱襞视为结膜边缘，并将其缝合。虽然不是严格意义上的结膜瘢痕，但半月皱襞前移、增生，持续呈肉色（图 14-6）。

图 14-6　累及半月皱襞的增生。*（译者注：资料来源见前页原文。）*

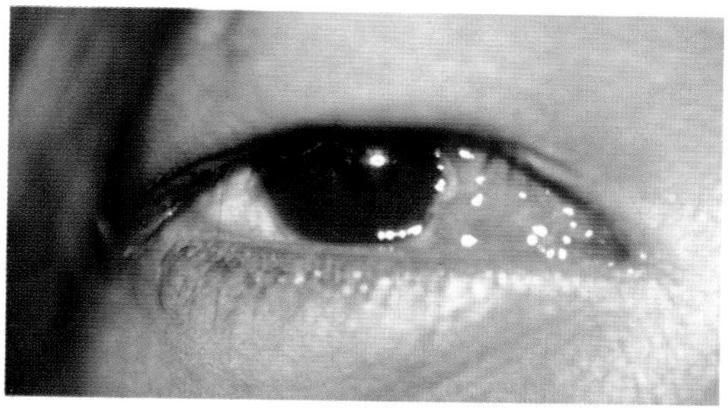

治疗方法包括结膜成形术联合结膜瘢痕切除术、邻近结膜移位术、结膜下纤维组织和瘢痕结膜切除术及羊膜移植术。

Adherence Syndrome

Tears in the Tenon capsule with prolapse of orbital fat into the sub-Tenon space can cause formation of a fibrofatty scar that may restrict ocular motility. Surgery involving the inferior oblique muscle is particularly prone to this complication because of the proximity of the fat space to the posterior border of the inferior oblique muscle. If recognized at the time of surgery, the prolapsed fat can be excised and the rent closed with absorbable sutures. Meticulous surgical technique usually prevents this serious complication.

Delle

A *delle (plural dellen)* is a shallow area of corneal thinning near the limbus. Dellen occur when raised abnormal bulbar conjunctiva prevents adequate lubrication of the cornea adjacent to the raised conjunctiva (Fig 14-7). Dellen are more likely to occur when the limbal approach to EOM surgery is used. They usually heal with time. Artificial tears or lubricants may be used until the chemosis subsides.

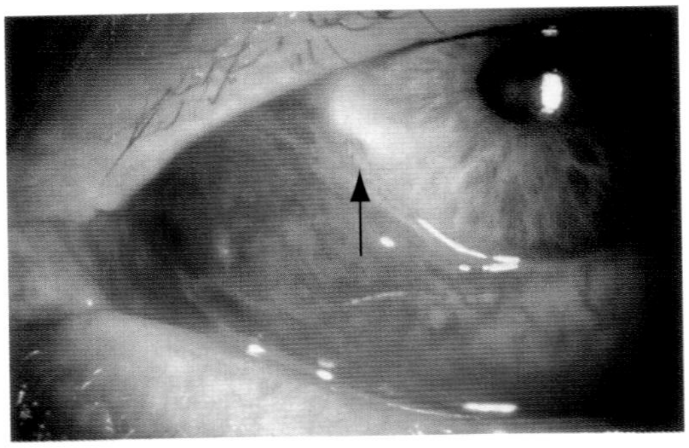

Figure 14-7 Corneal delle *(arrow)* subsequent to postoperative subconjunctival hemorrhage.

Anterior Segment Ischemia

The blood supply to the anterior segment of the eye is provided, in part, by the anterior ciliary arteries that travel with the 4 rectus muscles. Simultaneous surgery on 3 rectus muscles, or even 2 rectus muscles in patients with poor blood circulation, may therefore lead to anterior segment ischemia (ASI). The earliest signs of this complication are cells and flare in the anterior chamber. More severe cases are characterized by corneal epithelial edema, folds in the Descemet membrane, and an irregular pupil (Fig 14-8). This complication may lead to anterior segment necrosis and phthisis bulbi. No universally agreedupon treatment exists for ASI. Because the signs of ASI are similar to those of uveitis, most ophthalmologists treat with topical, subconjunctival, or systemic corticosteroids, although there is no firm evidence supporting this approach.

It is possible to recess, resect, or transpose a rectus muscle while sparing its anterior ciliary vessels. Though difficult and time consuming, this technique may be indicated in high-risk cases. Staging surgery, with an interval of several months between procedures, may also be helpful. Because the anterior segment is partially supplied by the conjunctival circulation through the limbal arcades, using fornix instead of limbal incisions may provide some protection against the development of ASI.

粘连综合征

Tenon 囊撕裂伴有眶脂肪脱入 Tenon 囊下间隙，可导致纤维脂肪瘢痕的形成，从而限制眼球运动。下斜肌手术特别容易出现这种并发症，因为眶脂肪间隙的远端与下斜肌的后缘毗邻。如果手术时发现，可切除脱垂的脂肪，并用可吸收缝线缝合裂口。精细的手术技巧常能预防这一严重的并发症。

角膜小凹

*角膜小凹*是角膜缘附近变薄的浅凹区域。当突起的异常结膜阻碍了邻近突起结膜的角膜的充分润滑时，就会发生角膜小凹（图 14–7）。当经角膜缘路经进行眼外肌（EOM）手术时，易发生角膜小凹，常随时间而愈合。可应用人工泪液或润滑液，直至结膜水肿消退。

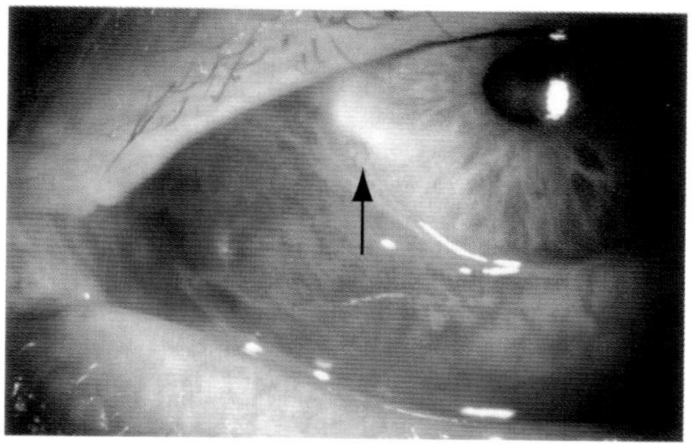

图 14–7　术后结膜下出血后的角膜小凹（*箭头*）。

眼前节缺血

眼前节的血液供应部分由睫状前动脉提供，其与 4 条直肌一起走行。因此，同时手术 3 条直肌或血液循环不良的患者仅行 2 条直肌，即可导致前节缺血（ASI）。这种并发症最早期的临床表现，是前房浮游细胞和闪辉，严重时角膜上皮水肿、后弹力层（Descemet 膜）褶皱和不规则瞳孔（图 14–8）。这种并发症可能导致前节坏死和眼球萎缩（眼球痨）。前节缺血（ASI）尚无公认的治疗方法，前节缺血（ASI）的症状与葡萄膜炎相似，多数眼科医生使用局部、结膜下或全身皮质类固醇治疗，这种方法还没有支持证据。

可在保留睫状肌前血管的同时，行直肌的后徙、切除或移位。尽管这项技术困难且耗时，但可用于高风险病例。可行分期手术，如间隔几个月可能有益。由于眼前节部分由角膜缘弓的结膜循环提供，可行穹窿切口，而不是角膜缘切口，以避免前节缺血（ASI）的发生。

Change in Eyelid Position

Change in the position of the eyelids is most likely to occur with surgery on the vertical rectus muscles. Pulling the inferior rectus muscle forward, as in a resection, advances the lower eyelid upward; recessing this muscle pulls the lower eyelid down, exposing sclera below the lower limbus (Fig 14-9). Surgery on the superior rectus muscle is less likely to affect upper eyelid position.

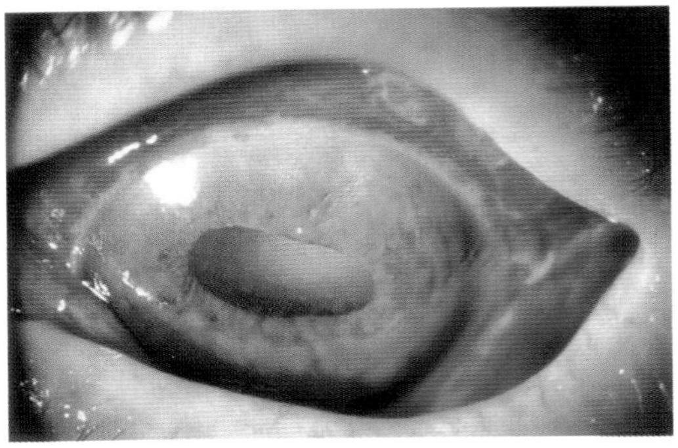

Figure 14-8 Superotemporal segmental anterior segment ischemia after simultaneous superior rectus muscle and lateral rectus muscle surgery following a scleral buckling procedure.

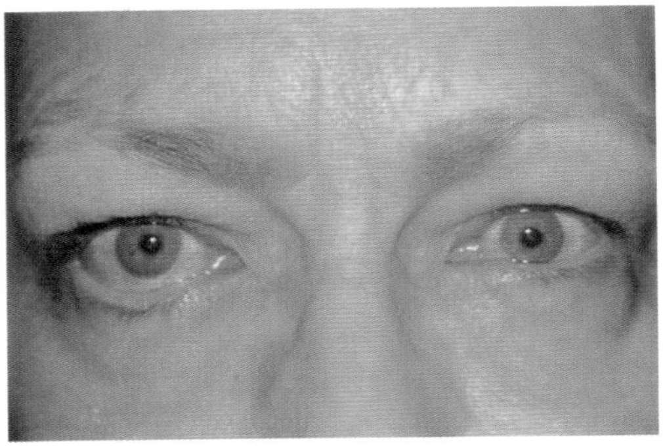

Figure 14-9 Patient treated for left hypertropia by recession of the right inferior rectus muscle, which pulled the right lower eyelid down, and resection of the left inferior rectus muscle, which pulled the left lower eyelid up.

Changes in eyelid position can be obviated somewhat by careful dissection. In general, all intermuscular septum and fascial connections of the vertical rectus muscle must be severed at least 12–15 mm posterior to the muscle insertion. Release of the lower eyelid retractors or advancement of the capsulopalpebral head is helpful to prevent lower eyelid retraction after inferior rectus muscle recession.

Refractive Changes

Changes in refractive error are most common when strabismus surgery is performed on 2 rectus muscles of an eye. An induced astigmatism of low magnitude usually resolves within a few months. Surgery on the oblique muscles can change the axis of preexisting astigmatism.

Kushner BJ. The effect of oblique muscle surgery on the axis of astigmatism. *J Pediatr Ophthalmol Strabismus.* 1986;23(6):277–280.

Anesthesia for Extraocular Muscle Surgery

Methods

In cooperative patients, topical anesthetic eyedrops alone (eg, tetracaine 0.5%, proparacaine 0.5%, lidocaine 2%) are effective for most steps in an EOM surgical procedure. Topical anesthesia is not effective for control of the pain produced by pulling on or against a restricted muscle or for cases in which exposure is difficult.

眼睑位置的变化

眼睑位置的改变最常发生在垂直直肌的手术中。将下直肌切除、向前拉时，使下睑向上移位，后徙下直肌将下睑向下拉，露出下角膜缘下方的巩膜（图 14–9）。上直肌手术较少影响上睑位置。

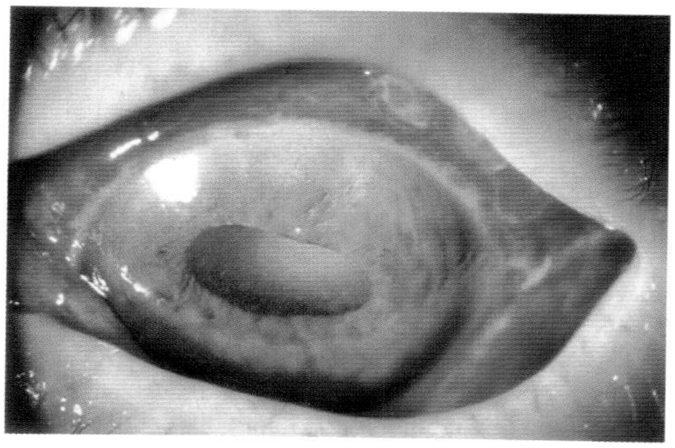

图 14–8　巩膜扣带术后，同时行上直肌和外直肌手术，导致颞上节段性前节缺血。

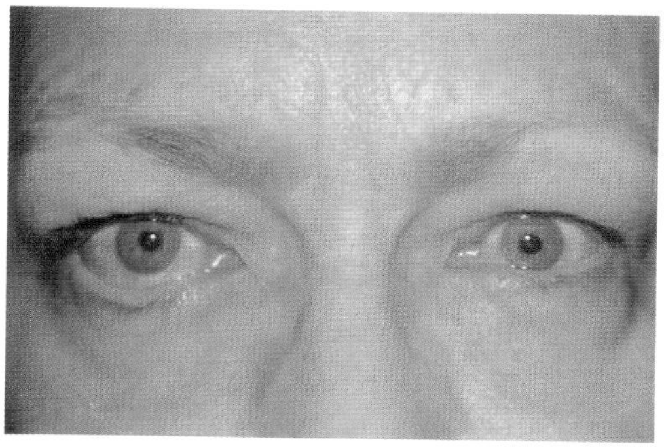

图 14–9　右下直肌后徙术治疗左眼上斜视，右眼下睑向下拉，左眼下直肌切除，左眼下睑向上拉。

手术中仔细分离，可以避免眼睑位置的变化。至少在肌肉附着点后 12 ~ 15 mm，切断所有垂直直肌肌间隔和筋膜连接。松解下眼睑收缩肌或前移睑伴前端，有助于防止下直肌后徙术后的下眼睑退缩。

屈光变化

当对眼睛的2条直肌进行斜视手术时，屈光不正的变化最常见。低度散光通常在几个月内消退。斜肌的手术可以改变先前存在的散光轴向。

Kushner BJ. The effect of oblique muscle surgery on the axis of astigmatism. *J Pediatr Ophthalmol Strabismus.* 1986;23(6):277–280.

眼外肌手术麻醉

方法

在合作的患者中，眼外肌（EOM）手术仅在局部表面麻醉下进行（如0.5% 丁卡因、0.5% 丙卡因、2% 利多卡因）。牵拉肌肉或暴露受限肌肉时，表面麻醉不能有效止痛。

Both peribulbar and retrobulbar anesthesia make most EOM procedures pain-free and should be considered in adults for whom general anesthesia may pose an undue hazard. The administration of a short-acting hypnotic by an anesthesiologist just before retrobulbar injection greatly improves patient comfort. Because injected anesthetics may influence alignment during the first few hours after surgery, suture adjustment is best delayed for at least half a day.

General anesthesia is necessary for children and is often used for adults as well, particularly those requiring bilateral surgery. Neuromuscular blocking agents such as succinylcholine, which are administered to facilitate intubation for general anesthesia, can temporarily affect the results of a traction test. Nondepolarizing agents, which do not have this effect, can be used instead.

Postoperative Nausea and Vomiting

Eye muscle surgery is a risk factor for postoperative nausea and vomiting. This risk can be reduced by prophylaxis with dexamethasone and serotonin type 3 (5-HT_3) antagonists (eg, ondansetron), propofol use, adequate hydration, and reduced use of inhalation anesthetics and opioid analgesia.

Oculocardiac Reflex

The oculocardiac reflex is a slowing of the heart rate caused by traction on the EOMs, particularly the medial rectus muscle. In its most severe form, the reflex can produce asystole. The surgeon should be aware of the possibility of inducing the oculocardiac reflex when manipulating a muscle and should be prepared to release tension if the heart rate drops excessively. Intravenous atropine and other agents can protect against this reflex.

Malignant Hyperthermia

Malignant hyperthermia (MH) is an important disorder for pediatric ophthalmologists because of its association with strabismus, myopathies, ptosis, and musculoskeletal abnormalities. MH is a defect of calcium binding by the sarcoplasmic reticulum of skeletal muscle that can occur sporadically or be dominantly inherited with incomplete penetrance. When MH is triggered by inhalational anesthetics or the muscle relaxant succinylcholine, unbound intracellular calcium concentration increases. This stimulates muscle contracture, causing massive acidosis. In its fully developed form, MH is characterized by extreme heat production, resulting from the hypermetabolic state.

MH can be fatal if diagnosis and treatment are delayed. The earliest sign is unexplained elevation of end-tidal carbon dioxide concentration. As soon as the diagnosis is made, surgery should be terminated, even if incomplete. Treatment is in the province of the anesthesiologist. See also BCSC Section 1, *Update on General Medicine.*

球周麻醉和球后麻醉可实现大多数无痛眼外肌（EOM）手术，用于成人手术，因为全身麻醉可能有危险。球后注射前，麻醉师可用短效安眠剂以改善患者的舒适度。因为麻药会影响术后几个小时的眼位，所以最好推迟半天进行缝线调整。

全身麻醉对儿童和成人都是必要的，特别是行双眼手术的成人。全身麻醉插管使用的神经肌肉阻滞剂，如琥珀酰胆碱，可能暂时影响牵拉试验的结果。可用无这种效果的非去极化剂替代。

术后恶心和呕吐

眼肌手术是术后恶心和呕吐的危险因素，通过使用地塞米松和5-羟色胺3型（5-HT_3）拮抗剂（如 ondansetron，昂丹司琼 / 枢复宁）、异丙酚、充分补水以及减少使用吸入性麻醉剂和阿片类镇痛药物，可以降低这种风险。

眼心反射

眼心反射是由于眼外肌（EOMs）引起的心率减慢，特别是内直肌牵拉。最严重的反射可以使心跳停止。进行眼肌手术时，医生应该注意可能诱发眼心反射，如果心率严重下降，应该放松对肌肉的牵张力。静脉注射阿托品和其他药物可以防止这种反射的发生。

恶性高热

对于小儿眼科医生来说，*恶性高热（MH）*是非常重要的疾病，因为它与斜视、肌病、上睑下垂和骨骼肌异常有关。恶性高热（MH）是骨骼肌的肌浆网结合钙的缺陷，呈偶发或不完全外显的显性遗传。当吸入麻醉剂或肌肉松弛剂琥珀胆碱时，诱发恶性高热（MH），未结合的细胞内钙浓度增加，刺激肌肉收缩，导致严重的酸中毒。完全表现时，由于代谢亢进状态导致的极端热量产生，即恶性高热（MH）的特征。

恶性高热（MH）诊断和治疗的延误，可危及生命。最早的症状是不明原因的潮气末二氧化碳浓度升高。一旦确诊，必须终止手术，即使是手术未完成。由麻醉师负责治疗。见 BCSC 第 1 册《*医学最新进展*》。

Chemodenervation Using Botulinum Toxin

Pharmacology and Mechanism of Action

Botulinum toxin type A paralyzes muscles by blocking the release of acetylcholine at the neuromuscular junction. This agent has a number of uses, but it was originally developed for the treatment of strabismus. Within 24–48 hours of injection, botulinum toxin is bound and internalized within local motor nerve terminals, where it remains active for many weeks. Paralysis of the injected EOM begins within 2–4 days of injection and lasts clinically for at least 5–8 weeks. This produces, in effect, a pharmacologic recession: the EOM lengthens while it is para lyzed by botulinum toxin, and its antagonist contracts. These changes may produce long-term improvement in the alignment of the eyes. The recent introduction of bupivacaine injection into the antagonist muscle to provide a chemical resection effect may extend the durability of the correction and expand the range of deviations in which chemodenervation can be successfully used.

Debert I, Miller JM, Danh KK, Scott AB. Pharmacologic injection treatment of comitant strabismus. *J AAPOS.* 2016;20(2):106–111.

Scott AB. Botulinum toxin injection of eye muscles to correct strabismus. *Trans Am Ophthalmol Soc.* 1981;79:734–770.

Indications, Techniques, and Results

Clinical trials using botulinum toxin for the treatment of strabismus have shown this agent to be most effective in the following conditions:

- small-to moderate-angle esotropia and exotropia (<40Δ)
- postoperative residual strabismus (2–8 weeks following surgery or later)
- acute paralytic strabismus (especially sixth nerve palsy; sometimes fourth nerve palsy), to eliminate diplopia while the palsy resolves
- active thyroid eye disease (Graves disease) or inflamed or pre-phthisical eyes, when surgery is inappropriate
- as a supplement to medial rectus muscle recession for large-angle infantile esotropia or lateral rectus muscle recession for large-angle exotropia

When used to treat patients with strabismus, the toxin is injected directly, with a small-gauge needle, into selected EOMs. Injections into the EOMs may be performed with the use of a portable electromyographic device, although experienced practitioners often dispense with electromyography. In adults, injections are performed with topical anesthetic; in children, general anesthesia is usually necessary (Videos 14-12, 14-13).

VIDEO 14-12 Strabismus surgery: botulinum medial rectus under general anesthetic.
Courtesy of John D. Ferris, FRCOphth, and Peter E. J. Davies, FRANZCO, MPH.

VIDEO 14-13 Strabismus surgery: botulinum medial rectus.
Courtesy of John D. Ferris, FRCOphth, and Peter E. J. Davies, FRANZCO, MPH.

肉毒杆菌毒素的化学去神经疗法

药理及作用机制

肉毒杆菌毒素 A 型，通过阻断神经肌肉交界处的乙酰胆碱释放，麻痹肌肉。这种药物有许多用途，但最初用于治疗斜视。在注射后的 24 ~ 48h 内，肉毒毒素在局部运动神经末梢内结合和内化，并保持数周的药学活性。注射 2 ~ 4d 后，眼外肌（EOM）麻痹，临床至少持续 5 ~ 8 周。药理学上，产生了药物性后徙：当肉毒杆菌毒素麻痹眼外肌（EOM）时，眼肌拉长，其拮抗肌会收缩。这些变化可长期改善眼位。最近采用将布比卡因注射到拮抗肌中，产生化学性切除效果，延长矫正时间，并增加化学去神经化的矫正偏斜的程度。

Debert I, Miller JM, Danh KK, Scott AB. Pharmacologic injection treatment of comitant strabismus. *J AAPOS.* 2016;20(2):106–111.

Scott AB. Botulinum toxin injection of eye muscles to correct strabismus. *Trans Am Ophthalmol Soc.* 1981;79:734–770.

适应证、技巧和结果

临床试验表明，以下情况中使用肉毒杆菌毒素治疗斜视最有效：

- 中小角度的内斜视和外斜视（<40Δ）
- 术后残余斜视（术后 2 ~ 8 周或更长）
- 急性麻痹性斜视（特别是Ⅵ颅神经麻痹，有时是Ⅳ颅神经麻痹），解决麻痹消除后的复视
- 活动性甲状腺眼病（Graves 病）或炎症眼或眼球痨，不宜手术时，补充大角度婴儿型内斜视时内直肌后徙或补充大角度外斜视时外直肌后徙

当用于治疗斜视患者时，用小针头将毒素直接注射到选定的眼外肌（EOM）中。经验丰富的医生不使用肌电图仪，但可用便携式肌电图仪进行注射。注射时，给成人用局部麻醉。儿童需全身麻醉（视频 14–12、14–13）。

视频14–12　斜视手术：全身麻醉下内直肌注射肉毒杆菌毒素。
（译者注：资料来源见前页原文。）

视频14–13　斜视手术：内直肌注射肉毒杆菌毒素。
（译者注：资料来源见前页原文。）

Multiple injections may be required, particularly in adults. As with surgical treatment, results are best when there is fusion to stabilize the alignment. Botulinum toxin injection is usually not effective in patients with large deviations, restrictive or mechanical strabismus (trauma, chronic thyroid eye disease), or secondary strabismus wherein a muscle has been overly recessed. Injection is in effec tive in A and V patterns, DVDs, and chronic paralytic strabismus. The long-term recovery rate for patients with acute sixth nerve palsy treated with observation alone is similar to that for patients who receive botulinum toxin.

Complications

The most common adverse effects of ocular botulinum toxin treatment are ptosis, lagophthalmos, dry eye, and induced vertical strabismus after horizontal muscle injection. These complications are usually temporary, resolving after several weeks. Rare complications include scleral perforation, retrobulbar hemorrhage, pupillary dilation, and permanent diplopia. Systemic botulism has been reported in animals and humans following massive injections of large muscle groups, but this has not been encountered in ophthalmologic use of botulinum toxin.

多次注射特别见于成年人。与手术治疗一样，有融合功能的效果最好。肉毒杆菌毒素注射对较大斜视、限制性或机械性斜视（外伤、慢性甲状腺眼病）或继发性斜视（肌肉过度切除）的患者无效。A 型和 V 型、DVD 和慢性麻痹性斜视时，注射治疗无效。单纯观察治疗急性Ⅵ颅神经麻痹患者的远期恢复率与接受肉毒杆菌毒素治疗的结果相似。

并发症

眼部肉毒杆菌毒素治疗最常见的副作用是眼睑下垂、睑裂闭合不全、干眼和水平肌肉注射后诱发的垂直斜视。这些并发症常是暂时的，几周后就会消失。罕见的并发症包括巩膜穿孔、球后出血、瞳孔扩大和持续性复视。在大量注射大肌肉群后，动物和人可出现全身肉毒毒素中毒，但眼科用肉毒杆菌毒素时并未有此报告。

（翻译　许志强　王文军　姚森 // 审校　石一宁 // 章节审校　石广礼）

PART II

Pediatric Ophthalmology

第二部分

小儿眼科

CHAPTER 15

Growth and Development of the Eye

Normal Growth and Development

The human eye undergoes dramatic anatomical and physiologic development throughout infancy and early childhood (Table 15-1). Ophthalmologists caring for pediatric patients should be familiar with the normal growth and development of the child's eye because departures from the norm may indicate pathology. See also BCSC Section 2, *Fundamentals and Principles of Ophthalmology.*

Table 15-1 Dimensions of Newborn and Adult Eyes

	Newborn	Adult
Axial length, mm	14.5–15.5	23.0–24.0
Corneal horizontal diameter, mm	9.5–10.5	12.0
K value, diopters	52.00	42.00–44.00

K = keratometry.

Dimensions of the Eye

Most of the growth of the eye takes place in the first year of life. Change in the eye's axial length occurs in 3 phases. The first phase (birth to age 2 years) is a period of rapid growth: the axial length increases by approximately 4 mm in the first 6 months of life and by an additional 2 mm during the next 6 months. During the second (age 2 to 5 years) and third (age 5 to 13 years) phases, growth slows, with axial length increasing by about 1 mm per phase.

Similarly, with growth of the globe, the corneal diameter increases rapidly during the first year of life. The average horizontal diameter of the cornea is 9.5–10.5 mm in newborns and increases to 12.0 mm in adults. The cornea also flattens in the first year such that keratometry values change markedly, from approximately 52.00 diopters (D) at birth, to 46.00 D by age 6 months, to adult measurements of 42.00–44.00 D by age 12 months. Mild corneal clouding may be seen in healthy newborns and is common in premature infants. It resolves as the cornea gradually becomes thinner, decreasing from an average central thickness of 691 μm at 30–32 weeks' gestation to 564 μm at birth.

The power of the pediatric lens decreases dramatically over the first several years of life—an important consideration when intraocular lens implantation is planned for infants and young children after cataract extraction. Lens power decreases from approximately 35.00 D at birth to about 23.00 D at age 2 years. Subsequently, the change is more gradual: lens power decreases to approximately 19.00 D by age 11 years, with little or no change thereafter.

Gordon RA, Donzis PB. Refractive development of the human eye. *Arch Ophthalmol.* 1985; 103(6):785–789.

Kirwan C, O'Keefe M, Fitzsimon S. Central corneal thickness and corneal diameter in premature infants. *Acta Ophthalmol Scand.* 2005;83(6):751–753.

第 15 章

眼的生长和发育

正常的生长与发育

在婴儿期和幼儿期，人眼的解剖和生理发育都发生了巨大变化（表 15–1）。对于小儿患者，眼科医生应该熟悉儿童眼的正常生长发育，因为偏离正常情况意味着病理性改变。见 BCSC 第 2 册《*眼科基础与原理*》。

表15–1 新生儿和成人的眼参数

	新生儿	成人
眼轴长度 / mm	14.5~15.5	23.0~24.0
角膜水平直径 / mm	9.5~10.5	12.0
K值 / D	52.00	42.00~44.00

K＝角膜曲率。

眼的大小

在出生后的第一年，眼睛就完成了大部分生长。眼球长度——眼轴的变化分 3 个阶段。第 1 阶段（出生 ~ 2 岁）是一个快速增长的时期：在出生后的前 6 个月，眼轴增长约 4mm，在接下来的 6 个月增长 2mm。在第 2 阶段（2 ~ 5 岁）和第 3 阶段（5 ~ 13 岁），生长速度变慢，每个阶段的眼轴增长约 1mm。

同样，伴随着眼球的增长，角膜直径在出生后的第 1 年也迅速增加。新生儿角膜水平直径平均为 9.5 ~ 10.5mm，成人增加至 12.0mm。角膜在第 1 年变平，角膜曲率值发生显著变化，从出生时的约 52.00D，到 6 个月的 46.00D，再到 12 个月 的 42.00 ~ 44.00D，接近成人测量值。轻度角膜混浊可见于健康的新生儿，在早产儿更常见，并随角膜逐渐变薄而消失。在妊娠 30 ~ 32 周，中心角膜厚度约 691 μ m，出生时减少到 564 μ m。

小儿晶状体的屈光度在出生后的最初几年急剧降低，这是婴幼儿白内障摘除后，人工晶状体植入术时需要认真考虑的重要因素。晶状体屈光度从出生时的 35.00D，下降到 2 岁时的 23.00D。随后，晶状体屈光度缓慢变化，至 11 岁下降到 19.00 D。此后几乎没有变化。

Gordon RA, Donzis PB. Refractive development of the human eye. *Arch Ophthalmol.* 1985; 103(6):785–789.

Kirwan C, O'Keefe M, Fitzsimon S. Central corneal thickness and corneal diameter in premature infants. *Acta Ophthalmol Scand.* 2005;83(6):751–753.

Refractive State

The refractive state of the eye changes as the eye's axial length increases and the cornea and lens flatten. In general, eyes are hyperopic at birth, become slightly more hyperopic until approximately age 7 years, and then experience a myopic shift until reaching adult dimensions, usually by about age 16 years (Fig 15-1). Emmetropization in the developing eye refers to the combination of changes in the refractive power of the anterior segment and in axial length that drive the eye toward emmetropia. The reduction in astigmatism that occurs in many infant eyes and the decreasing hyperopia that occurs after age 6–8 years are examples of emmetropization.

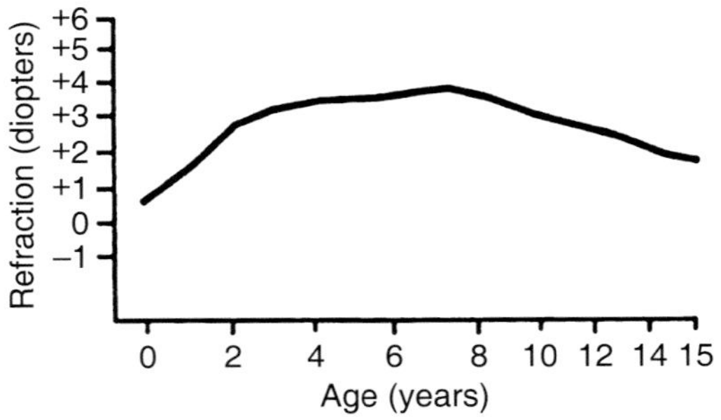

Figure 15-1 Change in mean refractive error as a function of age. *(Modified with permission from Eustis HS, Guthrie ME. Postnatal development. In: Wright KW, Strube YNJ, eds. Pediatric Ophthalmology and Strabismus. 2nd ed. New York: Springer-Verlag; 2003:49.)*

Race, ethnicity, and heredity play a role in the risk of particular types of refractive error. For example, myopia is more common among African American children compared with Hispanic children and non-Hispanic white children. Hyperopia is more common among non-Hispanic white children compared with African American and Hispanic children. Astigmatism is more common among Hispanic children and African American children than non-Hispanic white children.

Myopia is increasingly prevalent worldwide, and it is estimated that by 2050, 50% of the world population will be myopic. If myopia develops before age 10 years, there is a higher risk of eventual progression to myopia of 6.00 D or more. The etiology of increased myopia prevalence is unclear, but urbanization, increased near work, and decreased exposure to ultraviolet light are suggested influences. Low-dose (0.01%) atropine has been shown to significantly decrease myopic progression in Asian children.

Borchert MS, Varma R, Cotter SA, et al; Joint Writing Committee for the Multi-ethnic Pediatric Eye Disease Study and the Baltimore Pediatric Eye Disease Study Groups. Risk factors for hyperopia and myopia in preschool children: the Multi-ethnic Pediatric Eye Disease and Baltimore Pediatric Eye Disease Studies. *Ophthalmology.* 2011;118(10):1966–1973.

Chia A, Chua WH, Cheung YB, et al. Atropine for the treatment of childhood myopia: safety and efficacy of 0.5%, 0.1%, and 0.01% doses (Atropine for the Treatment of Myopia 2). *Ophthalmology.* 2012;119(2):347–354.

Holden BA, Fricke TR, Wilson DA, et al. Global prevalence of myopia and high myopia and temporal trends from 2000 through 2050. *Ophthalmology.* 2016;123(5):1036–1042.

McKean-Cowdin R, Varma R, Cotter SA, et al; Multi-ethnic Pediatric Eye Disease Study and the Baltimore Pediatric Eye Disease Study Groups. Risk factors for astigmatism in preschool children: the Multi-ethnic Pediatric Eye Disease and Baltimore Pediatric Eye Disease Studies. *Ophthalmology.* 2011;118(10):1974–1981.

屈光状态

随着眼轴长度增加、角膜和晶状体变平，眼睛的屈光状态也发生变化。一般来说，眼睛在出生时呈远视状态，7 岁时呈轻度远视；之后，经过近视化漂移，到 16 岁左右达到成人参数值（图 15-1）。发育中，眼的正视化过程是指在前节屈光力与眼轴长度的综合变化作用下，使眼向正视的方向发展。婴儿常见的散光逐渐减少，6 ~ 8 岁后的远视度数逐渐减少，都是正视化过程的例证。

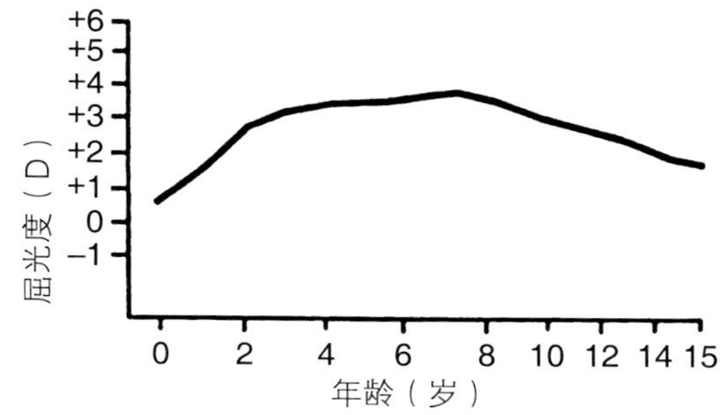

图 15-1　平均屈光度随年龄的变化。*（译者注：资料来源见前页原文。）*

人种、种族和遗传对某种类型的屈光不正的发展有作用。例如，与西班牙裔儿童和非西班牙裔白人儿童相比，近视在非洲裔美国儿童中更常见。与非洲裔美国人和西班牙裔儿童相比，远视在非西班牙裔白人儿童更常见。与非西班牙裔白人相比，散光在西班牙裔儿童和非洲裔美国儿童中更常见。

近视在世界范围内越来越普遍。据估计到 2050 年，50% 世界人口患有近视。如果 10 岁之前发生近视，那么近视最终发展成 6.00 D 以上的风险非常高。近视发病率增加的原因尚不清楚，但城市化、近距离工作增加和暴露于紫外线的机会减少可能对近视产生影响。已有研究表明，低浓度（0.01%）阿托品可显著降低亚洲儿童近视的进展。

Borchert MS, Varma R, Cotter SA, et al; Joint Writing Committee for the Multi-ethnic Pediatric Eye Disease Study and the Baltimore Pediatric Eye Disease Study Groups. Risk factors for hyperopia and myopia in preschool children: the Multi-ethnic Pediatric Eye Disease and Baltimore Pediatric Eye Disease Studies. *Ophthalmology*. 2011;118(10):1966–1973.

Chia A, Chua WH, Cheung YB, et al. Atropine for the treatment of childhood myopia: safety and efficacy of 0.5%, 0.1%, and 0.01% doses (Atropine for the Treatment of Myopia 2). *Ophthalmology*. 2012;119(2):347–354.

Holden BA, Fricke TR, Wilson DA, et al. Global prevalence of myopia and high myopia and temporal trends from 2000 through 2050. *Ophthalmology*. 2016;123(5):1036–1042.

McKean-Cowdin R, Varma R, Cotter SA, et al; Multi-ethnic Pediatric Eye Disease Study and the Baltimore Pediatric Eye Disease Study Groups. Risk factors for astigmatism in preschool children: the Multi-ethnic Pediatric Eye Disease and Baltimore Pediatric Eye Disease Studies. *Ophthalmology*. 2011;118(10):1974–1981.

Orbit and Ocular Adnexa

During infancy and childhood, orbital volume increases, and the orbital opening becomes less circular, resembling a horizontal oval. The lacrimal fossa becomes more superficial and the angle formed by the axes of the 2 orbits less divergent.

The palpebral fissure measures approximately 18 mm horizontally and 8 mm vertically at birth. Growth of the palpebral fissure is greater horizontally than vertically, resulting in the eyelid opening becoming less round and acquiring its elliptical adult shape. Most of the horizontal growth occurs in the first 2 years of life (see Chapter 17, Fig 17-1).

Cornea, Iris, Pupil, and Anterior Chamber

Central corneal thickness (CCT) decreases during the first 6–12 months of life (see the section Dimensions of the Eye). It then increases from approximately 553 µm at age 1 year to about 573 µm by age 12 years and stabilizes thereafter. CCT is similar in white and Hispanic children, whereas African American children tend to have thinner corneas.

Most changes in iris color occur over the first 6–12 months of life, as pigment accumulates in the iris stroma and melanocytes. Compared with the adult pupil, the infant pupil is relatively small. A pupil diameter less than 1.8 mm or greater than 5.4 mm is suggestive of an abnormality. The pupillary light reflex is normally present after 31 weeks' gestational age. At birth, the iris insertion is near the level of the scleral spur, but during the first year of life, the lens and ciliary body migrate posteriorly, resulting in formation of the angle recess.

Pediatric Eye Disease Investigator Group; Bradfield YS, Melia BM, Repka MX, et al. Central corneal thickness in children. *Arch Ophthalmol.* 2011;129(9):1132–1138.

Intraocular Pressure

Measurement of intraocular pressure (IOP) in infants can be difficult; results may vary depending on the method used and may not accurately represent the actual IOP. Nevertheless, normal IOP is lower in infants than in adults, and a pressure higher than 21 mm Hg should be considered abnormal. CCT influences the measurement of IOP, but this effect is not well understood in children. See Chapter 22 in this volume and BCSC Section 10, *Glaucoma*, for further discussion.

Extraocular Muscles

The rectus muscles of infants are smaller than those of adults; muscle insertions, on average, are 2.3–3.0 mm narrower, and the tendons are thinner in infants than in adults. In newborns, the distance from the rectus muscle insertion to the limbus is roughly 2 mm less than that in adults; by age 6 months, this distance is 1 mm less; and at 20 months, it is similar to that in adults.

Extraocular muscle function continues to develop after birth. Eye movements driven by the vestibular-ocular system are present as early as 34 weeks' gestational age. Conjugate horizontal gaze is present at birth, but vertical gaze may not be fully functional until 6 months of age. Intermittent strabismus occurs in approximately two-thirds of young infants but resolves in most by 2–3 months of age. Accommodation and fusional convergence are usually present by age 3 months.

眼眶和眼附属器

在婴儿期和儿童期，眼眶体积不断增大，眶口逐渐变小，呈水平椭圆形。泪腺窝逐渐变浅，两眼眶轴形成的开散夹角逐渐集合。

出生时，睑裂的水平方向长度约 18mm，垂直方向约 8mm。睑裂在水平向上的生长速度大于垂直方向的生长速度，这就导致随年龄增长，眼睑开口圆形逐渐改变，到成年时变为椭圆形。睑裂水平方向的生长多发生在 2 岁之前（见第 17 章，图 17–1）。

角膜、虹膜、瞳孔和前房

中央角膜厚度（CCT）在出生后 6 ～ 12 个月逐渐减小（见“眼的大小”一节）。随后，角膜厚度从 1 岁的 553μm 增加到 12 岁的 573μm，之后趋于稳定。白人和西班牙裔儿童的中央角膜厚度相似，而非洲裔美国儿童的角膜较薄。

虹膜颜色的变化大多发生在出生后 6 ～ 12 个月，是因为色素聚集在虹膜基质和黑色素细胞中。与成人的瞳孔相比，婴儿的瞳孔相对较小。瞳孔直径小于 1.8mm 或大于 5.4mm 均提示有异常。瞳孔光反射通常在妊娠 31 周后出现。出生时，虹膜附着点接近巩膜突的水平，但在出生后的一年内，晶状体和睫状体向后移动，最终形成房角隐窝。

Pediatric Eye Disease Investigator Group; Bradfield YS, Melia BM, Repka MX, et al. Central corneal thickness in children. *Arch Ophthalmol.* 2011;129(9):1132–1138.

眼压

测量婴儿眼压（IOP）很困难，其结果也可能因使用的方法不同而有差异，可能并不能准确地反映实际眼压。尽管如此，婴儿的正常眼压（IOP）低于成人，且眼压高于 21mmHg 应视为异常。中央角膜厚度（CCT）影响眼压的测量结果，但其对儿童的影响还未明确。进一步讨论见本册第 22 章和 BCSC 第 10 册《*青光眼*》。

眼外肌

婴儿的直肌比成人的小，肌肉附着点的宽度较成人约窄 2.3 ～ 3.0mm，且婴儿的肌腱比成人的薄。新生儿的直肌附着点到角膜缘的距离比成人约少 2mm，出生后 6 个月时，此差距缩小 1mm，20 岁时，与成人相同。

出生后，眼外肌的功能仍在发育完善。在前庭 – 眼系统作用下，眼球运动最早出现在妊娠 34 周。共轭水平凝视出生时即存在，但垂直凝视功能约到出生 6 个月时才能完成。约 2/3 的婴幼儿会有间歇性斜视，但大多数在出生后 2 ～ 3 个月会消失。调节和融像性集合在出生 3 个月时出现。

Retina

The macula is poorly developed at birth but changes rapidly during the first 4 years of life. Most significant are changes in macular pigmentation, development of the annular ring and foveal light reflex, and differentiation of cone photoreceptors. Improvement in visual acuity with age is due in part to development of the macula, specifically, differentiation of cone photoreceptors, narrowing of the rod-free zone, and an increase in foveal cone density (see Chapter 5). Retinal vascularization begins at the optic disc at 16 weeks' gestational age and proceeds to the peripheral retina, reaching the temporal ora serrata by 40 weeks' gestational age.

Hendrickson A, Possin D, Lejla V, Toth CA. Histologic development of the human fovea from midgestation to maturity. *Am J Ophthalmol.* 2012;154(5):767–778.

Visual Acuity and Stereoacuity

Visual acuity improvement in infancy and early childhood is attributable to neural development as well as ocular structural changes (see Chapter 16).

Two major methods are used to quantitate visual acuity in preverbal infants and toddlers: preferential looking (PL) and visual evoked potential (VEP). See Chapter 1 for a description of these methods. VEP studies show that visual acuity improves from approximately 20/400 in newborns to 20/20 by age 6–7 months. However, PL studies estimate the visual acuity of a newborn to be 20/600, improving to 20/120 by age 3 months and to 20/60 by 6 months. Further, PL testing shows that visual acuity of 20/20 is not reached until age 3–5 years. The discrepancy between measurements obtained by these 2 methods may be related to the higher cortical processing required for PL compared with VEP. Stereo acuity reaches 60 seconds of arc by about age 5–6 months (see Chapter 7).

Abnormal Growth and Development

Major congenital anomalies occur in 2%–3% of live births. Causes include chromosomal abnormalities, multifactorial disorders, and environmental agents, but many cases are idiopathic. Regardless of etiology, congenital anomalies may be categorized as shown in Table 15-2.

Table 15-2 Types of Congenital Anomalies

Anomaly	Defect	Ocular Example
Agenesis	Developmental failure	Anophthalmia
Hypoplasia	Developmental arrest	Optic nerve hypoplasia
Hyperplasia	Developmental excess	Distichiasis
Dysraphism	Failure to fuse	Choroidal coloboma
	Failure to divide or canalize	Congenital nasolacrimal duct obstruction
	Persistence of vestigial structures	Persistent fetal vasculature

视网膜

出生时，黄斑尚未发育完成，但在出生后 4 岁迅速发育。最显著的变化是黄斑色素化、环形圈和中心凹光反射的发育以及视锥细胞的分化。随着年龄的增长，视力的提高在一定程度上是由于黄斑的发育，具体来说，是视锥细胞的分化、无视杆细胞区的缩小以及视网膜中心凹视锥细胞密度的增加（见第 5 章）。在妊娠 16 周时，视网膜血管化从视盘起始，逐步扩展到周边视网膜，妊娠 40 周到达颞侧锯齿缘。

Hendrickson A, Possin D, Lejla V, Toth CA. Histologic development of the human fovea from midgestation to maturity. *Am J Ophthalmol.* 2012;154(5):767–778.

视力和立体视

婴儿期和儿童早期视力的改善主要是由于神经系统发育以及眼部结构的变化（见第 16 章）。

对于语前婴儿和刚刚学会走路的孩子，主要用 2 种方法来量化视力：优先注视法（PL）和视觉诱发电位（VEP）。有关这 2 种方法的描述见第 1 章。视觉诱发电位（VEP）研究表明，新生儿期的视力大约是 20/400，到 6 ~ 7 个月时视力提高到 20/20。然而，优先注视法（PL）研究也做出相应预估：新生儿的视力为 20/600，3 个月时提高到 20/120，6 个月时提高到 20/60。此外，优先注视法（PL）试验表明，人要到 3 ~ 5 岁时视力才能达到 20/20。这 2 种方法的测量值差异可能是由于与视觉诱发电位（VEP）研究法相比，优先注视法（PL）研究需要更高级的皮层处理。大约在 5 ~ 6 个月时，立体视达到 60 秒弧（见第 7 章）。

生长发育异常

2% ~ 3% 的存活婴儿可有先天性异常。原因包括染色体异常、多因素障碍和环境因素，但许多异常是特发性的。无论何种病因，先天异常的分类如表 15–2。

表15–2　先天性异常类型

异常现象	缺陷	眼部表现
发育不全	未发育	无眼症
发育不良	发育停止	视神经发育不良
发育过度	发育过剩	双行睫
闭合不全	未闭合	脉络膜缺损
	未能分离或管腔化	先天性鼻泪管阻塞
	退化结构的残留	永存性胚胎血管

A *malformation* implies a morphologic defect present from the onset of development or from a very early stage. A disturbance to a group of cells in a single developmental field may cause multiple malformations. Multiple etiologies may result in similar field defects and patterns of malformation. A single structural defect or factor can lead to a cascade, or domino effect, of secondary anomalies called a sequence. The Pierre Robin group of anomalies (cleft palate, glossoptosis, micrognathia, respiratory problems) may represent a sequence caused by underdevelopment of the mandible and is seen in disorders such as Stickler and fetal alcohol syndromes. A *syndrome* is a recognizable and consistent pattern of multiple malformations known to have a specific cause, which is usually a mutation of a single gene, a chromosome alteration, or an environmental agent. An association represents defects known to occur together in a statistically significant number of patients. An association may represent a variety of yet-unidentified causes. Two or more minor anomalies in combination significantly increase the likelihood of an associated major malformation.

Jones KL, Jones MC, del Campo M. *Smith's Recognizable Patterns of Human Malformation*. 7th ed. Philadelphia: Elsevier Saunders; 2013.

*畸形*是指发育开始或早期即出现的形态学异常。在某一发育部位的一组细胞的紊乱可能导致多种畸形。多种病因可能导致相似部位的异常和畸形。我们将某单一结构的缺陷或影响因素可以导致级联效应或多米诺骨牌效应的继发性异常，称为*后果*。Pierre Robin 综合征（腭裂、舌下垂、小颌畸形、呼吸道疾病）可能就是由于下颌骨发育不良而引起的一系列异常后果。还可见于 Stickler 综合征和胎儿酒精综合征等疾病。*综合征*是指可识别的、表现类型一致的、有特定病因的多种畸形的症候群，通常是单个基因突变、染色体改变或环境因素。关联症是指多种缺陷同时发生、且患者数量有统计学意义。一种关联症可能代表多种尚未明确的病因。联合 2 个或 2 个以上的微小异常增加了相关重大畸形发生的可能性。

Jones KL, Jones MC, del Campo M. *Smith's Recognizable Patterns of Human Malformation*. 7th ed. Philadelphia: Elsevier Saunders; 2013.

（翻译 姚森 朱丹 // 审校 石一宁 蒋宁 // 章节审校 石广礼）

CHAPTER 16

Decreased Vision in Infants and Pediatric Vision Rehabilitation

When an infant has not developed good visual attention or the ability to fixate on and follow objects by 3–4 months of age, the clinician must determine whether the decreased vision is due to an ocular or optic nerve (pregeniculate) condition, cerebral (retrogeniculate) visual impairment, or delayed visual maturation. This chapter discusses the classification of visual impairment in infants and children, as well as the evaluation and rehabilitation of these patients.

Visual Development in Young Infants

Visual development is a highly complex maturational process. Structural changes occur in both the eye and the central nervous system. Laboratory and clinical research has shown that normal vision develops as a result of both genetically programmed neural development and normal early visual experience.

A blink reflex to bright light should be present within a few days of birth. The pupillary light reflex is usually present after 31 weeks' gestation but can be difficult to evaluate in the early neonatal period because the newborn's pupils are miotic.

At approximately 6–8 weeks of age, the healthy full-term infant should be able to make and maintain eye contact with other humans and react with facial expressions. Infants aged 2–3 months should be interested in bright objects. By age 3–4 months, the nasal bias for smooth pursuit should have resolved, the eyes should be orthotropic, and fix-and-follow responses to a small (2–4 inches in diameter) toy should be present. Premature infants can be expected to reach these landmarks later, but there is not an exact week-for-week correlation for the attainment of these milestones.

Dysconjugate eye movements, skew deviation, and *sunsetting* (tonic downward deviation of both eyes) may be noted in healthy newborns but should not persist beyond approximately 3–4 months of age. Signs of poor visual development include searching eye movements, lack of response to familiar faces and objects, and nystagmus. Staring at bright lights and forceful rubbing or poking of the eyes (*oculodigital reflex*) in an otherwise visually disinterested infant are other signs of poor vision and suggest an ocular cause for the deficiency.

第 16 章

婴幼儿视力下降及儿童视力康复

当婴儿到 3 ～ 4 个月时，仍没有良好的视觉注意或固视和追随眼前物体的能力，临床医生必须要确定视力下降是否存在眼或视神经（膝状体前）、大脑（膝状体后）的视觉损害，或延迟视觉成熟。本章讨论婴幼儿和儿童视觉损害的分类，以及这些患者的视觉损害程度评估和视力康复。

婴幼儿的视觉发育

视觉发育是一个非常复杂的成熟过程。眼部和中枢神经系统都会发生相应的结构变化。实验和临床研究表明，在基因程序化下的神经系统发育和正常的早期视觉体验 2 个方面共同作用下，发育形成正常视力。

出生后几天内就出现对强光的瞬目反射。瞳孔光反射在妊娠 31 周后出现，但在新生儿早期很难判断，因为新生儿的瞳孔呈缩小状态。

出生后 6 ～ 8 周，健康足月婴儿能与他人进行眼神交流，并保持眼对视，且有面部表情反应。2 ～ 3 个月大的婴儿对明亮的物体感兴趣。3 ～ 4 个月，平滑追随注视的鼻侧眼位偏斜消失，呈现正眼位，具有对小型玩具（直径 2 ～ 4 英寸，1 英寸 =2.54cm）的固视和追随反应。早产儿发育达到上述标志性反应则需较长时间，但尚不能够确定具体到哪一周。

健康的新生儿可能出现眼球运动不协调、反向偏斜和*落日现象*（双眼张力性下偏视），但不会超过 3 ～ 4 个月。视觉发育不良的体征包括搜索性眼球运动、对熟悉的面孔和物体缺乏反应及眼球震颤。当婴儿视觉反应淡漠，而凝视明亮光照时使劲揉眼睛或戳指眼（*眼指反射*），即为另一种视力低下的体征，提示眼源性视觉障碍。

Classification of Visual Impairment in Infants and Children

The distinction between pregeniculate and cerebral visual impairment can be helpful in the context of infants who present with poor vision, although it should be recognized that some disorders cause both pregeniculate and retrogeniculate pathology. In addition, in some children, poor visual behavior normalizes over time, a phenomenon known as delayed visual maturation.

Pregeniculate Visual Impairment

Pregeniculate visual impairment results from pathology anterior to the lateral geniculate nucleus (the pregeniculate visual pathways). Causes of pregeniculate visual impairment in infants include corneal and lens opacities, glaucoma, retinal disorders, and optic nerve or optic tract abnormalities; these conditions are covered in detail elsewhere in this volume.

Cerebral Visual Impairment

Cerebral visual impairment (CVI; also termed *retrogeniculate visual impairment*) is the most frequent cause of childhood visual impairment in developed countries. The visual deficit results from pathology posterior to the lateral geniculate nucleus (retrogeniculate visual pathways). CVI is often referred to as cortical *visual impairment*, but the term *cerebral* is preferred because both subcortical (optic radiations) and cortical pathology can result in similar visual impairment. CVI can be transient or permanent and can be an isolated finding or associated with multiple neurologic deficits. Partial improvement in visual behavior may occur over the first few years of life.

CVI can be congenital or acquired. Prenatal and perinatal causes include intrauterine infection, structural central nervous system abnormalities, intracranial hemorrhage, periventricular leukomalacia (a prominent cause of visual impairment in premature children), hypoxia, seizures, and hydrocephalus. Acquired causes include accidental trauma, abusive head trauma, meningitis, and encephalitis.

Infants with CVI show variable degrees of impairment, from mildly decreased visual behavior to roving eye movements with complete absence of response to visual stimulation.

Delayed Visual Maturation

If normal visual fixation and tracking do not develop within the first 3–4 months of life, visual behavior may still normalize subsequently; this condition is termed *delayed visual maturation (DVM)*, or *cortical inattention*. There are 3 subgroups of infants with DVM: otherwise healthy infants; infants with systemic or neurologic abnormalities; and infants with associated ocular disorders presenting with poor vision out of proportion to the ocular condition.

In an otherwise healthy infant with suspected DVM, the following findings suggest a good visual and neurologic prognosis: some reaction to light, normal pupillary responses, no nystagmus, and normal ocular structures. If the visual behavior does not progress toward normal by 4–6 months of age, further investigation is warranted to assess for other causes of persistentvisual impairment.

Azmeh R, Lueder GT. Delayed visual maturation in otherwise normal infants. *Graefes Arch Clin Exp Ophthalmol.* 2013;251(3):941–944.

婴幼儿视觉损害的分类

区分膝状体前和脑性视觉损害有助于理解视力低下婴儿，尽管某些损害可以同时存在膝状体前和膝状体后的病变。此外，有些幼儿的视觉行为低下会随着时间正常化，这一现象被称为延迟视觉成熟。

膝状体前视觉损害

膝状体前视觉损害是由膝状体前到外侧膝状体核（膝状体前视觉传导通路）的病变引起。婴儿膝状体前视觉损害的病因，包括角膜和晶状体的混浊、青光眼、视网膜疾病、视神经或视束异常。具体讨论见本册其他部分。

脑性视觉损害

脑性视觉损害（CVI；也叫*膝状体后视觉损害*）是在发达国家儿童视觉损害的最常见原因。这种视力障碍是外侧膝状体核后的病变引起的（膝状体后视觉传导通路）。脑性视觉损害（CVI）通常又称为*脑皮质视觉损害*，但人们还是选用术语“*脑性*”，因为脑皮质下（视放射）和脑皮质的病变的视觉障碍表现相同。脑性视觉损害（CVI）呈短暂的，也可以是永久性的，可以是单一病变，也可以伴有多种神经性缺陷。在出生后几年内视觉行为可以部分改善。

脑性视觉损害（CVI）可以是先天性的，也可以是获得性的。孕期和围产期的病因包括宫内感染、中枢神经系统结构异常、颅内出血、脑室周白质软化症（早产儿视力损害的主要原因）、缺氧、癫痫和脑积水。获得性原因包括意外创伤、虐待性头部创伤、脑膜炎和脑炎。

患有脑性视觉损害（CVI）的婴儿可以表现为不同程度的视觉损害，可以是轻度的视觉行为低下，或是对视觉刺激完全无反应的巡回性眼球运动。

视觉发育迟缓

即使出生后 3 ~ 4 个月的婴儿没有发育形成正常的视觉固视和视觉追随，随后的视觉行为仍有可能恢复正常；这种现象称为*延迟视觉成熟（DVM）*或*皮质不注意*。延迟视觉成熟（DVM）分 3 个亚组：可能健康婴儿组、伴全身或神经系统异常的婴儿组和视力低下程度超出伴随眼部疾病的婴儿组。

在疑似延迟视觉成熟（DVM）的可能健康婴儿组中，以下发现提示视觉和神经系统预后良好：有一定的对光反应、正常瞳孔光反射、无眼球震颤及眼部结构正常。如果出生后 4 ~ 6 个月视觉行为向正常发育，则需要进一步评估持续性视觉损害的其他原因。

Azmeh R, Lueder GT. Delayed visual maturation in otherwise normal infants. *Graefes Arch Clin Exp Ophthalmol.* 2013;251(3):941–944.

Evaluation of the Infant With Decreased Vision

Family history may identify hereditary causes of pregeniculate visual impairment. Details of the pregnancy are important; factors such as in utero exposure to infection, drugs, alcohol, or radiation; trauma; and maternal diabetes mellitus may predispose to pregeniculate impairment and/or CVI. Perinatal problems such as prematurity, intrauterine growth retardation, fetal distress, bradycardia, meconium staining, and oxygen deprivation may be associated with CVI. In addition, the clinician should inquire about systemic abnormalities, delayed developmental milestones, and postnatal causes of brain injury.

Parental observations of the child's visual behavior should be noted. In a child with CVI, visual attentiveness may fluctuate widely; the family may report that the child sometimes seems to see and at other times does not appear to see at all.

Vision in the infant is assessed qualitatively by clinical appraisal and optokinetic nystagmus responses, and quantitatively by preferential looking tests—for example, Teller Acuity Cards II (Stereo Optical, Inc, Chicago, IL) or the Cardiff Acuity Test—and visual evoked potential (VEP); see Chapter 1 for a discussion of these quantitative tests. VEP results may be either normal or subnormal in CVI. Infants with ocular motor apraxia (see Chapter 12) may falsely appear to have poor vision due to impaired horizontal eye movements, but vertical movements are usually spared.

Pupillary responses are sluggish with certain pregeniculate causes of visual impairment such as retinal dystrophies and optic nerve abnormalities. Paradoxical pupils (pupillary constriction in response to darkness) can occur with these conditions. In contrast, pupillary responses are normal in infants with CVI.

In the setting of poor vision, nystagmus in infancy should raise suspicion for sensory nystagmus due to a pregeniculate disorder (see Chapter 13). Conversely, poor visual be havior with normal ocular examination results, normal pupillary responses, and no nystagmus by 3 months of age is more likely to represent CVI or DVM. Congenital motor nystagmus usually does not present with poor vision but is occasionally associated with DVM.

Anterior segment and fundus examinations may reveal a pregeniculate cause of the visual impairment, such as bilateral cataracts, bilateral macular colobomas or scars, bilateral optic nerve hypoplasia, bilateral optic atrophy, or foveal hypoplasia with or without albinism or aniridia. However, some retinal causes of pregeniculate visual impairment may not be associated with any visible abnormalities on fundus examination. Sometimes optic nerve abnormalities may be present even though the primary cause of visual impairment is CVI: descending optic atrophy (from transsynaptic degeneration) may coexist with CVI, and in preterm infants, optic disc cupping resembling that seen in glaucoma can occur as a result of transsynaptic degeneration, most commonly secondary to periventricular leukomalacia.

If the ocular examination is unrevealing yet suspicion is high for a pregeniculate cause of visual impairment (eg, when poor vision is accompanied by nystagmus), then electroretinography (ERG) may be indicated to diagnose a retinal dystrophy. ERG results are normal in CVI.

Neuroimaging studies in CVI may be normal, in which case the visual prognosis tends to be more favorable, or may reveal changes such as cerebral atrophy, porencephaly in the occipital (striate or parastriate) cortex, damage to the optic radiations, or periventricular leukomalacia.

视力低下婴儿的评估

家族史可以确定膝状体前视觉损害的遗传学病因。妊娠的细节很重要，宫内感染、药物、酒精或辐射、创伤、母体糖尿病，易发生膝状体前视觉损害和（或）脑性视觉损害（CVI）。围产期问题，如早产、宫内发育迟缓、胎儿窘迫、心动过缓、胎便染色、缺氧等，可能与脑性视觉损害（CVI）有关。此外，医生应了解全身系统异常、发育迟缓和产后脑损伤的原因。

应该重视父母对孩子视觉行为的观察。脑性视觉损害（CVI）儿童的视觉注意波动很大，家长会主诉孩子有时似乎能看见，有时则完全看不见。

婴儿视力可以通过临床和眼动性眼震反应进行定性评估，并通过优先注视试验，如，Teller 视力卡 II（Stereo Optical, Inc, Chicago, IL），或 Cardiff 敏敏度试验，或视觉诱发电位（VEP）进行定量评估。关于这些定量测试方法的讨论见第 1 章。脑性视觉损害（CVI）患儿的视觉诱发电位（VEP）正常，或低于正常。眼球运动失用的婴儿（见第 12 章），由于眼水平运动受损，可能出现假性视力低下，但仍保留眼垂直运动。

伴有某些膝状体前性的视觉损害的瞳孔光反应迟缓，如视网膜营养不良和视神经异常。在这些情况下，会出现矛盾性瞳孔常现象（即在黑暗环境下瞳孔缩小）。相反，脑性视觉损害（CVI）患儿的瞳孔光反射正常。

视力低下时的婴儿眼球震颤，应考虑系膝状体前疾病的感觉性眼球震颤（见第 13 章）。相反，眼科检查和瞳孔光反射正常，且出生后 3 个月无眼震的视觉低下者，则提示患有脑性视觉损害（CVI）或延迟视觉成熟（DVM）。先天性运动性眼球震颤不伴有视力低下，但偶尔伴有延迟视觉成熟（DVM）。

眼前节和眼底检查可诊断视觉损害的膝状体前的病因，如双眼白内障、双眼黄斑缺损或疤痕、双眼视神经发育不良、双眼视神经萎缩、伴或不伴白化病或无虹膜的中心凹发育不良。然而，有些膝状体前视觉损害的视网膜病变，眼底检查无明显异常。有时脑性视觉损害（CVI）是视觉损害的原发性病因，但视神经也有异常：如下行性视神经萎缩（源于跨突触变性）可能同时伴有脑性视觉损害（CVI）；早产儿可出现与青光眼相同的视杯，系跨突触变性，常继发于脑室周白质软化症。

如果眼部检查没有异常，但仍高度怀疑因膝状体前病变导致视觉损害（如视力低下伴眼球震颤），视网膜电图（ERG）可用于诊断视网膜营养不良。脑性视觉损害（CVI）患儿的视网膜电图（ERG）正常。

脑性视觉损害（CVI）患儿的神经影像检查可能正常，提示视觉预后较好；也可能会有改变，如脑萎缩、枕叶皮层（纹状体或纹旁区）的脑穿通畸形、视放射损伤或脑室周白质软化症。

Pediatric Low Vision Rehabilitation

Vision rehabilitation should be recommended when a child has a visual impairment that affects his or her ability to access the visual environment (as occurs with best-corrected visual acuity worse than 20/40 in the better-seeing eye, decreased visual field, central field loss, reduced contrast sensitivity, nyctalopia, or impaired visual processing). From diagnosis onward, the ophthalmologist plays an important role in recommending that children with low vision receive comprehensive vision rehabilitation. Early referral is essential for setting the family and child on a course to achieve optimal visual performance, access to instruction, and safe and in dependent mobility, and for enabling children with acquired visual impairment to adjust successfully to vision loss. Even though preschoolaged children may function well without any low vision aids, early-intervention programs can offer important stimulation and introduce strategies for transition to school.

Pediatric vision rehabilitation involves pediatric ophthalmologists, vision rehabilitation clinicians, teachers of the visually impaired (TVI), occupational therapists, teachers, orientation and mobility specialists, technology experts, state societies, and other professionals and Organizations. In the United States, a variety of approaches exist to educate children with visual impairments. Some states have state-funded residential schools for the visually impaired. Elsewhere, districts may cluster students with visual impairment into one school. More commonly, neighborhood schools work with itinerant TVI. An Individualized Education Plan (IEP) outlines the needs of an individual child in the school setting. The child's needs at home and in other nonacademic settings must be considered as well.

Many children can function well with partial sight, with the help of low vision aids, whereas others will benefit from braille literacy, which is most easily acquired in childhood. Because most children have large accommodative amplitudes, enabling them to hold a given object closer than normal to enlarge its retinal image, magnification may not be necessary for very young patients with low vision. However, accommodative amplitudes decrease and visual demands increase with age (as students are faced with smaller print size), so holding objects closer may not be a sustainable strategy for older children. Printed material can be enlarged, and dome-type magnifiers may be helpful for performing near work; video magnification can be used for near-or distance-vision tasks. For distance viewing, handheld monocular telescopes may help. Tablets, smartphones, e-textbooks, and text-to-speech conversion have greatly expanded the opportunities available to visually impaired children and have the benefit of being socially acceptable for older children trying to fit in with their peers. Table 16-1 lists sources of information on low vision.

The American Academy of Ophthalmology's Preferred Practice Pattern guidelines on vision rehabilitation outline the rehabilitation process for preschool-aged children to young adults. The availability of rehabilitation resources varies across communities, but the following online resources, which can be searched by location, may be helpful for clinicians and families in identifying such ser vices in their community: afb.org /directory.aspx (American Federation for the Blind) and tsbvi.edu / tagged-resources (Texas School for the Blind and Visually Impaired resources home page). To learn about the Academy's Initiative in Vision Rehabilitation, visit the Low Vision and Vision Rehabilitation page, which also offers a patient handout, available on the ONE Network at https://www.aao.org /low-vision-and-vision-rehab.

儿童低视力康复

当视觉损害影响到婴儿接触视觉环境的能力时（如较好眼的最佳矫正视力低于 20/40、视野缩小、中央视野缺损、对比敏感度下降、夜盲症或视觉通路损伤），建议进行视力康复。从诊断开始，眼科医生就对低视力儿童的综合视力康复具有重要的作用。早期转诊是至关重要的，其目的是为了使家长和患儿向实现最佳视觉功能的方向一起努力，并能够得到有效指导、安全独立的行走，并且使获得性视力障碍的儿童能够成功地适应视力丧失。即使学龄前儿童在不使用任何低视力辅助设备的情况下也可以正常生活，但在入学过渡期的早期干预能为他们提供重要的激励，并引入适应策略。

儿童视力康复需要小儿眼科医生、视力康复医师、视觉障碍教师（TVI）、职业治疗师、老师、定向与运动专家、技术人员、国家社会团体及其他的专业人士和组织。在美国，能够为视觉障碍儿童提供教育的途径很多。有些州还为视觉障碍儿童设立了政府资助的寄宿学校。其他地方会把分布在不同区域的视觉障碍学生集中到同一所学校。更常见的是，社区学校与巡回视觉障碍教师合作。个性化教育计划（IEP）提出学校中孩子的个性化需求。也要考虑孩子在家里和其他非学习环境中的需求。

在低视力辅助设备的帮助下，许多患儿即使仅有部分视力，也可以正常生活。没有辅助设备的患儿，可以采用 braille 盲文识字，这在儿童时期最容易获得。由于大多数儿童的调节幅度很大，低龄患者不需要放大效应，他们可以把物体拿到更近处，使视网膜成像放大。然而，随着年龄的增加，调节幅度降低、视觉需求增加（因为学生需要看更小的打印字体），大龄儿童不能持久把物体拿得很近，放大印刷材料、圆顶型放大镜可能有助于视近工作。视频放大器可以用于视近或视远工作。视远时，手持式单目望远镜会有帮助。平板电脑、智能手机、电子书以及文本 - 语音转换器等，大大地增加了视觉障碍儿童的视物机会，并有助于大龄患儿努力融入同龄人生活并为社会所接受。表 16-1 列出了低视力的信息来源。

美国眼科学会的视力康复临床指南，概述了学龄前儿童到青少年的康复过程。不同社区的康复资源可用性不同，但下面这些可以搜索到的在线资源，可以帮助临床医生和家人找到自己所在社区的此类服务 :afb.org/directory.aspx（美国盲人联合会）和 tsbvi.edu/tagged-resources（得克萨斯州盲人学校和视障资源主页）。要了解《学会视力康复倡议》，请访问“低视力和视力康复”页面，该页面还提供了患者手册，可访问 ONE Network https://www.aao.org/low-vision-and-vision-rehab。

Table 16-1 Sources of Information on Low Vision

American Council of the Blind; www.acb.org
American Foundation for the Blind; www.afb.org
American Printing House for the Blind, Inc; www.aph.org
Large-print and braille books, tapes, talking computer software, and low vision aids
Family Support America; www.familysupportamerica.org
For parent support groups in the United States
Learning Ally; www.learningally.org
Audiobooks for the blind and dyslexic
Lighthouse Guild; www.lighthouseguild.org
National Federation of the Blind; www.nfb.org
National Library Service for the Blind and Physically Handicapped, Library of Congress; https://www.loc.gov/nls
Free library program of braille and audio materials, including books and magazines
National Organization for Albinism and Hypopigmentation; www.albinism.org
Prevent Blindness; www.preventblindness.org
National Toll-Free Numbers
American Council of the Blind; (800) 424-8666
New York Times Large-Print Weekly; (800) 631-2580
Reader's Digest Large Print; (877) 732-4438

See also BCSC Section 3, *Clinical Optics*, for a detailed discussion of low vision aids.

American Academy of Ophthalmology Vision Rehabilitation Committee. Preferred Practice Pattern Guidelines. *Vision Rehabilitation.* San Francisco: American Academy of Ophthalmology; 2013. For the latest guidelines, go to https://www.aao.org/guidelines-browse?filter =preferredpracticepatterns.

表16－1　低视力患者的信息来源

美国盲人理事会; www.acb.org American
盲人基金会; www.afb.org
美国盲文出版社Inc; www.aph.org
大型印刷和盲文书籍、磁带、会说话的电脑软件和低视力辅助设备
家庭支持美国 ;www.familysupportamerica.org
美国家长支持团体
学习联盟; www.learningally.org
盲人和阅读困难者的有声读物
灯塔协会 ; www.lighthouseguild.org
全美盲人联合会; www.nfb.org
为盲人和残疾人士服务的国家图书馆，国会图书馆; https://www.loc.gov/nls
免费图书项目有盲文和有声资料，包括书和杂志
全国白化病和色素减退组织; www.albinism.org
防盲 ; www.preventblindness.org
全国免费电话号码
美国盲人理事会 ; (800) 424 - 8666
《纽约时报》大字周刊; (800)631 - 2580
读者文摘大字版; (877) 732 - 4438

有关低视力辅助设备的详细讨论见 BCSC 第 3 册《*临床光学*》。

American Academy of Ophthalmology Vision Rehabilitation Committee. Preferred Practice Pattern Guidelines. *Vision Rehabilitation.* San Francisco: American Academy of Ophthalmology; 2013. For the latest guidelines, go to https://www.aao.org/guidelines-browse?filter =preferredpracticepatterns.

（翻译 朱丹 // 审校 石一宁 蒋宁 // 章节审校 石广礼）

CHAPTER 17

Eyelid Disorders

This chapter includes a related video, which can be accessed by scanning the QR code provided in the text or going to www.aao.org/bcscvideo_section06.

Eyelid anatomy is described in BCSC Section 2, *Fundamentals and Principles of Ophthalmology*, and Section 7, *Oculofacial Plastic and Orbital Surgery*. Section 7 also discusses many of the eyelid disorders covered in this chapter.

Congenital Eyelid Disorders

Eyelid malformations can be isolated or associated with orbital malformations; they can also represent features of a syndrome. Because of these possibilities, systematic evaluation of the eyelids and ocular adnexa may be an important part of the clinical evaluation of a dysmorphic infant.

Morphologic measurements of the eyelids and orbit can be compared with normal reference measurements and may have clinical significance (Fig 17-1; see also Chapter 18). The *Farkas canthal index*, defined as the ratio of inner canthal distance to outer canthal distance, can also be used. A canthal index lower than 38 signifies *ocular hypotelorism* (smaller-than-average distance between the eyes), and a canthal index greater than 42 indicates *ocular hypertelorism* (greater-than-average distance between the eyes). Ethnic variations may occur.

Dystopia Canthorum

Dystopia canthorum is lateral displacement of both the inner canthi and the lacrimal puncta such that an imaginary vertical line connecting the upper and lower puncta crosses the cornea (Fig 17-2). The displacement is a characteristic feature of Waardenburg syndrome type 1.

Cryptophthalmos

Cryptophthalmos is a rare condition resulting from failed differentiation of eyelid structures. There is partial or complete absence of the palpebral fissure, as the skin extends uninterrupted from the forehead to the cheek, covering the eye (Fig 17-3). The adnexa are partially developed and fused to the anterior segment; the cornea is usually malformed.

第 17 章

眼睑疾病

本章包含一个相关视频，可通过扫描文本提供的二维码或者登录进行访问 www.aao.org/bcscvideo_section06。

眼睑解剖见 BCSC 第 2 册《*眼科学基础与原理*》及第 7 册《*眼面部整形与眼眶手术*》。第 7 册也讨论了本章所涵盖的许多眼睑疾病。

先天性眼睑疾病

眼睑畸形可与眼眶畸形有关或是无关，也可以表现为一种综合征的特征。由于这些可能性，对眼睑和眼附属器的系统评估是畸形婴儿临床评估的重要组成部分。

眼睑和眼眶的形态学测量可与正常参考值进行比较，可能具有临床意义（图 17–1; 见第 18 章）。也可以使用 *Farkas 眦指数*，其定义为内眦间距与外眦间距的比值。Canthal index 小于 38 表示*眼间距过短*（小于双眼之间的平均距离），Farkas 眦指数大于 42 表示*眼间距过长*（大于双眼之间的平均距离）。可存在种族差异。

内眦外移

内眦外移是指内眦部及泪小点的向外侧移位，连接上下泪小点的垂直线穿过角膜（图 17–2）。这种移位是 1 型 Waardenburg 综合征的特征。

隐眼

隐眼是由于眼睑结构未分化而导致的罕见病症。睑裂部分的或完全的缺失，皮肤从前额连续延伸到睑颊，覆盖眼部（图 17–3）。眼附属器部分发育，并融合到前节；角膜畸形。

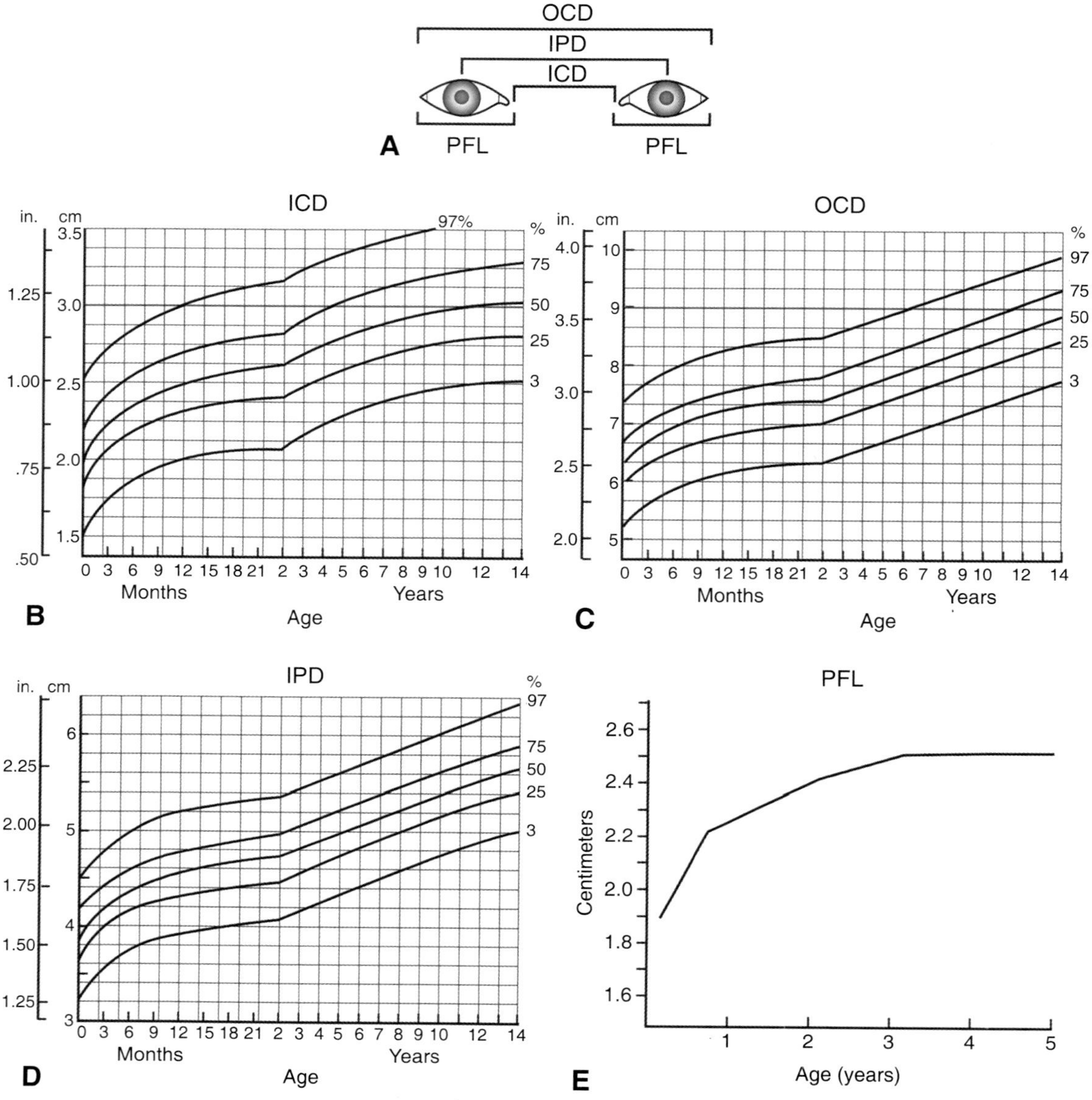

Figure 17-1 **A**, Schematic representation of measurements involved in the evaluation of the orbital region. OCD = outer canthal distance; IPD = interpupillary distance; ICD = inner canthal distance; PFL = palpebral fissure length. **B**, ICD measurements according to age. **C**, OCD measurements according to age. **D**, IPD measurements according to age. E, PFL measurements according to age. *(Modified with permission from Dollfus H, Verloes A. Dysmorphology and the orbital region: a practical clinical approach.* Surv Ophthalmol. *2004;49(6):549.)*

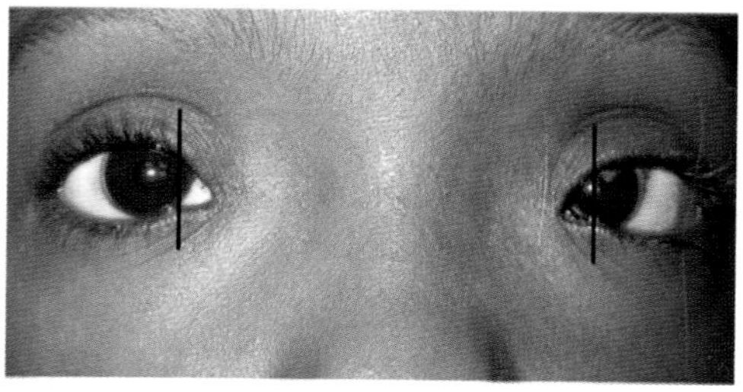

Figure 17-2 Dystopia canthorum in a patient with Waardenburg syndrome. Note that the *vertical lines* drawn through the puncta intersect the cornea. *(Courtesy of Amy Hutchinson, MD.)*

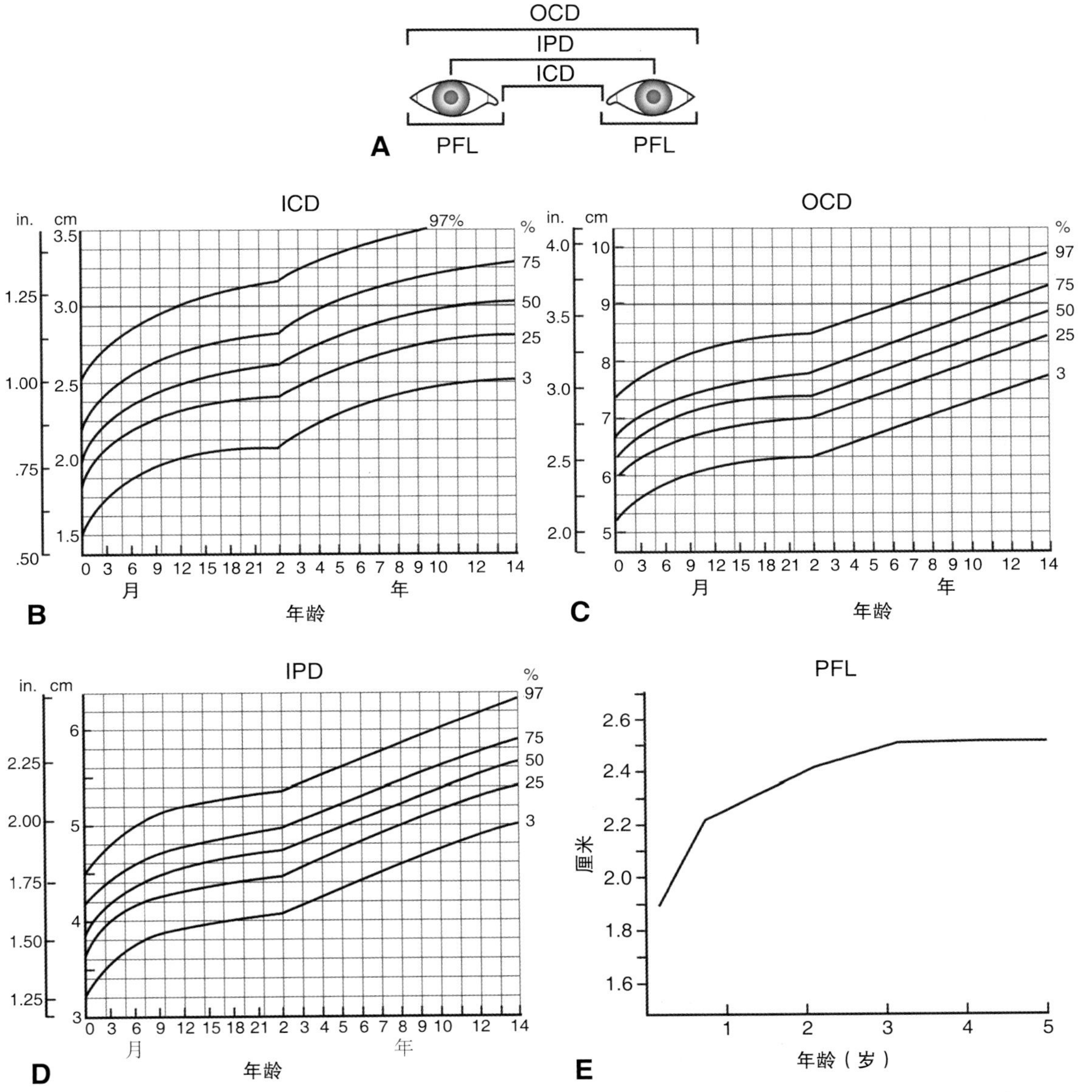

图 17–1　A. 眼眶区域评估的测量示意图。OCD= 外眦间距; IPD= 瞳距; ICD= 内眦间距; PFL= 睑裂长度。**B.** 随年龄变化的内眦间距（ICD）测量值。**C.** 随年龄变化的外眦间距（OCD）测量值。**D.** 随年龄变化的瞳距（IPD）测量值。E, 随年龄变化的睑裂长度（PFL）测量值。*（译者注：资料来源见前页原文。）*

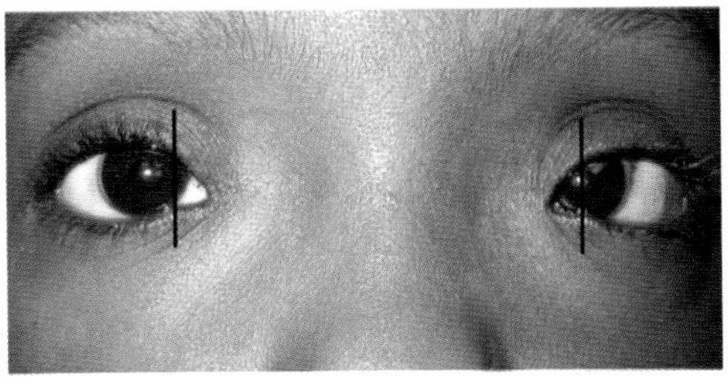

图 17–2　一位 Waardenburg 综合征患者的内眦外移。注意，连接泪小点的*垂直线*与角膜相交。*（译者注：资料来源见前页原文。）*

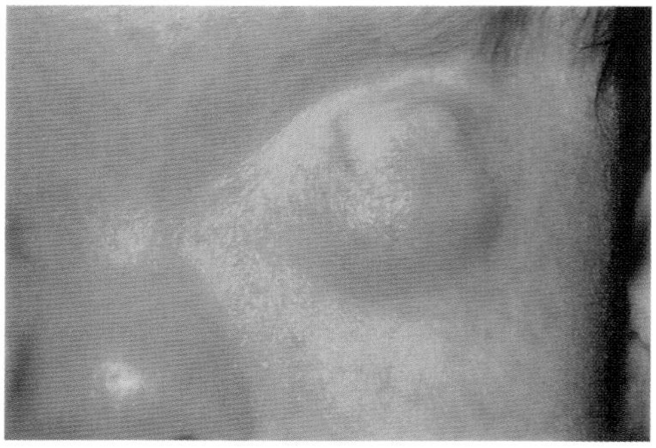

Figure 17-3 Cryptophthalmos, left eye.

Fraser syndrome, an autosomal recessive disorder characterized by partial syndactyly and genitourinary anomalies, may include unilateral or bilateral cryptophthalmos and other ocular malformations.

Ablepharon

Ablepharon, absence or severe hypoplasia of the eyelids, is very rare. Affected patients are at high risk for exposure keratopathy. Ablepharon is a characteristic feature of ablepharonmacrostomia syndrome.

Congenital Coloboma of the Eyelid

Congenital eyelid coloboma (eyelid cleft or notch) usually involves the upper eyelid and can range from a small notch to a defect encompassing the horizontal length of the eyelid. The eyelid may be fused to the globe (Fig 17-4). Eyelid colobomas are unrelated to other ocular colobomas and are commonly associated with Goldenhar syndrome or amniotic band syndrome. The eye of an infant with a congenital eyelid coloboma should be monitored for exposure keratopathy. Surgical closure of the eyelid defect is required in most cases.

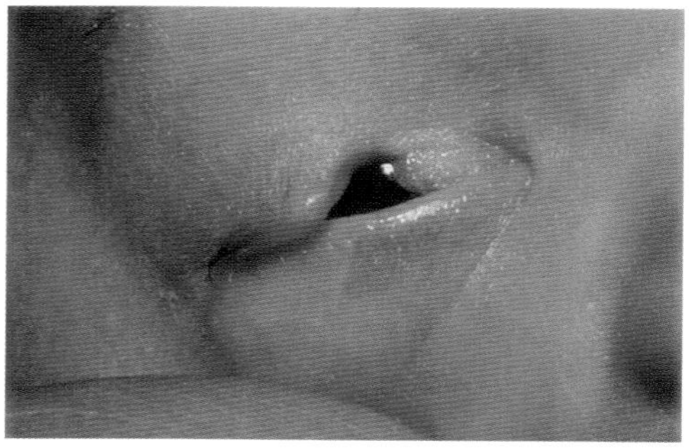

Figure 17-4 Congenital eyelid coloboma (cleft), right eye. The eyelid is fused to the globe.

Ankyloblepharon

Fusion of part or all of the eyelid margins is termed *ankyloblepharon*. This condition may be dominantly inherited. Treatment is surgical. In *ankyloblepharon filiforme adnatum*, avariant of ankyloblepharon, the margins of the upper and lower eyelids are joined by fine strands of tissue (Fig 17-5). This variant is seen in Hay-Wells syndrome (also known as *ankyloblepharon–ectodermal dysplasia–clefting syndrome*), a form of ectodermal dysplasia that includes cleft lip or palate. The eyelid adhesions in children with ankyloblepharon filiforme adnatum can often be easily separated in the office with blunt scissors and topical anesthesia.

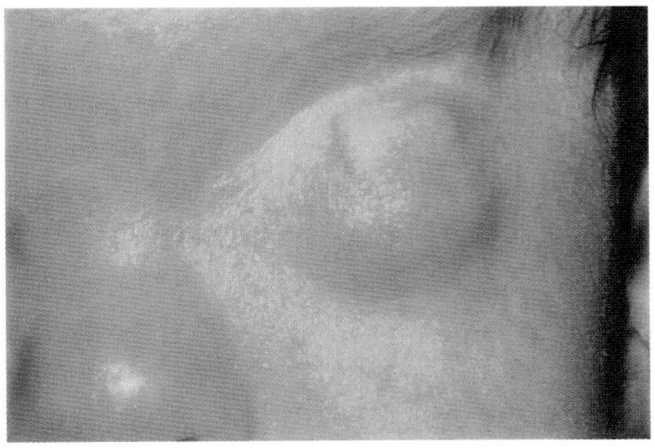

图 17–3　隐眼，左眼。

*Fraser 综合征*是一种常染色体隐性遗传病，以部分并指畸形和泌尿生殖系统异常为特征，可能包括单眼或双眼隐眼和其他眼部畸形。

无睑畸形

无睑畸形，即眼睑缺失或严重发育不全，是极为罕见的。受累患者极易并发暴露性角膜病变。无睑畸形是无睑 – 巨口综合征的特征。

先天性眼睑缺损

先天性眼睑缺损（眼睑裂开或缺口）通常累及上眼睑，缺损从一个小缺口到覆盖眼睑水平长度的缺损。眼睑可能与眼球融合（图 17–4）。眼睑缺损与其他眼部缺损无关联，通常与 Goldenhar 综合征或者羊膜带综合征有关。对于先天性眼睑缺损的婴儿应该要监测暴露性角膜病变。大多数情况下，眼睑缺损需要手术闭合。

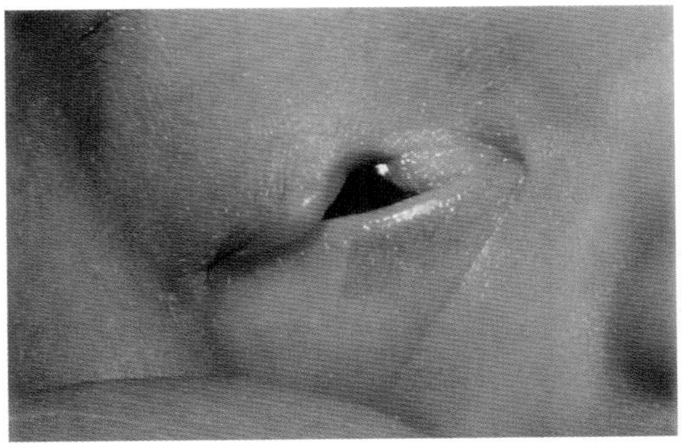

图 17–4　先天眼睑缺损（裂开），右眼。眼睑与眼球融合。

睑缘粘连

部分的或者全部的睑缘融合在一起称为*睑缘粘连*。主要是遗传性的。治疗是外科手术。在*丝状睑缘粘连*中，一种眼睑粘连的变异，上下睑缘由细小组织粘连在一起。这种变异见于 Hay-Wells 综合征（又称*睑叶 – 外胚层发育不全综合征*），这是外胚层发育不良的一种形式，包括唇裂或腭裂。丝状睑缘粘连患儿的眼睑融合常在门诊局麻下，用钝剪刀即可分离。

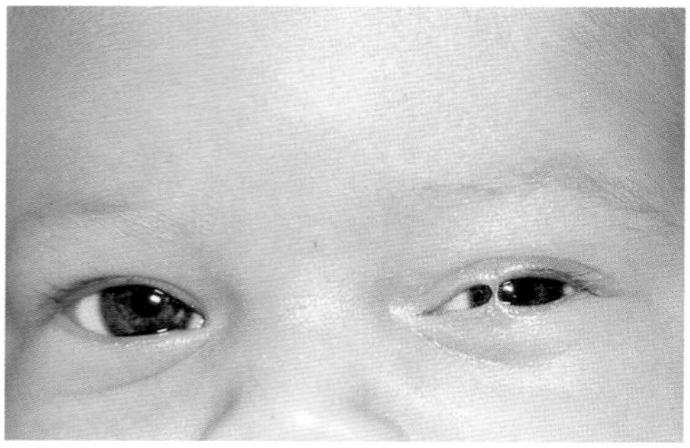

Figure 17-5 Ankyloblepharon filiforme adnatum. The eyelid margins are fused by a fine strand of tissue. *(Courtesy of Amy Hutchinson, MD.)*

Congenital Ectropion

Congenital ectropion is a rare abnormality characterized by eversion of the eyelid margin. It usually involves the lower eyelid and is secondary to a vertical deficiency of the skin. Lateral tarsorrhaphy may be effective for mild cases. More severe cases may require a skin flap or graft.

Congenital Entropion

Congenital entropion is a rare abnormality characterized by eyelid margin inversion. It does not resolve spontaneously. Surgery should be performed when corneal integrity is threatened.

Epiblepharon

Epiblepharon is a common congenital anomaly characterized by a horizontal fold of skin adjacent to the eyelid margin (most commonly the lower eyelid) that may turn the eyelashes inward, against the cornea (Fig 17-6). Infants' corneas often tolerate this condition surprisingly well. Unlike congenital entropion, epiblepharon often resolves spontaneously. Ocular lubricants may be beneficial. Surgical repair is required when the condition does not resolve or it causes chronic corneal irritation.

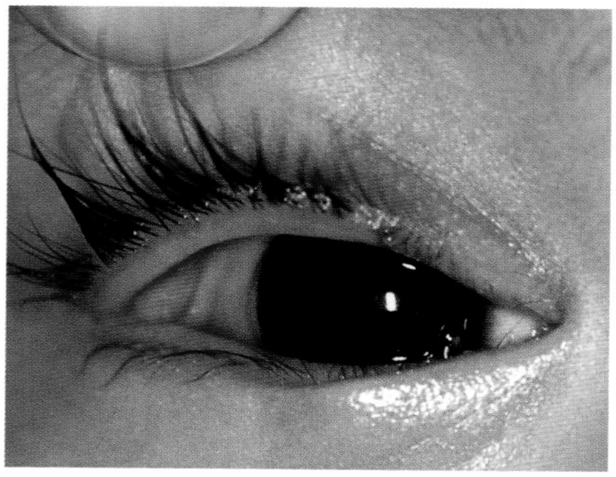

Figure 17-6 Epiblepharon, right eye. The medial lower eyelid eyelashes are turned inward, causing corneal irritation. *(Courtesy of Gregg T. Lueder, MD.)*

Congenital Tarsal Kink

In congenital tarsal kink, the tarsal plate of the upper eyelid is folded at birth, resulting in entropion. The cornea may be exposed and traumatized, leading to ulceration. The clinician can manage minor defects by manually unfolding the tarsus and taping the eyelid shut with a pressure dressing for 1–2 days. More severe cases require surgical incision of the tarsal plate or excision of a V-shaped wedge from the inner surface to permit unfolding.

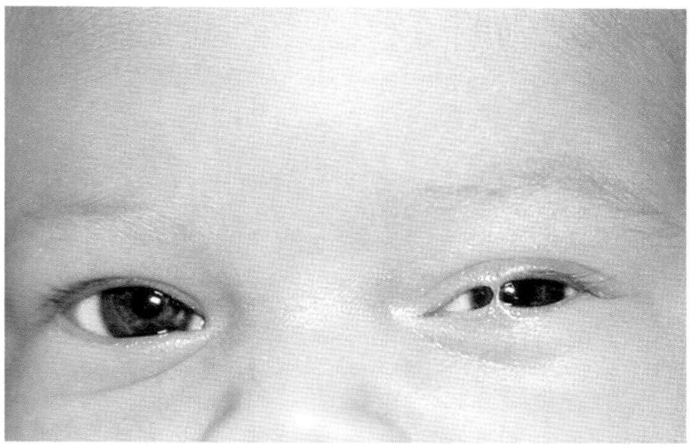

图 17–5　丝状睑缘粘连。眼睑边缘由细小组织粘连在一起。*（译者注：资料来源见前页原文。）*

先天性睑外翻

先天性睑外翻是一种罕见的以睑缘外翻为特征的畸形。通常累及下眼睑，继发于皮肤垂直缺损。外侧睑缘缝合术对轻度病例有效。更严重的病例需要皮瓣或移植物。

先天性睑内翻

先天性睑内翻是一种罕见的以睑缘内翻为特征的畸形，不会自发地恢复正常。当角膜完整性受损时，应进行手术。

眼睑赘皮

眼睑赘皮是一种常见的先天性异常，其特征是眼睑边缘（最常见的是下眼睑）附近的皮肤水平褶皱，可致睫毛内转，接触角膜（图 17–6）。婴儿的角膜对此有很好的耐受性。与先天性内翻不同，眼睑赘皮常自行消退。润眼液可能是有益的。当情况没有好转，或引起慢性角膜刺激症状时，需手术。

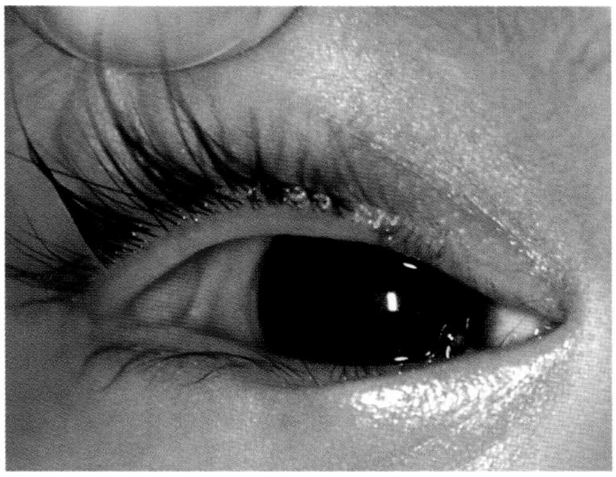

图 17–6　眼睑赘皮，右眼。下眼睑内侧的睫毛向内翻转，导致角膜刺激症状。*（译者注：资料来源见前页原文。）*

先天性睑板扭结

先天性睑板扭结，指出生时上睑板折叠，导致睑内翻。角膜可能会暴露和损伤，导致溃疡。对轻度扭结，医生可以通过手法使折叠的睑板展开，胶布粘贴使眼睑闭合，加压包扎 1 ~ 2d。严重的病例需手术切开睑板或从内表面行 V 形楔状切除，使其展开。

Distichiasis

In distichiasis, an extra (partial or complete) row of eyelashes arises from or slightly posterior to the meibomian gland orifices (Fig 17-7). The abnormal eyelashes tend to be thinner, shorter, softer, and less pigmented than normal cilia and are therefore often well tolerated. Removal of the abnormal eyelashes with electrolysis or cryotherapy, or eyelid surgery, may be indicated if chronic corneal irritation is present.

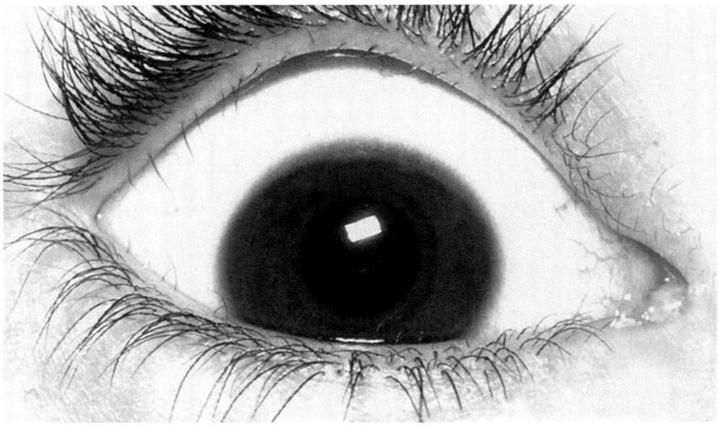

Figure 17-7 Distichiasis. An accessory row of eyelashes exits from the meibomian gland orifices. *(Reproduced with permission from Patil BB, Bell R, Brice G, Jeffery S, Desai SP. Distichiasis without lymphoedema? Eye (Lond). 2004;18(12):1270–1272.)*

Euryblepharon

In euryblepharon, the lateral aspect of the palpebral aperture is enlarged, with downward displacement of the temporal half of the lower eyelid. This condition gives the appearance of a very wide palpebral fissure or a droopy lower eyelid. Euryblepharon may occur in Kabuki syndrome. Most patients do not require treatment.

Epicanthus

Epicanthus refers to a crescent-shaped fold of skin running vertically between the eyelids and overlying the inner canthus (Fig 17-8). There are 4 types:

- *epicanthus tarsalis*: The fold is most prominent in the upper eyelid.
- *epicanthus inversus*: The fold is most prominent in the lower eyelid.
- *epicanthus palpebralis*: The fold is equally distributed between the upper and lower eyelids.
- *epicanthus supraciliaris*: The fold arises from the eyebrow and terminates over the lacrimal sac.

Epicanthus inversus may be isolated or associated with blepharophimosis–ptosis–epicanthus inversus syndrome or ptosis. Surgical correction is only occasionally required.

双行睫

在双行睫中，一排额外的（部分或完整的）睫毛从睑板腺孔或其稍后方出现（图 17–7）。与正常睫毛相比，异常睫毛更细、更短、更柔软、色素更少，因此可被较好耐受。若有慢性角膜刺激症状，可用电解、冷冻疗法或眼睑手术去除异常睫毛。

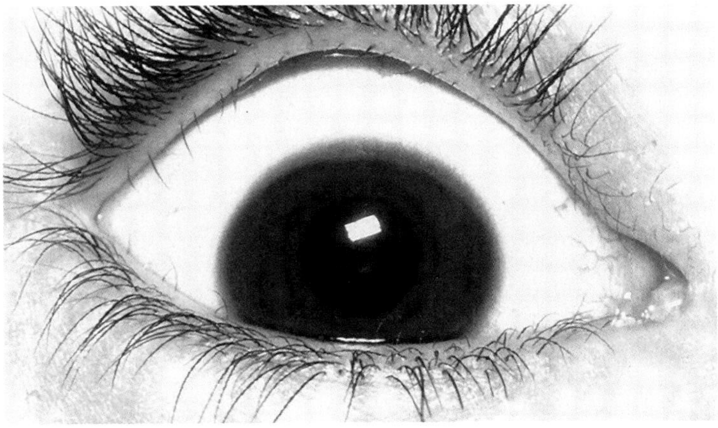

图 17–7　双行睫。一排附属睫毛从睑板腺孔中伸出。*（译者注：资料来源见前页原文。）*

阔睑裂

在阔睑裂中，睑裂外侧扩大，下睑颞侧向下移位。呈现出很宽的睑裂或下垂的下睑。阔睑裂可发生 Kabuki 综合征。大多数病人不需要治疗。

内眦赘皮

*内眦赘皮*是指一种月牙形的皮肤皱褶，垂直于眼睑之间，覆盖在内眦角上（图 17–8）。分为 4 型：

- *睑板型内眦赘皮*：上睑的褶皱最突出。
- *反向型内眦赘皮*：下睑的褶皱最突出。
- *睑型内眦赘皮*：褶皱均匀分布在上下眼睑。
- *眉型内眦赘皮*：褶皱从眉毛开始，到泪囊结束。

反向型内眦赘皮可独立存在，或与睑裂狭小 – 上睑下垂 – 反向型内眦赘皮综合征、上睑下垂共存。偶需手术矫正。

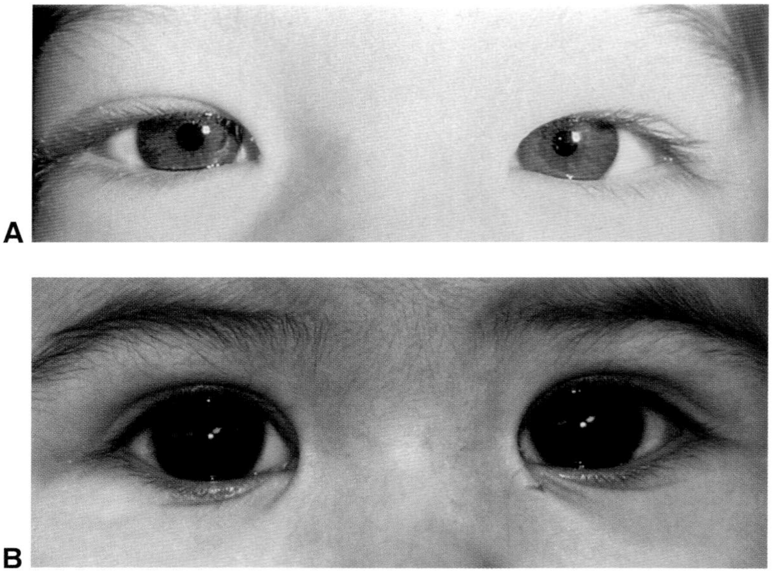

Figure 17-8 Epicanthus, bilateral. **A**, Epicanthus tarsalis. **B**, Epicanthus palpebralis. *(Part A reproduced with permission from Crouch E.* The Child's Eye: Strabismus and Amblyopia. *Slide script. San Francisco: American Academy of Ophthalmology; 1982. Part B courtesy of Robert W. Hered, MD.)*

Palpebral Fissure Slants

In the normal eye, the eyelids are generally positioned so that the lateral canthus is approximately 1 mm higher than the medial canthus. Slight upward or downward slanting of palpebral fissures normally occurs on a familial basis or in certain racial and ethnic groups (eg, Asians). An upward or downward slant is a characteristic feature of some craniofacial syndromes (eg, downward slant in Treacher Collins syndrome; see Chapter 18, Fig 18-9). Slanting of the palpebral fissures may be associated with A- or V-pattern strabismus (see Chapter 10).

Congenital Ptosis

Ptosis (ie, blepharoptosis) can be congenital or acquired. It is important to differentiate congenital ptosis from acquired cases with systemic associations (Table 17-1; see also BCSC Section 7, *Oculofacial Plastic and Orbital Surgery*). Congenital ptosis is usually caused by decreased levator muscle function. It may be familial. Anisometropic amblyopia and strabismus are common associations.

Table 17-1 Classification of Ptosis

- Pseudoptosis
- Congenital ptosis
- Acquired ptosis
  - Myogenic ptosis
    - Myasthenia gravis
    - Chronic progressive external ophthalmoplegia
  - Neurogenic ptosis
    - Horner syndrome
    - Third nerve palsy
  - Mechanical ptosis

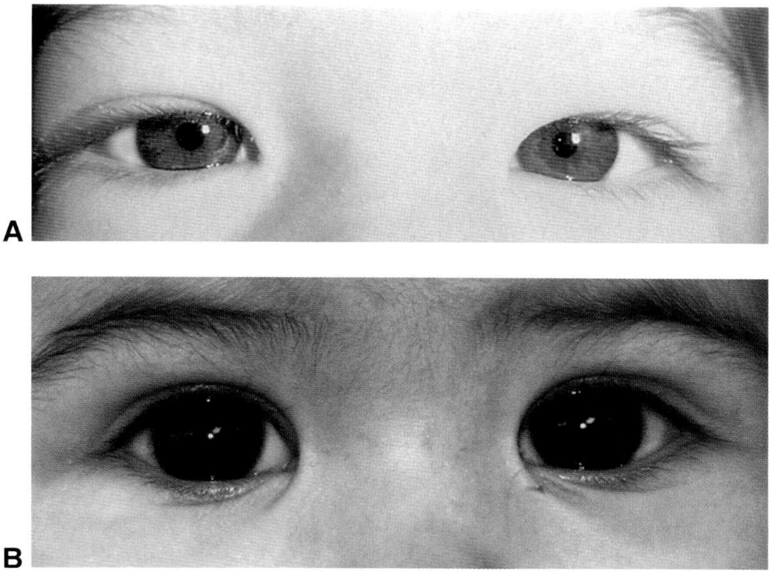

图 17-8　内眦赘皮，双眼。**A.** 睑板型内眦赘皮。**B.** 睑型内眦赘皮。*（译者注：资料来源见前页原文。）*

睑裂歪斜

在正常眼中，眼睑外眦角的位置比内眦角约高 1mm。睑裂轻微上斜或下斜多有家族史，或见于一些种族和民族（如亚裔）。睑裂上斜或下斜是一些颌面综合征的特征（例如，在 Treacher Collins 综合征中下斜，见第 18 章，图 18-9）。睑裂倾斜可伴有 A 型或 V 型斜视（见第 10 章）。

先天性上睑下垂

上睑下垂（即眼睑下垂）是先天性或后天性的。先天性与后天性上睑下垂重要的鉴别在于是否伴有全身系统性疾病（表 17-1，见 BCSC 第 7 册《*眼面部整形与眼眶手术*》）。先天性上睑下垂是由提上睑肌功能低下引起的，有家族史。常伴有屈光参差性弱视和斜视。

表17-1　上睑下垂分类

- 假性上睑下垂
- 先天性上睑下垂
- 后天性上睑下垂
    - 肌源性上睑下垂
        - 重症肌无力
        - 慢性进行性眼外肌麻痹综合征
    - 神经源性上睑下垂
        - 霍纳综合征
        - Ⅲ颅神经麻痹
    - 机械性上睑下垂

Evaluation of ptosis requires assessment of the upper eyelid crease, the palpebral fissure height, and levator muscle function. In severe congenital ptosis, the eyelid crease is usually absent. The clinician can determine the amount of ptosis by measuring the distance between the upper and lower eyelids and the margin–reflex distance (MRD). MRD_1 is the distance from the margin of the upper eyelid to the corneal light reflex when the eye is in primary position. Levator muscle function is assessed by measuring the distance that the upper eyelid moves when the patient shifts from downgaze to upgaze; during measurement, the examiner uses digital pressure on the brow to block recruitment of the frontalis muscle.

Tear function, corneal sensitivity, and the Bell phenomenon should also be evaluated because corneal exposure may occur after surgical repair, should it be necessary. Tear function can be assessed by evaluating the tear lake and tear breakup time, as well as checking for the presence of punctate keratitis. Corneal sensitivity can be assessed by the presence of a blink reflex when the cornea is touched with the tip of a cotton swab. In addition, the clinician should determine whether the globe is microphthalmic or whether a hypotropia is present, as either of these may produce pseudoptosis.

Marked congenital ptosis that obstructs vision must be corrected early in infancy to prevent deprivation amblyopia. Correction of severe ptosis usually requires frontalis suspension because of the lack of levator muscle function. Autologous or allogeneic fascia lata and synthetic material such as silicone rods are some of the materials used for suspension. Autologous fascia, however, cannot be obtained until the patient is 3 or 4 years old. Use of synthetic material or allogeneic fascia lata may lead to higher recurrence rates. Repair of mild or moderate ptosis can usually be performed when the patient is older, although the presence of a compensatory chin-up head position may justify earlier surgery. External levator muscle resection is typically performed for mild or moderate congenital ptosis.

Blepharophimosis–ptosis–epicanthus inversus syndrome

Blepharophimosis–ptosis–epicanthus inversus syndrome (BPES; also referred to as *congenital eyelid syndrome or blepharophimosis syndrome*) may occur as a sporadic or autosomal dominant disorder with features of blepharophimosis, epicanthus inversus, telecanthus, and ptosis. There are 2 types of BPES, both of which include abnormalities of the eyelid; type I also includes premature ovarian failure. Mutations in the *FOXL2* gene have been found in both types. The palpebral fissures are shortened horizontally and vertically (blepharophimosis), levator muscle function is poor, and no upper eyelid fold is present (Fig 17-9). The length of the horizontal palpebral fissure, normally 25–30 mm, is only 18–22 mm in these patients. Repair of the ptosis, usually with frontalis suspension procedures, may be necessary early in life. Because the epicanthus and telecanthus may improve with age, repair of these defects is often delayed.

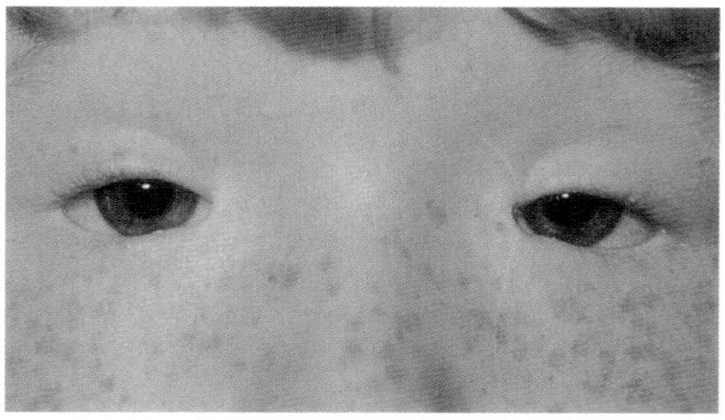

Figure 17-9 Blepharophimosis–ptosis–epicanthus inversus syndrome. Note telecanthus as well.

评估上睑下垂需要评估上睑皱褶、睑裂高度和提上睑肌功能。严重的先天性上睑下垂常没有眼睑皱褶。医生可以通过测量上下眼睑的距离和睑缘反射距离（MRD）来确定上睑下垂的程度。MRD_1 是眼睛处于第一眼位时，从上眼睑缘到角膜映光点的距离。评估提上肌功能，是测量患者从向下注视到向上注视时，上眼睑移动的距离。在测量过程中，检查者指压眉弓以阻止额肌参与。

必要时，泪液功能、角膜敏感性和 Bell 现象也应评估，因为手术修复后可能发生角膜暴露。泪液功能可通过评估泪湖和泪液破裂时间进行评估，以及检查是否存在点状角膜炎。角膜的敏感性可通过用棉签的尖端接触角膜时眨眼反射的存在进行评估。此外，医师应确定是否为小眼畸形或下斜视，因为这 2 种情况可导致假性上睑下垂。

明显的先天性上睑下垂影响视力时，须在婴儿期早期矫正，以防发生剥夺性弱视。由于严重上睑下垂的提上睑肌功能丧失，需额肌悬吊。自体或同种异体阔筋膜以及合成材料，如硅棒，是用于悬吊的材料。自体阔筋膜需要到 3 ~ 4 岁时才能获得。合成材料或同种异体阔筋膜的复发率较高。尽管代偿性下颌上抬头位需早期手术，但是轻度或中度上睑下垂的矫正可在患者年龄较大时进行。外路提上睑肌缩短术用于轻度或中度先天性上睑下垂患者。

睑裂狭小 – 上睑下垂 – 倒向型内眦赘皮综合征

睑裂狭小 – 上睑下垂 – 倒向型内眦赘皮综合征　睑裂狭小 – 上睑下垂 – 倒向型内眦赘皮综合征（BPES；*又称先天性眼睑综合征或先天性小睑裂综合征*）可能是一种散发性或常染色体显性疾病，具有睑裂狭小、倒向型内眦赘皮、内眦距增宽和上睑下垂的特征。睑裂狭小 – 上睑下垂 – 倒向型内眦赘皮综合征（BPES）有 2 型，都包括眼睑异常；I 型还包括卵巢功能早衰。2 型中都发现了 *FOXL2* 基因突变。睑裂水平性和垂直性缩短（小睑裂）、提上睑肌功能差、无上睑皱褶（图 17–9）。水平睑裂长度正常为 25 ~ 30mm，这些患者只有 18 ~ 22mm。幼儿上睑下垂的修复常用额肌悬吊术。由于内眦赘皮和内眦距过宽可随着年龄而改善，其修复应该推迟。

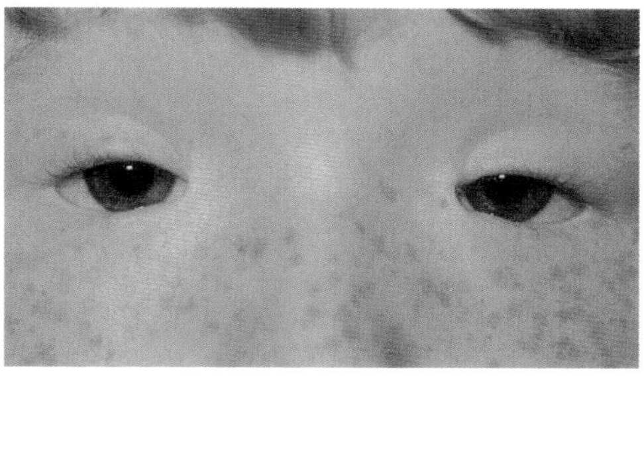

图 17–9　睑裂狭小 – 上睑下垂 – 倒向型内眦赘皮综合征。也要注意内眦距增宽。

Marcus Gunn jaw-winking syndrome

Marcus Gunn jaw-winking syndrome (also known as *co-contractive retraction with jaw–eyelid synkinesis syndrome [CCRS], type 5*) is a synkinetic syndrome in which the eyelid elevates with movement of the jaw; it may present with ptosis. In Video 17-1, note elevation of the left eyelid with movement of the jaw. The synkinesis is thought to be caused by aberrant connections between the motor division of cranial nerve V and the levator muscle. The clinician may test an infant for this condition by having the child suck on a bottle or pacifier. Many patients do not require treatment. If the ptosis is amblyogenic or a chin-up head position develops, ptosis surgery may be indicated.

VIDEO 17-1 Marcus Gunn jaw-winking ptosis.
Courtesy of Mary A. O'Hara, MD.
Access all Section 6 videos at www.aao.org /bcscvideo_section06.

Other Causes of Ptosis in Children

Ptosis may occur in children as a result of several other disorders, including third nerve palsy, monocular elevation deficiency, myasthenia gravis, congenital fibrosis of the extraocular muscles, chronic progressive external ophthalmoplegia, and Horner syndrome. It may also be associated with several systemic disorders, including Turner, Cornelia de Lange, and fetal alcohol syndromes. These entities are discussed elsewhere in this book and in other BCSC volumes.

Infectious and Inflammatory Eyelid Disorders

Inflammatory masses of the eyelids are common in children. *Chalazia* are caused by blockage of the meibomian glands, with secondary irritation due to lipid extravasation. *Hordeola* are localized infections of eyelid glands. Treatment of both disorders includes warm compresses and management of associated blepharitis. Supplements containing omega-3 fatty acids may be beneficial in some patients. Surgical treatment is reserved for large, painful, or chronic lesions.

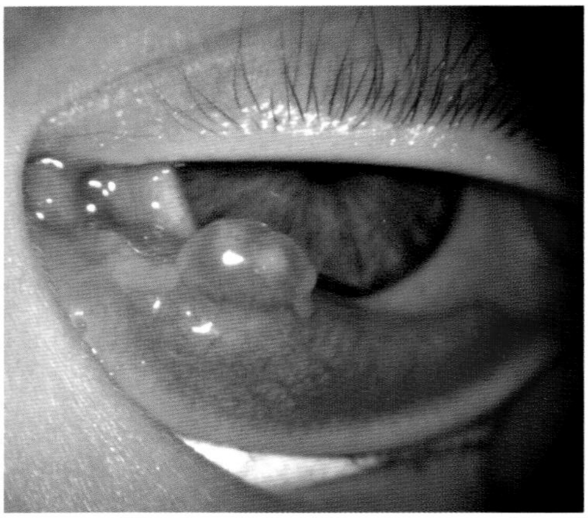

Figure 17-10 Pyogenic granuloma on tarsal conjunctiva at the site of a chalazion. *(Reproduced with permission from Lueder GT. Pediatric Practice Ophthalmology. New York: McGraw-Hill Professional; 2010:178.)*

Marcus Gunn 下颌 – 瞬目综合征

下颌瞬目综合征（也称为*痉挛性收缩伴下颌眼睑联动综合征 [CCRS]，5 型*）是一种联带运动综合征，眼睑随着下颌的运动而抬高；可存在上睑下垂。在视频 17–1 中，左眼睑随着下颌的运动而抬高。这种联带运动是 V 颅神经的运动支与提上睑肌间的异常连接引起的。医生可以让婴儿用奶瓶或奶嘴吮吸来检查婴儿是否患有这种疾病。许多病人无须治疗。如果上睑下垂形成弱视或者出现下颌上抬头位，可进行上睑下垂手术。

视频 17–1　下颌瞬目综合征。*（译者注：资料来源见前页原文。）*
大家可通过网站www.aao.org /bcscvideo_section06中访问所有的第6册视频。

儿童上睑下垂的其他原因

儿童上睑下垂可由其他疾病引发，包括Ⅲ颅神经麻痹、单眼上转缺陷、重症肌无力、先天性眼外肌纤维化、慢性进行性外眼肌麻痹综合征和 Horner 综合征。它也可能与一些系统性疾病相关，包括 Turner 综合征、Cornelia de Lange 综合征和胎儿乙醇综合征。这些疾病在本册其他章节和 BCSC 其他分册中讨论。

感染性和炎性眼睑疾病

儿童眼睑炎性包块很常见。*睑板腺囊肿*是由睑板腺阻塞引起的，脂质外溢引起继发性刺激症状。*睑腺炎*是眼睑腺体的局部感染。这 2 种疾病的治疗包括热敷和眼睑炎的治疗。补充 ω–3 脂肪酸可能会对一些患者有益。较大的、疼痛性的或者慢性的病变可手术治疗。

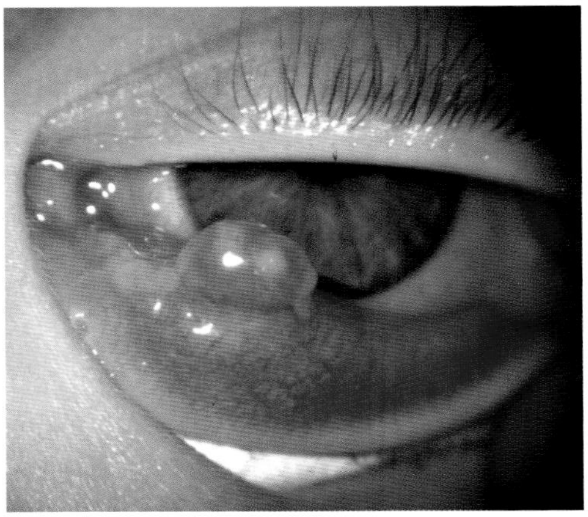

图 17–10　睑结膜上睑板腺囊肿位置的化脓性肉芽肿。*（译者注：资料来源见前页原文。）*

Pyogenic granuloma (lobular capillary hemangioma)—a pedunculated, fleshy pink hemangiomatous growth—can develop on the tarsal conjunctiva, overlying a chalazion or trauma site (Fig 17-10). Patients with *molluscum contagiosum* may present with characteristic lesions of the eyelids and secondary follicular conjunctivitis (see Chapter 20).

Vascular Eyelid Disorders

Port-Wine Stain

Port-wine stain (PWS; also known as *port-wine nevus* or *nevus flammeus*) is a congenital vascular malformation that manifests as a flat red or pink cutaneous lesion. It may lighten during the first year of life but then tends to become darker, thicker, and more nodular over time. PWS is associated with Sturge-Weber and Klippel-Trénaunay-Weber syndromes (see Chapter 28) and is seen in combination with ocular melanosis in phakomatosis pigmentovascularis. Glaucoma can occur in affected eyes (see Chapter 22). Lasers can be used to lighten the affected areas.

Eyelid Hemangioma

Hemangiomas are common vascular lesions that may involve the eyelid or orbit. They are discussed in Chapter 18.

Neoplasms and Other Noninflammatory Eyelid Lesions

Malignant tumors arising from eyelid skin or palpebral conjunctiva are extremely rare in children. Pediatric cases are likely to be associated with underlying systemic disorders that predispose to malignancy, such as basal cell nevus syndrome or xeroderma pigmentosum. Rhabdomyosarcoma infrequently presents as an eyelid or conjunctival mass (see Chapter 18). Eyelid and epibulbar lesions can develop in juvenile xanthogranuloma (see Chapter 21).

Pilomatricoma

Pilomatricomas (sometimes spelled *pilomatrixomas* or called *Malherbe calcifying epitheliomas*) are benign tumors that arise from hair matrix. They may present as solid, noninflamed lesions, often with a whitish appearance (Fig 17-11). Surgical excision is curative.

Epithelial Lesions

Numerous types of benign superficial lesions may arise on the eyelids, including squamous papillomas, epidermal inclusion cysts, verruca vulgaris, and milia. These are discussed in BCSC Section 7, *Oculofacial Plastic and Orbital Surgery.*

化脓性肉芽肿（小叶毛细血管瘤），一种带蒂的肉粉色血管瘤生长物，生长在睑结膜，覆盖在睑板腺囊肿或外伤的部位（图 17–10）。*传染性软疣*患者可能会出现眼睑特征性病变和继发性滤泡性结膜炎（见第 20 章）。

血管性眼睑疾病

鲜红斑痣

鲜红斑痣（PWS，*又称葡萄酒样痣或火焰痣*）是一种先天性血管畸形，表现为扁平的红色或粉色皮肤病变。出生后第一年颜色较浅，但随着时间会变得更黑、更厚，呈结节状。鲜红斑痣（PWS）伴有 Sturge–Weber 和 Klippel–Tr é naunay–Weber 综合征（见第 28 章），在色素血管性斑痣性错构瘤病中与眼黑素沉着病合并出现。受累眼可发生青光眼（见第 22 章）。激光治疗可使受病灶区域颜色变浅。

眼睑血管瘤

血管瘤是常见的血管病变，可累及眼睑或眼眶，见第 18 章讨论。

肿瘤和其他非炎症性眼睑病变

源于眼睑皮肤和睑结膜的恶性肿瘤在儿童中极为罕见。儿童肿瘤可能与潜在的易患恶性肿瘤的系统性疾病有关，如基底细胞痣综合征、着色性干皮病。横纹肌肉瘤很少表现为眼睑或结膜肿块（见第 18 章）。幼年黄色肉芽肿可发展为眼睑或眼表病变（见第 21 章）。

毛母质瘤

毛母质瘤（有时也拼写为 *pilomatrixomas* 或称为 *Malherbe 钙化上皮瘤*）是一种源自毛母质的良性肿瘤。它可能表现为实性、非炎性病变，呈白色外观（图 17–11）。手术切除可治愈。

上皮病变

眼睑可出现多种良性浅表病变，包括鳞状上皮乳头状瘤、表皮包涵囊肿、寻常疣和粟丘疹。见 BCSC 第 7 册《*眼面部整形与眼眶手术*》讨论。

Eyelid Nevi

Nevi arise from nevus cells, incompletely differentiated melanocytes in the epidermis and dermis and in the junction zone between these 2 layers, and are the third most common benign lesions encountered in the periocular region (after papillomas and epidermal inclusion cysts). The management of simple eyelid nevi in children is similar to that in adults (see BCSC Section 7, *Oculofacial Plastic and Orbital Surgery*).

Congenital nevocellular nevi

Congenital nevocellular (also called melanocytic) nevi can occur on the eyelids (Fig 17-12) and may cause visual deprivation amblyopia. They may undergo malignant transformation, the risk of which increases with the size of the lesion; large lesions (>20 cm) have a 5%–20% risk of malignant transformation. Observation is often recommended for small (<1.5 cm) and medium-sized (1.5–20.0 cm) lesions.

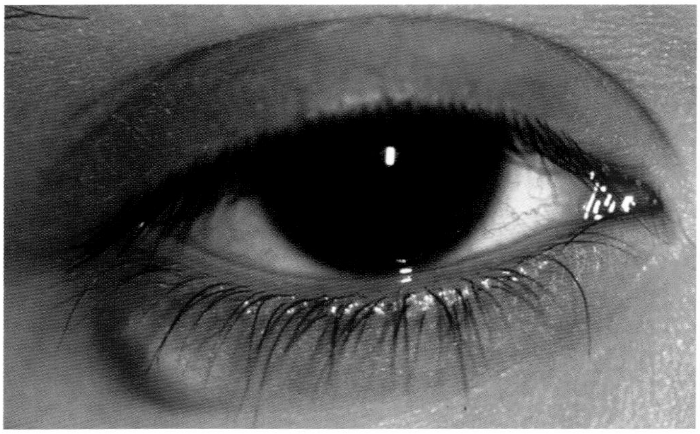

Figure 17-11 Pilomatricoma, right lower eyelid. Note the whitish center. *(Reproduced with permission from Lueder GT.* Pediatric Practice Ophthalmology. *New York: McGraw-Hill Professional; 2010:84.)*

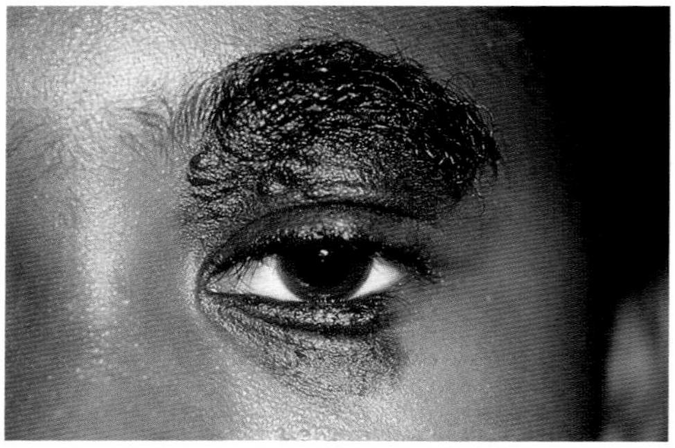

Figure 17-12 Congenital nevocellular nevus of the eyelid. *(Courtesy of Amy Hutchinson, MD.)*

Other Eyelid Conditions

Trichotillomania

Trichotillomania is characterized by the pulling out of one's hair, often including the eyebrows and eyelashes. It may be associated with obsessive-compulsive disorder. The characteristic appearance includes madarosis, broken hairs, and regrowth of hairs of varying lengths (Fig 17-13).

眼睑痣

痣起源于痣细胞，表皮和真皮层以及这两层之间的交界处存在的分化不完全的黑色素细胞，是眼周排名第三的最常见的良性病变（仅次于乳头状瘤和表皮包涵囊肿）。儿童单纯性眼睑痣的治疗与成人相似（见 BCSC 第 7 册《*眼面部整形与眼眶手术*》）。

先天性痣细胞痣

先天性痣细胞痣（也称为黑色素细胞痣）可发生在眼睑（图 17–12），并可导致视觉剥夺性弱视。其可转化为恶性，转化为恶性的风险随病灶的增大而增加，恶性转化的风险为 5% ~ 20%。建议对较小（<1.5 cm）和中等（1.5 ~ 20.0 cm）的病灶进行观察。

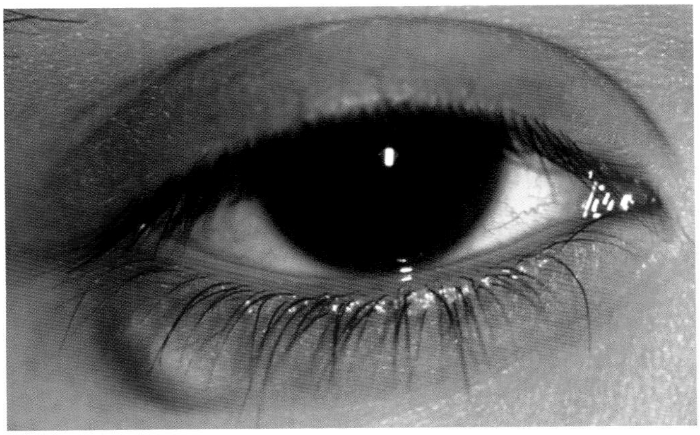

图 17–11　毛母质瘤，右眼下睑，白色的中心。*（译者注：资料来源见前页原文。）*

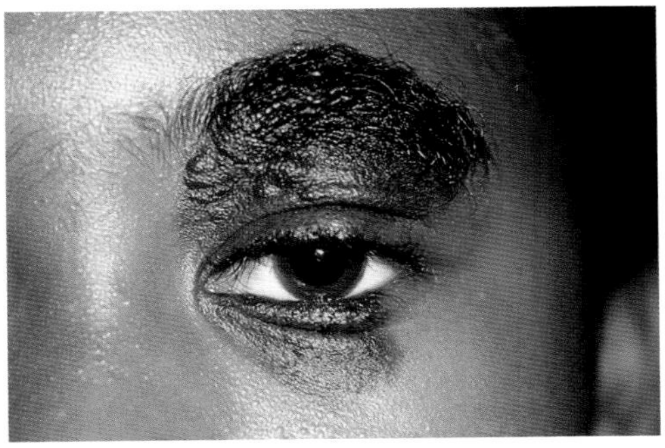

图 17–12　先天性眼睑痣细胞痣。*（译者注：资料来源见前页原文。）*

其他眼睑问题

拔毛癖

拔毛癖患者的特征是拔去自己的毛发，包括眉毛和睫毛，与强迫症有关。特征性外观包括睫毛脱落、断毛和不同长度的毛发再生（图 17–13）。

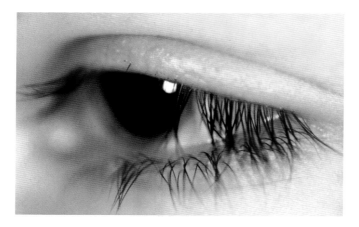

Figure 17-13 Trichotillomania. Note the segmental loss and irregular lengths of the eyelashes. *(Reproduced with permission from Lueder GT.* Pediatric Practice Ophthalmology. *New York: McGraw-Hill Professional; 2010;155.)*

Excessive Blinking

Excessive blinking is common in children. Causes include corneal and eyelid abnormalities, stress reactions, and tics. Ocular tics are usually benign and self-limited. Neurologic consultation may be indicated for patients with multiple tics to evaluate for Tourette syndrome. *Hemifacial spasm* causes unilateral forceful blinking and facial muscle contraction. Imaging is indicated in hemifacial spasm because the disorder may be caused by central nervous system lesions. See BCSC Section 7, *Oculofacial Plastic and Orbital Surgery*, for additional discussion of hemifacial spasm. Squinting may occur in patients with strabismus or uncorrected refractive errors.

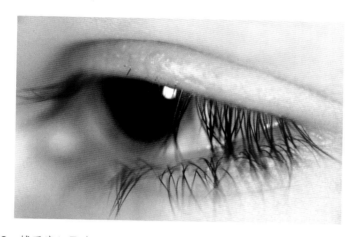

图 17–13　拔毛癖。见睫毛的节段性丢失和不等长度。*（译者注：资料来源见前页原文。）*

过度瞬目

过度瞬目儿童很常见。原因包括角膜和眼睑异常、应激反应和抽搐。眼部抽搐常是良性的和自限性的。多发性抽动症患者应进行神经系统咨询，评估是否患 Tourette 综合征。*半面痉挛*导致单侧强制瞬目和面部肌肉挛缩。半面痉挛可能是中枢神经系统病变引起的，应进行影像学检查。关于半面痉挛的进一步讨论见 BCSC 第 7 册《*眼面部整形与眼眶手术*》。眯眼见于斜视或未矫正的屈光不正患者。

（翻译 温龙波 白嘎丽 // 审校 石一宁 蒋宁 // 章节审校 石广礼）

CHAPTER 18

Orbital Disorders

Orbital anatomy is described in BCSC Section 2, *Fundamentals and Principles of Ophthalmology*, and Section 7, *Oculofacial Plastic and Orbital Surgery*. Many pediatric orbital disorders are also discussed in Section 7.

Abnormal Interocular Distance: Terminology and Associations

Telecanthus is characterized by a greater-than-normal distance between the inner canthi; it is distinct from, but may accompany, orbital hypertelorism (excessive distance between the medial orbital walls). In primary telecanthus, the abnormality is confined to the soft tissue, occurring without hypertelorism: the interpupillary distance is normal (see also Chapter 17 and Fig 17-1). When telecanthus is secondary to hypertelorism, the interpupillary distance is greater than normal. Telecanthus is common in many syndromes.

Orbital hypotelorism is smaller-than-normal distance between the medial orbital walls, with reduced inner and outer canthal distances. The finding is associated with more than 60 syndromes. Hypotelorism can be the result of skull malformation or a failure in brain development.

Exorbitism is variously defined as prominent eyes due to shallow orbits or as an increased angle of divergence of the orbital walls.

Congenital and Developmental Disorders: Craniofacial Malformations

Craniosynostosis

Cranial sutures are present throughout the skull, which is divided into 2 parts, the *calvarium* and the *skull base*, via an imaginary line drawn from the supraorbital rims to the base of the occiput (Fig 18-1). Cranial sutures normally fuse during the first 2 years of life. *Craniosynostosis* is the premature closure of one or more cranial sutures during the embryonic period or early childhood.

Bony growth of the skull occurs in osteoblastic centers located at the suture sites. Bone is laid down parallel and perpendicular to the direction of the suture (Fig 18-2). Premature suture closure prevents perpendicular growth but allows parallel growth. This growth pattern, called *Virchow's law*, results in clinically recognizable cranial bone deformations.

第 18 章

眼眶疾病

基础与临床科学教程 BCSC 第 2 册《*眼科学基础与原理*》和第 7 册《*眼面部整形与眼眶手术*》描述了眼眶解剖。第 7 册中讨论了许多儿童眼眶疾病。

异常双眼距：术语及相关概念

*内眦距过宽*是内眦之间的距离大于正常，它不同于眶距过宽（眼眶内侧壁之间的距离过大），但可与后者伴发。原发性内眦距过宽，仅局限于软组织，无眶距过宽：瞳孔间距正常（见第 17 章和图 17–1）。当内眦距过宽继发于眶距过宽时，瞳孔间距大于正常。内眦距过宽在许多综合征中很常见。

*眶距过窄*是指眼眶内壁之间的距离小于正常，伴随内眦和外眦距离减小。这一表现与 60 多种综合征有关。眶距过窄可能是颅骨畸形或大脑发育不良的结果。

*眼球突出*指由于眼眶较浅或眼眶壁开散角增加致眼球凸出。

先天性异常和发育异常：颅面畸形

颅骨缝早闭

颅骨缝贯穿整个颅骨，通过一条从眶上缘到枕骨底部的假想线（图 18–1），颅骨缝分为 2 部分，*颅盖*和*颅底*。颅骨缝在出生后的前 2 年融合。*颅骨缝早闭*是指在胚胎期或儿童早期，一个或多个颅缝未成熟闭合。

颅骨的骨生长发生在位于骨缝部位的成骨中心。骨平行且垂直于骨缝线方向（图 18–2）。过早的骨缝闭合阻止垂直生长，但可以平行生长。这种生长模式导致临床上可识别的颅骨畸形，称为 *Virchow 定律*。

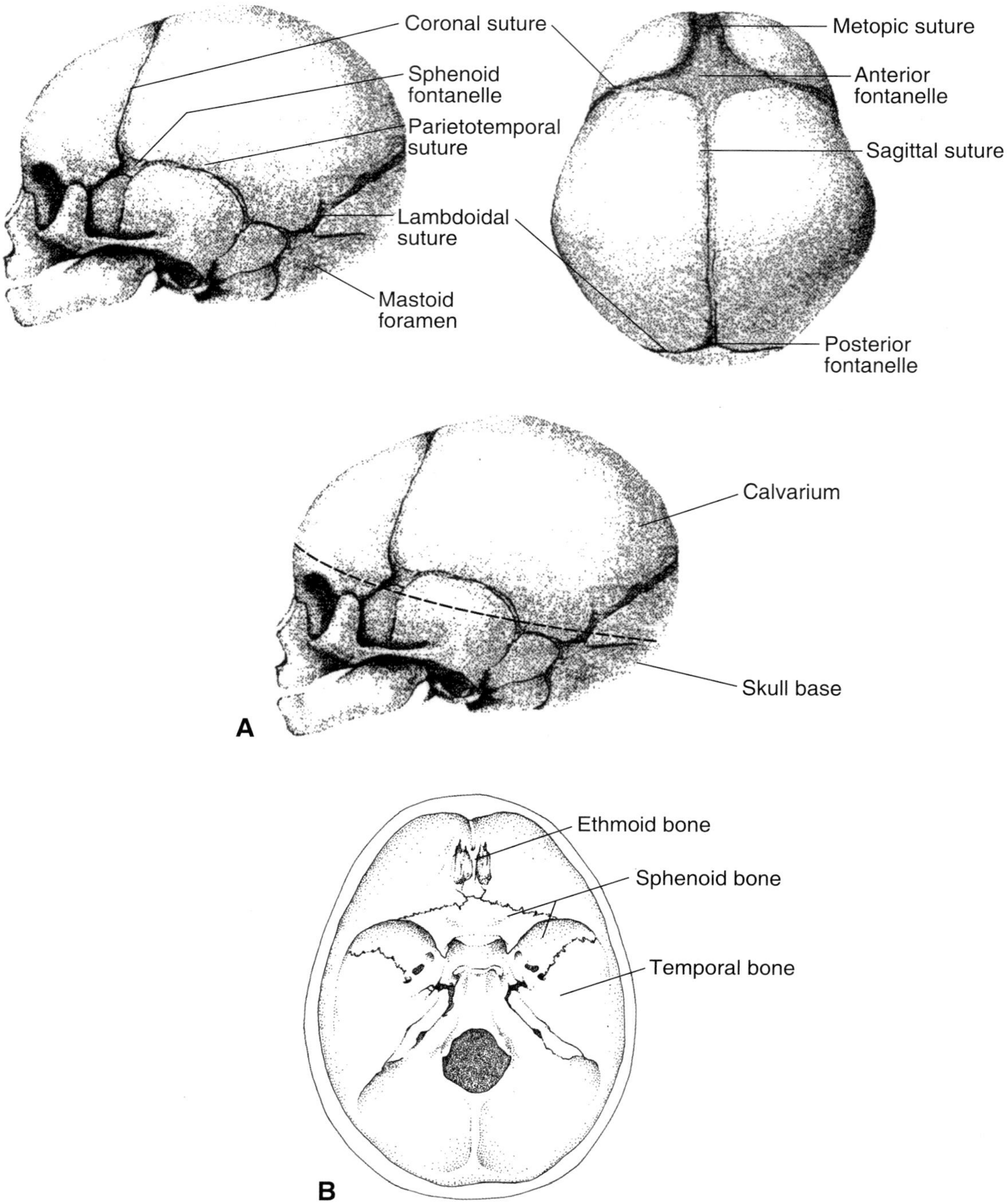

Figure 18-1 **A**, Normal sutures and fontanelles of the fetal skull. **B**, Adult cranial base, complete with sutures. *(Illustration by C. H. Wooley.)*

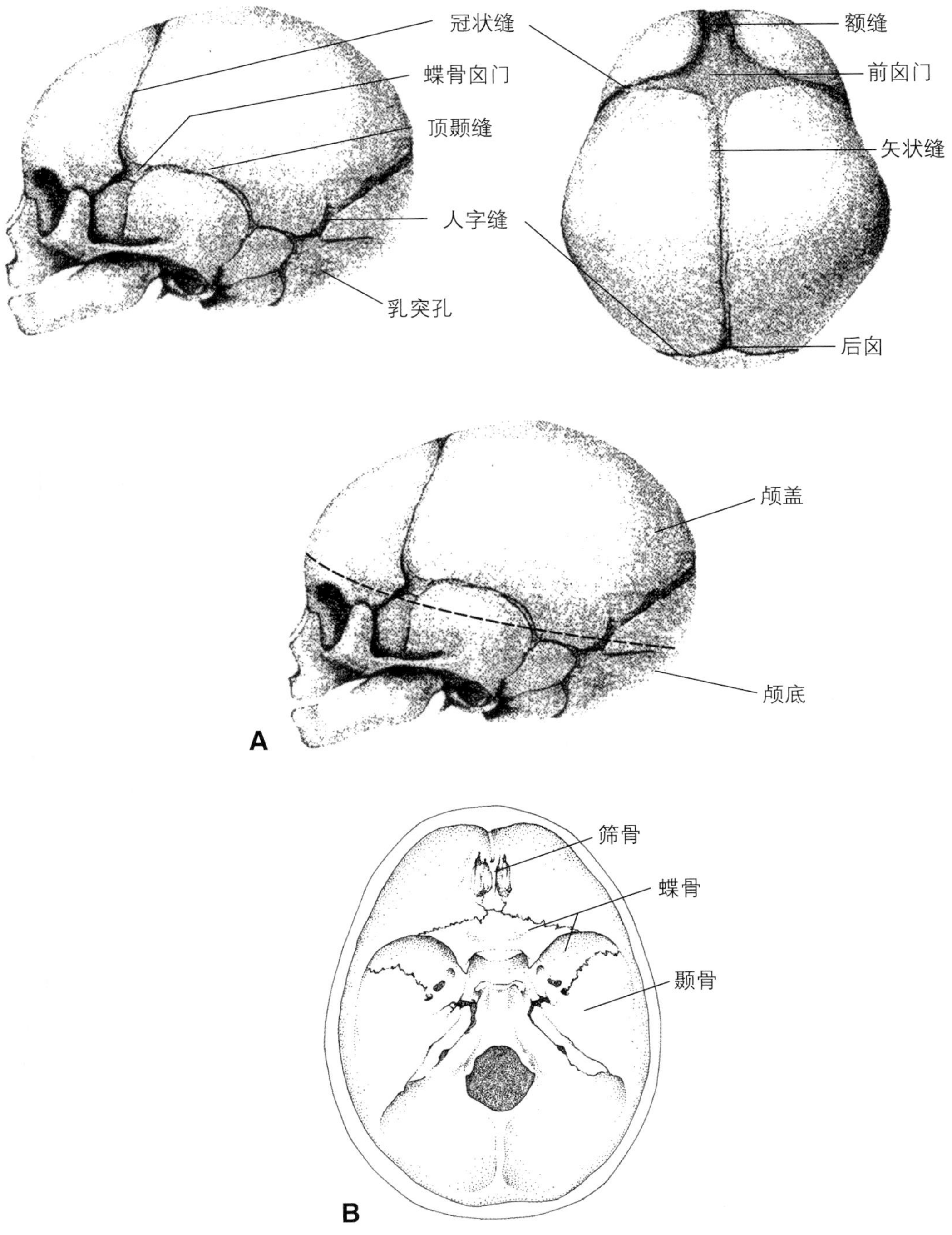

图 18-1　**A.** 正常的胎儿颅骨缝和囟门。**B.** 成人颅底，骨缝完整。*（译者注：资料来源见前页原文。）*

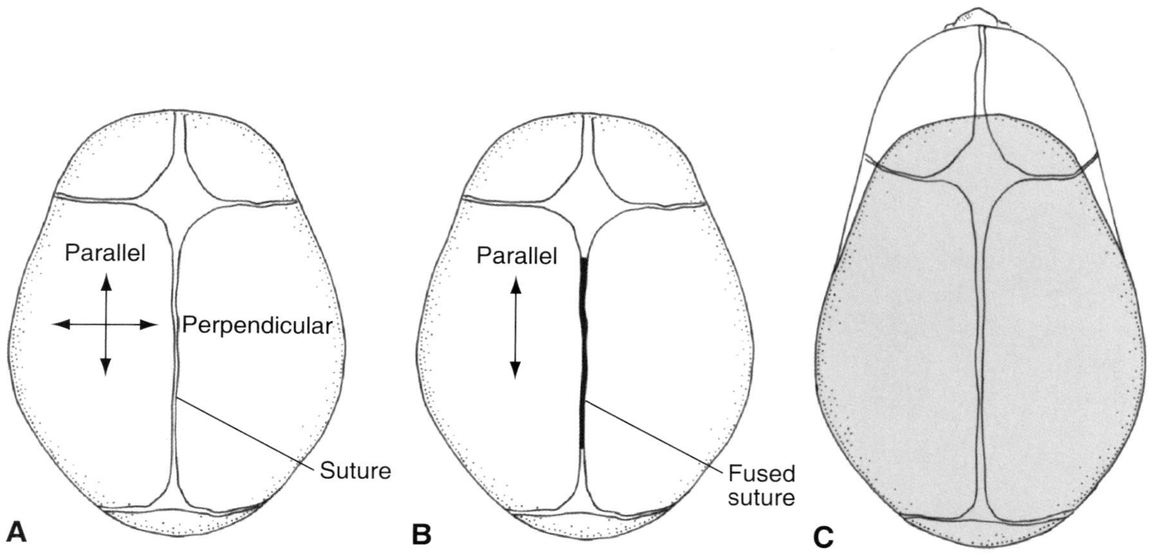

Figure 18-2 **A,** Normal sutures. Bone growth occurs at the suture, with bone laid down parallel and perpendicular to the direction of the suture. **B**, Virchow's law. Prematurely fused sutures allow bone growth only in the parallel direction; perpendicular growth is inhibited. **C**, An example of Virchow's law. Premature closure of the sagittal suture produces scaphocephaly (boatlike skull); the shaded area shows the normal skull shape. *(Illustration by C. H. Wooley.)*

The following are types of abnormal head shapes in infants, listed in order of decreasing frequency:

Plagiocephaly Most often plagiocephaly (Greek, *plagio*, "oblique"; *kephale,* "head") is deformational, the consequence of external compressive forces, occurring prenatally or during infancy. Deformational plagiocephaly due to intrauterine constraint (eg, oligohydramnios) is characterized by ipsilateral occipital flattening with contralateral forehead flattening. This condition may also be caused by unilateral coronal suture synostosis. On the synostotic side, the forehead and supraorbital rim are retruded (depressed), the interpalpebral fissure is wider, and the orbit is often higher than on the nonsynostotic side. The nonsynostotic side displays a protruding or bulging forehead, a lower supraorbital rim, a narrower interpalpebral fissure, and frequently a lower orbital position.

Brachycephaly Brachycephaly (literally, "short head") is frequently the result of bilateral closure of the coronal sutures. Limited growth along the anterior-posterior axis results in a comparatively short head. Most often, the forehead is wide and flat.

Scaphocephaly Scaphocephaly (literally, "boat head") is usually a result of premature closure of the sagittal suture. There is anteroposterior elongation of the skull, along with bitemporal narrowing.

Dolichocephaly In patients with dolichocephaly (literally, "long head"), the skull shape is similar to that in scaphocephaly.

Kleeblattschädel The skull shape is trilobar. Kleeblattschädel ("cloverleaf skull") is typically the result of synostosis of the coronal, lambdoidal, and sagittal sutures.

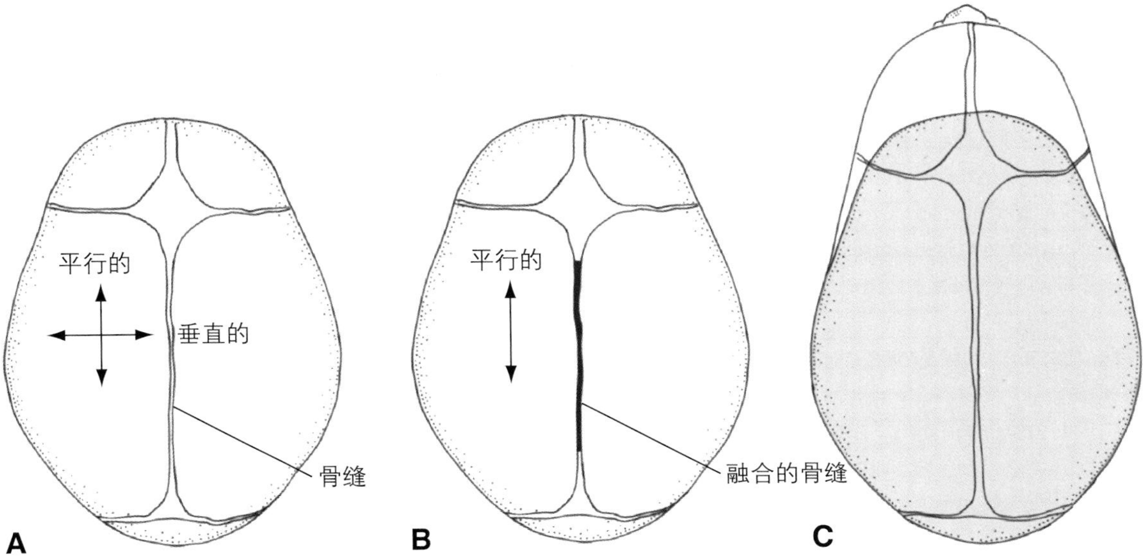

图 18–2　A. 正常骨缝线。骨生长发生在骨缝处，颅骨与骨缝方向平行和垂直。**B.** Virchow 定律，过早融合的骨缝线只允许骨骼在平行方向生长；垂直生长受到抑制。**C.** Virchow 定律的病例。矢状缝过早闭合导致舟状颅骨；阴影部分显示的是正常的颅骨形状。*（译者注：资料来源见前页原文。）*

以下是婴儿头部形状异常的类型，按发生率递减的顺序排列：

斜头畸形　大多数斜头畸形（希腊语，*plagio* 意为“斜”； *kephale* 意为“头”）是外部压缩力所致的变形，发生于产前或婴儿期。宫内限制所致（如羊水过少）的变形性斜头畸形，其特点是同侧枕叶变平，对侧前额变平。这种情况也可能是由于单侧冠状缝骨性连结。在骨性连结处，前额和眶上缘向后收缩（凹陷），眼睑间隙较宽，眼眶常高于非骨性连结侧。非骨性连结表现出从颞侧前额突出或膨出，眶上缘较低，睑间裂较窄，而且经常处于较低的眶位。

短头畸形　短头畸形（词义为“短头”）通常是冠状缝双侧闭合的结果。前后轴生长受限，导致头部相对较短。大多数情况下，前额宽而平。

舟头畸形　舟头畸形（词义为“舟状头”）通常是矢状缝过早闭合的结果。颅骨前后延伸，伴随着双颞骨的狭窄。

长头畸形　（词义为“长头”）在长头畸形的患者中，颅骨形状类似于舟状头畸形。

三叶草形头颅　颅骨的形状是三叶形。三叶草形头颅（“分叶状颅”）通常是冠状缝、人字缝和矢状缝骨性连结的结果。

Etiology of craniosynostosis

Early suture fusion can be sporadic and occur as an isolated abnormality (eg, sagittal suture synostosis and most cases of unilateral coronal suture synostosis), or it can be part of a genetic syndrome, associated with other abnormalities. Craniosynostosis syndromes are usually autosomal dominant conditions, often with associated limb abnormalities. Many of these syndromes have overlapping features, making accurate diagnosis based on clinical findings difficult. Identification of specific mutations may be diagnostic. Mutations in the fibroblast growth factor receptor genes (*FGFRs*) or in the *TWIST* gene are found in most patients with syndromic craniosynostosis.

Craniosynostosis syndromes

Common systemic features of the craniosynostosis syndromes include fusion of multiple calvarial sutures and skull base sutures. Syndactyly (partial fusion of the digits) and brachydactyly (short digits), ranging in severity, are hallmarks of these syndromes, the exception being Crouzon syndrome. The following sections discuss the most common types of craniosynostosis syndromes. All are autosomal dominant.

Crouzon syndrome Crouzon syndrome is the most common craniosynostosis syndrome. Calvarial bone synostosis often includes both coronal sutures, resulting in a broad, retruded forehead; brachycephaly; and a tower-shaped skull. The skull base sutures are also involved, leading to varying degrees of **midfacial retrusion**. There is marked variability of the skull and facial features, with milder cases escaping diagnosis through multiple generations. Hypertelorism and proptosis, with inferior scleral show, are the most frequent features of Crouzon syndrome (Fig 18-3). Hydrocephalus is common, but intelligence is usually normal. Typically, findings are limited to the head. Unlike in the other syndromes, patients with Crouzon syndrome do not have anomalies of the hands and feet; thus, the presence or absence of these anomalies in a patient can aid diagnosis.

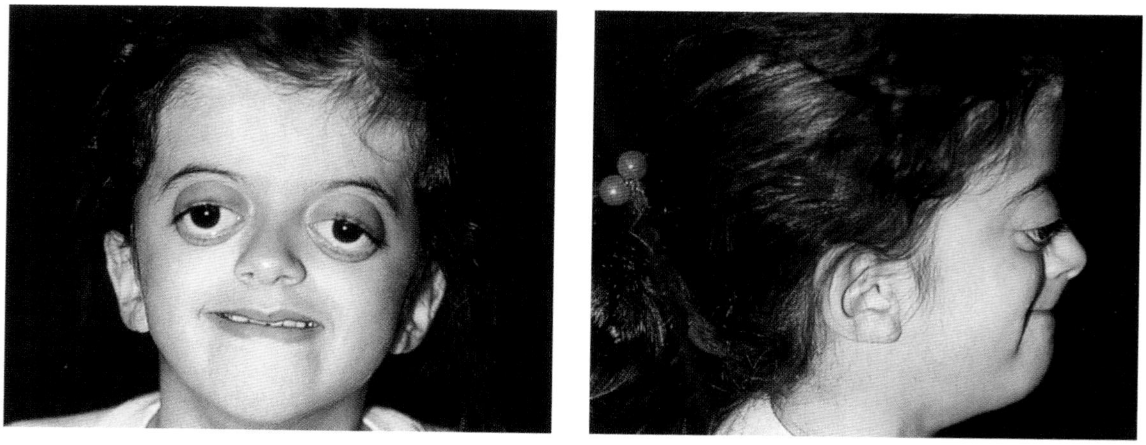

Figure 18-3 Crouzon syndrome. This patient exhibits brachycephaly and a "tower" skull with **forehead retrusion**; proptosis; inferior scleral show; and a small, beaklike nose. Also visible is the emerging midfacial hypoplasia. *(Reproduced with permission from Katowitz JA, ed.* Pediatric Oculoplastic Surgery. *New York: Springer; 2002:fig 31-23.)*

颅缝早闭的病因分析

早期骨缝融合可以偶发,并呈孤立的异常(如矢状缝骨性连结和大多数单侧冠状缝骨性连结),也可能是遗传综合症的一部分，伴有其他异常。颅缝早闭综合征常为常染色体显性遗传，常伴有肢体异常。许多这些综合症状具有重叠的特点，根据临床症状不易做出准确诊断。特异性突变的鉴定可能具有诊断意义。在大多数颅缝早闭综合征患者中，都有发现成纤维细胞生长因子受体基因（*FGFRs*）或 *TWIST* 基因的突变。

颅缝早闭综合征

颅缝早闭综合征的常见全身特征包括多个颅顶骨缝和颅底骨缝的连结。严重程度不等的并指（趾）（手指 / 脚趾部分融合）和短指（趾）（手指 / 脚趾短）是综合征的特征，Crouzon 综合征除外。下面几节讨论最常见的颅缝早闭综合征类型。其均为常染色体显性遗传。

Crouzon 综合征　（Crouzon syndrome）是最常见的颅缝早闭综合征。颅顶骨的骨性连结常包括 2 条冠状缝，导致宽而后缩的前额、短头畸形，和塔状颅骨。颅底缝的连结受累时，不同程度的中面部后缩。颅骨和面部特征变异较大，较轻的病例在几代人中未能做出诊断。双眼眶距过宽和眼球突出，伴下巩膜暴露，是 Crouzon 综合征最常见的特征（图 18-3）。脑积水很常见，但智力正常，病变仅限于头部。与其他综合征不同，Crouzon 综合征没有手脚异常；因此，患者是否伴发这些异常有助于诊断。

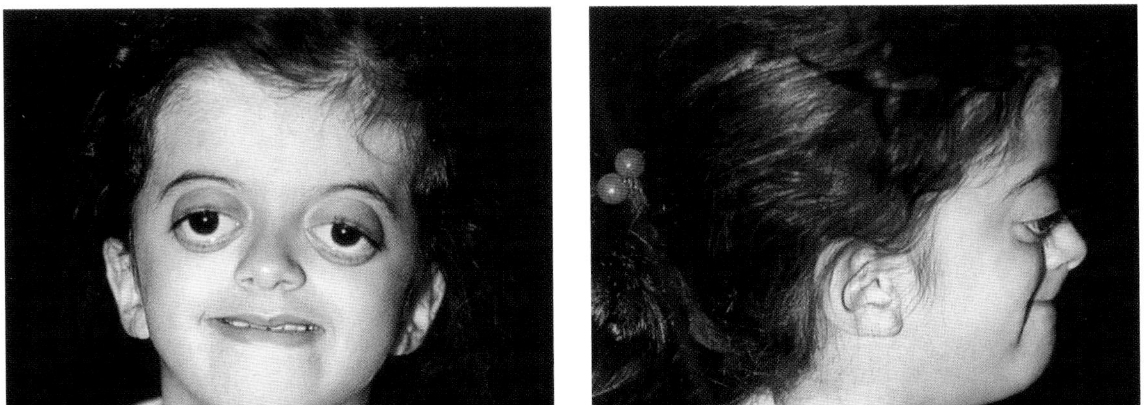

图 18-3　Crouzon 综合征。病人表现为短头畸形和“塔状”颅骨，伴前额后缩、眼球突出、下巩膜暴露，以及喙状小鼻子。同样可见的是正在出现的面部中部发育不良。*（译者注：资料来源见前页原文。）*

Apert syndrome Fusion of multiple calvarial sutures, most often both coronal sutures, and skull base suture fusion are usually found in patients with Apert syndrome. The skull shape and facial features of these patients resemble those of Crouzon patients. Apert syndrome, however, is associated with an often extreme amount of syndactyly (Fig 18-4), in which most or all digits of the hands and feet are completely fused (*mitten deformity*). Apert syndrome is likely to be associated with internal organ (cardiovascular and genitourinary) malformations and mental deficiency. Hydrocephalus is less common in this syndrome than in Crouzon syndrome.

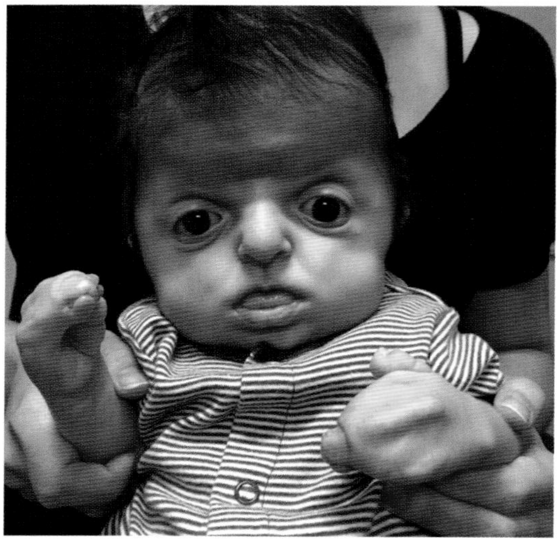

Figure 18-4 Broad forehead, midfacial retrusion, and marked syndactyly in a patient with Apert syndrome. *(Courtesy of Robert W. Hered, MD.)*

Pfeiffer syndrome Patients with Pfeiffer syndrome have craniofacial abnormalities resembling those of Apert patients but often have more severe craniosynostosis, resulting in a cloverleaf skull. There is a high risk of hydrocephalus. The syndactyly is much less severe, and patients have characteristic short, broad thumbs and toes.

Saethre-Chotzen syndrome The features of Saethre-Chotzen syndrome are much milder than those of other craniosynostosis syndromes; this syndrome is therefore underdiagnosed. Early suture fusion is not a constant feature but, when present, typically involves 1 coronal suture (plagiocephaly), resulting in facial asymmetry. Other common features are ptosis, low hairline, and ear abnormalities. Abnormalities of the hands and feet include brachydactyly and mild syndactyly (Fig 18-5). Intelligence is usually normal.

Ocular complications of craniosynostosis

Proptosis Proptosis (or exorbitism) results from the reduced volume of the bony orbit. The severity of the proptosis in patients with craniosynostosis is not uniform and frequently increases with age because of the impaired growth of the bony orbit.

Corneal exposure Because the eyelids may not close completely over the proptotic globes, corneal exposure may occur, with possible development of exposure keratitis. Aggressive lubrication may be necessary to prevent corneal drying. Tarsorrhaphy can reduce the exposure. Surgically expanding the orbital volume, thereby eliminating the proptosis, may be indicated in extreme cases.

Apert 综合征　多发颅骨缝融合，最常见的是冠状缝和颅底缝融合，常见于 Apert 综合征。颅骨形状和面部特征与 Crouzon 综合征相似，而 Apert 综合征常有多处并指畸形（图 18–4），其中手和脚的大部分或所有手指 / 脚趾完全融合（*连指畸形*）。Apert 综合征可伴有内脏器官（心血管和泌尿生殖系统）畸形和智力缺陷。与 Crouzon 综合征相比，脑积水少见。

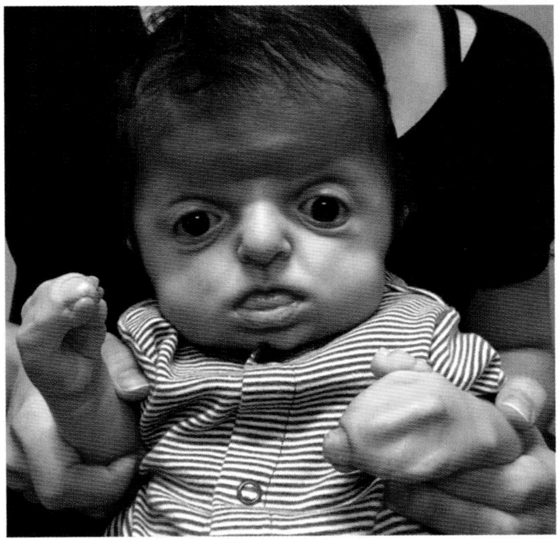

图 18–4　Apert 综合征病人，宽前额，中面部后缩，有明显的并指。*（译者注：资料来源见前页原文。）*

Pfeiffer 综合征　患者的颅面畸形与 Apert 患者相似，但颅缝早闭更严重，导致三叶形颅骨。脑积水的风险很高，并指的程度较轻，拇指和脚趾短而宽。

Saethre–Chotzen 综合征　Saethre–Chotzen 综合征的颅缝早闭综合征较轻，因此多漏诊。早期颅骨缝连结不具特征性，即使出现，也仅累及 1 条冠状缝（斜头畸形），导致面部两侧不对称。其他常见的特征是上睑下垂、低发际线和耳部异常。手脚异常包括短指（趾）和轻度并指（趾）（图 18–5）。智力通常是正常的。

颅缝早闭的眼部并发症

眼球突出症　眼球突出症（或突眼）是眼眶体积缩小所致。伴颅缝骨性连结的眼球突出的严重程度不一，并且因为系骨性眼眶的发育异常，眼球突出常会随着年龄的增长而增加。

角膜暴露　由于眼球突出使眼睑不能完全闭合，可发生角膜暴露，并可发展为暴露性角膜炎。大量眼液可以防止角膜干燥。睑缘缝合术可以减少角膜暴露。在极端情况下，可以通过手术扩大眼眶体积，从而消除眼球突出。

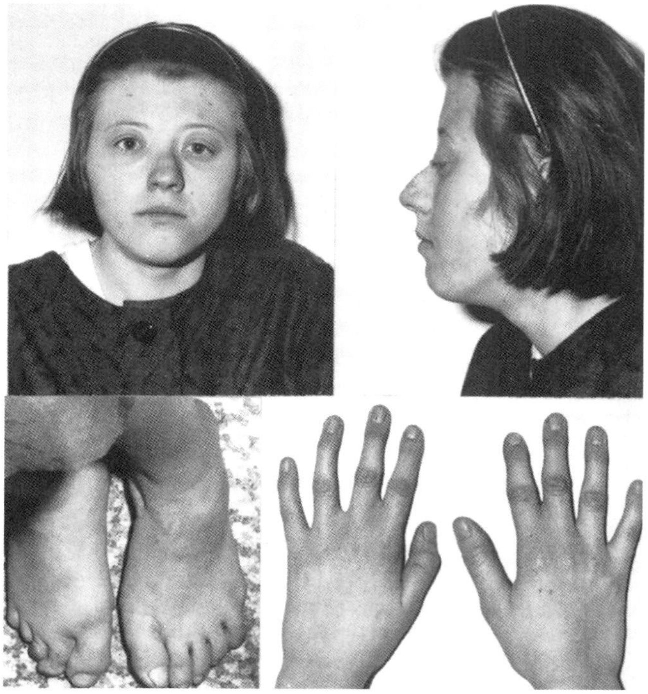

Figure 18-5 Patient with Saethre-Chotzen syndrome. Note the facial asymmetry, flat forehead, low hairline, mild left ptosis, lateral deviation of the great toes, shortened toes, and partial syndactyly of fingers 2 and 3. *(Courtesy of the March of Dimes.)*

Globe luxation In patients with extremely shallow orbits, globe luxation may occur when the eyelids are manipulated or when there is increased pressure in the orbits, such as occurs with a Valsalva maneuver. The globe is luxated forward, the eyelids closing behind the equator of the globe. The condition is very painful and can cause corneal exposure. It may also compromise the blood supply to the globe, which is a medical emergency. Physicians and patients (or their caregivers) should quickly reposition the globe behind the eyelids. The best technique for doing this is to place a fin ger and thumb over the conjunctiva within the interpalpebral fissure and exert gentle but firm pressure; this technique does not damage the cornea. For recurrent luxation, the short-term solution is tarsorrhaphy; the long-term solution is orbital volume expansion.

Strabismus Patients with craniosynostosis show a variety of horizontal deviations in primary position; exotropia is the most frequent. The most consistent finding, however, is a marked V pattern (see Chapter 10). This V pattern is often accompanied by a marked overelevation in adduction, especially when 1 or both coronal sutures are fused, as occurs in unilateral coronal suture synostosis and Apert (Fig 18-6) and Crouzon syndromes. The apparent overaction (often pseudo-overaction) of the inferior oblique muscle on the side of the coronal suture fusion may be due to one of the following: orbital and globe extorsion, which converts the medial rectus muscle into an elevator when the eye is in adduction; superior oblique trochlear retrusion (because of superior orbital rim retrusion), which induces superior oblique underaction and secondary true inferior oblique overaction; anomalous extraocular muscle insertions or agenesis; or orbital pulley abnormalities (see Chapter 3).

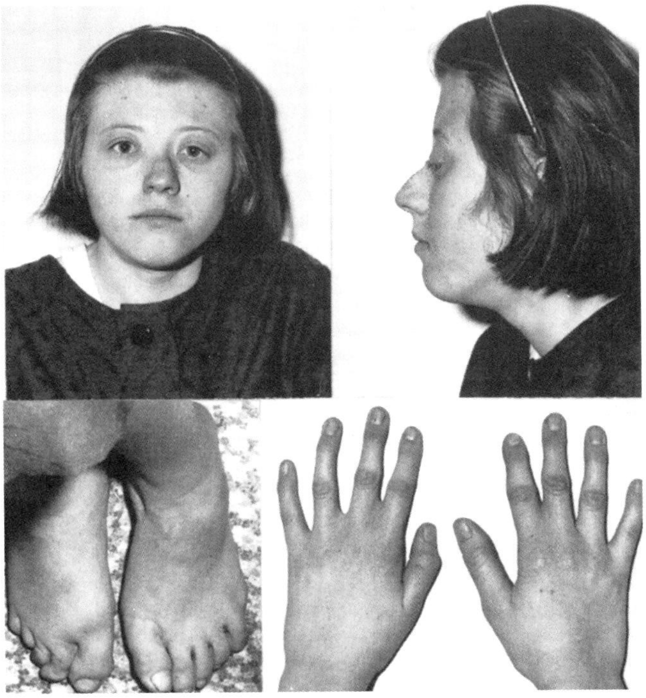

图 18-5　Saethre-Chotzen 综合征。面部不对称，前额扁平，发际线低，轻度左上睑下垂，大脚趾侧倾，短趾，手指 2、3 指部分并指。*（译者注：资料来源见前页原文。）*

眼球脱位　在眼眶极浅的患者中，眼球脱位可能发生在眼睑操作或眼眶内压力增加时，如采用 Valsalva 手法。眼球向前脱位，眼睑在眼球赤道后闭合，病人剧痛，可导致角膜暴露，它也可能危及眼球的血液供应，属急诊。医生和患者（或他们的护理人员）应迅速将眼球重新放置在眼睑后面。最佳方法是将手指和拇指放在睑裂间隙的结膜上，施加温和而有力的压力，不损伤角膜。对于复发性脱位，短期的解决方案是睑缘缝合术，长期的解决方案是眼眶体积扩张。

斜视　颅缝早闭的患者在第一眼位有各种水平眼位偏斜，多见外斜视，而 V 征最常见（见第 10 章）。V 征常伴有明显的内转时眼球上转过度，特别是当 1 个或 2 个冠状缝连结时，如单侧冠状缝连结、Apert 综合征（图 18-6）和 Crouzon 综合征。冠状缝融合侧下斜肌的过度运动（通常为假性过度运动）可能是由于以下原因之一引起的：眼眶和眼球外旋，当眼内收时，将内直肌转换成上转肌；上斜肌滑车后缩（由于上眶缘后缩），引起上斜肌功能不足和继发性下斜肌功能亢进；异常眼外肌附着点或发育不全；或眼眶滑车结缔组织异常（见第 3 章）。

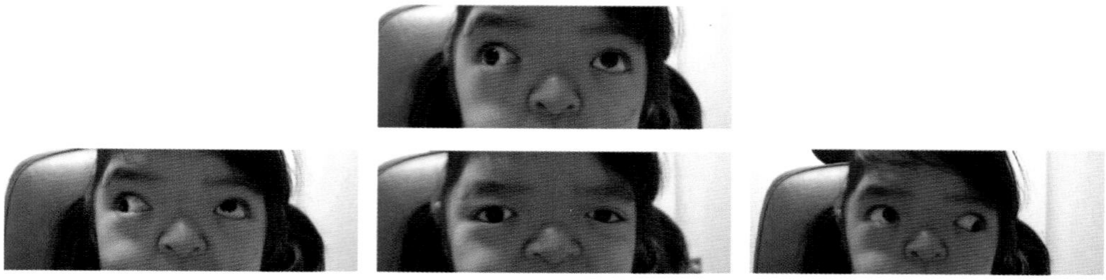

Figure 18-6 Strabismus in a patient with Apert syndrome. Note the good alignment in primary position with marked overelevation in adduction and exotropia in upgaze (V pattern). *(Courtesy of John Simon, MD.)*

Optic nerve abnormalities Optic nerve damage may occur for several reasons in patients with craniosynostosis. Optic nerve function may deteriorate in patients with chronically elevated intracranial pressure (ICP), which may result from hydrocephalus or be caused by crowding of the intracranial contents due to synostosis. In patients with midfacial retrusion, sleep apnea may develop and can cause idiopathic intracranial hypertension. In rare cases, optic nerve damage can occur secondary to compression stemming from synostosis of the optic foramina. Optic atrophy may occur with or without antecedent papilledema. Because children with elevated ICP may not report headache, a common symptom of this condition, young patients with multiple fused sutures should be monitored for this complication.

Ocular adnexal abnormalities Common ocular adnexal abnormalities include orbital hypertelorism, telecanthus, abnormal slant of the palpebral fissures secondary to superior displacement of the medial canthi, ptosis, and nasolacrimal abnormalities. Epiphora is common and may be secondary to nasolacrimal duct obstruction, poor blink secondary to proptosis, obliquity of the palpebral fissures, or ocular irritation from corneal exposure.

Surgical management of craniosynostosis

Reconstructive surgery for severe craniofacial malformation is frequently extensive and involves en bloc movement of the facial structures. The status of the visual system should be documented preoperatively and monitored postoperatively, with appropriate treatment as indicated. Procedures that involve moving the orbits may significantly change the degree or type of strabismus. Because of this, deferring treatment of strabismus until craniofacial surgery is completed may be appropriate.

Nonsynostotic Craniofacial Conditions

Many craniofacial syndromes do not involve synostosis. Nonsynostotic syndromes and conditions of particular importance to the ophthalmologist are discussed in the following sections.

Anophthalmia

Anophthalmia (anophthalmos), the absence of tissues of the eye (Fig 18-7), is the most severe and rare phenotypic expression of a spectrum of abnormalities that includes typical coloboma and microphthalmia (see also Chapter 21). These conditions may be isolated, but they are frequently associated with other congenital anomalies. Anophthalmia and severe microphthalmia are associated with hypoplastic orbits and eyelids. Various techniques have been utilized for orbital expansion. The best results are achieved with early treatment.

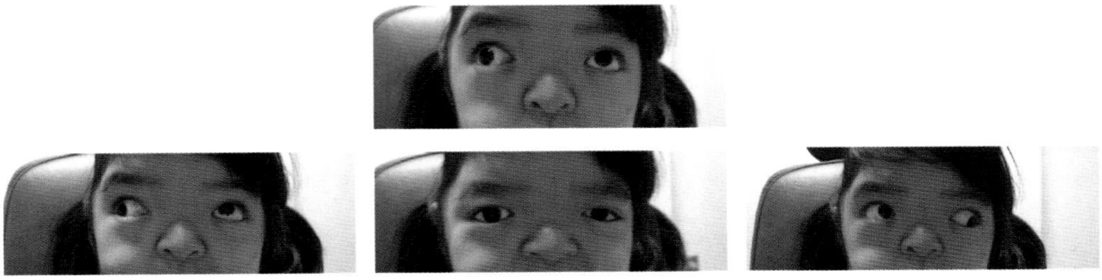

图 18-6　Apert 综合征伴斜视。第一眼位正位，内转时眼球上转过度，上转外斜视（V 征）。*（译者注：资料来源见前页原文。）*

视神经异常　在颅缝早闭患者中，视神经损伤的发生有多种原因。慢性颅内压升高（ICP）使视神经功能恶化，由脑积水引起，或由于颅骨连结使颅内容积拥挤引起的。中面部后缩时，睡眠呼吸暂停可能发展并可引起特发性颅内高压。在极少数情况下，视神经损伤可能继发于视神经孔的骨性连结。视神经性萎缩发生前可没有视乳头水肿。因为颅内压升高（ICP）时，儿童不会告知头痛，而头痛是颅内压升高的常见症状，低龄患者有多发骨缝连结时，应监测这种并发症。

眼附件异常　常见的眼附件异常包括眼眶距过宽、内眦距过宽、继发于内眦向上移位的睑裂异常倾斜、上睑下垂和鼻泪管异常。常见的溢泪继发于鼻泪管阻塞，继发于眼球突出的瞬目差、睑裂倾斜或角膜暴露引起眼刺激征。

颅缝早闭的手术治疗

严重颅面畸形的重建手术适应证广泛，包括面部结构的整体运动。术前应记录视觉系统的状态，术后进行监测，并进行适当的治疗。眶移位手术可能会显著改变斜视的程度或类型。因此，斜视治疗需待颅面手术完成后进行。

非骨连结性颅面异常

许多颅面部综合征不涉及骨性连结，与眼科相关的重要非骨性连结综合征和特征将在以下章节中讨论。

无眼（畸形）

*无眼症*是指眼球组织缺失（图 18-7），是包括典型眼组织残缺和小眼症在内的一系列异常的、最严重的和罕见的表型表达（见第 21 章）。这些情况可能是孤立的，但往往与其他先天性异常有关。无眼症和小眼症与眼眶和眼睑发育不良有关。各种技术已被应用于眼眶扩张。早期治疗效果最好。

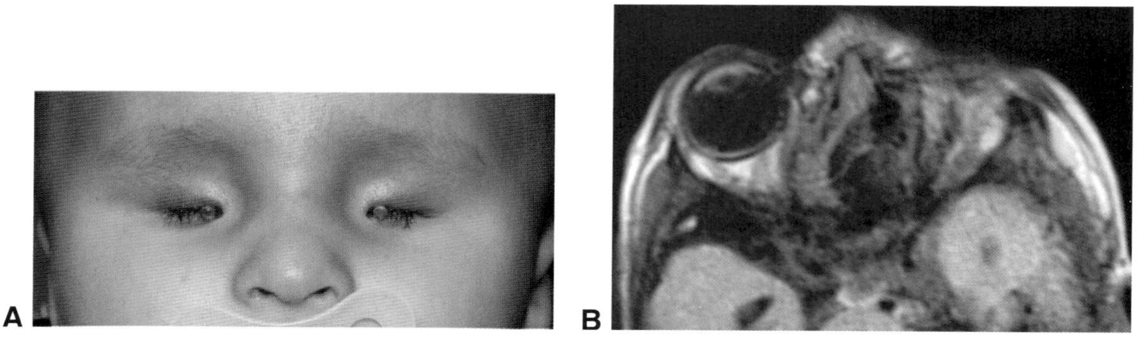

Figure 18-7 **A**, Anophthalmia, both eyes. **B**, Magnetic resonance image from a patient with unilateral anophthalmia shows absence of ocular structures. *(Part A courtesy of Steven Couch, MD; part B courtesy of Alice Bashinsky, MD.)*

Branchial arch syndromes

Branchial arch syndromes are caused by disruptions in the embryonic development of the first 2 branchial arches, which are responsible for formation of the maxillary and mandibular bones, the ear, and facial musculature. The *oculoauriculovertebral spectrum (OAVS)*, which includes hemifacial microsomia and Goldenhar syndrome, and Treacher Collins syndrome are the best-known branchial arch syndromes. Hemifacial microsomia is a milder form of OAVS. Patients with OAVS may have vertebral abnormalities such as hemivertebrae and vertebral hypoplasia. They may also have neurologic, cardiovascular, and genitourinary abnormalities. Most cases are sporadic.

Goldenhar syndrome Patients with Goldenhar syndrome have hemifacial microsomia (unilateral or bilateral) and characteristic ophthalmic abnormalities (Fig 18-8). Most cases are sporadic.

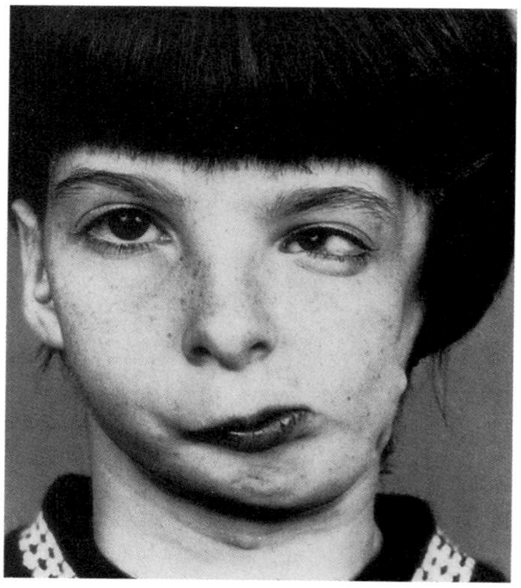

Figure 18-8 Goldenhar syndrome with hemifacial microsomia. The patient has facial asymmetry, a hypoplastic left ear (microtia), an ear tag near the right ear, epibulbar dermolipoma in the left eye, and esotropia. The patient also has Duane retraction syndrome, left eye.

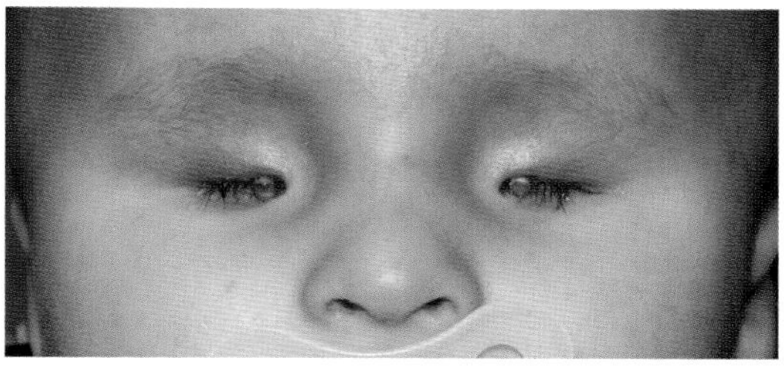

A

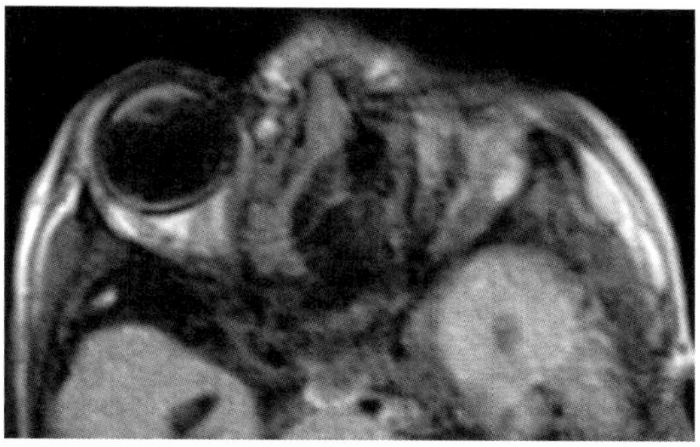

B

图 18-7　A. 无眼（畸形），双眼。**B.** 单侧无眼症患者的磁共振图像，显示眼结构缺如。*（译者注 资料来源见前页原文。）*

鳃弓综合征

鳃弓综合征是由第一二鳃弓在胚胎发育中中断引起的，鳃弓负责上颌和下颌骨骼、耳朵和面部肌肉组织的形成。*眼耳脊椎系列（OAVS）*包括半侧颜面短小畸形以及 Goldenhar 综合征，Treacher Collins 综合征，是最主要的鳃弓综合征。半侧颜面短小畸形是较轻的眼耳脊椎系列（OAVS）。眼耳脊椎系列（OAVS）患者可伴有椎体异常，如半椎体和椎体发育不良。也可伴有神经、心血管和泌尿生殖系统异常。大多数病例是散发的。

Goldenhar 综合征　患者有半侧颜面短小畸形（单侧或双侧）和特征性眼病（图 18-8）。大多数病例是散发的。

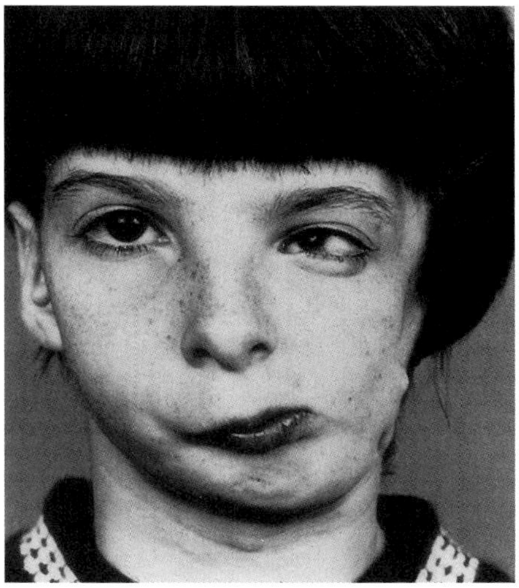

图 18-8　Goldenhar 综合征伴半侧颜面短小畸形。面部不对称，左耳发育不全（小耳），右耳附近有耳标，左眼有结膜（角膜缘）皮样瘤和内斜视。还患有 Duane 后退综合征，左眼。

Epibulbar (limbal) dermoids and dermolipomas are characteristic ocular signs. Dermolipomas (also termed *lipodermoids*) usually occur in the temporal quadrant, covered by conjunctiva and often hidden by the lateral upper and lower eyelids. Epibulbar limbal dermoids occur more frequently than dermolipomas and can be bilateral (approximately 25% of cases). They occasionally impinge on the visual axis but more commonly interfere with vision by causing astigmatism and anisometropic amblyopia. Eyelid colobomas may occur. Other ocular conditions include microphthalmia, cataract, and iris abnormalities. Duane retraction syndrome is more common in patients with Goldenhar syndrome.

Treacher Collins syndrome Treacher Collins syndrome (mandibulofacial dysostosis) is caused by abnormal growth of the first and second branchial arches, with underdevelopment and even agenesis of the zygoma and malar eminences. The lateral orbital rims are depressed and the palpebral fissures slant downward because of lateral canthal dystopia (Fig 18-9). Pseudocolobomas (uncommonly, true colobomas) occur in the outer third of the lower eyelids. Meibomian glands may be absent. The cilia of the lower eyelid medial to the pseudocoloboma may also be absent. The ears are malformed and hearing loss is common. The mandible is typically hypoplastic, leading to micrognathia. Intelligence is normal. The syndrome is inherited in an autosomal dominant fashion. Most affected patients have a mutation in the *TCOF1* gene.

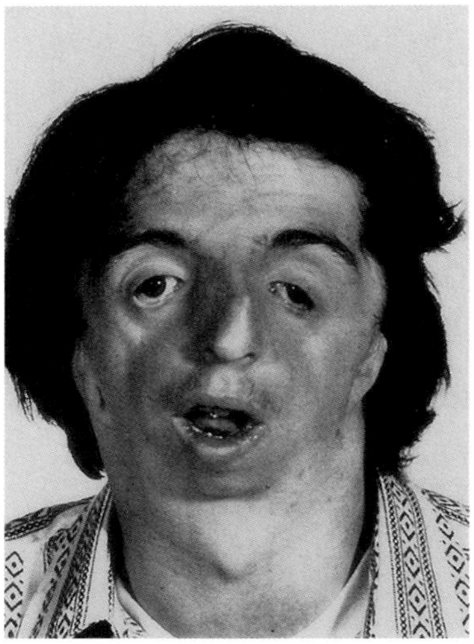

Figure 18-9 Treacher Collins syndrome (mandibulofacial dysostosis). Note the downward slant of the palpebral fissure, low-set abnormal ears, notch or curving of the inferotemporal eyelid margin, and maxillary and mandibular hypoplasia. *(Reproduced with permission from Peyman GA, Sanders DR, Goldberg MF. Principles and Practice of Ophthalmology. Philadelphia: Saunders; 1980:2411.)*

Pierre Robin sequence

The Pierre Robin sequence (also *anomaly, deformity*) is characterized by micrognathia, glossoptosis, and cleft palate. The sequence is a frequent finding in Stickler syndrome. Associated ocular anomalies include retinal detachment, microphthalmia, congenital glaucoma, cataracts, and high myopia.

Fetal alcohol syndrome

Fetal alcohol syndrome is caused by in utero exposure to ethanol. It is characterized by prenatal and postnatal growth retardation, central nervous system and craniofacial abnormalities, and intellectual disability.

眼表（角膜缘）皮样瘤和皮脂瘤是典型的眼部症状。皮脂瘤（也称为*脂皮样囊肿*）通常发生在颞象限，被覆结膜，常被外侧上眼睑和下眼睑遮盖。眼表（角膜缘）皮样瘤比皮脂瘤更常见，且为双侧的（约占 25%）。偶尔会累及视轴，但更常见的是引起散光和屈光参差性弱视，进而影响视力。可有眼睑缺损。其他眼部疾病包括小眼球、白内障和虹膜异常。Duane 后退综合征更常见于 Goldenhar 综合征患者中。

Treacher Collins 综合征　Treacher Collins 综合征（下颌面发育不良）是由第一、二鳃弓发育异常引起的，伴颧骨和颧骨弓发育不全、甚至不发育。眼眶外侧缘发育不良，外眦异位致睑裂向下倾斜（图 18-9）。下睑外 1/3 可有假性眼睑缺损（真性缺损不常见）。伴睑板腺缺如。下睑假性眼睑缺损的内侧有睫毛缺失。耳部畸形，听力丧失。下颌骨发育不良，出现小颌畸形。智力正常。该综合征是常染色体显性遗传，大多数患者有 *TCOF1* 基因突变。

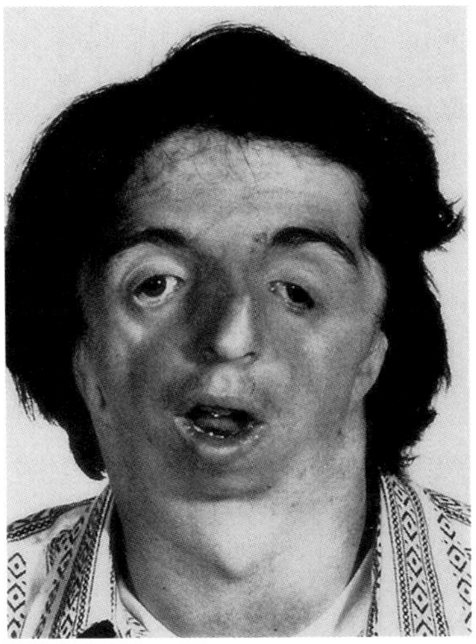

图 18-9　Treacher Collins 综合征（下颌面发育不良）。向下倾斜的睑裂，异常低耳位，颞下睑缘切迹或弯曲，上颌骨和下颌骨发育不良。*（译者注：资料来源见前页原文。）*

Pierre Robin 序列

Pierre Robin 序列（亦称*异常*、*畸形*）以小颌、舌下垂、腭裂为特征，常见于 Stickler 综合征。伴随的眼部异常包括视网膜脱离、小眼球、先天性青光眼、白内障和高度近视。

胎儿酒精综合征

胎儿酒精综合征是由胎儿期宫腔内暴露接触乙醇引起的，其特点是宫内和产后发育迟缓、中枢神经系统和颅面畸形以及智力障碍。

The classic ocular features of fetal alcohol syndrome are short palpebral fissures, telecanthus, epicanthus, ptosis, microphthalmia, and esotropia (Fig 18-10). Anterior segment dysgenesis, optic nerve hypoplasia, and high refractive errors have been reported. Fifty percent of children with this underdiagnosed syndrome have some form of visual impairment.

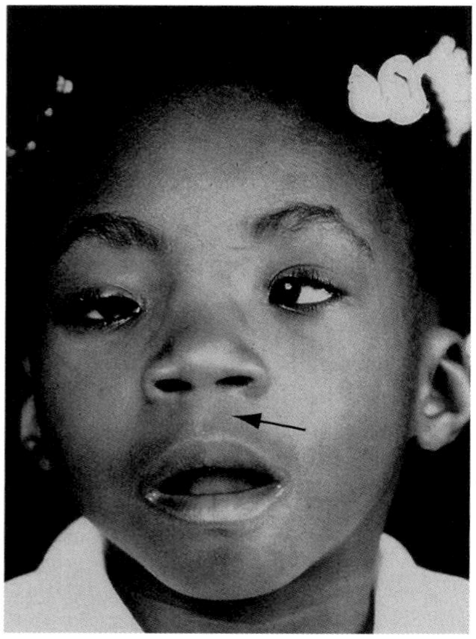

Figure 18-10 Fetal alcohol syndrome. Asymmetric ptosis; telecanthus; strabismus; long, flat philtrum (*arrow*); anteverted nostrils. This child also had Peters anomaly, left eye, and myopia, right eye. *(Reproduced with permission from Miller MT, Israel J, Cuttone J. Fetal alcohol syndrome.* J Pediatr Ophthalmol Strabismus. 1981;18(4):6–15.)

Nonsynostotic disorders of bone growth

Infantile malignant osteopetrosis In this rare and severe autosomal recessive form of osteopetrosis, proliferation of bone results in narrowing of the foramina of the skull. Stenosis of the optic canal increases the risk of compressive optic neuropathy. Bone marrow transplant has been reported to reverse the stenosis.

Craniometaphyseal dysplasia Craniometaphyseal dysplasia is a rare disorder of osteoclast resorption that causes hyperostosis of the cranial bones. The typical facial appearance includes frontal and paranasal bossing. Progressive stenosis of cranial nerve foramina can result in compressive optic neuropathy.

Infectious and Inflammatory Conditions

Preseptal and orbital cellulitis usually progress more rapidly and are more severe in children than in adults. See also BCSC Section 7, *Oculofacial Plastic and Orbital Surgery*.

Preseptal Cellulitis

Preseptal cellulitis, a common infection in children, is an inflammatory process involving the tissues anterior to the orbital septum. Eyelid edema may extend into the forehead. The periorbital skin becomes taut and inflamed, and edema of the contralateral eyelids may appear. Proptosis is not a feature of preseptal cellulitis, and the globe remains uninvolved. Full ocular motility and absence of pain on eye movement help distinguish preseptal from orbital cellulitis.

胎儿酒精综合征的典型眼部特征为短睑裂、内眦距过宽、内眦赘皮、上睑下垂、小眼球、内斜视（图 18–10）。可伴有眼前节发育不良、视神经发育不全、高度屈光不正。50% 的漏诊患者会有视力损害。

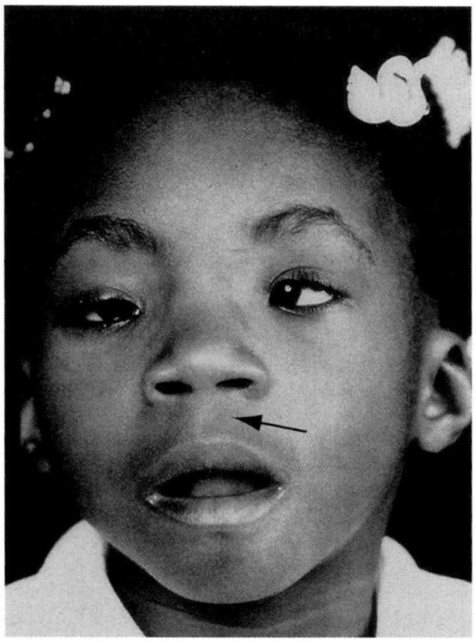

图 18–10　胎儿酒精综合征。不对称上睑下垂，内眦距过宽，斜视，长而平的人中（*箭头*），前仰鼻孔。患儿同时患有左眼 Peter 异常，右眼近视。*（译者注：资料来源见前页原文。）*

骨生长的非骨性连结疾病

婴儿恶性骨硬化病　这种罕见严重的常染色体隐性骨硬化、骨增殖导致颅骨孔的狭窄。视神经管狭窄增加了压迫性视神经病变的风险。有报道称骨髓移植可以逆转视神经管狭窄。

颅骨骺端发育不良　颅骨骺端发育不良是一种罕见的破骨细胞吸收障碍，可导致颅骨骨增生。典型的面部特征包括额部和鼻旁部结节，颅神经孔进行性狭窄导致压迫性视神经病变。

感染及发炎

儿童的眶前和眶蜂窝织炎比成人进展更快、后果更严重。见 BCSC 第 7 册《*眼面部整形与眼眶手术*》。

眶前蜂窝织炎

眶前蜂窝织炎是一种常见的儿童感染，是一种累及眶隔前组织的炎症，眼睑水肿可扩展至前额，眶周皮肤肿胀发炎，可出现对侧眼睑水肿。眶前蜂窝织炎一般不累及眼球，不伴眼球突出。眼球运动不受限和不伴眼部转动疼痛可与眶蜂窝织炎鉴别。

Preseptal cellulitis typically develops in 1 of 3 ways:

- following puncture, insect bite, or laceration of the eyelid skin (posttraumatic cellulitis): In these cases, organisms found on the skin, such as *Staphylococcus* or *Streptococcus* species, are most commonly responsible for the infection.
- in conjunction with severe conjunctivitis such as epidemic keratoconjunctivitis or methicillin-resistant *Staphylococcus aureus* (MRSA) conjunctivitis, or with skin infection such as impetigo or herpes zoster.
- secondary to upper respiratory tract or sinus infection: *Streptococcus pneumoniae* and other streptococcal species, and *S aureus* are the most common causative organisms.

Children with nonsevere preseptal infections can be treated with oral antibiotics as outpatients. Broad-spectrum drugs effective against the most common pathogens, such as cephalosporins or ampicillin–clavulanic acid combination, are usually effective. Particularly with eyelid abscesses, clindamycin may be an appropriate choice because of the increasing prevalence of MRSA, which should also be considered in patients who do not improve with treatment. Eyelid abscesses may require urgent incision and drainage.

For young infants or patients with signs of systemic illness such as sepsis or meningeal involvement, hospital admission may be indicated for appropriate cultures, imaging of the sinuses and orbits, and intravenous (IV) antibiotics. In newborns, dacryocystocele should be considered in the differential diagnosis (see Chapter 19).

Orbital Cellulitis

Orbital cellulitis involves the tissues posterior to the orbital septum. It is most commonly associated with ethmoid or frontal sinusitis but can also occur following penetrating injuries of the orbit.

Most young children with orbital cellulitis have infections caused by a single aerobic pathogen. In the neonate, *S aureus* and gram-negative bacilli are most common. In older children and adults, *S aureus*, *Streptococcus pyogenes*, and *S pneumoniae* are common etiologic agents. Concurrent infections with multiple pathogens, including gram-negative and anaerobic organisms, can occur in older or immunosuppressed patients.

Early signs and symptoms of orbital cellulitis include lethargy, fever, eyelid edema, rhinorrhea, headache, orbital pain, and tenderness on palpation. The nasal mucosa becomes hyperemic, with a purulent nasal discharge. Increased venous congestion may cause elevated intraocular pressure. Proptosis, chemosis, and limited ocular movement suggest orbital involvement.

The differential diagnosis of orbital cellulitis includes nonspecific orbital inflammation, benign orbital tumors such as lymphatic malformation and hemangioma, and malignant tumors such as rhabdomyosarcoma, leukemia, and metastases.

Paranasal sinusitis is the most common cause of bacterial orbital cellulitis (Fig 18-11). In children younger than 10 years, the ethmoid sinuses are most frequently involved. If orbital cellulitis is suspected, orbital imaging is indicated to confirm orbital involvement, to document the presence and extent of sinusitis and a subperiosteal abscess (Fig 18-12), and to rule out a foreign body in a patient with a history of trauma.

眶前蜂窝织炎的病程发展有以下 3 种情况：

- 眼睑皮肤刺伤、昆虫咬伤或划伤（外伤后蜂窝组织炎）：在这些情况下，细菌培养可以为阳性，*葡萄球菌*和*链球菌*是最常见的致病菌。

- 常伴发严重结膜炎，如流行性角膜结膜炎或耐甲氧西林*金黄色葡萄球菌*（MRSA）结膜炎，或脓疱疮或带状疱疹等皮肤感染。

- 继发于上呼吸道或鼻窦感染：*肺炎链球菌*、其他链球菌和*金黄色葡萄球菌*是最常见的病原菌。

轻中度感染的儿童可口服抗生素治疗，门诊随诊。对常见病原体，广谱抗生素通常有效，如头孢菌素或克拉维酸－氨苄西林。考虑到 MRSA 越来越常见，对于治疗无效的眼睑脓肿患者，可选择克林霉素。眼睑脓肿可根据需要切开、引流。

对于婴幼儿或有全身受累（如败血症或脑膜受累）的患者，可住院治疗，培养病原体，行鼻窦和眼眶影像学检查，静脉注射抗生素。新生儿患者需与泪囊膨出相鉴别（见第 19 章）。

眶蜂窝织炎

眶蜂窝织炎累及眶隔后组织。常见于筛窦炎或额窦炎，但也见于眶穿通裂伤之后。

大多数儿童眶蜂窝织炎都是单一需氧病原体引起的感染。在新生儿中，金黄色葡萄球菌和革兰阴性杆菌最为常见。在年龄较大的儿童和成人中，*金黄色葡萄球菌*、*化脓性链球菌*和*肺炎链球菌*是常见的病原体。老年或免疫抑制使用的患者，可以发生包括革兰氏阴性菌和厌氧菌在内的各种病原体的混合感染。

眶蜂窝组织炎的早期症状和体征包括嗜睡、发烧、眼睑水肿、流鼻涕、头痛、眼眶疼痛和触痛。鼻腔黏膜充血伴脓性分泌物。静脉充血可引起眼压升高。眼球突出、球结膜水肿和眼球运动受限提示眶内受累。

眼窝蜂窝织炎的鉴别诊断包括非特异性眶部炎症、良性眶部肿瘤（如淋巴畸形和血管瘤）以及恶性肿瘤（如横纹肌肉瘤、白血病和转移癌）。

鼻窦炎是细菌性眶蜂窝织炎最常见的病因（图 18–11）。10 岁以下的儿童患者常伴有筛窦炎。一旦怀疑眶蜂窝组织炎，需要行眶部影像学检查以明确眶部受累情况，是否伴有鼻副窦炎及其程度，是否有骨膜下脓肿（图 18–12），对于有外伤史患者，还要排除眶内异物可能。

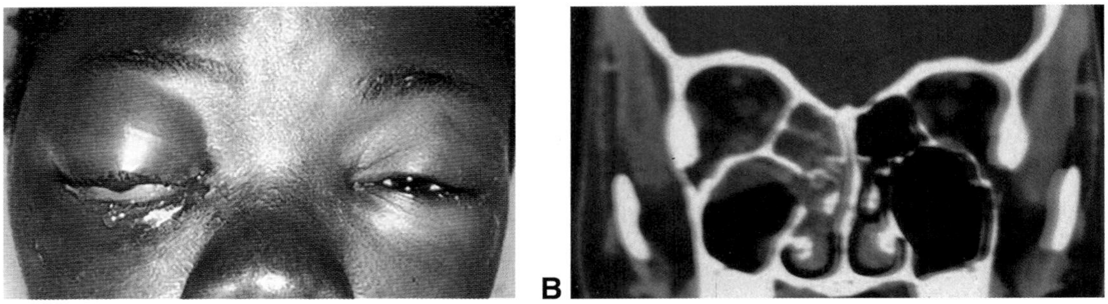

Figure 18-11 Bacterial orbital cellulitis with proptosis **(A)** secondary to sinusitis **(B)**. *(Courtesy of Jane Edmond, MD.)*

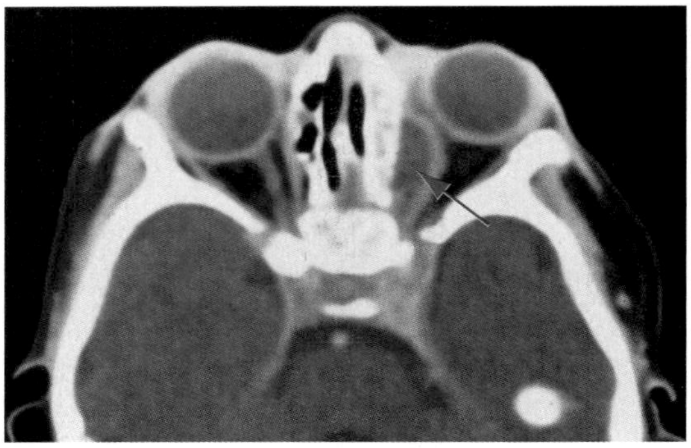

Figure 18-12 Axial computed tomography (CT) image showing a medial subperiosteal abscess (*arrow*) of the left orbit associated with ethmoid sinusitis. *(Courtesy of Jane Edmond, MD.)*

It is crucial to distinguish orbital cellulitis from preseptal cellulitis because the former requires hospital admission and treatment with IV broad-spectrum antibiotics. Choice of IV antibiotic is based on the most likely pathogens until results from cultures are known. If associated sinusitis or subperiosteal abscess is present, pediatric otolaryngologists should be consulted. The patient should be observed closely for signs of visual compromise. Many subperiosteal abscesses in children younger than 9 years resolve with medical management. Emergency drainage of a subperiosteal abscess is indicated for a patient of any age with either of the following:

- evidence of optic nerve compromise (decreasing vision, relative afferent pupillary defect) and an enlarging subperiosteal abscess
- an abscess that does not resolve within 48–72 hours of administration of antibiotics

Intraconal orbital abscesses are much less common than subperiosteal abscesses in children and require urgent surgical drainage.

Complications of orbital cellulitis include cavernous sinus thrombosis and intracranial extension (subdural or brain abscesses, meningitis, periosteal abscess), which may result in death. Cavernous sinus thrombosis can be difficult to distinguish from simple orbital cellulitis. Paralysis of eye movement in cavernous sinus thrombosis is often out of proportion to the degree of proptosis. Pain on motion and tenderness on palpation are absent. Decreased sensation along the maxillary division of cranial nerve V (trigeminal) supports the diagnosis. Bilateral involvement is virtually diagnostic of cavernous sinus thrombosis.

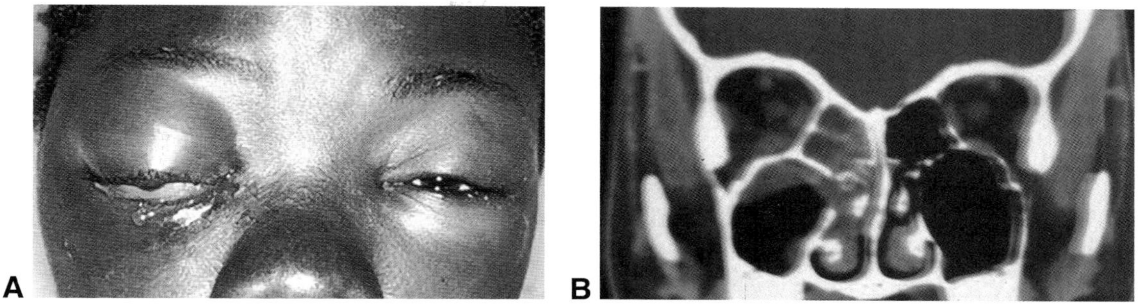

图 18–11　细菌性眶蜂窝组织炎伴眼球突出（**A**），继发于筛窦炎（**B**）。*（译者注：资料来源见前页原文。）*

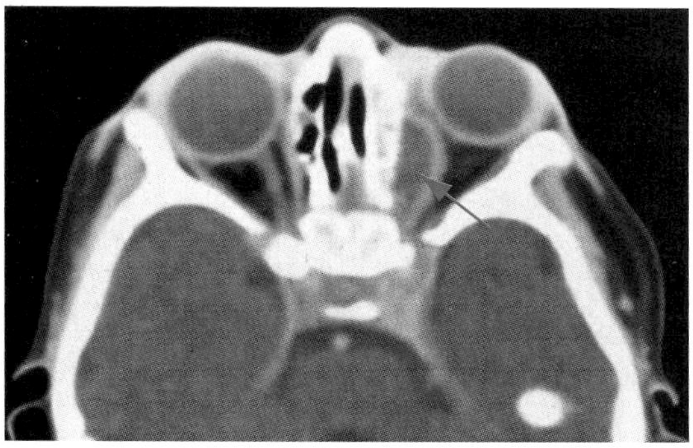

图 18–12　轴性 CT 影像提示左侧筛窦相关的鼻侧骨膜下脓肿（*箭头*）。*（译者注：资料来源见前页原文。）*

眶蜂窝织炎和眶前蜂窝织炎的鉴别至关重要，因为前者需要住院和静脉应用广谱抗生素。静脉注射抗生素的选择先根据临床经验选择，培养结果出来后再根据培养结果调整。如果伴有鼻窦炎或骨膜下脓肿，需要儿童耳鼻喉科会诊。应该密切观察病人视力变化。9 岁以下儿童的骨膜下脓肿多数可通过药物治疗缓解，但如果出现下述情况，需要考虑行急诊切开引流：

- 视神经损害（视力下降，相对传入性瞳孔障碍）和骨膜下脓肿增大。
- 使用抗生素后 48 ~ 72h 内未消退的脓肿。

儿童眶内脓肿比骨膜下脓肿少见得多，需要行急诊手术引流。

眼窝蜂窝织炎的并发症包括海绵窦血栓形成和颅内扩散（硬膜下或脑脓肿、脑膜炎、骨膜脓肿），可导致死亡。海绵窦血栓和单纯的眼窝蜂窝织炎非常难鉴别，海绵窦血栓形成引起的眼球运动麻痹与眼球突出程度不成比例，不伴有眼球运动痛和压痛，第 V 颅神经上颌支分布区域感觉减退有助于诊断。双眼受累即可确诊海绵窦血栓形成。

Other complications of orbital cellulitis include corneal exposure with secondary ulcerative keratitis, neurotrophic keratitis, secondary glaucoma, septic uveitis or retinitis, exudative retinal detachment, optic nerve edema, inflammatory neuritis, infectious neuritis, central retinal artery occlusion, and panophthalmitis.

Liao JC, Harris GJ. Subperiosteal abscess of the orbit: evolving pathogens and the therapeutic protocol. *Ophthalmology*. 2015;122(3):639–647.

Related conditions

Fungal orbital cellulitis (mucormycosis) occurs most frequently in patients with ketoacidosis or severe immunosuppression. The infection causes thrombosing vasculitis with ischemic necrosis of involved tissue (Fig 18-13). Cranial nerves often are involved, and extension into the central nervous system is common. Smears and biopsy of the involved tissues reveal the fungal organisms. Treatment includes debridement and systemic administration of antifungal medication. Allergic fungal sinusitis is a less fulminant condition that frequently presents with orbital signs, including proptosis from remodeling of the bony orbit. See BCSC Section 7, *Oculofacial Plastic and Orbital Surgery*, for further discussion.

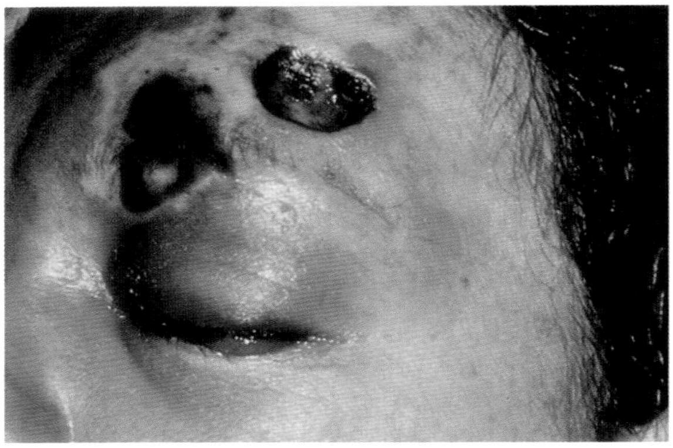

Figure 18-13 Mucormycosis, left orbit.

Childhood Orbital Inflammation

Several noninfectious, nontraumatic disorders cause orbital inflammation in children that may simulate infection or an orbital mass lesion. Thyroid eye disease, the most common cause of proptosis in adults, rarely occurs in prepubescent children but occasionally affects adolescents. Bilateral orbital inflammation may occur with sarcoidosis.

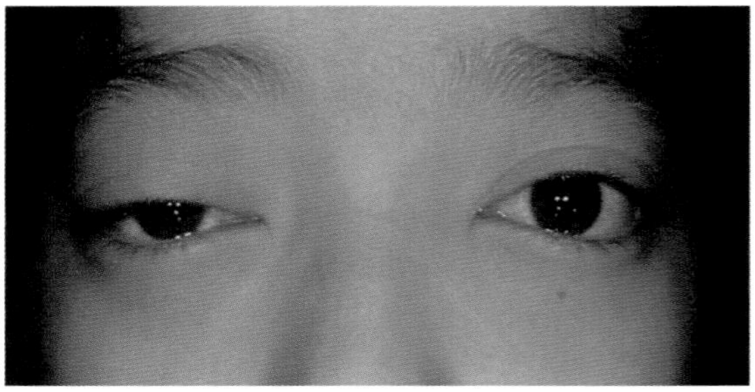

Figure 18-14 Bilateral nonspecific orbital inflammation (orbital pseudotumor) in an 11-year-old boy with a 1-week history of eye pain. Ocular rotation was markedly limited in all directions. CT confirmed proptosis and showed enlargement of all extraocular muscles. Laboratory workup was negative for thyroid disease and rheumatologic disorders. Complete resolution occurred after 1 month of corticosteroid treatment.

眼窝蜂窝织炎的其他并发症包括角膜暴露继发溃疡性角膜炎、神经营养性角膜炎、继发性青光眼、感染性葡萄膜炎或视网膜炎、渗出性视网膜脱离、视神经水肿、炎性神经炎、感染性神经炎、视网膜中央动脉阻塞和全眼炎。

Liao JC, Harris GJ. Subperiosteal abscess of the orbit: evolving pathogens and the therapeutic protocol. *Ophthalmology*. 2015;122(3):639–647.

相关疾病

*真菌性眶蜂窝织炎（毛霉菌病）*最常发生在酮症酸中毒患者或严重的免疫抑制患者身上。感染引起血栓性血管炎，进而导致组织缺血性坏死（图 18–13）。颅神经常累及，并扩散到中枢神经系统。组织涂片和切片检查提示真菌感染。治疗包括清创和全身应用抗真菌药物。过敏性真菌性鼻窦炎是一种症状相对较轻的疾病，常伴有眼眶症状，包括眶骨重塑引起的眼球突出。见 BCSC 第 7 册《*眼面部整形与眼眶手术*》。

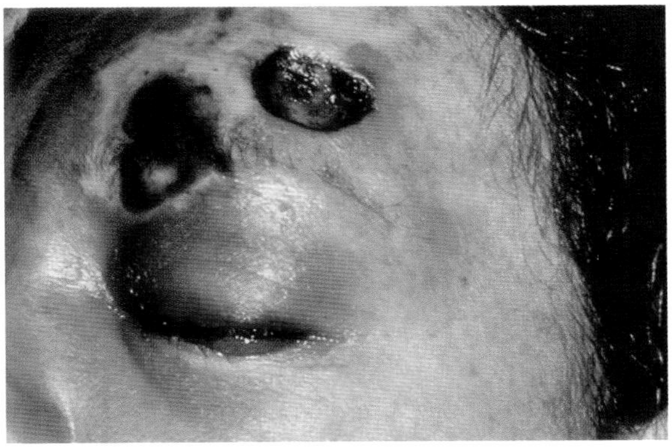

图 18–13　毛霉菌病，左眼框。

儿童眶部感染

有一些非感染性、非创伤性疾病引起的儿童眶部炎症与眶部感染或眼眶肿物表现非常相似。甲状腺相关眼病是成人眼球突出最常见的原因，学龄期儿童很少发生，但偶尔会发生在青春期孩子身上。双眼眶部炎症可见于结节病。

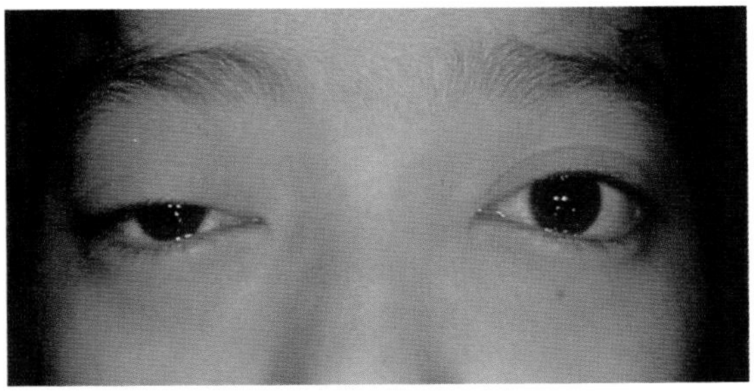

图 18–14　双侧非特异性眼眶炎症（炎性假瘤）：11 岁男孩主诉眼疼 1 周。眼球转动各个方向受限。CT 显示眼球突出和所有眼外肌肥大。实验室检查提示无甲状腺病和风湿。经过 1 个月的糖皮质激素的治疗，炎症完全消除。

Nonspecific orbital inflammation

Nonspecific orbital inflammation (NSOI) (also known as *orbital pseudotumor, idiopathic orbital inflammatory syndrome*) is an inflammatory cause of proptosis in childhood that differs significantly from the adult form. The typical pediatric presentation is acute and painful, more closely resembling orbital cellulitis than tumor or thyroid eye disease (Fig 18-14). NSOI is often bilateral and may be associated with systemic manifestations such as headache, nausea, vomiting, and lethargy. Uveitis is frequently present and occasionally constitutes the dominant manifestation. Imaging studies may show increased density of orbital fat, thickening of posterior sclera and the Tenon layer, or enlargement of extraocular muscles. The lacrimal gland is often involved. Sinusitis is typically not present. Systemic treatment with a corticosteroid usually provides prompt and dramatic relief. Recurrent disease is common. A slow tapering of corticosteroid dosage is usually required to prevent recurrence.

Orbital myositis Orbital myositis describes NSOI that is confined to one or more extraocular muscles. The clinical presentation depends on the amount of inflammation. Diplopia, conjunctival chemosis, and orbital pain are common. Symptoms can be subacute or progress rapidly. Vision is rarely impaired unless massive muscle enlargement is present. Imaging studies show diffusely enlarged muscles with the enlargement extending all the way to the insertion (unlike in thyroid myopathy, which mainly involves the muscle belly). Corticosteroid treatment usually produces rapid relief of symptoms. Prolonged treatment is often necessary, and recurrence is common.

Neoplasms

Several pediatric malignancies may occur in the orbit. Benign adnexal masses, which may threaten vision, are common in the pediatric population.

Differential Diagnosis

Diagnosis of space-occupying lesions in the orbit is particularly challenging because the clinical manifestations are both nonspecific and relatively limited:

- proptosis or other displacement of the globe
- swelling or discoloration of the eyelids
- palpable subcutaneous mass
- ptosis
- strabismus

Many orbital processes may cause rapid onset of symptoms. These include trauma, which may occur without a reliable history. Mild or moderate proptosis can be difficult to detect in an uncooperative child with associated eyelid swelling. Nevertheless, typical presentations of the more common benign orbital and periorbital masses in infants and children (eg, hemangioma and dermoid cyst, discussed later) are sufficiently distinctive to permit confident clinical diagnosis in most cases. A malignant process should be suspected when proptosis and eyelid swelling suggestive of cellulitis are not accompanied by signs of inflammation or when periorbital ecchymosis or hematoma develops in the absence of a history of trauma. Pseudoproptosis can result when the volume of the globe exceeds the capacity of the orbit (eg, patients with primary congenital glaucoma or high myopia).

非特异性眶部炎症

非特异性眼眶炎症（NSOI）（也称为*眼眶假性肿瘤*，*特发性眼眶炎症综合征*）是一种可以引起儿童眼球突出的炎性疾病，其临床表现与成人眼球突出有明显差异。儿童的典型表现发病急，伴疼痛，更像是眶蜂窝织炎，而不是眶肿瘤或甲状腺眼病的表现（图 18–14）。非特异性眼眶炎症（NSOI）常为双侧发病并伴有全身症状，如头痛、恶心、呕吐和嗜睡。常伴有葡萄膜炎，偶尔以葡萄膜炎为主要表现。影像学显示眶脂肪密度增加、后巩膜和 Tenons 囊增厚或眼外肌肥大。泪腺常受累，少见鼻窦。全身应用糖皮质激素治疗常能快速有效地缓解症状，但容易复发。糖皮质激素逐渐减量可以防止复发。

眼眶肌炎　眼眶肌炎是非特异性眼眶炎症 (NSOI) 的一种，仅局限于一条或多条眼外肌。临床表现取决于炎症严重程度。常见复视、结膜水肿及眶周疼痛，可表现为亚急性或急性进展。除非有肿大的肌肉，视力很少受影响。影像学表现显示弥漫性眼外肌肥大，直至肌肉止点 (而甲状腺相关性眼病仅累及肌腹)。糖皮质激素治疗可快速有效地缓解症状，需继续维持用药，因为易复发。

肿瘤

眼眶内可发生多种小儿恶性肿瘤。小儿良性眼附属器肿物，也常危及视力。

鉴别诊断

眼眶占位性病变的诊断具有挑战性，因为其临床表现既非特异性又相对局限：

- 眼球突出或异位
- 眼睑肿胀或变色
- 眼睑皮下肿物
- 上睑下垂
- 斜视

许多眼眶疾病病程发展迅速。如眼眶外伤，发病史不清，轻度或中度的眼球突出伴眼睑肿胀时，因孩子哭闹不合作，很难检查。如果能够提供儿童原发良性眶内或眶周肿物的情况 (如血管瘤和皮样囊肿，稍后讨论)，则对明确诊断有很大帮助。当表现为类似蜂窝织炎的眼球突出和眼睑肿胀但又不伴有炎症体征，或表现有眶周的瘀斑或血肿但又没有明确的外伤史时，应怀疑恶性肿瘤。当眼球体积明显超过眶容积时可以表现为假性眼球突出（如先天性青光眼或高度近视）。

High-quality imaging allows orbital masses to be differentiated noninvasively in many cases. Magnetic resonance imaging (MRI) is the preferred modality for most patients. Computed tomography (CT) is superior at detecting bone abnormalities but exposes the child to radiation and thus should be avoided unless necessary. Ultrasonography may be useful.

Definitive diagnosis often requires biopsy. A pediatric oncologist should be consulted when appropriate. A metastatic workup should be considered prior to orbital surgery, because other, more easily accessible sites can sometimes be biopsied.

Primary Malignant Neoplasms

Malignant diseases of the orbit include primary and metastatic tumors. Most primary malignant tumors of the orbit in childhood are sarcomas. Tumors of epithelial origin are extremely rare.

Rhabdomyosarcoma

The most common primary orbital malignant tumor in children is rhabdomyosarcoma, which is thought to originate from undifferentiated mesenchymal cells. The incidence of this disease (which is found in approximately 5% of pediatric orbital biopsies) exceeds that of all other sarcomas combined. The orbit is the origin of 10% of rhabdomyosarcomas; 25% of these tumors arise elsewhere in the head and neck, occasionally involving the orbit secondarily. The average age at onset is 5–7 years, but rhabdomyosarcoma can occur at any age. Rhabdomyosarcoma in infancy is more aggressive and carries a poorer prognosis.

Although ocular rhabdomyosarcoma usually originates in the orbit, it occasionally arises in the conjunctiva, eyelid, or anterior uveal tract. Presenting signs and symptoms include proptosis (80%–100% of cases), globe displacement (80%), blepharoptosis (30%–50%) (Fig 18-15), conjunctival and eyelid swelling (60%), palpable mass (25%), and pain (10%). Onset of symptoms and signs is usually rapid. Acute, rapidly progressive proptosis with an absence of pain are suggestive of orbital rhabdomyosarcoma. Imaging shows an irregular but well-circumscribed mass of uniform density.

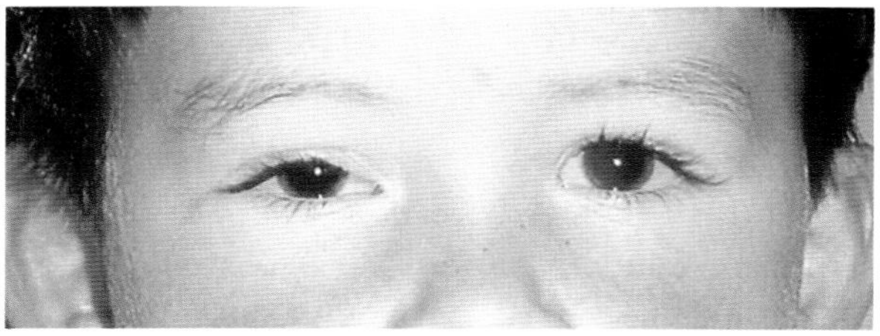

Figure 18-15 Rhabdomyosarcoma in a 4-year-old boy presenting with right upper eyelid ptosis of 3 weeks' duration and a palpable subcutaneous mass.

A biopsy is required for confirmation of the diagnosis whenever rhabdomyosarcoma is suspected. The most common histologic type is embryonal, which shows few cells containing characteristic cross-striations. Second in frequency is the prognostically unfavorable alveolar pattern, showing poorly differentiated tumor cells compartmentalized by orderly connective tissue septa. Botryoid (grapelike) or well-differentiated pleomorphic tumors are rarely found in the orbit but may originate in the conjunctiva.

Small encapsulated or otherwise well-localized rhabdomyosarcomas should be totally excised when possible. Usually, chemotherapy and radiation are used in conjunction with surgery. Exenteration of the orbit is seldom indicated. Primary orbital rhabdomyosarcoma has a relatively good prognosis. The 5-year survival rates are 74% and 94% for patients with alveolar cell type and those with embryonal cell type, respectively.

高分辨率影可以无创鉴别多数眼眶肿物。核磁共振成像（MRI）是首选方式。计算机断层扫描（CT）检测骨骼异常有优势，但会使儿童暴露于辐射线，因此应避免使用。超声检查有助于诊断。

确诊需要进行活检。必要时需请儿科肿瘤专家会诊。眼眶手术前应排除转移灶，因为有时可能对更容易操作的其他部位进行活检。

原发性恶性肿瘤

眼眶恶性疾病包括原发性和转移性肿瘤，儿童眼眶原发性恶性肿瘤多为肉瘤，上皮源性肿瘤极为罕见。

横纹肌肉瘤

儿童最常见的原发性眼眶恶性肿瘤是横纹肌肉瘤，它被认为起源于未分化的间质细胞。这种疾病的发生率（约 5% 的儿童是在眼眶活检中发现的）超过所有其他肉瘤的总和，在横纹肌肉瘤中，源发于眼眶的占 10%，源于头部和颈部等部位的占 25%，偶见继发累及眼球。平均发病年龄为 5~7 岁，也见于其他年龄段。婴儿期即出现的横纹肌肉瘤进展快，预后较差。

眼部横纹肌肉瘤常源于眼眶，偶见脱结膜、眼睑或前部葡萄膜，其症状和体征包括眼球突出（80%~100%）、眼球脱位（80%）、眼睑下垂（30%~50%）（图 18-15）、结膜和眼睑肿胀（60%）、眼睑肿物（25%）和疼痛（10%）。症状和体征常进展迅速。急性、迅速进展的无痛性眼球突出提示眶横纹肌肉瘤。影像学表现为不规则但界限清楚的均匀密度肿块。

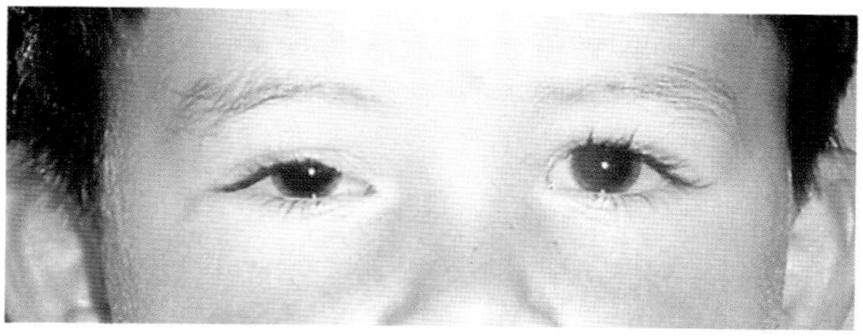

图 18-15 4 岁男孩横纹肌肉瘤在 3 周内呈现右眼上睑下垂，并可触及皮下包块。

当怀疑横纹肌肉瘤时，需要进行活检以确定诊断。最常见的组织学类型是胚胎细胞型，只有很少细胞具有典型的横纹状外观。其次是预后较差的肺泡型横纹肌肉瘤，细胞分化程度较低，有规则的组织间隔。葡萄状或分化较好的多形性肿瘤在眼球横纹肌肉瘤中很少见，但偶见于结膜横纹肌肉瘤。

小结节状或其他比较局限的横纹肌肉瘤应尽可能彻底切除。通常，结膜囊内化疗和放疗治疗与手术同步开展。眶剜除术罕见。原发眼球横纹肌肉瘤预后相对良好。肺泡细胞型和胚胎细胞型 5 年生存率分别为 74% 和 94%。

Other sarcomas

Osteosarcoma, chondrosarcoma, and fibrosarcoma can develop in the orbit during childhood. The risk of sarcoma is increased in children with a history of heritable retinoblastoma, particularly when external-beam radiation treatment has been given.

Metastatic Tumors

The orbit is the most common site of ocular metastasis in children, in contrast to adults, in whom the uvea is the most frequent site.

Neuroblastoma

Neuroblastoma is the most frequent source of orbital metastasis in childhood. This disorder is discussed in Chapter 28.

Ewing sarcoma

Ewing sarcoma is composed of small round cells and usually originates in the long bones of the extremities or in the axial skeleton. Among solid tumors, Ewing sarcoma is the second most frequent source of orbital metastasis. Treatment regimens involving surgery, radiation, and chemotherapy allow long-term survival in many patients with disseminated disease.

Hematopoietic, Lymphoproliferative, and Histiocytic Neoplasms

Leukemia

Leukemic infiltration of the orbit is relatively uncommon and more characteristic of acute myelogenous leukemia. Orbital involvement may be difficult to distinguish from bacterial or fungal orbital cellulitis. Orbital infiltration can cause proptosis, eyelid swelling, and ecchymosis. It may be best managed by radiation therapy. *Granulocytic sarcoma*, or *chloroma* (in reference to the greenish color of involved tissue), is a localized accumulation of myeloid leukemic cells; the tumor may occur anywhere in the body, including in the orbit. This lesion may develop several months before leukemia becomes evident hematologically. Leukemia is discussed in Chapter 28.

Lymphoma

In contrast with lymphoma in adults, lymphoma in children very rarely involves the orbit. Burkitt lymphoma, endemic to East Africa and uncommon in North America , is the most likely form to involve the orbit.

Langerhans cell histiocytosis

Langerhans cell histiocytosis (*LCH*; formerly called *histiocytosis X*) is the collective term for a group of disorders, usually arising in childhood, that involve abnormal proliferation of histiocytes, often within bone. The disorders are classified as unifocal eosinophilic granuloma of the bone, multifocal eosinophilic granuloma of the bone, and diffuse soft-tissue histiocytosis.

其他肉瘤

儿童眼眶也可以发生骨肉瘤、软骨肉瘤和纤维肉瘤等。患儿有遗传性视网膜母细胞瘤病史时发生肉瘤的概率会增加，特别是曾行外放射治疗的患儿。

转移性肿瘤

眼眶是儿童最常见的眼部转移性肿瘤部位，而成人最常见的转移性肿瘤部位是葡萄膜。

神经母细胞瘤

神经母细胞瘤是儿童最常见的眶内转移瘤。我们将在第 28 章进行讨论。

Ewing 肉瘤

Ewing 肉瘤由小的圆细胞组成，常源于四肢长骨或中轴骨骼。在实体肿瘤中，Ewing 肉瘤是第二大眶部常见转移瘤。手术、放射治疗和化学治疗等治疗方案联合应用可使许多播散性肿瘤患者获得长期生存。

造血、淋巴增生性和组织细胞性肿瘤

白血病

白血病浸润眶部相对少见，是急性髓性白血病的特征性表现，眼眶受累时的临床表现可能与细菌性或真菌性眶蜂窝织炎难以区分。眼眶浸润可引起眼球突出、眼睑肿胀和瘀斑，最好采用放射治疗。*粒细胞肉瘤*或*绿色瘤*（受累组织呈绿色）是髓性白细胞的局部聚集表现，肿瘤可出现在全身任何地方，包括眶部。可先于血液异常几个月出现。白血病将在第 28 章讨论。

淋巴瘤

与成人淋巴瘤表现不同，儿童淋巴瘤极少累及眶部。Burkitt 淋巴瘤较容易累及眶部，其多见于东非人，少见于北美人。

Langerhans 细胞组织细胞增生症

Langerhans *细胞组织细胞增多症*（*LCH*，以前称为*组织细胞增多症 X*）是一组疾病的统称，通常发生在儿童时期，涉及组织细胞异常增殖，常发生在骨骼内。这些疾病可分为单灶性骨嗜酸性肉芽肿、多灶性骨嗜酸性肉芽肿和弥漫性软组织组织细胞增多症。

Unifocal eosinophilic granuloma, the most localized and benign form of LCH, produces a bone lesion that involves the orbit, skull, ribs, or long bones in childhood or adolescence. Signs and symptoms may include proptosis, ptosis, and periorbital swelling; localized pain and tenderness are relatively common. CT characteristically shows sharply demarcated osteolytic lesions without surrounding sclerosis (Fig 18-16). Treatment consists of observation of isolated asymptomatic lesions, excision or curettage, systemic or intralesional corticosteroid administration, or low-dose radiation therapy. All modalities have a high rate of success.

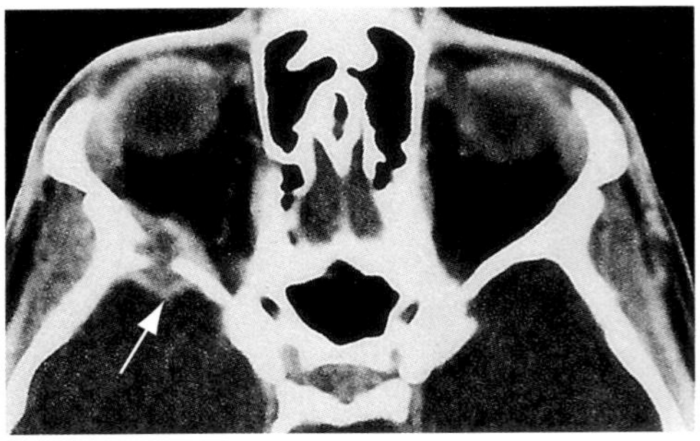

Figure 18-16 Axial CT image showing unifocal eosinophilic granuloma with partial destruction of the right posterior lateral orbital wall (*arrow*) in a 15-year-old boy, who presented with retrobulbar pain and mild edema and erythema of the right upper eyelid.

Multifocal eosinophilic granuloma of the bone is a disseminated and aggressive form of LCH. It usually presents between 2 and 5 years of age and may produce proptosis from involvement of the bony orbit. Diabetes insipidus is common. Chemotherapy is often required, but the prognosis is generally good.

Diffuse soft-tissue histiocytosis, the most severe form, usually affects infants younger than 2 years. It is characterized by soft-tissue lesions of multiple viscera (liver, spleen) but rarely involves the eye.

Benign Tumors

Vascular lesions: hemangiomas

The current classification of vascular lesions establishes clinical, histologic, and prognostic differences between hemangiomas and vascular malformations. The older terms *capillary* and *strawberry hemangioma* have been replaced by the single term *hemangioma*. Cavernous hemangiomas, port-wine stains, and lymphangiomas are classified as "malformations." This nomenclature has not been used consistently in the ophthalmologic literature.

Hemangiomas are hamartomatous growths composed of proliferating capillary endothelial cells. Periocular hemangiomas can be classified as follows:

- preseptal, involving the skin and preseptal orbit
- intraorbital, involving the postseptal orbit
- compound/mixed, involving the preseptal and postseptal orbit

Hemangiomas occur in 1%–3% of term newborns and are more common in premature infants, in females, and after chorionic villus sampling. Most hemangiomas are clinically insignificant at birth. They can be inapparent or can appear as an erythematous macule or a telangiectasia. The Natural history is one of rapid proliferation and growth over the first several months of life, rarely lasting beyond 1 year. Periocular lesions may cause amblyopia by inducing astigmatism or obstructing the visual axis. After the first year of life, the lesions usually begin to regress, although the rate and degree of involution vary.

单灶性骨嗜酸性肉芽肿，是 Langerhans 细胞组织细胞增多症（LCH）中局灶化良性病变且多局灶化，表现为儿童或青少年眶部、头颅、肋骨、四肢长骨的骨质局限性病灶。症状和体征包括眼球突出、上睑下垂和球周组织水肿。常见局部肿胀和疼痛。CT 显示界清的溶骨性改变，不伴病灶周围硬化（图 18–16）。治疗包含观察孤立的无症状肿物变化，肿瘤切除或者刮除，全身应用激素、肿瘤局部激素注射，或低剂量放射治疗。各种方法都有较高成功率。

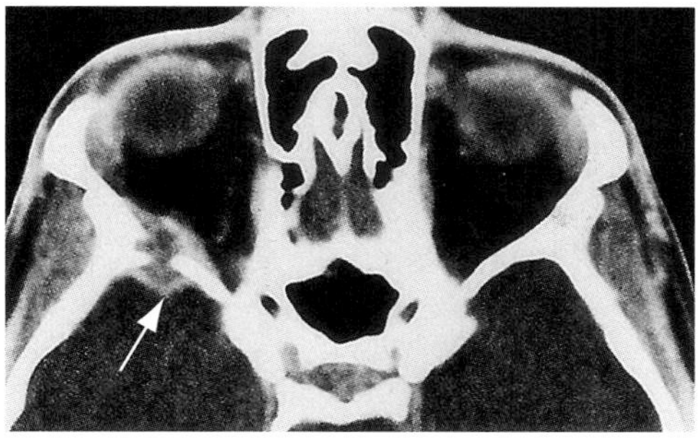

图 18–16　15 岁男孩述球后痛和右上眼睑轻度水肿和充血，轴向 CT 显示单灶性骨嗜酸性肉芽肿，伴右后颞侧眶壁部分破坏（*箭头*）。

*骨多灶嗜酸性肉芽肿*是一种弥漫性进行性 Langerhans 细胞组织细胞增多症（LCH）。常见于 2~5 岁儿童，当眶骨受累时可出现眼球突出。尿崩症常见。常需化学治疗，预后较好。

*弥漫性软组织组织细胞增多症*是最严重的一种 Langerhans 细胞组织细胞增多症（LCH），常见于 2 岁以下婴儿，其特征是多脏器（肝、脾）的软组织损害，但很少累及眼睛。

良性肿瘤

血管病变：肝血管瘤

新的血管病变分类从临床表现、组织学和预后差异对血管瘤和血管畸形进行鉴别。以前的*毛细血管瘤*和*草莓状血管瘤*名称已被统一称为*血管瘤*。海绵状血管瘤、斑疹性斑疹和淋巴管瘤称为“血管畸形”。这一命名在眼科文献中并没有得到很好的应用。

血管瘤是由增生的毛细血管内皮细胞组成的错构瘤。眼周血管瘤可分为以下几类：

- 隔前，包括皮肤和隔前眼眶
- 眶内，包括眶隔后眶部
- 复合 / 混合，包括眶隔前和眶隔后眶部

血管瘤发生在 1%~3% 的新生儿中，在早产儿、女性和绒毛膜绒毛取样后婴儿中更常见。大多数血管瘤出生时的临床意义不大，可能不明显可见或表现为红色的斑点或毛细血管扩张。在出生的头几个月里快速生长和扩大，但很少持续超过 1 年，球周的病变可能由于散光或遮挡视轴而导致弱视。1 年后，肿瘤自然消退，但消退的程度和速度不相同。

Systemic disease associated with hemangiomas *PHACE* is an acronym for posterior fossa malformations, hemangiomas, arterial lesions, and cardiac and eye anomalies. The eye abnormalities include increased retinal vascularity, microphthalmia, optic nerve hypoplasia, proptosis, choroidal hemangiomas, strabismus, colobomas, cataracts, and glaucoma. The PHACE syndrome should be considered in any infant presenting with a large, segmental, plaquelike facial hemangioma involving one or more dermatomes (Fig 18-17).

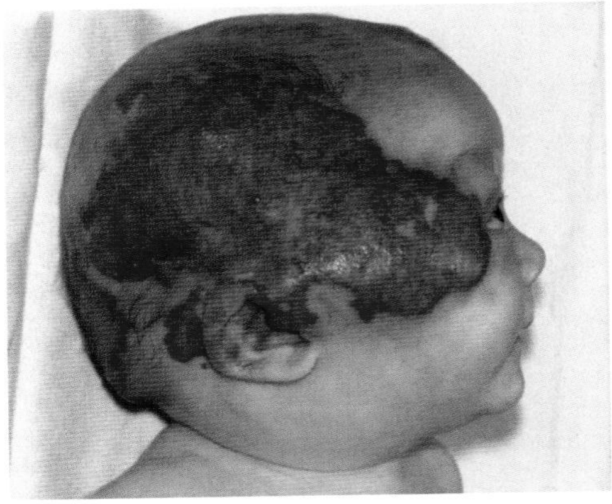

Figure 18-17 Plaque hemangioma in a child with PHACE (posterior fossa malformations, hemangiomas, arterial lesions, and cardiac and eye anomalies) syndrome. *(Courtesy of Ken K. Nischal, MD.)*

Kasabach-Merritt syndrome is a thrombocytopenic coagulopathy with a high mortality rate. It is caused by sequestration of platelets within a vascular lesion.

Diffuse neonatal hemangiomatosis is a potentially lethal condition that occurs in infants, with multiple small cutaneous hemangiomas associated with visceral lesions affecting the liver, gastrointestinal tract, and brain. These hemangiomas are initially asymptomatic but can lead to cardiac failure and death within weeks. Infants with more than 3 cutaneous lesions should be evaluated for visceral lesions.

Treatment of hemangiomas The diagnosis of hemangiomas is usually obvious from the clinical presentation. MRI or ultrasonography is sometimes helpful in establishing the diagnosis and delineating the posterior extent of the lesion.

Observation is indicated when hemangiomas are small and there is no risk of amblyopia.

Propranolol, a nonselective β-adrenergic blocking agent, induces involution of most hemangiomas (Fig 18-18). The risks of systemic treatment with β-blockers in infants include bradycardia, hypotension, hypoglycemia, and bronchospasm, but the medication is usually well tolerated. Particular caution should be taken when propranolol is used in children with PHACE syndrome, because this drug may increase their risk of stroke. Timolol maleate solution applied topically may be effective in treating superficial hemangiomas. Pulsed dye laser can treat superficial hemangiomas with few complications, but it has little effect on deeper components of the tumor.

Surgical excision of periocular hemangiomas is feasible for some well-localized lesions or for lesions that do not respond to propranolol.

Drolet BA, Frommelt PC, Chamlin SL, et al. Initiation and use of propranolol for infantile hemangioma: report of a consensus conference. *Pediatrics*. 2013;131(1):128–140.

与血管瘤相关的全身性疾病　*PHACE* 是后颅窝畸形、血管瘤、动脉病变、心脏和眼睛异常的首字母缩写。眼部异常包括视网膜血管增生、小眼球、视神经发育不良、眼球突出、脉络膜血管瘤、斜视、组织缺损、白内障和青光眼。任何婴儿出现一片或多片皮肤上大的、节段的、片状的面部血管瘤时，都应考虑 PHACE 综合征（图 18–17）。

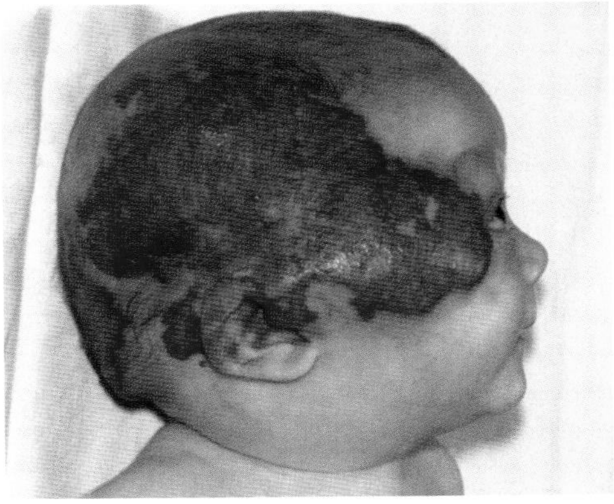

图 18–17　伴 PHACE 综合征（后颅窝畸形、血管瘤、动脉病变、心脏和眼睛异常）患儿的斑块状血管瘤。*（译者注：资料来源见前页原文。）*

*Kasabach–Merritt 综合征*是一种高死亡率的血小板减少性凝血病，由血管病变内的血小板聚集引起。

*弥漫性新生儿血管瘤病*是一种发生在婴儿身上的潜在致命疾病，多发的小片状皮肤血管瘤伴有影响肝脏、胃肠道和大脑的内脏病变。这些血管瘤最初无症状，但可在数周内导致心力衰竭和死亡。婴儿身上有超过 3 处的皮肤血管瘤即应该考虑排除内脏病变。

血管瘤的治疗　血管瘤的诊断通常从临床表现上就很容易明确，MRI 或超声检查有时有助于确定诊断和描述病变的严重程度。

血管瘤小的时候以观察为主，无弱视危险。

普萘洛尔，一个非选择性 β 肾上腺素能阻滞剂，可以导致大多数血管瘤退化（图 18–18）。在婴儿全身应用的风险包括心动过缓、低血压、低血糖、支气管痉挛，但一般来说，患者是可以耐受的。普萘洛尔在 PHACE 综合征患儿身上应用时应特别小心谨慎，因为这种药物可能增加其患中风的风险。马来酸噻吗洛尔溶液局部使用对浅表血管瘤有效。脉冲激光治疗浅表血管瘤并发症少，但对肿瘤深部成分影响很小。

一些良性的眼周局部血管瘤或对普萘洛尔治疗没有反应的眼周血管瘤可以手术切除。

Drolet BA, Frommelt PC, Chamlin SL, et al. Initiation and use of propranolol for infantile hemangioma: report of a consensus conference. *Pediatrics*. 2013;131(1):128–140.

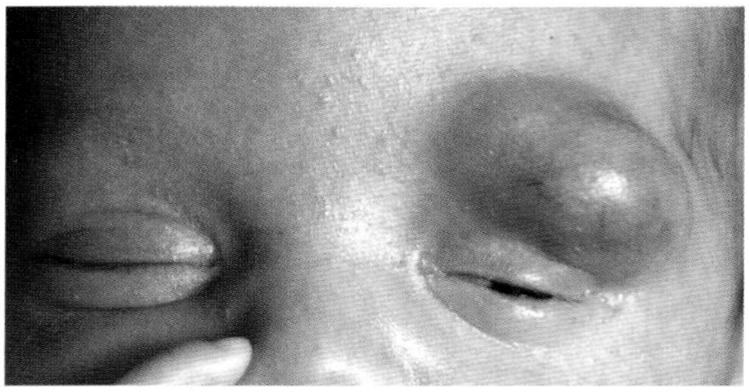

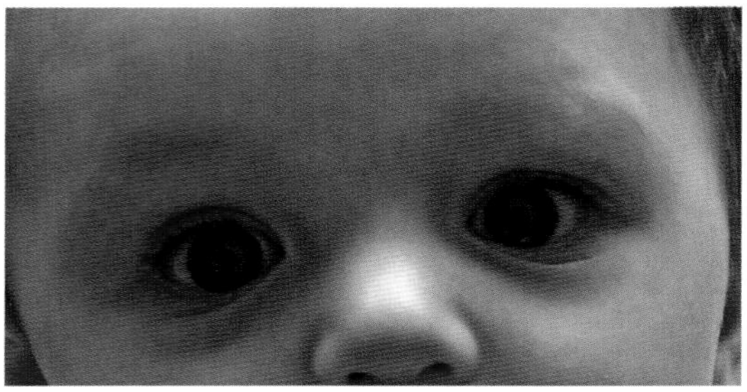

Figure 18-18 **A**, Two-month-old infant with a large hemangioma above the left eye. **B**, Resolution of the lesion following treatment with propranolol. *(Courtesy of Gregg T. Lueder, MD.)*

Vascular lesions: malformations

Vascular malformations are developmental anomalies derived from capillary venous, arterial, or lymphatic vessels. In contrast to hemangiomas, vascular malformations remain relatively static. The age at onset and mode of clinical presentation vary. Cutaneous vascular malformations such as port-wine stains are evident from birth, but many vascular malformations do not manifest until later in life.

Orbital lymphatic malformation Orbital lymphatic malformation, previously known as lymphangioma, may produce proptosis in infancy, but usually does not until the second decade of life or later. Unilateral smaller cornea, anomalous anterior segment vessels, and abnormal retinal vessel branching in association with orbital lymphatic malformation represent a unique malformation syndrome. Lymphatic malformation of the orbit is best managed conservatively. Exacerbations tend to occur during upper respiratory tract infections and may be managed with a short course of systemic corticosteroids. Rapid expansion may be seen in cases of intralesional hemorrhage (Fig 18-19). Partial resection and drainage may be required if vision is threatened. Because of the infiltrative character of this malformation, complete removal is usually impossible. Newer treatments include oral sildenafil and intralesional injection of sclerosing agents.

Khan AO, Ghadhfan FE. Small cornea with anomalous anterior segment and retinal vasculature associated with lymphangioma. *J AAPOS.* 2009;13(1):82–84.

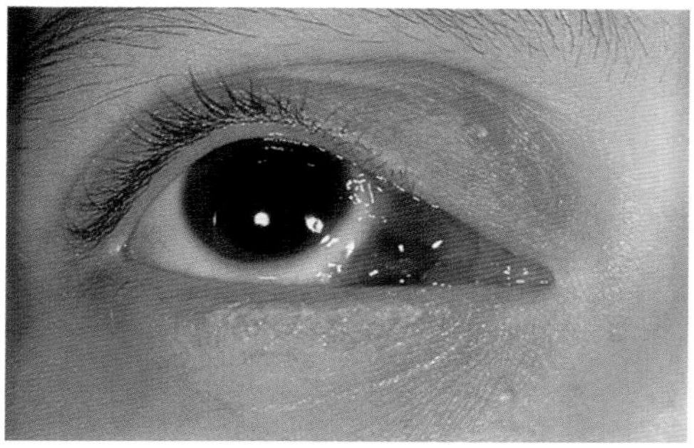

Figure 18-19 Lymphatic malformation with hemorrhage involving the right orbit, upper eyelid, and conjunctiva in a 15-year-old girl.

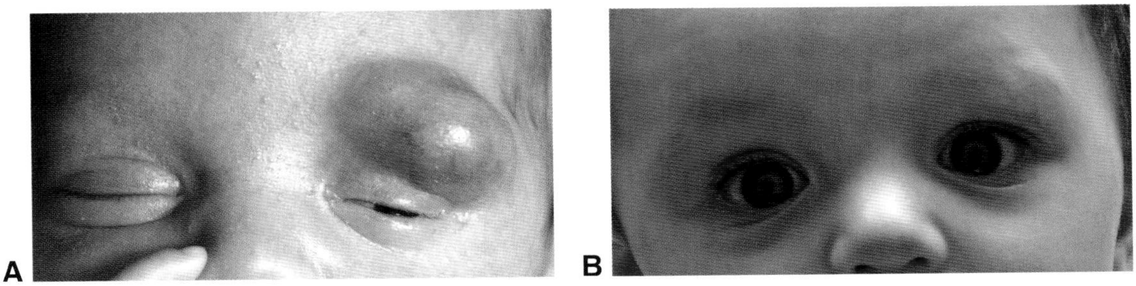

图 18-18　**A.** 2 个月大的婴儿，左眼上方有一个巨大的血管瘤。**B.** 普萘洛尔治疗后病灶的消退情况。*（译者注：资料来源见前页原文。）*

血管病变：畸形

血管畸形是源于毛细血管静脉、动脉或淋巴管的发育异常。与血管瘤相比，血管畸形相对稳定。发病年龄和临床表现形式各不相同。皮肤血管畸形，如葡萄酒斑，出生时就很明显，但许多血管畸形直到晚年才表现出来。

眼眶淋巴管畸形　眼眶淋巴管畸形，以前称为淋巴管瘤，可导致婴儿时期出现眼球突出，但通常眼球突出要到 20 岁或以后才会出现。单侧小角膜和与眼眶淋巴管畸形有关的眼前节血管异常和视网膜脉络膜血管分支异常，构成一种独特的畸形综合征。眼眶淋巴畸形最好保守治疗。病情恶化往往发生在上呼吸道感染期间，可通过短期的全身皮质类固醇激素治疗。病灶内出血的病例可见瘤体快速增大（图 18-19）。如果视力受到影响，需要部分切除和引流。由于这种肿瘤呈浸润生长，不可能完全切除。较新的治疗方法包括口服西地那非和局部注射硬化剂。

Khan AO, Ghadhfan FE. Small cornea with anomalous anterior segment and retinal vasculature associated with lymphangioma. *J AAPOS.* 2009;13(1):82–84.

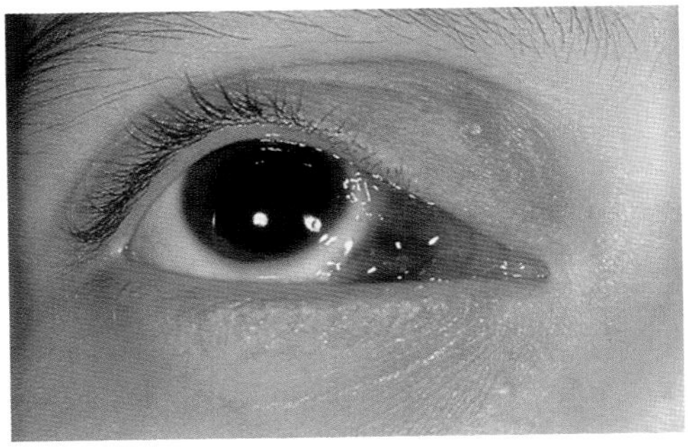

图 18-19　15 岁女童右侧眼眶、上眼睑和结膜淋巴畸形合并出血。

Orbital venous malformations Orbital venous malformations, or varices, can be divided into 2 types: primary and secondary. The primary type is confined to the orbit and is not associated with arteriovenous malformations (AVMs). Secondary orbital varices occur as a result of intracranial AVM shunts that cause dilation of the orbital veins. Orbital venous malformations usually become symptomatic after years of progressive congestion and rarely manifest before the second decade of life. Treatment is reserved for highly symptomatic lesions.

Orbital arteriovenous malformations AVMs isolated within the orbit are extremely rare. Patients with congenital AVMs of the retina and midbrain (*Wyburn-Mason syndrome;* see Chapter 28) may have orbital involvement. AVMs of the bony orbit rarely manifest in childhood but when present are characterized by pulsatile proptosis, chemosis, congested conjunctival vessels, and elevated intraocular pressure. AVMs may be treated by embolization, surgical resection, or both.

Tumors of bony origin

During the early years of life, a variety of uncommon benign orbital tumors of bony origin can present with gradually increasing proptosis. *Fibrous dysplasia and juvenile ossifying fibroma* are similar disorders in which normal bone is replaced by fibro-osseous tissue. In both conditions, orbital CT shows varying degrees of lucency and sclerosis.

Fibrous dysplasia has a slow progression that ceases when skeletal maturation is complete. The most serious complication is vision loss caused by optic nerve compression, which may occur acutely. Periodic assessment of vision, pupil function, and optic disc appearance is indicated. Surgical treatment is indicated for functional deterioration or disfigurement.

Juvenile ossifying fibroma is distinguished histologically by the presence of osteoblasts. It tends to be more locally invasive than fibrous dysplasia; some authorities recommend early excision.

Brown tumor of bone is an osteoclastic giant cell reaction resulting from hyperparathyroidism. *Aneurysmal bone cyst* is a degenerative process in which normal bone is replaced by cystic cavities containing fibrous tissue, inflammatory cells, and blood, producing a characteristic radiographic appearance.

Tumors of connective tissue origin

Benign orbital tumors originating from connective tissue are rare in childhood. *Juvenile fibromatosis* may present as a mass in the inferoanterior part of the orbit. These tumors, sometimes called *myofibromas* or *desmoid tumors*, are composed of relatively mature fibroblasts. They tend to recur locally after excision and can be difficult to control, but they do not metastasize.

Tumors of neural origin

Optic pathway glioma is the most important orbital tumor of neural origin in childhood. Optic pathway gliomas are usually low-grade pilocytic astrocytomas, but the rate of growth with or without therapeutic intervention is unpredictable. Management of these tumors is controversial and depends largely on their location. Approximately 30% of optic pathway gliomas are associated with neurofibromatosis type 1. *Plexiform neurofibroma* nearly always occurs in the context of neurofibromatosis and frequently involves the eyelid and orbit. See Chapter 28 for further discussion of plexiform neurofibroma and optic pathway glioma. Orbital *meningioma* and *schwannoma* (neurilemoma, neurinoma) are rare in childhood.

眼眶静脉畸形 眼眶静脉畸形或静脉曲张可分为原发性和继发性两种类型。原发性局限于眶内，与动静脉畸形（AVMs）无关。继发性眼眶静脉曲张是由于颅内静脉分流导致眼眶静脉扩张所致。眼眶静脉畸形通常在多年的进行性充血后出现症状，在 20 岁之前很少出现。病情严重者采取保留治疗。

眼眶动静脉畸形 眼眶内孤立的动静脉畸形（AVMs）极其罕见。先天性视网膜和中脑动静脉畸形（AVMs）患者（*Wyburn- Mason 综合征*；见第 28 章）可累及眼眶。骨性眼眶动静脉畸形在儿童时期很少出现，特征性表现为搏动性眼球突出、结膜水肿、结膜充血和眼压升高。动静脉畸形（AVMs）可以通过栓塞、手术切除或两者联合治疗。

骨源性肿瘤

各种罕见的良性骨源性眶肿瘤可出现在生命早期，眼球逐渐突出。骨纤维异常增殖症和幼年骨化性纤维瘤是相似的疾病，正常骨被纤维骨组织所取代。在这两种情况下，眼眶 CT 显示不同程度的透明和硬化。

骨纤维异常增殖症进展缓慢，当骨骼成熟时停止。最严重的并发症是由视神经急剧性受压引起的视力丧失，需要定期评估视力、瞳孔功能和视盘形态。当功能退化或外观畸形改变时需手术治疗。

幼年骨化纤维瘤的显著性组织学特征是成骨细胞的存在。比骨纤维异常增殖症的局部畸形增长更快，一些专家建议早期切除。

*骨棕色瘤*是由甲状旁腺功能亢进引起的破骨巨细胞反应。*动脉瘤性骨囊肿*是一种退行性的过程，正常的骨被含有纤维组织、炎症细胞和血液的囊腔所取代，形成一种特征性的影像学表现。

结缔组织源性肿瘤

起源于结缔组织的良性眼眶肿瘤在儿童中很少见。*青少年纤维瘤病*可在眼眶前下方形成肿块。这些由相对成熟的成纤维细胞构成的肿瘤有时被称为*肌纤维瘤*或*硬纤维瘤*。切除后复发，且很难控制，但不转移。

神经源性肿瘤

*视路胶质瘤*是儿童眼眶最重要的神经源性肿瘤。视路神经胶质瘤通常是低度毛细胞星形细胞瘤，但无论是否干预治疗，其生长速度都是不可预测的。这些肿瘤的治疗是有争议的，很大程度上取决于其位置。大约 30% 的视神经通路胶质瘤与 1 型神经纤维瘤病有关。*丛状神经纤维瘤*总是发生在神经纤维瘤病的患者，常累及眼睑和眼眶。关于丛状神经纤维瘤和视路胶质瘤的进一步讨论见第 28 章。眼眶*脑膜瘤*和*神经鞘瘤*（neurilemoma，neurinoma）在儿童中很少见。

Ectopic Tissue Masses

The term *choristoma* is applied to growths consisting of tissue that is histologically normal but present in an abnormal location. The growths may result from abnormal sequestration of germ layer tissue during embryonic development or from faulty differentiation of pluripotential cells. Masses composed of such ectopic tissue that are growing in the orbit can also be a consequence of herniation of tissue from adjacent structures.

Cystic Lesions

Dermoid and epidermoid cysts

Dermoid cysts are the most common space-occupying orbital lesions of childhood. They are benign developmental choristomas that arise from primitive dermal and epidermal elements sequestered in fetal skull suture lines. The tissue forms a cyst lined with keratinized epithelium and dermal appendages, including hair follicles, sweat glands, and sebaceous glands. Cysts containing squamous epithelium without dermal appendages are called *epidermoid cysts.*

Orbital dermoid cysts in childhood most commonly arise in the superotemporal and superonasal quadrants (Fig 18-20) but sometimes extend into the bony suture line. Clinically, they present as painless, smooth masses that are mobile and unattached to overlying skin. Inflammation may occur with ruptures of the cyst and extrusion of cyst contents. Most patients have no visual symptoms. Clinical examination is often sufficient for diagnosis. In some cases, imaging is indicated to identify and delineate the extent of the cyst. Imaging reveals a well-circumscribed lesion with a low-density lumen and often bony remodeling (Fig 18-21).

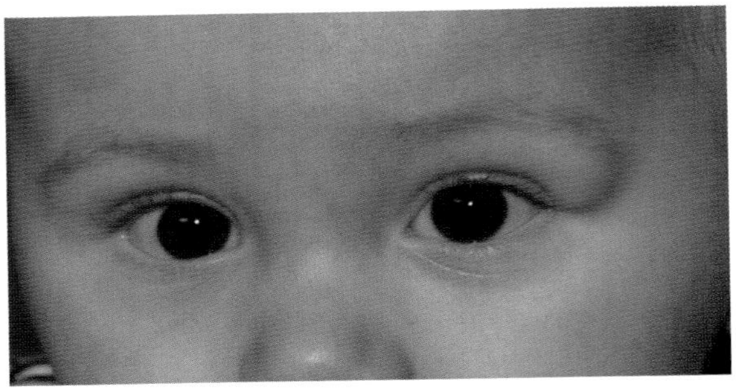

Figure 18-20 Eight-month-old boy with a periorbital dermoid cyst, left eye, with typical superotemporal location. (*Courtesy of Robert W. Hered, MD.*)

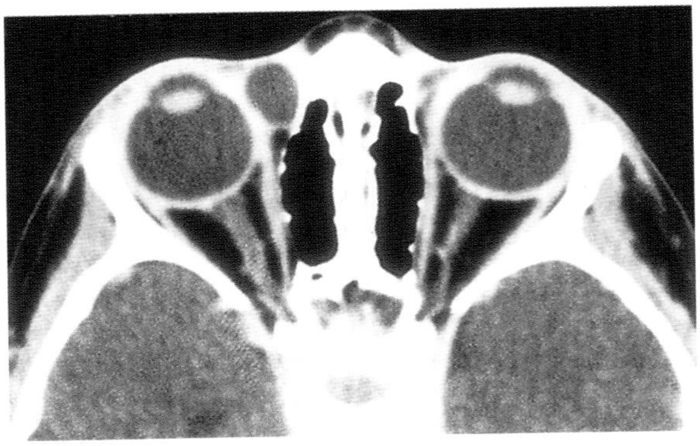

Figure 18-21 Axial CT image showing a dermoid cyst of the superonasal anterior orbit, right eye, in a 6-year-old boy.

异位组织包块

迷芽瘤是指由组织学正常但位置异常的组织构成的肿瘤。胚胎发育过程中胚层组织的异常隔离或多能干细胞的分化错误可能导致其生长。由这些生长在眶内的异位组织组成的肿块也可能是邻近结构组织疝出的结果。

囊性病变

皮样囊肿和表皮样囊肿

*皮样囊肿*是儿童最常见的眼眶占位性病变。它们是良性发育性迷芽瘤，起源于胎儿颅骨缝合线中隔离的原始真皮和表皮成分。该组织形成一个囊肿，内衬角化上皮和真皮附属物，包括毛囊、汗腺和皮脂腺。含有鳞状上皮而无真皮附属物的囊肿称为*表皮样囊肿*。

儿童眼眶皮样囊肿最常见于颞上和鼻上象限（图 18–20），但有时可延伸至骨缝合线。临床表现为无痛、光滑的肿块，可移动且不附着于其上覆盖的皮肤，在囊肿破裂和囊肿内容物挤出时可发生炎症。大多数患者没有视觉症状。临床检查可以诊断。在某些情况下，影像学可用于鉴别和确定囊肿的范围。影像学显示为边界清楚的低密度腔样结构，常伴有骨重建（图 18–21）。

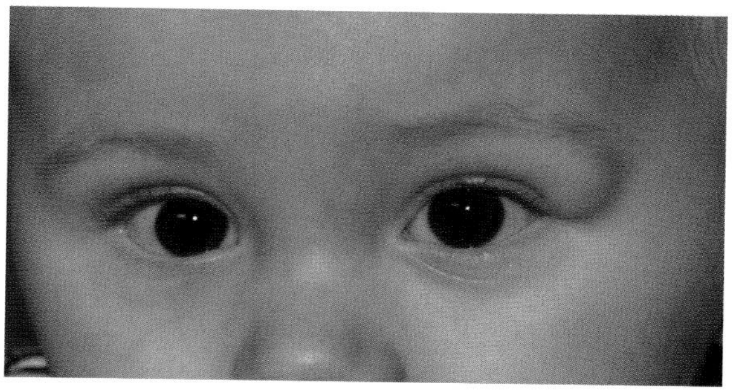

图 18–20　8 个月大的男孩，典型的左眼眶颞上皮样囊肿。*（译者注：资料来源见前页原文。）*

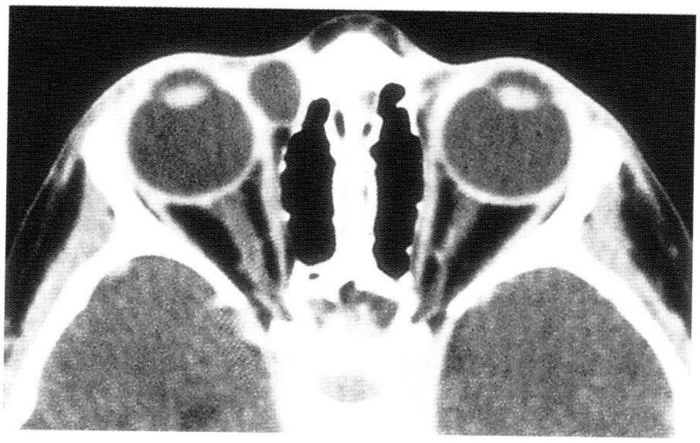

图 18–21　轴向 CT 影像显示 6 岁男童鼻上眼眶前皮样囊肿。

Management of dermoid cysts is surgical. Early excision can reduce the risk of traumatic rupture and subsequent inflammation. An infrabrow or eyelid crease incision is used, and the cyst is carefully dissected. If possible, rupture of the cyst at the time of surgery is avoided to limit lipogranulomatous inflammation and scarring. If the cyst is entered, the intraluminal material should be thoroughly removed. Sutural cysts sometimes cannot be removed intact because of their extension into or through bone. To limit the possibility of recurrence, the surgeon must attempt removal of all remaining cyst lining.

Microphthalmia with cyst

Microphthalmia with cyst (also known as colobomatous cyst) is characterized by a small, malformed globe with posterior segment coloboma and a cyst composed of tissues originating from the eye wall of the globe. Most fundus colobomas show some degree of scleral ectasia. In extreme cases, a bulging globular appendage grows to become as large as or larger than the globe itself, which is invariably microphthalmic, sometimes to a marked degree.

Microphthalmia with cyst may occur either as an isolated congenital defect or in association with a variety of intracranial or systemic anomalies. Frequently, the fellow eye shows evidence of coloboma as well. The usual location of the cyst is inferior or posterior to the globe, with which the cyst is always in contact.

Whether posteriorly located cysts cause proptosis depends on the size of the globe and the cyst. Inferiorly located cysts present as a bulging of the lower eyelid or a bluish subconjunctival mass (Fig 18-22). If fundus examination does not make the diagnosis obvious, orbital imaging may reveal a cystic lesion that is attached to the globe and has the uniform internal density of vitreous. The goal of treatment is to promote normal growth of the orbit; methods include aspiration or surgical excision of the cyst, and use of orbital expanders and conformers.

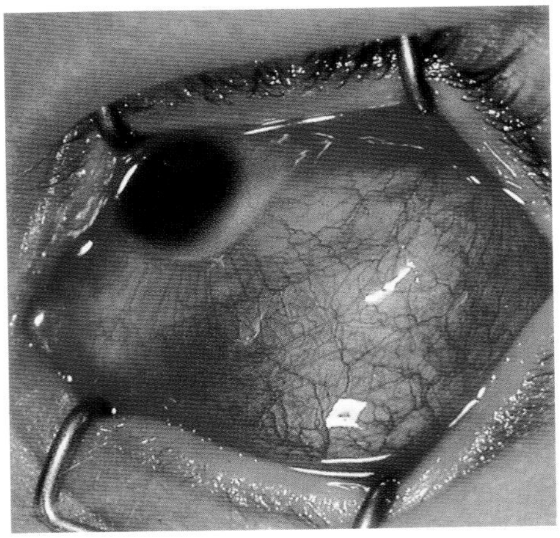

Figure 18-22 Microphthalmia with cyst (colobomatous cyst), left eye.

Mucocele

Mucoceles are cystic lesions that originate from obstructed paranasal sinus drainage. They may expand over time, potentially causing destruction of bone and eroding into the orbit or intracranial space. These lesions most commonly arise from the frontal or anterior ethmoid sinuses, resulting in inferior or medial displacement of the globe. The differential diagnosis includes encephalocele with skull base deformity. Treatment involves reestablishing normal sinus drainage and removing the cyst wall.

皮样囊肿可手术切除。早期切除可以降低外伤性破裂和炎症的风险采用眉下或重睑线切口，仔细分离囊肿。手术时尽量避免囊肿破裂，从而抑制脂肪肉芽肿性炎症和瘢痕形成。如果囊肿已破裂，应彻底清除腔内物质。骨缝的囊肿有时不能完整地切除，因为它们延伸至骨或穿过骨。为了降低复发的可能性，术者须尽量切除所有残留的囊膜内衬。

先天性小眼球伴囊肿

先天性小眼球伴囊肿（又称缺损性囊肿）的特征是一个小的畸形眼球，伴眼后节缺损，囊肿组织源于眼球壁。大多数眼底缺损表现为一定程度的巩膜扩张。在极端的情况下，膨出物会长得和小眼球本身一样大，甚至会长成巨大囊肿。

伴囊肿的先天性小眼球可以是一种孤立的先天性缺陷，也可与多种颅内或全身异常有关。通常，另一眼睛也常有缺损。囊肿常在下方或后方与眼球相邻。

球后的囊肿是否引起眼球突出取决于眼球和囊肿的大小。位于下眼睑的囊肿表现为下眼睑隆起或结膜下蓝色肿块（图 18–22）。如果眼底检查不能明确诊断，影像学检查可见附着于眼球的囊性病变，内部为密度均匀的玻璃体。治疗的目的是促进眼眶的正常生长，方法包括抽吸或手术切除囊肿，使用眼眶扩张器和植入填充物。

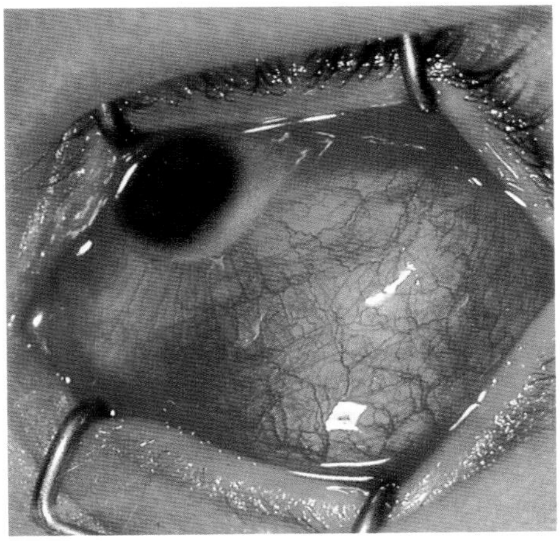

图 18–22　左眼先天性小眼球伴囊肿（缺损性囊肿）。

黏液囊肿

黏液囊肿是一种源于鼻窦引流阻塞的囊性病变。随着时间的推移，瘤体会逐渐扩大，可破坏周围骨质并累及眼眶或颅内。病变最常发生在额窦或筛窦前部，导致眼球向下或内移位。鉴别诊断包括颅底畸形的脑膨出。治疗方法为重建正常的窦腔引流和切除囊壁。

Encephalocele and meningocele

Encephaloceles and meningoceles in the orbital region may result from a congenital bony defect that allows herniation of intracranial tissue, or they may develop after trauma that disrupts the bone and dura mater of the anterior cranial fossa. An intraorbital location leads to proptosis or downward displacement of the globe. Anterior presentation takes the form of a subcutaneous mass that can be misdiagnosed as a dacryocystocele. However, encephaloceles and meningoceles are typically located above the medial canthal tendon; dacryocystoceles are typically located below it (see Chapter 19). Pulsation of the globe or the mass from the transmission of intracranial pulse pressure is characteristic. Neuroimaging confirms the diagnosis. Surgical repair is usually performed by neurosurgeons.

Teratoma

Choristomatous tumors that contain multiple tissues derived from all 3 germinal layers (ectoderm, mesoderm, and endoderm) are referred to as *teratomas*. Most teratomas are partially cystic, with varying fluid content. Orbital teratomas account for a very small fraction of both orbital tumors and teratomas in general. The clinical presentation of orbital teratomas may be particularly dramatic, with massive proptosis evident at birth (Fig 18-23). In contrast with teratomas in other locations, which tend to show malignant growth, most orbital lesions are benign. Surgical excision, facilitated by prior aspiration of fluid, can often be accomplished without sacrificing the globe. Permanent optic nerve damage from stretching and compression may cause poor vision in the involved eye.

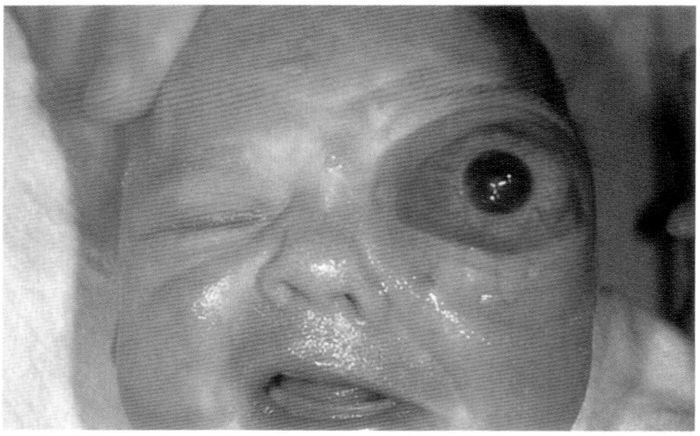

Figure 18-23 Congenital cystic teratoma originating in the left orbit of a 1-day-old girl.

Ectopic Lacrimal Gland

These are rare choristomatous lesions that may present with proptosis in childhood. Cystic enlargement and chronic inflammation sometimes aggravate the condition.

脑膨出和脑脊膜膨出

眶区脑膨出和脑膜膨出可能是先天性骨缺损导致颅内组织疝出，也可能是外伤破坏了前颅窝的骨质和硬脑膜造成的。框内膨出导致眼球突出或向下移位。在眼眶前部膨出表现为皮下肿块，可误诊为泪囊囊肿。然而，脑膨出和脑膜膨出常位于内眦肌腱上方，泪囊囊肿常位于内眦肌腱下（见第 19 章）。由于颅内脉压差可见性特征性的眼球或包块的搏动。影像学检查可以确诊。手术修复由神经外科医生进行。

畸胎瘤

迷芽瘤是由 3 个胚层（外胚层、中胚层和内胚层）、多个组织形成的，称为*畸胎瘤*。大多数畸胎瘤是部分囊性的，含有不同程度的液体。一般来说，眼眶畸胎瘤只占眼眶肿瘤和畸胎瘤的很小一部分。眼眶畸胎瘤的临床表现可能特别明显，在出生时有明显的巨大眼球突出（图 18–23）。与其他部位的往往呈恶性生长的畸胎瘤相比，大多数眼眶病变是良性的。手术切除前，先负压抽吸囊液，不会伤及眼球。但拉伸和压迫造成的永久性视神经损伤可导致受累眼视力下降。

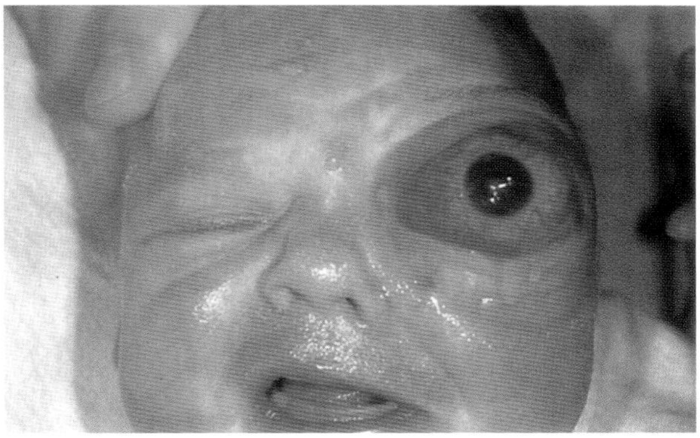

图 18–23　先天性囊性畸胎瘤，位于一个 1 天大的女婴的左眼眶。

异位泪腺

异位泪腺是罕见的迷芽瘤性病变，可能在儿童期出现眼球突出。瘤体囊性增大和慢性炎症有时会加重病情。

（翻译 白嘎丽 吴捷 叶璐 // 审校 石一宁 蒋宁 // 章节审校 石广礼）

CHAPTER 19

Lacrimal Drainage System Abnormalities

Nasolacrimal duct obstruction (NLDO) can be congenital or acquired. Congenital NLDO (CNLDO) is the most common lacrimal system disorder encountered in pediatric ophthalmology. This chapter discusses CNLDO, including nonsurgical and surgical management, as well other congenital and developmental anomalies of the lacrimal system that may be treated by the ophthalmologist. Acquired NLDO is discussed in BCSC Section 7, *Oculofacial Plastic and Orbital Surgery.*

Anatomical features of the lacrimal drainage system and their development are discussed in BCSC Section 2, *Fundamentals and Principles of Ophthalmology,* and Section 7, *Oculofacial Plastic and Orbital Surgery.*

Congenital and Developmental Anomalies

Atresia of the Lacrimal Puncta or Canaliculi

Atresia of the lacrimal puncta or canaliculi refers to failure of canalization during development of the upper lacrimal system structures. Patients with atresia usually present with overflow of clear tears; there is no infection because bacteria cannot reach the lacrimal sac to produce one. The presence of mucopurulent discharge in a patient with atresia of either the upper or lower canaliculus usually indicates concomitant obstruction of the distal NLD, with reflux of discharge through the normal canaliculus.

There are 2 main causes of upper lacrimal system obstruction. One is a thin membrane that obstructs the lacrimal puncta, which are otherwise normal. Simple puncture of the membrane with a punctal dilator eliminates this obstruction. For concomitant obstruction of the distal NLD, probing of the distal system is necessary.

The second cause of upper lacrimal system obstruction is atresia of the puncta and canaliculi. In affected patients, no puncta can be seen (Fig 19-1). If only 1 of the canaliculi is atretic and there is mucopurulent discharge, probing of the distal duct through the patent canaliculus may be curative. If both the upper and the lower canaliculi are absent, an incision through the eyelid margin at the expected location of the canaliculi may reveal structures that can be cannulated. However, many patients ultimately require conjunctivodacryocystorhinostomy (CDCR), a procedure that creates a complete bypass of the lacrimal drainage system. CDCR is usually deferred until these patients are older. See BCSC Section 7, *Oculofacial Plastic and Orbital Surgery,* for a discussion of this procedure.

第 19 章
泪道系统异常

鼻泪管阻塞（NLDO）可以是先天性的，也可以是获得性的。先天性鼻泪管阻塞（CNLDO）是小儿眼科最常见的泪道系统疾病。本章讨论的先天性鼻泪管阻塞（CNLDO），包括非手术和手术治疗，以及其他可由眼科医生治疗的先天性和发育性泪道系统异常。获得性 NLDO 在 BCSC 第 7 册《*眼面部整形与眼眶手术*》中讨论。

泪道排水系统的解剖学特征及其发育在 BCSC 第 2 册《*眼科学基础与原理*》和第 7 册《*眼面部整形与眼眶手术*》进行了讨论。

先天性疾病和发育异常

泪小点或泪小管闭锁

泪小点或泪小管闭锁是指上泪道系统结构发育过程中未能管腔化。泪点闭锁患者常伴有明显的泪液溢出、没有感染，因为细菌无法进入泪囊而产生感染。上泪小管或下泪小管闭锁患者出现黏液脓性分泌物，提示鼻泪管远端梗阻伴有正常泪小管返流。

上泪道系统阻塞的主要原因有 2 个。一个原因是泪小点覆盖一层薄膜，其他部位正常。用泪点扩张器对薄膜进行简单的穿刺可以消除这种阻塞。同时伴有远端鼻泪管阻塞时，需要远端泪道系统探通。

上泪道系统阻塞的第 2 个原因是泪小点和泪小管闭锁。患者没有泪小点（图 19–1）。如果只有 1 个泪小管闭锁并有黏液脓性分泌物，经可见的泪小管探通远端泪道，可以治愈。如果没有上下泪小管，在泪小管可能的位置切开睑缘，找到插管的管腔结构。但许多患者需行结膜 – 泪囊鼻腔吻合术（CDCR），即建立完整泪道排水系统旁路的手术。结膜 – 泪囊鼻腔吻合术（COCR）多用于年龄较大患者。关于此手术过程的讨论见 BCSC 第 7 册《*眼面部整形与眼眶手术*》。

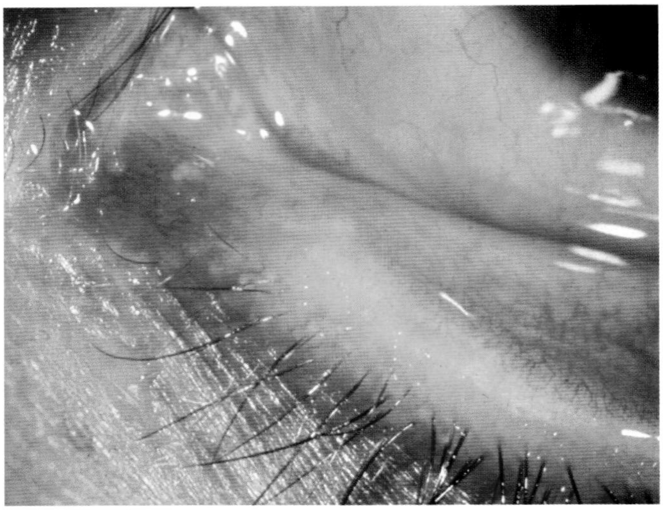

Figure 19-1 Atresia of the lacrimal puncta. No indentation is visible at the site of the normal punctal opening. *(Reproduced with permission from Lueder GT. Neonatal lacrimal system anomalies. Semin Ophthalmol. 1997;12(2):109.)*

Congenital Lacrimal Fistula

Congenital lacrimal fistula (lacrimal–cutaneous fistula) is an epithelium-lined tract extending from the common canaliculus or lacrimal sac to the overlying skin surface. It usually presents as a small dimple medial to the eyelids and may be difficult to detect in the absence of symptoms (Fig 19-2). It is not always patent. If the patient is asymptomatic, no treatment is necessary. Discharge from the fistula is often associated with distal NLDO and may cease after probing of the distal obstruction. If discharge persists despite a patent lacrimal duct, surgical excision of the fistula between the skin and normal lacrimal structures is required.

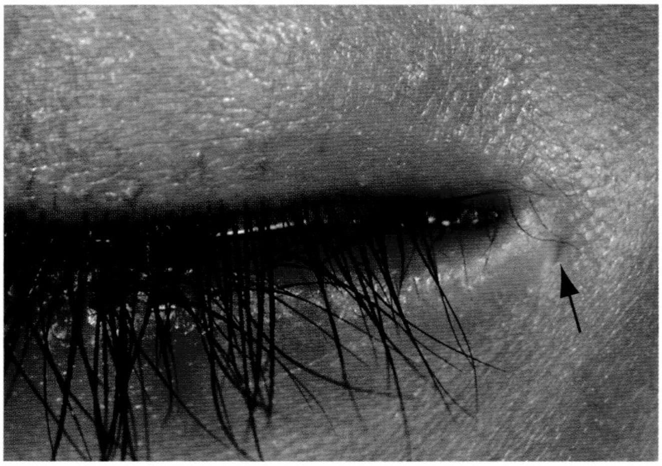

Figure 19-2 Lacrimal fistula. *(Reproduced with permission from Lueder GT. Neonatal lacrimal system anomalies.* Semin Ophthalmol. *1997;12(2):109.)*

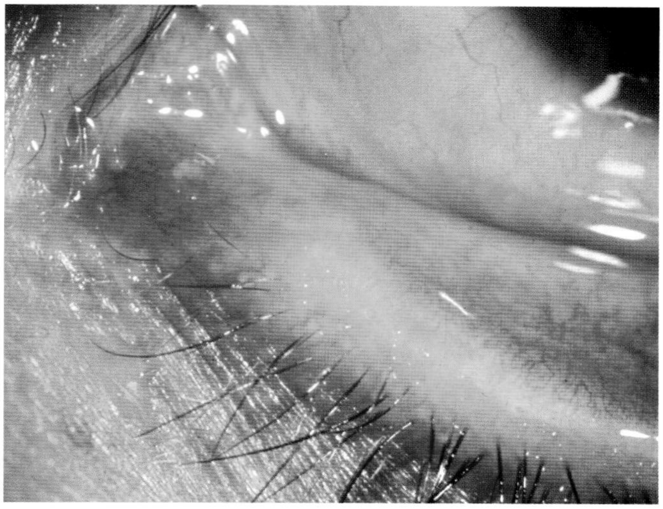

图 19–1　泪点闭锁。正常泪点开口处无凹陷。*（译者注：资料来源见前页原文。）*

先天性泪道瘘

先天性泪道瘘（泪道 – 皮肤瘘）是内衬上皮细胞的泪管，从泪总管或泪囊延伸至皮肤表面。常表现为眼睑内侧的一个浅凹，没有症状时很难发现（图 19–2）。它常无症状。没有症状时无须治疗。瘘管排出分泌物常与远端鼻泪管阻塞有关，在探通远端阻塞后则不再有分泌物。如果泪道可见，但仍有分泌物，则需手术切除皮肤和正常泪道结构之间的瘘管。

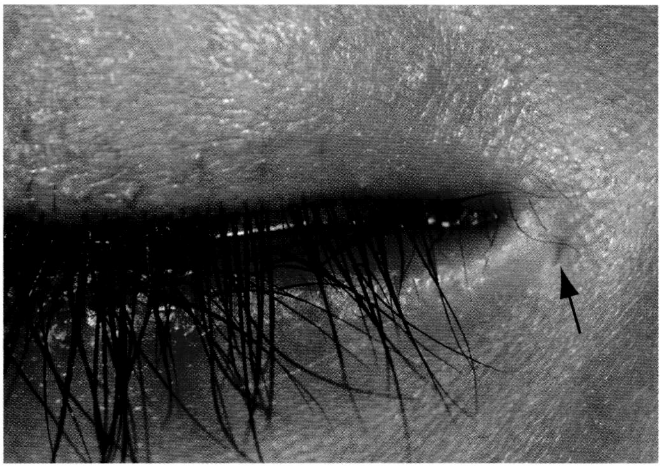

图 19–2　泪道瘘。*（译者注：资料来源见前页原文。）*

Dacryocystocele

Congenital dacryocystocele (dacryocele, mucocele, amniotocele) is present in approximately 3% of infants with NLDO. It develops when a distal blockage causes distention of the lacrimal sac. The valve of Rosenmüller can act as a one-way valve, thereby preventing decompression of the lacrimal sac. Most patients with dacryocystoceles have associated cysts of the distal NLD, which may be seen beneath the inferior turbinate. Involvement is bilateral in 20%–30% of cases.

Clinical features and diagnosis

Dacryocystocele presents at birth or within the first few days of life as a bluish swelling just below and nasal to the medial canthus. The differential diagnosis includes hemangioma, dermoid cyst, and encephalocele. Hemangiomas are not typically present at birth. They have a vascular appearance and are generally less firm than dacryocystoceles. Dermoid cysts and encephaloceles present most often above the medial canthal tendon. The diagnosis is clinically apparent when a newborn has a nasal mass beneath the medial canthus that is associated with symptoms of NLDO (discussed later in the chapter); imaging is usually not required in this case.

Dacryocystoceles are prone to infection, and acute dacryocystitis usually develops. The skin over the distended lacrimal sac becomes erythematous (Fig 19-3), and pressure applied on the sac may produce reflux of purulent material.

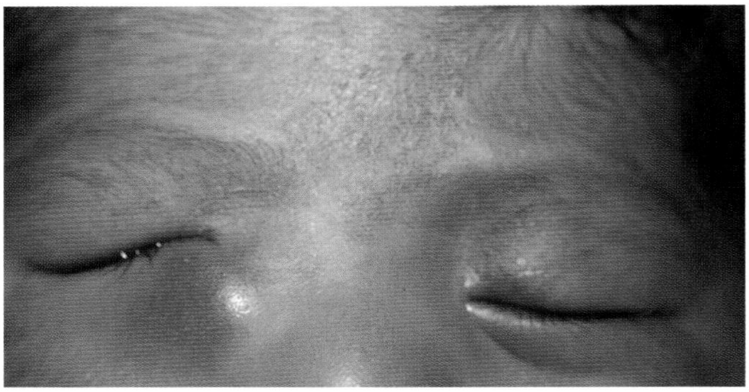

Figure 19-3 Infected congenital dacryocystocele, right eye, in a newborn. Note the typical location and erythema overlying the distended lacrimal sac. *(Courtesy of Edward L. Raab, MD.)*

Infants who have large intranasal cysts may present with respiratory symptoms because infants are obligate nasal breathers. Symptoms range from difficulty during feeding (due to obstruction of the mouth) to respiratory distress.

Management

Early treatment of dacryocystoceles is advised to prevent complications related to infection. Infants are relatively immunocompromised and are therefore at risk for local or systemic spread of infection. Digital massage may be attempted to decompress the dacryocystocele, as the condition occasionally resolves without surgery.

泪囊囊肿

约 3% 的鼻泪管阻塞的患儿存在先天性泪囊囊肿（泪囊囊肿、黏液囊肿、泪囊羊水囊肿）。发生于远端阻塞引起泪囊扩张。Rosenmüller 瓣膜的作用呈单向阀，防止泪囊减压。大多数泪囊囊肿患者伴有远端鼻泪管阻塞的囊肿，可见于下鼻甲。20%~30% 双侧受累。

临床特点及诊断

泪囊囊肿表现为，在出生时或出生后几天内，内眦鼻下方皮下的浅蓝色的肿胀。鉴别诊断包括血管瘤、皮样囊肿和脑膨出。血管瘤在出生时并不常见，有血管的外观，没有泪囊囊肿坚硬。皮样囊肿和脑囊肿最常见于内眦肌腱上方。当新生儿的内眦下鼻侧肿块伴有鼻泪道阻塞症状时（本章稍后讨论），临床诊断明确，不需行影像学检查。

泪囊囊肿易受感染，常发生急性泪囊炎。肿胀的泪囊区皮肤红肿（图 19–3），按压泪囊区有脓性物质溢出。

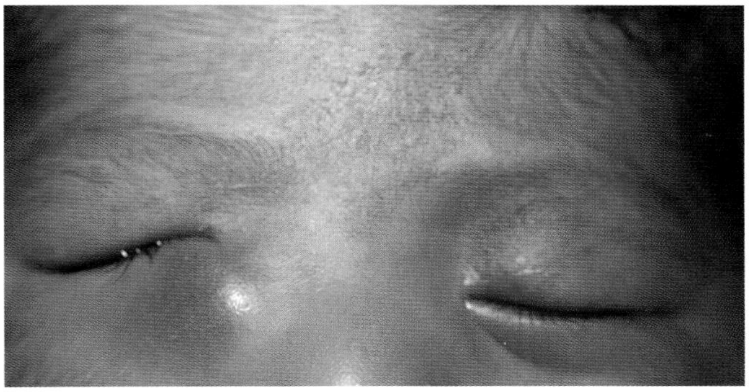

图 19–3　新生儿先天性泪囊囊肿（右眼）。注意扩张泪囊的典型位置和红肿。*（译者注：资料来源见前页原文。）*

鼻内囊肿较大的婴儿会出现呼吸道症状，因为婴儿仅用鼻呼吸。轻者出现进食困难（由于口腔的阻塞），重者出现呼吸窘迫。

治疗

为了预防与感染有关的并发症，建议尽早治疗泪囊囊肿。婴儿的免疫功能相对较差，因此有局部或全身感染扩散的风险。手指按摩可减小泪囊囊肿的压力，使少数患儿避免手术治疗。

Dacryocystoceles associated with acute respiratory distress require immediate surgical intervention. If the lesions do not resolve within the first 1–2 weeks of life or if there is acute infection of the dacryocystocele, surgery is necessary. NLD probing alone may be curative, but in approximately 25% of patients, the condition persists after probing. NLD probing in conjunction with nasal endoscopy and intranasal cyst removal is effective in more than 95% of infants. Because approximately 20%–30% of patients have bilateral nasal cysts, sometimes without visible dacryocystoceles, bilateral endoscopy is appropriate. Systemic antibiotics should be used perioperatively if acute dacryocystitis is present. Surgical treatment of an infected dacryocystocele via a skin incision should be avoided because of the risk of creating a persistentfistulous tract.

Lueder GT. The association of neonatal dacryocystoceles and infantile dacryocystitis with nasolacrimal duct cysts (an American Ophthalmological Society thesis). *Trans Am Ophthalmol Soc.* 2012;110:74–93.

Congenital Nasolacrimal Duct Obstruction

Congenital nasolacrimal duct obstruction (CNLDO) (dacryostenosis) is the most common lacrimal system disorder encountered in pediatric ophthalmology, occurring in approximately 5% of infants, and is more common in patients with Down syndrome (22%) and in those with midfacial abnormalities.

CNLDO can be classified as simple or complex. Simple CNLDO is caused by a thin mucosal membrane at the distal end of the NLD, at the valve of Hasner (Fig 19-4). Complex CNLDO is due to diffuse obstruction or bony obstruction, as is frequently found in patients with midfacial abnormalities.

Excessive tearing due to CNLDO must be differentiated from epiphora due to infantile glaucoma, which has additional features, including photophobia, blepharospasm, ocular hypertension, corneal clouding with or without enlargement, and breaks in Descemet membrane (see Chapter 22). Besides infantile glaucoma, the differential diagnosis of CNLDO includes conjunctivitis, and epiblepharon with irritation due to trichiasis. A thorough examination is necessary to rule out other ocular abnormalities. A cycloplegic refraction should be performed as results of some studies suggest that there is an increased rate of anisometropia and amblyopia in patients with CNLDO.

Clinical Features and Examination

Infants with CNLDO usually present within the first month of life with epiphora, recurrent periocular crusting, or both (Fig 19-5). They do not have photophobia or blepharospasm. Symptoms are usually chronic and worse with nasal congestion; bilateral involvement is common. Applying digital pressure to the lacrimal sac usually results in retrograde discharge of mucoid or mucopurulent material.

Nonsurgical Management

There is a high rate of spontaneous resolution of CNLDO, with approximately 90% of patients improving within the first 9–12 months of life. For this reason, conservative treatment is recommended initially for these patients.

泪囊囊肿伴急性呼吸窘迫需立即手术治疗。如果病变在出生后 1~2 周内没有消退，或有急性泪囊囊肿感染，则需手术治疗。单纯的鼻泪管探通可能有效，但约 25% 的患者在探通后症状仍然存在。95% 以上的婴儿进行鼻泪管探通联合鼻内窥镜和鼻内囊肿清除术是有效的。20%~30% 的患儿有双侧鼻腔囊肿，尽管有时并不明显可见，则应考虑行双侧内窥镜检查。急性泪囊炎的围手术期应使用全身抗生素。应避免通过皮肤切口对感染期的泪囊囊肿进行手术，因为这可能造成永久性瘘道。

Lueder GT. The association of neonatal dacryocystoceles and infantile dacryocystitis with nasolacrimal duct cysts (an American Ophthalmological Society thesis). *Trans Am Ophthalmol Soc.* 2012;110:74–93.

先天性鼻泪管阻塞

先天性泪道阻塞（CNLDO）（泪管狭窄）是小儿眼科最常见的泪道系统疾病，约 5% 的婴儿患有此病，在 Down 综合征（22%）和中面部异常患儿中更为常见。

先天性泪道阻塞（CNLDO）可以分为单纯性和复杂性。单纯性先天性泪道阻塞（CNLDO）是由鼻泪管远端、Hasner 瓣膜处的一薄层黏膜引起的（图 19–4）。复杂性先天性泪道阻塞（CNLDO）是由于弥漫性阻塞或骨性阻塞引起的，这常见于中面部异常的患者。

先天性泪道阻塞的溢泪需与婴儿型青光眼的流泪相鉴别，青光眼伴有其他体征，包括畏光、眼睑痉挛、高眼压、伴有或不伴有角膜扩张的角膜混浊、Descemet 膜破裂（见第 22 章）。除了婴儿型青光眼，先天性泪道阻塞的鉴别诊断还包括结膜炎和内眦赘皮导致的倒睫对角膜的刺激。需要全面检查，以排除其他眼部异常。应行睫状肌麻痹验光检查，研究表明，先天性泪道阻塞患儿的屈光参差和弱视的发生率较高。

临床特点及检查

先天性泪道阻塞患儿常在出生后 1 个月内出现溢泪、反复眼周分泌物结痂，或两者同时出现（图 19–5）。没有畏光或眼睑痉挛。症状呈慢性，鼻塞时加重；也可累及双眼。按摩泪囊区常会导致黏液样或黏液性脓性物质的溢出。

非手术治疗

先天性泪道阻塞（CNLDO）的自愈率很高，约 90% 的患儿在出生后 9~12 个月内得到改善。因此建议这些患者保守治疗。

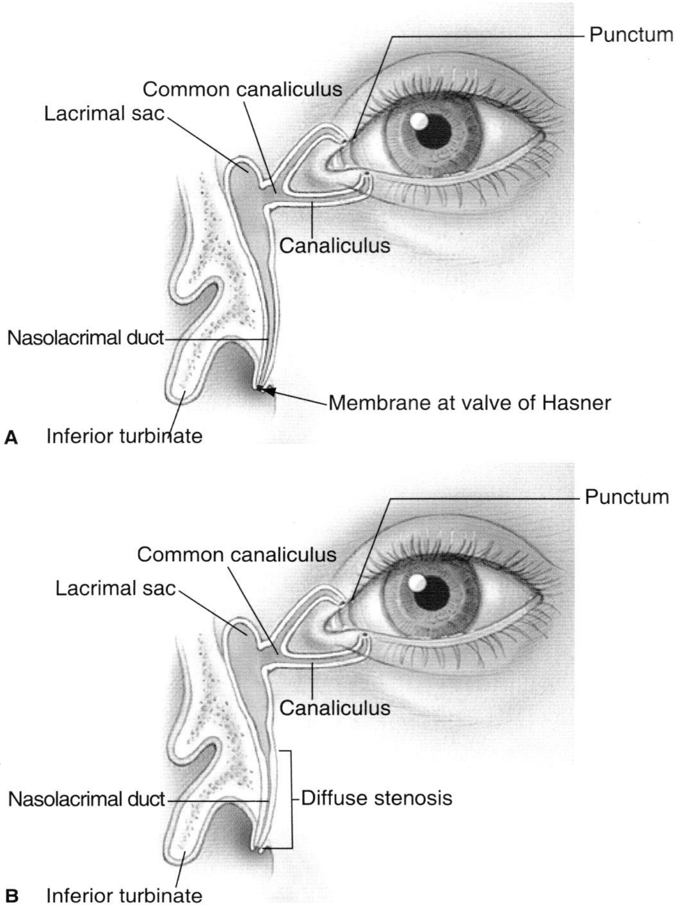

Figure 19-4 **A**, Typical location of the membrane causing simple nasolacrimal duct obstruction (NLDO) (*arrow*). **B**, Diffuse stenosis of the distal NLD. *(Adapted from an illustration by Christine Gralapp.)*

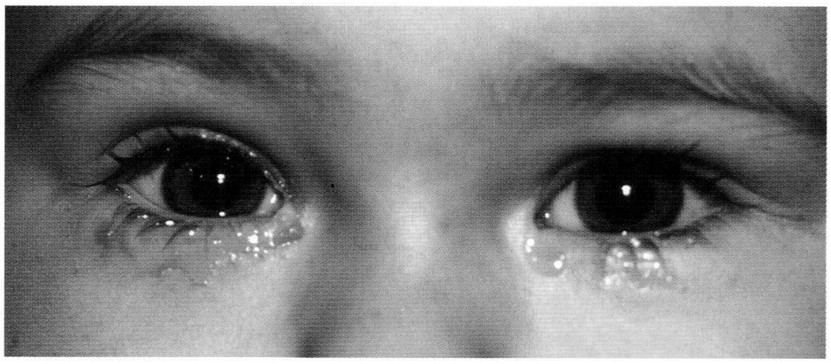

Figure 19-5 Bilateral NLDO. Note epiphora and periocular crusting without evidence of inflammation. *(Reproduced with permission from Lueder GT.* Pediatric Practice Ophthalmology. *New York: McGraw-Hill Professional; 2011:55.)*

Conservative treatment includes lacrimal sac massage and use of topical antibiotics. Massage serves 2 purposes: it empties the sac, thereby reducing the opportunity for bacterial growth, and it applies hydrostatic pressure to the obstruction, which may open the duct and resolve the condition. Massage is performed by applying pressure to the lacrimal sac, at the medial canthus, a few times per day. This is the only location where application of external pressure on the lacrimal sac can be effective. Passing the fin ger along the nares, which is often recommended by primary care providers, is not effective because the NLD is covered by bone at this site.

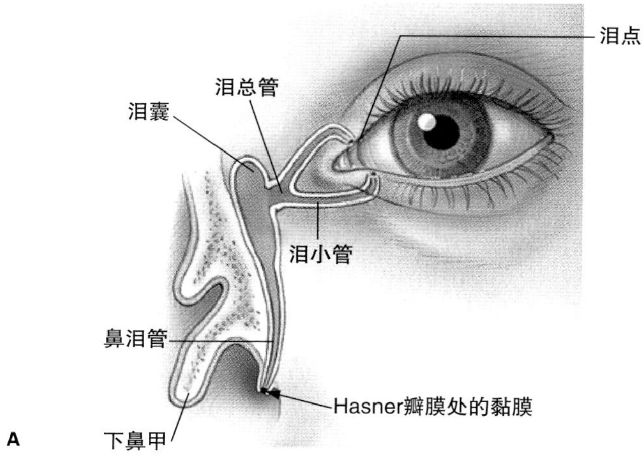

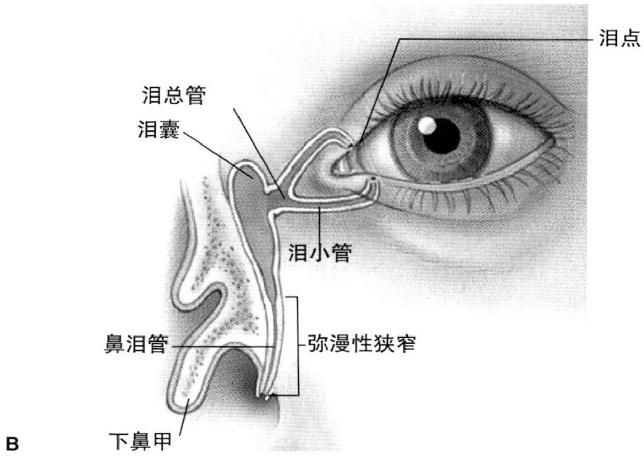

图 19-4　A. 造成单纯性鼻泪管阻塞(NLDO)的典型瓣膜位置(*箭头*)。**B.** 末端鼻泪管阻塞的弥漫性狭窄。*(译者注：资料来源见前页原文。)*

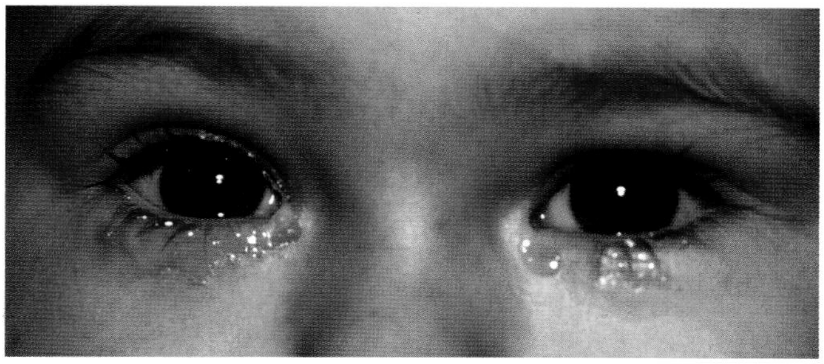

图 19-5　双侧先天性泪道阻塞。有溢泪和眼周结痂，但是无炎症迹象。*(译者注：资料来源见前页原文。)*

保守治疗包括泪囊区按摩和局部使用抗生素。按摩有 2 个目的：排空泪囊，从而减少细菌滋生的机会；同时对阻塞施加静水压，以开放阻塞的泪道。按摩是在内眦处对泪囊区加压，每天按摩几次。这是外部压力作用于泪囊的唯一有效的位置。初级保健人员推荐的采用手指沿着鼻孔按摩是无效的，因为在这个位置处鼻泪管是被骨头覆盖的。

Topical antibiotics are often recommended if patients have significant periocular discharge. There are 3 important points with regard to topical antibiotic use in this disorder. First, the antibiotics do not cure the obstruction but may reduce the amount of mucopurulent discharge. Second, the infection in CNLDO is due to stasis of fluid within the lacrimal sac; therefore, almost any bacteria, including normal flora, may cause infection. Most broad-spectrum antibiotics are effective in reducing the associated symptoms, so culturing the mucoid or mucopurulent material is usually not necessary. Third, antibiotic use for a few days often produces improvement, and prolonged use may not be necessary. Parents may be instructed to administer the antibiotics as needed when the amount of discharge increases.

Surgical Management

Nasolacrimal probing is one of the most common procedures performed by pediatric ophthalmologists and is very effective in treating CNLDO. It is used to treat infants with CNLDO whose symptoms do not resolve over time with conservative treatment. There are 2 common approaches to the surgical management of this disorder. Some ophthalmologists recommend in-office probing of young infants, whereas others prefer to delay treatment and perform surgery in the operating room on older infants. The advantages of early in-office probing are that it avoids general anesthesia, resolves symptoms earlier, and is likely more cost effective. The disadvantages are that a painful procedure is performed on an awake infant and that surgery is performed on many infants who would have spontaneously improved without surgery. The advantages of later surgery in the operating room are that fewer infants require treatment and the procedure is performed in a more controlled environment in which additional procedures can be performed concurrently. Either of these approaches is acceptable.

Surgical procedures for CNLDO are also discussed in BCSC Section 7, *Oculofacial Plastic and Orbital Surgery.*

Pediatric Eye Disease Investigator Group. A randomized trial comparing the costeffectiveness of 2 approaches for treating unilateral nasolacrimal duct obstruction. *Arch Ophthalmol.* 2012;130(12):1525–1533.

Probing

When nasolacrimal probing is to be performed in the operating room, placement of an oxymetazoline-soaked pledget beneath the inferior turbinate before surgery may decrease intraoperative bleeding. The initial step in nasolacrimal probing is dilation of the puncta and proximal canaliculi. Punctal membranes and atretic canaliculi are sometimes not recognized until surgery. Their management is discussed earlier in this chapter. Because the lacrimal system cannot be visualized beyond the puncta, knowledge of the anatomy and normal course of the lacrimal excretory system is essential for passing lacrimal probes properly. The probes are initially inserted in the puncta, perpendicular to the eyelid. Within 1–2 mm of the eyelid margin, the canaliculi turn approximately 90°; the probes are therefore turned almost immediately and passed along the course of the canaliculi until the nasal bone is encountered on the medial side of the lacrimal sac. The probes are held flat on the patient's face and rotated and passed gently into the distal duct (Fig 19-6A). With simple CNLDO, most surgeons feel a slight popping sensation as the probe passes through the membrane causing the obstruction. With complex CNLDO (see the following section), the surgeon's probe may encounter a firmer obstruction or a tight passage throughout the length of the NLD.

如果患儿有明显的眼周分泌物，可局部使用抗生素。抗生素的使用有 3 个要点。首先，抗生素不能治愈阻塞，但可减少黏液脓性分泌物的量。其次，先天性泪道阻塞感染是由于泪囊内液体滞留所致；因此，几乎任何细菌，包括正常菌群，都可引起感染。大多数广谱抗生素对减轻症状有效，不需要对黏液或黏液脓性分泌物进行培养。第三，抗生素使用几天后即可改善症状，不需要长期使用。当分泌物增加时，可指导父母使用抗生素。

手术治疗

鼻泪管探通术是小儿眼科医生最常用的方法之一，对先天性鼻泪管阻塞（CNLDO）的治疗非常有效，用于治疗保守治疗未愈的先天性鼻泪管阻塞（CNLDO）患儿。有 2 种常见的手术方法，一些眼科医生在治疗室行幼小婴儿的泪道探通，而另一些医生则推迟治疗，在手术室对较大婴儿进行手术治疗。早期治疗泪道探通的优点是避免了全身麻醉，更早地解决了症状，可能更经济有效。其缺点是，需要对清醒的婴儿进行痛苦的手术，但有许多婴儿可能不经手术即可自愈。推迟在手术室中进行手术的优点是：需要治疗的婴儿较少，而且手术是在更可控的环境中进行的，还可以同时进行其他手术。这 2 种方法都是可以选择的。

先天性鼻泪管阻塞（CNLDO）的手术过程在 BCSC 第 7 册《*眼面部整形与眼眶手术*》中进行讨论。

Pediatric Eye Disease Investigator Group. A randomized trial comparing the costeffectiveness of 2 approaches for treating unilateral nasolacrimal duct obstruction. *Arch Ophthalmol*. 2012;130(12):1525–1533.

泪道探通术

在手术室内行鼻泪管探通术时，术前在下鼻甲下放置羟甲唑啉浸泡脱脂棉，可以减少术中出血。鼻泪管探通术的第一步是扩张泪小点和近端的泪小管。有时到手术时才发现泪小点膜闭和泪小管闭锁，本章前面讨论了相关治疗。除泪小点外，泪道系统不可直视，因此泪液排泄系统的解剖学和正常经行知识的掌握对于正确探通泪道至关重要。探针最初是垂直于眼睑进入泪小点，在距睑缘 1~2mm 处泪小管呈 90° 转弯，探针也随之转，继续沿着泪小管走行，直到在泪囊内侧碰到鼻骨。此时探针平放在患儿脸上，然后旋转着轻轻进入远端泪道（图 19-6A）。对于简单的先天性鼻泪管阻塞（CNLDO），大多数手术医生在探针穿过阻塞的膜时会有轻微的爆裂感。对于复杂的先天性鼻泪管阻塞（CNLDO）（见下一节），手术医生的探针可能会在整个鼻泪管中遇到更坚硬的阻塞或管径更狭窄。

A wide variety of techniques are used for probing in NLDO. Most surgeons begin with a size 0 or 1 Bowman probe, and some pass successively larger probes to enlarge the distal duct. Introducing a second metal probe into the nares and making direct contact with the previously placed lacrimal probe verifies the position of the latter (Fig 19-6B). Alternatively, direct inspection with a nasal speculum and headlamp or with a nasal endoscope can precisely determine the position of the probe. Irrigation may be performed following probing in order to verify that the system is patent. **Infracture of the inferior turbinate** may be used to widen the area where the fluid drains beneath the inferior turbinate. The surgeon A B accomplishes this by placing a small periosteal elevator beneath the turbinate or by grasping it with a hemostat and then rotating the instrument.

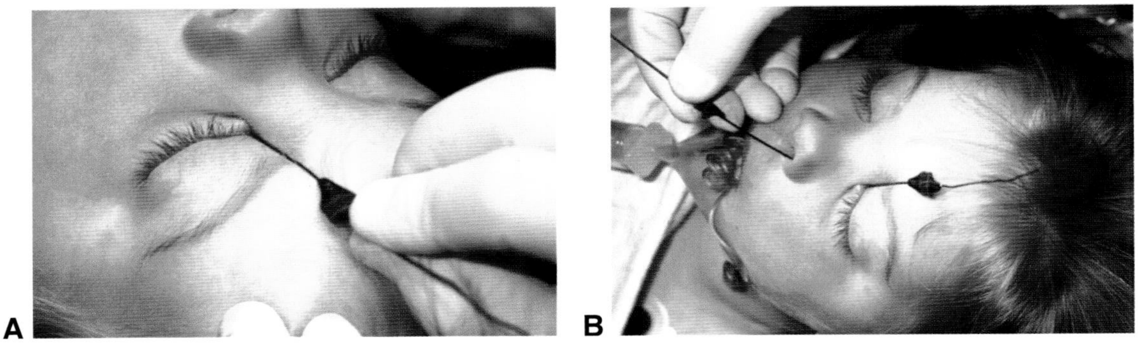

Figure 19-6 Probing for NLDO. **A,** The probe is advanced through the lacrimal sac and NLD, in this instance via the lower canaliculus. **B,** A second probe introduced into the nares is used to verify the position of the probe tip. *(Courtesy of Edward L. Raab, MD.)*

Postoperatively, minor bleeding from the nose or into the tears commonly occurs and usually requires no treatment. Optional postoperative medications include antibiotic drops, corticosteroid drops, or both instilled 1–4 times daily for 1–2 weeks. Phenylephrine or oxymetazoline nasal spray may be used to control nasal bleeding or congestion. Because transient bacteremia can occur after probing, systemic antibiotic prophylaxis should be considered for patients with cardiac disease.

Resolution of signs after probing may not occur until 1 week or more postoperatively. Recurrence after unsuccessful probing is usually evident within 1–2 months. The success rate of properly performed initial probing for CNLDO exceeds 80% in infants younger than 15 months.

Significant complications of probing are rare. In some patients, mild epiphora occurs occasionally, particularly outdoors in cold weather or in conjunction with an upper respiratory tract infection. This epiphora is probably attributable to a patent but narrow lacrimal drainage channel. Usually no additional treatment is required.

各种各样的技术应用于鼻泪管阻塞探通术。大多数手术医生从 0 号或 1 号 Bowman 探针开始，有些医生则通过较粗的探针来扩张远端泪道。将第 2 个金属探针进入鼻腔，并与先前放置的泪道探针直接接触，确定后者的位置（图 19–6B）。另外，直接用鼻镜和头灯或鼻内窥镜检查，可以精确确定探针的位置。探通后可进行泪道冲洗。下鼻甲不全切除术可用于扩大下鼻甲下引流液体区域。手术医生通过在鼻甲下放置一个小的骨膜分离器或用止血器抓住它，然后旋转仪器完成下鼻甲不全切除术。

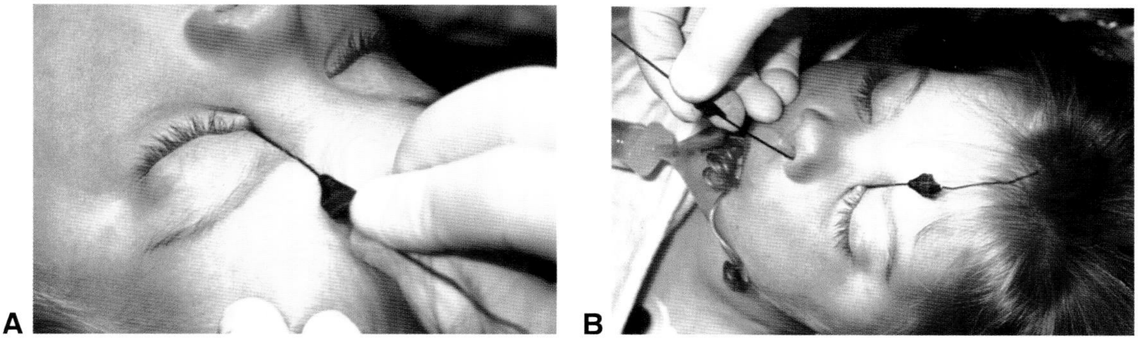

图 19–6　鼻泪管阻塞探通术。**A.** 探针经下泪导管，通过泪囊和鼻泪管。**B.** 第 2 个探针进入鼻腔，确定探针尖的位置。*（译者注：资料来源见前页原文。）*

术后常发生轻微的鼻血或泪中带血，通常不需要治疗。术后可选用的药物包括抗生素滴剂、皮质类固醇滴剂，或两者同时使用，每日 1~4 次，持续 1~2 周。苯肾上腺素或羟甲唑啉鼻腔喷雾剂可用于控制鼻出血或充血。由于探通术后能发生一过性菌血症，心脏病患儿应预防性全身使用抗生素。

体征缓解可能要到泪道探通术后 1 周或更长时间才会出现。复发常发生在探通失败后的 1~2 个月内。在 15 个月以下的先天性鼻泪管阻塞（CNLDO）婴儿中，首次正确实施泪道探通术的成功率超过 80%。

严重的探通术后并发症是罕见的。在一些患者中，偶尔会出现轻微的溢泪，特别是在寒冷的室外或伴有上呼吸道感染的婴儿中。这种溢泪很可能是由于明显狭窄的泪道造成的，通常不需要额外的治疗。

Patients with complex CNLDO or persistent symptoms after initial probing

A variety of treatment options are available for patients with complex CNLDO (usually discovered at the time of initial surgery) or those with symptoms that persist following initial probing. Some surgeons may choose to perform balloon dacryoplasty or NLD stenting as the initial procedure in patients they believe are at risk for recurrence of CNLDO. Recurrent NLDO is more likely in persons with chronic rhinitis, those older than 36 months, or patients with complex CNLDO. Balloon dacryoplasty or intubation is more successful than probing alone for persistent NLDO after initial probing. The selection of intubation or balloon dacryoplasty is based on surgeon preference. Infracture of the inferior turbinate has not been shown to improve surgical outcomes. Perioperative systemic antibiotics and steroids may be beneficial in children at risk for recurrence.

Pediatric Eye Disease Investigator Group. Balloon catheter dilation and nasolacrimal duct intubation for treatment of nasolacrimal duct obstruction after failed probing. *Arch Ophthalmol.* 2009;127(5):633–639.

Silbert DI, Matta N. Congenital nasolacrimal duct obstruction. *Focal Points: Clinical Practice Perspectives*. San Francisco: American Academy of Ophthalmology; 2016, module 6.

Balloon dacryoplasty Balloon dacryoplasty (balloon catheter dilation) is performed by passing a catheter into the distal NLD and inflating its balloon at the site of obstruction (Fig 19-7). This procedure is particularly useful for patients with diffuse, rather than localized, obstruction of the distal duct.

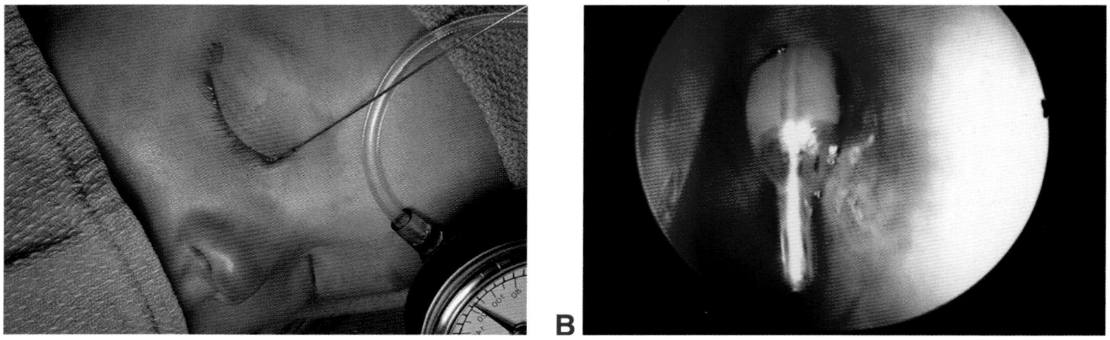

A B

Figure 19-7 Balloon dacryoplasty. **A,** Passing the balloon into the NLD. **B,** Inflated balloon, endoscopic view. *(Part B courtesy of Eric Paul Purdy, MD.)*

Intubation Intubation of the lacrimal system is usually recommended when probing or balloon dacryoplasty has failed. Several methods of intubation are available. Bicanalicular intubation is performed by passing stents through the upper and lower canaliculi and recovering them in the nares. Most surgeons secure the stents in the nares by using a **bolster** or by suturing the stents to the nasal mucosa. Monocanalicular stents are placed by passing them through either the upper or lower canaliculus or sometimes by passing separate stents through both canaliculi.

Complications associated with stents include elongation of the lacrimal puncta, dislodging and protrusion of the stents, and corneal abrasions. In some cases, the stent can be repositioned, but early

复杂性先天性鼻泪管阻塞（CNLDO）或初次探通术后有持续性症状的患者
对于复杂性先天性鼻泪管阻塞（CNLDO）患儿（通常在初次手术时发现），或在初次探通后症状仍然存在的患儿有多种治疗方案。一些手术医生对有先天性鼻泪管阻塞（CNLDO）复发风险的患儿首次即行球囊泪道成形术或鼻泪管支架。复发性鼻泪管阻塞（NLDO）多发生在慢性鼻炎、年龄大于 36 月龄或伴有复杂先天性鼻泪管阻塞（CNLDO）的患儿。初次泪道探通术后持续性鼻泪管阻塞（NLDO）时，球囊泪道成形术或插管术比单独探通术成功率高。根据手术医生的习惯来选择插管术或球囊泪道成形术。下鼻甲不全切除术并不能改善手术结果。围手术期全身使用抗生素和类固醇可能对有复发风险的儿童有益。

Pediatric Eye Disease Investigator Group. Balloon catheter dilation and nasolacrimal duct intubation for treatment of nasolacrimal duct obstruction after failed probing. *Arch Ophthalmol.* 2009;127(5):633–639.

Silbert DI, Matta N. Congenital nasolacrimal duct obstruction. *Focal Points: Clinical Practice Perspectives*. San Francisco: American Academy of Ophthalmology; 2016, module 6.

球囊泪道成形术　球囊泪道成形术（球囊导管扩张术）是将导管置入远端鼻泪管（NLD），并在阻塞处充气球囊（图 19–7）。这一手术特别适用于弥漫性阻塞患儿，而非局限性远端泪道阻塞患儿。

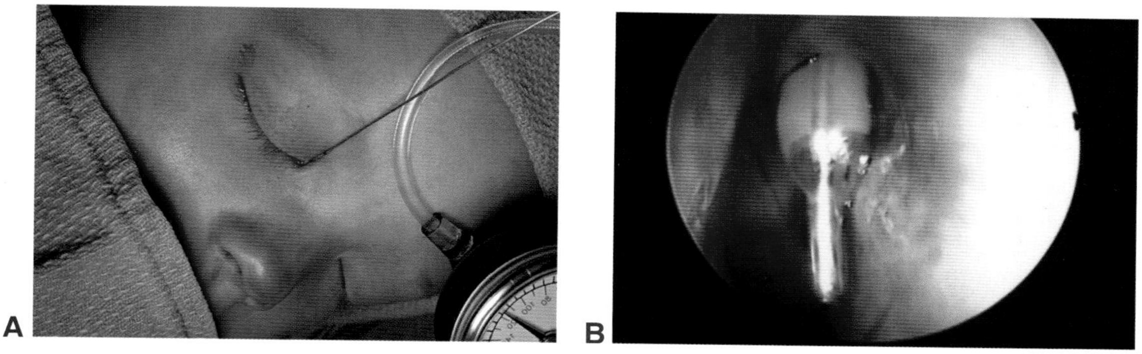

图 19–7　球囊泪道成形术。**A.** 把球囊送到鼻泪管（NLD）处。**B.** 充气球囊，内窥镜所见。*（译者注：资料来源见前页原文。）*

泪道插管术　当探通术或球囊泪道成形术失败时，可行泪道插管术。泪道插管有几种方法，双泪小管插管是过支架穿过上泪小管和下泪小管，并置于鼻腔内。多数手术医生通过栓或缝合支架到鼻黏膜上，以使支架固定在鼻腔内。单泪小管支架是通过上泪小管或下泪小管放置，有时通过 2 个泪小管分别放置支架。

与支架相关的并发症包括泪小管延长、支架移位和突出以及角膜擦伤。有时可以重新放置支架，必要时也可早期取出。

removal may be necessary.

Stents are usually left in place for 2–6 months, but shorter periods can be successful. The technique used for stent removal depends on the age of the patient, the measure employed to secure the stent, and the position of the stent (in place or partially dislodged).

Nasal endoscopy Anatomical abnormalities of the distal NLD account for some of the failures of initial probing. These abnormalities include cysts similar to those seen in infants with dacryocystoceles and flaccid mucosal membranes obstructing the distal duct. In addition, there may be false passages, which may be recognized endoscopically; in these cases, probing may be repeated. Removal of abnormal structures is performed under endoscopic guidance. Endoscopy may be performed by the ophthalmologist alone or in conjunction with an otolaryngologist.

Older children with NLDO

There is some controversy in the literature regarding success rates for NLD surgery in older children. The Pediatric Eye Disease Investigator Group (PEDIG) found a high success rate for simple probing in children up to 36 months of age. Many older children have simple NLDO; they have the same membranous obstruction of the distal duct found in younger children with NLDO (see Fig 19-4A). As previously mentioned, this obstruction is identified by a distinct popping sensation as the probe is passed into the distal duct. Probing in older patients with this finding has a success rate similar to that in younger children. Because probing is less likely to be successful in complex NLDO, particularly in older children, balloon dacryoplasty or stent placement should be considered as the initial surgical procedure.

Pediatric Eye Disease Investigator Group; Repka MX, Chandler DL, Beck RW, et al. Primary treatment of nasolacrimal duct obstruction with probing in children younger than 4 years. *Ophthalmology.* 2008;115(3):577–584.

Dacryocystorhinostomy

Dacryocystorhinostomy involves creation of a new opening between the lacrimal sac and the nasal cavity. It is an option when the procedures described in the preceding sections are unsuccessful and NLDO persists or recurs. The decision of when to perform this procedure is affected by the severity of the signs and symptoms of obstruction. See BCSC Section 7, *Oculofacial Plastic and Orbital Surgery,* for further discussion of this procedure.

支架通常放置 2~6 个月，但短一些时间也可以成功。取出支架技术的选择取决于患儿的年龄、固定支架的方法及支架的位置（原位或部分移位）。

鼻内窥镜 远端鼻泪管（NLD）的解剖异常是导致初次探通失败的原因之一，这些异常包括与在婴儿泪囊囊肿相似的囊肿以及松弛的黏膜阻塞远端泪道。另外，还有内窥镜下的假道，这需要再次进行探通。在内窥镜引导下切除异常结构。鼻内窥镜检查可以由眼科医生单独进行，也可以与耳鼻喉科医生联合进行。

患有鼻泪管阻塞（NLDO）的大龄儿童

文献中关于大龄儿童鼻泪管（NLD）手术的成功率存有争议。儿童眼病研究小组（PEDIG）发现，单纯泪道探通术在 36 月龄幼儿的成功率很高。许多大龄儿童有单纯的鼻泪管阻塞（NLDO）；其远端泪道中有与低龄鼻泪管阻塞（NLDO）儿童相同的膜性阻塞（见图 19-4A）。如前所述，当探针进入远端泪道时，可通过明显的破裂感来确定阻塞。有这一体征的大龄儿童，其探通术成功率与低龄儿童相似。在复杂的鼻泪管阻塞（NLDO）患儿中，尤其是在大龄儿童中，探通术成功率低，所以应该将球囊泪道成形术或支架置入术作为首选的手术方式。

Pediatric Eye Disease Investigator Group; Repka MX, Chandler DL, Beck RW, et al. Primary treatment of nasolacrimal duct obstruction with probing in children younger than 4 years. *Ophthalmology*. 2008;115(3):577–584.

泪囊鼻腔吻合术

泪囊鼻腔吻合术是在泪囊和鼻腔之间造一个新的开口，当上述几种手术方式不成功、鼻泪管阻塞（NLDO）持续存在或复发时，这是一种选择。选择进行该手术时机取决于阻塞症状和体征的严重程度。详细讨论参见 BCSC 第 7 册《*眼面部整形与眼眶手术*》。

（翻译 叶璐 王眪 // 审校 石一宁 蒋宁 // 章节审校 石广礼）

CHAPTER 20

External Diseases of the Eye

This chapter focuses on external diseases of the eye that are seen in the pediatric population. Many of the topics covered in this chapter are also discussed in BCSC Section 8, *External Disease and Cornea.*

Infectious Conjunctivitis

Bacterial and viral infections are the most common causes of infectious conjunctivitis in children in developed countries. Presenting symptoms of infectious conjunctivitis commonly include burning, stinging, and foreign-body sensation; signs include conjunctival hyperemia, ocular discharge, and matting of the eyelids. Symptoms and signs may be present unilaterally or bilaterally. The character of the discharge is diagnostically helpful and may be serous, mucopurulent, or purulent. Purulent discharge suggests a polymorphonuclear response to a bacterial infection, mucopurulent discharge suggests a viral or chlamydial infection, and a serous or watery discharge suggests a viral or allergic reaction. Membrane or pseudomembrane formation may occur in severe viral or bacterial conjunctivitis, Stevens-Johnson syndrome, ligneous conjunctivitis, and chemical burns. Table 20-1 lists common causes of conjunctival hyperemia, or *red eye,* in infants and children.

Table 20-1 Common Causes of Conjunctival Hyperemia in Infants and Children

Infectious conjunctivitis
Bacterial infection
Chlamydial infection
Viral infection
Blepharitis
Allergic conjunctivitis
Trauma
Foreign body
Drug, toxic, or chemical reaction
Iritis
Episcleritis or scleritis
Epiblepharon

Ophthalmia Neonatorum

Ophthalmia neonatorum refers to conjunctivitis occurring in the first month of life. This condition can be caused by bacterial, viral, or chemical agents. Widespread effective prophylaxis has diminished its occurrence to very low levels in industrialized countries, but ophthalmia neonatorum remains a significant cause of ocular infection, blindness, and even death in medically underserved areas around the world.

第 20 章

眼表疾病

本章主要讨论儿童常见的眼表疾病。本章涉及的内容在 BCSC 第 8 册《*外眼疾病与角膜*》中进行讨论。

感染性结膜炎

细菌和病毒感染是发达国家儿童结膜炎常见的病因。感染性结膜炎的常见症状包括灼烧、刺痛和异物感；体征包括结膜充血、眼部分泌物和上下眼睑粘在一起。症状和体征可以单眼或双眼出现。分泌物可以是浆液性、黏液脓性或脓性，其特征对诊断有帮助。脓性分泌物提示对细菌感染的多形核白细胞反应，黏液脓性分泌物提示病毒或衣原体感染，浆液或水性分泌物提示病毒感染或过敏反应。严重病毒性或细菌性结膜炎、Stevens–Johnson 综合征、木样结膜炎和化学性烧伤可形成膜或假膜。表 20–1 列出了婴幼儿结膜充血或*红眼*的常见原因。

表20–1　婴儿及儿童结膜充血的常见病因

感染性结膜炎
细菌感染
衣原体感染
病毒感染
睑缘炎
过敏性结膜炎
外伤
异物
药物、毒性或化学反应
虹膜炎
表层巩膜炎或深层巩膜炎
内眦赘皮

新生儿眼炎

*新生儿眼炎*是指新生儿出生后第 1 个月内发生的结膜炎，可能由细菌、病毒或化学制剂引起。在工业化国家，广泛有效的预防已将其发生率降到非常低，但新生儿眼炎仍然是医疗资源不足地区眼部感染、失明甚至死亡的一个重要原因。

Epidemiology and etiology

Worldwide, the incidence of ophthalmia neonatorum is greater in areas with high rates of sexually transmitted disease and poor health care. The prevalence ranges from 0.1% in highly developed countries with effective prenatal and perinatal care to 10% in areas such as East Africa. Because a mother may have multiple sexually transmitted diseases, infants with one type of ophthalmia neonatorum should be screened for other such diseases. Public health authorities should be contacted to initiate evaluation and treatment of other maternal contacts in cases of sexually transmitted diseases.

The causative organism usually infects the infant through direct contact during passage through the birth canal. Infection can ascend to the uterus, especially if there is prolonged rupture of membranes, so even with cesarean delivery, infants can be infected.

Neisseria gonorrhoeae Ophthalmia neonatorum caused by *Neisseria gonorrhoeae* typically presents in the first 3–4 days of life. Patients may present with mild conjunctival hyperemia and ocular discharge. In severe cases, there is marked chemosis, copious discharge, and potentially rapid corneal ulceration and perforation (Fig 20-1). Systemic infection can cause sepsis, meningitis, and arthritis.

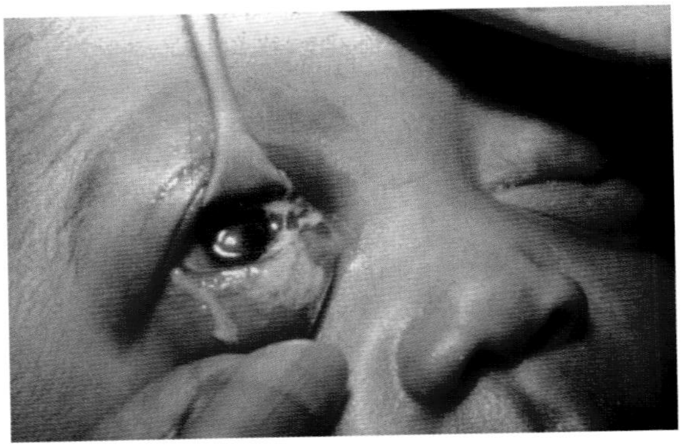

Figure 20-1 Neisseria gonorrhoeae conjunctivitis. *(Courtesy of Jane C. Edmond, MD.)*

Gram stain of the conjunctival exudate showing gram-negative intracellular diplococci allows a presumptive diagnosis of *N gonorrhoeae* infection; treatment should be started immediately. Ophthalmia neonatorum from *Neisseria meningitidis* has also been reported. Definitive diagnosis is based on culture of the conjunctival discharge. Treatment of gonococcal ophthalmia neonatorum includes systemic ceftriaxone and topical irrigation with saline. Topical antibiotics may also be indicated if there is corneal involvement.

Chlamydia trachomatis *Chlamydia trachomatis* is an obligate intracellular bacterium that can cause neonatal inclusion conjunctivitis. Onset of conjunctivitis usually occurs around 1 week of age, although it may be earlier, especially in cases with premature rupture of membranes. Eye infection is characterized by minimal to moderate filmy discharge, mild swelling of the eyelids, and hyperemia with a papillary reaction of the conjunctiva (Fig 20-2). Severe cases may be accompanied by more copious discharge and pseudomembrane formation. Chlamydial infection in infants differs from that in adults in several ways: in infants, membrane formation may occur, the amount of mucopurulent discharge is greater, and there is no follicular response.

流行病学及病因学

世界范围内，新生儿眼炎在性传播疾病发病率高和卫生保健差的地区发病率更高。发达国家产前和围产期检查较好，其患病率为 0.1%，而东非等地区达 10%。由于母亲可能患有多种性传播疾病，因此患有一种类型新生儿眼炎的婴儿应筛查其他此类疾病。此外，还应与公共卫生部门联系，对性传播疾病产妇的其他接触者进行评估和治疗。

病原体通常是婴儿经产道时直接接触感染的。感染可以逆行到子宫，特别是在伴有长时间的胎膜破裂时，即使行剖宫产，新生儿也有可能被感染。

淋病奈瑟球菌　淋病奈瑟球菌引起的新生儿眼炎通常在出生后 3~4d 出现。患儿可出现轻度结膜充血和眼部分泌物。严重球结膜高度水肿、大量的分泌物及潜在的快速角膜溃疡和穿孔（图 20–1）。全身感染可引起败血症、脑膜炎和关节炎。

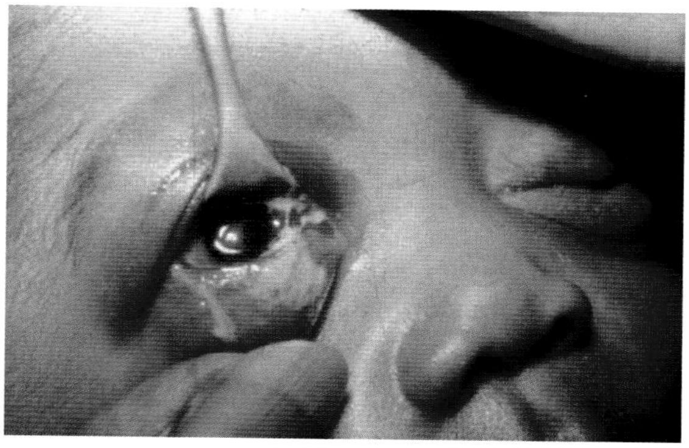

图 20–1　淋病奈瑟球菌性结膜炎。*（译者注：资料来源见前页原文。）*

结膜分泌物的革兰氏染色提示革兰氏阴性细胞内双球菌可推断诊断为*淋病奈瑟球菌*感染；应立即开始治疗。有报道*脑膜炎奈瑟球菌*导致的新生儿眼炎，结膜分泌物的培养是确诊的重要依据。新生儿淋病奈瑟球菌性眼炎的治疗包括全身性头孢曲松治疗和局部盐水冲洗。如果角膜受累，也可局部使用抗生素。

沙眼衣原体　*沙眼衣原体*是一种专性细胞内细菌，可引起新生儿包涵体结膜炎。结膜炎的发病通常发生在 1 周龄，特别是胎膜早破时可能发生得更早。眼部感染的特征是轻度到中度的膜性分泌物，眼睑轻度肿胀以及充血并伴有结膜乳头样改变（图 20–2）。严重的病例可能伴有较多的分泌物和假膜形成。婴儿衣原体感染与成人衣原体感染的不同之处在于：婴儿可发生膜的形成，黏液脓性分泌物较多，无滤泡反应。

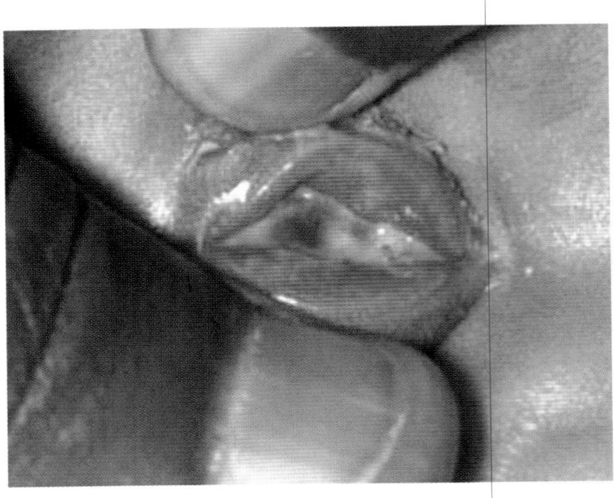

Figure 20-2 Chlamydial ophthalmia neonatorum. *(Courtesy of Jane C. Edmond, MD.)*

Chlamydial infections can be diagnosed by culture of conjunctival scrapings, polymerase chain reaction, direct fluorescent antibody tests, and enzyme immunoassays. Systemic treatment of neonatal chlamydial disease is indicated because of the risk of pneumonitis and otitis media. The treatment of choice is oral erythromycin, 50 mg/kg per day in 4 divided doses for 14 days. Topical erythromycin ointment may be used in addition to but not as a replacement for oral therapy.

Herpes simplex virus Infection with herpes simplex virus (HSV) is usually secondary to HSV type 2 and typically presents later than infection with *N gonorrhoeae* or *C trachomatis*, frequently in the second week of life. See the discussion of congenital HSV infection in Chapter 28.

Chemical conjunctivitis

Chemical conjunctivitis refers to a mild, self-limited irritation and redness of the conjunctiva occurring in the first 24 hours after instillation of silver nitrate, a preparation used for ophthalmia neonatorum prophylaxis. This condition improves spontaneously by the second day of life.

Ophthalmia neonatorum prophylaxis

Originally, 2% silver nitrate was used as prophylactic treatment of gonorrheal ophthalmia neonatorum. However, it is not effective against *C trachomatis* and has largely been supplanted by agents that are effective against both *N gonorrhoeae* and *C trachomatis*, such as erythromycin and tetracycline ointments and 2.5% povidone-iodine solution. Silver nitrate is still used in some parts of the world.

Bacterial Conjunctivitis in Children and Adolescents

The most common causes of bacterial conjunctivitis in school-aged children are *Streptococcus pneumoniae*, *Haemophilus* species, *Staphylococcus aureus*, and *Moraxella*. The incidence of infection from *Haemophilus* has decreased because of widespread immunization, whereas the incidence of methicillin-resistant *S aureus* (MRSA) conjunctivitis has increased. More severe forms of bacterial conjunctivitis accompanied by copious discharge suggest infection with more virulent organisms, including *N gonorrhoeae* and *N meningitidis*.

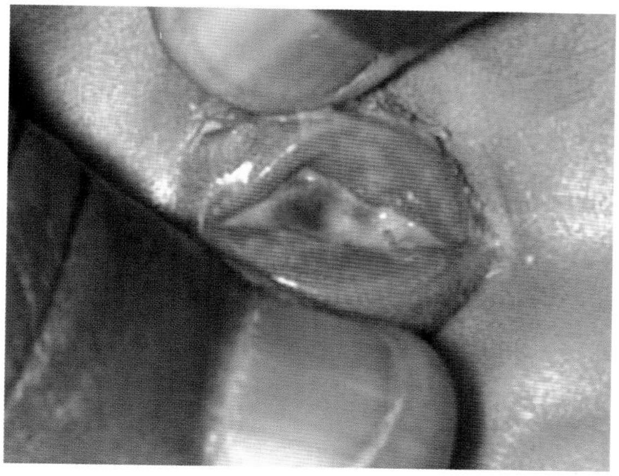

图 20–2　新生儿衣原体眼炎（*译者注：资料来源见前页原文。*）

衣原体感染可通过结膜刮片培养、聚合酶链反应、直接荧光抗体检测和酶免疫分析确诊。有肺炎和中耳炎危险时，新生儿衣原体感染需全身治疗。治疗方法可以选择口服红霉素，50mg/（kg · d），分 4 次服用，共 14d。局部红霉素软膏可作为口服治疗的补充，但不能替代口服治疗。

单纯疱疹病毒　单纯疱疹病毒（HSV）感染通常继发于单纯疱疹病毒（HSV）2 型感染，比*淋病奈瑟球菌*或*沙眼衣原体*感染发生得晚，常出现在出生后的第 2 周。参见第 28 章先天性单纯疱疹病毒（HSV）感染的讨论。

化学性结膜炎

化学性结膜炎是指硝酸银滴眼后 24h 内发生的一种轻度、自限性的结膜刺激反应和发红，硝酸银滴眼液用于预防治疗新生儿眼炎这种情况在第 2 天即可自发改善。

新生儿眼炎的预防

2% 硝酸银最初用于预防治疗新生儿淋病奈瑟球菌性眼炎，而对*沙眼衣原体*没有效果，因此已被对*淋病奈瑟球菌*和*沙眼衣原体*都有效的药物所取代，如红霉素、四环素软膏和 2.5% 聚维酮碘溶液。然而硝酸银仍在一些地区使用。

儿童和青少年细菌性结膜炎

学龄儿童细菌性结膜炎最常见的病因是*肺炎链球菌*、*嗜血杆菌*、*金黄色葡萄球菌*和*莫拉杆菌*。由于广泛的免疫接种，*嗜血杆菌*感染的发生率有所下降，而耐甲氧西林*金黄色葡萄球菌*（MRSA）结膜炎的发生率有所上升。伴有大量分泌物的、严重的细菌性结膜炎，提示感染的微生物毒性较强，包括*淋病奈瑟球菌*和*脑膜炎奈瑟球菌*。

Diagnosis is by clinical presentation. Culture to identify the offending agent is usually not necessary in mild cases but should be performed in severe cases. If the infection is untreated, symptoms are self-limited but may last up to 2 weeks. A broad-spectrum topical ophthalmic drop or ointment should shorten the course to a few days. Topical medications that are usually effective include polymyxin combinations, aminoglycosides, erythromycin, bacitracin, fluoroquinolones, and azithromycin. Fluoroquinolones may be considerably more expensive than other medications and may increase the risk of promoting drug-resistant organisms. Patients with *N meningitidis* conjunctivitis, and others exposed to these patients, require systemic treatment because of the high risk of meningitis.

Parinaud oculoglandular syndrome

Parinaud oculoglandular syndrome (POS) manifests as unilateral granulomatous conjunctivitis associated with preauricular and submandibular lymphadenopathy that can be very marked (Fig 20-3). MRSA conjunctivitis can have a similar presentation. *Bartonella henselae,* a pleomorphic gram-negative bacillus that is endemic in cats and causes cat-scratch disease, is the most common cause of POS. Other causative organisms include *Mycobacterium tuberculosis, Mycobacterium leprae, Francisella tularensis, Yersinia pseudotuberculosis, Treponema pallidum,* and *C trachomatis.* Cat-scratch disease is usually associated with a scratch from a kitten, but a cat bite or even touching the eye with a hand that has been licked by an infected kitten can cause the disease.

Serologic testing is an effective means of diagnosing POS. Presence of antibodies to *B henselae,* detected by indirect fluorescent antibody testing or enzyme immunoassay, can confirm a diagnosis of cat-scratch disease. Treatment can be supportive in mild cases of cat-scratch disease because the disease is self-limited. In more severe cases systemic treatment, usually with azithromycin, may be indicated. Appropriate systemic antibiotics are used to treat the other organisms that cause POS.

A 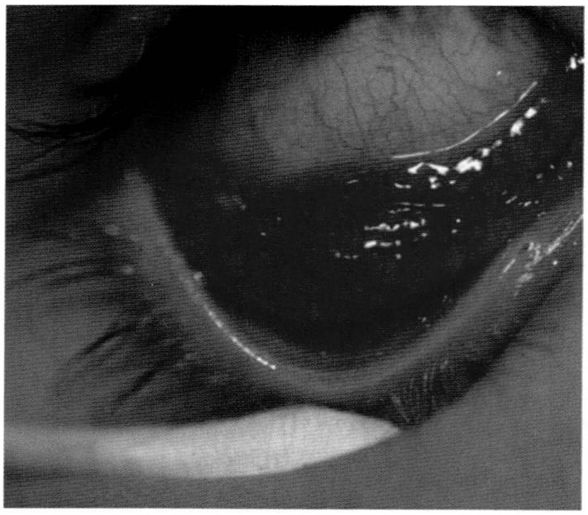

B 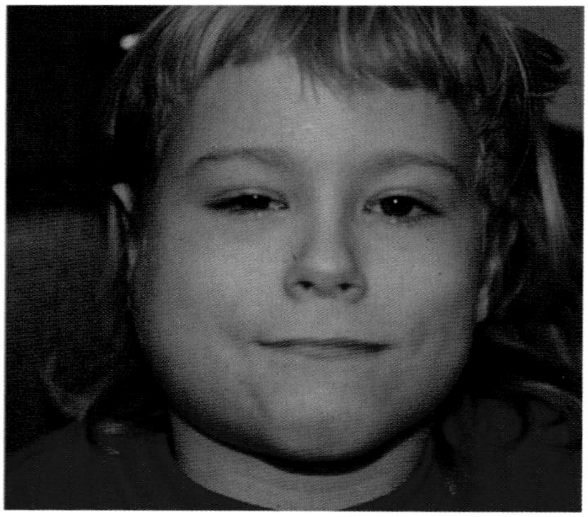

Figure 20-3 Parinaud oculoglandular syndrome. **A,** Marked follicular reaction in the lower fornix. **B,** Massive enlargement of submandibular lymph node on the affected right side. *(Courtesy of David A. Plager, MD.)*

Chlamydial infections

Two different diseases can be caused by *C trachomatis* in children and adolescents: trachoma (serotypes A–C) and adult inclusion conjunctivitis (serotypes D–K).

临床表现可为诊断依据。常不需要培养来鉴别轻度感染的致病因子，重度感染应进行培养。感染未经治疗，症状呈自限性，但可能持续 2 周左右。局部使用广谱滴眼液或眼药膏可缩短病程至几日。有效的局部药物有多黏菌素复合剂、氨基糖苷类、红霉素、杆菌肽、氟喹诺酮类和阿奇霉素。氟喹诺酮类比其他药物贵，同时也有增加耐药性的风险。因为*脑膜炎奈瑟球菌*型结膜炎患儿及与其有接触的人需要全身治疗，患脑膜炎的风险较高。

Parinaud 眼 – 腺综合征

Parinaud 眼 – 腺综合征（POS）表现为单侧肉芽肿性结膜炎，伴明显耳前淋巴结肿大和下颌下淋巴结肿大（图 20–3）。耐甲氧西林金黄色葡萄球菌（MRSA）结膜炎也有类似的表现。*Bartonella 体*是一种多形性革兰氏阴性杆菌，在猫中流行，可引起猫抓病，是引起 Parinaud 眼 – 腺综合征（POS）的最常见原因。其他致病微生物包括*结核分枝杆菌*、*麻风分枝杆菌*、*土热拉杆菌*、*假结核耶尔森菌*、*梅毒螺旋体*和*沙眼衣原体*。猫抓病通常与小猫抓伤有关，但被猫咬伤或用被感染小猫舔过的手触摸眼睛都可能导致这种疾病。

血清学检查是诊断 Parinaud 眼 – 腺综合征（POS）的有效手段。通过间接荧光抗体检测或酶免疫分析法检测 *Bartonella 体*抗体的存在，即可确诊猫抓病。因猫抓病属于自限性疾病，故对于轻症患儿，可采取支持性疗法。重症患儿需全身性治疗，常规用阿奇霉素。其他致病微生物引起的 Parinaud 眼 – 腺综合征（POS），选用适当的全身性抗生素。

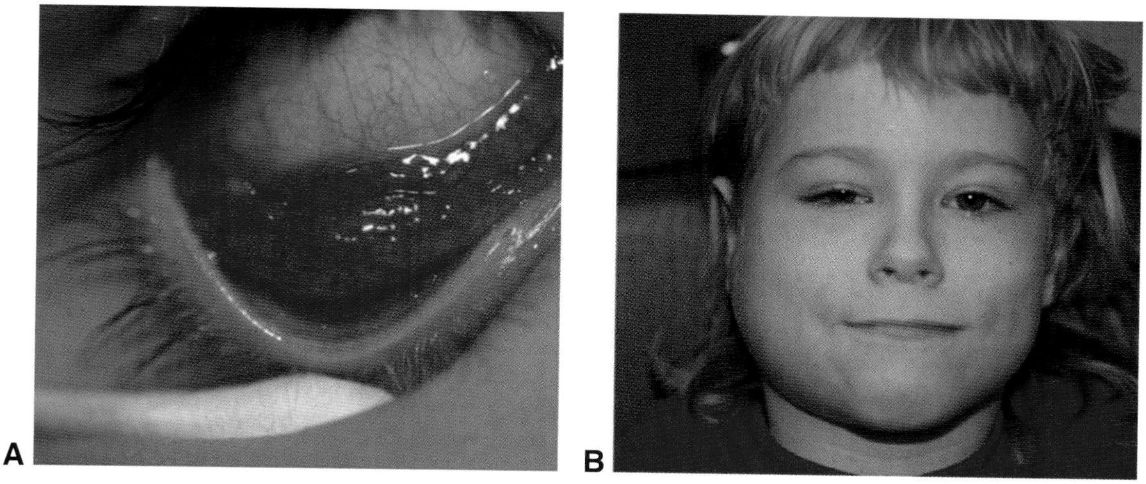

图 20–3　Parinaud 眼 – 腺综合征 **A.** 下穹窿有明显的滤泡反应。**B.** 受累右侧下颌下淋巴结肿大。*（译者注：资料来源见前页原文。）*

衣原体感染

儿童和青少年*沙眼衣原体*可引起 2 种不同的疾病：沙眼（血清型 A~C）和成人包涵体结膜炎（血清型 D~K）。

Trachoma Trachoma is the most common cause of preventable blindness in the world. This disease is uncommon in Europe and the United States, except in areas of the southern United States and on Native American reservations. It is caused by poor hygiene and inadequate sanitation and is spread from eye to eye or by flies or fomites. Clinical manifestations include acute purulent conjunctivitis, a follicular reaction, papillary hypertrophy, vascularization of the cornea, and progressive cicatricial changes of the cornea and conjunctiva. Diagnosis is made by Giemsa stain, cell culture, or polymerase chain reaction. Treatment includes both topical and systemic erythromycin. Tetracycline can be used in children 8 years of age and older.

Adult inclusion conjunctivitis Adult inclusion conjunctivitis is a sexually transmitted disease that can be found in sexually active adolescents in association with chlamydial urethritis or cervicitis. However, there are nonsexual modes of transmission, including shared eye cosmetics and contaminated swimming pools. Patients present with follicular conjunctivitis, scant mucopurulent discharge, and preauricular lymphadenopathy. There is no membrane formation. This condition can be diagnosed by culture of conjunctival scrapings, polymerase chain reaction, direct fluorescent antibody tests, and enzyme immunoassays. If untreated, inclusion conjunctivitis resolves spontaneously in 6–18 months. The recommended treatment is oral tetracycline, doxycycline, azithromycin, or erythromycin. The clinician should consider whether the patient has been sexually abused, especially if adult inclusion conjunctivitis is found in a young child.

Viral Conjunctivitis in Infants and Children

Adenovirus

Viral conjunctivitis is most often caused by an adenovirus, a DNA virus that can cause a range of human diseases, including upper respiratory tract infection and gastroenteritis. The following adenoviral diseases are listed with their associated serotypes: epidemic keratoconjunctivitis (serotypes 8, 19, and 37, subgroup D), pharyngoconjunctival fever (serotypes 3 and 7), acute hemorrhagic conjunctivitis (serotypes 11 and 21), and acute follicular conjunctivitis (serotypes 1, 2, 3, 4, 7, and 10). Contact precautions are especially important during the examination of infants. Outbreaks of adenoviral conjunctivitis have been associated with retinopathy of prematurity examinations in neonatal intensive care units. In neonates, adenoviral pneumonia can be fatal or lead to serious morbidity.

Haas J, Larson E, Ross B, See B, Saiman L. Epidemiology and diagnosis of hospitalacquired conjunctivitis among neonatal intensive care unit patients. *Pediatr Infect Dis J.* 2005;24(7):586–589.

Epidemic keratoconjunctivitis Epidemic keratoconjunctivitis (EKC) is a highly contagious conjunctivitis that tends to occur in epidemic outbreaks. This infection is an acute bilateral follicular conjunctivitis that is usually unilateral at onset and associated with preauricular lymphadenopathy. Initial symptoms are foreign-body sensation and periorbital pain. A diffuse superficial keratitis is followed by focal epithelial lesions that stain. After 11–15 days, subepithelial opacities begin to form beneath the focal epithelial infiltrates. The epithelial component fades by day 30, but the subepithelial opacities may remain for up to 2 years. In severe infections, particularly in infants, a conjunctival membrane forms and marked swelling of the eyelids occurs; these signs must be differentiated from those of orbital or preseptal cellulitis. In severe cases, complications include persistent subepithelial opacities and conjunctival scar formation.

沙眼　沙眼是世界上最常见的可预防盲的病。其在欧洲和美国（美国南部地区和美洲土著保留地除外）已不常见。它是由卫生条件差和卫生设施不足，由眼－眼传播或由苍蝇及污染物传播。临床表现包括急性化脓性结膜炎、滤泡增生、乳头肥大、角膜血管化以及角膜和结膜的进行性瘢痕性改变。通过 Giemsa 染色、细胞培养或聚合酶链反应进行诊断。治疗方法包括局部和全身应用红霉素。四环素可用于 8 岁及以上儿童。

成人包涵体性结膜炎　成人包涵体性结膜炎是一种性传播疾病，可见于性生活活跃的青年人，与衣原体性尿道炎或宫颈炎有关。除性传播途径外，也有非性传播方式，包括共用眼部化妆品及污染的游泳池。患者表现为滤泡性结膜炎，黏液脓性分泌物较少，耳前淋巴结肿大，没有膜形成。可通过结膜刮取物培养、聚合酶链反应、直接荧光抗体试验和酶免疫检测进行诊断。未经治疗的成人包涵体性结膜炎会在 6~18 个月内自行消退。建议口服四环素、多西环素、阿奇霉素或红霉素。临床医生还应该考虑患者是否遭受过性虐待，特别是幼儿患病时。

婴幼儿及儿童病毒性结膜炎

腺病毒

病毒性结膜炎最常见的病因是腺病毒感染，腺病毒是一种 DNA 病毒，该病毒可导致包括上呼吸道感染和胃肠炎在内的多种人类疾病。腺病毒疾病及其相关血清类型有：流行性角结膜炎（血清型 8，19 和 37 型，亚组 D）、咽结膜热（血清型 3 和 7 型）、急性出血性结膜炎（血清型 11 和 21 型）和急性滤泡结膜炎（血清型 1，2，3，4，7 和 10 型）。在婴幼儿检查期间，接触预防措施甚为重要。腺病毒性结膜炎的院内爆发与新生儿重症监护病房中的早产儿视网膜病变检查相关。在新生儿中，腺病毒性肺炎是致命的，或导致严重并发症。

Haas J, Larson E, Ross B, See B, Saiman L. Epidemiology and diagnosis of hospitalacquired conjunctivitis among neonatal intensive care unit patients. *Pediatr Infect Dis J.* 2005;24(7):586–589.

流行性角结膜炎　流行性角结膜炎（EKC）是一种高度传染性结膜炎，常见爆发性流行。流行性角结膜炎（EKC）是一种急性双侧滤泡性结膜炎，在发病初期仅累及单眼，伴耳前淋巴结肿大。初始症状为异物感及眶周围疼痛。弥漫性浅表性角膜炎，随后是染色的局灶性上皮病变。发病 11~15d 后，在局部上皮浸润下，形成角膜上皮下混浊。上皮浸润在第 30d 消退，但上皮下混浊仍可持续 2 年。在严重感染中，特别是在婴儿中，结膜膜状物形成，并伴有明显的眼睑肿胀，这需与眼眶或隔前蜂窝织炎相鉴别。在严重的病例中，并发症还包括持续性上皮下混浊和结膜瘢痕形成。

Because EKC is easily transmitted, contact precautions must be maintained for up to 2 weeks. Isolation areas should be designated for examination of patients known or suspected to have adenoviral infections.

Diagnosis is usually based on clinical presentation but can be confirmed in the office by a rapid immunodetection assay. The organism can be recovered from the eyes and throat for 2 weeks after onset, demonstrating that patients are infectious during this period. Treatment is supportive in most cases. Artificial tears and cold compresses can provide symptomatic relief. Topical corticosteroids may be used judiciously to decrease symptoms in severe cases and in cases of decreased vision secondary to subepithelial opacities; such agents may prolong the time to full recovery. Corticosteroid use in adenoviral infection is seldom indicated in children.

Pharyngoconjunctival fever Pharyngoconjunctival fever presents with conjunctival hyperemia, subconjunctival hemorrhage, conjunctival edema, epiphora, and eyelid swelling, accompanied by sore throat and fever. Within a few days, a follicular conjunctival reaction and preauricular lymphadenopathy develop. Symptoms may last for 2 weeks or more. Treatment is supportive because no topical or systemic treatment alters the course of the disease.

Herpes simplex virus

Conjunctivitis caused by HSV type 1 is covered in BCSC Section 8, *External Disease and Cornea.*

Varicella-zoster virus

Varicella-zoster virus (VZV) is a herpesvirus that can cause varicella and herpes zoster.

Varicella Varicella (chickenpox) is a contagious viral exanthem of childhood caused by primary infection with VZV. Varicella vaccine is very effective in preventing severe disease, but immunized children exposed to VZV may have mild symptoms. Clinical manifestations of primary VZV infection include fever and characteristic vesicular lesions of the skin and mucous membranes. Except for eyelid vesicles and follicular conjunctivitis, ocular involvement is uncommon. Treatment of conjunctival disease is usually not necessary. Intravenous or oral acyclovir is recommended by the American Academy of Pediatrics in the treatment of immunocompromised children with varicella.

Herpes zoster Reactivation of latent VZV in dorsal root and cranial nerve ganglia results in herpes zoster. Vesicular lesions may erupt on the periorbital skin and are localized to a single dermatome, with subsequent ocular involvement (Fig 20-4). Keratitis and anterior uveitis are most likely to occur if the nasociliary branch of cranial nerve V is affected.

Oral acyclovir is indicated in healthy children to shorten the course of the illness and decrease the risk of bacterial superinfection. Intravenous antiviral agents (famciclovir, valacyclovir, acyclovir) are indicated in immunocompromised patients or individuals with severe disseminated disease. Antiviral medications should be started within 72 hours of onset of symptoms.

由于流行性角结膜炎（EKC）易于传播，所以接触性预防措施需维持 2 周。应在指定隔离区检查确诊或疑似腺病毒感染者。

流行性角结膜炎（EKC）通常以临床表现作为诊断依据，或在诊室中进行快速免疫检测法确认。腺病毒可在发病后 2 周内的眼部及咽喉部分离出来，提示患者在此期间仍具有传染性。在大多数情况下，该病主要采取支持性治疗。人工泪液和冷敷可以缓解症状。局部使用皮质类固醇可有效减轻严重病例的症状及上皮下混浊所致视力下降，但会延长完全恢复的时间。儿童腺病毒感染很少使用糖皮质激素治疗。

咽结膜热　咽结膜热患者伴有结膜充血、结膜下出血、结膜水肿、溢泪及眼睑肿胀，并伴有咽喉痛和发热症状。患者在发病几天内，会出现结膜滤泡和耳前淋巴结肿大。其症状可能持续 2 周或更长时间。多采取支持性治疗，因为任何局部或全身性治疗都不会改变病程。

单纯疱疹病毒

有关单纯疱疹病毒（HSV）1 型引起的结膜炎，请参阅 BCSC 第 8 册《*外眼疾病与角膜*》。

水痘 – 带状疱疹病毒

水痘 – 带状疱疹病毒（VZV）是一种能引起水痘和带状疱疹的疱疹病毒。

水痘　水痘是儿童时期由水痘 – 带状疱疹病毒（VZV）感染引起的一种传染性病毒疹。水痘疫苗对预防重症患儿非常有效，但接种疫苗的儿童可有轻微的症状。原发性水痘 – 带状疱疹病毒（VZV）感染的临床表现有发热、皮肤及黏膜特征性水泡性病变。除眼睑小泡和滤泡性结膜炎外，一般不累及眼部其他结构。结膜病变不需要治疗。美国儿科学会建议，免疫功能低下的水痘患儿可静脉注射或口服阿昔洛韦。

带状疱疹　带状疱疹是由背根和颅神经节中潜伏的水痘 – 带状疱疹病毒（VZV）被重新激活所导致。患者眶周皮肤可能出现水泡性病变，并局限于单个皮区，随后出现眼部受累（图 20–4）。如果患者Ⅱ颅神经的鼻睫状支受到感染，可引发角膜炎和前葡萄膜炎。

健康儿童可口服阿昔洛韦，缩短病程，降低细菌的双重感染风险。免疫功能低下的患者或患有严重播散性疾病的患者应静脉注射抗病毒药物（泛昔洛韦、伐昔洛韦、阿昔洛韦）适用于抗病毒药物应在症状出现后 72h 内开始使用。

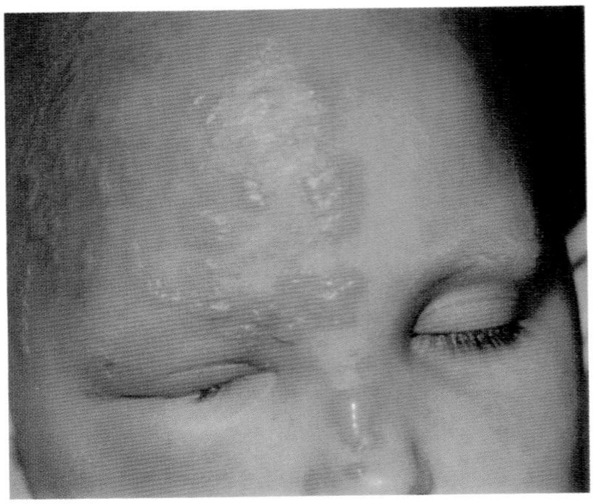

Figure 20-4 Herpes zoster.

Epstein-Barr virus

Epstein-Barr virus is a herpesvirus that can cause infectious mononucleosis, a benign and self-limited disease that occurs most commonly between ages 15 and 30 years. Findings include fever, widespread lymphadenopathy, pharyngitis, hepatic involvement, and the presence of atypical lymphocytes in the circulating blood. Conjunctivitis is the most common ocular finding. Nummular keratitis may also occur. The diagnosis is confirmed with detection of immunoglobulin M antibodies to viral capsid antigens or with a positive result on the heterophile antibody test. Ocular treatment is cool compresses to the eyes.

Molluscum contagiosum

Molluscum contagiosum is caused by a DNA poxvirus and usually presents as numerous umbilicated skin lesions (Fig 20-5A). Lesions on or near the eyelid margin can release viral particles onto the conjunctival surface, resulting in a follicular conjunctivitis (Fig 20-5B). Most lesions do not require treatment because they tend to resolve spontaneously; however, resolution can take months or years. Lesions causing conjunctivitis can be treated by incising each lesion and debriding the central core; in young children, such treatment usually requires general anesthesia.

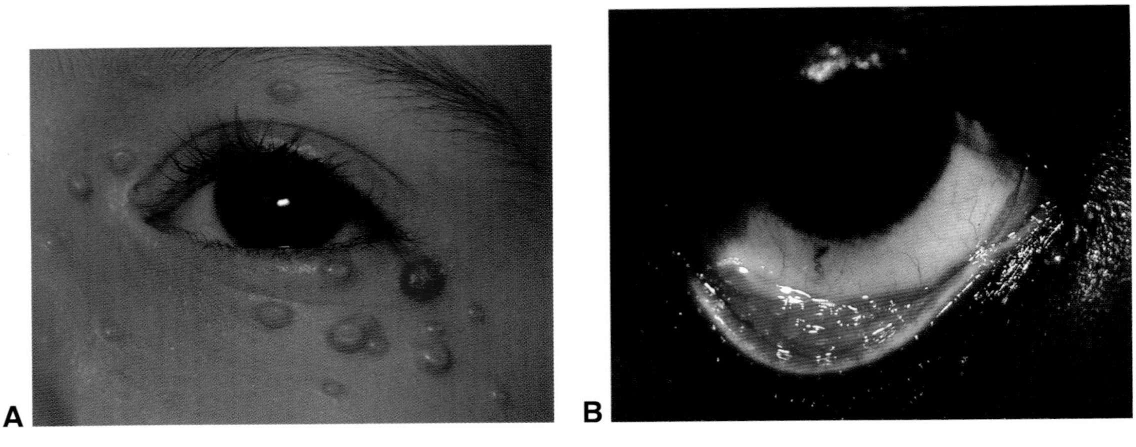

Figure 20-5 Molluscum contagiosum. **A,** Eyelid lesions. **B,** Secondary follicular conjunctivitis. *(Part A courtesy of Edward L. Raab, MD; part B courtesy of Gregg T. Lueder, MD.)*

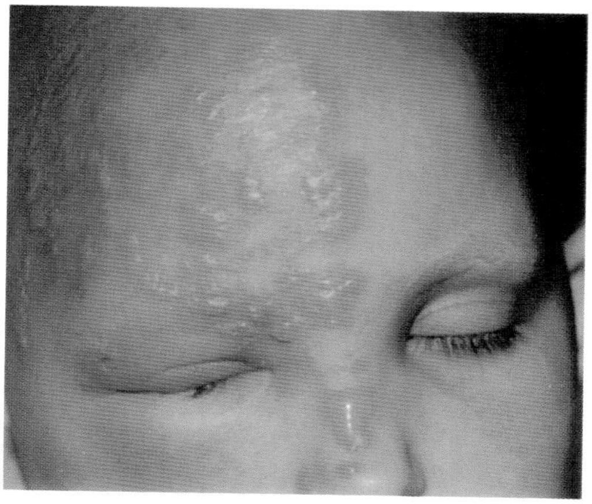

图 20-4 带状疱疹。

EB 病毒

EB 病毒是一种疱疹病毒，能引起传染性单核细胞增多症，这是一种良性及自限性疾病，最常见于 15~30 岁人群。可引起发热、广泛的淋巴结病、咽炎、肝脏受累及循环血液中存在非典型淋巴细胞。结膜炎是最常见的眼部表现。可出现钱币状角膜炎。检测出病毒衣壳抗原的免疫球蛋白 M 抗体及嗜异性抗体试验阳性即可确诊。眼部可冷敷。

传染性软疣

传染性软疣是由 DNA 痘病毒引起，表现为大量的皮肤肚脐状病灶（图 20-5A）。眼睑边缘或其附近的病变可将病毒颗粒释放到结膜表面，从而导致滤泡性结膜炎（图 20-5B）。病变会自行消退，多数病变不需治疗，但完全自愈需数月或数年时间。引起结膜炎的病灶，可单个切除每个病灶并清除其中心核，幼儿患者治疗时需全身麻醉。

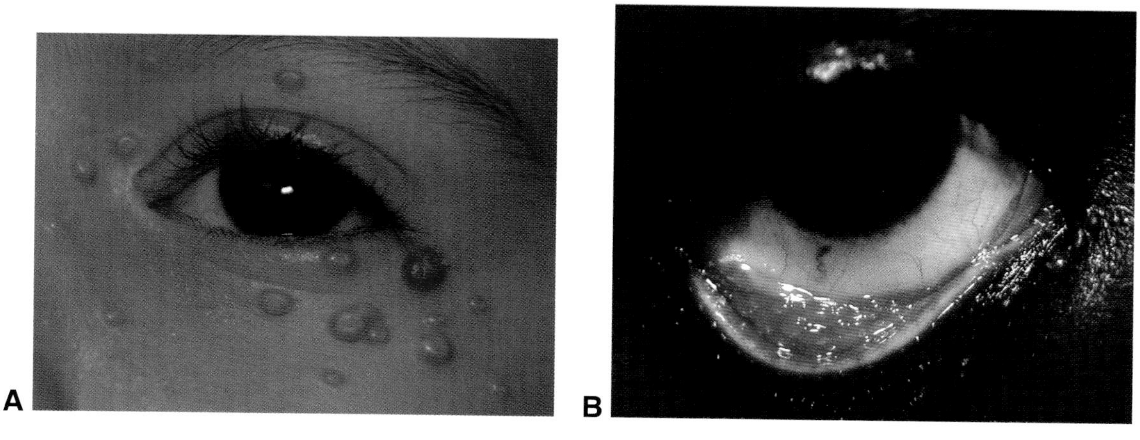

图 20-5 传染性软疣 **A.** 眼睑病变 **B.** 继发滤泡性结膜炎。*（译者注：资料来源见前页原文。）*

Inflammatory Disease

Blepharitis

Blepharitis is a common cause of chronic conjunctivitis in children. The signs and symptoms of blepharitis in children are similar to those in adults and include ocular irritation, conjunctival hyperemia, morning eyelid crusting, eyelid margin erythema, and meibomian gland obstruction (Fig 20-6). Intermittent blurred vision may occur because of tear film instability. Inferior keratitis may develop in more severe cases, leading to epithelial disruption and fluorescein staining, corneal scarring, and permanent vision loss (Figs 20-7, 20-8).

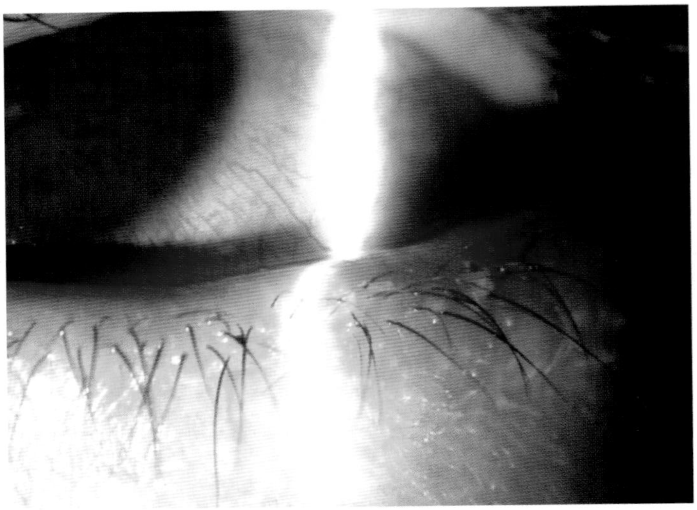

Figure 20-6 Blepharitis with meibomian gland dysfunction, scurf, and telangiectasias. *(Courtesy of Steven Safran, MD.)*

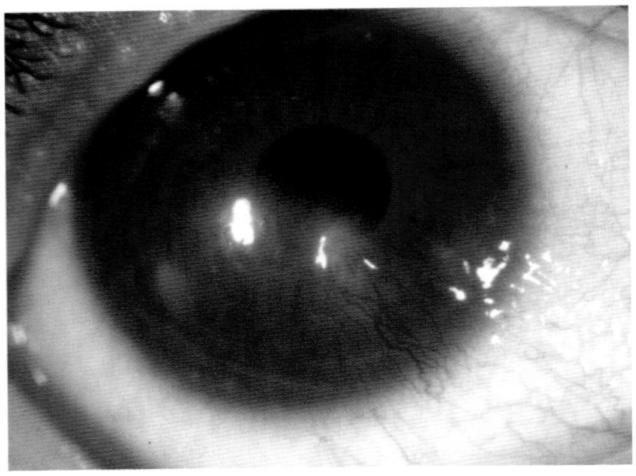

A

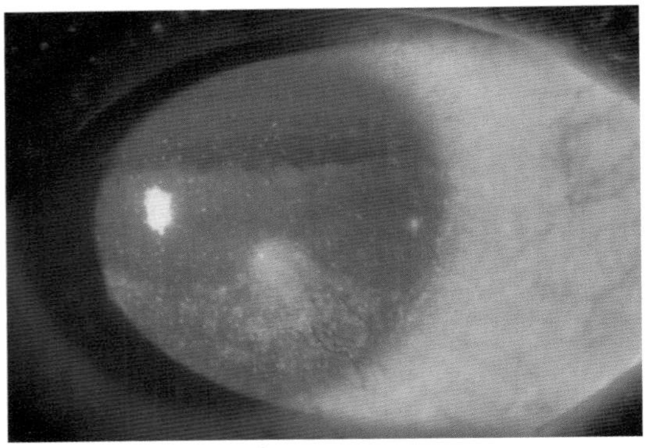

B

Figure 20-7 **A,** Inferior keratitis secondary to severe blepharitis. **B,** Fluorescein staining of keratitis *(same patient as in part A). (Courtesy of Robert W. Hered, MD.)*

炎性疾病

睑缘炎

睑缘炎是儿童慢性结膜炎的常见原因。其症状和体征与成人相似，包括眼部刺激、结膜充血、晨起睑结痂、睑缘红斑及睑板腺阻塞（图 20–6）。因泪膜不稳定，患儿出现间歇性视力模糊。严重时可引起下方角膜炎，导致上皮损伤、荧光素染色、角膜瘢痕及永久视力丧失（图 20–7，20–8）。

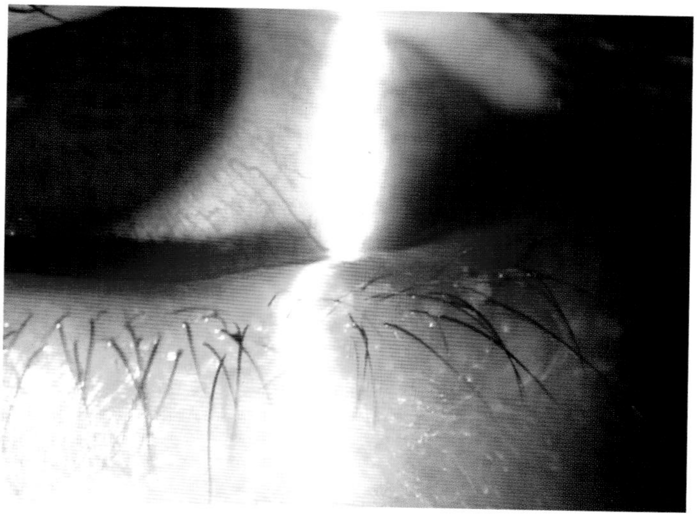

图 20–6　睑缘炎伴有睑板腺功能障碍、皮屑和毛细血管扩张。*（译者注：资料来源见前页原文。）*

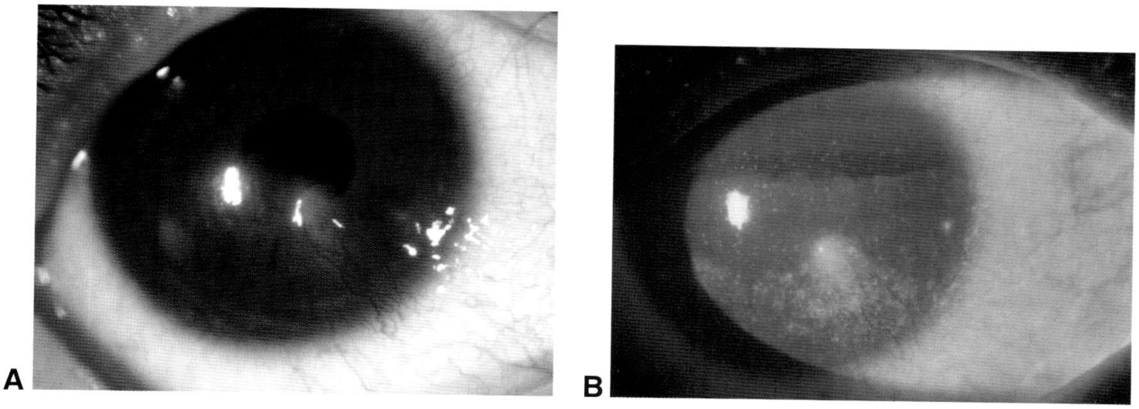

图 20–7　**A.** 继发于严重睑缘炎的下方角膜炎。**B.** 角膜炎的荧光素染色（B 图与 A 图为同一患者）。*（译者注：资料来源见前页原文。）*

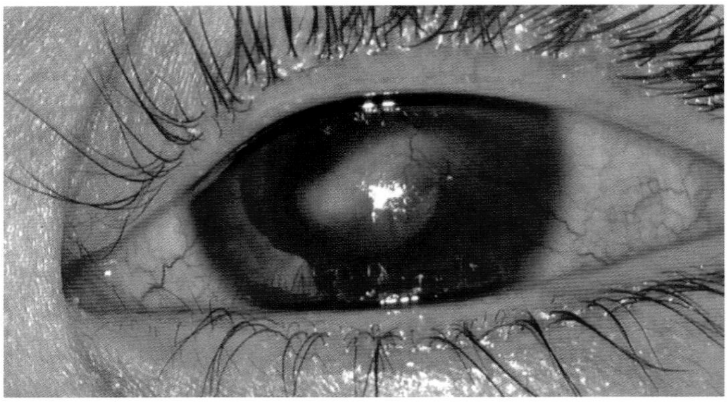

Figure 20-8 Severe corneal scarring secondary to keratitis caused by blepharitis. *(Courtesy of Erin Stahl, MD.)*

Recurrent chalazia in children may indicate underlying blepharitis. Acne rosacea in children may be manifested by chronic blepharitis and facial telangiectasias, papules, and pustules. *Demodex* (human mites that inhabit the hair follicles) may play a role in the pathogenesis of blepharitis and should be considered when blepharitis does not respond to treatment. Patients with demodicosis typically present with a waxy, sleevelike buildup at the base of eyelashes. Demodicosis may respond to dilute tea tree oil applied to lash bases.

Initial treatment of blepharitis includes warm compresses, eyelid scrubs with baby shampoo, and erythromycin or bacitracin ophthalmic ointment or azithromycin ophthalmic solution, 1%. Severe cases may benefit from oral antibiotic use. Tetracyclines (tetracycline, doxycycline, minocycline) and macrolides (erythromycin, azithromycin) may be helpful. Macrolides are most commonly used in children younger than 8 years to avoid the potential dental staining associated with use of tetracyclines. Judicious use of topical corticosteroids may be indicated in patients with corneal disease. Dietary supplementation with omega-3 fatty acids may benefit some patients.

Hammersmith KM. Blepharoconjunctivitis in children. *Curr Opin Ophthalmol.* 2015; 26(4):301–305.

Ocular Allergy

Allergies are thought to affect approximately 20% of the US and European populations; more than 50% of patients who seek treatment for allergies present with ocular symptoms. Allergic ocular disease is a common problem in children and is often associated with asthma, allergic rhinitis, and atopic dermatitis. Marked itching and bilateral conjunctival inflammation of a chronic, recurrent, and possibly seasonal nature are hallmarks of external ocular disease of allergic origin. Other signs and symptoms may be nonspecific and include tearing, stinging, burning, and photophobia.

Four specific types of ocular allergy are discussed in this section: seasonal and perennial allergic conjunctivitis, vernal keratoconjunctivitis (VKC), and atopic keratoconjunctivitis (AKC). All have some element of a type I hypersensitivity reaction caused by the interaction between an allergen and specific immunoglobulin E antibodies on the surface of mast cells in the conjunctiva. This interaction initiates a cascade of biochemical events involved in mediation of the allergic response. Among the mediators released is histamine, which causes much of the itching, vasodilation, and edema that are characteristic of the ocular allergic response.

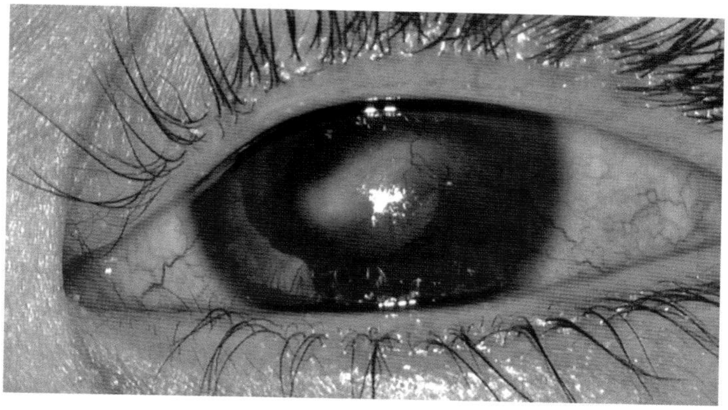

图 20–8　由睑缘炎引起的角膜炎继发严重的角膜瘢痕。*（译者注：资料来源见前页原文。）*

儿童复发性霰粒肿常伴有睑缘炎。儿童痤疮表现为慢性睑缘炎、面部毛细血管扩张、丘疹及脓疱。当睑缘炎治疗无效时，应考虑*蠕形螨*（毛囊的人类螨虫）可能是睑缘炎的致病原。蠕形螨病患者的睫毛根部常有蜡状及袖套状的堆积物。在睫毛根部涂抹稀释的茶树油对蠕形螨病有一定的疗效。

睑缘炎的初始治疗包括温敷、用婴儿洗发水擦洗眼睑以及局部使用的红霉素或杆菌肽眼用软膏及阿奇霉素眼药水，浓度为 1%。严重时口服抗生素，四环素类（四环素、多西环素、米诺环素）和大环内酯类（红霉素、阿奇霉素）。大环内酯类药物最常用于 8 岁以下儿童，以避免四环素类的牙齿染色。伴角膜病变时慎用皮质类固醇药物。膳食补充 ω–3 脂肪酸对一些患者有益。

Hammersmith KM. Blepharoconjunctivitis in children. *Curr Opin Ophthalmol.* 2015; 26(4):301–305.

眼部过敏

在美国及欧洲，大约有 20%的人患有过敏。而在寻求治疗过敏症状的患者中，有 50%以上的人存在眼部症状。过敏性眼病是儿童常见的疾病，常伴有哮喘、过敏性鼻炎及特应性皮炎。明显的瘙痒及伴有慢性、复发性、季节性的双眼结膜炎是外眼过敏性疾病的特征。其他体征和症状如流泪、刺痛、灼热及畏光等则是非特异性的。

本章节讨论了 4 种特殊类型的眼部过敏反应：季节性和常年性过敏性结膜炎、春季角结膜炎（VKC）及特应性角结膜炎（AKC）。以上 4 种过敏反应均存在 I 型超敏反应的共同特征，由结膜肥大细胞表面的过敏原与特异性免疫球蛋白 E 抗体相互作用，引发过敏反应调节的生化级联反应。该反应所释放的介质中的组胺引起瘙痒、血管扩张及水肿，这是眼部过敏反应的特征。

Seasonal and perennial allergic conjunctivitis

Seasonal allergic conjunctivitis is a common clinical entity that affects approximately 40 million people in the United States, including many children. It occurs in the spring and fall and is triggered by environmental contact with specific airborne allergens such as pollens from grasses, flowers, weeds, and trees. Patients typically present with red and watery eyes, boggy-appearing conjunctiva, and ocular itching (Fig 20-9). Blue-gray to purple discoloration of the lower eyelids, termed *allergic shiners*, can occur secondary to venous stasis from nasal congestion.

The signs, symptoms, and presentation of perennial allergic conjunctivitis are similar to those of seasonal allergic conjunctivitis. Perennial allergic conjunctivitis is a type I hypersensitivity reaction that occurs after contact with ubiquitous house hold allergens, such as dust mites and dander from domestic pets. This condition is diagnosed based on the history and clinical presentation.

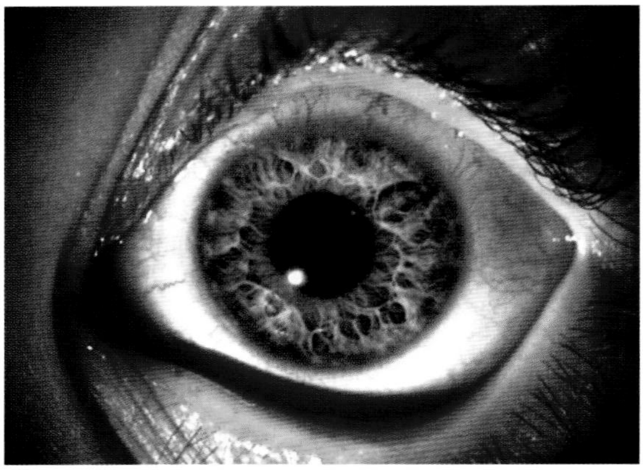

Figure 20-9 Seasonal allergic conjunctivitis. *(Courtesy of Albert W. Biglan, MD.)*

Treatment of all ocular allergy disorders is fundamentally similar to that of other allergy-related disorders. The most effective treatment is to avoid offending allergens or remove them from the patient's environment. Unfortunately, avoidance may not be possible and complete removal may not be adequate to alleviate the patient's symptoms. Medical treatment can be systemic or topical. Although oral antihistamines may be less effective at relieving specific ocular symptoms, they are often better tolerated in children, who may not accept eyedrops.

Topical medications include mast-cell stabilizers, H_1-receptor antagonists, antihistamines, vasoconstrictors, corticosteroids, or combinations of these drugs (Table 20-2). H_1-receptor antagonists can be used on an as-needed basis, but mast-cell stabilizers must be used for a few days before an effect is seen. In addition, mast-cell stabilizers should be used continuously through the allergy season to maximize their effectiveness. Nonsteroidal anti-inflammatory drops should be used with caution; cases of corneal perforation, though rare, have been reported. Topical corticosteroid drops used in pulsed doses can effectively reduce severe allergic ocular symptoms, but patients must be closely monitored for adverse effects, including glaucoma and cataracts.

季节性和常年性过敏性结膜炎

季节性过敏性结膜炎是一种常见的临床疾病，美国约有 4,000 万人罹患此病，其中就包括了许多儿童。该病发生在春、秋季节，由接触特定的空气过敏原引起，如牧场、花、杂草及树木的花粉。患者出现红眼及流泪，结膜水肿及眼部瘙痒典型症状（图 20–9）。由于鼻充血引起的静脉瘀滞，导致下眼睑呈蓝灰色至紫色，称为*过敏性眼圈*。

常年性过敏性结膜炎的体征、症状和临床表现与季节性过敏性结膜炎相似，属于 I 型超敏反应，当患者接触到家中无所不在的过敏原后发生，如尘螨及家养宠物身上的毛皮垢屑。根据患者病史和临床表现即可诊断。

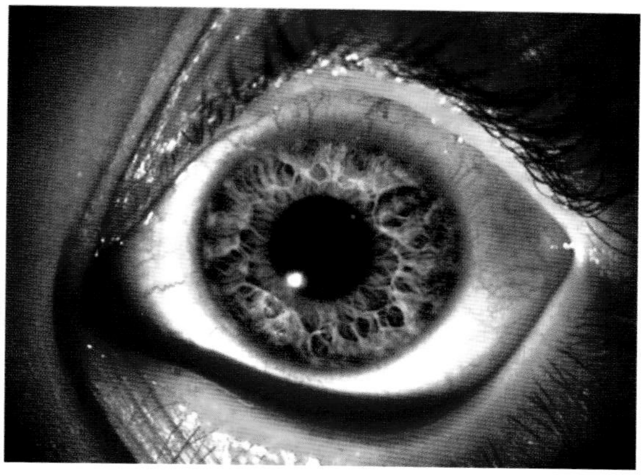

图 20–9　季节性过敏性结膜炎。*（译者注：资料来源见前页原文。）*

所有的眼部过敏性疾病的治疗，与其他过敏性疾病类似。其中，最为有效的治疗方法是脱离过敏原或移除周围环境中的致敏物。但完全避免致敏物不大可能，且完全移除致敏物也不能缓解患者的症状。药物治疗包括全身性或局部性治疗。虽然口服抗组胺药在缓解特定眼部症状方面效果较差，但容易被患儿接受，滴眼药常不被儿童接受。

局部药物包括肥大细胞稳定剂、H_1 受体拮抗剂、抗组胺药、血管收缩剂、皮质类固醇或联合用药（表 20–2）。H_1 受体拮抗剂的使用可视需要而定，而肥大细胞稳定剂须使用数天后方能见效。此外，肥大细胞稳定剂应在过敏季节持续使用，以最大限度地提高药物有效性。非甾体类抗炎药应谨慎使用，因偶有报道角膜穿孔。局部皮质类固醇滴眼液的冲击剂量可有效地减轻眼部重度过敏症状，但需严格监测青光眼和白内障等副作用。

Table 20-2 Topical Drops for Treatment of Allergic Ocular Disorders

Over-the-counter antihistamines/vasoconstrictors
Naphazoline/antazoline (Vasocon-A)
Naphazoline/pheniramine (Naphcon-A, Opcon-A, Visine-A)
Mast-cell stabilizers
Cromolyn sodium 2% (Opticrom)
Cromolyn sodium 4% (Crolom)
Lodoxamide tromethamine 0.1% (Alomide)
Nedocromil sodium 2% (Alocril)
Pemirolast potassium 0.1% (Alamast)
H_1-receptor antagonist
Cetirizine 0.24% (Zerviate)
Emedastine difumarate 0.05% (Emadine)
Drops with both mast-cell stabilizer and H_1-antagonist
Alcaftadine 0.25% (Lastacaft)
Azelastine hydrochloride 0.05% (Optivar)
Bepotastine besilate 1.5% (Bepreve)
Epinastine hydrochloride 0.05% (Elestat) [also H_2 blocker]
Ketotifen fumarate 0.025% (Alaway, Zaditor)
Olopatadine hydrochloride 0.1% (Patanol)
Olopatadine hydrochloride 0.2% (Pataday)
Olopatadine hydrochloride 0.7% (Pazeo)
Corticosteroids
Fluorometholone 0.1% (FML, Fluor-Op)
Fluorometholone 0.25% (FML Forte)
Loteprednol etabonate 0.2% (Alrex)
Loteprednol etabonate 0.5% (Lotemax)
Medrysone 1% (HMS)
Prednisolone acetate 0.12% (Pred Mild)
Prednisolone acetate 1% (Pred Forte, Econopred Plus)
Rimexolone 1% (Vexol)
Nonsteroidal anti-inflammatory drug
Ketorolac tromethamine 0.5% (Acular)
Anti-inflammatory drug
Cyclosporine 0.05% (Restasis)

Vernal keratoconjunctivitis

Vernal keratoconjunctivitis (VKC) is caused by type I and type IV hypersensitivity reactions. This condition most commonly affects males in the first 2 decades of life and, like seasonal allergic conjunctivitis, usually occurs in the spring and fall. There are 2 forms of VKC: palpebral and limbal (or bulbar). Both types manifest with severe itching. The limbal form is more common in patients of African or Asian descent and is more prevalent in warm, subtropical climates.

Clinically, the palpebral form of VKC preferentially affects the tarsal conjunctiva of the upper eyelid. In the early stages, the eye may be diffusely injected, with little discharge. There may be no progression beyond this stage. However, papillae may multiply, covering the tarsal area with a mosaic of flat papules (Fig 20-10). A thick, ropy, whitish discharge may be present.

The limbal form of VKC manifests early with thickening and opacification of the conjunctiva at the limbus, usually most marked at the upper margin of the cornea. The discrete limbal nodules that appear are gray, jelly-like, elevated lumps with vascular cores. A whitish center filled with eosinophils and epithelioid cells may appear in the raised lesion. This complex is called a Horner-Trantas dot. Limbal nodules may increase in number and become confluent (Fig 20-11). They persist as long as the seasonal exacerbation of the disease lasts.

表20-2　治疗过敏性眼部疾病的局部滴眼液

非处方药物	**抗组胺药/血管收缩剂**
萘甲唑啉/安他唑啉(Vasocon - A)	
萘甲唑啉/非尼拉敏(Naphcon - A, Opcon - A, Visine - A)	
肥大细胞稳定剂	
2%色甘酸钠（Opticrom）	
4%色甘酸钠 (Crolom)	
0.1%洛度沙胺氨丁三醇 (Alomide)	
2%尼多考米钠 (Alocril)	
0.1% 吡嘧司特钾 (Alamast)	
H_1受体拮抗剂	
0.24%西替利嗪 (Zerviate)	
0.05%二富马酸依美斯汀 (Emadine)	
肥大细胞稳定剂联合H_1受体拮抗剂类药物	
0.25%阿卡他定 (Lastacaft)	
0.05% 盐酸氮卓斯汀(Optivar)	
1.5% 苯磺酸贝他斯汀(Bepreve)	
0.05% 盐酸依匹斯汀(Elestat) [亦属于H_2阻滞剂]	
0.025% 富马酸酮替芬(Alaway, Zaditor)	
0.1%盐酸奥洛他定(Patanol)	
0.2%盐酸奥洛他定 (Pataday)	
0.7% 盐酸奥洛他定(Pazeo)	
皮质类固醇激素	
0.1%氟米龙 (FML, Fluor - Op)	
0.25%氟米龙 (FML Forte)	
0.2% 氯替泼诺(Alrex)	
0.5% 氯替泼诺(Lotemax)	
1%甲羟松 (HMS)	
0.12% 醋酸泼尼松龙(Pred Mild)	
1%醋酸泼尼松龙 (Pred Forte, Econopred Plus)	
1% 利美索龙(Vexol)	
非甾体抗炎药	
0.5% 酮咯酸氨丁三醇(Acular)	
抗炎药	
0.05% 环孢菌素(Restasis)	

春季角结膜炎

春季角结膜炎（VKC）是由Ⅰ型和Ⅳ型超敏反应引起的。该病常见于 20 岁以下男性，与季节性过敏性结膜炎一样，常在春季和秋季发病。春季角结膜炎（VKC）有 2 种临床表现类型：眼睑型和角膜缘型（球结膜型）。2 型都表现为严重的瘙痒症状。角膜缘型在非洲裔或亚裔中更常见，且多见于温暖的亚热带气候。

临床上，眼睑型春季角结膜炎（VKC）较易影响到上睑板结膜。早期眼部弥漫充血，不伴有分泌物，病情也不加重而乳头继续增多，在睑板结膜上形成扁平丘疹状的马赛克（图 20-10）。有时可见到浓厚丝状的白色分泌物。

角膜缘型春季角结膜炎（VKC）的早期表现为角膜缘结膜增厚及混浊，常在角膜上缘最为明显。可有散在的角膜缘结节，呈灰色、果冻状、隆起的团块，伴血管性核，隆起的病灶中可见充满嗜酸性粒细胞和上皮样细胞的白色中心，被称为 Horner-Trantas 结节。角膜缘结节的数量增加并融合（图 20-11）。只要引起春季角结膜炎（VKC）的季节性因素存在，病程一直持续。

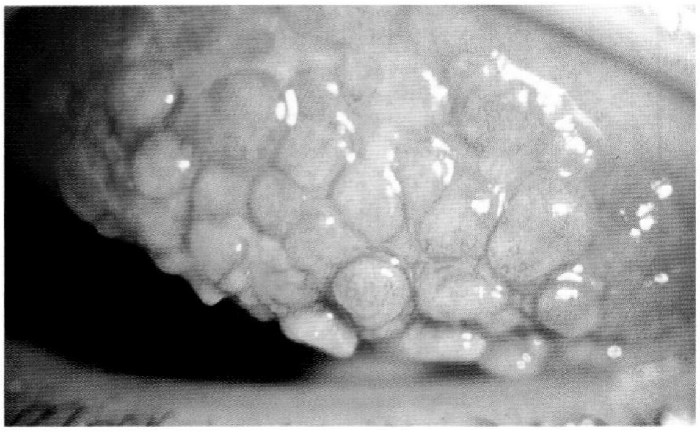

Figure 20-10 Palpebral vernal keratoconjunctivitis (VKC), upper eyelid. *(Courtesy of Ken K. Nischal, MD.)*

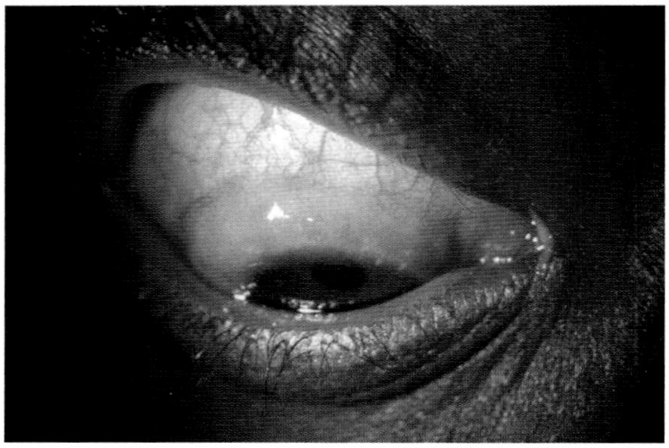

Figure 20-11 Limbal VKC with Horner-Trantas dots. *(Courtesy of Stephen P. Christiansen, MD.)*

The cornea may become involved, with punctate epithelial erosions, especially superiorly. Corneal involvement may progress to a large, confluent epithelial defect, typically in the upper half of the cornea, called a shield ulcer. The ulcer is sterile and clinically resembles an ovoid corneal abrasion (Fig 20-12).

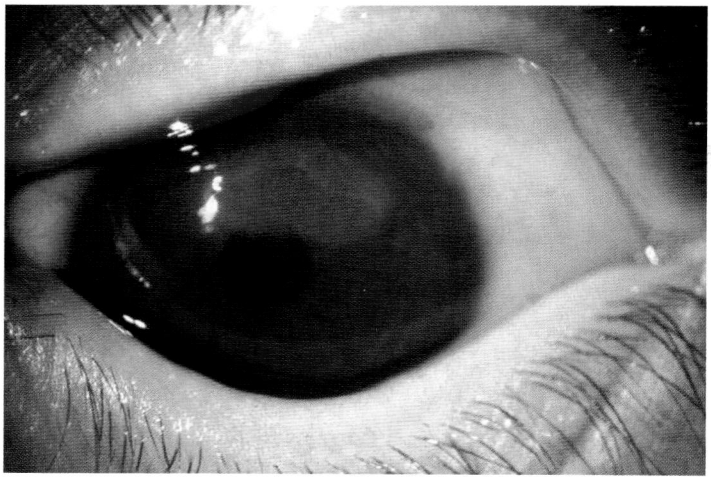

Figure 20-12 VKC with shield ulcer. *(Courtesy of Stephen P. Christiansen, MD.)*

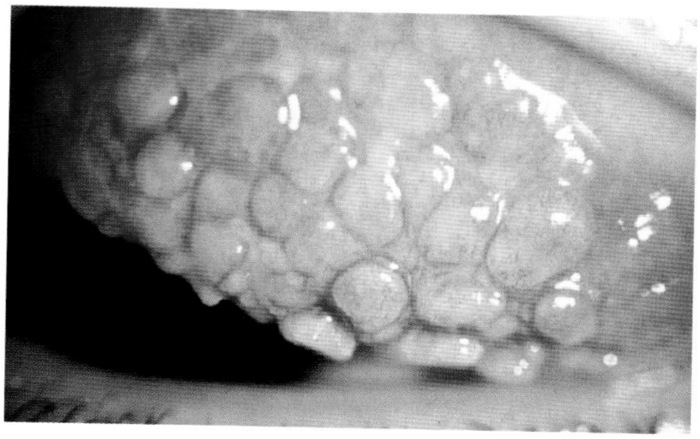

图 20-10 眼睑型春季角结膜炎（VKC），上眼睑。*（译者注：资料来源见前页原文。）*

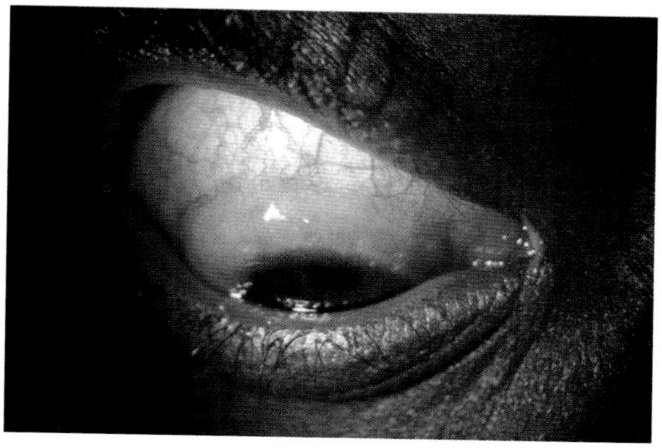

图 20-11 角膜缘型春季角结膜炎（VKC）的 Horner-Trantas 结节。*（译者注：资料来源见前页原文。）*

患者角膜可能受累，出现点状上皮糜烂，多见于上方角膜。角膜的点状上皮糜烂可发展为大的融合性上皮缺损，缺损常位于角膜的上半部分，称为盾形溃疡。溃疡是无菌的，类似于卵圆形角膜擦伤（图 20-12）。

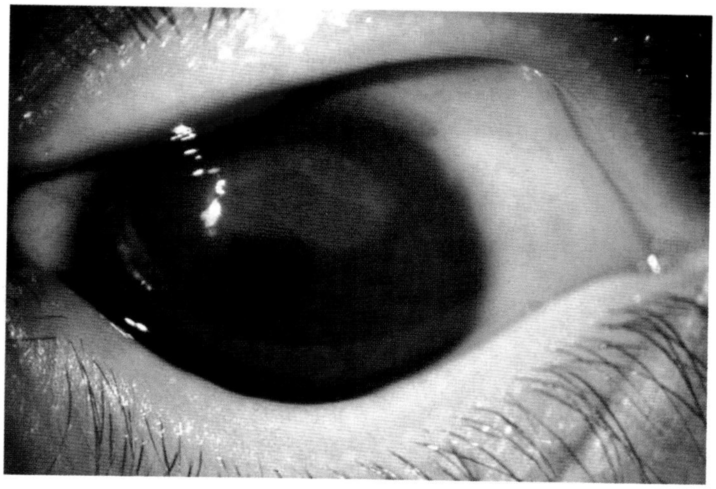

图 20-12 春季角结膜炎（VKC）的盾形溃疡。*（译者注：资料来源见前页原文。）*

Treatment of VKC is usually less effective than that of seasonal allergic conjunctivitis. Eyedrops combining a mast-cell stabilizer and an H1-receptor antagonist may be used initially. In addition, treatment of VKC often requires topical steroids or topical cyclosporine. Supratarsal injection of corticosteroids may be used in patients with refractory palpebral VKC.

Atopic keratoconjunctivitis

Atopic keratoconjunctivitis is a nonseasonal disorder that occurs in patients with atopic disease. It is relatively rare in children. See BCSC Section 8, *External Disease and Cornea*, for further discussion.

Ligneous Conjunctivitis

Ligneous conjunctivitis is a rare bilateral chronic disorder characterized by firm ("woody"), yellowish, fibrinous pseudomembranes on the palpebral conjunctiva. It is thought to be secondary to severe deficiency in type I plasminogen and can affect persons of all ages. No single treatment is consistently effective. Surgical removal, amniotic membrane transplantation, fresh frozen plasma, and heparin have been used.

Other Conjunctival and Subconjunctival Disorders

Papillomas

Papillomas are benign epithelial proliferations that usually appear as sessile masses at the limbus or as pedunculated lesions of the caruncle, fornix, or palpebral conjunctiva. They may be transparent, pale yellow, or salmon colored and are sometimes speckled with red dots. Papillomas in children usually result from viral infection. They often resolve spontaneously. Oral cimetidine can induce papilloma regression. Carbon dioxide laser or surgical incision is indicated when symptoms are severe or if new lesions continue to appear. Seeding may follow excision, leading to recurrence.

Conjunctival Epithelial Inclusion Cysts

Conjunctival inclusion cysts are clear, fluid-filled cysts on the conjunctiva. These cysts are often noted in patients who had ocular surgery or trauma. Excision is indicated if the cyst causes irritation.

Conjunctival Nevi

Conjunctival nevi are relatively common in childhood. Nevocellular nevi of the conjunctiva consist of nests or more diffuse infiltrations of benign melanocytes. Histologically, most of these nevi are compound (nevus cells found in both epithelium and substantia propria); others are junctional (nevus cells confined to the interface between epithelium and substantia propria). The lesions are occasionally noted at birth. More commonly, they develop during later childhood or adolescence. The lesions may be flat or elevated. Nevi are typically brown, but approximately one-third are nonpigmented and have a pinkish appearance (Fig 20-13). Removal may be indicated if significant growth occurs, although transformation to malignant melanoma is extremely rare in childhood.

春季角结膜炎（VKC）的治疗效果不如季节性过敏性结膜炎。一开始即可使用肥大细胞稳定剂和 H_1 受体拮抗剂的复合滴眼液进行治疗。此外，春季角结膜炎（VKC）的治疗还需局部使用类固醇或环孢菌素。难治性眼睑型春季角结膜炎（VKC）患者可睑板上注射皮质类固醇。

特应性角结膜炎

特应性角结膜炎是非季节性疾病，发生在特应性疾病患者中。罕见于儿童中。有关该病进一步的讨论，请参阅 BCSC 第 8 册《*外眼疾病与角膜*》。

木样结膜炎

木样结膜炎是一种罕见的双眼慢性疾病，其特征为睑结膜上的坚硬木状物质，黄色，伴有纤维蛋白假膜，由于Ⅰ型纤溶酶原严重缺乏所致，各年龄段均可发病。手术切除、羊膜移植、应用新鲜冷冻血浆和肝素等治疗方式均有报道，尚无有效的治疗方法。

结膜及结膜下其他疾病

乳头状瘤

乳头状瘤是一种良性上皮增生，常表现为角膜缘无蒂包块或在泪阜、结膜穹隆部及睑结膜的有蒂病灶。乳头状瘤呈透明、浅黄色或三文鱼肉色，瘤体上可伴红色斑点。儿童乳头状瘤常由病毒感染所致。口服西咪替丁可使乳头状瘤消退。当症状严重或继续出现新的病变时，可使用二氧化碳激光治疗或手术切除。瘤体切除时可能会播散，导致复发。

结膜上皮包涵体囊肿

结膜包涵体囊肿是结膜上透明、充满液体的结膜囊肿。常发生于眼科手术或外伤患者。如果囊肿引起眼部刺激症状，则手术切除。

结膜色素痣

结膜色素痣儿童常见，是良性黑色素细胞的聚集或弥散性浸润。组织学上，多数痣呈复合性（上皮层和固有层都含有色素痣细胞），其余则是交界性的（色素痣细胞局限于上皮层和固有层之间的界面）。色素痣偶见于新生儿，但更多的色素痣是在儿童后期或青少年时期形成。色素痣形状呈扁平的或稍隆起，常为棕色，但大约 1/3 的色素痣并无色素呈粉红色（图 20-13）。虽然儿童色素痣罕见恶化，但明显生长的色素痣仍需手术切除。

Figure 20-13 Pigmented nevus of the bulbar conjunctiva, right eye.

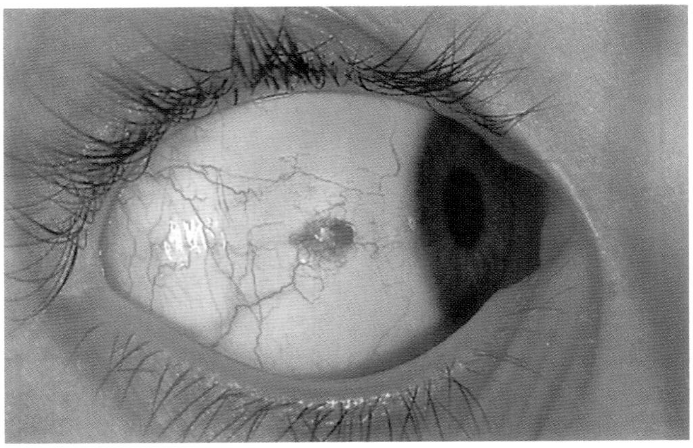

Ocular Melanocytosis

Ocular melanocytosis (*melanosis oculi*) is a congenital focal proliferation of subepithelial melanocytes characterized by unilateral patchy but extensive slate-gray or bluish discoloration of the episclera (Fig 20-14). Intraocular pigmentation is also increased, which is associated with a higher incidence of glaucoma and risk of malignant melanoma. Some patients, particularly persons of Asian ancestry, may have associated involvement of eyelid and adjacent skin with dermal hyperpigmentation that produces brown, bluish, or black discoloration without thickening (*oculodermal melanocytosis, nevus of Ota*). Small patches of slate-gray scleral pigmentation, typically bilateral and without clinical significance, are common in black and Asian children. Melanosis of skin and sclera is occasionally associated with Sturge-Weber syndrome and Klippel-Trénaunay-Weber syndrome.

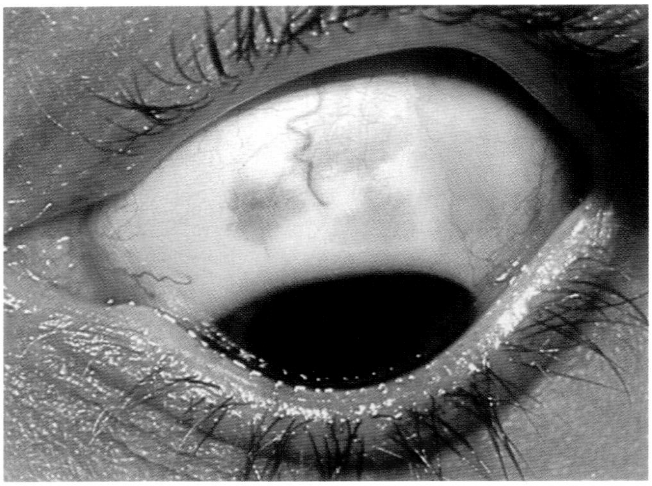

Figure 20-14 Ocular melanocytosis.

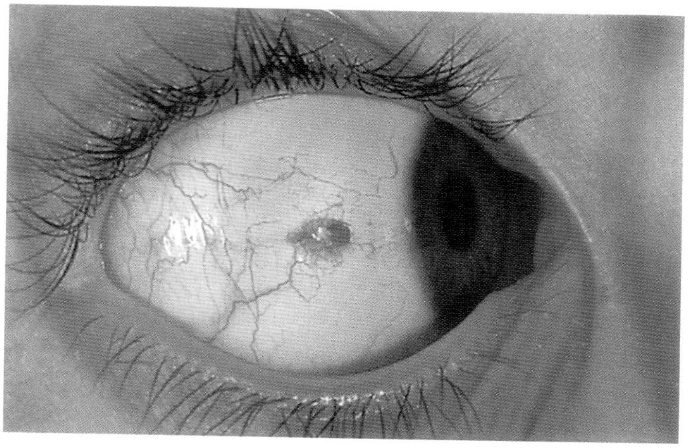

图 20–13　右眼球结膜色素痣。

眼黑素细胞增多症

眼黑素细胞增多症（*眼球黑变病*）是一种先天性局灶性上皮下黑色素细胞增生，单眼表层巩膜呈片状且弥漫的灰白色或蓝色（图 20–14）。同时，眼内色素也增加，这与青光眼的高发病率、恶性黑色素瘤的发生风险相关。一些患者，特别是亚洲血统的患者，可能伴有眼睑和邻近皮肤的色素沉着过度，产生褐色、蓝色或黑色变，但其并没有组织增厚（*眼皮肤黑素细胞增多症，Ota 痣*）。双眼的小片状的灰色巩膜色素沉着在黑人和亚洲儿童中很常见，但无临床意义。皮肤和巩膜的黑变病偶伴发 Sturge–Weber 综合征和 Klippel–*Trénaunay*–Weber 综合征。

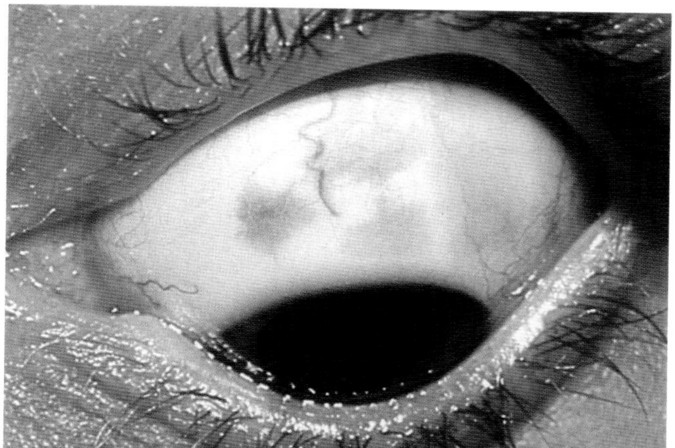

图 20–14　眼黑素细胞增多症。

Stevens-Johnson Syndrome and Toxic Epidermal Necrolysis

Stevens-Johnson syndrome (SJS) and toxic epidermal necrolysis (TEN) are rare hypersensitivity reactions that affect skin and mucous membranes. The most common etiologies of SJS and TEN in children are medications (usually anticonvulsants and sulfonamides) and infections (usually *Mycoplasma* species or herpes simplex virus). The pathogenesis of SJS and TEN is discussed in BCSC Section 8, *External Disease and Cornea.*

Systemic manifestations range from mild to severe. A prodrome of fever, malaise, and upper respiratory tract infection is followed by bullous mucosal and skin lesions. These lesions rupture, ulcerate, and become covered by gray-white membranes and a hemorrhagic crust.

Ocular involvement, which occurs in as many as 50% of patients, varies from mild mucopurulent conjunctivitis to severe perforating corneal ulcers. Ocular involvement in SJS and TEN begins with edema, erythema, and crusting of the eyelids. The palpebral conjunctiva becomes hyperemic, and distinct vesicles or bullae may occur. In many instances, epithelial defects or ulcers involving the tarsus and fornices develop. In severe cases, membranous or pseudomembranous conjunctivitis may occur (Fig 20-15) and lead to symblepharon formation. Superinfection, most commonly with *Staphylococcus* species, may develop.

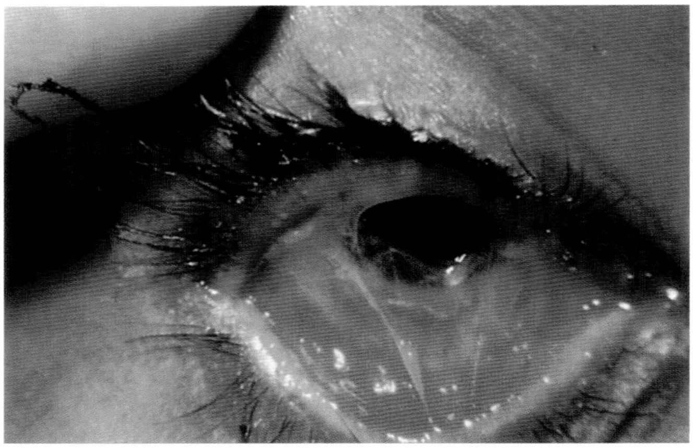

Figure 20-15 Stevens-Johnson syndrome. Early, severe involvement of the conjunctiva, right eye.

Late ocular complications, possibly accompanied by a decrease in vision, occur in approximately 27% of pediatric patients. These complications include anomalies of eyelid position (ectropion and entropion), dry eye disease, trichiasis, chronic conjunctivitis, corneal defects, corneal vascularization, and symblepharon formation.

SJS and TEN are considered a disease continuum, distinguished by severity. The current nomenclature is based on the amount of skin involvement, with SJS being of lesser severity; TEN, greater severity; and SJS-TEN in between these. They are diagnosed based on clinical presentation and skin biopsy results. Initial management includes treatment of any underlying infection and discontinuation of any inciting drug. Systemic therapy with corticosteroids or intravenous immunoglobulin is controversial. The mortality rate for these conditions is much lower in children than in adults: 0% in SJS, 4% in SJS-TEN, and 16% in TEN. A full discussion of systemic treatment is beyond the scope of this book. A dermatologist and a specialist in pediatric infectious diseases should be consulted.

Stevens-Johnson 综合征与毒性表皮坏死松解症

Stevens-Johnson 综合征（SJS）与毒性表皮坏死松解症（TEN）是累及皮肤与黏膜的罕见过敏反应。儿童发病最常见的病因是药物（抗惊厥药和磺胺类药物）和感染（*支原体*类或单纯疱疹病毒）。Stevens-Johnscn 综合征（SJS）和毒性表皮坏死松解症（TEN）的发病机制详见 BCSC 第 8 册《*外眼疾病与角膜*》。

全身表现轻重不等。其前驱症状为发烧、不适和上呼吸道感染，继而出现、黏膜和皮肤水疱样病灶。这些病变破裂、形成溃疡，并被覆灰白色膜和血痂。

50% 的患者眼部受累，表现从轻度的黏液脓性结膜炎到严重的穿孔性角膜溃疡。Stevens-Johnscn 综合征（SJS）和毒性表皮坏死松解症（TEN）的眼部病变始于水肿、红斑和眼睑结痂。睑结膜充血，可出现明显的小泡或大泡。在许多情况下，形成累及睑板和结膜穹窿部的上皮缺损或溃疡。严重时，可发生膜性或假膜性结膜炎（图 20-15），导致睑球粘连。可发生双重感染，最常见的是*葡萄球菌*。

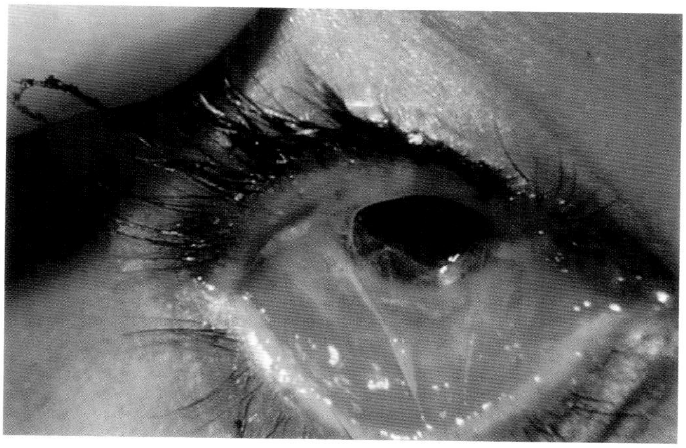

图 20-15 Stevens-Johnson 综合征。早期，严重累及结膜，右眼。

约 27% 的患儿发生晚期眼部并发症，伴视力下降。并发症包括眼睑位置异常（睑外翻和睑内翻）、干眼症、倒睫、慢性结膜炎、角膜上皮缺损、角膜新生血管和睑球粘连。

Stevens-Johnscn 综合征（SJS）和毒性表皮坏死松解症（TEN）是一个疾病严重程度的接续。目前的命名是基于皮肤受累的程度，Stevens-Johnscn 综合征（SJS）的严重程度较轻，毒性表皮坏死松解症（TEN）的程度更严重，而 Stevens-Johnscn 综合征（SJS）和毒性表皮坏死松解症（TEN）的严重程度介于两者之间。根据临床表现和皮肤活检结果对这 3 个阶段进行诊断。早期方法包括所有潜在的感染和停用刺激性药物。使用皮质激素或静脉注射免疫球蛋白进行全身治疗目前尚有争议。该病的儿童死亡率成人低得多：其中 Stevens-Johnscn 综合征（SJS）期死亡率为 0%，Stevens-Johnscn 综合征（SJS）和毒性表皮坏死松解症（TEN）期死亡率为 4%，TEN 期死亡率为 16%。关于系统治疗的讨论超出了本书的范围，应请皮肤科医生和儿科传染病专家会诊。

Early intervention is important for preventing the late ocular complications of SJS, SJS-TEN, and TEN. Ocular lubrication with artificial tears and ointments (preferably preservative-free) should be applied frequently. Associated microbial infections should be treated. The fornices may be swept to lyse adhesions, although some ophthalmologists believe that doing so may stimulate inflammation and cause further scarring. In severe cases, a symblepharon ring may be useful in cooperative patients. In patients with significant ocular disease, a corneal ban dage device using amniotic membrane or amniotic membrane grafting should be considered early to decrease the risk of late ocular complications.

Hsu DY, Brieva J, Silverberg NB, Paller AS, Silverberg JI. Pediatric Stevens-Johnson syndrome and toxic epidermal necrolysis in the United States. *J Am Acad Dermatol.* 2017;76(5): 811–817.

Jain R, Sharma N, Basu S, et al. Stevens-Johnson syndrome: the role of an ophthalmologist. *Surv Ophthalmol.* 2016;61(4):369–399.

早期干预对预防 Stevens–Johnscn 综合征（SJS）、Stevens–Johnscn 综合征（SJS）和毒性表皮坏死松解症（TEN）和毒性表皮坏死松解症（TEN）的晚期眼部并发症非常重要。应经常使用人工泪液和眼膏（最好不含防腐剂）进行眼部润滑。应治疗相关的细菌感染。需清理穹窿结膜以解除粘连，但一些眼科医生认为这可能会刺激炎症反应，造成疤痕的加重。在严重的病例中，睑球粘连环可能对配合较好的病人有效。对于有严重眼部疾病的患者，应尽早考虑使用羊膜制的角膜绷带镜或羊膜移植术，以降低晚期眼部并发症的风险。

Hsu DY, Brieva J, Silverberg NB, Paller AS, Silverberg JI. Pediatric Stevens-Johnson syndrome and toxic epidermal necrolysis in the United States. *J Am Acad Dermatol.* 2017;76(5): 811–817.

Jain R, Sharma N, Basu S, et al. Stevens-Johnson syndrome: the role of an ophthalmologist. *Surv Ophthalmol.* 2016;61(4):369–399.

（翻译 王昞 陈琳 何元浩 // 审校 刘陇黔 石一宁 蒋宁 // 章节审校 石广礼）

CHAPTER 21

Disorders of the Anterior Segment

Disorders of the anterior segment include a wide spectrum of conditions involving the cornea, iris, anterior chamber angle, and lens. Pediatric glaucoma and lens disorders are discussed in Chapters 22 and 23, respectively. Anatomy of the anterior segment and its development are discussed in BCSC Section 2, *Fundamentals and Principles of Ophthalmology*. See also Section 8, *External Disease and Cornea*, for detailed discussion of some of the disorders covered in this chapter.

Abnormalities of Corneal Size or Shape

Megalocornea

Primary megalocornea is characterized by bilateral congenitally enlarged corneas, with an increased horizontal corneal diameter and a deep anterior chamber (Fig 21-1); it is often associated with iris transillumination. On biometry, the ratio of anterior chamber depth to total axial length is typically 0.19 or greater, a feature that is useful for distinguishing this anomaly from buphthalmos. Late changes include corneal mosaic degeneration (shagreen), arcus juvenilis, presenile cataracts, and glaucoma. The phenotype is often caused by X-linked recessive mutation in *CHRDL1*. *Secondary megalocornea* is typically a result of increased intraocular pressure.

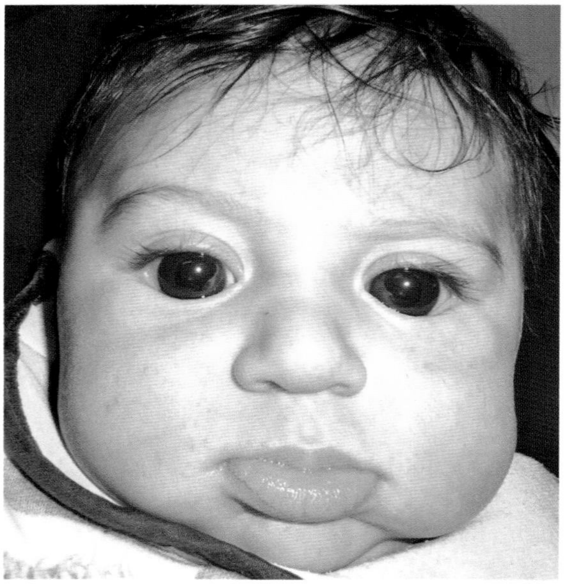

Figure 21-1 Megalocornea. The depth of the anterior chamber in this male infant was more than 19% of total axial length, a feature that is useful for distinguishing the anomaly from buphthalmos. *(Courtesy of Arif O. Khan, MD.)*

第 21 章

眼前节疾病

眼前节的疾病包括累及角膜、虹膜、前房角以及晶状体的相关疾病。儿童青光眼和晶状体的疾病分别在第 22 章、第 23 章中讨论。关于眼前节的解剖与发育已在 BCSC 第 2 册《*眼科学基础与原理*》中讨论。关于本章所涉及的一些疾病的详细讨论，见第 8 册《*外眼疾病与角膜*》。

角膜大小或形态异常

大角膜

*原发性大角膜*的特征是双眼先天性角膜增大，水平角膜直径增大及前房加深 (图 21–1)。在生物统计学方面，前房深度占眼轴长度的比例一般为 0.19 或更大，这个特征能用于区别大角膜与水眼。晚期病变包括角膜镶嵌样变性（shagreen）、青年环、早发性白内障及青光眼。该表型通常由 *CHRDL1* 中的 X - 连锁隐性突变引起。*继发性大角膜*一般是由于高眼内压引起的。

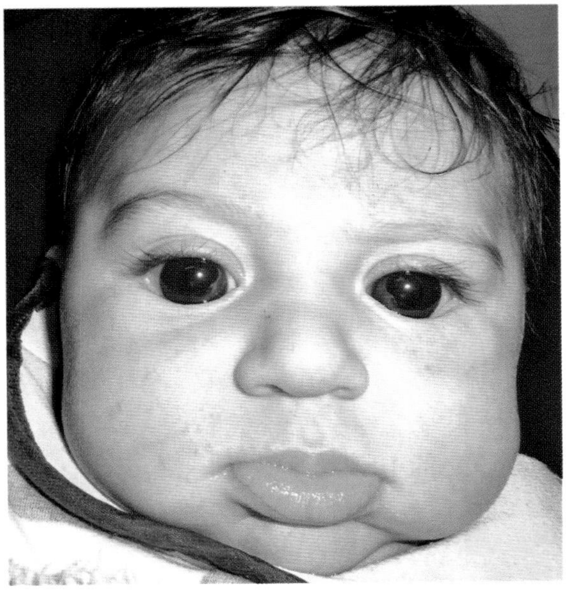

图 21–1 大角膜。这个男婴的前房深度占了整个眼轴长度的 19%，这个特征有助于与牛眼相区别。*（译者注：资料来源见前页原文。）*

Davidson AE, Cheong SS, Hysi PG, et al. Association of *CHRDL1* mutations and variants with X-linked megalocornea, Neuhäuser syndrome and central corneal thickness. *PLoS One*. 2014; 9(8):e104163.

Microcornea

Microcornea is characterized by a horizontal corneal diameter of 9 mm or less at birth and less than 10 mm after 2 years of age (Fig 21-2). It is often a component of ocular malformations such as microphthalmia and persistent fetal vasculature and of syndromes such as oculodentodigital, Nance-Horan, and Lenz syndromes.

Keratoglobus

Keratoglobus is characterized by a steep corneal curvature, peripheral corneal thinning, and a very deep anterior chamber. The phenotype can be due to brittle cornea syndrome, which is the result of biallelic mutations in *ZNF469* or *PRDM5*. Spontaneous breaks in Descemet membrane may produce acute corneal edema. Because the cornea can be ruptured by minor blunt trauma, wearing protective spectacles full time is appropriate.

Keratoconus

Keratoconus is characterized by central or paracentral corneal bulging and progressive thinning. It may present and progress during adolescence and is often familial. Keratoconus is more common in Down syndrome, atopic diseases, Leber congenital amaurosis, and chronic eye rubbing. Iron lines (Fleischer rings), stress lines (Vogt striae), and apical scarring are often noted. Tears in Descemet membrane can occur and cause acute corneal edema (hydrops).

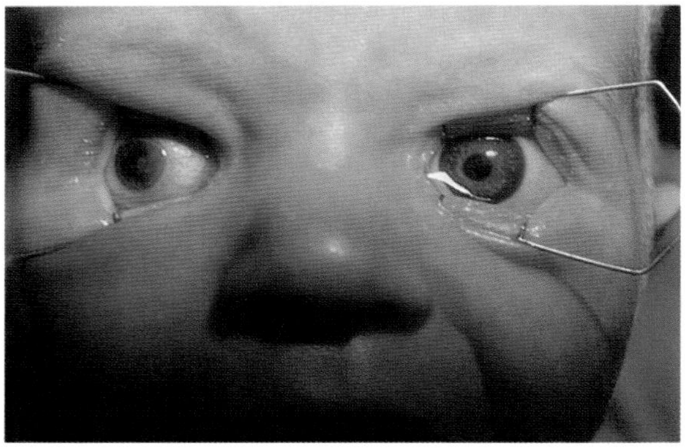

Figure 21-2 Microcornea, right eye.

Abnormalities of Peripheral Corneal Transparency

Posterior Embryotoxon

Posterior embryotoxon (prominent Schwalbe line) represents a thickening and anterior displacement of the Schwalbe line, causing the anomaly to be seen as an irregular white line just concentric with and anterior to the limbus (Fig 21-3). It is a common isolated finding (occurring in 15% of healthy patients) but is often seen in Axenfeld-Rieger syndrome, arteriohepatic dysplasia (Alagille syndrome), and velocardiofacial syndrome (22q11 deletion syndrome).

Davidson AE, Cheong SS, Hysi PG, et al. Association of *CHRDL1* mutations and variants with X-linked megalocornea, Neuhäuser syndrome and central corneal thickness. *PLoS One*. 2014; 9(8):e104163.

小角膜

*小角膜*的特征是水平角膜直径在出生时≤ 9mm 或 2 岁时< 10mm (图 21–2)。它是眼部畸形的一部分，如小眼球与持续性胚胎血管症以及综合征，如眼齿指发育不良综合征、Nance–Horan 综合征和 Lenz 综合征。

球形角膜

*球形角膜*的特征是角膜曲率变陡、周边角膜变薄及前房加深。该表型是由脆性角膜综合征引起，这是双等位基因 *ZNF469* 或 *PRDM5* 突变的结果。Descemet 膜（后弹力层）的自发破裂可导致急性角膜水肿，因为轻微的钝挫伤会导致角膜破裂，所以需全天候戴防护眼镜。

圆锥角膜

*圆锥角膜*的特征是中央或旁中央角膜膨出和逐渐变薄，在青春期出现并发展，通常是家族性的。圆锥角膜常见于 Down 综合征、特应性疾病、Leber 先天性黑矇和长期揉眼。常见铁线（Fleischer 环）、张力线（Vogt 条纹）以及圆锥顶部瘢痕。Descemet 膜（后弹力层）破裂可导致急性角膜水肿。

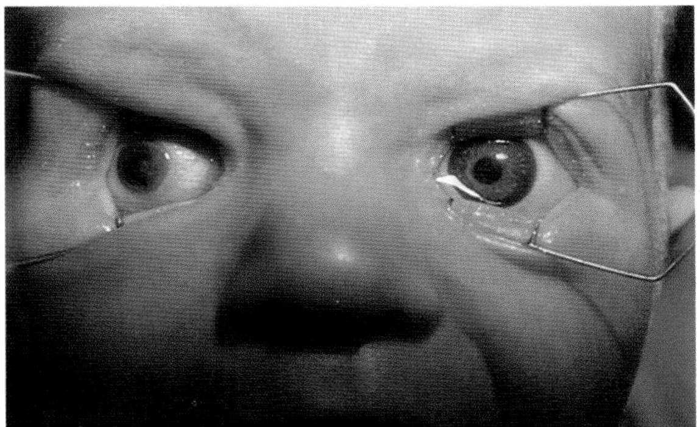

图 21–2　小角膜，右眼。

周边角膜透明度异常

角膜后胚胎环

*角膜后胚胎环（Schwalbe 线凸出）*主要特征为 Schwalbe 线增粗和前移，临床可见一条位于角巩膜缘前的同心性不规则白线（图 21–3）。常为孤立的临床表现（15% 为正常人），也常见于 Axenfeld - Rieger 综合征、肝动脉发育不良（Alagille 综合征）及颚 – 心 – 脸综合征（22q11 缺失综合征）。

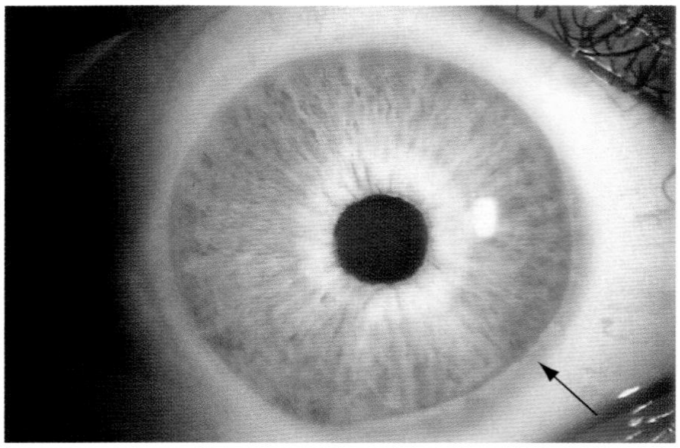

Figure 21-3 Posterior embryotoxon (*arrow*) in Axenfeld-Rieger syndrome.

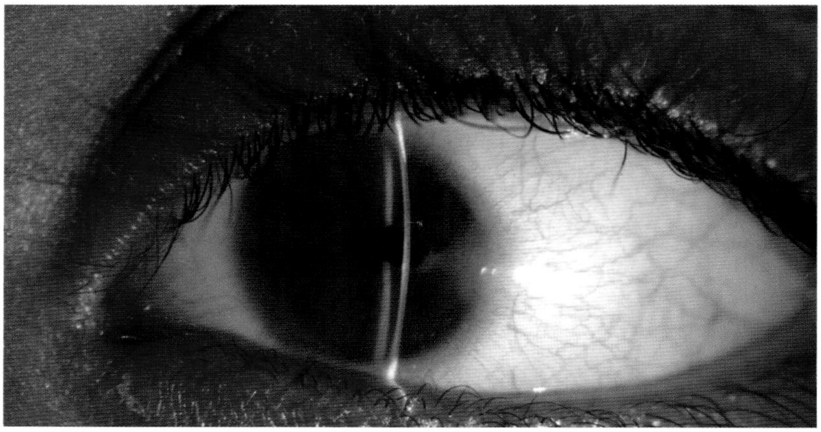

Figure 21-4 An extremely flat cornea is apparent in this child with cornea plana. Also note the indistinct limbus and irregular pupil. *(Reproduced with permission from Khan AO. Ocular genetic disease in the Middle East. Curr Opin Ophthalmol. 2013;24(5):369–378.)*

Cornea Plana

Cornea plana is a pathognomonic phenotype of flat cornea, indistinct limbus, shallow anterior chamber, hyperopia, and associated accommodative esotropia (Fig 21-4); it is specific for biallelic *KERA* mutations. Refractive correction and monitoring for glaucoma, which may develop later in life, are the mainstays of treatment.

Khan AO, Aldahmesh M, Meyer B. Recessive cornea plana in the Kingdom of Saudi Arabia. *Ophthalmology.* 2006;113(10):1773–1778.

Epibulbar Dermoid

An epibulbar (limbal) dermoid is a choristoma composed of fibrofatty tissue covered by keratinized epithelium; it may contain hair follicles, sebaceous glands, or sweat glands. The dermoid often straddles the limbus (typically inferotemporally) or, less frequently, resides more centrally in the cornea. It is typically less than 10 mm in diameter, with minimal postnatal growth. The dermoid may extend into the corneal stroma and adjacent sclera but seldom encompasses the full thickness (Fig 21-5). Often, a lipoid infiltration of the corneal stroma is noted at the leading edge. Sometimes the lesion is continuous with epibulbar dermolipomas that involve the lateral quadrant of the eye.

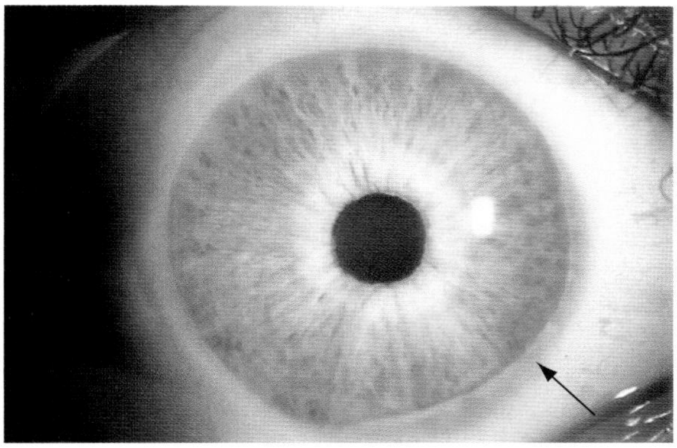

图 21–3　AxenfeldRieger 综合征中的角膜后胚胎环（*箭头*）。

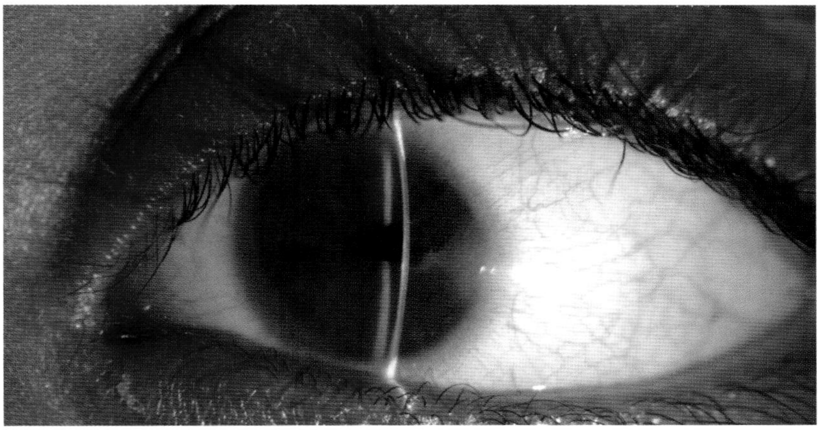

图 21–4　患儿角膜极其平坦，同时角膜缘边界不清以及瞳孔不规则。*（译者注：资料来源见前页原文。）*

扁平角膜

*扁平角膜*是一组症状的病理表型，包括有角膜平坦、角膜缘边界不清、浅前房、远视及相关调节性内斜视的 (图 21–4)，是双等位基因 *KERA* 突变特有的。治疗主要包括屈光矫正和对青光眼的监测，后者可在成年后发病。

Khan AO, Aldahmesh M, Meyer B. Recessive cornea plana in the Kingdom of Saudi Arabia. *Ophthalmology*. 2006;113(10):1773–1778.

眼球表层皮样瘤

*眼球表层（角膜缘）皮样瘤*是由角质化上皮覆盖的纤维脂肪组织构成的迷芽瘤，它可能含有毛囊、皮脂腺或汗腺。皮样瘤通常跨在角膜缘上 (典型的位于颞下方)，少见位于角膜中央。常< 10mm，出生后几乎不再生长。皮样瘤可延伸至角膜基质层和邻近的巩膜，但很少覆盖全层 (图 21–5)。通常，在累及角膜的前缘可见脂质浸润。有时与累及眼外侧象限的眼球表层皮肤脂肪瘤相连续。

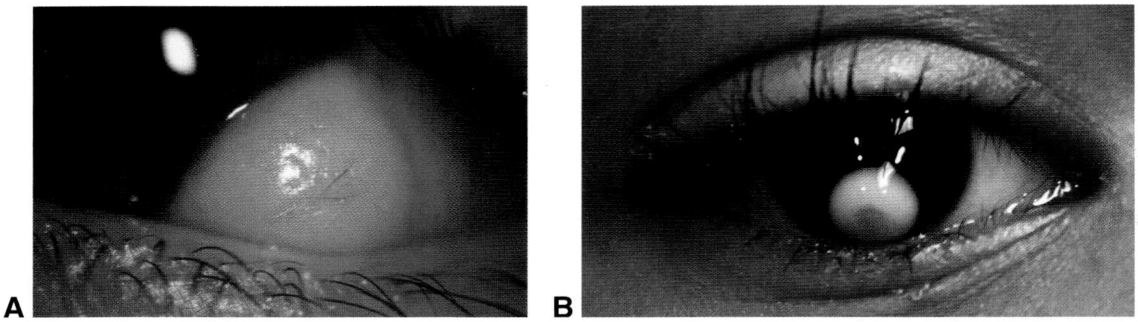

Figure 21-5 **A,** Epibulbar limbal dermoid with hair growing in the center. **B,** Corneal dermoid. *(Part A courtesy of Ken K. Nischal, MD; part B courtesy of Robert W. Hered, MD.)*

Epibulbar dermoids may be seen in Goldenhar syndrome (see also Chapter 18). Patients with Goldenhar syndrome may have one or more of a variety of anomalies, including ear deformities or periauricular tags, maxillary or mandibular hypoplasia, vertebral deformities, eyelid colobomas, or Duane retraction syndrome.

Epibulbar dermoids can produce astigmatism with secondary anisometropic amblyopia. Large epibulbar dermoids can block the visual axis. Surgical excision may be indicated if they cause ocular irritation or amblyopia, but the procedure may result in scarring and astigmatism, which can also lead to amblyopia. Although excision will not eliminate the preexisting astigmatism, surgery may be useful for treating very elevated lesions. Tumor removal involves excising the episcleral portion flush with the plane of surrounding tissue. In general, the surgeon need not remove underlying clear corneal tissue, mobilize surrounding tissue, or apply a patch graft over the resulting surface defect; however, because some lesions extend into the anterior chamber, tissue should be available in the event that a patch graft is required. The cornea and conjunctiva heal within a few days to several weeks, generally with some scarring and imperfect corneal transparency; nevertheless, the appearance can be improved considerably.

Dermolipoma

A *dermolipoma* is an epibulbar choristoma composed of adipose and dense connective tissue. Often, dermal tissue, including hairs, has replaced a portion of the overlying conjunctiva. Dermolipomas can be extensive, involving orbital tissue, the lacrimal gland, extraocular muscle, or a combination of these. Like limbal dermoids, dermolipomas can be associated with Goldenhar syndrome (see Chapter 18).

Dermolipomas rarely require excision. If surgery is undertaken, the surgeon should attempt to remove only the portion of the lesion that is visible within the palpebral fissure, disturbing the conjunctiva and the Tenon layer as little as possible to minimize scarring and the risks of strabismus and dry eye. Cicatrization may occur even with a conservative operative approach.

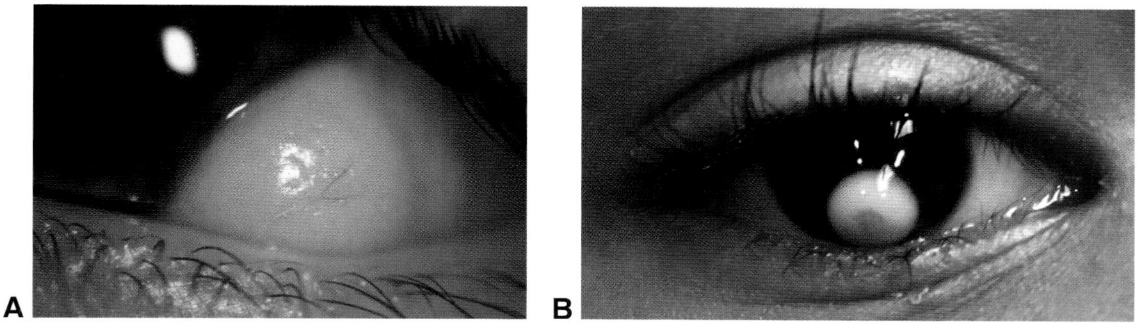

图 21–5　**A.** 眼球表层角膜缘皮样瘤，中央有毛发生长。**B.** 角膜皮样瘤。*（译者注：资料来源见前页原文。）*

眼球表层皮样瘤可见于 Goldenhar 综合征 (参见第 18 章)。Goldenhar 综合征可有一种或多种异常，包括耳畸形或副耳、上颌或下颌发育不良、椎体畸形、眼睑缺损或 Duane 后退综合征。

眼球表层皮样瘤可造成散光，继而引起屈光参差性弱视。较大的眼球表层皮样瘤可遮挡视轴。如果引起眼刺激症状或弱视，则需手术切除，但手术可导致瘢痕和散光，这也会形成弱视。虽然切除不能消除之前存在的散光，但对明显突出的病变是有用的。切除肿瘤的表层巩膜部分，至与周围组织齐平 / 等高。手术不需要切除至透明角膜组织、移行周围组织或在缺损区表面移植片，但有些病变可能扩展到前房，应准备移植片。角膜和结膜能在几天到几周内愈合，一般会留有瘢痕和角膜透明度不佳；但是外观可以得到极大地改善。

皮肤脂瘤

*皮肤脂瘤*是由脂肪和致密结缔组织构成的眼部迷芽瘤。包括毛发在内的皮肤组织取代了覆盖的结膜。皮肤脂瘤的生长范围可以很大，可累及至眼眶组织、泪腺、眼外肌或全部。和角膜缘皮样瘤一样，皮肤脂瘤也伴有 Goldenhar 综合征 (见第 18 章)。

皮肤脂瘤不需要切除。如果进行手术，应尽量切除睑裂内可见的病变部分，尽可能不影响结膜和 Tenon 囊，以减少瘢痕、斜视和干眼的风险。即使采用保守的手术方法，也可能发生瘢痕化。

Abnormalities of Central and Diffuse Corneal Transparency

The mnemonic *STUMPED* refers to sclerocornea, tears in Descemet membrane (usually owing to forceps trauma or congenital glaucoma), *u*lcers (infection; see Chapter 28), *m*etabolic disorders (eg, mucopolysaccharidosis), *P*eters anomaly, edema (eg, congenital hereditary endothelial dystrophy [CHED], *p*osterior polymorphous corneal dystrophy [PPCD], congenital hereditary stromal dystrophy [CHSD], glaucoma), and *d*ermoid (Table 21-1). Although this mnemonic has been used when the differential diagnosis of corneal opacity in young patients is considered, an alternative and more useful classification of corneal opacities is based on whether they are primary or secondary (Table 21-2).

Table 21-1 Differential Diagnosis of Infantile Corneal Opacities

Entity	Location and Description of Opacity	Other Signs	Method of Diagnosis
Sclerocornea (total corneal opacification)	Peripheral opacity, clearest centrally; unilateral or bilateral; often vascularized	Flat cornea	Inspection; anterior segment imaging
Forceps injury	Central opacity; unilateral	Breaks in Descemet membrane	History
Posterior corneal defect	Central opacity; unilateral or bilateral	Iris adherence to cornea; posterior keratoconus	Inspection
Infection	Central or diffuse opacity; unilateral or bilateral	Dendrites, infiltrate, ulceration	Culture, polymerase chain reaction, serologic tests
Mucopolysaccharidosis	Diffuse opacity; bilateral	Smooth epithelium	Biochemical testing
Congenital hereditary stromal dystrophy (CHSD)	Diffuse opacity; bilateral	Stromal opacities; normal thickness; normal epithelium	Examination of family members for autosomal dominance
Congenital hereditary endothelial dystrophy (CHED)	Diffuse opacity; bilateral	Thickened cornea	Inspection
Infantile glaucoma	Diffuse opacity; unilateral or bilateral	Enlarged cornea; breaks in Descemet membrane	Tonometry for elevated intraocular pressure
Dermoid	Inferotemporal opacity; unilateral; elevated; surface hair; keratinized; usually limbal	Associated with Goldenhar syndrome	Inspection

角膜中央及弥漫性透明度异常

缩写 *STUMPED* 代表*巩膜*化角膜（sclerocornea）、Descemet 膜（后弹力层）*撕裂*（tears in Descemet membrane，常系钳外伤或先天性青光眼所致）、*溃疡*（ulcers，感染，详见第 28 章）、*代谢缺陷*（metabolic disorders，如黏多糖累积病）、*Peters* 异常（Peters anomaly），*水肿* [edema，如先天性遗传性角膜内皮营养不良（CHED），后多形性角膜营养不良（PPCD），先天性遗传性角膜基质营养不良（CHSD），青光眼] 以及*皮样瘤*（Dermoid）（表 21–1）。虽然这种助记方法已用于患儿角膜混浊的鉴别诊断，但另一种角膜混浊分类方法更有帮助，是根据原发性或继发性而分类的（表 21–2）。

表21–1 婴儿期角膜混浊的鉴别诊断

诊断	混浊的位置与类型	其他指征	诊断方法
巩膜化角膜（全角膜不透明）	周边混浊，中央透明度最佳，单眼或双眼，常有新生血管	角膜平坦	检查，眼前节照相
钳外伤	中央混浊，单眼	后弹力层被破裂	病史
后角膜缺损	中央混浊，单眼或双眼	虹膜角膜粘连，后圆锥角膜	检查
感染	中央或弥漫状混浊，单眼或双眼	树枝状、浸润、溃疡	培养，聚合酶链反应，血清检测
黏多糖累积病	弥漫状混浊，双眼	上皮光滑	生化检测
先天性遗传性角膜基质层营养不良(CHSD)	弥漫状混浊，双眼	基质混浊，厚度正常，上皮正常	检查家庭成员：常染色体显性遗传
先天性遗传性角膜内皮营养不良(CHED)	弥漫状混浊，双眼	角膜增厚	检查
婴幼儿型青光眼	弥漫状混浊，单眼或双眼	角膜扩张，Descemet 膜（后弹力层）破裂	测量眼压
皮样瘤	颞下方混浊，单眼，凸起，表面有毛发，角化状，好发于角膜缘处	与Goldenhar综合征相关	检查

Table 21-2 Primary and Secondary Corneal Opacities: An Alternative Classification

Primary
- Corneal dystrophies (eg, CHED, PPCD, CHSD)
- Corneal dermoid

Secondary
- Posterior corneal depression
- Kerato-irido-lenticular dysgenesis (KILD)
  - Iridocorneal adhesions only (Peters anomaly type 1)
  - Failure of lens to separate from cornea (Peters anomaly type 2)
  - Lens separation but failure to form thereafter (sclerocornea)
  - Failure of lens to form (sclerocornea)
- Congenital or infantile glaucoma
- Traumatic breaks in Descemet membrane
- Infection
- Metabolic causes

CHED = congenital hereditary endothelial dystrophy; CHSD = congenital hereditary stromal dystrophy; PPCD = posterior polymorphous corneal dystrophy.

Adapted with permission from Nischal KK. A new approach to the classification of neonatal corneal opacities. Curr Opin Ophthalmol. 2012;23(5):344–354.

Primary Causes

Congenital hereditary endothelial dystrophy

In CHED, the cornea is diffusely and uniformly edematous (thick), often with a mosaic haze (Fig 21-6). The phenotype is specific for biallelic *SLC4A11* mutations. On measurement, intraocular pressure is sometimes falsely elevated, which can lead to the misdiagnosis of glaucoma. Deafness presents later in some cases (Harboyan syndrome).

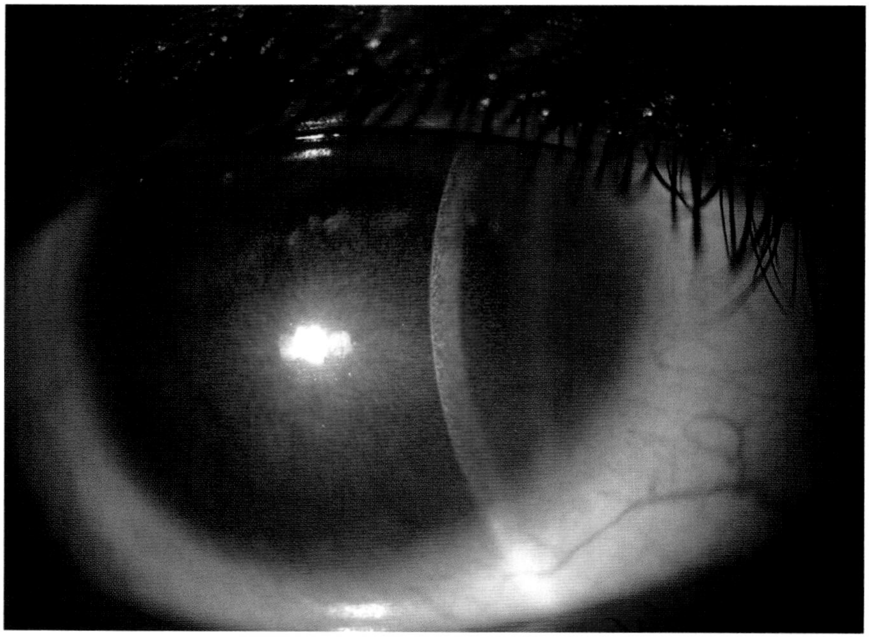

Figure 21-6 Congenital hereditary endothelial dystrophy. Note the diffuse mosaic haze, bluish discoloration, and thickness of the cornea. *(Courtesy of Arif O. Khan, MD.)*

表21-2　原发性和继发性角膜混浊

原发性	
角膜营养不良（例如CHED, PPCD, CHSD）	
角膜皮样瘤	
继发性	
后角膜凹陷	
角膜-虹膜-晶状体发育不良（KILD）	
仅角膜虹膜粘连（Peters异常1型）	
晶状体未与角膜分离（Peters异常2型）	
晶状体分离后但未成形（巩膜化角膜）	
晶状体未成形（巩膜化角膜）	
先天型或婴幼儿型青光眼	
外伤性Descemet膜（后弹力层）破裂	
感染	
代谢性疾病	

CHED=先天性遗传性角膜内皮营养不良，CHSD=先天性遗传性角膜基质营养不良，PPCD=后多形性角膜营养不良

（译者注：资料来源见前页原文。）

原发性病因

先天性遗传性角膜内皮营养不良

先天性遗传性角膜内皮营养不良 CHED 的角膜呈弥漫性均匀水肿（增厚），常伴有镶嵌的 / 马赛克雾状混浊（图 21-6）。是双等位基因 *SLC4A11* 突变的特异性表型。检查时有时会出现眼内压假性升高，可误诊为青光眼。部分患儿随后会出现耳聋（Harboyan 综合征）。

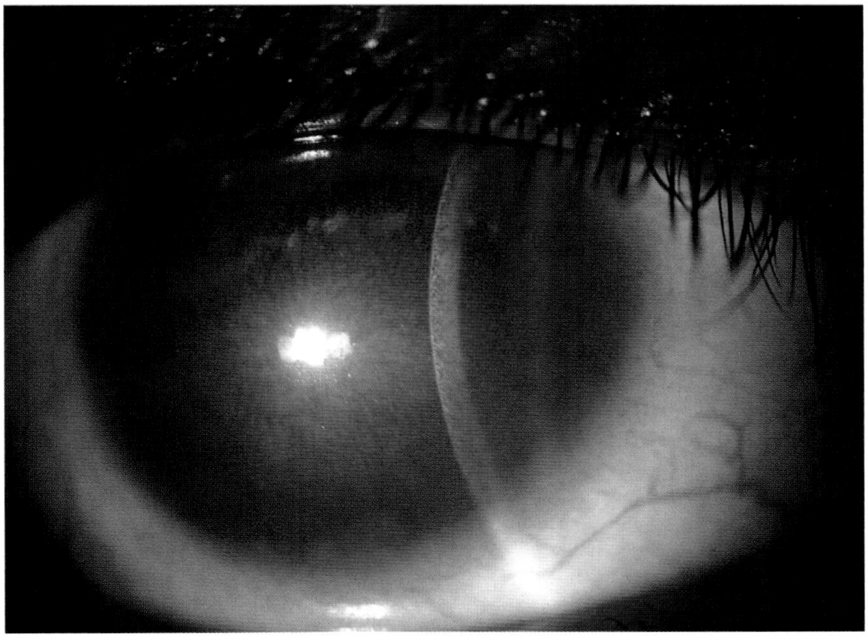

图 21-6　先天性遗传性角膜内皮营养不良。可见角膜弥漫性镶嵌的 / 马赛克雾状混浊、蓝色及水肿。

（译者注：资料来源见前页原文。）

Congenital hereditary stromal dystrophy

An autosomal dominant condition, CHSD is extremely rare. It is characterized by a smooth, normal epithelium with flaky or feathery clouding of the stroma, which is of normal thickness.

Weiss JS, Møller HU, Aldave AJ, et al. IC3D classification of corneal dystrophies—edition 2. *Cornea.* 2015;34(2):117–159. [Erratum appears in *Cornea.* 2015;34(10):e32.]

Secondary Causes

Posterior corneal depression

Posterior corneal depression (central posterior keratoconus; von Hippel internal ulcer) is a discrete posterior corneal indentation with a normal anterior curvature; it can be considered a variant of Peters anomaly (see the following section). Pigment deposits sometimes are seen on the border of the defect. An abnormal red reflex is noted during examination with a retinoscope or direct ophthalmoscope. If refractive correction is not successful, Descemet stripping endothelial keratoplasty (DSEK) can be considered.

Peters anomaly

Peters anomaly (kerato-irido-lenticular dysgenesis) is characterized by a posterior corneal defect with an overlying stromal opacity, often accompanied by adherent iris strands (Peters anomaly type 1; Fig 21-7A). A more severe phenotype includes adherence of the lens to the cornea at the site of the central defect (Peters anomaly type 2; Fig 21-7B). The corneal opacity ranges from a dense to mild central leukoma (Fig 21-7C). In severe cases, the central leukoma may be vascularized and protrude above the level of the cornea. In rare cases, a membrane may form posterior to the posterior corneal defect, causing the appearance of a central cyst in an opacified cornea (Fig 21-7D). The stromal opacity may decrease with time in some cases. Lysis of adherent iris strands has been reported to improve corneal clarity in some cases.

Peters anomaly can arise from a variety of gene mutations (eg, heterozygous *PAX6* mutation, biallelic *CYP1B1* mutations) or from in utero insult (eg, congenital rubella). Unilateral cases are usually isolated. Bilateral cases warrant a complete genetic evaluation. One Peters anomaly syndrome is *Peters-plus syndrome*, which is caused by biallelic *B3GLCT* mutations. Peters-plus syndrome is associated with short stature, a distinct craniofacial appearance, shortened fin gers and toes, and intellectual disability. In this syndrome, the stromal opacity may diminish with time.

Bhandari R, Ferri S, Whittaker B, Liu M, Lazzaro DR. Peters anomaly: review of the literature. *Cornea.* 2011;30(8):939–944.

Khan AO, Al-Katan H, Al-Gehedan S, Al-Rashed W. Bilateral congenital stromal cyst of the cornea. *J AAPOS.* 2007;11(4):400–401.

Nischal KK. genetics of congenital corneal opacification—impact on diagnosis and treatment. *Cornea.* 2015;34(Suppl 10):S24–S34.

先天性遗传性角膜基质层营养不良

先天性遗传性角膜基质营养不良（CHSD）是常染色体显性遗传，十分罕见。其特征是上皮细胞光滑且正常，但基质层有片状或羽状混浊，厚度正常。

Weiss JS, Møller HU, Aldave AJ, et al. IC3D classification of corneal dystrophies—edition 2. *Cornea.* 2015;34(2):117–159. [Erratum appears in *Cornea.* 2015;34(10):e32.]

继发性病因

后角膜凹陷

*后角膜凹陷（中央后圆锥角膜，von Hippel 眼内溃疡）*是散在的后角膜凹陷，前角膜曲率正常。可视为是Peters异常的变体(见下一节)。病灶边缘有时可见色素沉积。检影镜或直接检眼镜下，可见异常红色反光。如果无法屈光矫正，可考虑行后弹力层剥离角膜内皮移植术（DSEK）。

Peters 异常

*Peters 异常（角膜－虹膜－晶状体发育不良）*的特征是后角膜缺损，相应基质混浊，常伴有粘连的虹膜条索（Peters 异常 1 型，图 21–7A）。更严重的表型包括晶状体与角膜中心缺损区黏附（Peters 异常 2 型，图 21–7B）。角膜混浊呈致密的到轻度的中央白斑（图 21–7C）。严重时，中央角膜白斑血管化，并突出于角膜。罕见后角膜缺损后方可形成一层膜，导致混浊的角膜出现中央囊肿（图 21–7D）。有时基质混浊可随时间而减轻。有报告，松解粘连的虹膜条索可改善角膜透明度。

Peters 异常可由多种基因突变(如杂合 *PAX6* 突变、双等位基因 *CYP1B1* 突变)或宫内感染(如先天性风疹)所致。单眼发病常是孤立的，双眼发病需行全面的基因评估。Peters 异常综合征之一是 *Peters–plus 综合征*，由双等位基因 *B3GLCT* 突变引起。Peters–plus 综合征伴身材矮小、特征性颅面、短手指 / 脚趾以及智力障碍，其基质混浊可随着时间而减轻。

Bhandari R, Ferri S, Whittaker B, Liu M, Lazzaro DR. Peters anomaly: review of the literature. *Cornea.* 2011;30(8):939–944.

Khan AO, Al-Katan H, Al-Gehedan S, Al-Rashed W. Bilateral congenital stromal cyst of the cornea. J *AAPOS.* 2007;11(4):400–401.

Nischal KK. genetics of congenital corneal opacification—impact on diagnosis and treatment. *Cornea.* 2015;34(Suppl 10):S24–S34.

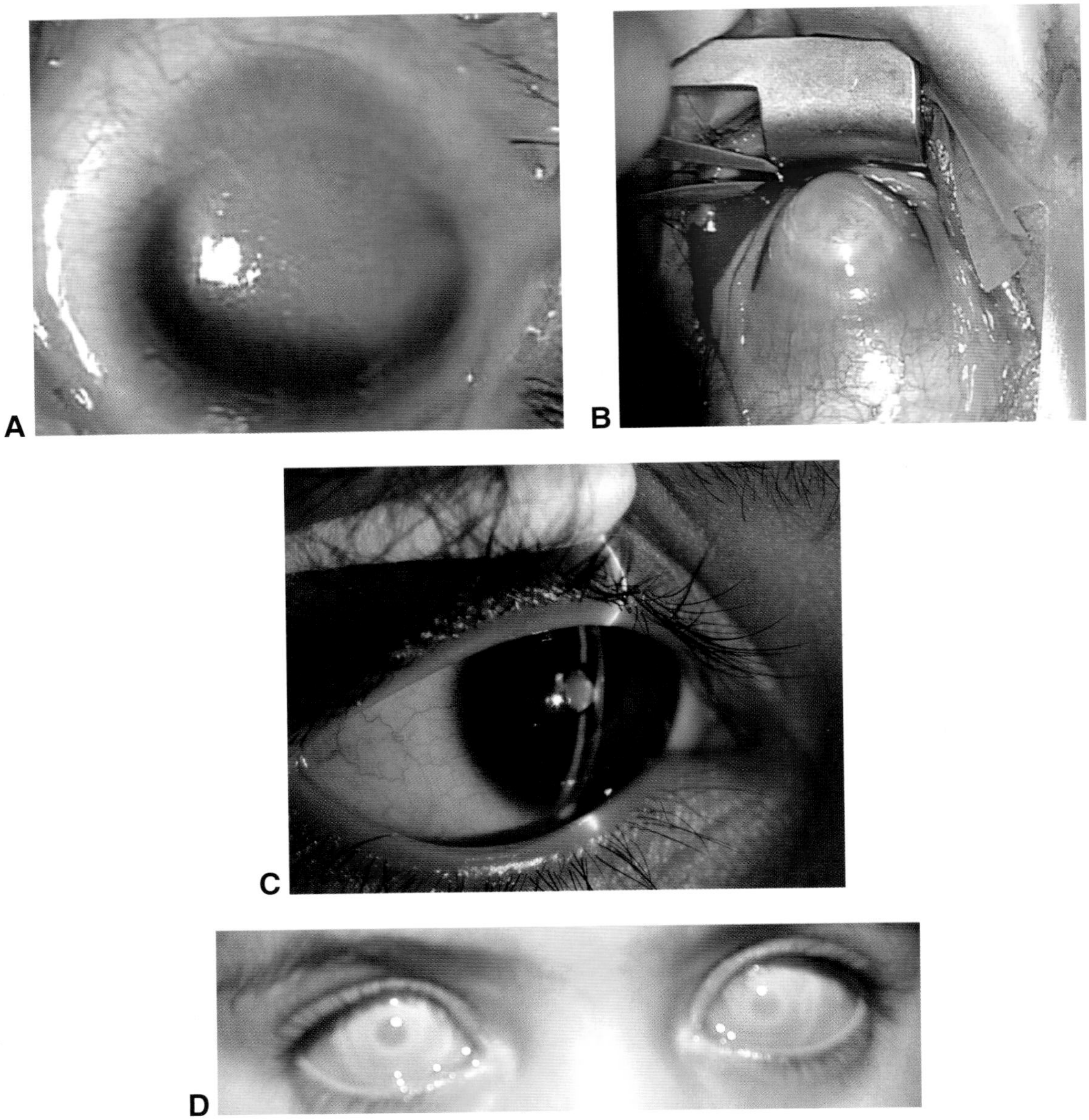

Figure 21-7 **A,** Corneal opacity secondary to iridocorneal adhesion (Peters anomaly type 1). **B,** Corneal opacity secondary to keratolenticular adhesion (Peters anomaly type 2). **C,** A Peters phenotype of central lens opacity with keratolenticular adhesion. **D,** Bilateral posterior corneal defect with a thin posterior membrane, causing the appearance of a central cyst in an opacified cornea. *(Parts A and B courtesy of Ken K. Nischal, MD; parts C and D courtesy of Arif O. Khan, MD.)*

Sclerocornea

Sclerocornea (total corneal opacification) is a descriptive term for a congenitally opaque cornea resembling sclera (Fig 21-8). As it is a vague term that does not suggest causation, its use should be avoided.

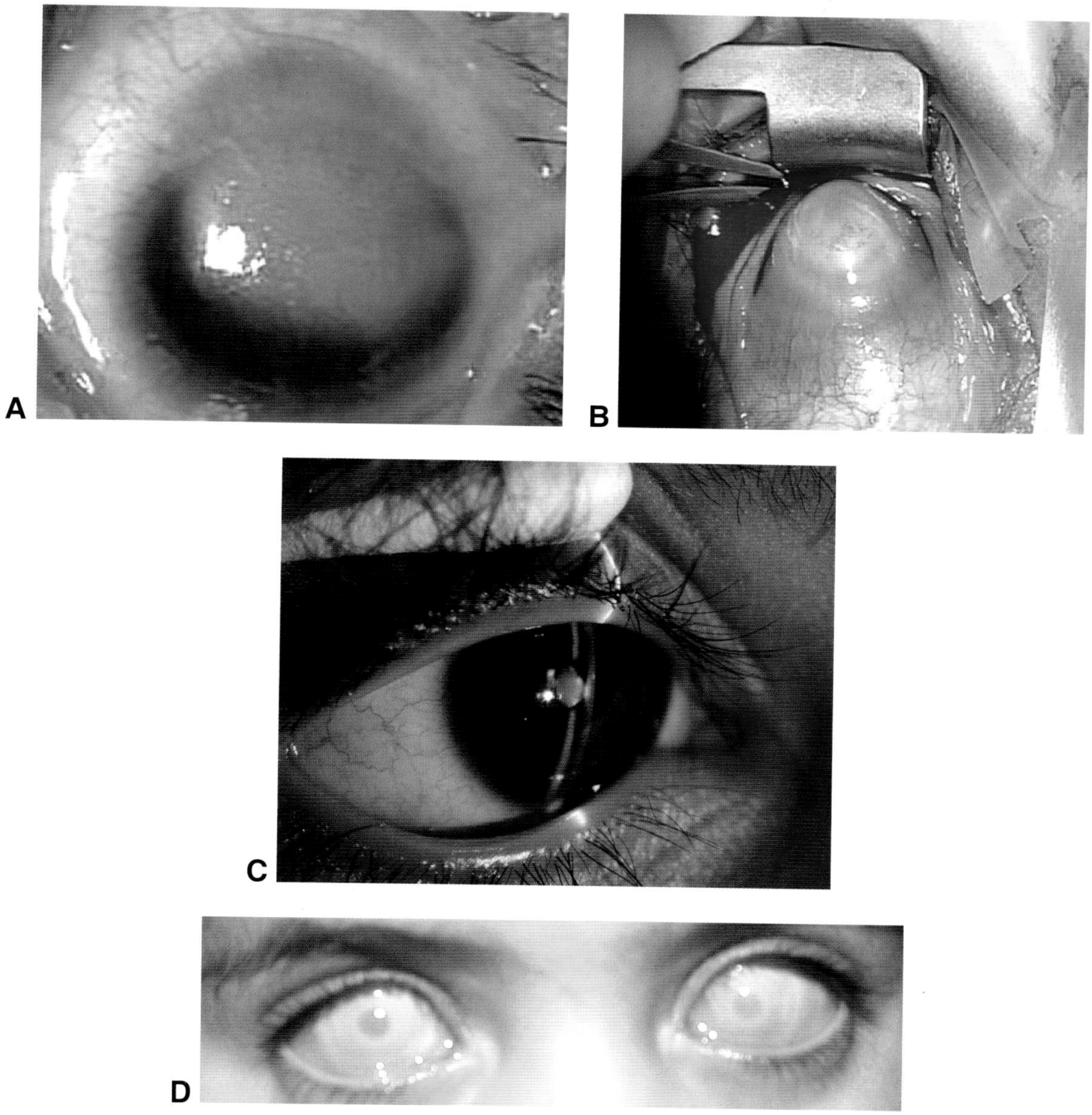

图 21–7　**A.** 虹膜角膜粘连继发的角膜混浊（Peters 异常 1 型）。**B.** 角膜晶状体粘连继发的角膜混浊（Peters 异常 2 型）。**C.** 中央晶状体混浊伴角膜晶状体粘连的 Peters 表型。**D.** 双眼后角膜缺损后方薄膜，呈混浊角膜的中央囊肿。*（译者注：资料来源见前页原文。）*

巩膜化角膜

*巩膜化角膜（全角膜混浊）*是一个描述性的术语，表示先天性角膜混浊如同巩膜一样（图 21–8）。它是一个含混的术语、没有提示发病原因，应避免使用。

Congenital or infantile glaucoma

Glaucoma in young children can cause the cornea to become edematous, cloudy, and enlarged. Breaks in Descemet membrane from glaucomatous enlargement are termed *Haab striae* (Figs 21-9, 21-10). See Chapter 22 for further discussion.

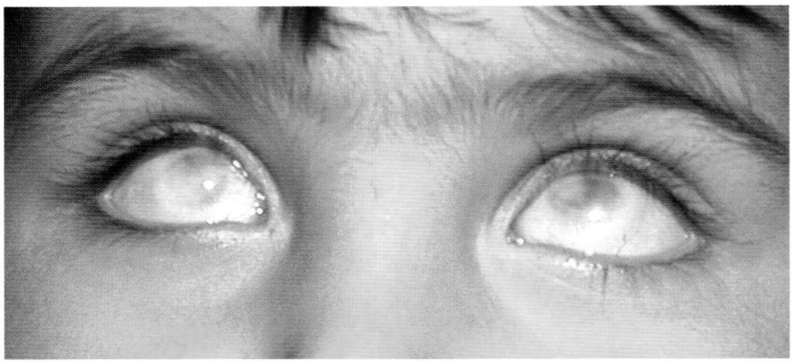

Figure 21-8 Bilateral sclerocornea. *(Courtesy of Arif O. Khan, MD.)*

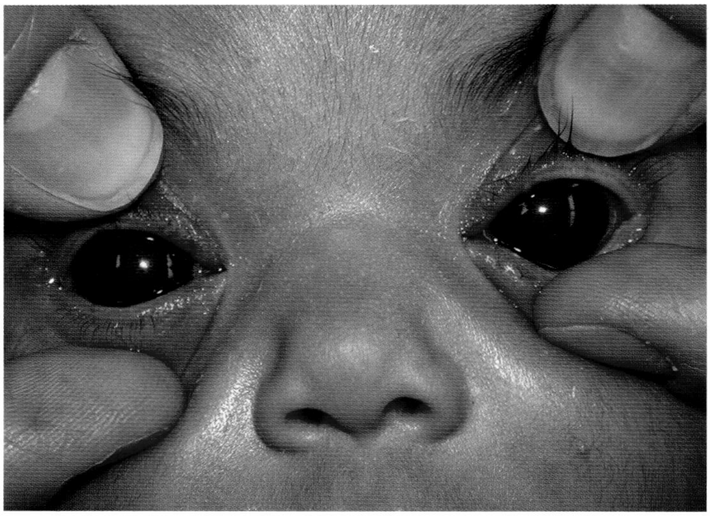

Figure 21-9 Primary congenital glaucoma. *(Reproduced with permission from Khan AO. Genetics of primary glaucoma. Curr Opin Ophthalmol. 2011;22(5):347–355.)*

Traumatic breaks in Descemet membrane

Traumatic breaks in Descemet membrane can be caused by forceps trauma during delivery. Other signs of trauma are frequently apparent on the child's head. Traumatic breaks are usually vertical and linear, unlike the curvilinear and often horizontal Haab striae of congenital glaucoma. Acute rupture leads to stromal and sometimes epithelial edema. Acute stromal and epithelial edema regresses, but the edges of the broken Descemet membrane persist and can be seen as ridges protruding slightly from the posterior corneal surface. Amblyopia may result from prolonged corneal opacity or, more commonly, from induced anisometropic astigmatism. In patients with brittle cornea syndrome, a disorder of corneal fragility caused by biallelic mutations in *ZNF469* or *PRDM5*, minor trauma can cause traumatic breaks in Descemet membrane (Fig 21-11).

Khan AO. Conditions that can be mistaken as early childhood glaucoma. *Ophthalmic Genet*. 2011;32(3):129–137.

先天性或婴幼儿型青光眼
儿童期的青光眼可引起角膜水肿、混浊和扩张。青光眼的角膜扩张导致 Descemet 膜（后弹力层）破裂，形成 *Haab 纹*（图 21–9，21–10）。进一步讨论见第 22 章。

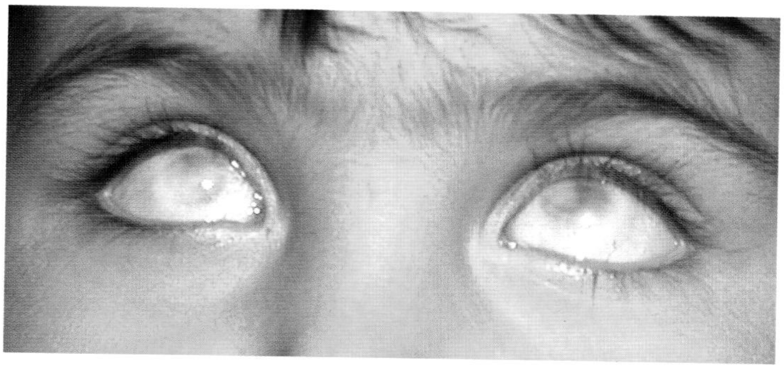

图 21–8　双眼巩膜化角膜。*（译者注：资料来源见前页原文。）*

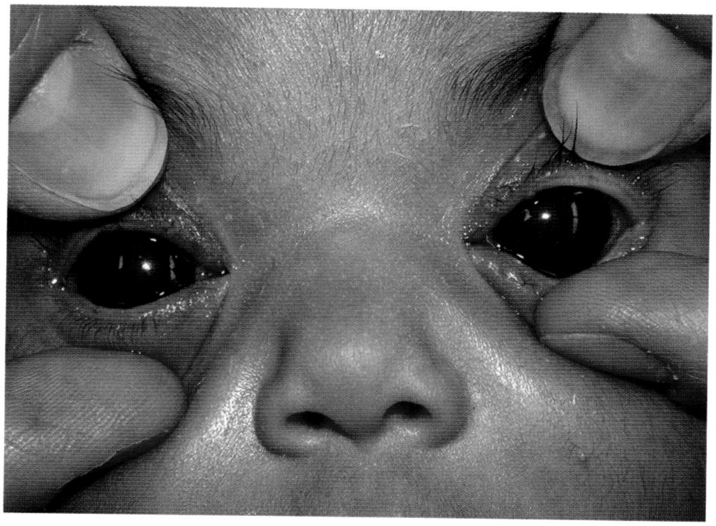

图 21–9　原发性先天性青光眼。*（译者注：资料来源见前页原文。）*

外伤性角膜 Descemet 膜（后弹力层）破裂
在分娩过程中，产钳损伤可引起角膜 Descemet 膜（后弹力层）的创伤性破裂。孩子的头上可见其他创伤的痕迹。外伤性破裂常呈垂直性和线性，这有别于先天性青光眼的曲线、常为水平的 Haab 纹。急性破裂可导致基质水肿，有时致上皮水肿。急性基质水肿和上皮水肿消退后，角膜 Descemet 膜破裂的边缘仍存在，从角膜后表面可以看到轻微的脊状突起。长时间的角膜混浊会导致弱视，更常见的是屈光参差性散光导致的弱视。脆性角膜综合征是由于双等位基因 *ZNF469* 或 *PRDM5* 突变而导致角膜脆弱，轻微的创伤可导致 Descemet 膜（后弹力层）的外伤性破裂（图 21–11）。

Khan AO. Conditions that can be mistaken as early childhood glaucoma. *Ophthalmic Genet*. 2011;32(3):129–137.

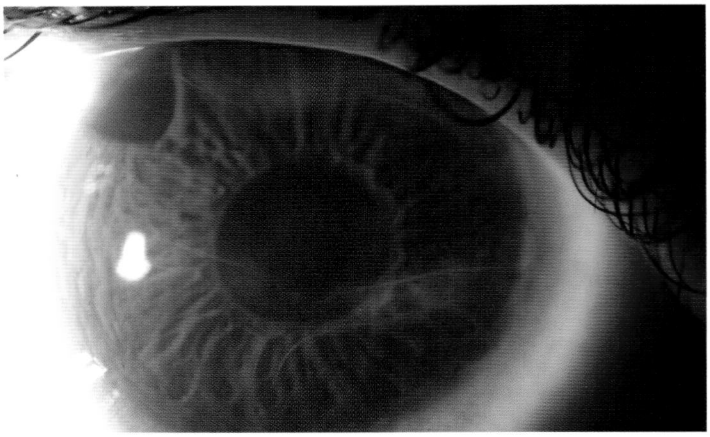

Figure 21-10 Haab striae in an eye that underwent peripheral iridectomy related to prior glaucoma surgery. *(Courtesy of Arif O. Khan, MD.)*

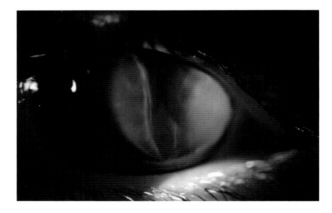

Figure 21-11 Descemet tears from minor trauma in a child with brittle cornea syndrome. *(Courtesy of Arif O. Khan, MD.)*

Corneal ulcers

Congenital corneal ulcers are rare and may be caused by herpes simplex keratitis or other infection (see Chapter 28).

Treatment of Corneal Opacities

If bilateral dense opacities are present, early keratoplasty can be considered for 1 eye so that deprivation amblyopia can be minimized. Coexistent anterior segment disease must be considered before keratoplasty is undertaken. If the opacity is unilateral, the decision is more difficult. Keratoplasty should be undertaken only if the family and the ophthalmologists involved in the child's care are prepared for the significant commitment of time and effort needed to deal with corneal graft rejection, which occurs often in children, as well as with amblyopia. The team should include ophthalmologists skilled in pediatric corneal surgery, pediatric glaucoma, and amblyopia. Contact lens expertise is important for the care of infants with small eyes and large refractive errors. Repeated examinations under anesthesia are often required.

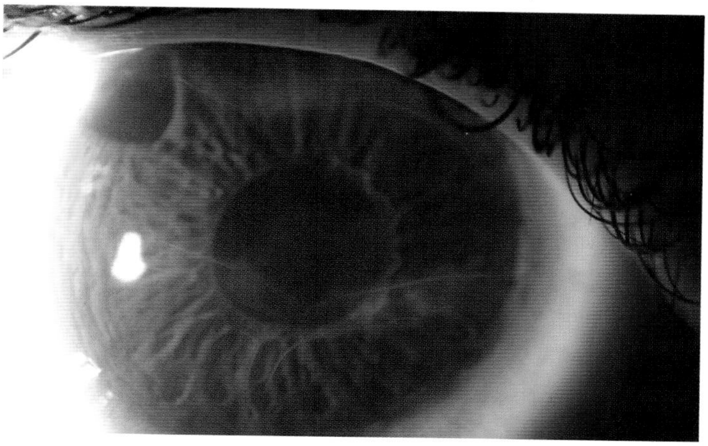

图 21–10　青光眼手术（虹膜周边切除术）后的 Haab 纹。*（译者注：资料来源见前页原文。）*

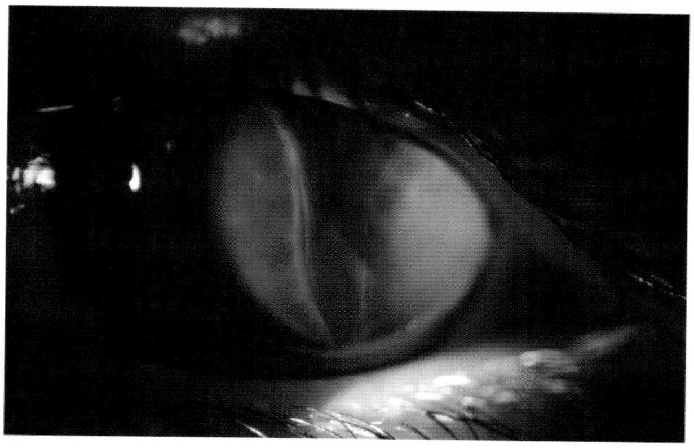

图 21–11　脆性角膜综合征患儿受到轻微外伤所致的 Descemet 膜（后弹力层）破裂。*（译者注：资料来源见前页原文。）*

角膜溃疡

先天性角膜溃疡较为罕见，可是单纯疱疹角膜炎或其他感染所致（见第 28 章）。

角膜混浊的治疗

如果双眼存在致密混浊，可对一眼行早期角膜移植，以减少剥夺性弱视。角膜移植术前必须考虑合并的眼前节病变。如果只有一眼角膜不透明，则更难做出决定。角膜移植手术前，患儿的家庭和眼科医生需有思想准备，在手术后需花费大量时间和精力，处理常发生于儿童的角膜移植排斥反应以及弱视。技术团队应包括擅长儿童角膜手术、儿童青光眼和弱视的眼科医生。对于小眼球和高度的屈光不正儿童来说，接触镜专业知识特别重要，常需要在麻醉下反复检查。

In addition to traditional penetrating keratoplasty, treatment options include optical iridectomy, deep anterior lamellar keratoplasty (DALK; used for stromal disease with healthy endothelium), DSEK (used to replace diseased endothelium or Descemet membrane), and keratoprostheses.

Ashar JN, Ramappa M, Vaddavalli PK. Paired-eye comparison of Descemet's stripping endothelial keratoplasty and penetrating keratoplasty in children with congenital hereditary endothelial dystrophy. *Br J Ophthalmol.* 2013;97(10):1247–1249.

Harding SA, Nischal KK, Upponi-Patil A, Fowler DJ. Indications and outcomes of deep anterior lamellar keratoplasty in children. *Ophthalmology.* 2010;117(11):2191–2195.

Congenital and Developmental Anomalies of the Globe

Microphthalmia, Anophthalmia, and Coloboma

Microphthalmia, anophthalmia, and coloboma (MAC) is a spectrum that may be isolated or syndromic. It has been associated with mutations in numerous genes, including *CHX10, MAF, PAX6, PAX2, RAX, SHH, SIX3*, and *SOX2*.

Microphthalmia

Microphthalmia is a small, disor ga nized globe that can be associated with cystic outpouching of the posteroinferior sclera.

Anophthalmia

Anophthalmia is absence of any ocular globe tissue (see Chapter 18). It is very rare; usually, when anophthalmia is clinically suspected, the child actually has severe microphthalmia.

Coloboma

Coloboma is the most common and least severe manifestation of the MAC spectrum. It is typically an inferonasal gap in the iris or retina. Coloboma results from failure of the embryonic fissure to close in the fifth week of gestation.

Nanophthalmos

Nanophthalmos is a small eye, typically with an axial length of 18 mm or less and with associated high hyperopia. The cornea is abnormally steep in the recessive form, distinguishing it from ordinary hyperopia. The lens-to-eye ratio is high, with a shallow anterior chamber and risk for angle-closure glaucoma. Another distinguishing feature is a characteristic papillomacular fold. The phenotype can result from biallelic mutations in *PRSS56* or *MFRP* or from heterozygous mutations in *TMEM98*. When the anterior segment is of grossly normal depth, the phenotype is termed *posterior microphthalmos*.

Nowilaty SR, Khan AO, Aldahmesh MA, Tabbara KF, Al-Amri A, Alkuraya FS. Biometric and molecular characterization of clinically diagnosed posterior microphthalmos. *Am J Ophthalmol.* 2013;155(2):361–372.e7.

除了传统的穿透性角膜移植外，治疗方法还包括光学虹膜切除术、深层前板层角膜移植（DALK，用于内皮健康的基质混浊）、后弹力层剥离角膜内皮移植术（DSEK，用于替换病变的内皮或 Descemet 膜）和人工角膜。

Ashar JN, Ramappa M, Vaddavalli PK. Paired-eye comparison of Descemet's stripping endothelial keratoplasty and penetrating keratoplasty in children with congenital hereditary endothelial dystrophy. *Br J Ophthalmol.* 2013;97(10):1247–1249.

Harding SA, Nischal KK, Upponi-Patil A, Fowler DJ. Indications and outcomes of deep anterior lamellar keratoplasty in children. *Ophthalmology.* 2010;117(11):2191–2195.

先天性与发育性眼球异常

小眼症、无眼症和眼组织缺损

小眼症、无眼症和眼组织缺损（MAC）是一个序列，可能是孤立的或综合征候群，与许多基因的突变有关，包括 *CHX10*、*MAF*、*PAX6*、*PAX2*、*RAX*、*SHH*、*SIX3* 和 *SOX2*。

小眼症

*小眼症*是一种小而组织紊乱的眼球，可伴后下方巩膜囊性外翻。

无眼症

*无眼症*是眼球的组织完全缺如（见第 18 章），非常罕见，临床上的无眼症常是严重的小眼症。

眼组织缺损

*眼组织缺损*是小眼症 – 无眼症 – 眼组织缺损序列（MAC）中最常见、较轻的表现，常表现为虹膜或视网膜的鼻下方缺损。眼组织缺损是由于妊娠第 5 周胚胎裂未闭合。

小眼球

*小眼球*的特点是眼轴长度 ≤ 18mm，并伴有高度远视。隐性小眼球表现为角膜曲率异常高，晶状体与眼之比很高、前房较浅及有患闭角型青光眼的风险。另一个显著的特征是视盘 – 黄斑皱襞，此表型可由双等位基因 *PRSS56* 或 *MFRP* 突变或 *TMEM98* 杂合突变引起。当眼前段深度非常正常时，其表型被称为后小眼球。

Nowilaty SR, Khan AO, Aldahmesh MA, Tabbara KF, Al-Amri A, Alkuraya FS. Biometric and molecular characterization of clinically diagnosed posterior microphthalmos. *Am J Ophthalmol.* 2013;155(2):361–372.e7.

Congenital and Developmental Anomalies of the Iris or Pupil

Abnormalities of the Iris

Persistent pupillary membrane

Persistent pupillary membrane (Fig 21-12) is the most common developmental abnormality of the iris; it can be seen in approximately 95% of newborns. Remnants are common in older children and adults. Persistent pupillary membranes are rarely visually significant. If especially prominent, they can adhere to the anterior lens capsule, causing a small anterior polar cataract. They may be associated with other anterior segment abnormalities.

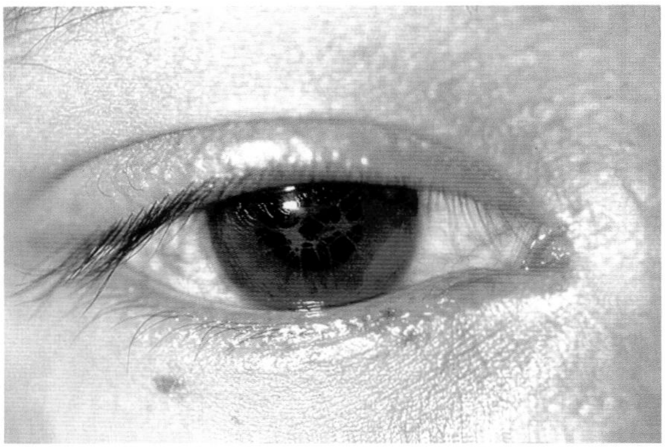

Figure 21-12 Persistent pupillary membrane. Uncorrected visual acuity was 20/40.

Iris hypoplasia

Iris hypoplasia refers to an underdeveloped iris stroma. It may be focal (iris coloboma) or diffuse (aniridia). If only the posterior pigment epithelium is underdeveloped, iris transillumination occurs.

Axenfeld-Rieger syndrome *Axenfeld-Rieger syndrome (ARS)* is the commonest cause of iris (stromal) hypoplasia. Characteristic findings include posterior embryotoxon with attached iris strands and iris hypoplasia. These patients have a 50% lifetime risk of glaucoma (Figs 21-13, 21-14, 21-15). ARS is a spectrum that shows phenotypic and genetic heterogeneity. Conditions previously considered distinct—such as Axenfeld anomaly, Rieger anomaly or syndrome, iridogoniodysgenesis anomaly or syndrome, iris hypoplasia, and familial glaucoma iridogoniodysplasia—are now recognized as part of the spectrum of ARS.

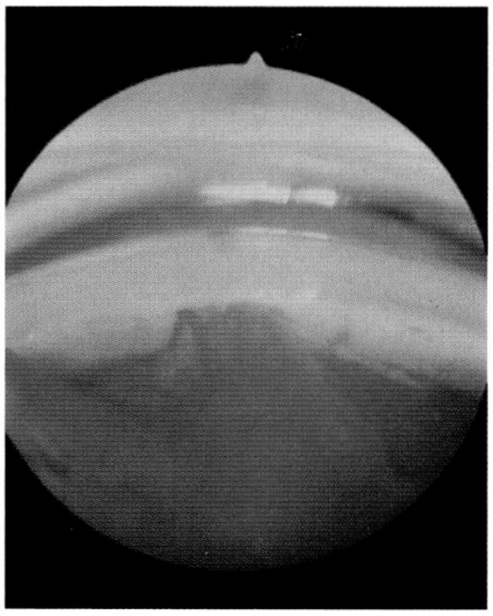

Figure 21-13 Gonioscopic view in Axenfeld-Rieger syndrome.

先天性与发育性虹膜或瞳孔异常

虹膜异常

瞳孔膜残留 / 永久性瞳孔膜

瞳孔膜残留 / 永久性瞳孔膜（图 21–12）是最常见的虹膜发育异常，约 95% 的新生儿可见，在大龄儿童和成人亦常见。瞳孔膜残留很少影响视觉，特别突出时会附着在晶状体前囊上，造成小的前极性白内障。可伴有其他眼前节异常。

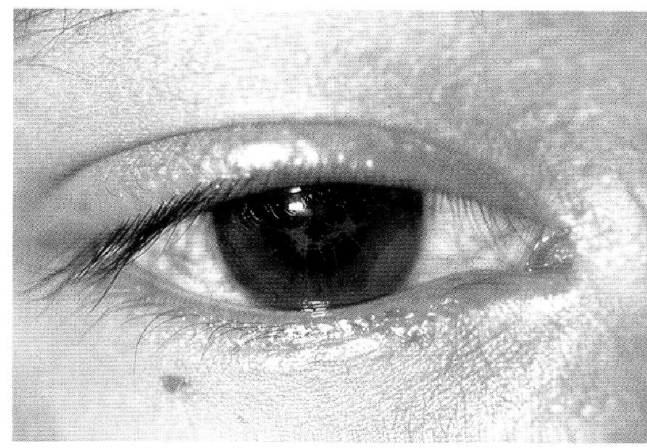

图 21–12　瞳孔膜残存，裸眼视力 20/40（0.5）。

虹膜发育不全

*虹膜发育不全*是指虹膜基质发育不全，可呈局灶性（虹膜缺损）或弥漫性（无虹膜）。如果仅是后色素上皮发育不全，可见虹膜透视。

Axenfeld–Rieger 综合征　*Axenfeld-Rieger 综合征（ARS）*是虹膜（基质）发育不全最常见的原因，特征有与虹膜条索附着的后胚胎环和虹膜发育不全。这些患者终生存在 50% 的青光眼风险（图 21–13, 图 21–14, 图 21–15)。Axenfeld–Rieger 综合征是一个序列，具有表型和遗传异质性。以前视为特殊疾病，如 Axenfeld 异常、Rieger 异常或综合征、虹膜性腺发育不全或综合征、虹膜发育不全和家族性青光眼虹膜性腺发育不全，现在均视为是 Axenfeld–Rieger 综合征序列的一部分。

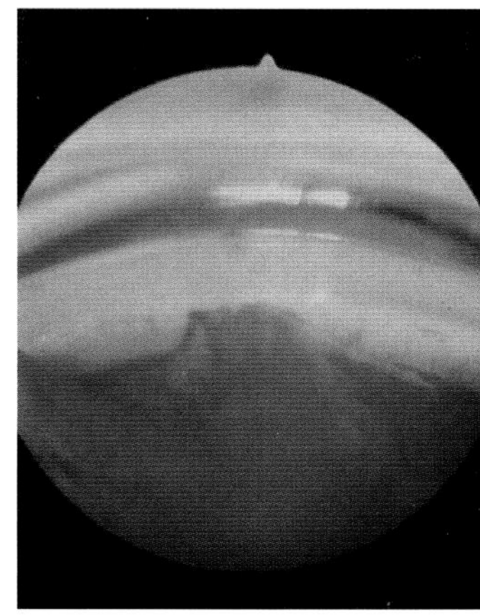

图 21–13　前房角镜下的 Axenfeld–Rieger 综合征。

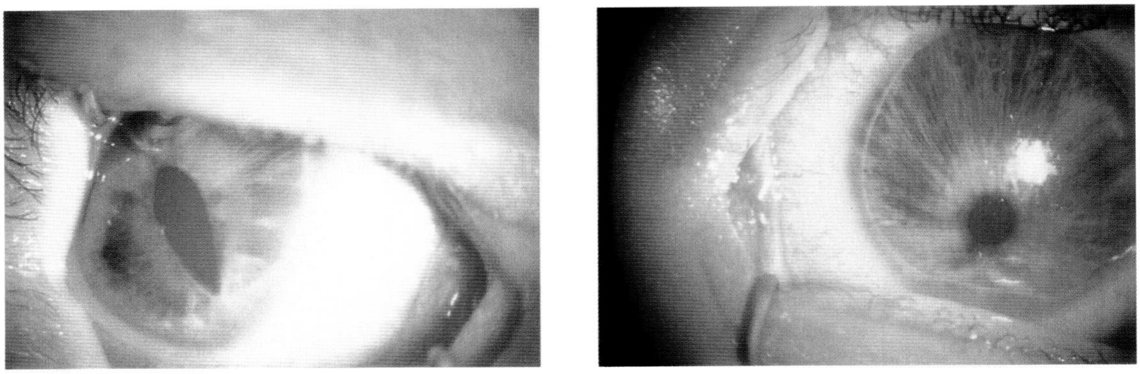

Figure 21-14 Axenfeld-Rieger syndrome, bilateral.

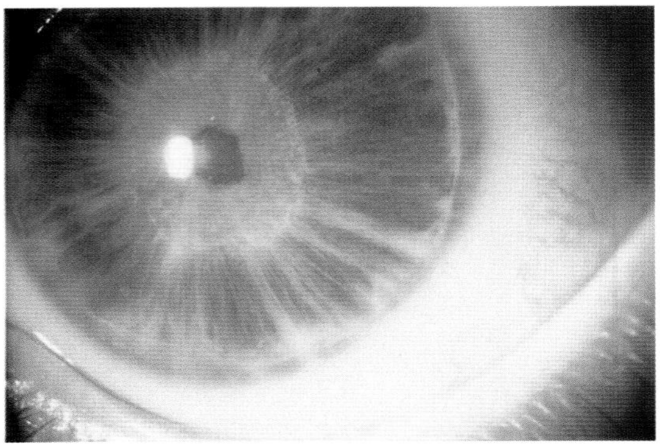

Figure 21-15 Axenfeld-Rieger syndrome. Note variation compared with Figures 21-13 and 21-14. *(Courtesy of Jane D. Kivlin, MD.)*

The features of ARS range from a smooth, cryptless iris surface to a phenotype that mimics aniridia. Examples include mild stromal thinning, marked atrophy with hole formation, corectopia, and ectropion uveae. Posterior embryotoxon, megalocornea (secondary to glaucoma), or microcornea may occur. Associated nonocular abnormalities include abnormal teeth, distinct facies, redundant periumbilical skin, hypospadias, cardiac valve abnormalities, and pituitary abnormalities. Heterozygous mutations in *PITX2* or *FOXC1*, homeobox genes that regulate other ocular developmental genes, are the most common identifiable cause.

Iris transillumination *Iris transillumination* results from the absence of pigment in the posterior epithelial layers (albinism) or from iris hypoplasia (as part of anterior segment dysgenesis, as in ARS). Iris transillumination has also been reported in Marfan syndrome, Prader-Willi syndrome, ectopia lentis et pupillae, X-linked megalocornea, and microcoria. Patchy areas of transillumination can also be seen after trauma, surgery, or uveitis. Scattered iris transillumination defects may be a normal variant in individuals with very lightly pigmented irides.

Coloboma of the iris With a typical inferonasal iris coloboma, the pupil is shaped like a lightbulb, keyhole, or inverted teardrop (Fig 21-16). Typical colobomas may also involve the lens, ciliary body, choroid, retina, or optic nerve and are part of the MAC spectrum (discussed previously in this chapter). Parents of an affected child may have small, previously undetected chorioretinal or iris defects in an inferonasal location; thus, careful examination of family members is indicated.

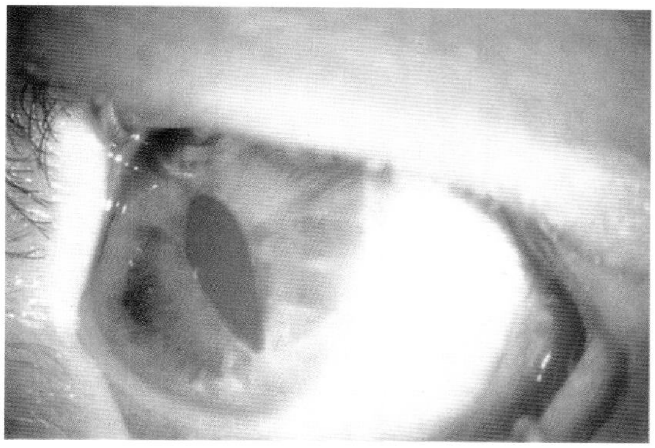
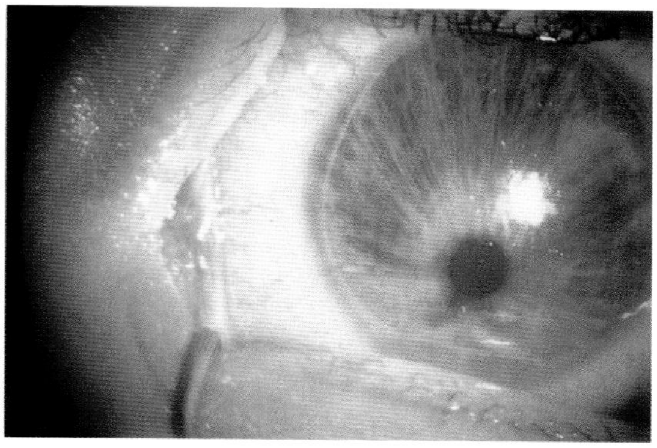

图 21-14　Axenfeld-Rieger 综合征，双眼。

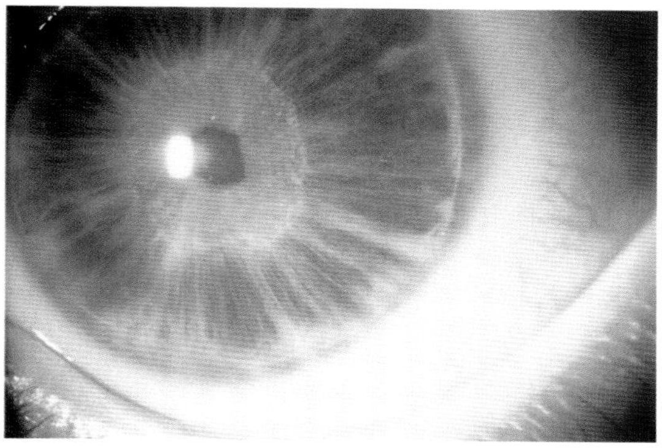

图 21-15　Axenfeld-Rieger 综合征，对比与图 21-13 和图 21-14 的变化。*（译者注：资料来源见前页原文。）*

Axenfeld-Rieger 综合征（ARS）表现为虹膜表面平滑、无隐窝，也可呈类似无虹膜的表型。如有基质变薄、明显萎缩伴孔的形成、瞳孔异位和色素层外翻，也可有后胚胎环、大角膜（继发于青光眼）或小角膜。伴有的非眼部异常有牙齿异常、相异 / 特殊面容、脐周皮肤冗余、尿道下裂、心瓣膜异常和垂体异常。调节其他眼部发育基因的同源盒基因——*PITX2* 或 *FOXC1* 的杂合突变是最常见的确诊原因。

虹膜透照　*虹膜透照*是由于后上皮层色素缺乏（白化病）或虹膜发育不全（为前节发育不良的一部分，如 Axenfeld-Rieger 综合征 ARS）所致。Marfan 综合征、Prader-Willi 综合征、晶状体瞳孔异位、X - 连锁大角膜和小眼球也有虹膜透照的报道。创伤 / 外伤、手术或葡萄膜炎后也能看到斑片状透照区。在虹膜色素极少的正常变异时，可出现散在的虹膜透照缺陷。

虹膜缺损　典型的鼻下方虹膜缺损，瞳孔形状呈灯泡状、钥匙孔样或倒置的泪滴（图 21-16），可累及晶状体、睫状体、脉络膜、视网膜或视神经，属于小眼症 - 无眼症 - 眼组织缺损 MAC 序列的一部分（本章前面已讨论）。患儿的父母可有未被检查的微小的鼻下方脉络膜视网膜或虹膜缺损。因此，患儿童的家人亦应仔细检查。

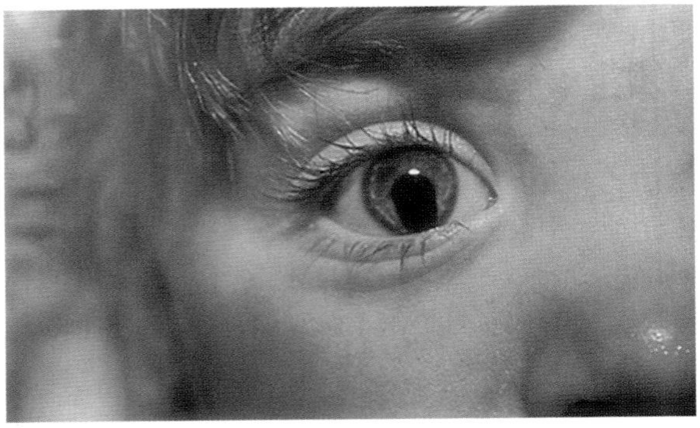

Figure 21-16 Typical iris coloboma, right eye.

Atypical iris colobomas occur in areas other than the inferonasal quadrant and are not usually associated with posterior uveal colobomas. These colobomas probably result from fibrovascular remnants of the anterior hyaloid system and pupillary membrane.

Aniridia Classic *aniridia* is a panocular bilateral disorder. The term is a misnomer, however, because at least a rudimentary iris is always present. The degree of iris formation ranges from almost total absence to only mild hypoplasia, overlapping with ARS. The typical presentation is an infant with nystagmus who appears to have absent irides or dilated, unresponsive pupils. Examination findings commonly include small anterior polar lens opacities, at times with attached strands of Persistent pupillary membranes (Fig 21-17). Foveal hypoplasia is usually present, with visual acuity often less than 20/100. Glaucoma, typically juvenile, and optic nerve hypoplasia are common. Corneal opacification often develops later in childhood and may lead to progressive deterioration of visual acuity. The corneal abnormality is due to a stem cell deficiency; therefore, keratolimbal allograft stem cell transplantation may be a more effective treatment than corneal transplantation.

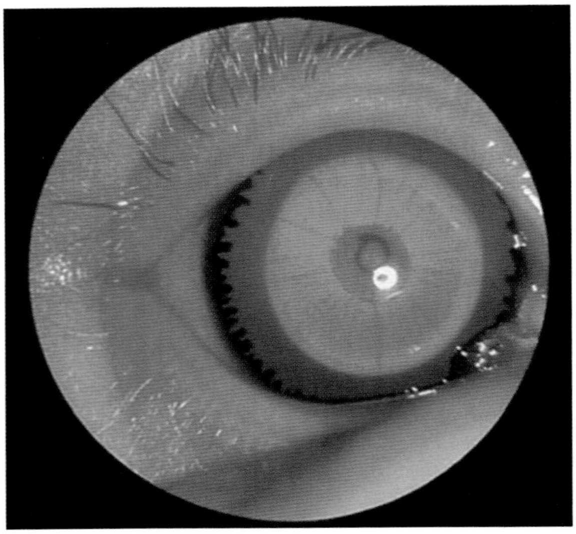

Figure 21-17 Aniridia in an infant. Both the ciliary processes and the edge of the lens are visible. Also present are persistent pupillary membrane fibers and a small central anterior polar cataract.

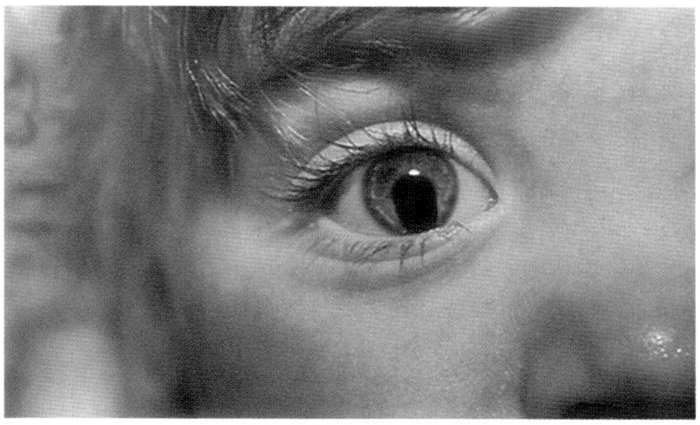

图 21–16 典型的虹膜缺损。

非典型性虹膜缺损可发生在鼻下象限以外的区域，常不伴有后葡萄膜缺损。这些缺损可能是由前玻璃体系统和瞳孔膜的纤维血管残余所致。

无虹膜症 典型的*无虹膜症*常是双眼的全眼病变，这个术语用词不当，但至少虹膜发育不全始终存在。虹膜的发育可完全缺如，或呈轻度发育不全，与 Axenfeld–Rieger 综合征 ARS 部分重叠。典型的表现为婴儿眼球震颤，伴虹膜缺如或瞳孔扩大且对光反射迟钝。检查见小的前极性晶状体混浊，有时伴有附着的瞳孔膜残留（图 21–17）；黄斑中心凹多发育不全，视力低于 20/100（0.2）；常见青少年型青光眼和视神经发育不良；儿童后期常发生角膜混浊，并导致视力逐渐下降。角膜异常系干细胞缺乏所致，因此，异体角膜缘干细胞移植可能比角膜移植更有效。

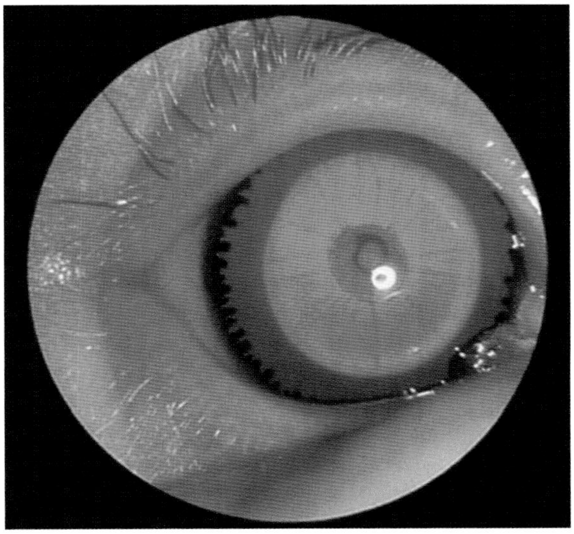

Figure 21-17 婴儿无虹膜症。睫状突和晶状体边缘都可见，同时见瞳孔膜残留纤维和小的中央前极白内障。

Heterozygous *PAX6* gene mutations (11p13) cause classic aniridia, particularly nonsense mutations (haploinsufficiency). Missense mutations are more likely associated with variable expressivity and partial phenotypes. Most (approximately two-thirds) aniridic children have the familial form. The *PAX6* gene is a homeotic eye morphogenesis control gene involved in complex interactions between the optic cup, surface ectoderm, and neural crest during formation of the iris and other ocular structures.

Approximately one-third of aniridia cases result from new deletions that, if large enough, can also affect the contiguous *WT1* gene (a contiguous gene syndrome); such patients are therefore at risk for Wilms tumor (nephroblastoma) before 5 years of age. This phenotype is part of the WAGR syndrome (Wilms tumor, aniridia, genitourinary malformations, and mental retardation). All children with sporadic aniridia should undergo chromosomal deletion analysis of 11p13 to exclude increased Wilms tumor risk. Familial aniridia does not carry a significant risk, although there have been rare reports of Wilms tumor associated with familial aniridia.

Congenital iris ectropion

Ectropion of the posterior pigment epithelium onto the anterior surface of the iris is sometimes termed *ectropion uveae,* but this is a misnomer because posterior iris epithelium is derived from neural ectoderm and is not considered part of the uvea. Congenital iris ectropion can occur as an acquired tractional abnormality, often associated with rubeosis iridis, or as a congenital nonprogressive abnormality, which can be associated with later glaucoma. It may occur in patients with neurofibromatosis, facial hemihypertrophy, or Prader-Willi syndrome. *Congenital iris ectropion syndrome* is a constellation of unilateral congenital iris ectropion, a glassy-smooth cryptless iris surface, a high iris insertion, dysgenesis of the drainage angle, and glaucoma risk, often with ptosis.

Abnormalities in the Size, Shape, or Location of the Pupil

Dyscoria

Dyscoria is an abnormal pupil shape, typically resulting from congenital malformation such as ARS (see Fig 21-14).

Congenital miosis

Congenital miosis (microcoria) may represent an absence or malformation of the dilator pupillae muscle. It can also occur secondary to contracture of fibrous material on the pupil margin owing to remnants of the tunica vasculosa lentis or neural crest cell anomalies. The pupil rarely exceeds 2 mm in diameter, is often eccentric, and reacts poorly to my driatic drops. Severe cases require surgical pupilloplasty. *Ectopia lentis et pupillae* refers to eccentric microcoria with lens subluxation, often from biallelic *ADAMTSL4* mutations (also see the section "Corectopia").

Congenital mydriasis

Many cases of *congenital mydriasis (iridoplegia)* fall within the aniridia spectrum, especially if the central iris structures from the collarette to the pupillary sphincter are absent. Congenital cardiovascular defects may be associated with congenital mydriasis in patients with heterozygous ACTA2 mutation, which sometimes causes an alternate phenotype of prominent iris flocculi rather than iridoplegia. Other causes include iris sphincter trauma, pharmacologic mydriasis, and acquired neurologic disease that affects parasympathetic innervation.

PAX6 杂合基因突变 (11p13)， 特别是无义突变 (单倍体功能不全)，可引起典型的无虹膜症。错义突变可能与表型的变异和不全表型有关。大多数 (约 2/3) 无虹膜症的儿童有家族性。*PAX6* 基因是一种同源的眼形态发生控制基因，在虹膜和其他眼部结构形成过程中，参与视杯、表面外胚层和神经嵴之间复杂的相互作用。

大约 1/3 的无虹膜症由新的基因缺失引起，如果缺失足够大，还会影响相邻的 *WT1* 基因（一种相邻基因综合征），5 岁前有患 Wilms 肿瘤（肾母细胞瘤）的风险。这种表型是 WAGR 综合征的一部分 [*W*ilms 肿瘤、无虹膜症（*a*niridia）、*泌尿*生殖系统畸形（genitourinary malformations）和智力发育*迟缓*（mental retardation）的缩写]。所有散发性无虹膜症患儿需行 11p13 染色体缺失分析，以排除 Wilms 肿瘤风险。家族性无虹膜症没有明显的风险，但也偶有关于 Wilms 肿瘤伴家族性无虹膜症的报告。

先天性虹膜外翻

后色素上皮向虹膜前表面的外翻有时称为*葡萄膜外翻*，但这是一个错误命名，因为后虹膜上皮源于神经外胚层，而不是葡萄膜的一部分。先天性虹膜外翻可发生在获得性牵拉异常时，常伴虹膜红变；先天性虹膜外翻亦可为一种先天性非进行性异常，可伴迟发性青光眼。可见于神经纤维瘤病、面部偏侧肥大或 Prader-Willi 综合征患者。*先天性虹膜外翻综合征*指一组综合征，包括单眼先天性虹膜外翻、光滑无隐窝虹膜表面、虹膜高位附着、房角引流发育不良和青光眼风险，常伴有上睑下垂。

瞳孔大小、形态或位置异常

瞳孔变形

*瞳孔变形*是指异常的瞳孔形态，常由先天性畸形所致，如 Axenfeld-Rieger 综合征（ARS）.（见图 21-14）。

先天性小瞳孔

*先天性小瞳孔*可能系瞳孔开大肌缺如或畸形，由于晶状体血管膜残留或神经脊细胞异常，继发性瞳孔边缘纤维收缩。瞳孔直径＜ 2mm，常偏位，对扩瞳药反应差。严重时需行瞳孔成形术。*晶状体瞳孔异位*是指偏位小瞳孔伴晶状体半脱位，常由双等位基因 *ADAMTSL4* 突变引起（也见“瞳孔异位”一节）。

先天性大瞳孔

许多*先天性大瞳孔*（*虹膜麻痹*）属无虹膜序列，特别是从虹膜领 / 卷缩轮到瞳孔括约肌的虹膜中心结构缺如。先天性心血管缺陷伴先天性大瞳孔的患者有杂合 *ACTA2* 突变，这时呈现突出的虹膜小叶表型，而不是虹膜麻痹。其他原因包括虹膜括约肌损伤、药物性扩瞳和影响副交感神经支配的获得性神经病变。

Milewicz DM, Østergaard JR, Ala-Kokko LM, et al. Denovo *ACTA2* mutation causes a novel syndrome of multisystemic smooth muscle dysfunction. *Am J Med Genet A*. 2010;152A(10): 2437–2443.

Corectopia

Normally, the pupil is located approximately 0.5 mm inferonasally from the center of the iris. Minor deviations of up to 1.0 mm are usually cosmetically insignificant and are not considered abnormal; displacement greater than this is considered *corectopia*. Sector iris hypoplasia or other colobomatous lesions can lead to corectopia. Vision can be good.

Isolated noncolobomatous, autosomal dominant corectopia has been reported. Progressive corectopia can be associated with ARS or, in adults, with iridocorneal endothelial (ICE) syndrome.

Ectopia lentis et pupillae is corectopia associated with lens subluxation. It is often due to biallelic *ADAMTS4* mutations. The pupils and lenses are displaced in opposite directions. The pupils may be very small and misshapen; they often dilate poorly (see Chapter 23).

Polycoria and pseudopolycoria

True *polycoria* (in which each pupil has a sphincter mechanism) is very rare. Most accessory iris openings are *pseudopolycoria*. These iris holes may be congenital or may develop in response to progressive corectopia and iris hypoplasia in ARS (Fig 21-18) or, in adults, in ICE syndrome. Pseudopolycoria can also result from trauma, surgery, or Persistent pupillary membranes.

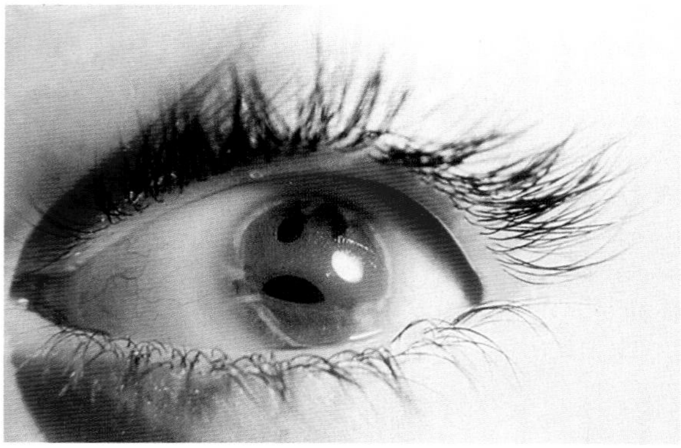

Figure 21-18 Pseudopolycoria secondary to Axenfeld-Rieger syndrome. *(Courtesy of John W. Simon, MD.)*

Acquired Corneal Conditions

Keratitis

Keratitis may be epithelial, stromal, peripheral, or, in rare cases, endothelial.

Infectious causes

Congenital syphilis Interstitial keratitis may occur in the first decade of life secondary to congenital syphilis (discussed in Chapter 28). The keratitis presents as a rapidly progressive corneal edema followed by abnormal vascularization in the deep stroma adjacent to Descemet membrane. Intense vascularization may give the cornea a salmonpink color—hence the term *salmon patch.* Blood flow through these vessels gradually ceases over several weeks to several months, leaving empty "ghost" vessels in the corneal stroma. Immune-mediated uveitis, arthritis, and hearing loss may also develop and may recur even after treatment of syphilis. Immunosuppression may be necessary to diminish sequelae.

Milewicz DM, Østergaard JR, Ala-Kokko LM, et al. Denovo *ACTA2* mutation causes a novel syndrome of multisystemic smooth muscle dysfunction. *Am J Med Genet A*. 2010;152A(10): 2437–2443.

瞳孔异位

正常情况下，瞳孔位于虹膜中心鼻下方约 0.5mm 处。1mm 以内的微小偏差外观上无影响，也不视为异常，但大于 1mm 的移位则视为*瞳孔异位*。扇形虹膜发育不全或其他虹膜缺损病变可导致瞳孔异位。视力正常。

有报告孤立的、无缺损、常染色体显性瞳孔异位。进展性瞳孔异位伴有 Axenfeld–Rieger 综合征（ARS），成人可伴有虹膜角膜内皮综合征（ICE）有关。

*晶状体瞳孔异位*是伴有晶状体半脱位的瞳孔异位，常是由于双等位基因 *ADAMTS4* 突变。瞳孔和晶状体呈反方向移位。瞳孔很小且变形，不易散大（见第 23 章）。

多瞳症与假多瞳症

真正的*多瞳症*非常罕见（即每个瞳孔都有括约肌）。出现的虹膜孔多是*假多瞳症*。这些虹膜孔可是先天性的，也可是 Axenfeld–Rieger 综合征 ARS 的进行性瞳孔异位和虹膜发育不良（图 21–18)，或是成人的虹膜角膜内皮综合征 ICE。假性多瞳症也可由外伤、手术或瞳孔膜残留所致。

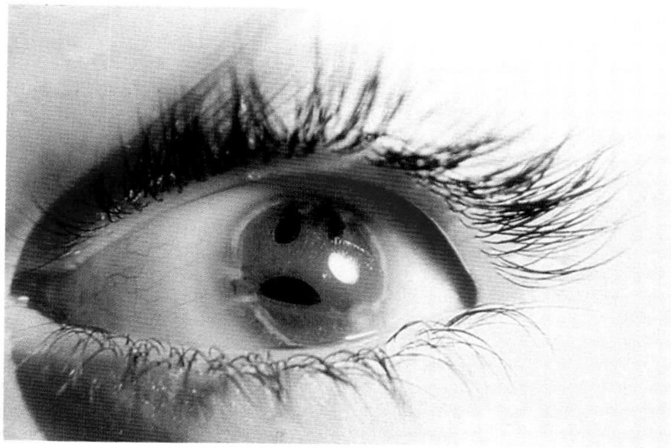

图 21–18　继发于 Axenfeld–Rieger 综合征的多瞳症。*（译者注：资料来源见前页原文。）*

获得性角膜病变

角膜炎

角膜炎分为上皮性、基质性、周边性，以及罕见的内皮性。

感染性

先天性梅毒　间质性角膜炎可能发生在 10 岁前，继发于先天性梅毒（第 28 章讨论）。角膜炎表现为一种快速进展的角膜水肿，随之在毗邻 Descemet 膜（后弹力层）的深层基质出现异常血管化。密集的血管使角膜呈鲑鱼粉红色——因此称*鲑鱼斑*。血管的血液几周 ~ 几个月逐渐消失，在角膜基质中留下空的“影子”血管。即使经梅毒治疗，免疫介导的葡萄膜炎、关节炎和听力损失也可能发展和复发。为减少后遗症，需用免疫抑制。

Herpes simplex infection Eye involvement in congenital herpes simplex virus (HSV) infection can include conjunctivitis, keratitis, retinochoroiditis, and cataracts. Congenital HSV infection is discussed in Chapter 28.

Adenovirus infection Punctate epithelial keratitis is most often seen after adenoviral infection; it is due to subepithelial immune complex deposition. See BCSC Section 8, *External Disease and Cornea*, for further discussion.

Noninfectious causes

Punctate epithelial erosions are most commonly seen in patients with lagophthalmos or dry eye disease. Peripheral (marginal) keratitis is usually associated with blepharokeratoconjunctivitis secondary to meibomian gland disease.

Thygeson superficial punctate keratitis The etiology of *Thygeson superficial punctate keratitis* is unclear, but it is thought to be immune-mediated. It can occur in children and presents with tearing, photophobia, and reduced vision. The condition is bilateral but often asymmetric. Characteristic features include slightly elevated gray corneal epithelial lesions with negative staining. It is treated with mild corticosteroids (eg, fluorometholone 0.1%) or topical cyclosporine 0.05%.

Cogan syndrome This syndrome is a rare vasculitis that presents with ocular, audiovestibular, and systemic features. Interstitial keratitis, uveitis, conjunctivitis, episcleritis, or a combination of these features may be seen.

Systemic Diseases Affecting the Cornea or Iris

Metabolic Disorders Affecting the Cornea or Iris

See also Chapter 28, Ocular Manifestations of Systemic Disease, and Table 28-2.

Mucopolysaccharidosis

The mucopolysaccharidoses (MPSs) are a group of lysosomal storage diseases. Ocular manifestations can include corneal haze from incompletely degraded glycosaminoglycan. Corneal haze may be present in early life in MPS IH (Hurler syndrome), MPS IS (Scheie syndrome), and MPS IV (Morquio syndrome). Treatment options for significant opacities include penetrating keratoplasty and DALK. Enzyme replacement therapy is available for certain forms of these lysosomal storage diseases. See BCSC Section 8, *External Disease and Cornea*, for further discussion.

Cystinosis

Cystinosis is caused by biallelic *CTNS* mutations. The infantile form includes failure to thrive, rickets, and progressive renal failure, resulting in Fanconi syndrome.

Iridescent, elongated corneal crystals appear at approximately age 1 year, first in the peripheral cornea and the anterior stroma. Crystals also present in the uvea and on the surface of the iris. Corneal crystals result in severe photophobia. There are reports of angleclosure glaucoma secondary to crystal deposition in the ciliary body.

单纯疱疹病毒感染　先天性单纯疱疹病毒（HSV）感染可导致结膜炎、角膜炎、视网膜脉络膜炎和白内障。第 28 章讨论先天性 HSV 感染。

腺病毒感染　点状上皮性角膜炎最常见于腺病毒感染后，是由于上皮下免疫复合物沉积所致。进一步讨论见 BCSC 第 8 册《*外眼疾病与角膜*》。

非感染性

角膜上皮点状糜烂最常见于睑闭合不全或干眼症。周边(边缘)性角膜炎是继发与睑板腺疾病，常伴睑 – 角膜 – 结膜炎。

Thygeson 表层点状角膜炎　*Thygeson 表层点状角膜炎*的病因尚不清楚，可能是免疫介导的。常见于儿童，表现为流泪、畏光和视力下降。累及双眼，但不对称。特点是轻度高起的灰色角膜上皮病灶，但染色阴性。低浓度皮质类固醇（如 0.1% 氟米龙）或局部使用 0.05% 环孢霉素进行治疗。

Cogan 综合征　该综合征是一种罕见的血管炎伴眼部、听觉前庭和全身病变，可见间质性角膜炎、葡萄膜炎、结膜炎、表层巩膜炎或同时出现上述多种症状。

影响角膜或虹膜的全身性疾病

影响角膜或虹膜的代谢紊乱

见第 28 章“系统性疾病的眼部表现”以及表 28–2。

黏多糖贮积症

黏多糖贮积症（MPSs）是一类溶酶体贮积症，眼部表现为角膜混浊，是不完全降解的葡萄糖胺聚糖所致。角膜混浊还出现于一些综合征的早期，如黏多糖贮积症 MPS IH（Hurler 综合征）、黏多糖贮积症 MPS IS （Scheie 综合征）和黏多糖贮积症 MPS IV （Morquio 综合征）。严重患者的治疗有穿透性角膜移植术和深层前板层角膜移植 DALK。酶替代疗法可用于某些类型的溶酶体贮积症。进一步讨论见 BCSC 第 8 册《*外眼疾病与角膜*》。

胱氨酸贮积症

*胱氨酸贮积症*是双等位基因 CTNS 突变引起的。婴儿型包括发育不良、佝偻病和进行性肾功能衰竭，导致 Fanconi 综合征。

1 岁时，首先在周边角膜和前基质出现彩色长条状的结晶体。结晶体也出现于葡萄膜和虹膜表面。角膜上的结晶体导致严重的畏光。有报道，结晶体沉积于睫状体，导致继发性闭角型青光眼。

Oral cysteamine alleviates systemic problems but not the corneal crystal deposition. Topical cysteamine can reduce corneal crystal deposition but requires frequent application, may be difficult to obtain, and has an unpleasant odor.

Tyrosinemia type II

Tyrosinemia type II (Richner-Hanhart syndrome) results from biallelic *TAT* mutations and is associated with photophobia, pseudodendritic ulcers on the cornea, and ulceration on the palms and soles. Systemic problems include liver and kidney dysfunction. Dietary restriction of phenylalanine and tyrosine is the mainstay of treatment.

Wilson disease

In *Wilson disease (hepatolenticular degeneration)*, there is excess copper deposition in the liver, kidneys, and basal ganglia of the brain, leading to cirrhosis, renal tubular damage, and a Parkinson-like disorder of motor function. The phenotype results from biallelic *ATP7B* mutations. The characteristic Kayser-Fleischer ring—a golden-brown, ruby-red, or green pigment ring consisting of copper deposits—is limited to Descemet membrane, can be several millimeters in width, and may resolve with treatment. Laboratory tests for serum copper and ceruloplasmin are better than an eye examination for early diagnosis because the ring can develop late.

Fabry disease

Fabry disease is an X-linked lysosomal storage disease with variable systemic manifestations. It is due to α-galactosidase deficiency (hemizygous *GLA* mutations). Vortex keratopathy (verticillata) can be seen in affected males and in female carriers.

Schnyder corneal dystrophy

Schnyder corneal dystrophy is a predominantly local disorder of corneal lipid metabolism arising from biallelic *UBIAD1* mutations. Although crystalline keratopathy is characteristic, stromal haze without crystals is a common presentation.

Other Systemic Diseases Affecting the Cornea or Iris

Familial dysautonomia

Familial dysautonomia (Riley-Day syndrome) is a disorder of autonomic dysfunction characterized by relative insensitivity to pain, temperature instability, and absence of the fungiform papillae of the tongue. The phenotype occurs largely in children of Eastern Euro pean Jewish (Ashkenazic) descent and results from biallelic *IKBKAP* mutations. Failure to respond with a wheal and flare to intradermal injection of 1:1000 histamine solution is characteristic. Exposure keratitis and corneal ulcers with secondary opacification are frequent. Treatment includes artificial tears and tarsorrhaphy.

Waardenburg syndrome

Waardenburg syndrome is a rare neurocristopathy characterized by Hirschsprung disease; deafness; and depigmentation of hair (a white forelock), skin, and iris. Ophthalmic findings include telecanthus and dystopia canthorum (see Chapter 17).

口服半胱胺可以减轻全身症状，但对角膜结晶体沉积无效。局部滴半胱胺可减少角膜结晶体沉积，但需经常使用，且不易购买、有异味。

酪氨酸血症 II 型

*酪氨酸血症 II 型（Richner–Hanhart 综合征）*是由双等位基因 *TAT* 突变引起的，伴畏光、角膜假性树枝状溃疡以及手掌和脚底溃疡，全身疾病有肝肾功能障碍。治疗的主要方法是限制苯丙氨酸和酪氨酸饮食摄入。

Wilson 病（肝豆状核变性）

在 *Wilson 病（肝豆状核变性）*中，肝脏、肾脏和大脑基底神经节中有过多的铜沉积，导致肝硬化、肾小管损害和 Parkinson 样运动功能障碍。该表型由双等位基因 *ATP7B* 突变引起。Kayser–Fleischer 环是铜沉淀形成的色素环，呈金棕色的、红宝石红色的或绿色的，其局限于 Descemet 膜（后弹力层），宽度可达几毫米，治疗后可以消失。实验室检测血清铜和铜蓝蛋白有助于早期诊断，优于眼部检查，因为此色素环的形成较晚。

Fabry 病

*Fabry 病*是一种 X– 连锁溶酶体贮积症，有多种全身表现，是 α – 半乳糖苷酶缺乏 (半合子 *GLA* 突变)。男性患病者和女性携带者可见涡旋性角膜病变 (野葵样)。

Schnyder 角膜营养不良

*Schnyder 角膜营养不良*是一种双等位基因 *UBIAD1* 突变引起的角膜局部脂代谢紊乱。无结晶的基质混浊常见，结晶性角膜病变也是其特征性改变。

其他影响角膜或虹膜的全身性疾病

家族性自主神经机能异常

*家族性自主神经机能异常（Riley–Day 综合征）*是一种自主神经功能障碍，其特征为对疼痛相对不敏感、体温不稳定以及舌部菌状乳头缺乏。这种表型多见于东欧犹太裔（德裔）儿童，主要是由于双等位基因 *IKBKAP* 变异。皮内注射 1 ∶ 1000 组氨溶液，无风团和潮红反应。常见继发于角膜混浊的暴露性角膜炎和角膜溃疡。治疗方法包括人工泪液和睑缝合术。

Waardenburg 综合征

*Waardenburg 综合征*是一种罕见神经嵴 / 分泌性疾病，其临床特征为 Hirschsprung 病（先天性巨结肠）、耳聋、头发脱色（一撮白额发）、皮肤脱色以及虹膜色素缺失。眼部表现有内眦距过宽和内眦异位（见第 17 章）。

Tumors of the Anterior Segment

Cornea

Tumors of the cornea are extremely rare in children, but squamous cell carcinomas have been reported in cases of xeroderma pigmentosum.

Iris

Nodules

Lisch nodules *Lisch nodules* occur in patients with neurofibromatosis and are discussed in Chapter 28.

Juvenile xanthogranuloma *Juvenile xanthogranuloma* is a nonneoplastic histiocytic proliferation that develops in infants younger than 2 years. It is characterized by the presence of Touton giant cells. Skin involvement—consisting of one or more small, round, orange or tan papules—is typically but not always present. Iris lesions are relatively rare and virtually always unilateral. The fleshy, yellow-brown masses may be small and localized or may diffusely infiltrate the entire iris, resulting in heterochromia. Spontaneous bleeding with hyphema is a characteristic clinical presentation. Secondary glaucoma may cause acute pain, photophobia, and vision loss. Those at greatest risk for ocular involvement are children with multiple skin lesions.

Juvenile xanthogranuloma is a self-limited condition that usually regresses spontaneously by age 5 years, but to avoid complications, treatment is indicated for ocular involvement. Topical corticosteroids and pharmacologic agents to lower intraocular pressure, given as necessary, are generally sufficient to control the problem. Surgical excision or radiation should be considered if intractable glaucoma is present.

Iris mammillations *Iris mammillations* may be unilateral or bilateral. They appear as numerous tiny, diffuse, pigmented nodules on the surface of the iris (Fig 21-19). They are more common in darkly pigmented eyes and are usually the same color as the iris. These nodules may be bilateral, autosomal dominant, and isolated, or they may be associated with oculodermal melanocytosis or phakomatosis pigmentovascularis type IIb (nevus flammeus with persistent, aberrant mongolian spots). Iris mammillations have also been reported in cases of ciliary body tumor and choroidal melanoma. They must be differentiated from Lisch nodules; mammillations are usually dark brown, smooth, uniformly distributed, and equal in size or slightly larger near the pupil. The incidence of iris mammillations is higher among patients with neurofibromatosis type 1.

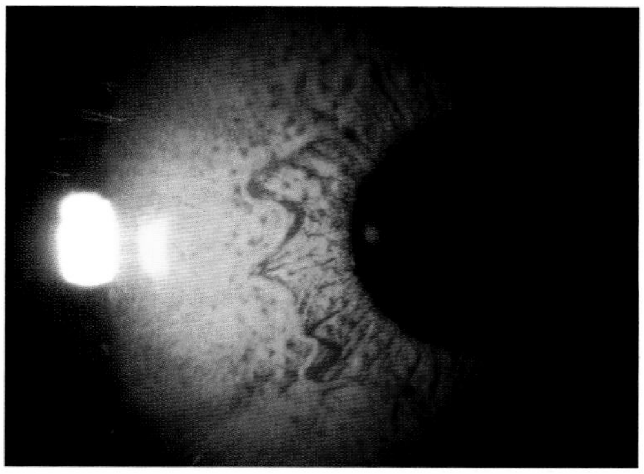

Figure 21-19 Iris mammillations. The nodules are diffuse and are the same color as the iris (Lisch nodules, by contrast, are lighter or darker than the surrounding iris). *(Courtesy of Arlene Drack, MD.)*

眼前节肿瘤

角膜

角膜肿瘤在儿童当中极其罕见，但有报道着色性干皮病发生鳞状细胞癌的病例。

虹膜

结节

Lisch 结节　*Lisch 结节*发生于神经纤维瘤，见第 28 章中讨论。

幼年性黄色肉芽肿　*幼年性黄色肉芽肿*是一种非肿瘤性组织细胞增生，发生于 2 岁以下的婴儿，其特点是 Touton 巨细胞的存在。典型的临床表现为皮肤受累，包括一个或多个小的、圆形的、橙色或棕褐色丘疹，但并不是所有患儿都会存在。虹膜病变较罕见，且单眼发病，呈肉质的、黄褐色、小的肿块，局部或弥漫的浸润整个虹膜，形成虹膜异色症。自发性出血伴前房积血也是特征性的临床表现。继发性青光眼可能会引起急性疼痛，畏光和视力丧失。有多处皮肤病变的儿童眼部受累的风险最大。

幼年性黄色肉芽肿是一种自限性疾病，常在 5 岁时自行消退，但为了避免眼部并发症，需要及时治疗。局部皮质类固醇和降眼压常可有效控制病情。如果存在顽固性青光眼，应考虑手术切除或放射治疗。

虹膜乳头样突起　*虹膜乳头样突起*可单眼或双眼发病，虹膜表面呈现微小的、弥漫性、色素沉着结节（图 21–19）。在色素较深的眼睛中更常见，且与虹膜同色。结节呈双眼孤立的，常染色体显性遗传，亦可伴眼 – 皮肤黑色素细胞增多症，或 IIb 型色素血管性斑痣性错构瘤病（持续性焰色痣，异常蒙古斑）。有报道，虹膜乳头样突起亦可出现在睫状体肿瘤和脉络膜黑色素瘤中。该病需与 Lisch 结节鉴别：乳头样突起常为深褐色、光滑，均匀分布，近瞳孔时可略大。神经纤维瘤病 1 型患者虹膜乳头样突起发病率较高。

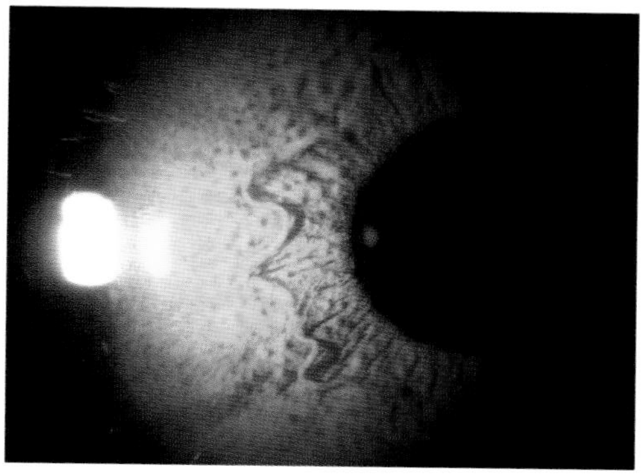

图 21–19　虹膜乳头样突起。与虹膜颜色一样弥漫性分布的结节（Lisch 结节，与周围虹膜相比，颜色稍淡或稍暗）。*（译者注：资料来源见前页原文。）*

Brushfield spots Focal areas of iris stromal hyperplasia surrounded by relative hypoplasia occur in up to 90% of patients with Down syndrome; in such patients, these areas are known as *Brushfield spots*. They are hypopigmented. Similar lesions, known as *Wolfflin nodules*, occur in up to 24% of healthy individuals. Neither condition is visually significant.

Cysts

Primary iris cysts These cysts may originate from the iris pigment epithelium or the iris stroma.

CYSTS OF IRIS PIGMENT EPITHELIUM Spontaneous cysts of the iris pigment epithelium result from a separation of the 2 layers of epithelium anywhere between the pupil and ciliary body (Fig 21-20). These cysts tend to be stable and rarely cause ocular complications. They are usually not diagnosed until the teenaged years.

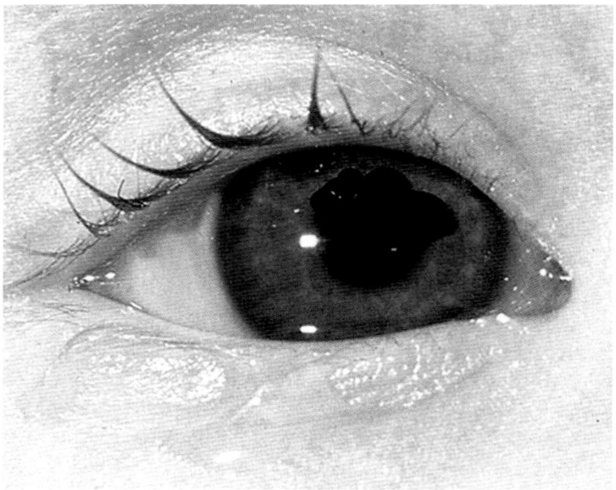

Figure 21-20 Cysts of the iris pigment epithelium at the pupillary border (flocculi).

CENTRAL CYSTS Pigment epithelial cysts at the pupillary border, also termed *iris flocculi*, are sometimes hereditary. In rare cases, they may be from an *ACTA2* mutation (see the section "Congenital mydriasis"). They are usually diagnosed in infancy. The cysts may enlarge slowly but generally remain asymptomatic and rarely require treatment. Cholinesteraseinhibiting eyedrops such as echothiophate may produce similar pupillary cysts, especially in young phakic eyes. Discontinuation of the drug or concomitant administration of phenylephrine generally results in improvement.

CYSTS OF IRIS STROMA Primary iris stromal cysts are often diagnosed in infancy. They are most likely caused by sequestration of epithelium during embryologic development. The epithelium-lined stromal cysts usually contain goblet cells, and they may enlarge, causing obstruction of the visual axis, glaucoma, corneal decompensation, or iritis from cyst leakage.

Numerous treatments have been described, including cyst aspiration and photocoagulation or photodisruption, but the sudden release of cystic contents may result in transient iritis and glaucoma. Because of these potential complications and frequent cyst recurrence, surgical excision may be the preferred treatment method. Iris stromal cysts account for approximately 16% of childhood iris cysts. The visual prognosis is guarded.

Brushfield 斑点 局灶虹膜基质增生周围，环绕相对发育不全，即色素减少，称为*Brushfield 斑点*，90%的 Down 综合征患儿有此症。24%的健康个体中可有类似改变，称为 *Wolfflin 结节*。这两种情况对视力没有影响。

囊肿

原发性虹膜囊肿 囊肿可源于虹膜色素上皮细胞或虹膜基质。

虹膜色素上皮囊肿 虹膜色素上皮自发性囊肿是指瞳孔至睫状体之间的 2 层上皮分离（图 21–20）。囊肿稳定，少有眼部并发症，常在十几岁被确诊。

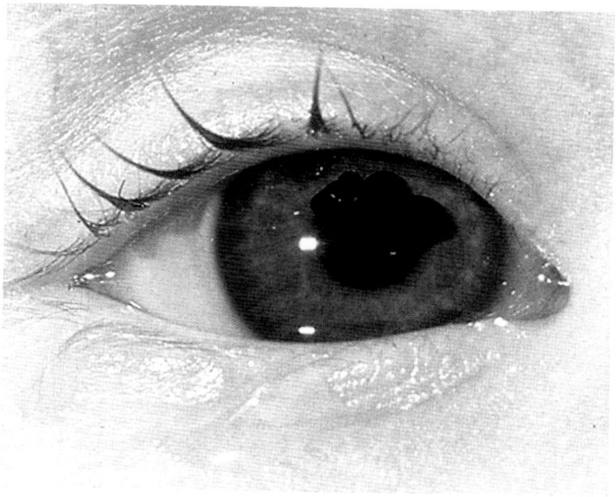

图 21–20 瞳孔边缘的虹膜色素上皮细胞囊肿（絮状）。

虹膜中心囊肿 瞳孔缘的色素上皮囊肿，也称为*虹膜絮状物*，有遗传性。在极少数情况下，系 *ACTA2* 基因突变（见“先天性大瞳孔”一节）。婴儿期确诊，囊肿缓慢增大，无症状，很少需治疗。胆碱酯酶抑制剂滴眼液，如乙膦硫胆碱 / 依可酯可产生类似的瞳孔囊肿，特别是儿童有晶状体眼，停药或同时用去氧肾上腺素可减小囊肿。

虹膜基质囊肿 原发性虹膜基质囊肿常在婴儿期诊断。可能是胚胎发育过程中上皮细胞的隔离。内衬上皮的基质囊肿可见杯状细胞，囊肿增大可遮挡视轴、导致青光眼、角膜失代偿或囊肿渗漏引发虹膜炎。

治疗方法有囊肿抽吸术和光凝术或光致破裂术，但囊肿内容物的突然释放可导致一过性虹膜炎和青光眼。由于存在上述潜在的并发症和囊肿的复发，应首选手术切除。虹膜基质囊肿占儿童虹膜囊肿的 16%，应注意视力预后。

Secondary iris cysts Secondary iris cysts have been reported in childhood after trauma; they are also associated with tumors and iris nevi.

Ciliary Body

Medulloepithelioma

A *medulloepithelioma (diktyoma)* originates from the nonpigmented epithelium of the ciliary body and most often presents as an iris mass during the first decade of life. Secondary glaucoma, hyphema, and ectopia lentis et pupillae or sectoral cataract (Fig 21-21) are less frequent initial manifestations. This rare lesion shows a spectrum of clinical and pathologic characteristics, ranging from benign to malignant. Although distant metastasis is rare, local invasion can lead to death. Teratoid elements are often present. Enucleation is usually required and is curative in most cases.

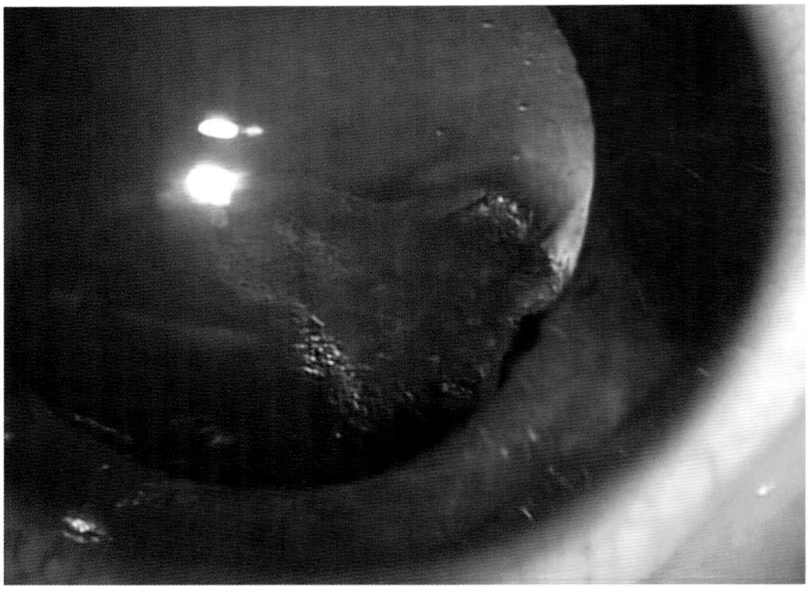

Figure 21-21 Sectoral cataract adjacent to medulloepithelioma. *(Courtesy of Ken K. Nischal, MD.)*

Miscellaneous Clinical Signs

Pediatric Iris Heterochromia

The differential diagnosis of pediatric iris heterochromia is extensive. Causes can be classified based on whether the condition is congenital or acquired and whether the affected eye is hypopigmented or hyperpigmented (Fig 21-22, Table 21-3). Trauma, chronic iridocyclitis, intraocular surgery, and use of topical prostaglandin analogues are important causes of acquired hyperpigmented heterochromia. Whether congenital or acquired, hypopigmented heterochromia that is associated with a more miotic pupil and ptosis on the ipsilateral side should prompt a workup for Horner syndrome.

继发性虹膜囊肿　有报道儿童外伤后继发虹膜囊肿。还可发生在肿瘤和虹膜痣。

睫状体

髓上皮瘤

*髓上皮瘤（视网膜胚瘤）*起源于睫状体无色素上皮，常在 10 岁前表现为虹膜肿块。最初很少发生继发性青光眼、前房出血和晶状体瞳孔异位或扇形白内障（图 21–21）。此病罕见，临床和病理特征呈现出从良性到恶性的一个序列。虽然很少远处转移，但局部侵及可致死。常有畸胎瘤成分。常需摘除眼球，且多数可治疗。

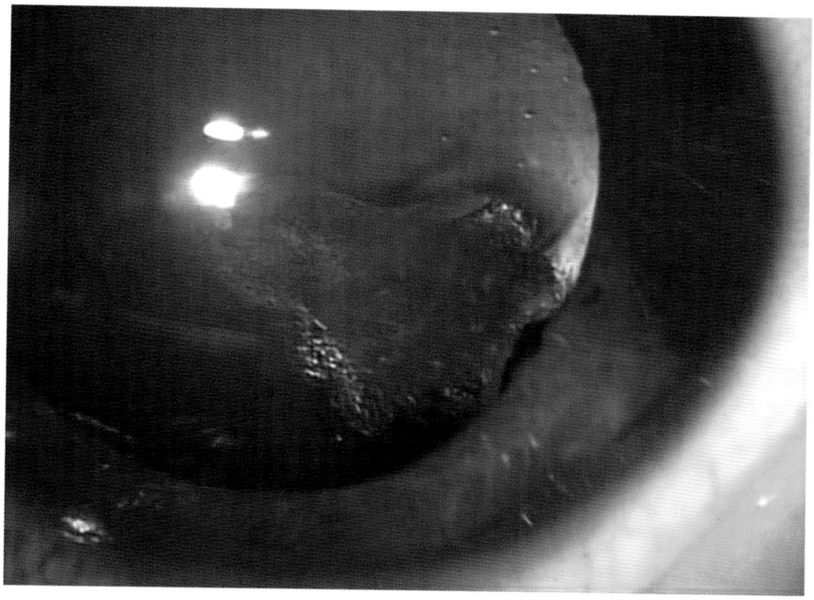

图 21–21　与髓上皮瘤相邻的扇形白内障。*（译者注：资料来源见前页原文。）*

其他临床体征

小儿虹膜异色症

小儿虹膜异色症的鉴别诊断很广泛。根据先天性或获得性、受累眼色素减少或色素沉着，进行分类（图 21–22，表 21–3）。外伤、慢性虹膜睫状体炎、眼内手术和局部前列腺素类药引起获得性色素沉着异色症。无论是先天性还是获得性色素减少异色症，同时伴有瞳孔缩小和同侧上睑下垂时，应做 Horner 综合征的相关检查。

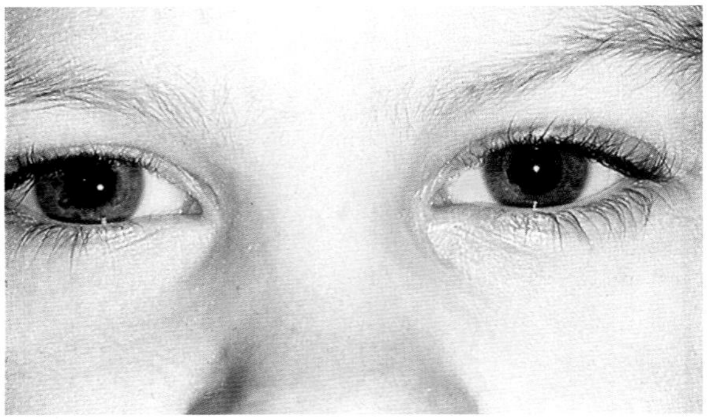

Figure 21-22 Iris heterochromia. The left iris has become darker since development of a traumatic cataract. *(Courtesy of John W. Simon, MD.)*

Table 21-3 Causes of Pediatric Iris Heterochromia

Hypochromic heterochromia
Horner syndrome (congenital or early in life)
Incontinentia pigmenti (Bloch-Sulzberger syndrome; rare)
Fuchs heterochromia
Waardenburg syndrome
Nonpigmented tumors
Hypomelanosis of Ito
Hyperchromic heterochromia
Oculodermal melanocytosis (associated with glaucoma in nonwhite adults)
Pigmented tumors
Siderosis
Iris ectropion syndrome
Extensive rubeosis
Port-wine stain
Trauma
Chronic iridocyclitis
Intraocular surgery
Topical prostaglandin analogues

Modified with permission from Roy FH. *Ocular Differential Diagnosis.* 3rd ed. Philadelphia: Lea & Febiger; 1984.

Anisocoria

In equality in the diameters of the 2 pupils is called anisocoria. For a detailed discussion of anisocoria and the following conditions, see BCSC Section 5, *Neuro-Ophthalmology.*

Physiologic anisocoria

Physiologic anisocoria is a common cause of a difference in size between the 2 pupils. This difference is usually less than 1 mm and can vary from day to day in an individual. The in equality does not change significantly when the patient is in dim light or bright light.

Tonic pupil

Features of a tonic pupil include anisocoria that is greater in bright light and a pupil that is sluggishly and segmentally responsive to light and more responsive to near effort. Greaterthan-normal constriction in response to dilute pilocarpine is diagnostic. Possible etiologic causes in children include varicella-zoster virus infection and Adie syndrome with absence of deep tendon reflexes.

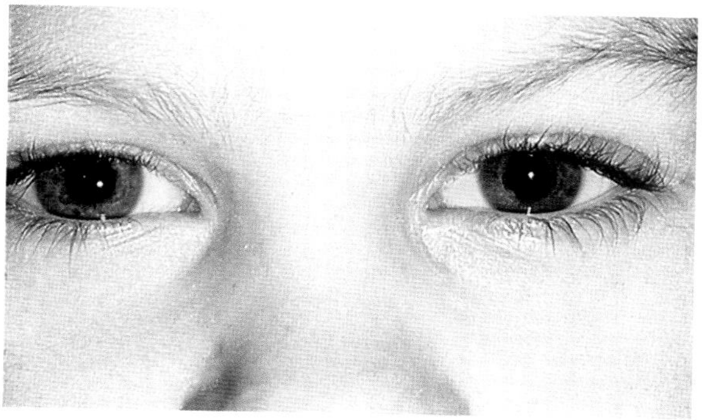

图 21-22　虹膜异色症。左眼虹膜颜色随着外伤性白内障的进展逐渐变深。*（译者注：资料来源见前页原文。）*

表21-3　小儿虹膜异色症常见原因

低色素异色症
Horner综合征（先天性或早期）
色素失调症（Bloch - Sulzberger综合征；罕见）
Fuchs异色症
Waardenburg综合征
非色素性肿瘤
Ito色素减少症
高色素异色症
眼–皮肤黑素细胞增多症（与非白人成年人青光眼有关）
色素瘤
铁质沉着症
虹膜外翻综合征
广泛虹膜红变
焰色痣
外伤
慢性虹膜睫状体炎
内眼手术
局部前列腺素类药

（译者注：资料来源见前页原文。）

瞳孔不等大

双眼瞳孔直径不一致称为瞳孔不等大。关于瞳孔不等大的详细讨论，见 BCSC 第 5 册《*神经眼科学*》。

生理性瞳孔不等大

常见的双眼瞳孔大小差异原因是生理性瞳孔不等大，这种差异小于 1mm，并随时间而不同。在暗处或强光下，瞳孔大小不会显著改变。

强直性瞳孔

强直性瞳孔的特征包括：在明亮光线下瞳孔不等大明显，瞳孔对光反应缓慢且呈节段状，瞳孔近反射更敏感。对稀释的毛果芸香碱的“大于正常的”收缩反应即可确诊。儿童可能的病因有水痘 – 带状疱疹病毒感染和伴有深腱反射缺如的 Adie 综合征。

Horner syndrome

A lesion at any location along the oculosympathetic pathway may lead to *Horner syndrome.* Affected patients have anisocoria that is greater in dim light and ptosis secondary to paralysis of the Müller muscle. Congenital cases may be associated with iris heterochromia in which the affected iris is lighter in color. However, the heterochromia may not be present in infants because the normal iris needs time to acquire pigment.

The diagnosis of Horner syndrome can be confirmed with the use of topical cocaine or apraclonidine drops. Apraclonidine reverses the anisocoria, causing dilation of the affected (smaller) pupil and having no effect on the normal pupil. This agent should be used with caution in young children, as it may cause excessive sedation owing to its central nervous system effects. Additional pharmacologic testing may not be necessary in the presence of typical clinical findings.

Horner syndrome in children may be idiopathic or may be caused by trauma, surgery, or the presence of neuroblastoma affecting the sympathetic chain in the chest. For children with acquired Horner syndrome but no history of trauma or surgery that could explain the anisocoria, evaluation should include imaging studies of the brain, neck, and chest. The value of measuring catecholamine excretion has been questioned because some patients with normal catecholamine measurements have been found to have neuroblastomas.

***Horner* 综合征**

沿眼交感神经通路的任何部位病变均可导致 *Horner 综合征*。受累患儿在暗光线下双眼瞳孔不等大明显，继发于 Müller 肌麻痹性眼睑下垂。先天性患儿伴虹膜异色症，其受累虹膜颜色变浅。但虹膜异色症不发生于婴儿，因为正常的虹膜需要时间以获取色素。

Horner 综合征的诊断是通过局部使用可卡因或阿拉可乐定进行确诊。阿拉可乐定使得受累（较小）瞳孔扩张，而对正常瞳孔则无影响，从而逆转瞳孔不等大。该药在幼儿应谨慎使用，因为对中枢神经系统产生过度镇静作用。临床表现典型时，不需额外的药理学试验。

儿童 Horner 综合征可能是特发性的，也可能由外伤、手术或累及胸交感神经链的神经母细胞瘤引起。若没有解释瞳孔不等大的外伤或手术史时，获得性 Horner 综合征的儿童需行脑、颈部和胸部的影像学检查和评估。有人质疑测量儿茶酚胺排泄的意义，因为一些神经母细胞瘤的患者具有正常的儿茶酚胺浓度。

（翻译　何元浩　吴以凡　陈娜 // 审校　刘陇黔　石一宁 // 章节审校　石广礼）

CHAPTER 22

Pediatric Glaucomas

This chapter includes related videos, which can be accessed by scanning the QR codes provided in the text or going to www.aao.org/bcscvideo_section06.

Pediatric glaucomas are a heterogeneous group of diseases that may result from an isolated congenital abnormality of the aqueous outflow pathways (primary glaucoma) or from abnormalities affecting other regions of the eye (secondary glaucoma). A variety of systemic conditions are associated with pediatric glaucoma. See BCSC Section 10, *Glaucoma*, for additional discussion of topics covered in this chapter.

Classification

In 2013, an international classification system for childhood glaucoma was established by the Childhood Glaucoma Research Network and the World Glaucoma Association. In the classification system, *childhood glaucoma* is defined as intraocular pressure (IOP)–related damage to the eye as opposed to IOP-related damage to the optic nerve, which defines adult glaucoma. This classification is summarized in Table 22-1, and an algorithm for classifying a patient with childhood glaucoma using these criteria is presented in Figure 22-1.

Beck AD, Chang TCP, Freedman SF. Definition, classification, differential diagnosis. In: Weinreb RN, Grajewski AL, Papadopoulos M, Grigg J, Freedman S, eds. Childhood Glaucoma. Amsterdam: Kugler Publications; 2013:3–10. *World Glaucoma Association Consensus Series—9.*

Table 22-1 Classification of Childhood Glaucoma

Primary childhood glaucoma
Primary congenital glaucoma (PCG)
Neonatal or newborn onset (age 0–1 month)
Infantile onset (age 1–24 months)
Late-onset or late-recognized (age ≥24 months)
Juvenile open-angle glaucoma (JOAG)
Secondary childhood glaucoma
Glaucoma associated with nonacquired ocular anomalies
Glaucoma associated with nonacquired systemic disease or syndrome
Glaucoma associated with acquired condition
Glaucoma following cataract surgery

Information from Beck AD, Chang TCP, Freedman SF. Definition, classification, differential diagnosis. In: Weinreb RN, Grajewski AL, Papadopoulos M, Grigg J, Freedman S, eds. *Childhood Glaucoma.* Amsterdam: Kugler Publications; 2013:3–10. *World Glaucoma Association Consensus Series—9.*

第 22 章

小儿青光眼

本章包含的相关视频可通过扫描文中的二维码或登陆网址 www.aao.org/bcscvideo_section06 观看。

小儿青光眼是不同病因所致的一组疾病，可以是单纯的房水流出通道的先天性异常（原发性青光眼），或其他累及眼部的异常（继发性青光眼）。多种全身性疾病与小儿青光眼有关。本章的其他讨论见 BCSC 第 10 册《*青光眼*》。

分类

2013 年，儿童青光眼研究网站和世界青光眼协会建立了儿童青光眼国际分类系统。在分类系统中，*儿童青光眼*的定义为与眼内压相关的眼损伤，与成人青光眼的定义不同，成人青光眼是与眼内压相关的视神经损伤。分类的汇总见表 22–1，在图 22–1 中给出了使用这些标准对儿童青光眼进行分类的步骤。

Beck AD, Chang TCP, Freedman SF. Definition, classification, differential diagnosis. In: Weinreb RN, Grajewski AL, Papadopoulos M, Grigg J, Freedman S, eds. Childhood Glaucoma. Amsterdam: Kugler Publications; 2013:3–10. *World Glaucoma Association Consensus Series—9.*

表22–1　儿童青光眼的分类

原发性儿童青光眼
原发性先天性青光眼（PCG）
新生儿或婴儿发病（0～1月）
婴幼儿发病（1～24个月）
晚期发病或晚期发现（≥24个月）
青少年性开角型青光眼（JOAG）
继发性儿童青光眼
伴非获得性眼部异常的青光眼
伴非获得性系统性疾病的青光眼
伴获得性疾病的青光眼
白内障术后青光眼

（译者注：资料来源见前页原文。）

Genetics

Although primary congenital glaucoma (PCG) usually occurs sporadically, it may be inherited as an autosomal recessive trait. When no other family history of PCG exists, the chance of an affected parent having a child with PCG is approximately 2%. Four chromosomal loci for PCG have been identified: GLC3A on band 2p21, GLC3B on 1p36, GLC3C on 14q24.3, and GLC3D on 14q24.3. Mutations in *CYP1B1* (at the GLC3A locus) have been shown to cause PCG. Populations in which consanguinity is common, especially those in which the carrier rate of the *CYP1B1* gene is high, have higher incidences of PCG. Individuals who carry the *CYP1B1* gene but who are nonpenetrant for PCG remain at higher risk for adult-onset glaucoma. *LTBP2* mutations (at the GLC3D locus) cause a primary megalocornea with zonular weakness, forward displacement of the lens, and a secondary glaucoma that responds poorly to standard angle surgery. In this condition, the preferred treatment is lens removal.

Juvenile open-angle glaucoma is inherited as an autosomal dominant trait and has been linked to the GLC1A myocilin gene (*MYOC*), which is also responsible for some forms of adult open-angle glaucoma.

The genetic causes of many conditions associated with secondary childhood glaucoma have been identified; they are discussed in the chapters associated with their primary conditions.

Khan AO, Aldahmesh MA, Alkuraya FS. Congenital megalocornea with zonular weakness and childhood lens-related secondary glaucoma—a distinct phenotype caused by recessive LTBP2 mutations. *Mol Vis.* 2011;17:2570–2579.

Primary Childhood Glaucoma

Primary Congenital Glaucoma

Primary congenital glaucoma (PCG; also called *congenital or infantile glaucoma*) is the most common form of childhood glaucoma. The incidence of PCG varies in different populations, ranging from 1 in 1250 live births to 1 in 68,000. PCG occurs more frequently in males (65% of cases), and it is bilateral in about two-thirds of patients. PCG results in blindness in 2%–15% of cases, and visual acuity remains worse than 20/50 in at least 50% of cases.

Although the diagnosis is made at birth in only 25% of affected infants, disease onset occurs within the first year of life in more than 80% of cases. Neonatal-onset and laterecognized PCG are associated with guarded prognoses.

Pathophysiology

The basic pathologic defect is increased resistance to aqueous outflow through the trabecular meshwork due to abnormal development of neural crest–derived tissue of the anterior chamber angle. The anomaly occurs late in embryologic development.

基因

虽然原发性先天性青光眼（PCG）偶尔发生，但可能为常染色体隐性遗传。即使无原发性先天性青光眼（PCG）家族史，但如果父母中有 1 位患病，则其孩子的患病率约为 2%。已确定 4 个原发性先天性青光眼（PCG）的染色体位点：2p21 上的 GLC3A，1p36 上的 GLC3B，14q24.3 上的 GLC3C 和 14q24.3 上的 GLC3D。已证实 *CYP1B1*（在 GLC3A 上）基因突变导致的原发性先天性青光眼（PCG）。有血缘关系的，特别是在携带 *CYP1B1* 基因的人群中，其原发性先天性青光眼（PCG）的发病率较高。*CYP1B1* 基因携带，但并无外显的个体，仍存在成人期发病的高风险。*LTBP2* 基因突变（在 GLC3D 上）可致原发性大角膜，伴悬韧带脆弱、晶状体前脱位和继发性青光眼（常规手术效果不佳），此症的首选治疗是晶状体摘除。

青少年开角型青光眼为常染色体显性遗传，并与 GLC1A 肌纤蛋白基因（*MYOC*）相关，这也导致部分类型的成人开角型青光眼。

继发性儿童型青光眼与许多疾病的遗传基因有关，讨论见相关原发性疾病的章节。

Khan AO, Aldahmesh MA, Alkuraya FS. Congenital megalocornea with zonular weakness and childhood lens-related secondary glaucoma—a distinct phenotype caused by recessive LTBP2 mutations. *Mol Vis.* 2011;17:2570–2579.

原发性儿童青光眼

原发性先天性青光眼

原发性先天性青光眼（PCG，亦称*先天性或婴幼儿型青光眼*）是最常见的儿童青光眼。原发性先天性青光眼 PCG 的发病率在不同人群中有所不同，为 1/68000 ~ 1/1250，男性更常见（65%），约 2/3 双眼发病，2% ~ 15%的患儿失明，50%的患者视力低于 20/50。

25%的婴儿在出生时确诊，80%在 1 岁内发病。新生儿发病和晚期发现的原发性先天性青光眼（PCG）的预后不佳。

病理生理

基本的病理改变是前房角神经嵴组织发育异常，房水经小梁网流出的阻力增加，多发生在胚胎发育后期。

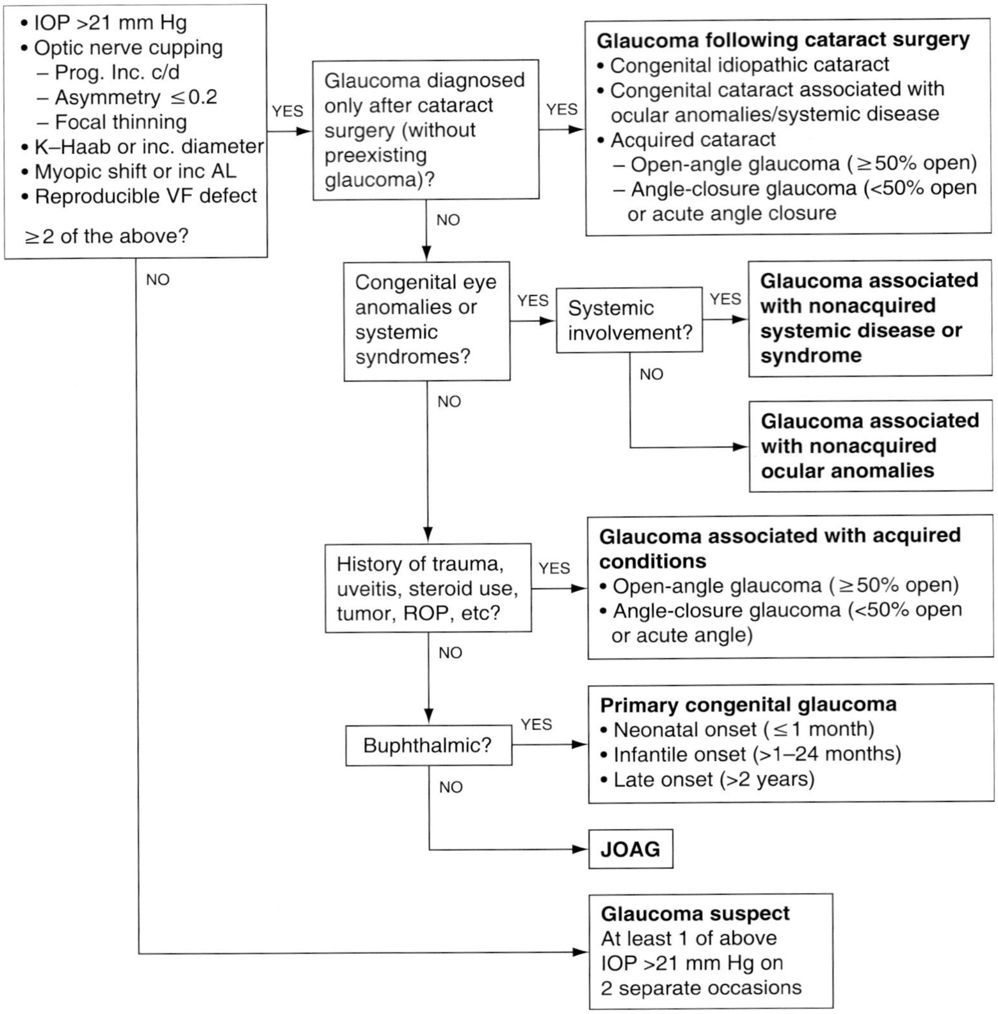

Figure 22-1 Childhood Glaucoma Research Network/World Glaucoma Association algorithm for the classification of childhood glaucoma. AL = axial length; C/D = cup–disc; JOAG = juvenile open-angle glaucoma; ROP = retinopathy of prematurity; VF = visual field. *(Courtesy of Allen Beck, MD, and Ta Chen Peter Chang, MD; www.gl-foundation.org/.)*

Clinical manifestations

Primary congenital glaucoma usually presents in the neonatal period or within the first 2 years of life (*infantile PCG*), but it can present or be recognized after 2 years of age (*late-onset* or *late-diagnosed PCG*). Epiphora, photophobia, and blepharospasm constitute the classic clinical triad of PCG. A red eye may be present. Other signs include clouding and enlargement of the cornea (Fig 22-2).Corneal edema results from elevated IOP and may be gradual or sudden in onset.

Corneal edema is often the presenting sign in infants younger than 3 months and is responsible for the clinical triad. Microcystic edema initially involves the corneal epithelium but later extends into the stroma, often accompanied by one or more curvilinear breaks in Descemet membrane (*Haab striae*) (Fig 22-3). Although the edema may resolve with IOP reduction, the split in Descemet membrane persists. Significant corneal scarring and persistent opacification may require penetrating keratoplasty. Corneal enlargement occurs with gradual stretching of the cornea as a result of elevated IOP.

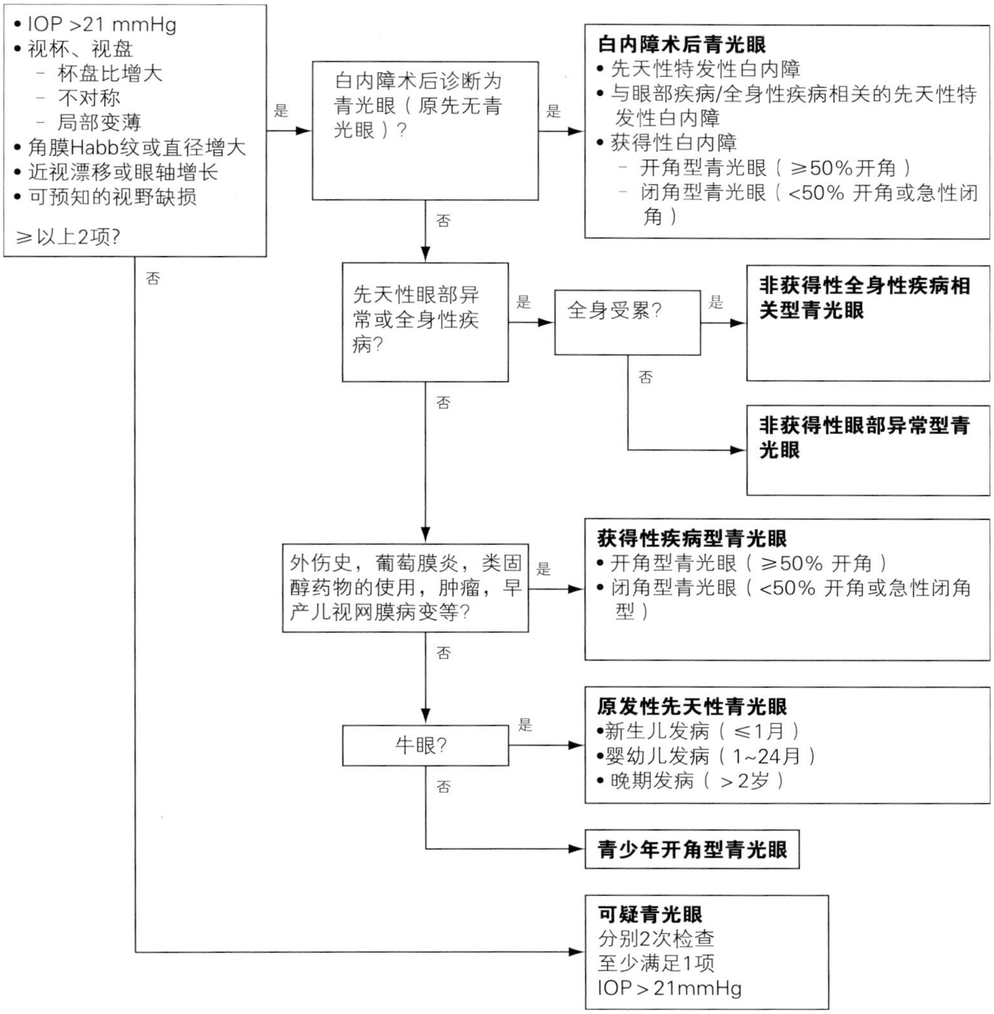

图 22–1　儿童青光眼研究网站 / 世界青光眼协会的儿童青光眼分类步骤。AL = 眼轴，C/D = 杯 / 盘比，JOAG = 青少年性开角型青光眼，ROP = 早产儿视网膜病变，VF = 视野。*（译者注：资料来源见前页原文。）*

临床表现

原发性先天性青光眼通常出现在新生儿期或出生后的 2 年内［*婴幼儿型原发性先天性青光眼（PCG）*］，但可在 2 岁后出现或发现［*晚期发病或晚期诊断的原发性先天性青光眼（PCG）*］。流泪、畏光和眼睑痉挛是原发性先天性青光眼（PCG）的典型临床三联征，也可有红眼。其他体征有角膜混浊和角膜扩张（图 22–2）。

角膜水肿是由于眼压（IOP）升高所致，可逐渐出现或突然发生。角膜水肿常发生于 3 个月以下的婴儿，是产生临床三联征的原因。微囊样水肿最初仅累及角膜上皮，逐渐扩展至基质层，常伴有 Descemet 膜 / 后弹力层 1 个或多个曲线断裂（*Haab 纹*）（图 22–3）。降低眼压则水肿消退，但 Descemet 膜 / 后弹力层的断裂仍存在。严重的角膜瘢痕和持续性角膜混浊需行穿透性角膜移植术。眼压（IOP）升高使角膜逐渐扩展，致使角膜扩张 / 增大。

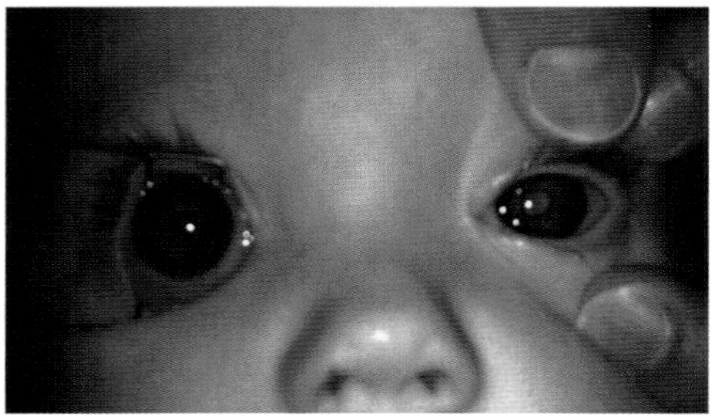

Figure 22-2 Primary congenital glaucoma, right eye. The cornea is enlarged. *(Courtesy of Gregg T. Lueder, MD.)*

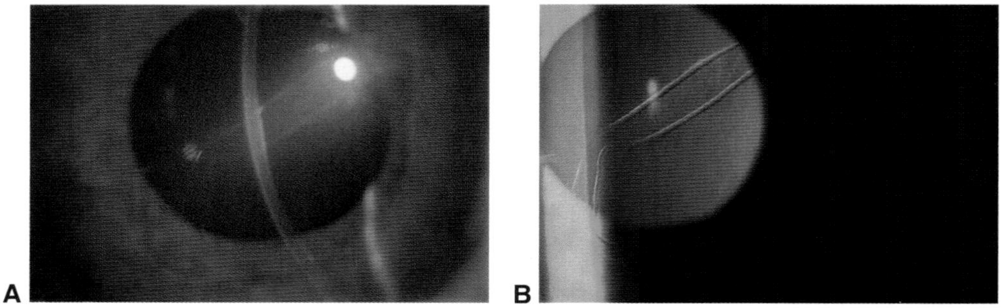

Figure 22-3 **A,** Breaks in Descemet membrane (Haab striae), right eye. **B,** Retroillumination, same eye.

The signs and symptoms of PCG can occur in infants with other forms of glaucoma as well. Nonglaucomatous conditions may also cause some of the signs and symptoms seen in PCG (Table 22-2).

Diagnostic examination

A full ophthalmologic examination of every child suspected of having glaucoma is imperative, despite the challenges. Both office examination and examination under general anesthesia are usually required. Although visual field testing is helpful in following disease progression in older children, results of these tests are rarely reliable in children younger than 6–8 years. Vision is usually poorer in the affected eye in unilateral cases and may be poor in both eyes when glaucoma is bilateral. Fixation and following behavior and the presence of nystagmus should be noted. Refraction, when possible, often reveals myopia and astigmatism from eye enlargement and corneal irregularity.

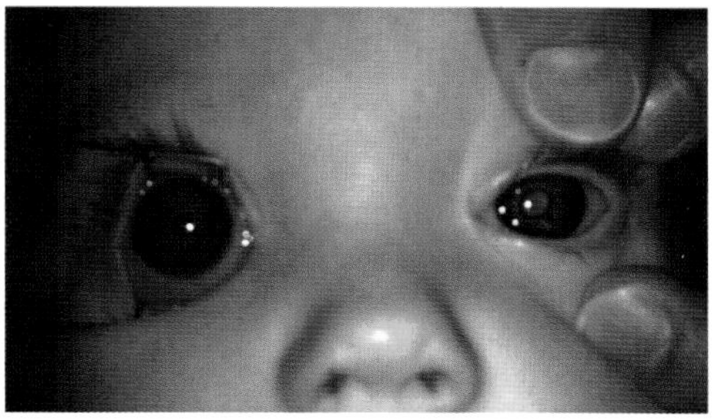

Figure 22–2　右眼原发性先天性青光眼。角膜扩张。*（译者注：资料来源见前页原文。）*

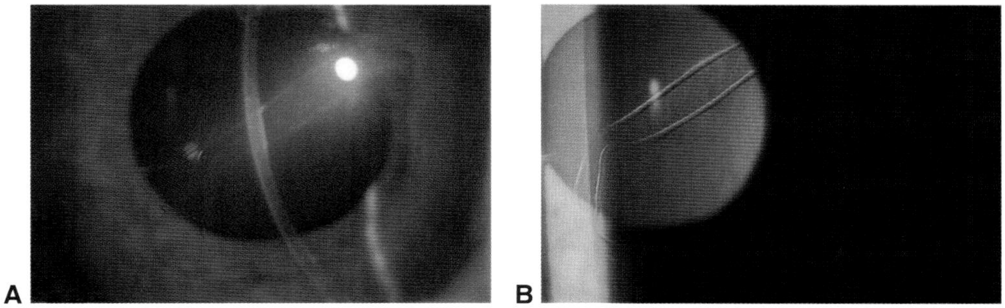

图 22–3　**A.** 右眼角膜后弹力层膜破裂（Haab 纹）。**B.** 右眼，后照法。

原发性先天性青光眼（PCG）的体征和症状亦可出现在其他类型青光眼，而非青光眼疾病也可能出现青光眼的症状和体征（表 22–2）。

诊断性检查

尽管儿童的眼科检查有些困难，但应对每个青光眼疑似儿童进行全面的眼科检查，可在门诊和全身麻醉下进行。视野检查有助于大龄儿童病情发展的随访，但 6 ~ 8 岁以下的儿童检查结果多不可信。单眼受累时受累眼的视力常较差，双眼受累时受累眼的视力都差，要注意观察眼的固视、追随行为和眼球震颤。屈光检查表现为近视和散光，系眼球扩张和角膜不规则所致。

Table 22-2 Differential Diagnosis of Signs in Primary Congenital Glaucoma

Conditions sharing signs of epiphora and red eye
Conjunctivitis
Congenital nasolacrimal duct obstruction
Corneal epithelial defect/abrasion
Keratitis
Ocular inflammation (eg, due to uveitis, trauma, foreign body)
Epiblepharon with eyelash touch
Conditions sharing sign of corneal edema or opacification
Corneal dystrophies: congenital hereditary endothelial dystrophy, posterior polymorphous dystrophy
Obstetric birth trauma with Descemet tears
Storage diseases: mucopolysaccharidoses, cystinosis, sphingolipidosis
Congenital anomalies: sclerocornea, Peters anomaly, choristomas
Keratitis (eg, secondary to maternal rubella, herpes, phlyctenules)
Keratomalacia (from vitamin A deficiency)
Skin disorders affecting the cornea: congenital ichthyosis, congenital dyskeratosis
Idiopathic (diagnosis of exclusion only)
Conditions sharing sign of corneal enlargement
Axial myopia
Megalocornea
Conditions sharing sign of optic nerve cupping (real or apparent)
Physiologic optic nerve cupping
Cupping associated with prematurity, periventricular leukomalacia
Optic nerve coloboma or pit
Optic atrophy
Optic nerve hypoplasia
Optic nerve malformation

Adapted with permission from Buckley EG. Primary congenital open-angle glaucoma. In: Kahook M, Schuman J, eds. *Chandler and Grant's Glaucoma.* 5th ed.Thorofare, NJ: Slack Incorporated; 2013.

Cornea The cornea should be examined for size, clarity, and Haab striae. In newborns, the normal horizontal diameter of the cornea is 9.5–10.5 mm; a diameter greater than 11.5 mm suggests glaucoma. By age 1 year, the normal corneal diameter is 10.0–11.5 mm; a diameter greater than 12.5 mm suggests abnormality. Glaucoma should be suspected in any child with a corneal diameter greater than 13.0 mm. A difference as small as 0.5 mm between the 2 eyes may be significant. Haab striae are best seen against the red reflex after pupil dilation (see Fig 22-3B).

Central corneal thickness Portable ultrasonic pachymeters may be used to measure central corneal thickness (CCT), which is typically higher in infants with glaucoma. CCT affects the IOP measurement, but current evidence is inadequate to quantify these effects. See also Chapter 15.

Tonometry If the child is struggling during measurement of IOP, pressure readings may be falsely elevated. Examination under sedation or anesthesia may be necessary in children for accurate assessment, but IOP can also be unpredictably altered (usually lowered) with anesthetics and sedation. A useful technique to avoid these issues is to have the parent bottle-feed the infant during pressure measurement. In infants and young children, the most commonly used tonometers are Icare (Icare Finland Oy, Helsinki, Finland), Tono-Pen (Reichert Technologies, Depew, NY), and Perkins (Haag-Streit USA, Mason, OH). Goldmann applanation readings are preferred when a child is old enough to cooperate.

表22-2　原发性先天性青光眼体征的鉴别诊断

有泪溢和红眼体征的疾病
- 结膜炎
- 先天性鼻泪管阻塞
- 角膜上皮缺损/磨损
- 角膜炎
- 眼部炎症（例如，由葡萄膜炎、外伤、异物引起）
- 内眦赘皮伴睫毛后倾

有角膜水肿或者混浊体征的疾病
- 角膜营养不良：先天性遗传性内皮营养不良，后部多形性营养不良
- 产科分娩创伤伴后弹力层破裂
- 贮积病：黏多糖贮积病、胱氨酸病、鞘脂沉着症
- 先天性异常：硬化性角膜、Peters 异常（角膜基质中角膜细胞分化及细胞外基质异常）、脉络膜瘤
- 角膜炎（如：继发于母体风疹、疱疹、小水泡）
- 角膜软化症（由维生素A缺乏引起）
- 影响角膜的皮肤病：先天性鱼鳞病、先天性角化不良
- 特发性（仅排除诊断）

有角膜扩大体征的疾病
- 轴性近视
- 大角膜

有视杯增大体征的疾病（真实的或明显的）
- 生理性大视杯
- 早产或脑室周围白质软化症相关的大视杯
- 视神经缺或坑
- 视神经萎缩
- 视神经发育不全
- 视神经畸形

（译者注：资料来源见前页原文。）

角膜　需检查角膜的大小、透明度和 Haab 条纹。新生儿的正常角膜水平直径为 9.5 ~ 10.5mm，> 11.5mm 提示有青光眼。1 岁时的正常角膜直径为 10.0 ~ 11.5mm，> 12.5mm 提示异常。角膜直径> 13.0mm 的儿童都应怀疑青光眼。双眼角膜直径相差 0.5mm 的具有显著差异性。瞳孔散大后，使用红光反射法最容易观察到 Haab 条纹（见图 22-3B）。

中央角膜厚度　便携式超声波测厚仪可用于测量中央角膜厚度（CCT），青光眼婴儿的中央角膜厚度（CCT）较厚。中央角膜厚度（CCT）影响眼压（IOP）测量，但目前尚不能量化这些影响。见第 15 章。

眼压测量　如果测量眼压（IOP）时孩子不配合，眼压读数会错误性地偏高。为了准确评估，需使用镇静剂或麻醉，但麻醉或镇静下的眼压改变亦无法预测（常降低）。避免这些问题的有效方法是，在测量眼压时给婴儿喂奶。婴幼儿最常用的眼压计是 Icare（Icare Finland Oy, Helsinki, Finland），Tono-Pen（Reichert Technologies, Depew, NY）和 Perkins（Haag-Streit USA, Mason, OH）。当孩子可以配合时，最好使用 Goldmann 压平式眼压计。

The normal mean IOP in infants and young children is lower than that in adults: between 10 and 12 mm Hg in newborns and approximately 14 mm Hg by age 7–8 years. In PCG, IOP commonly ranges between 30 and 40 mm Hg, and it is usually greater than 20 mm Hg even with the patient under anesthesia. Asymmetric IOP readings in a quiet or anesthetized child should raise suspicion of glaucoma.

Anterior segment A portable slit lamp enables detailed examination of the anterior seg-ment. An abnormally deep anterior chamber and hypoplasia of the peripheral iris stroma are common findings in PCG.

Gonioscopy provides important information about the mechanism of glaucoma. A direct (Koeppe-type) goniolens is preferred for examining children. The anterior chamber angle of a normal infant eye (Fig 22-4A) differs from that of an adult's eye in the following ways:

- The trabecular meshwork is more lightly pigmented.
- The Schwalbe line is often less distinct.
- The uveal meshwork is translucent, so the junction between the scleral spur and the ciliary body band is often not well seen.

In an eye with PCG, the iris often shows a more anterior insertion compared with the insertion in a normal infant eye, and the translucence of the uveal meshwork is altered, making the ciliary body band, trabecular meshwork, and scleral spur indistinct (Fig 22-4B). The scalloped border of the iris pigment epithelium is often unusually prominent, especially when peripheral iris stromal hypoplasia is present.

Optic nerve In PCG, the optic nerve, when visible, usually shows increased cupping. Generalized enlargement of the optic cup in very young patients with glaucoma has been attributed to stretching of the optic canal and backward bowing of the lamina cribrosa. In most eyes with PCG, the cup–disc ratio exceeds 0.3, whereas in most normal newborn eyes, the cup–disc ratio is less than 0.3. Cup–disc asymmetry greater than 0.2 between the 2 eyes is also suggestive of glaucoma. In young children, optic nerve cupping may be reversible if IOP is lowered (Fig 22-5). Whenever possible, photographs should be taken of the optic disc for comparison during later examinations.

Axial length Serial measurement of axial length is useful for monitoring disease progression in infant eyes. Excessive axial length in an eye, especially compared with the fellow eye, may indicate inadequate IOP control.

Optical coherence tomography Newer methods of optic nerve and retinal nerve fiber analysis, such as optical coherence tomography (OCT), are being used as objective tools for follow-up of children with elevated IOP and glaucoma. Macular thickness, retinal nerve fiber layer thickness, and optic nerve topography have been shown to vary with race, axial length, and age in children, but normative data are becoming available, which should further increase the usefulness of OCT in the assessment of pediatric glaucoma.

婴幼儿正常的平均眼压低于成人，为 10 ~ 12mmHg；7 ~ 8 岁时的眼压约为 14mmHg。原发性先天性青光眼 PCG 的眼压常在 30 ~ 40mmHg，即使在麻醉下，眼压亦高于 20mmHg。安静或麻醉状态下，眼压读数有差异应怀疑青光眼。

眼前节　便携式裂隙灯可对眼前节进行详细检查。原发性先天性青光眼（PCG）可见前房异常加深和周边虹膜基质发育不全。

前房角镜检查提供青光眼发病机制的重要信息。检查儿童时最好使用直接型前房角镜(Koeppe 型)。正常婴儿的前房角（图 22-4A）与成人的差别体现在以下方面：

- 小梁网颜色较浅。
- Schwalbe 线常不明显。
- 葡萄膜小梁网呈半透明，巩膜突和睫状体带之间的连接常不易看到。

与正常婴幼儿相比，原发性先天性青光眼（PCG）的虹膜附着前移，葡萄膜小梁网半透明改变，使睫状体带、小梁网和巩膜突模糊不清（图 22-4B）。虹膜色素上皮的扇形边缘异常突出，特别是在有周边虹膜基质发育不良时。

视神经　原发性先天性青光眼（PCG）可见视神经的增大视杯。婴幼儿青光眼的视杯普遍增大，是由于视神经管的伸展和筛板的后弯所致。多数原发性先天性青光眼（PCG）的杯盘比＞ 0.3，而多数正常新生儿的杯盘比＜ 0.3。双眼杯盘比的差异＞ 0.2 也提示青光眼。如果眼压降低，则儿童的视杯增大可逆（图 22-5）。尽可能拍视盘照片，以便日后进行比较。

眼轴　连续眼轴测量有助于监控婴幼儿病情的进展。单眼眼轴过长，特别是比较对侧眼时，提示眼压控制不佳。

光学相干断层扫描　新的视神经和视网膜神经纤维层分析方法，如光学相干断层扫描（OCT）等客观检测，已用于随访高眼压和青光眼的儿童。在不同种族、眼轴长度和年龄的儿童中，黄斑厚度、视网膜神经纤维层厚度和视神经形态有所不同，现已有标准数据库，这进一步提高了 OCT 在儿童青光眼评估中的应用。

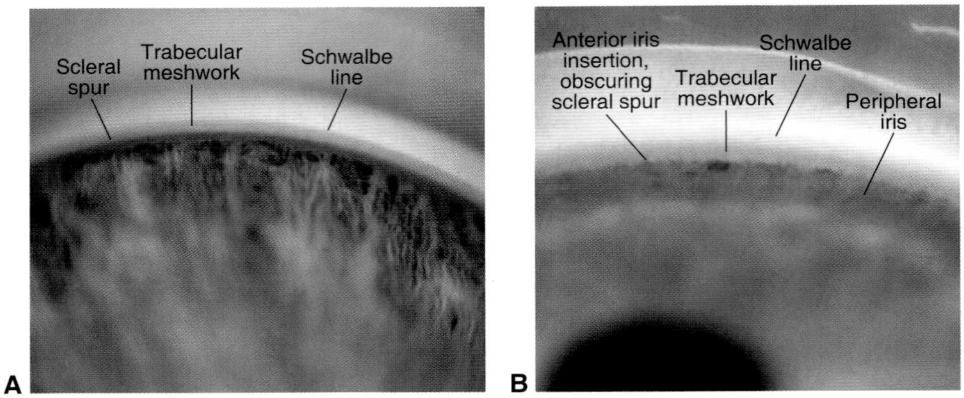

Figure 22-4 **A**, The anterior chamber angle of a normal infant eye, as seen by direct gonioscopy with a Koeppe lens. **B**, Typical appearance of the anterior chamber angle of an infant with primary congenital glaucoma. Note the scalloped appearance of the peripheral iris. The anterior iris insertion obscures the scleral spur. *(Courtesy of Ken K. Nischal, MD.)*

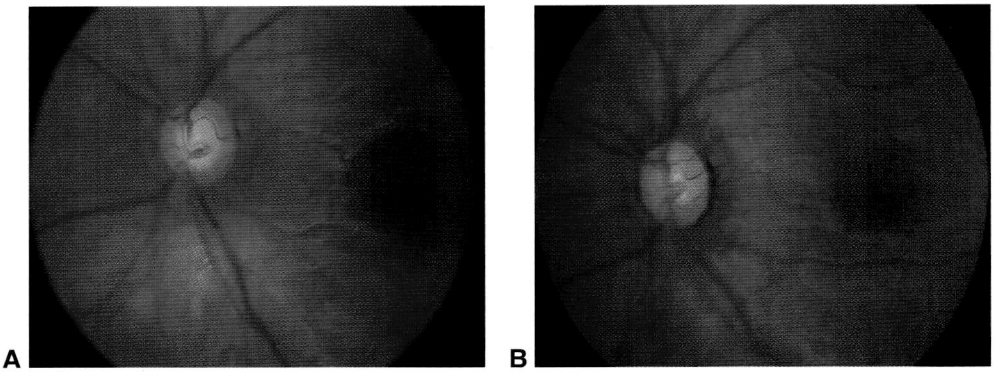

Figure 22–5 Optic nerve changes after treatment of congenital glaucoma. A, Preoperative enlarged optic disc cup. B, Reduction in disc cupping after intraocular pressure is reduced by goniotomy. *(Reproduced from Mochizuki H, Lesley AG, Brandt JD. Shrinkage of the scleral canal during cupping rever-sal in children. Ophthalmology. 2011;118(10):2009.)*

El-Dairi MA, Asrani SG, Enyedi LB, Freedman SF. Optical coherence tomography in the eyes of normal children. *Arch Ophthalmol.* 2009;127(1):50–58.

Prakalapakorn SG, Freedman SF, Lokhnygina Y, et al. Longitudinal reproducibility of optical coherence tomography measurements in children. *J AAPOS.* 2012;16(6):523–528.

Natural history

Untreated PCG almost always progresses to blindness. The cornea irreversibly opacifies and may vascularize. It may continue to enlarge through the first 2–3 years of life, reaching a diameter of up to 17 mm. As the entire eye enlarges, pseudoproptosis and an "ox eye" appearance (buphthalmos) may result. Scleral thinning and myopic fundus changes may occur, and spontaneous lens dislocation can result. Optic nerve damage progresses, leading to complete blindness. However, rare cases of spontaneous resolution have been reported.

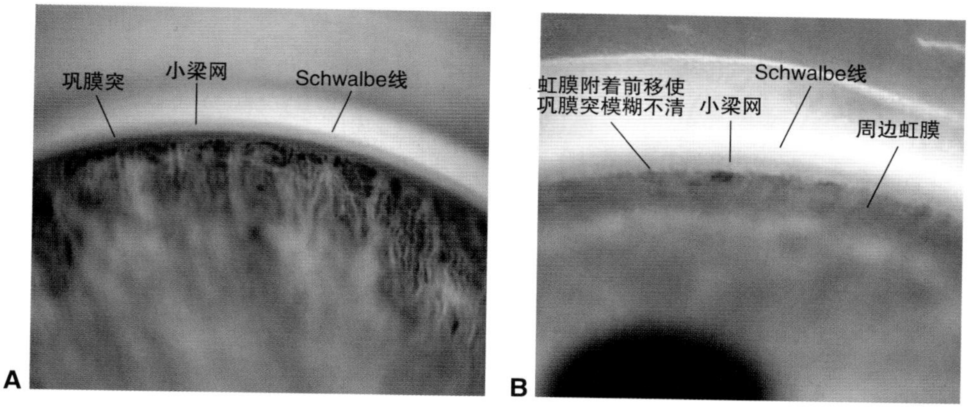

图 22-4 **A.** 使用直接前房角镜及 Koeppe 镜观察正常婴儿的眼前房角。**B**. 原发性先天性青光眼婴儿前房角的典型表现。注意周边虹膜的扇形外观，虹膜附着前移使巩膜突模糊不清。*（译者注：资料来源见前页原文。）*

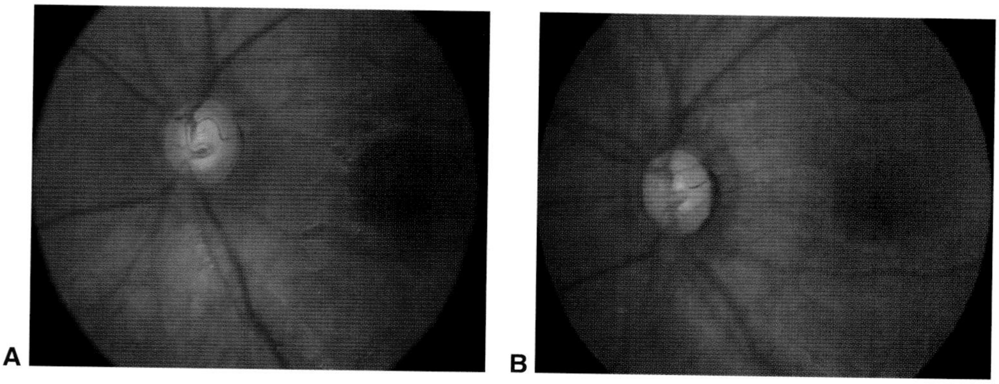

图 22-5 先天性青光眼治疗后的视神经改变。**A.** 术前视盘视杯扩大。**B.** 前房角切开术后眼压降低，扩大的视杯减小。*（译者注：资料来源见前页原文。）*

El-Dairi MA, Asrani SG, Enyedi LB, Freedman SF. Optical coherence tomography in the eyes of normal children. *Arch Ophthalmol*. 2009;127(1):50–58.

Prakalapakorn SG, Freedman SF, Lokhnygina Y, et al. Longitudinal reproducibility of optical coherence tomography measurements in children. *J AAPOS*. 2012;16(6):523–528.

自然病程

未经治疗的原发性先天性青光眼（PCG）基本失明，角膜混浊不可逆，并血管化。在出生后的前 2 ~ 3 年，角膜继续扩大，直径可达 17mm。当整个眼球扩张时，最终会呈现假性眼球突出和“牛眼”外观（牛眼），巩膜变薄和近视性眼底改变，以及自发性晶状体脱位。视神经进行性损害，导致完全失明。也罕见自发性消退的病例报道。

Juvenile Open-Angle Glaucoma

uvenile open-angle glaucoma (JOAG) is an autosomal dominant condition that presents after 4 years of age. Unlike in late-recognized PCG, the cornea is not enlarged, Haab striae are not present, and the anterior chamber angle usually appears normal. Management of JOAG is similar to that of adult primary open-angle glaucoma, but the condition frequently requires surgery. See BCSC Section 10, *Glaucoma*, for management of adult glaucoma.

Secondary Childhood Glaucoma

Glaucoma caused by other ocular anomalies (congenital or acquired) or associated with systemic disease or syndromes is considered secondary. Table 22-3 lists nonacquired ocular anomalies and systemic diseases and syndromes associated with secondary glaucoma.

Secondary Glaucoma Associated With an Acquired Condition

In children, as in adults, glaucoma may develop secondary to corticosteroid use, uveitis, infection, or ocular trauma. The anticonvulsant and antidepressant medication topira-mate can cause acute, usually bilateral, angle-closure glaucoma secondary to ciliary ef-fusion. The ciliochoroidal effusion causes relaxation of zonules, resulting in extreme anterior displacement of the lens–iris complex, which leads to secondary angle-closure glaucoma and high myopia. Peripheral iridectomy is not effective as treatment, but timely cessation of the medication is.

Table 22-3 Nonacquired Conditions Associated With Secondary Glaucoma

Ocular Anomalies	Systemic Disease or Syndrome
Anterior segment abnormalities	Sturge-Weber syndrome
Aniridia	Neurofibromatosis type 1
Axenfeld-Rieger syndrome	Lowe (oculocerebrorenal) syndrome
Congenital iris ectropion	Lens-associated disorders
Microcornea	Homocystinuria
Microspherophakia	Marfan syndrome
Peters anomaly	Weill-Marchesani syndrome
Sclerocornea	
Tumors of the iris	
Posterior segment abnormalities	
Familial exudative vitreoretinopathy	
Persistent fetal vasculature	
Retinopathy of prematurity	
Tumors of the retina or ciliary body	

Glaucoma Following Cataract Surgery

Aphakic glaucoma is a common form of secondary glaucoma in childhood. The reported incidence of open-angle aphakic glaucoma after congenital cataract surgery varies from 15% to 50% or higher. Aphakic glaucoma often develops years after cataract surgery, but it can occur within weeks to months of surgery and remains a lifelong risk. Consequently, patients who have undergone cataract surgery in childhood require regular ophthalmic examination. The children at highest risk for glaucoma development following cataract surgery are those who have surgery during infancy, and the risk appears to be even higher in patients with microcornea or persistentfetal vasculature.

青少年开角型青光眼

青少年开角型青光眼（JOAG）是常染色体显性遗传，4 岁后发病，与晚期原发性先天性青光眼（PCG）不同，没有角膜扩张、没有 Habb 条纹及前房角正常。青少年开角型青光眼（JOAG）的治疗与成年原发性开角型青光眼相同，多需手术治疗。成人青光眼的治疗见 BCSC 第 10 册《*青光眼*》。

儿童继发性青光眼

其他眼部异常（先天性或获得性）、伴全身性疾病或综合征相关的青光眼视为继发性。表 22-3 列出了伴继发性青光眼的非获得性眼病、全身性疾病和综合征。

继发性青光眼伴获得性疾病

与成人一样，儿童青光眼可继发于使用皮质类固醇药、葡萄膜炎、感染或眼外伤。抗惊厥和抗抑郁的托吡酯会使得睫状体渗漏，导致双眼继发性急性闭角型青光眼。睫状体脉络膜渗漏会使悬韧带松弛、晶状体 - 虹膜复合体严重前移位，导致继发性闭角型青光眼和高度近视。周边虹膜切除术治疗无效，但及时停止使用抗惊厥和抗抑郁药物有效。

表22-3　伴继发性青光眼的非获得性疾病

眼部异常	全身性疾病或综合征
前节异常	Sturge-Weber综合征
虹膜缺失	1型神经纤维瘤病
Axenfeld-Rieger综合征	Lowe（眼脑肾）综合征
先天性虹膜外翻	晶状体相关疾病
小角膜	高胱氨酸尿症
球形晶状体	Marfan综合征
Peters 异常	Weill-Marchesani综合征
角膜硬化	
虹膜肿瘤	
后节异常	
家族性渗出性玻璃体视网膜病变	
持续性胎儿血管化	
早产儿视网膜病变	
视网膜或睫状体肿瘤	

白内障术后青光眼

无晶状体青光眼是儿童继发性青光眼的常见类型。有报道称，先天性白内障手术后无晶状体开角型青光眼的发病率为 15% ~ 50%。无晶状体青光眼常在白内障手术数年后出现，也可在手术数周至数月内发生，且终生存在风险，因此，白内障手术的患儿需定期进行眼科检查。白内障手术后青光眼发生率风险最高的情况是在婴儿期接受手术，而小角膜或持续性胎儿血管化 / 永久性胎儿血管的青光眼风险更高。

The mechanism of aphakic glaucoma is unclear. The anterior chamber angle usually appears open on gonioscopy; the outflow channels are compromised by some combination of abnormal development of the anterior chamber angle and perhaps susceptibility of the infant eye to surgically induced inflammation, loss of lens support, retained lens epithelial cells, or vitreous factors.

Acute or subacute angle closure with iris bombé is a rare form of aphakic glaucoma. Although it usually occurs soon after surgery, onset can be delayed by a year or more. The diagnosis should be apparent with a slit lamp, but examination at the slit lamp may be difficult in young children. Treatment consists of anterior vitrectomy to relieve the pupillary block, often with surgical iridectomy and goniosynechialysis.

Freedman SF, Lynn MJ, Beck AD, Bothun ED, Örge FH, Lambert SR; Infant Aphakia Treatment Study Group. Glaucoma-related adverse events in the first 5 years after unilateral cataract removal in the Infant Aphakia Treatment Study. *JAMA Ophthalmol.* 2015;133(8):907–914.

Treatment

The primary treatment for most types of childhood glaucoma is surgery. PCG is usually effectively treated with angle surgery (goniotomy or trabeculotomy). Although angle surgery may be used to treat some forms of secondary pediatric glaucoma—most notably, those associated with Axenfeld-Rieger syndrome, Sturge-Weber Syndrome, and aniridia—the outcome is often less successful. The treatment of most forms of secondary childhood glaucoma (see Table 22-3) is similar to that of open-angle or secondary glaucoma in adults. Medical treatment often has value prior to surgery and may have long-term benefit, particularly in JOAG and some secondary childhood glaucomas.

Surgical Therapy

Surgical intervention is the treatment of choice for PCG. Goniotomy or trabeculotomy is the preferred initial procedure. In a *goniotomy*, an incision is made, under direct gonioscopic visualization, across the trabecular meshwork (Fig 22-6, Video 22-1).

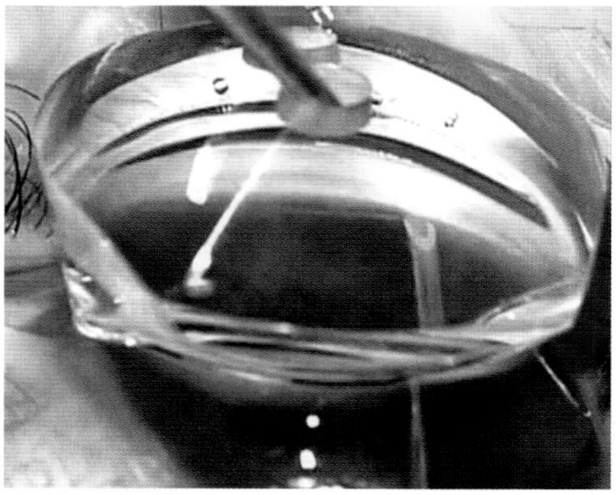

Figure 22-6 Goniotomy needle with its tip in the trabecular meshwork. The trabecular meshwork to the left of the needle has been incised. *(Courtesy of Ken K. Nischal, MD.)*

VIDEO 22-1 Goniotomy.
Courtesy of Ken K. Nischal, MD.
Access all Section 6 videos at www.aao.org/bcscvideo_section06.

无晶状体青光眼的发病机制尚不清楚。前房角镜检查时房角是开角的，但房水流出通道受阻受多种因素的共同影响，如房角发育异常和婴儿对手术引发的炎症易感性、晶状体支架的丧失、残留晶状体上皮细胞或玻璃体的影响。

急性或亚急性房角关闭伴虹膜膨隆是无晶状体青光眼的罕见形式。常在术后即发病，但也可延迟 1 年后发病。裂隙灯下即可确诊，但婴幼儿很难行裂隙灯检查。治疗包括前玻璃体切除术联合虹膜切除术和房角分离术，以缓解瞳孔阻滞状况。

Freedman SF, Lynn MJ, Beck AD, Bothun ED, Örge FH, Lambert SR; Infant Aphakia Treatment Study Group. Glaucoma-related adverse events in the first 5 years after unilateral cataract removal in the Infant Aphakia Treatment Study. *JAMA Ophthalmol.* 2015;133(8):907–914.

治疗

儿童青光眼的治疗主要是手术治疗。原发性先天性青光眼（PCG）采用房角手术（前房角切开术或小梁切开术）可得到有效治疗。房角手术亦可用于某些类型的继发性儿童青光眼，但伴 Axenfeld - Rieger 综合征、Sturge - Weber 综合征及无虹膜症时，房角手术的疗效不佳。大多数继发性儿童青光眼（见表 22–3）的治疗方法与成人开角型或继发性青光眼相同。手术前应行药物治疗，并可能需要长期使用，特别是青少年开角型青光眼（JOAG）和一些继发性儿童青光眼。

手术治疗

原发性先天性青光眼（PCG）首选手术治疗，首先采用前房角切开术或小梁切开术。在行*前房角切开术*时，在直接前房角镜下，经小梁网做一个切口（图 22–6，视频 22–1）。

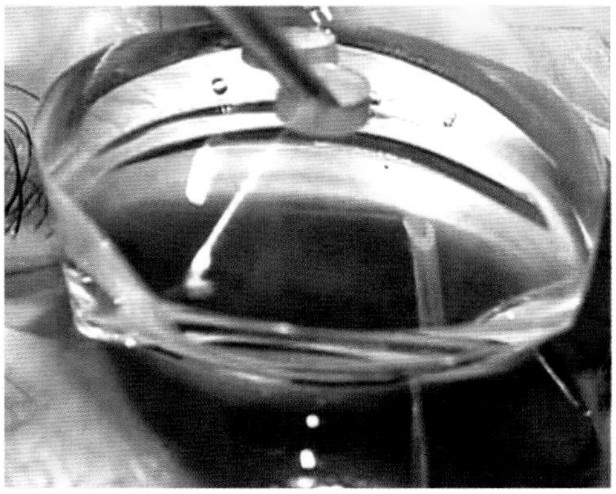

图 22–6　前房角切开针位于小梁网内。针左侧的小梁网已被切开。*（译者注：资料来源见前页原文。）*

视频 22-1　房角切开术。*（译者注：资料来源见前页原文。）*

可登陆网站观看www.aao.org/bcscvideo_section06观看第6册中的所有视频。

VIDEO 22-2 Trabeculotomy.
Courtesy of Young H. Kwon, MD, PhD.

In *trabeculotomy*, an external approach is used to identify and cannulate the Schlemm canal, and then connect it with the anterior chamber through incision of the trabecular meshwork (Fig 22-7, Video 22-2).

A modification of this technique uses a 6-0 polypropylene monofilament suture or illuminated microcatheter to cannulate and open the Schlemm canal for its entire 360° circumference in one surgery (Video 22-3).

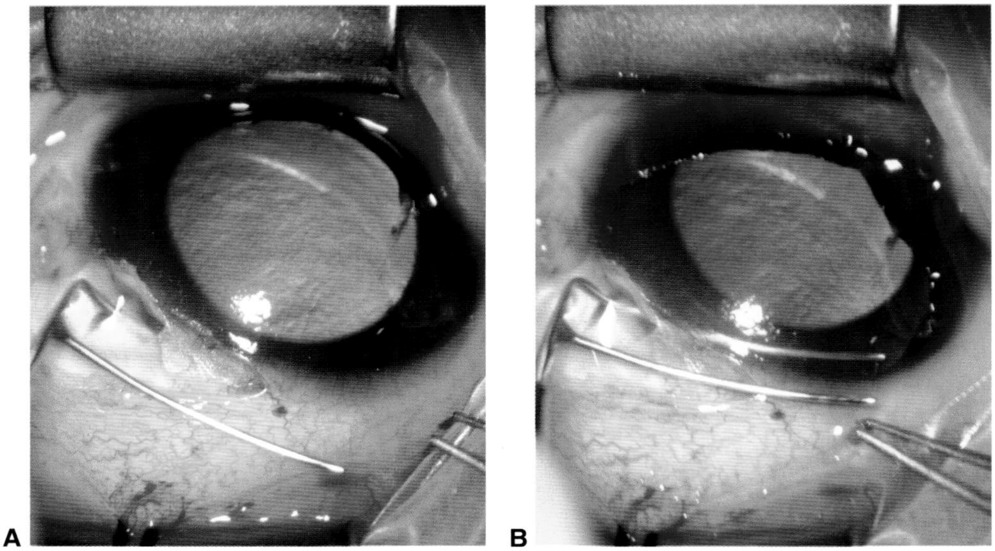

Figure 22-7 Trabeculotomy. **A,** The trabeculotome has entered the Schlemm canal. **B,** The trabeculotome has been rotated into the anterior chamber. *(Courtesy of Steven M. Archer, MD.)*

VIDEO 22-3 Illuminated microcatheter–assisted 360-degree trabeculotomy.
Courtesy of Brenda L. Bohnsack, MD, PhD.

If the cornea is clear, either a goniotomy or a trabeculotomy can be performed at the surgeon's discretion. Preoperative glaucoma medications or stripping of edematous epithelium from the cornea can temporarily clear the cornea. If the view through the cornea is compromised, trabeculotomy or combined trabeculotomy-trabeculectomy can be performed.

In approximately 80% of infants with PCG presenting from 3 months to 1 year of age, IOP is controlled with 1 or 2 angle surgeries. If the first procedure is not sufficient, at least 1 additional angle surgery is usually performed before a different procedure is used.

视频 22-2　小梁切开术。*（译者注：资料来源见前页原文。）*

行*小梁切开术*时，经外路识别，并于 Schlemm 管插入导管；然后通过小梁网切口将其与前房连接（图 22–7，视频 22–2）。

改良技术是用 6–0 聚丙烯单丝缝合或带照明微导管插管，Schlemm 管 360° 一次性打开 (视频 22–3)。

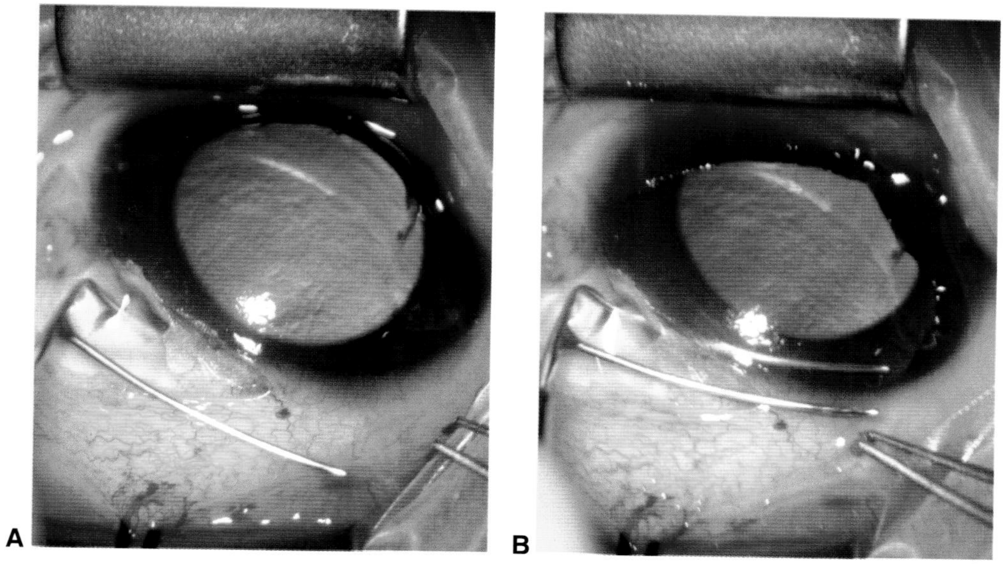

图 22–7 小梁切开术。**A.** 小梁切开刀已经进入 Schlemm 管。**B.** 小梁切开刀已经旋转到前房。*（译者注：资料来源见前页原文。）*

视频 22-3　带照明的微导管引导下的360° 小梁切开术。*（译者注：资料来源见前页原文。）*

如果角膜透明，手术医生则会决定行房角切开术或小梁切开术。术前青光眼药物治疗或剥离角膜水肿上皮可暂时使角膜透明。如果通过角膜的视野受损，可以实行小梁切开术或小梁切开术联合小梁切除术。

婴儿原发性先天性青光眼（PCG）的 80% 在 3 个月 ~ 1 岁发病，需 1 ~ 2 次房角手术才能控制眼压。如果第一次手术的效果不佳，在采用不同术式前，应再做一次房角手术。

When angle surgery is not successful in a child or is not indicated (as is the case in many forms of secondary glaucoma) and medical therapy is inadequate, additional surgical options include trabeculectomy with or without antifibrotic therapy (eg, mitomycin C [MMC]), tube shunt implantation, and cyclodestructive procedures.

Reported success rates for trabeculectomy vary considerably by surgical technique and type of glaucoma and decrease as the length of follow-up increases. Patients younger than 1 year and those who are aphakic are more prone to treatment failure. Although the success rate of trabeculectomy improves with the use of antifibrotics such as MMC, the long-term risk of bleb leaks and endophthalmitis also increases. Long-term risk is reduced by using a fornix-based rather than a limbus-based conjunctival flap. Ab interno trabeculectomy using a mechanical device such as Trabectome (NeoMedix, Tustin, CA) has been described in the treatment of pediatric glaucoma, but its use is still evolving.

The reported success rate of tube shunt implantation surgery with Molteno (Molteno Ophthalmic Limited, Dunedin, New Zealand), Baerveldt (Johnson & Johnson Vision, Santa Ana, CA), and Ahmed (New World Medical, Rancho Cucamonga, CA) devices varies between 54% and 85%. Although most children with implanted tube shunts must remain on adjunct topical medical therapy to control IOP after surgery, their blebs are thicker and are less prone to leaking and infection than those of patients who have undergone MMC-augmented trabeculectomy. Potential complications include shunt failure, tube erosion or migration, tube–cornea touch, cataract, restrictive strabismus, and endophthalmitis.

Laser cyclodestruction and cyclocryotherapy are generally reserved for resistant cases or those not amenable to other surgical procedures. These techniques decrease ciliary body production of aqueous humor, which results in lower IOP. *Cyclocryotherapy* (freez-ing the ciliary processes through the sclera) may be successful, but the complication rate is high. Repeated applications are often necessary, and the risk of phthisis and blindness is significant (approximately 10%). *Transscleral cyclophotocoagulation* with the Nd:YAG or diode laser has a lower risk of complications. The short-term success rate is approximately 50%. Patients usually require more than one treatment.

Endoscopic cyclophotocoagulation (ECP) has been used in children with glaucomas that are difficult to treat. In ECP, a microendoscope applies laser energy to the ciliary processes under direct visualization (Fig 22-8). Success rates of up to 50% have been reported. Although this is an intraocular procedure, the complication rate may be lower than that of external cyclodestructive procedures. Use of the microendoscope is advantageous in eyes with abnormal anterior segment anatomy. Some studies have shown encouraging results for patients with aphakic glaucoma.

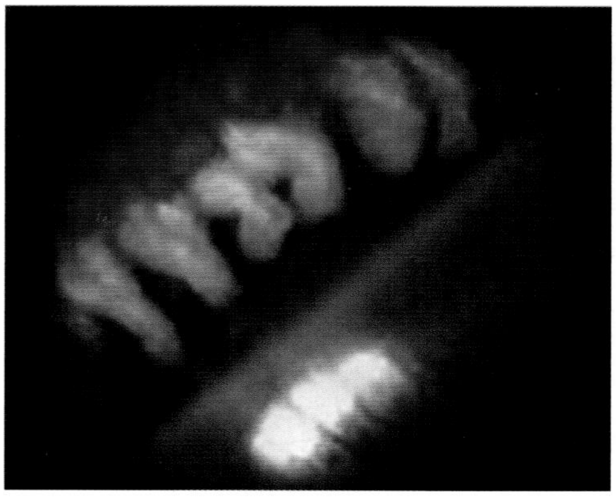

Figure 22-8 Endoscopic view of the ciliary processes during endoscopic cyclophotocoagulation. The white structure at the bottom right of the photo is the lens. *(Courtesy of Endo Optiks, Little Silver, NJ.)*

当儿童的房角手术不成功或不是适应证时（如有些类型的继发性青光眼），且不宜进行药物治疗时，手术应选择小梁切除术联合或不联合抗纤维化药物［如丝裂霉素 C（MMC）］、分流管植入和睫状体破坏性手术。

因手术技巧和青光眼类型的不同，小梁切除术的成功率的文献报告差异较大，且随着随访时间的延长而降低。1 岁以下患儿和无晶状体患儿更不易成功。虽然小梁切除术的成功率随着抗纤维化药物的使用而提高，如丝裂霉素 C（MMC），但滤泡渗漏和眼内炎的长期风险也随之增加。以穹窿为基底的结膜瓣较以角膜缘为基底的结膜瓣的远期风险降低。使用器械如 Trabectome （NeoMedix, Tustin, CA）进行内路小梁切除术如小梁消融术已用于治疗儿童青光眼，但这种方法仍在进行改进。

使用 Molteno（Molteno Ophthalmic Limited, Dunedin, New Zealand）、Baerveldt（Johnson & Johnson Vision,Santa Ana, CA）和 Ahmed（New World Medical, Rancho Cucamonga, CA）等装置行分流管植入术的成功率在 54% ~ 85% 之间。多数行分流管植入术的儿童，手术后仍需点药来控制眼压。与联合丝裂霉素 C（MMC）的增强小梁切除术相比，分流管植入术的滤泡壁较厚、不易渗漏和感染。潜在的并发症包括分流失败、导管侵蚀或移位、分流管接触角膜、白内障、限制性斜视和眼内炎。

激光睫状体破坏和睫状体冷冻治疗只用于难治性或不适合其他手术的病例。该技术可减少睫状体房水的产生，降低眼压。*睫状体冷冻治疗*（经巩膜冷冻睫状突）可能奏效，但并发症高发，需多次重复，眼球痨和失明的风险较大（约为 10%）。掺钕钇铝榴石激光（Nd : YAG）或二极管激光*经巩膜睫状体光凝术*的并发症发生率较低，近期成功率约为 50%，常需治疗数次。

*内窥镜下睫状体光凝术（ECP）*已用于难治性儿童青光眼。手术中使用显微内窥镜，在直视下将激光作用于睫状突（图 22–8），成功率可达 50%。尽管属内眼手术，但并发症的发生率低于外路睫状体破坏术。眼前节解剖异常时，显微内窥镜的应用是其优点。有报告称其对无晶状体青光眼的治疗效果亦较好。

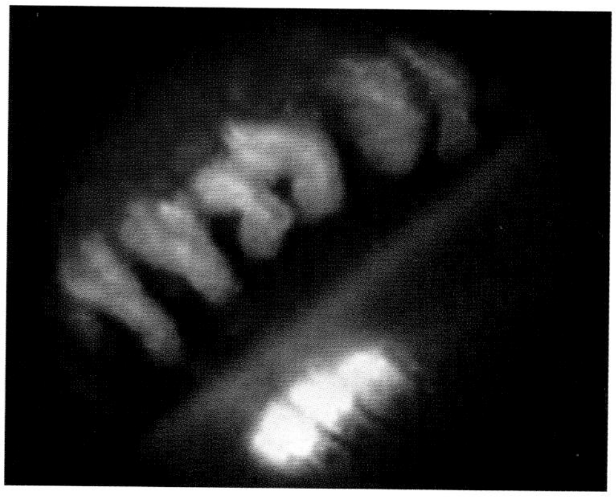

图 22–8　内窥镜下睫状体光凝术中的内视睫状突。图右下方的白色结构是晶状体。*（译者注：资料来源见前页原文。）*

Chen TC, Chen PP, Francis BA, et al. Pediatric glaucoma surgery: a report by the American Academy of Ophthalmology. *Ophthalmology.* 2014;121(11):2107–2115.

Jayaram H, Scawn R, Pooley F, et al. Long-term outcomes of trabeculectomy augmented with mitomycin C undertaken within the first 2 years of life. *Ophthalmology.* 2015;122(11):2216–2222.

Medical Therapy

Generally, medical therapy for childhood glaucoma has lower success rates and greater risks than medical therapy for adult glaucomas. However, it serves several important purposes in preoperative, postoperative, and long-term management, particularly in childhood glaucoma other than PCG. For example, medications can be used to lower IOP before surgery in order to reduce corneal edema and improve visualization during surgery. They may also be used after surgical procedures in order to provide additional IOP lowering.

Medical therapy for pediatric glaucoma also carries unique risks (Table 22-4) because of the greater dose per body weight and the limited number of controlled clinical trials in children. Although punctal occlusion may be used to reduce systemic absorption of topical medications, it may be impractical in many young children. Limiting the frequency of eyedrop administration in young children may enhance adherence.

Topical medications

Therapy with topical β-adrenergic antagonists, or β-blockers, may reduce IOP by 20%–30%. The major risks of this therapy are respiratory distress (caused by apnea or bronchospasm) and bradycardia, both of which occur mostly in small infants and in children with a history of bronchospasm. Betaxolol, a cardioselective β_1-adrenergic antagonist, may be safer than a nonselective β-blocker for use in patients with asthma, but its pressure-lowering effect is less than that of nonselective agents.

Topical carbonic anhydrase inhibitors (CAIs) are effective in children, but they produce a smaller reduction in IOP (<15%) than do β-blockers. Corneal edema is a risk of topical CAIs; thus, they should be used with caution in children with coexisting corneal disease.

Prostaglandin analogues are effective in many pediatric patients. Their low systemic risk and once-daily dosing are advantageous.

Miotics are rarely used in children; perioperative pilocarpine, however, may facilitate angle surgery. Pilocarpine and echothiophate may be effective in patients with aphakic glaucoma.

Chen TC, Chen PP, Francis BA, et al. Pediatric glaucoma surgery: a report by the American Academy of Ophthalmology. *Ophthalmology*. 2014;121(11):2107–2115.

Jayaram H, Scawn R, Pooley F, et al. Long-term outcomes of trabeculectomy augmented with mitomycin C undertaken within the first 2 years of life. *Ophthalmology*. 2015;122(11):2216–2222.

药物治疗

一般来说，儿童青光眼的药物治疗较成人的效果差且风险更大。但在术前、术后和远期治疗中具有重要作用，特别是儿童青光眼［原发性先天性青光眼（PCG）除外］。如术前用药可降低眼压、减少角膜水肿、提高术中的可视程度；术后使用药物也可进一步降低眼压。

儿童青光眼的药物治疗也有特殊风险（表 22–4），单位体重的剂量更大，且儿童的临床对照试验有限。虽然泪小点阻塞可减少局部药物的全身吸收，但在许多幼儿中无法实施。限制儿童眼药水的使用频率可增强其依从性。

局部用药

局部使用 β – 肾上腺素能受体拮抗剂或 β – 阻滞剂可以降低眼压 20% ~ 30%，其主要风险是呼吸窘迫（由窒息或支气管痉挛引起）和心动过缓，多见于小婴儿和有支气管痉挛病史的儿童。倍他洛尔是一种心脏选择性 $β_1$ 肾上腺素能受体拮抗剂，可应用于伴有哮喘的患者，较非选择性的 β – 受体阻滞剂安全，但其降低眼压的作用比非选择性药物小。

儿童局部使用碳酸酐酶抑制剂有效，但降低眼压的作用比 β – 受体阻滞剂小（<15%）。局部使用碳酸酐酶抑制剂的风险是角膜水肿，因此伴角膜疾病的儿童中慎用。

前列腺素类似物对许多儿童患者有效，其优点是全身性风险较低和每日仅使用 1 次。

缩瞳剂很少用于儿童，围手术期毛果云香碱的使用有助于房角手术。毛果云香碱和乙膦硫胆碱对无晶状体青光眼有效。

Table 22-4 Systemic and Ocular Adverse Effects of Glaucoma Medications in Children

Drug	Adverse Effects	Precautions
β-Adrenergic antagonists		
Betaxolol, carteolol, levobunolol, metipranolol, timolol hemihydrate, timolol maleate	Hypotension, bradycardia, bronchospasm, apnea Hallucinations Masking of hypoglycemia in diabetic children	Avoid in premature or small infants Use with caution in infants, children with asthma or cardiac disease Select lower concentrations Use punctal occlusion Consider cardioselective β-blocker to reduce risk of bronchospasm
Prostaglandin analogues		
Bimatoprost, latanoprost, latanoprostene bunod, tafluprost, travoprost	May exacerbate uveitis Risk of retinal detachment in Sturge-Weber syndrome Low systemic risk, possible sleep disturbance or exacerbation of asthma	Avoid in patients with uveitis Use with caution following intraocular surgery
α_2-Adrenergic agonists		
Apraclonidine, brimonidine	Apraclonidine: tachyphylaxis, allergy Apraclonidine and brimonidine: hypotension, bradycardia, hypothermia, CNS depression, coma Risks are greater with brimonidine	Brimonidine relatively contraindicated in children <2 years of age Caution in children <6 years of age or <20 kg Use low dosage Avoid in patients with cardiovascular disease, hepatic or renal impairment
Topical CAIs		
Brinzolamide, dorzolamide	Metabolic acidosis (rare) Stevens-Johnson syndrome Corneal edema	Contraindicated in infants with renal insufficiency Contraindicated in sulfonamide hypersensitivity Monitor infant feeding, weight gain Caution in corneal disease
Oral CAIs		
Acetazolamide, methazolamide	Metabolic acidosis Stevens-Johnson syndrome Headache, nausea, dizziness, paresthesia Growth suppression, failure to thrive, weight loss Bed-wetting	Contraindicated in renal insufficiency, hypokalemia, hyponatremia Contraindicated in sulfonamide hypersensitivity Monitor for metabolic acidosis Monitor infant feeding, weight gain
Parasympathomimetic agents (miotics)		
Echothiophate, pilocarpine	Risk of pupillary block Paradoxical rise in IOP Echothiophate: diarrhea, urinary incontinence, cardiac arrhythmia, weakness, headache, fatigue, iris cysts Pilocarpine: bronchospasm, hypertension, vomiting, diarrhea, dizziness, weakness, headache	Avoid in patients with uveitis Use with caution in cardiac disease, asthma, urinary tract obstruction Limit dosage and use lower concentrations Echothiophate: avoid succinylcholine Consider stopping before general anesthesia

CAIs = carbonic anhydrase inhibitors.

表22-4　儿童青光眼药物的全身和眼部不良反应

药物	不良反应	预防措施
β-肾上腺素能受体拮抗剂		
倍他洛尔（贝特舒）、卡替洛尔（美开朗）、左不诺洛尔（贝他根）、美替洛尔、噻吗洛尔半水合物、马来酸噻吗洛尔	低血压、心动过缓、支气管痉挛、呼吸暂停 幻视、幻听 掩盖糖尿病儿童的低血糖症	避免用于早产儿或婴儿 婴儿、儿童哮喘或心脏病慎用 选择低浓度 使用泪小点阻塞 考虑用心脏选择性β-阻滞剂滴眼液来减少支气管痉挛风险
前列腺素类似物		
贝美前列腺素、拉坦前列腺素、布诺-拉坦前列烯、他氟前列腺素、曲伏前列腺素	可加重葡萄膜炎 Sturge - Weber综合征有视网膜脱离的风险	避免用于葡萄膜炎患者 眼内手术后慎用
α_2-肾上腺素能受体激动剂		
可乐定、溴莫尼定	阿拉可乐定：快速抗药反应、过敏 阿拉可乐定和溴莫尼定：低血压、心动过缓、低体温症、中枢神经系统抑郁症、昏迷 溴莫尼定的风险更大	溴莫尼定的相对禁忌证为2岁以下儿童 6岁以下或20kg以下儿童慎用 使用低剂量 避免用于有心血管疾病、肝肾损害的患儿
局部使用CAIs		
布林佐胺（派立明）、杜噻酰胺（添素得）	代谢性酸中毒 Stevens - Johnson综合征 角膜水肿	肾功能不全的患儿禁用 磺胺过敏禁用 监测婴儿喂养、体重增加的状况 角膜疾病慎用
口服CAIs		
乙酰唑胺、醋甲唑胺	代谢性酸中毒 Stevens - Johnson综合征 头痛、恶心、头晕、感觉异常 生长抑制、发育不良、体重减轻 遗尿	肾功能不全、低钾血症、低钠血症禁用 磺胺过敏禁用 监测代谢性酸中毒 监测婴儿喂养、体重增加的状况
拟胆碱能药物（缩瞳剂）		
乙膦硫胆碱、毛果芸香碱	存在瞳孔阻滞风险 眼压的反常上升 乙膦硫胆碱：腹泻,尿失禁,心律失常,虚弱,头痛，疲劳，虹膜囊肿 毛果云香碱：支气管痉挛,高血压、呕吐、腹泻、头晕、虚弱、头痛	避免用于葡萄膜炎患者 心脏病、哮喘、尿路阻塞慎用 限制剂量，使用较低的浓度 乙膦硫胆碱：避免同时使用琥珀胆碱 考虑在全身麻醉前停止使用

CAIs表示碳酸酐酶抑制剂。

The α_2-adrenergic agonist apraclonidine may be useful for shortterm IOP reduction, but there is a high incidence of tachyphylaxis and allergy with use of this drug in young children. Brimonidine, another α_2-adrenergic agonist, effectively reduces IOP in some cases of pediatric glaucoma. Both medications can produce somnolence and respiratory depression in infants and young children. Infants and young children are particularly susceptible to brimonidine's adverse effects. Therefore, brimonidine should be used with caution in children younger than 6 years, and it is relatively contraindicated in children younger than 2 years because of the risk of respiratory depression. There are similar limitations for the use of fixed-dose combination drugs such as brimonidine/timolol and brinzolamide/brimonidine in the pediatric population.

Oral medications

Oral CAIs may be used effectively in children, particularly to delay the need for surgery or to clear the cornea before goniotomy. Their usefulness may be limited because of their systemic adverse effects (see Table 22-4).

Prognosis and Follow-Up

The prognosis for control of IOP and preservation of vision is poor for patients with PCG who present at birth; at least half of these patients become legally blind. If the horizontal diameter of the cornea is greater than 14 mm at diagnosis, the visual prognosis is simi-larly poor. Up to 90% of cases in the "favorable prognostic group" (onset at 3–12 months of age) can be controlled with angle surgery and medications. The remaining 10%, and many of the remaining cases of primary and secondary glaucomas, often present a lifelong challenge.

Vision loss in childhood glaucoma is multifactorial. It may result from corneal scarring and opacification, optic nerve damage, myopic astigmatism, and associated anisometropic and strabismic amblyopia. Myopia results from axial enlargement of the eye in the setting of high IOP; astigmatism may result from unequal expansion of the anterior segment or from corneal scarring. Careful treatment of refractive errors and amblyopia is necessary to optimize outcomes.

All cases of childhood glaucoma, as well as suspected but unconfirmed glaucoma, require diligent follow-up. After any surgical intervention or change in medical therapy, control of IOP should be assessed within a few weeks. Examination under sedation or anesthesia is often necessary in children for accurate assessment. The IOP should be considered not as an isolated finding but rather in conjunction with other measurements obtained from the examination, including refractive error (measured serially), corneal diameter, axial length, and cup–disc ratio. If the IOP is less than 20 mm Hg under anesthesia but clinical evidence shows persistentcorneal edema or enlargement, progressive optic nerve cupping, or myopic progression, further intervention should be pursued despite the IOP reading. In contrast, a young child who has an IOP of about 20 mm Hg but shows evidence of clinical improvement may be observed carefully.

Long-term follow-up of children with glaucoma is important. Relapse can occur years later, with elevated IOP and subsequent vision loss. Parents, and patients themselves as they become older, should be educated about the need for lifelong monitoring and management.

α_2- 肾上腺素能受体激动剂阿拉可乐定，短时降眼压有效，但低龄儿童的快速抗药反应和过敏的发生率较高。溴莫尼定是另一种 α_2- 肾上腺素能受体激动剂，对一些儿童青光眼可有效降低眼压。这 2 种药物都能导致婴幼儿嗜睡和呼吸抑制。婴幼儿对溴莫尼定的副作用特别敏感，6 岁以下的儿童应慎用，2 岁以下的儿童相对禁忌，因为有呼吸抑制风险。在儿童中使用固定联合制剂，如溴莫尼定 / 噻吗洛尔和布林唑胺 / 溴莫尼定也有类似的限制。

口服药物

口服碳酸酐酶抑制剂对儿童应用有效，特别是可推迟手术时间，或在房角切开术前可使角膜透明。因为全身性不良反应会使其应用受限（见表 22-4）。

预后和随访

出生时发病的原发性先天性青光眼（PCG）患儿，其控制眼压和视力保持的预后较差，至少有 1/2 的患儿为法定盲。如果诊断时角膜水平直径＞ 14mm，视力预后亦较差。在“预后良好组”(3 ~ 12 个月发病) 中，90% 的患儿经房角手术和药物治疗后病情可控制。其余 10% 的患者和其他的原发性和继发性青光眼的患者需终生治疗。

多种因素致儿童青光眼视力丧失，如角膜瘢痕和混浊、视神经损伤、近视性散光及屈光参差性和斜视性弱视。近视是高眼压下眼轴增长所致，散光是眼前节扩张不均匀或角膜瘢痕所致。精心治疗屈光不正和弱视是获得最好结果的必要条件。

所有儿童青光眼以及疑似未确诊的青光眼患儿，都需积极的随访。任何手术后，或治疗方案变动时，均应用数周时间评估眼压的控制效果。儿童的检查常在镇静或麻醉状态下进行，以准确地评估。眼压不能孤立考量，应该结合其他检查结果，包括屈光不正（连续测量）、角膜直径、眼轴长度及杯盘比。如果麻醉状态下眼压低于 20mmHg，但临床呈持续性角膜水肿或增大、进行性杯盘比增加，或为进行性近视，即便眼压读数正常，也应做进一步干预。但如果低龄儿童的眼压高于 20mmHg、各项临床体征有好转，则应该严密观察。

对青光眼患儿的长期随访很重要的，青光眼复发可发生在数年之后，伴眼压升高和进行性视力下降。随着患儿年龄的增加，应对家长和患儿进行科普教育，病情的终生监控和管理非常必要。

（翻译　陈娜　李世金　张令仪 // 审校　刘陇黔　石一宁　蒋宁 // 章节审校　石广礼）

CHAPTER 23

Childhood Cataracts and Other Pediatric Lens Disorders

Disorders of the pediatric lens include cataract and abnormalities in lens shape, size, and location. Such abnormalities constitute a significant source of visual impairment in children. The incidence of lens abnormalities ranges from 1:4000 to 1:10,000 live births per year worldwide.

See BCSC Section 11, *Lens and Cataract*, for additional discussion of many of the topics covered in this chapter.

Pediatric Cataracts

Cataracts are responsible for nearly 10% of all vision loss in children worldwide. Pediatric cataracts can be

- isolated or associated with a systemic condition or other ocular anomalies
- congenital (infantile) or acquired
- inherited orsporadic
- unilateral or bilateral
- partial or complete
- stable or progressive

General Features

Cataracts in children can be isolated, or they can be associated with a number of conditions, including chromosomal abnormalities, systemic syndromes and diseases, infection, trauma, and radiation exposure. In almost all cases of cataract associated with systemic disease, the cataracts are bilateral (Table 23-1); many bilateral cataracts, however, are not associated with systemic disease. Significant asymmetry can be present in bilateral cases.

Cataracts can also be associated with other ocular anomalies, including persistentfetal vasculature, anterior segment dysgenesis, aniridia, and retinal disorders (eg, coloboma, detachment).

Pediatric cataracts can be congenital or acquired. Congenital cataracts are present at birth, although they may not be identified until later. Infantile cataracts are present during the first year of life. The terms *congenital* and *infantile cataract* are typically used syn-onymously. In general, the earlier the onset, the more amblyogenic the cataract will be, particularly in unilateral cases. Lens opacities that are visually significant before 2–3 months of age are the most likely to be detrimental to vision.

第 23 章

儿童白内障和其他小儿晶体相关疾病

儿童晶状体疾病包括白内障和晶状体形状、大小和位置的异常，是导致儿童视力损伤的重要原因。在全世界的新生儿中，晶状体异常的发生率在 1 ： 4000 ~ 1 ： 10000。

关于本章的更多讨论见 BCSC 第 11 册《*晶状体与白内障*》。

儿童白内障

白内障是全世界的近 10% 儿童视力丧失的原因。儿童白内障可以是

- 孤立的，伴全身性疾病或其他眼部异常
- 先天性（婴儿）或获得性
- 遗传性或散发
- 单眼或双眼
- 部分性或完全性
- 稳定的或进行性

一般特征

儿童白内障可孤立出现，也可伴多种疾病，包括染色体异常、全身综合征和疾病、感染、外伤和辐射暴露。所有伴全身性疾病的白内障病均是双眼的（表 23–1），但双眼性白内障与全身性疾病无关，双眼白内障可明显不对称。

白内障也可伴其他眼部异常，包括永久性胎儿血管、前节发育不良、无虹膜和视网膜疾病（如缺损、视网膜脱离）。

儿童白内障可以是先天性的，或获得性的。先天性白内障出生时即发病，有时为以后才确诊。婴儿性白内障都在出生后 1 年内确诊。*先天性白内障*和*婴儿性白内障*是同义词。一般来说，发病越早，白内障的弱视越重，特别是单眼时。2 ~ 3 个月龄前的影响视觉的晶状体混浊对视力的损害最大。

Table 23-1 Etiology of Pediatric Cataracts

Bilateral cataracts
- Idiopathic
- Familial (hereditary), usually autosomal dominant; also X-linked; rarely autosomal recessive
- Chromosomal abnormality
  - Trisomy 21 (Down syndrome), 13, 18
  - Other translocations, deletions, and duplications
- Craniofacial syndromes
  - Hallermann-Streiff, Rubinstein-Taybi, Smith-Lemli-Opitz, others
- Musculoskeletal disorders
  - Albright syndrome, Conradi-Hünermann syndrome, myotonic dystrophy
- Renal syndromes
  - Alport syndrome, Lowe syndrome
- Metabolic diseases
  - Cerebrotendinous xanthomatosis, diabetes mellitus, Fabry disease, galactosemia, mannosidosis, Wilson disease
- After intrauterine infection
  - Cytomegalovirus
  - Rubella
  - Syphilis
  - Toxoplasmosis
  - Varicella
- Ocular anomalies
  - Aniridia
  - Anterior segment dysgenesis
- Iatrogenic
  - Corticosteroid use
  - Radiation exposure

Unilateral cataracts
- Idiopathic
- Ocular anomalies
  - Persistent fetal vasculature
  - Posterior lenticonus, lentiglobus
  - Posterior segment tumor
  - Retinal detachment (from any cause) or coloboma
- Trauma (including child abuse)
- Radiation exposure

Most hereditary cataracts show an autosomal dominant mode of transmission, and they are almost always bilateral. X-linked and autosomal recessive inheritance may occur; the latter is more common in consanguineous populations. *OMIM (Online Mendelian Inheritance in Man*; omim. org) includes the most up-to-date information on genetic dis-orders with lens involvement.

Morphology

Cataracts can involve the entire lens (*total*, or *complete*, cataract) or only part of the lens structure. The location in the lens and morphology of the cataract provide information about etiology (Table 23-2), onset, and prognosis. Important types and causes of cataract in children are discussed in the following sections.

表23-1　小儿白内障的病因

双眼白内障
- 特发性
- 家族性（遗传性），通常是常染色体显性；也是X-连锁的；很少见常染色体隐性遗传。
  - 13，18，21三体（唐氏综合征）
  - 其他易位、缺失和重复
- 颅面部综合征
  - Hallermann-Streiff综合征，Rubinstein-Taybi综合征，Smith-Lemli-Opitz综合征，其他综合征
- 骨骼肌肉疾病
  - 奥尔布赖特综合征，斑点状软骨发育异常综合征，肌强直性营养不良
- 肾综合征
  - Alport综合征，Lowe综合征
- 代谢疾病
  - 脑腱性黄瘤病、糖尿病、Fabry病、半乳糖血症、甘露糖苷贮积症、威尔逊病
- 宫内感染
  - 巨细胞病毒风疹
  - 梅毒
  - 弓形虫感染
  - 水痘
- 眼部缺损
  - 无虹膜
  - 前节发育不全
- 医疗处理不当
  - 皮质类固醇使用
  - 辐射暴露

单眼白内障
- 特发性
- 眼部异常
  - 永久性胎儿血管
  - 晶状体后圆锥
  - 球后段肿瘤
  - 视网膜脱离（任何原因引起的）或者缺失
- 外伤（包括虐待儿童）
- 辐射暴露

大多数遗传性白内障表现为常染色体显性遗传、双眼。亦有X-连锁和常染色体隐性遗传，后者在近亲中更常见。*OMIM*（*Online Mendelian Inheritance in Man;omim*.org）提供与晶状体相关的遗传性疾病的最新信息。

形态学

白内障可累及整个晶状体（*全部*或*完全*，白内障）或部分晶状体。白内障在晶状体中的位置和形态提示有关病因信息（表23-2）、发病及预后。下面将讨论儿童白内障的重要类型和病因。

Table 23-2 Morphology and Etiology of Select Pediatric Cataracts

Cataract Morphology	Etiology	Other Possible Findings
Spokelike	Fabry disease	Corneal whorls
	Mannosidosis	Hepatosplenomegaly
Vacuolar	Diabetes mellitus	Elevated blood glucose level
Multicolored flecks	Hypoparathyroidism	Low serum calcium level
	Myotonic dystrophy	Characteristic facial features, tonic "grip"
Green "sunflower"	Wilson disease	Kayser-Fleischer ring
Thin disciform	Lowe syndrome	Hypotonia, glaucoma

Anterior polar cataract

Anterior polar cataracts (APCs) are common and usually less than 3 mm in diameter, appearing as small white dots in the center of the anterior lens capsule (Fig 23-1). They are congenital, usually sporadic opacities. APCs can be unilateral or bilateral. They are usually nonprogressive and visually insignificant, perhaps more appropriately termed *anterior lens opacities*. However, unilateral APCs are associated with anisometropia, which may cause amblyopia; thus, careful refraction and follow-up are indicated. *Anterior pyramidal cataracts*, as the name suggests, have a pyramidal shape and project into the anterior chamber. This cataract is a larger, more severe form of APC. It is often associated with cortical changes that can be progressive and amblyogenic, depending on the size of the opacity.

Infantile nuclear cataract

Nuclear cataracts are opacities that involve the center, or nucleus, of the lens. They are usually approximately 3 mm in diameter, but the irregularity of the lens fibers can extend more peripherally. Density and size can vary. Infantile nuclear cataracts may not be sig-nificantly dense at birth (Fig 23-2). They can be inherited or sporadic and are more com-monly bilateral. These opacities are usually stable, but they can progress. Eyes with nuclear cataracts may be smaller than normal.

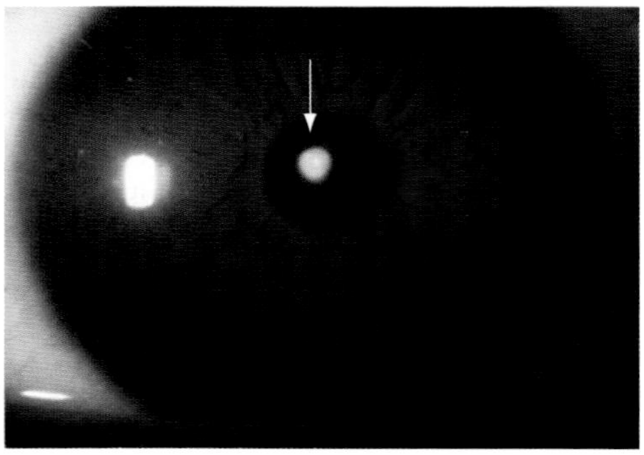

Figure 23-1 Anterior polar cataract (*arrow*). *(Courtesy of Gregg T. Lueder, MD.)*

Lamellar cataract

Lamellar (*zonular*) cataracts affect one or more of the layers of the developing lens cortex surrounding the nucleus. Affected lenses have a clear center, a discrete lamellar opacity, and a clear peripheral cortex. Larger than nuclear cataracts, these opacities are typically 5 mm or more in diameter (Fig 23-3). They can be unilateral but are more often bilateral. The size and corneal diameter of affected eyes are normal. Lamellar cataracts are often less dense than other forms of infantile cataracts, and therefore the visual prognosis is usually better.

表23-2　儿童白内障的形态学和病因学

白内障形态学	病因学	其他
尖刺样的	Fabry病	角膜轮状
	甘露糖苷贮积症	肝脾肥大
气泡样	糖尿病	血糖升高
彩色斑点	甲状旁腺功能减退	低血钙
	肌强直性营养不良	特殊面部特征，强直性肌肉紧张
绿色“向日葵”	肝豆状核变性	Kayser - Fleischer环
薄盘形	眼脑肾综合征	肌张力减退，青光眼

前极性白内障

前极性白内障（APCs）常见，直径＜ 3mm，呈晶状体前囊中心的小白点（图 23–1），为先天性、散发性混浊。前极性白内障（APCs）可以是单眼的或双眼的，非进行性的，不影响视力，定义为*前晶状体混浊*可能更恰当。而单眼前极性白内障（APCs）伴屈光参差，可导致弱视，因此，需注意屈光状态和严密随访。*前锥体型白内障*，顾名思义呈锥体状，向前房突出，是一种混浊范围较大、更严重的前极性白内障，常伴晶状体皮质的变化，是进行性的，是否伴弱视取决于混浊的大小。

婴儿核性白内障

核性白内障累及晶状体中心，即核的混浊，直径通常在 3mm 左右，但不规则的晶状体纤维可向周边扩展。混浊的密度和大小可有变异。婴儿核性白内障在出生时可能不明显（图 23–2），属遗传的或散发的，常见双眼，核性混浊不变化，但亦可进展。核性白内障患者的眼球比正常人的小。

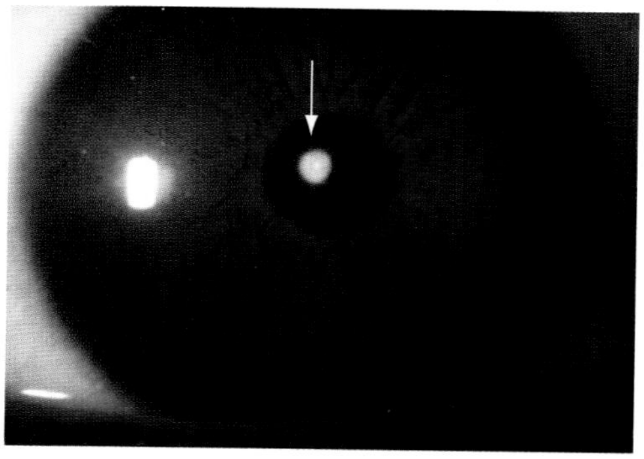

图 23–1　前极性白内障（*箭头*）。*（译者注：资料来源见前页原文。））*

板层性白内障

板层性白内障（*绕核性白内障*）累及 1 层或多层、围绕着核的、发育中的晶状体皮质，晶状体中心透明，与核分离的板层混浊及透明的周边皮质。比核性白内障的混浊范围大，直径在 5mm 以上（图 23–3）。可为单眼，但双眼多见。眼的大小和角膜直径均正常。与其他类型的婴儿性白内障相比，板层性白内障的密度较低，视觉预后较好。

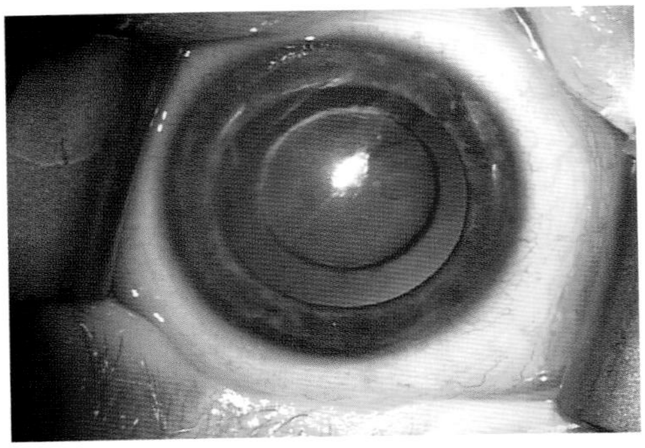

Figure 23-2 Congenital nuclear cataract. *(Cour-tesy of Ken K. Nischal, MD.)*

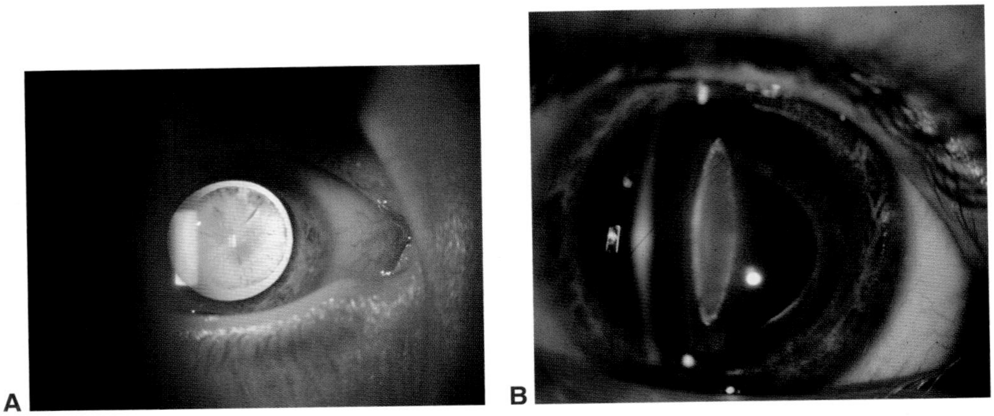

Figure 23-3 Lamellar cataract. **A,** Retroillumination shows the size of the lamellar opacity. **B,** Slit-lamp view shows a lamellar opacity surrounding clear nucleus. *(Courtesy of David A. Plager, MD.)*

Posterior lenticonus

Posterior lenticonus is a cone-shaped deformation of the posterior lens surface caused by progressive thinning of the central capsule (Fig 23-4A); when the deformation is spherical, it is referred to as lentiglobus. This thinning initially causes the lens to have an "oil droplet" appearance on red reflex examination. As the outpouching of the lens progresses, the surrounding cortical fibers gradually opacify (Fig 23-4B). This process can take many years, but if the capsule develops a small tear, rapid, total opacification of the lens can occur (Fig 23-4C).

The opacities are almost always unilateral, and the affected eye is normal in size. Although the weakness in the posterior capsule may be congenital, the cataract does not usually form until later and thus behaves like an acquired cataract. The visual prognosis after cataract surgery is usually favorable.

Posterior subcapsular cataract

Posterior subcapsular cataracts (PSCs) are less common in children than in adults. They are usually acquired and are often bilateral. PSCs tend to progress. Causes of PSC include corticosteroid use, uveitis, retinal abnormalities, radiation exposure, and trauma. PSCs can be seen in association with neurofibromatosis type 2 and may be the first observed manifestation of this disorder.

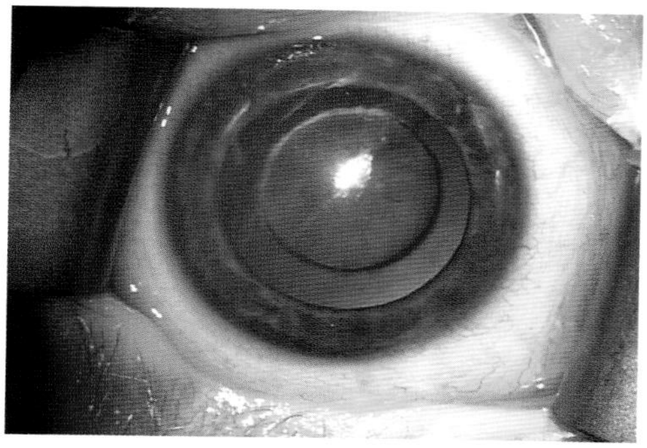

图 23–2　先天性核性白内障。*（译者注：资料来源见前页原文。）*

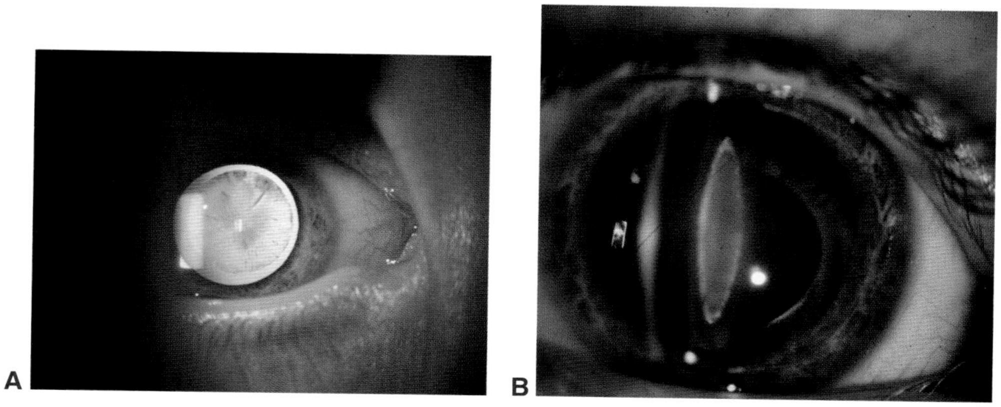

图 23–3　板层性白内障。**A.** 后照明法显示板层混浊的大小。**B.** 裂隙法显示透明核周围有板层状混浊。*（译者注：资料来源见前页原文。）*

后圆锥形晶状体

后圆锥形晶状体是后晶状体表面因中央囊逐渐变薄而引起的锥状变形（图 23–4A）；当变形是球形的，它被称为*球形晶状体*。这种变薄最初导致晶状体有一个“油滴”出现在红光反射检查中。随着晶状体外部囊袋状的进展，周围的皮质纤维逐渐混浊（图 23–4B）。这个过程可能需要很多年，但如果后囊形成一个小的撕裂，可能会迅速发展成完全混浊的晶状体（图 23–4C）。

混浊均是单眼，受累眼大小正常。后囊膜薄弱是先天性的，但白内障形成较晚，故表现为获得性白内障。白内障手术后，视觉预后良好。

后囊下白内障

后囊下白内障（PSCs）在儿童中的发生率低于成人，常是获得性的，且累及双眼，呈进行性。后囊下白内障（PSCs）的原因包括皮质类固醇的使用、葡萄膜炎、视网膜异常、辐射暴露和外伤。伴 2 型神经纤维瘤病时，后囊下白内障（PSCs）可能是观察到的第一个临床表现。

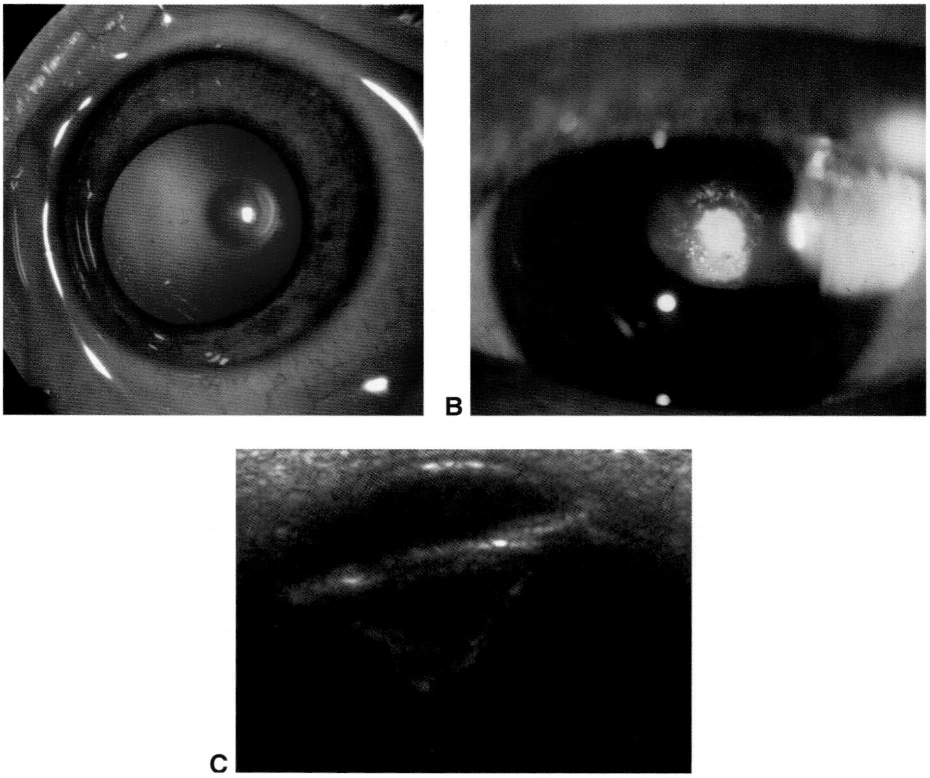

Figure 23-4 Posterior lenticonus. **A,** Early clear defect in the central posterior capsule. **B,** Opacification of the central defect. C, Ultrasound biomicroscopy of advanced posterior lenticonus. *(Part A courtesy of Edward L. Raab, MD; part B, David A. Plager, MD; part C, Ken K. Nischal, MD.)*

Sectoral cataract

Wedge-shaped cortical cataracts are occasionally seen in children. These opacities may be idiopathic, or they may be associated with occult posterior segment tumor, previous blunt trauma, vitreoretinopathies, or retinal coloboma with fibrous bands attached to the posterior lens capsule. Careful posterior segment examination is indicated to rule out these associated pathologies.

Peripheral vacuolar cataract

These asymptomatic peripheral lens vacuoles are sometimes seen in premature infants. The cataracts are most often encountered during examination for retinopathy of prematurity. They are rarely visually significant and usually resolve spontaneously.

Persistentfetal vasculature

Persistentfetal vasculature (PFV; previously called *persistenthyperplastic primary vitreous*) is the most common cause of a unilateral cataract. PFV is typically an isolated, sporadic ocular malformation, but bilateral cases may be associated with systemic or neurologic abnormalities. Usually, affected eyes are smaller than normal.

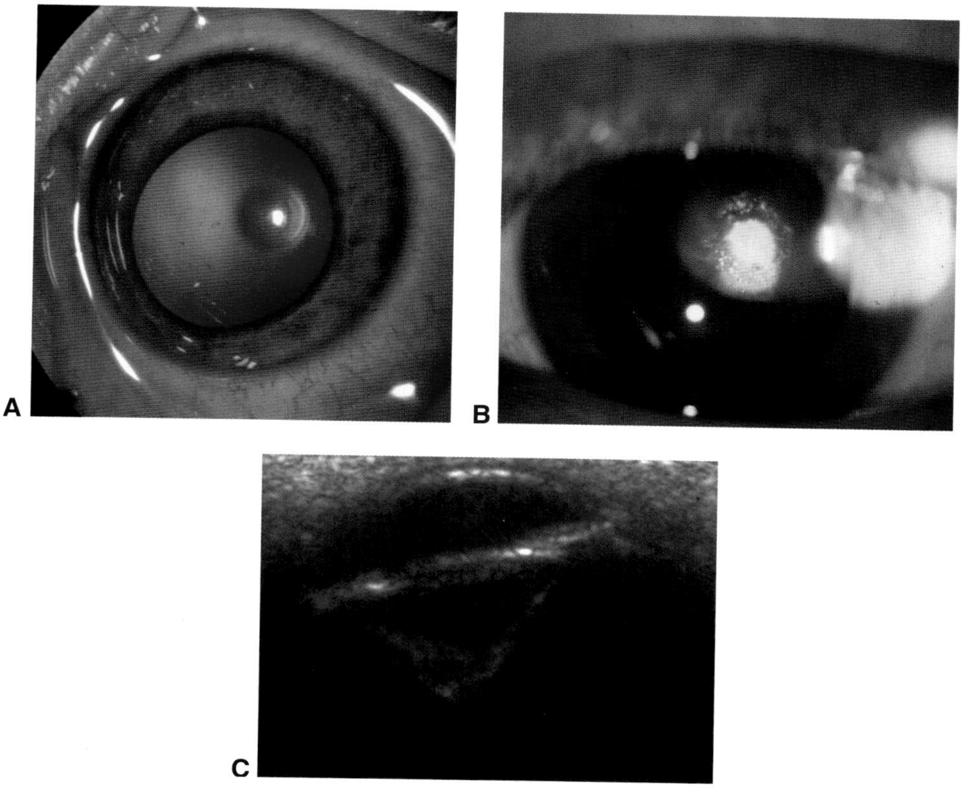

图 23–4　后圆锥形晶状体。**A.** 后囊中央早期明显病灶。**B.** 中央混浊。**C.** 晚期后圆锥的超声生物显微镜图像。
（译者注：资料来源见前页原文。）

楔形皮质性白内障

楔形皮质性白内障偶见于儿童，混浊可能是特发性的，也可伴隐匿性后节肿瘤、钝挫伤、玻璃体视网膜病变或有纤维带附着在后晶状体囊上的视网膜缺损等病变，应进行仔细的后节检查，以排除相关疾病。

周边空泡性白内障

无症状的周边晶状体空泡见于早产儿，对早产儿视网膜病变检查时确诊，很少影响视觉，且常可自愈。

永久性胎儿血管

永久性胎儿血管（PFV，曾称为*永久性原始玻璃体增生*）是单眼白内障的最常见原因。永久性胎儿血管（PFV）是一种孤立的散发性眼部畸形，但双眼多伴全身性或神经系统异常。受累眼睛比正常的小。

PFV ranges in severity from mild to severe (Fig 23-5). Features of mild PFV are prominent hyaloid vessel remnants, a large Mittendorf dot, and Bergmeister papilla. At the other end of the spectrum are microphthalmic eyes with dense retrolental plaques; a thick, fibrous persistenthyaloid artery; elongated ciliary processes (classic for PFV), which may be visible through the dilated pupil; and prominent radial iris vessels. Traction on the optic disc may cause distortion of the posterior retina. Varying degrees of lens opacification occur. The opacity usually consists of a retrolental plaque that is densest centrally and may contain cartilage and fibrovascular tissue.

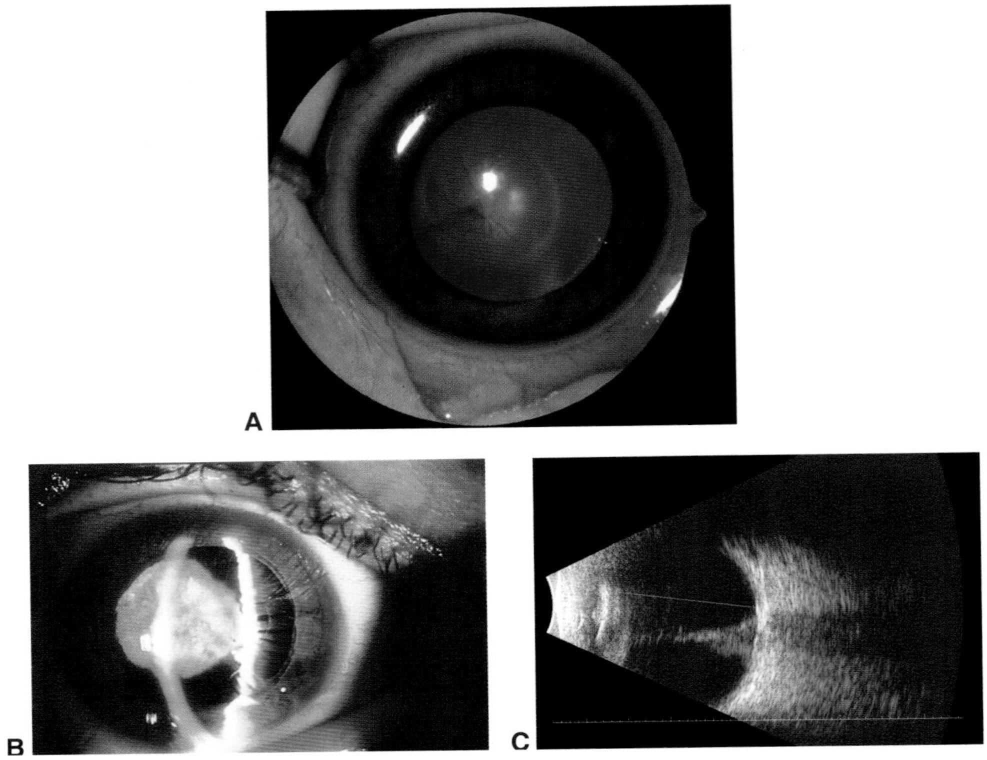

Figure 23-5 Persistent fetal vasculature (PFV). **A,** Mild variant with central retrolental membrane. **B,** Elongated ciliary processes are adherent to the lens. Note the dense fibrous plaque on the posterior lens capsule. **C,** Ultrasonogram of an eye with PFV. Note the dense stalk arising from the optic nerve and attaching to the posterior lens. *(Part A courtesy of David A. Plager, MD; part C courtesy of Edward L. Raab, MD.)*

The natural history of more severely affected eyes is usually one of progressive cataract formation and anterior chamber shallowing, causing secondary glaucoma. The glaucoma can occur acutely because of rapid, total lens opacification and swelling, or it may develop gradually, over years. Congenital retinal nonattachment, ciliary body detachment, vitreous hemorrhage, and optic nerve dysmorphism are other features of severe PFV.

Retinoblastoma may be part of the initial differential diagnosis of PFV because of leukocoria. The presence of microphthalmia and cataract are important factors in the differentiation of these disorders, as retinoblastoma is rarely found in microphthalmic eyes, and cataracts are very unusual in retinoblastoma.

永久性胎儿血管（PFV）的严重程度不同（图 23–5），永久性胎儿血管（PFV）轻度者仅呈玻璃体血管残留，大的Mittendorf点和Bergmeister乳突。重度则呈小眼球、晶状体后致密斑、粗大的纤维性永久性玻璃体动脉、拉长的睫状突（典型的永久性胎儿血管）——散大瞳孔即可见，并可见明显的放射状虹膜血管。视盘上的牵引可引起视网膜后部的变形。晶状体有不同程度的混浊，混浊由中央密集的晶状体后致密斑和含软骨及纤维血管的组织构成。

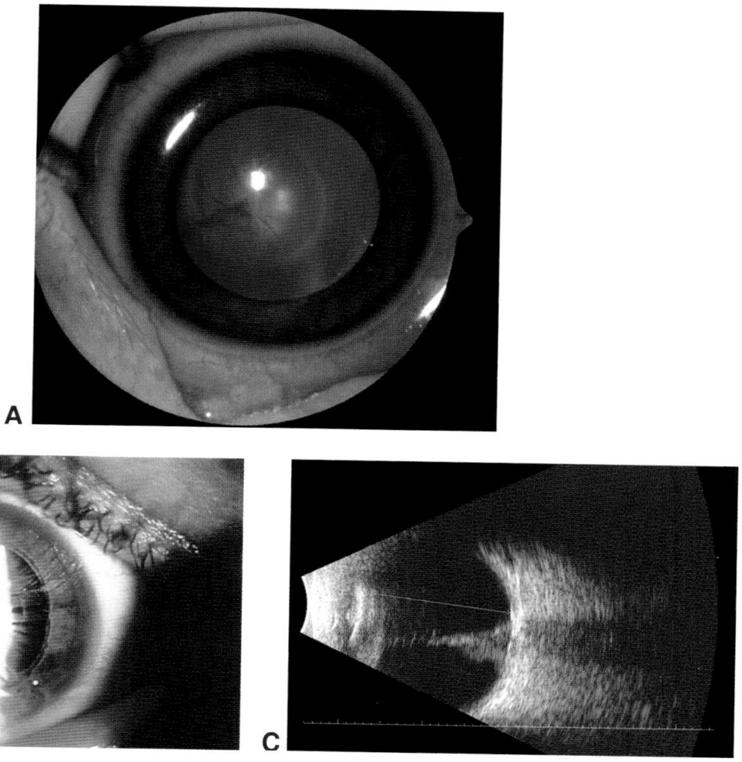

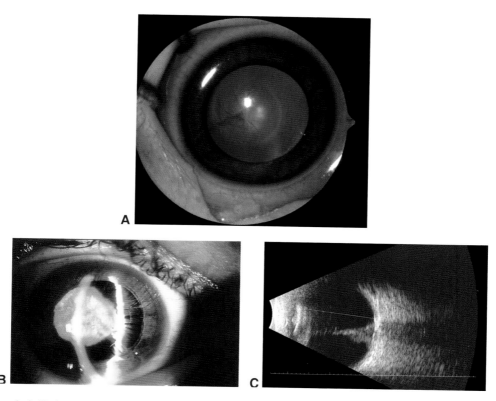

图 23–5　永久性胎儿血管（PFV）。**A.** 轻度的表现为中央晶状体后膜。**B.** 拉长的睫状突附着在晶状体上。晶状体后囊上有致密的纤维斑。**C.** 超声检查。视神经上发出密集的茎柄，并附着于晶状体后。*（译者注：资料来源见前页原文。）*

受累较严重的眼表现为白内障进行性加重、前房变浅，导致继发性青光眼。青光眼可急性发作，表现为晶状体迅速地完全混浊和肿胀，亦可随着时间的推移，逐步发展。严重永久性胎儿血管（PFV）的其他病变有先天性视网膜无附着、睫状体脱离、玻璃体积血和视神经畸形。

作为白瞳症，永久性胎儿血管（PFV）需首先与视网膜母细胞瘤相鉴别，小眼球和白内障是鉴别这些病症的重要指标，因为视网膜母细胞瘤很少出现在小眼球中，而白内障在视网膜母细胞瘤中则非常罕见。

Evaluation of Pediatric Cataracts

All newborns should have a screening eye examination performed by their primary care provider, including an evaluation of the red reflex. Retinoscopy through an undilated pupil is helpful for assessing the potential visual significance of an axial lens opacity in a preverbal child. Table 23-3 summarizes the evaluation of pediatric cataracts.

Table 23-3 Evaluation of Pediatric Cataracts

Family history (autosomal dominant, X-linked, autosomal recessive, reduced penetrance, variable expressivity; associated anomalies may be indicative of chromosomal translocation, balanced in the parent, unbalanced in the child)
Detailed history of the child's growth, development, and systemic disorders
Pediatric physical examination
Genetics evaluation
Ocular examination, including
Visual function
Corneal diameter
Iris configuration
Anterior chamber depth
Lens position
Cataract morphology
Posterior segment
Rule out posterior mass.
Rule out retinal detachment.
Rule out stalk between optic nerve and lens.
Intraocular pressure
Laboratory studies to consider for bilateral cataracts of unknown etiology
Disorders of galactose metabolism: urine for reducing substances; galactose-1-phosphate uridyltransferase; galactokinase
Infectious diseases: TORCH and varicella titers, VDRL test
Metabolic diseases: urine amino acids test (Lowe syndrome); serum calcium (low in hypoparathyroidism), phosphorus (high in hypoparathyroidism), glucose (high in diabetes mellitus), and ferritin (high in hyperferritinemia)

TORCH = toxoplasmosis, rubella, cytomegalovirus, herpes simplex virus.

History

The clinician should obtain a history of the child's growth, development, and systemic disorders, in addition to a family history, as this information can help guide the evaluation. For example, a patient with acquired cataract and intractable diarrhea should be evaluated for the treatable metabolic disorder cerebrotendinous xanthomatosis. A slit-lamp examination of immediate family members can reveal previously undiagnosed lens opacities that are visually insignificant but that may indicate an inherited cause for the child's cataracts. Congenital posterior sutural cataracts, for example, develop in female carriers of X-linked Nance-Horan syndrome, and mild lenticular opacities develop in female carriers of Lowe (oculocerebrorenal) syndrome by puberty.

Examination

Visual function

The mere presence of a cataract does not suggest that surgical removal is necessary. That determination requires assessment of the visual significance of the lens opacity.

小儿白内障的评估

所有新生儿都应该接受初级保健的眼部检查，包括红光反射的评估。评估语前儿童存在的轴向晶状体混浊，是否造成视觉损害，应用小瞳下检影很有帮助。表 23-3 总结了儿童白内障的评估。

表23-3　儿童白内障的评估

家族史（常染色体显性、X-连锁、常染色体隐性、外显率降低、表型变异；伴随的异常提示染色体易位，父母中平衡、孩子不平衡）
儿童生长发育及全身疾病的详细病史
儿科查体
遗传学评价
眼部检查包括
　视觉功能
　角膜直径
　虹膜形态
　前房深度
　晶状体位置
　白内障形态学
　后节
　　排除后部肿块
　　排除视网膜脱离
　　排除视神经和晶状体之间的茎柄
　眼压
病因不明的双眼白内障的实验室检测
　半乳糖代谢紊乱：尿中还原物质；半乳糖-1-磷酸尿嘧啶转移酶；半乳糖激酶
　传染病：TORCH和水痘滴度，VDRL试验
　代谢疾病：尿氨基酸试验（Lowe综合征）；血清钙（甲状旁腺功能减退症较低）、磷（甲状旁腺功能减退症较高）、葡萄糖（糖尿病较高）和铁蛋白（高铁质血症较高）

TORCH=弓形虫病、风疹、巨细胞病毒、单纯疱疹病毒。

病史

除了家族史外，医生还应询问孩子成长发育史和全身疾病史，这些信息有助于指导评估，如对于获得性白内障和难治性腹泻的患儿应评估代谢性疾病的脑腱黄瘤病，其为可治性疾病，并立即对直系亲属行裂隙灯检查，可发现未被诊断的晶状体混浊，这些混浊可能不影响视觉，但提示儿童白内障的遗传性。如先天性后缝性白内障发生在 X- 连锁 Nance-Horan 综合征的女性携带者，以及 Lowe（前脑硬化）综合征的青春期女性携带者，后者仅呈现轻度晶状体混浊。

检查

视功能

单纯的白内障不一定是手术指征，视晶状体混浊对视觉的影响而定。

In healthy infants aged 2 months or younger, the fixation reflex may not be fully developed; thus, its absence in this group of patients is not necessarily abnormal. In general, anterior capsule opacities are not visually significant unless they occlude the entire pupil. Central or posterior lens opacities of sufficient density that are greater than 3 mm in diameter are usually visually significant. Opacities that have a large area of surrounding normal red reflex or that have clear areas within them may allow good visual development. Strabismus associated with a unilateral cataract and nystagmus associated with bilateral cataracts indicate that the opacities are visually significant. Although these signs may also indicate that the optimal time for treatment has passed, cataract surgery may still improve visual function.

In preverbal children older than 2 months, standard clinical assessment of fixation behavior, fixation preference, and objection to occlusion provide additional evidence of the visual significance of the cataract(s). For bilateral cataracts, assessment of the child's visual behavior and the family's observations of the child at home help determine the level of visual function. Preferential looking tests and visual evoked potentials can provide quantitative information (see Chapter 1). In older children, particularly those with lamellar or posterior subcapsular cataracts, glare testing may be useful for assessing decreased vision.

Ocular examination

Slit-lamp examination can help classify the morphology of the cataract and reveal associated abnormalities of the anterior segment. If the cataract allows some view of the posterior segment, the optic nerve and fovea should be examined. If no such view is possible, B-scan ultrasonography should be performed to assess for anatomical abnormalities of the posterior segment. The presence of retinal or optic nerve abnormalities cannot be definitively ruled out, however, until the posterior pole can be visualized directly. See Table 23-3 for additional information.

Workup

Unilateral cataracts are not usually associated with systemic disease; laboratory tests are therefore not warranted in these cases. In contrast, bilateral cataracts are associated with many metabolic or other systemic diseases. If the child has a positive family history of isolated congenital or childhood cataract or if examination of the parents shows lens opacities (and there are no associated systemic diseases to explain their cataracts), systemic evaluation and laboratory tests are not necessary. A basic laboratory evaluation for bilateral cataracts of unknown etiology is outlined in Table 23-3.

Further workup should be directed by the presence of other systemic abnormalities. Evaluation by a geneticist may be helpful for determining whether there are associated disorders and for counseling the patient's family regarding recurrence risks. Next-generation gene sequencing, which analyzes large portions of the genome, is of increasing utility, even in cases without evidence of systemic disease.

Cataract Surgery in Pediatric Patients

Timing of the Procedure

In general, the younger the child, the greater the urgency to remove the cataract, because of the risk of deprivation amblyopia. For optimal visual development, a visually significant unilateral cataract should be removed before age 6 weeks; visually significant bilateral cataracts, before age 10 weeks.

2 个月或更小的健康婴儿的注视反射发育不完全，所以没有注视并不一定是异常的。一般来说，前囊混浊没有遮盖整个瞳孔时，不影响视觉。当中心或后晶状体混浊密度高、直径大于 3mm 时，则会影响视觉。有大范围晶状体混浊环绕红光反射区或者红光反射区有足够清晰的区域时，其视觉发育良好。斜视伴单眼白内障和眼球震颤伴双眼白内障提示晶状体混浊影响视觉，虽然这表明已经错过了最佳的治疗时间，但白内障手术仍可改善视功能。

2 个月以上的语前儿童，评价其注视行为、注视偏好以及拒绝遮盖等行为，有助于进一步判断白内障对视觉的影响程度。评估双眼白内障儿童的视觉行为和家长对患儿在家中相关行为的观察情况，有助于医生确定患儿的视功能状态。优先注视试验和视觉诱发电位（VEP）技术可以定量分析（见第 1 章）。在较大的儿童中，特别是板层白内障或后囊下白内障，眩光试验可以更有效地评估其视力损害。

眼部检查

裂隙灯检查可以用于鉴别判断白内障的形态，以及发现与前段相关的异常。如果白内障可观察到后段，则应检查视神经和中央凹。如果不能看到后端，则应进行 B 超检查，以评估后段的解剖异常。除非眼后段的状况可见，否则不能明确地排除视网膜或视神经的异常。附加的相关信息见表 23–3。

检查

单眼白内障常与全身性疾病无关，不需行实验室检查。而双眼白内障伴有多种代谢性或其他全身性疾病。如果患儿家族史有孤立性先天性或儿童白内障，或父母晶状体混浊（并不伴白内障相关的全身性疾病），也不需行全身性评估和实验室检查。表 23–3 列出了病因不明的双眼白内障的基本实验室评估。

进一步检查的指征是存在全身性异常。遗传学家的评估有助于确定是否存在相关的疾病，并提示患儿家庭可能会发生的风险。新一代的基因测序可分析大部分的基因组，特别是对于没有系统性疾病表现有实用价值。

儿童白内障的手术

手术时机

一般来说，年龄越小的儿童，越急需摘除白内障，因为存在形觉剥夺性弱视的风险。为了使视觉发育达到最佳状态，明显的单眼白内障应在 6 周龄之前摘除，明显的双眼白内障应在 10 周龄之前摘除。

For older children with bilateral cataracts, surgery is indicated when the level of visual function interferes with the child's visual needs. Although children with best-corrected visual acuity of roughly 20/70 may function relatively well in early grade school, their participation in activities such as unrestricted driving may be restricted. Surgery should be considered when visual acuity decreases to 20/40 or worse.

For older children with unilateral cataract, cataract surgery is indicated when visual acuity cannot be improved beyond 20/40.

Intraocular Lens Use in Children

The choice of optical device for correction of aphakia depends primarily on the age of the patient and the laterality of the cataract. Intraocular lens (IOL) implantation in children aged 1–2 years and older is widely accepted. The use of IOLs in younger infants, however, is associated with a higher rate of complications and larger shifts in refractive error with age. Early surgical intervention followed by consistent contact lens wear and patching of the uninvolved eye usually allows development of some useful vision. In most infants who are left aphakic, secondary IOL implantation can be performed after 1–2 years of age.

Infants with mild PFV have a higher incidence of adverse events after lensectomy compared with children with other forms of unilateral cataract, but visual outcomes are similar in both groups.

Management of the Anterior Capsule

To enable access to the lens nucleus and cortex during cataract surgery, a *capsulorrhexis* is performed. Because the tearing characteristics of the pediatric capsule are quite different from those of the adult capsule, lens removal techniques are modified for pediatric patients so that the risk of inadvertent extension of the tear is minimized. The elasticity of the capsule is greatest in younger patients, especially infants, making continuous curvilinear capsulorrhexis more difficult. The pulling force should be directed nearly perpendicular to the direction of intended tear, and the capsule should be regrasped frequently to maintain optimal control over the direction of tear. An alternative to capsulorrhexis in infants is *vitrectorhexis*, the creation of an anterior capsule opening using a vitrectomy instrument. In children with dense cataracts that obscure the red reflex, visibility of the anterior capsule can be enhanced with application of trypan blue ophthalmic solution 0.06% to the capsule.

Lensectomy Without Intraocular Lens Implantation

In children who will be left aphakic, lensectomy is done through a small peripheral corneal, limbal, or pars plana incision with a vitreous-cutting instrument (vitrector). Irrigation can be provided by an integrated infusion sleeve or by a separate anterior chamber cannula. Ultrasonic phacoemulsification is not required, as the lens cortex and nucleus are generally soft in children of all ages. Removing all cortical material is important because of the propensity for reproliferation of pediatric lens epithelial cells. Tough, fibrotic plaques (eg, in severe PFV) may require manual excision with intraocular scissors and forceps.

Because posterior capsule opacification occurs rapidly in young children, a controlled posterior capsulectomy and anterior vitrectomy should be performed at the time of cataract surgery. This technique allows rapid, permanent establishment of a clear visual axis for retinoscopy and prompt fitting and monitoring of the aphakic optical correction. If possible, sufficient peripheral lens capsule should be left to facilitate secondary posterior chamber IOL implantation later.

对于年龄较大的双眼白内障，视功能水平影响到其视觉需求时，需要手术治疗。尽管学龄期低年级儿童的最佳矫正视力在 20/70，但参加驾驶等非限制性活动时可能会受到影响，视力下降到 20/40 以下时应考虑手术治疗。

对于年龄较大的单眼白内障患儿，矫正视力低于 20/40 时应行白内障手术。

人工晶体在儿童中的使用

无晶状体眼的光学矫正方法选择取决于患儿的年龄和白内障累及的眼。普遍认可对 1 ~ 2 岁及以上儿童实施人工晶体（IOL）植入。而对年幼的婴儿人工晶体（IOL）植入，其并发症的发生率较高，随年龄的增大会发生较大屈光不正漂移。早期白内障手术后，持续配戴角膜接触镜，并遮盖未受累眼，常能使有用视力得以发育。大多数无晶状体眼患儿，可在 1 ~ 2 岁后行二次人工晶体（IOL）植入术。

与其他单眼白内障患儿相比，伴轻度永久性胎儿血管（PFV）的患儿术后并发症的发生率较高，但 2 组的视力结果相似。

前囊的处理

白内障手术中，先行*撕囊*，之后才进入晶状体核和皮质。与成人的晶状体囊膜不同，儿童晶状体的囊膜易撕裂，因此需对儿童晶状体摘除技术进行改进，以便将囊膜撕裂意外的风险降至最低。低龄儿童的囊膜弹性最大，特别是婴儿，这使得连续环形撕囊术更加困难。用力方向应垂直于撕囊方向，同时需不断重新抓住囊膜，以保持对撕囊方向的最佳控制。婴儿撕囊术的另一种替代方法是*玻璃体切除头撕囊术*，即使用玻璃体切除器械切开前囊。儿童白内障致密可遮盖红光反射，为了增强前囊的可视性，可使用 0.06% 的台盼蓝眼液。

无人工晶体植入的晶状体摘除术

对于术后无晶状体眼的儿童，通过周边角膜、角膜缘、睫状体平坦部的小切口，用玻璃体切头行晶状体切除术。由一体化灌注套管或独立的前房灌注管提供灌注。不需要超声乳化，因为儿童的晶状体皮质和核较软。清除所有皮质非常重要，因为儿童晶状体的上皮细胞有再增殖的倾向。坚硬的纤维化膜［如严重永久性胎儿血管（PFV）］需用眼内剪和镊子手动切除。

儿童的后囊膜混浊可迅速发生，因此行白内障手术时应行有限的后囊膜切除术和前玻璃体切除术，这种技术可快速、永久地形成清晰的视轴区，便于视网膜检影，快速确定屈光度和监测无晶体眼屈光矫正。尽可能地留下足够的周边晶状体囊膜，以便二期后房型人工晶体（IOL）植入。

Lensectomy With Intraocular Lens Implantation

Single-piece foldable acrylic IOLs, which can be placed through a 3-mm clear corneal or scleral tunnel incision, have become popular in pediatric cataract surgery, although larger single-piece polymethyl methacrylate (PMMA) lenses are also still used. Silicone lenses have not been well studied in children.

If an IOL is to be placed at the time of cataract extraction, 2 basic techniques can be used for the lensectomy, depending on whether the posterior capsule will be left intact. Many pediatric cataract surgeons leave the posterior capsule intact if the child is approaching the age when an Nd:YAG laser capsulotomy in an awake patient could be performed (usually 5 years of age). Primary capsulectomy is usually preferred for younger children. Studies have shown that in early childhood, the lens capsule opacifies, on average, within 18–24 months of surgery, but this can vary considerably.

Technique with posterior capsule intact

After the cortex is aspirated, the clear corneal or scleral tunnel incision is enlarged to allow placement of the IOL. Placement in the capsular bag is desirable, but ciliary sulcus fixation is acceptable. Viscoelastic material should be removed to prevent a postoperative spike in intraocular pressure. Closure of 3-mm clear corneal incisions with absorbable suture is safe and does not induce astigmatism in children.

Techniques for primary posterior capsulectomy

Posterior capsulectomy/vitrectomy before IOL placement After lensectomy, the vitrector settings should be set to the low-suction, high-cutting rate appropriate for vitreous surgery. A posterior capsulectomy with anterior vitrectomy is then performed. The anterior capsule is enlarged, if necessary, to an appropriate size for the IOL, and the lens is implanted in the capsular bag or the ciliary sulcus. The surgeon must take care to ensure that the capsulotomy does not extend, the IOL haptics do not go through the posterior opening, and vitreous does not become entangled with the IOL or enter the anterior chamber.

Posterior capsulectomy/vitrectomy after IOL placement Some surgeons prefer to place the IOL in the capsular bag, close the anterior incision, and approach the posterior capsule through the pars plana. Irrigation can be maintained through the same anterior chamber infusion cannula used during lensectomy. A small conjunctival opening is made over the pars plana, and a sclerotomy is made with a microvitreoretinal blade 2.5–3.0 mm posterior to the limbus. This provides good access to the posterior capsule, and a wide anterior vitrectomy can be performed.

人工晶体植入的晶状体摘除术

单片式可折叠丙烯酸酯人工晶体（IOL）可通过 3mm 宽透明角膜或巩膜隧道切口植入，已被广泛用于儿童白内障手术，但较大的单片式聚甲基丙烯酸甲酯（PMMA）晶体也在使用。对于硅胶人工晶体在儿童中的应用研究较少。

如果在白内障摘除的同时植入人工晶体（IOL），可根据后囊是否完整，采用 2 种基本技术进行晶状体摘除术。如果儿童可接受清醒状态下的 Nd:YAG 激光囊膜切开术（通常在 5 岁），许多儿童白内障手术医生会保留完整的后囊膜。一期囊膜切除术常用于幼儿。研究表明，儿童早期的晶状体囊膜混浊发生在术后的 18 ~ 24 个月，但变异很大。

后囊膜完整的技术

吸出皮质后，扩大透明角膜或巩膜隧道切口，植入人工晶体（IOL）。最好植入囊袋内，也可睫状沟固定。取出黏弹剂，以防止术后一过性眼压升高。用可吸收缝线行 3mm 透明角膜切口缝合比较安全，而且不会引起散光。

一期后囊膜切除术技术

人工晶体（IOL）植入术前的后囊膜切除术 / 玻璃体切除术　晶状体摘除后，设置玻璃体切割机为低吸力、高切割率的玻璃体手术模式，然后行后囊膜切除和前玻璃体切除。将前囊扩大至适合人工晶体（IOL）的适当大小，将晶状体植入囊袋或睫状沟。医生须确保囊膜切开术不会扩大、人工晶体（IOL）不会穿过后囊开口，且玻璃体不与 IOL 缠绕或进入前房。

人工晶体（IOL）植入后的后囊膜切除术 / 玻璃体切除术　有些手术医生喜欢将人工晶状体植入囊袋内，闭合角膜切口，经睫状体扁平部接近后囊。维持晶状体摘除的前房灌注管冲洗。在睫状体扁平部处做 1 个结膜小切口，用微型玻璃体视网膜刀，在角膜缘后 2.5~3.0 mm 处行巩膜切开。这样后囊膜易于接近，并可行较广泛的前玻璃体切除。

Intraocular lens implantation issues

Because the eye continues to elongate throughout the first decade of life and beyond, selecting an appropriate IOL power is complicated. Power calculations in infants and young children may be unpredictable for several reasons, including widely variable growth of the eye, difficulty obtaining accurate keratometry and axial length measurements, and use of power formulas that were developed for adults rather than children. Studies have shown that in aphakic pediatric eyes, a variable myopic shift in refractive error of approximately 7.00–8.00 D occurs from 1 year to 10 years of age, with a wide standard deviation. This suggests that if a child is made emmetropic with an IOL at 1 year of age, refractive error at 10 years of age can be −8.00 D or greater. Refractive change in children younger than 1 year is even more unpredictable. This assumes that the presence of an IOL does not alter the normal growth curve of the aphakic eye, an assumption that may not be valid based on results of both animal and early human studies.

Lens implantation in children requires consideration of the age of the child, the target refractive error at the time of surgery, and the refractive error of the contralateral eye. Some surgeons implant IOLs with powers that are expected to be required in adulthood, allowing the child to grow into the selected lens power. Thus, the child initially requires hyperopic correction. Other surgeons aim for emmetropia at the time of lens implantation, especially in unilateral cases, believing that this approach improves the treatment of amblyopia and facilitates development of binocular function by decreasing anisometropia in the early childhood years. These children usually become progressively more myopic and may eventually require a second procedure to address the increasing anisometropia.

Postoperative Care

Medical therapy

If all cortical material is adequately removed, postoperative inflammation is usually mild in a child without a lens implant. Topical antibiotics, corticosteroids, and cycloplegics are commonly applied for a few weeks after surgery. Topical corticosteroids should be used more aggressively in children who have undergone IOL implantation. Some surgeons administer intracameral corticosteroids at the time of surgery, and others use oral corticosteroids postoperatively, especially in very young children and in children with heavily pigmented irides. Some surgeons administer intracameral antibiotics in addition to topical antibiotics.

Amblyopia management

Amblyopia therapy should begin as soon as possible after surgery. For aphakic patients, contact lenses or glasses should be dispensed within a few weeks of surgery.

For infants with bilateral aphakia, glasses are the safest and simplest method of correction. They can be easily changed according to the refractive shifts that occur with growth of the eye. Until the child can use a bifocal lens properly, the power selected should make the eye myopic, because most of an infant's visual activity occurs at near. Contact lenses may also be used in bilaterally aphakic patients, but they require more effort on the part of both the caregiver and the physician than do glasses.

人工晶状体植入

直至 10 岁前后，眼睛一直在增长，所以很难选择合适的人工晶体（IOL）。婴儿和幼儿的屈光度无法预测，因为眼睛的生长变异很大、难以获得精准的角膜曲率和眼轴长度检测，而且屈光度计算公式是针对成人的，而不是针对儿童的。研究表明，在 1 ~ 10 岁之间，无晶状体眼儿童的屈光度会发生 7.00 ~ 8.00D 的近视飘移，且标准差较大。这提示儿童在 1 岁时用 IOL 使其成为正视眼，10 岁时屈光度可达 -8.00D 或更高。1 岁以下儿童的屈光度变化更不可预测。由此可以推测，人工晶体（IOL）的存在并不会改变无晶状体眼的正常生长曲线，这一假设不同于基于动物和早期人类研究的结果。

儿童的晶体植入需考虑儿童的年龄、手术时的目标屈光度和对侧眼的屈光度。一些手术医生植入的人工晶体（IOL）是成年后所需的屈光度，使儿童屈光状态向所选择的晶状体屈光度发育，因此，儿童最初需要进行远视矫正。另一些手术医生则以植入的人工晶体呈正视为既定目标，特别是单眼白内障，认为通过这种方法减少儿童早期的屈光参差，可以改善弱视的治疗、促进双眼功能的发展。这些儿童常发生进行性近视，需二次手术治疗逐渐加重的屈光参差。

术后护理

药物治疗

如果充分清除所有的皮质，儿童在无人工晶体植入的白内障术后炎症通常很轻。手术后需使用数周的局部抗生素、皮质类固醇和睫状肌麻痹剂。儿童行人工晶体植入术时，应大量使用局部皮质类固醇。一些手术医生在手术时使用球内皮质类固醇激素，一些手术医生，特别是对低龄儿童和虹膜颜色深的儿童，术后使用口服皮质类固醇激素，另一些手术医生除了局部使用抗生素外，还使用球内抗生素。

弱视的治疗

手术后应尽早开始弱视治疗。无晶状体眼患儿应在手术后几周内配戴接触镜或框架眼镜。

双眼无晶状体眼的婴儿，配戴框架眼镜是最安全、最简单的矫正方法，可根据眼睛的生长过程中发生的屈光变化而随时更换。因为婴儿的大部分视觉活动在近处，在孩子能够正确配戴双焦镜之前，应选择呈近视状态的屈光度。接触镜也可以用于双眼无晶状体患儿，但与使用框架眼镜相比，护理人员和医生需要付出更多。

For infants with unilateral aphakia, contact lenses are the most common method of correction. Advantages of contact lenses include relatively easy power changes and the potential for extended wear with certain lenses. Disadvantages include easy displacement by eye rubbing, the expense of replacement, and the risk of microbial keratitis. Aphakic glasses are occasionally used in infants with unilateral aphakia who are unable to tolerate contact lenses, but these glasses are suboptimal owing to the amblyogenic effect of aniseikonia and the difficulty of wearing glasses that are much heavier on one side.

After optical correction of aphakia, patching of the better eye is necessary in patients with unilateral cataract and in some patients with bilateral cataracts if the visual acuity is asymmetric. The amount of patching is based on the degree of amblyopia and the age of the child. Avoidance of full-time occlusion in the neonatal period may allow stimulation of binocular vision and may help prevent strabismus.

Complications Following Pediatric Cataract Surgery

Strabismus is very common in children following surgery for either unilateral or bilateral cataracts. The risk of glaucoma is increased in children who have cataract surgery in infancy and in those with small eyes (see Chapter 22), but glaucoma often does not develop until several years after surgery. Corneal decompensation is very rare in children. Retinal detachments are also rare and are most likely to occur when other ocular abnormalities are present. The incidence of macular edema is unknown, as it is difficult to detect ophthalmoscopically in young children and optical coherence tomography is usually not possible. Postoperative endophthalmitis rarely occurs in children after cataract surgery.

Visual Outcome After Cataract Extraction

Visual outcome after cataract surgery depends on many factors, including age at onset and type of cataract, timing of surgery, choice of optical correction, and treatment of amblyopia. Early surgery by itself does not ensure a good outcome. Optimal vision requires careful, long-term postoperative management, particularly regarding amblyopia. Even when congenital cataracts are detected late (after age 4 months), cataract removal combined with a strong postoperative vision rehabilitation program can achieve good vision in some eyes.

Structural or Positional Lens Abnormalities

Congenital Aphakia

Congenital aphakia, the absence of the lens at birth, is rare. This condition is usually associated with a markedly abnormal eye.

Spherophakia

A lens that is spherical and smaller than normal is termed *spherophakic*. This condition is usually bilateral. The lens may dislocate and prolapse into the anterior chamber, causing secondary glaucoma.

单眼无晶状体眼的婴儿，配戴接触镜是最常见的矫正方法。接触镜的优点有：相对容易改变屈光度，某些类型的接触镜可长期配戴。缺点有：容易因揉搓眼睛而导致移位、更换的费用和微生物角膜炎的风险。框架眼镜偶用于无法耐受接触镜的单眼无晶状体眼婴儿，但仅是个次选的方案，因为双眼不等像性弱视，以及一侧眼镜的重量过重会使得戴镜困难。

单眼白内障和视力不对称的双眼白内障患儿，对无晶状体眼进行光学矫正后，还需要对视力较好眼进行遮盖。遮盖的时间取决于弱视的程度和孩子的年龄。新生儿避免全天候遮盖，这样有助于刺激双眼视觉，并预防斜视。

儿童白内障术后的并发症

斜视在儿童单眼或双眼白内障术后很常见。婴儿期行白内障手术的儿童和小眼球的儿童患青光眼的风险增加（见第 22 章），但青光眼常在白内障手术后数年才会发生。儿童角膜失代偿的状况很少见。视网膜脱离也很少见，且多发生在伴有其他眼部异常的情况。黄斑水肿的发生率尚未知，因为很难对儿童进行眼底镜检查和光学相干断层扫描。眼内炎很少发生在儿童白内障术后。

白内障术后的视力

白内障手术后的视力取决于许多因素，包括发病年龄、白内障类型、手术时机、光学矫正的方法以及对弱视的治疗。早期手术本身并不能保证获得良好的视力。理想的视力康复需要仔细、长期的术后管理，特别是弱视。即使先天性白内障发现较晚（4 个月龄后），白内障摘除联合术后严格的视力康复计划也能使一些眼睛获得良好的视力。

晶状体结构或位置异常

先天性无晶状体眼

先天性无晶状体眼罕见，是指出生时晶状体缺失的状况，常伴有明显的眼睛异常。

球形晶状体

晶状体呈球形，且比正常小，称为*球形晶状体*，常为双眼。晶状体可能脱位和脱入前房，导致继发性青光眼。

Coloboma

A lens coloboma involves flattening or notching of the lens periphery (Fig 23-6). It may be associated with a coloboma of the iris, optic nerve, or retina, all of which are caused by abnormal closure of the embryonic fissure. The term *lens coloboma* is a misnomer because the lens defect is caused by absence or stretching of the zonular fibers in the affected area (usually inferonasally) and is not directly due to abnormal embryonic fissure closure. In more significant colobomatous defects, lens dislocations may occur superiorly and temporally. Most colobomatous lenses do not progressively worsen.

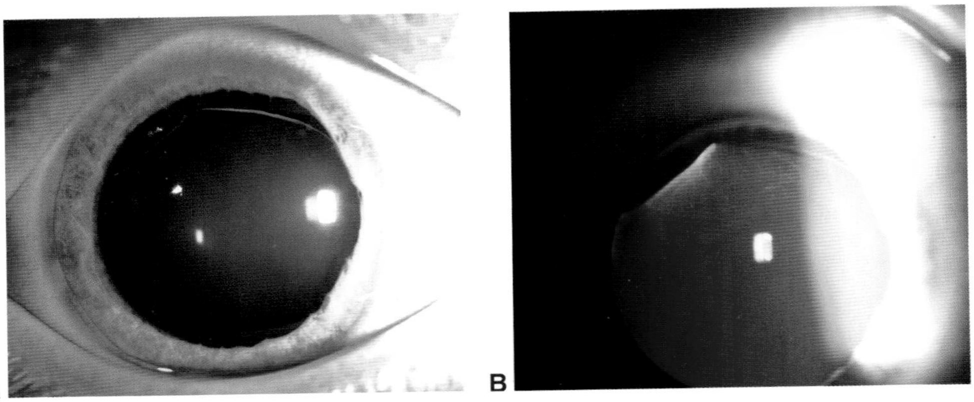

Figure 23-6 Lens coloboma, viewed with slit-beam illumination **(A)** and retroillumination **(B).** The lens is subluxated inferonasally, and there is a notch in the superotemporal portion of the lens where zonules are lacking. *(Courtesy of Gregg T. Lueder, MD.)*

Dislocated Lenses in Children

When the lens is not in its normal position, it is said to be *dislocated. Subluxated* (or *subluxed*) lenses are partly dislocated. *Luxated* (or *luxed*), or *ectopic*, lenses are completely detached from the ciliary body; they are free in the posterior chamber (Fig 23-7), or they have prolapsed into the anterior chamber. The amount of dislocation can vary, from slight displacement with minimal *iridodonesis* (tremulousness of the iris) to severe displacement in which the lens periphery is not visible through the pupillary opening. Lens dislocation can be familial or sporadic. It can be associated with gene mutations that specifically affect the eye, with multisystem disease, and with inborn errors of metabolism (Table 23-4). Lens dislocation can occur with trauma, usually involving significant injury to the eye, but this is not common. Spontaneous lens dislocation has been reported in aniridia, buphthalmos associated with congenital glaucoma, and congenital megalocornea with zonular weakness (due to mutations in latent transforming growth factor beta-binding protein 2 *[LTBP2]).*

Khan AO, Aldahmesh MA, Alkuraya FS. Congenital megalocornea with zonular weakness and childhood lens-related secondary glaucoma—a distinct phenotype caused by recessive LTBP2 mutations. *Mol Vis.* 2011;17:2570–2579.

缺损

晶状体缺损包括晶状体周边部变平或出现缺口（图 23–6），可伴虹膜、视神经或视网膜缺损，这些均是由胚胎裂闭合异常所致。但晶状体缺损一词有误，因为晶状体缺损是由于受影响区域（常位于鼻下侧）的悬韧带缺失或拉伸引起的，并不是直接由胚胎裂隙闭合异常引起的。缺损严重时，晶状体可能脱位到上方和颞侧。多数晶状体缺损不会出现进行性恶化。

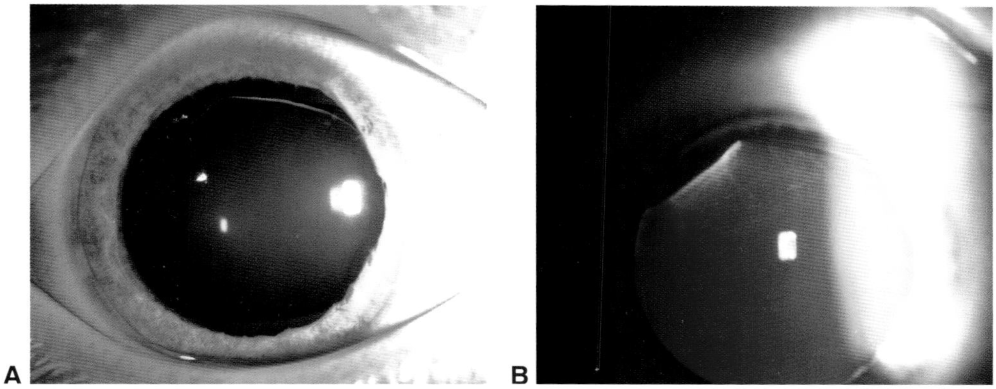

图 23–6　在裂隙灯下观察晶状体缺损的弥散光照法（**A**）和后部照射法（**B**）。晶状体鼻下方不全脱位和颞上方有一缺口，其悬韧带缺如。*（译者注：资料来源见前页原文。）*

儿童晶状体脱位

晶状体不在其正常的解剖位置称为*脱位*。*半脱位*晶状体是指部分脱位。*脱位*或*异位*是指晶状体完全脱离睫状体，游离在后房（图 23–7），或脱入前房。脱位的程度不一，从轻微的*虹膜震颤*（虹膜颤动）到严重的异位，经瞳孔窥不到晶状体的边缘）。晶状体脱位可呈家族性，或呈偶发性。可伴有特定影响眼的基因突变、多系统疾病和先天性代谢异常（表 23–4）。外伤也可引发晶状体脱位，常为严重的眼外伤，并不常见。有报道称，在无虹膜症、伴随悬韧带薄弱先天性青光眼的牛眼症中，发生自发性晶状体脱位［这是由于潜在转化生长因子 β 结合蛋白 2（*LTBP2*）的突变］。

Khan AO, Aldahmesh MA, Alkuraya FS. Congenital megalocornea with zonular weakness and childhood lens-related secondary glaucoma—a distinct phenotype caused by recessive LTBP2 mutations. *Mol Vis.* 2011;17:2570–2579.

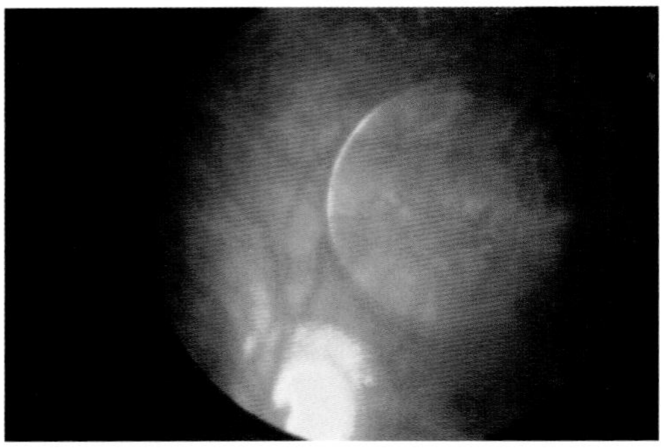

Figure 23-7 Lens dislocation into vitreous.

Table 23-4 Conditions Associated With Dislocated Lenses

Systemic conditions	Ocular conditions
Marfan syndrome	Aniridia
Homocystinuria	Iris coloboma
Weill-Marchesani syndrome	Trauma
Sulfite oxidase deficiency	Hereditary ectopia lentis
	Congenital megalocornea with zonular weakness

Isolated Ectopia Lentis

In simple ectopia lentis, the lens is displaced superiorly and temporally. The condition is usually bilateral and symmetric. Most commonly, it is inherited as an autosomal dominant trait. Onset can be at birth or later in life. Glaucoma is common in the late-onset type.

Some patients with heterozygous mutations in *FBN1*, which cause Marfan syndrome (discussed later), do not have the systemic findings associated with this syndrome and have only ectopia lentis.

Ectopia Lentis et Pupillae

Ectopia lentis et pupillae is a rare autosomal recessive condition in which there is bilateral displacement of the pupil, usually inferotemporally, and dislocation of the lens in the opposite direction (Fig 23-8A) (see Chapter 21). The condition is characterized by small, round lenses (microspherophakia); miosis; and poor pupillary dilation with mydriatics. Ectopia lentis et pupillae may be the result of a membrane extending from a posterior origin to attach to the proximal pupil margin (Fig 23-8B).

A B

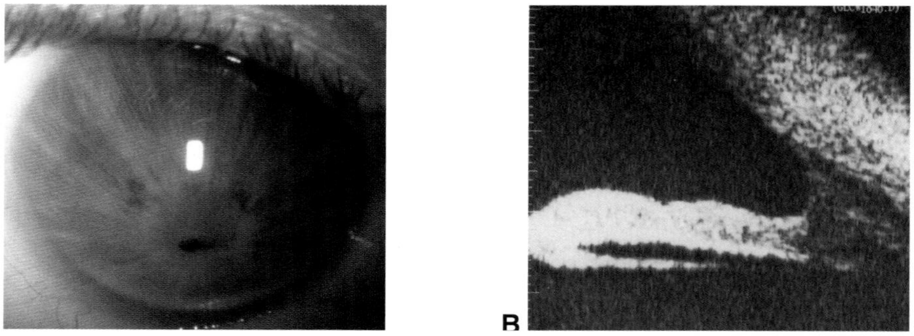

Figure 23-8 **A,** Ectopia lentis et pupillae. **B,** Ultrasonography shows a membrane posterior to the iris attaching at the pupil margin. *(Part A reproduced from Byles DB, Nischal KK, Cheng H. Ectopia lentis et pupillae. A hypothesis revisited. Ophthalmology. 1998;105(7):1331–1336. Part B courtesy of Ken K. Nischal, MD.)*

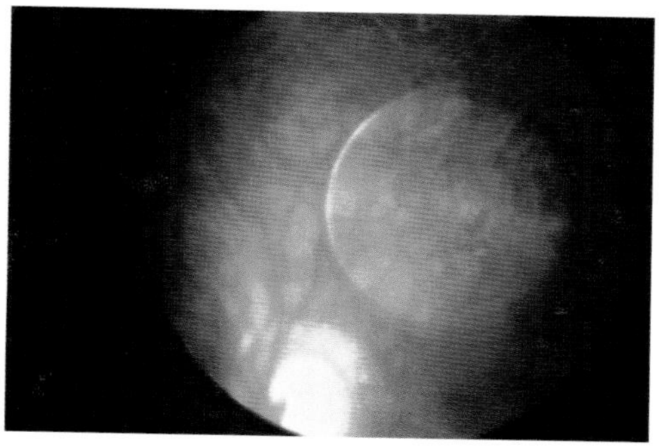

图 23-7　晶状体脱位到玻璃体。

表 23-4 伴晶状体脱位的疾病

系统性疾病	眼部疾病
Marfans综合征	无虹膜症
同型胱氨酸尿症	虹膜缺损
Weill - Marchesani综合征	外伤
亚硫酸氧化酶缺乏症	遗传性晶状体异位
	先天性巨角膜伴随悬韧带脆弱

孤立性晶状体异位

在单纯性晶状体异位中，晶状体会异位到上方和颞侧，常是双眼和对称的。最常见的是常染色体显性遗传。可出生时发病或迟发，青光眼常见于迟发型。

FBN1 杂合突变可导致 Marfans 综合征（稍后讨论），伴有这种突变的患儿并没有该综合征的相关系统性疾病，仅表现为晶状体脱位。

晶状体瞳孔异位

晶状体瞳孔异位是一种罕见的常染色体隐性遗传病，其表现为双眼瞳孔移位，常向颞下方移位，晶状体则向相反方向脱位（图 23-8A）（见第 21 章）。其特征是晶状体小而圆（小球形晶状体）、瞳孔缩小、瞳孔不易散大。形成晶状体瞳孔异位可能是由于有一层膜从后部延伸到了近端瞳孔边缘（图 23-8B）。

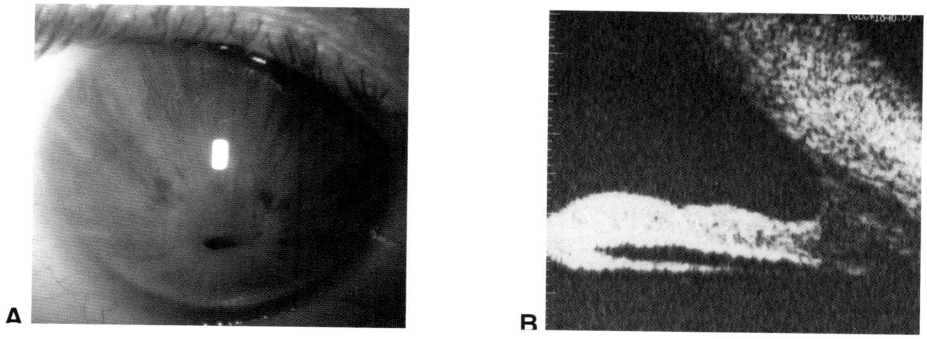

图 23-8　**A.** 晶状体瞳孔异位。**B.** 超声显示一层膜附着于虹膜后的瞳孔边缘。*（译者注：资料来源见前页原文。）*

Marfan Syndrome

Marfan syndrome is the systemic disease most commonly associated with subluxated lenses. The syndrome consists of abnormalities of the cardiovascular, musculoskeletal, and ocular systems. It is inherited as an autosomal dominant trait, but family history is negative in 15% of cases. Marfan syndrome is caused by mutations in *FBN1*, which provides instructions for making the protein fibrillin-1, the major constituent of extracellular microfibrils. Affected patients are characteristically tall, with long limbs and fin gers (*arachnodactyly*) (Fig 23-9); loose, flexible joints; scoliosis; and chest deformities. Cardiovascular abnormalities are a source of significant mortality and manifest as enlargement of the aortic root, dilation of the descending aorta, dissecting aneurysm, and floppy mitral valve. The life expectancy of patients with Marfan syndrome is about half that of the normal population.

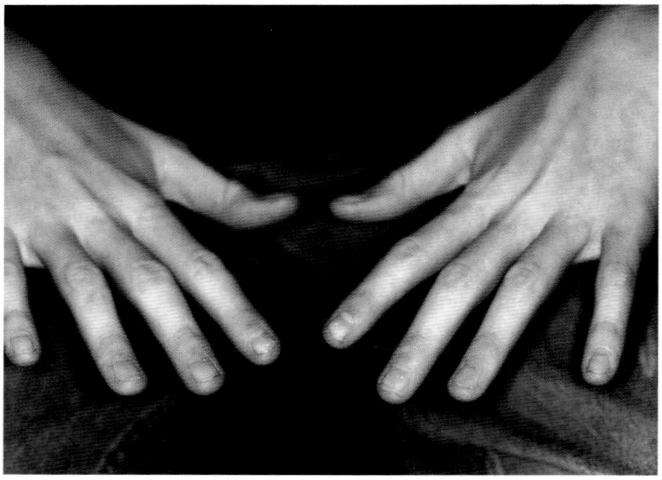

Figure 23-9 Long, slender digits in a patient with Marfan syndrome. *(Reproduced with permission from Lueder GT. Pediatric Practice: Ophthalmology. New York: McGraw-Hill Education; 2010: 222.)*

Ocular abnormalities occur in more than 80% of affected patients, with lens subluxation being the most common (Fig 23-10). In approximately 75% of cases, the lens is subluxated superiorly. Typically, the zonules that are visible are intact and unbroken. Examination of the iris usually shows iridodonesis and may reveal transillumination defects near the iris base. The pupil is small and dilates poorly. The corneal curvature is often decreased. The axial length is increased, and affected patients are frequently myopic. Retinal detachment can occur spontaneously, usually in the second and third decades of life.

Homocystinuria

Homocystinuria is a rare autosomal recessive condition, occurring in approximately 1 in 100,000 births. The classic form is usually caused by mutations in the gene encoding cystathionine β-synthase, which causes homocysteine to accumulate in the plasma and to be excreted in the urine.

Marfan 综合征

Marfan 综合征是一种全身性疾病，常伴有晶状体半脱位。该综合征包括心血管、肌肉骨骼和眼部异常，属于一种常染色体显性遗传，但 15% 的病例中家族史为阴性。Marfan 综合征是由 *FBN1* 基因突变引起的，该基因提供制造细胞外微纤维的主要成分原纤维蛋白 -1 的指令。患者的特征是身材高大、四肢和手指较长（*蜘蛛样指 / 趾*）（图 23–9）、松弛灵活的关节、脊柱侧弯及胸部畸形。心血管异常是重要的致死原因，表现为主动脉根部扩大、降主动脉扩张、夹层动脉瘤和二尖瓣下垂。Marfan 综合征患者的寿命约为正常人的一半。

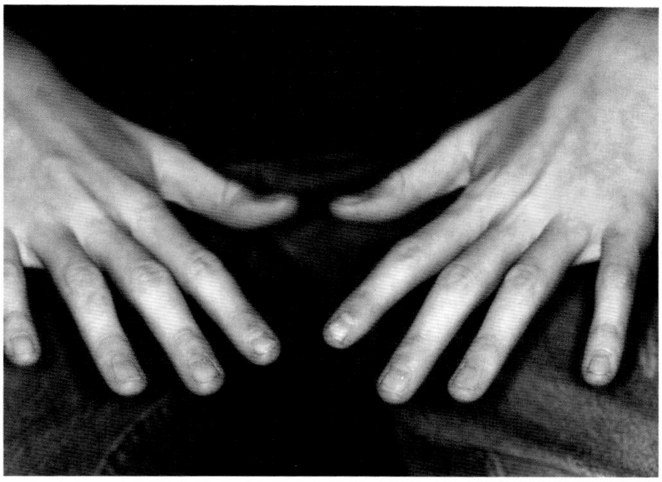

图 23–9　Marfan 综合征患者细长的手指。*（译者注：资料来源见前页原文。）*

80% 以上的患者有眼部异常，最常见的是晶状体半脱位（图 23–10）。在约 75% 的病例中，晶状体上方脱位，悬韧带完整无缺损。虹膜检查显示虹膜震颤，虹膜基底的透光缺失。瞳孔小，且不易散大。角膜曲率降低，眼轴增长，患者表现为近视。视网膜脱离在 20 ~ 30 岁时自发发生。

同型胱氨酸尿症

同型半胱氨酸尿症是一种罕见的常染色体隐性遗传疾病，新生儿的发病率约为 1/10 万。典型的形式是胱硫氨 β 合成酶的编码基因突变，导致血浆同型半胱氨酸堆积，并由尿液排出。

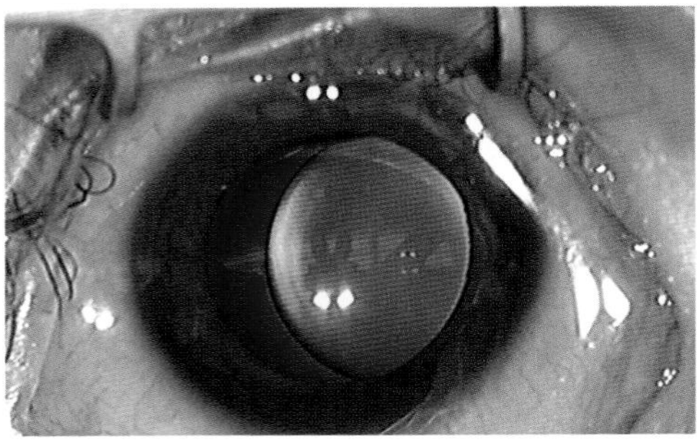

Figure 23-10 Lens subluxation in a patient with Marfan syndrome. *(Courtesy of Gregg T. Lueder, MD.)*

The clinical manifestations of homocystinuria vary; the eye, skeletal system, central nervous system, and vascular system can be affected. Most of the abnormalities develop after birth and become progressively worse with age. The ophthalmologist may see patients with this disorder before the systemic diagnosis is made. The skeletal features are similar to those of Marfan syndrome. Affected patients are usually tall and have osteoporosis, scoliosis, and chest deformities. Central nervous system abnormalities occur in approximately 50% of patients; intellectual disability and seizures are the most common.

Vascular complications are common and secondary to thrombotic disease, which affects large or medium-sized arteries and veins anywhere in the body. Hypertension and cardiomegaly are also common. Anesthesia carries a higher risk for patients with homocystinuria because of thromboembolic phenomena; thus, this disorder should be identified before patients undergo general anesthesia.

The main ocular finding is lens subluxation, most frequently inferiorly, but the direction of subluxation is not diagnostic. Subluxation typically begins between the ages of 3 and 10 years. The lenses may dislocate into the anterior chamber, a finding suggestive of homocystinuria (Fig 23-11). The zonular fibers are frequently broken, in contrast with those in Marfan syndrome.

The diagnosis is confirmed by the detection of disulfides, including homocystine, in the urine. Medical management of homocystinuria is directed toward normalizing the biochemical abnormality. Dietary management (low-methionine diet and supplemental cysteine) may be attempted. Supplementation with the coenzyme pyridoxine (vitamin B_6) diminishes systemic problems in approximately 50% of cases.

Weill-Marchesani Syndrome

Patients with Weill-Marchesani syndrome can be thought of as clinical opposites of patients with Marfan syndrome in that the former are characteristically short, with brachydactyly and short limbs. Inheritance can be autosomal dominant or recessive. Mutations in the *ADAMTS10* gene have been identified in patients with this disorder. The lenses are microspherophakic. With time, the lenses may dislocate into the anterior chamber and cause pupillary block glaucoma. For this reason, prophylactic laser peripheral iridectomy or lensectomy may be indicated.

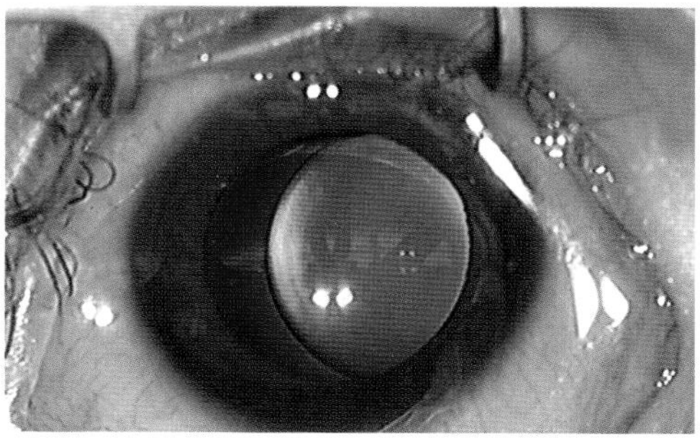

图 23-10　晶状体半脱位的 Marfan 综合征。*（译者注：资料来源见前页原文。）*

同型胱氨酸尿症的临床表现不一，眼睛、骨骼系统、中枢神经系统和血管系统都会受累。大多数异常发生在出生后，并随着年龄的增长而逐渐恶化。眼科医生可能在全身病诊断之前接诊患儿。骨骼特征类似于 Marfan 综合征，患儿身材高大、骨质疏松症、脊柱侧弯和胸部畸形。约 50% 的患者有中枢神经系统异常，最常见的是智力障碍和癫痫。

血管并发症常见，继发于血栓性疾病，累及全身动、静脉的大、中血管。高血压和心脏肥大也常见。由于形成了血栓栓塞，同型半胱氨酸尿症患者进行麻醉时风险较大，因此，患者全身麻醉之前应明确此病是否存在。

主要的眼部表现是晶状体半脱位，最常见的是向下方脱位，但半脱位的方向不能用作诊断依据。半脱位出现在 3 ~ 10 岁。晶状体可脱位进入前房，这一表现提示同型胱氨酸尿症（图 23-11）。与 Marfan 综合征相反，其悬韧带是断裂的。

通过检测尿液中的二硫化物，包括同型半胱氨酸，即可确诊。同型胱氨酸尿症的治疗可以使生化异常值正常化。可试行饮食疗法（低蛋氨酸饮食和补充半胱氨酸）。补充辅酶吡哆醇（维生素 B_6）可减少约 50% 的全身性疾病。

Weill - Marchesani 综合征

与 Marfan 综合征的临床表现相反，Weill-Marchesani 综合征的特点是身材矮小、短指和短肢。为常染色体显性遗传或隐性遗传。检测到 *ADAMTS10* 基因突变。晶状体呈小球形，随着时间的推移，晶状体可能脱入前房，导致瞳孔阻滞型青光眼。因此，需行预防性激光虹膜周边切开术或晶状体切除术。

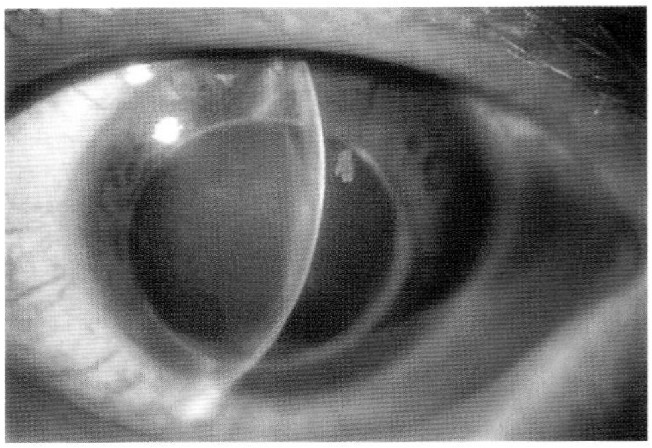

Figure 23-11 Homocystinuria. The lens may dislocate into the anterior chamber and cause acute pupillary block glaucoma.

Sulfite Oxidase Deficiency

Sulfite oxidase deficiency (molybdenum cofactor deficiency) is a very rare hereditary disorder of sulfur metabolism manifested by severe neurologic disorders and ectopia lentis. The enzyme deficiency interferes with conversion of sulfite to sulfate, resulting in increased excretion of sulfite in the urine. The diagnosis can be confirmed by the absence of sulfite oxidase activity in skin fibroblasts. Neurologic abnormalities include infantile hemiplegia, choreoathetosis, and seizures. Irreversible brain damage and death usually occur by 5 years of age.

Treatment

Optical correction

Optical correction of the refractive error caused by lens dislocation is often difficult. With mild subluxation, the patient may be only myopic, and corrected visual function may be good. More severe dislocation causes optical distortion, because the patient is looking through the far periphery of the lens. Because the resultant myopic astigmatism is difficult to measure accurately by retinoscopy or automated refractometry, using an aphakic correction may provide the patient with better vision, as long as the subluxated lens does not fill the pupillary space. Refraction before and after pupil dilation is often helpful for selecting the best type of optical correction. If satisfactory visual function cannot be achieved with glasses or if visual function worsens, lens removal should be considered.

Surgery

Subluxated lenses can be removed either from the anterior segment through a limbal incision or posteriorly through the pars plana. In most circumstances, complete lensectomy is indicated. Lens removal is easier when the lens is not severely subluxated.

In the United States, contact lenses or glasses are usually used for postoperative vision rehabilitation, with good visual results. Anterior chamber or scleral-fixated IOLs are sometimes implanted. The latter should be used with caution if sutures are used for fixation because of the high rate of suture breakage. Iris-claw lenses (Artisan; OPHTEC BV, Groningen, the Netherlands) are widely used in other countries and are currently under investigation in the United States.

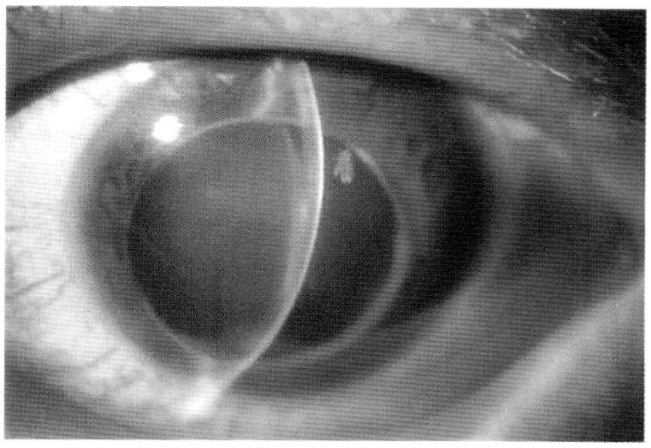

图 23-11　同型胱氨酸尿症。晶状体脱位进入前房，并引起急性瞳孔阻滞型青光眼。

亚硫酸盐氧化酶缺乏症

亚硫酸盐氧化酶缺乏症（钼辅助因子缺乏症）是一种罕见的硫代谢遗传性疾病，表现为严重的神经功能障碍和晶状体脱位。酶缺乏会干扰亚硫酸盐转化为硫酸盐，导致亚硫酸盐在尿液中的排泄量增加。如果皮肤成纤维细胞中的亚硫酸盐氧化酶缺乏活性，即可确诊。神经系统异常包括婴儿偏瘫、舞蹈徐动症和癫痫，常在 5 岁之前出现不可逆的脑损伤和死亡。

治疗

光学矫正

晶状体脱位引起的屈光不正不易矫正。轻度半脱位仅表现为近视，矫正视力较好。严重的脱位会导致光学畸变，患者通过晶状体的远周边部来视物，由此产生的近视性散光很难通过视网膜检影或自动验光仪来精确测量。当半脱位的晶状体没有占据整个瞳孔，使用无晶状体眼矫正的方法可使患者获得较好的视力。散瞳前后的屈光度有助于选择最佳的光学矫正方法。如果戴眼镜无法获得令人满意的视力，或视力下降，应考虑摘除晶状体。

手术

半脱位的晶状体可以通过角膜缘的切口从前节摘除，也可以通过睫状体的扁平部从后节摘除。在大多数情况下，需要行完全的晶状体切除术。当没有严重半脱位时，晶状体摘除较为容易。

美国常采用接触镜或框架眼镜行术后视力康复，效果良好，有时植入前房或巩膜固定型人工晶体，后者应谨慎使用，因为固定缝线的断线率较高。虹膜夹持晶体（Artisan; OPHTEC BV， Groningen， the Netherlands）在其他国家被广泛使用，目前美国正在审查中。

（翻译 张令仪 仁千格麦 // 审校 刘陇黔 石一宁 蒋宁 // 章节审校 石广礼）

CHAPTER 24

Uveitis in the Pediatric Age Group

Uveitis is broadly defined as inflammation of the uvea, including the iris, ciliary body, and choroid. See BCSC Section 9, *Uveitis and Ocular Inflammation*, for a more detailed description of the clinical features and inflammatory mechanisms of the conditions discussed in this chapter.

Epidemiology

The prevalence of pediatric uveitis varies among studies, with pediatric cases accounting for 2%–14% of all uveitis cases. The distribution between the sexes is similar to that of uveitis in adults, showing a slight female preponderance. The mean age at diagnosis is 8–9 years, and 75% of patients have bilateral disease. In the United States, approximately 62% of pediatric patients with uveitis are white. The 2 major etiologies of uveitis in children are idiopathic (25%–54% of cases) and juvenile idiopathic arthritis (15%–47% of cases). Most types of uveitis are not inherited.

Classification

As in adults, uveitis in children can be classified according to several factors, including anatomical location, pathology (granulomatous or nongranulomatous), course (acute, chronic, or recurrent), or etiology (traumatic, immunologic, infectious [exogenous or endogenous], masquerade, or idiopathic). This chapter categorizes and describes uveitic entities using the basic anatomical classification of uveitis into 4 groups: anterior, intermediate, posterior, and panuveitis. Anatomical location of the uveitis can be helpful in determining etiology (Table 24-1). Results of a recent claims-based study of uveitis in the United States showed that anterior uveitis accounted for 75% of pediatric uveitis cases, with posterior uveitis and panuveitis accounting for the remaining 25%.

Thorne JE, Suhler E, Skup M, et al. Prevalence of noninfectious uveitis in the United States: a claims-based analysis. *JAMA Ophthalmol.* 2016;134(11):1237–1245.

第 24 章

儿童葡萄膜炎

*葡萄膜炎*广义为葡萄膜的炎症，包括虹膜、睫状体和脉络膜。详见 BCSC 第 9 册《*葡萄膜炎与眼部炎症*》，本章将更详细地描述临床特征和相应的炎症机制。

流行病学

儿童葡萄膜炎的患病率在不同的研究中有所不同，儿童患者占所有葡萄膜炎患者的 2% ~ 14%。男、女儿童葡萄膜炎的患病率分布与成人相似，女性占比稍大。儿童葡萄膜炎的平均诊断年龄为 8 ~ 9 岁，75% 的患儿为双眼发病。在美国，约有 62% 的儿童葡萄膜炎是白人。儿童葡萄膜炎的 2 个主要病因是特发性葡萄膜炎（25% ~ 54%）和幼年特发性关节炎（15% ~ 47%）。大多数类型的葡萄膜炎为非遗传性。

分类

与成人一样，儿童葡萄膜炎可根据几个因素进行分类，包括解剖部位、病理学（肉芽肿或非肉芽肿）、病程（急性、慢性或复发性）、病因学［外伤性、免疫性、传染性（外源性、内源性）、伪装性或特发性］。本章根据葡萄膜炎发病的解剖部位将葡萄膜炎分为 4 类：前、中间、后和全葡萄膜炎。明确葡萄膜炎发病的解剖部位有助于确定病因（表 24-1）。美国最近的一项葡萄膜炎认证研究结果显示，在儿童葡萄膜炎中，前葡萄膜炎占 75%，后葡萄膜炎和全葡萄膜炎占 25%。

Thorne JE, Suhler E, Skup M, et al. Prevalence of noninfectious uveitis in the United States: a claims-based analysis. *JAMA Ophthalmol.* 2016;134(11):1237–1245.

Table 24-1 Differential Diagnosis of Uveitis in Children

Anterior uveitis
Juvenile idiopathic arthritis
Trauma
Sarcoidosis
Tuberculosis
Syphilis
Lyme disease
Herpes virus
Kawasaki disease
Tubulointerstitial nephritis and uveitis syndrome
Behçet disease
Inflammatory bowel disease
Granulomatosis with polyangiitis (Wegener granulomatosis)
Nonspecific orbital inflammation (orbital pseudotumor)
Idiopathic anterior uveitis
Intermediate uveitis
Sarcoidosis
Tuberculosis
Syphilis
Lyme disease
Multiple sclerosis
Idiopathic intermediate uveitis (pars planitis)
Posterior uveitis and panuveitis
Toxoplasmosis
Toxocariasis
Sarcoidosis
Tuberculosis
Syphilis
Lyme disease
Herpes virus
Rubella or measles
Sympathetic ophthalmia
Bartonella henselae infection (cat-scratch disease)
Candida albicans infection
Familial juvenile systemic granulomatosis (Blau syndrome)
Diffuse unilateral subacute neuroretinitis
Vogt-Koyanagi-Harada syndrome
Behçet disease
Idiopathic posterior uveitis or panuveitis

Anterior Uveitis

Anterior uveitis primarily involves inflammation of the iris and ciliary body. When the anterior chamber is the primary site where inflammation is observed, the term *iritis* may be used for this inflammation. When inflammation is also observed in the anterior vitreous, the term *iridocyclitis* may be used.

Juvenile Idiopathic Arthritis

Juvenile idiopathic arthritis (JIA) (formerly, *juvenile rheumatoid arthritis*) is the most common identifiable etiology of childhood anterior uveitis. JIA is defined as arthritis of at least 6 weeks' duration without an identifiable cause in children younger than 16 years. There are several subtypes of JIA, which are listed in Table 24-2.

表24-1　儿童葡萄膜炎的鉴别诊断

前葡萄膜炎
幼年特发性关节炎
外伤
结节病
结核病
梅毒
Lyme 病
疱疹病毒
Kawasaki病（川崎病）
肾小管间质性肾炎和葡萄膜炎综合征
Behçet病
炎症性肠病
肉芽肿性多血管炎（Wegener肉芽肿病）
非特异性眼眶炎症（眼眶假瘤）
特发性前葡萄膜炎
中间葡萄膜炎
结节病
结核病
梅毒
Lyme病
多发性硬化症
特发性中间葡萄膜炎（扁平部炎）
后葡萄膜炎和全葡萄膜炎
弓形虫病
弓蛔虫病
结节病
结核病
梅毒
Lyme 病
疱疹病毒
风疹或麻疹
交感性眼炎
*巴尔通体*感染（猫抓病）
*白色念珠菌*感染
家族性幼年全身性肉芽肿（Blau综合征）
弥漫性单眼亚急性神经视网膜炎
Vogt - Koyanagi - Harada综合征（Vogt-小柳原田综合征）
Behçet病
特发性后葡萄膜炎或全葡萄膜炎

前葡萄膜炎

前葡萄膜炎是主要累及虹膜和睫状体的炎症。当前房是发现炎症的初始部位时，称*虹膜炎*。同时也在前部玻璃体观察到炎症时，称*虹膜睫状体炎*。

幼年特发性关节炎

幼年特发性关节炎（*JIA*）（曾称为*幼年类风湿性关节炎*）是儿童前葡萄膜炎最常见的病因。幼年特发性关节炎（JIA）的定义为16岁以下儿童的关节炎，持续时间至少为6周，无明确原因。幼年特发性关节炎（JIA）有几个亚型，如表24-2所示。

Table 24-2 Subtypes of Juvenile Idiopathic Arthritis

I. Systemic arthritis
II. Pauciarticular arthritis
III. Polyarticular arthritis
IV. Spondyloarthritis
  A. Enthesitis-related arthritis
  B. Juvenile psoriatic arthritis
  C. Juvenile ankylosing spondylitis
  D. Enteropathic arthritis
  E. Reactive arthritis
  F. Undifferentiated spondyloarthritis
V. Undifferentiated arthritis

Overall, the prevalence of uveitis in JIA varies from 2% to 34%. The subtypes of JIA that are particularly associated with uveitis are pauciarticular (oligoarthritis), polyarticular, psoriatic arthritis, and enthesitis-related arthritis. Uveitis almost never occurs in children with systemic arthritis and is very rare in those with rheumatoid factor–positive polyarticular subtype. In contrast to most forms of anterior uveitis, the uveitis associated with pauciarticular JIA and polyarticular JIA is initially asymptomatic. It has been described as "white iritis" because of the absence of a red eye. Screening for uveitis among children with JIA is therefore of great importance.

Pauciarticular is the most frequent type of JIA in children in North America and Europe. By definition, pauciarticular JIA affects 4 or fewer joints during the first 6 months of the disease. It occurs predominantly in young girls. Anterior uveitis is most likely to occur with this type of arthritis, developing in 10%–30% of patients. Laboratory markers include a high prevalence of antinuclear antibodies (ANA). Rheumatoid factor is almost always absent.

Children with *polyarticular* JIA show involvement of more than 4 inflamed joints during the first 6 months of the disease. This disease is more common in girls, and the mean age at onset is higher compared with pauciarticular JIA. Uveitis occurs in approximately 10% of these children. Affected patients may have a positive ANA test result, which is associated with an increased risk of uveitis. Human leukocyte antigen (HLA) associations have not been consistently documented.

The pathogenesis of the anterior uveitis associated with JIA is unknown, but it is likely to have an immunologic basis. The risk for development of uveitis is highest during the first 4 years after diagnosis of JIA. Among patients with JIA, 90% of uveitis cases develop within 7 years of onset of arthritis. Occasionally, uveitis is diagnosed before or at the onset of joint symptoms; in these cases, unfortunately, the prognosis is often poorer because the initially asymptomatic nature of the ocular inflammation often delays diagnosis and thus treatment. A shorter interval between the onset of arthritis and uveitis is also associated with a more aggressive course.

JIA-associated uveitis is usually bilateral and nongranulomatous with fine to mediumsized keratic precipitates, but a minority of children, especially African Americans, may have granulomatous precipitates. Chronic inflammation may produce band keratopathy (Fig 24-1), posterior synechiae, ciliary membrane formation, hypotony, cataract, glaucoma, and phthisis. Vitritis and macular edema occur infrequently.

表24-2　幼年特发性关节炎的亚型

I. 全身性关节炎
II. 少关节的关节炎
III. 多关节的关节炎
IV. 脊柱炎
　A.附着点相关性关节炎/关节囊相关性关节炎
　B.幼年银屑病关节炎
　C.幼年强直性脊柱炎
　D.肠病性关节炎
　E.反应性关节炎
　F.未分化型脊柱炎
V. 未分化型关节炎

总体来说，幼年特发性关节炎（JIA）中间葡萄膜炎的患病率从 2% 到 34% 不等。与葡萄膜炎特别相关的幼年特发性关节炎（JIA）亚型有少关节的（少关节炎）、多关节的、银屑病关节炎和附着点相关性关节炎。葡萄膜炎几乎从未发生在全身性关节炎的儿童中，在类风湿因子阳性的多关节亚型的儿童中也罕见。与大多数类型的前葡萄膜炎不同，伴少关节型和多关节型幼年特发性关节炎（JIA）的葡萄膜炎最初是无症状的。因为无红眼症状，被称为“白色虹膜炎”，所以，对患有幼年特发性关节炎（JIA）的儿童进行葡萄膜炎的筛查是非常重要的。

*少关节炎*是北美和欧洲地区儿童最常见的幼年特发性关节炎（JIA）类型。根据定义，在患病的前 6 个月，少关节幼年特发性关节炎（JIA）累及 4 个或更少的关节，多见于幼女。前葡萄膜炎中最多见于此型，占 10% ~ 30%。实验室标记物有抗核抗体（ANA）的高检出率，类风湿因子几乎不存在。

*多关节型*幼年特发性关节炎（JIA）的儿童，患病的前 6 个月，有 4 个以上的关节发炎，女孩多见，发病的平均年龄大于少关节型幼年特发性关节炎（JIA）。约 10% 有葡萄膜炎。患者的抗核抗体 ANA 试验结果呈阳性，提示患葡萄膜炎的风险增加。而人类白细胞抗原（HLA）的相关性尚未完全证实。

与幼年特发性关节炎（JIA）相关的前葡萄膜炎的发病机制尚不清楚，可能与免疫有关。在诊断为幼年特发性关节炎（JIA）后的前 4 年，葡萄膜炎的发病风险最高。在幼年特发性关节炎（JIA）患者中，90% 在发病的 7 年内发生葡萄膜炎。偶见葡萄膜炎在关节症状开始之前或开始时即被诊断，但其预后往往较差，因为最初无症状的眼部炎症常常延误诊断和治疗。关节炎和葡萄膜炎的发病间隔较短，也提示其病情进展更快。

幼年特发性关节炎（JIA）相关性葡萄膜炎常为双眼和非肉芽肿性，呈细小到中等大小的角膜后沉着物，但少数儿童，特别是非裔美国人可见肉芽肿沉着物。慢性炎症可导致带状角膜病变（图 24-1）、后粘连、睫状体膜形成、低血压、白内障、青光眼和眼球痨。很少发生玻璃体炎和黄斑水肿。

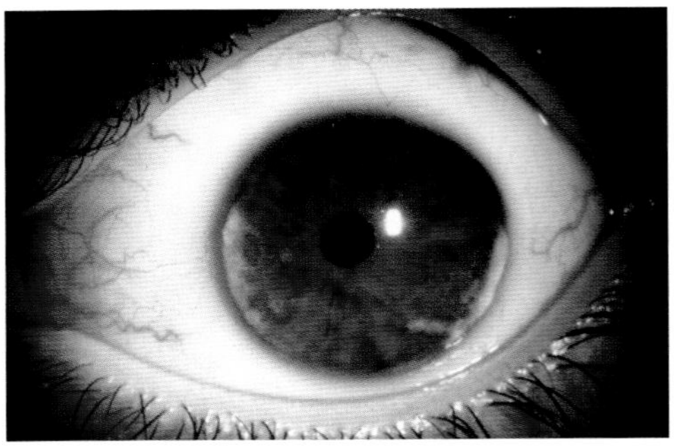

Figure 24-1 Slit-lamp photograph from a patient with uveitis associated with juvenile idiopathic arthritis (JIA). As is typical in pauciarticular or polyarticular JIA, the conjunctiva is "white." Band keratopathy is present. *(Courtesy of Amy Hutchinson, MD.)*

Screening for uveitis

Recognition of the importance of screening for uveitis in children with JIA has resulted in an improved prognosis for this disorder. However, visual impairment has been reported in up to 40% of children with JIA-associated uveitis, and blindness may occur in as many as 10% of affected eyes. Screening guidelines continue to undergo revision but are based on 4 factors that are associated with an increased risk of uveitis:

- category of arthritis
- age at onset of arthritis
- presence of ANA positivity
- duration of the disease

Table 24-3 outlines the eye examination schedule for pauciarticular and polyarticular JIA, as recommended by the American Academy of Pediatrics. After 4 years, the eye examinations become less frequent. Although female sex is associated with a higher incidence of uveitis, this factor is not incorporated in the guidelines. Initial ophthalmologic examination should occur within 6 weeks of diagnosis.

Table 24-3 Frequency of Eye Examination in Patients With Pauciarticular or Polyarticular JIA

Age at Onset of JIA, y	Duration of Disease, y	Eye Examination Frequency (mo) for ANA-Positive, ANA-Negative Patients	
		ANA+	ANA−
≤6	≤4	3	6
≤6	>4 to ≤7	6	12
≤6	>7	12	12
>6	≤4	6	12
>6	>4	12	12

ANA = antinuclear antibody; JIA = juvenile idiopathic arthritis.

Frequencies are for the first 4 years after diagnosis.

Information from Cassidy J, Kivlin J, Lindsley C, Nocton J; Section on Rheumatology; Section on Ophthalmology. Ophthalmologic examinations in children with juvenile rheumatoid arthritis. *Pediatrics.* 2006;117(5):1844.

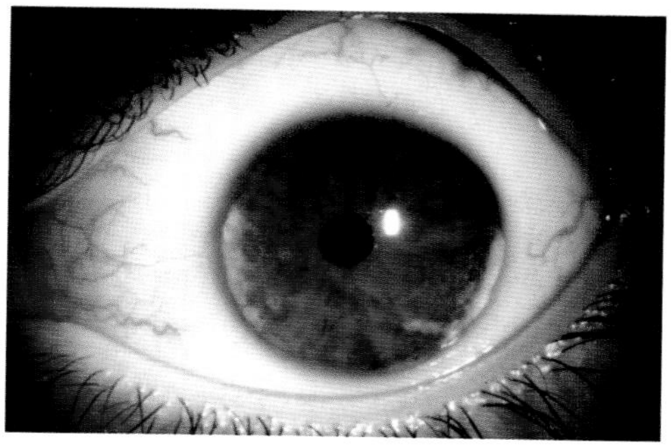

图 24–1　幼年特发性关节炎（JIA）葡萄膜炎的裂隙灯照片。呈少关节或多关节的典型表现，结膜为“白色”，有带状角膜病变。（*译者注：资料来源见前页原文。*）

葡萄膜炎的筛查

对幼年特发性关节炎（JIA）患儿进行葡萄膜炎筛查的重要性认知，可改善疾病的愈后。但有报道称，高达 40% 的幼年特发性关节炎（JIA）相关性葡萄膜炎患儿出现视力损害，10% 的受累眼失明。筛查指南仅针对增加葡萄膜炎患病风险的 4 个相关因素进行修订：

- 关节炎的类别
- 关节炎的发病年龄
- 抗核抗体 ANA 阳性
- 疾病持续时间

表 24–3 概述了美国儿科学会推荐的少关节和多关节幼年特发性关节炎（JIA）的眼科检查方案。4 年后，眼部检查的频率降低。尽管女性的葡萄膜炎发病率较高，但并未纳入指南中。初次眼科检查应在诊断后 6 周内进行。

表 24–3　多关节型或少关节型幼年特发性关节炎患儿的眼部检查频率

JIA发病年龄/岁	病程持续时间/年	ANA阳性、ANA阴性患儿的眼部检查频率（月）	
		ANA+	ANA –
≤6	≤4	3	6
≤6	>4 且 ≤7	6	12
≤6	> 7	12	12
> 6	≤4	6	12
> 6	>4	12	12

ANA = 抗核抗体；JIA = 幼年特发性关节炎。
频率是针对在确诊以后的4年内。
（*译者注：资料来源见前页原文。*）

Juvenile Spondyloarthropathies

Juvenile spondyloarthropathies are a group of HLA-B27–associated disorders and are associated with uveitis in 25% of affected individuals. Boys are more commonly affected than girls, and the disease onset is usually in early adolescence. There are differentiated and undifferentiated forms. Differentiated types include enthesitis-related arthritis, juvenile ankylosing spondylitis, juvenile psoriatic arthritis, reactive arthritis, and the arthritis associated with inflammatory bowel disease (enteropathic) (Table 24-4). A unifying feature of the differentiated forms is enthesitis, an inflammation of the sites where the ligaments, tendons, and joint capsules attach to bone. Enthesitis most commonly affects the insertions of the patellar ligament at the inferior patella, plantar fascia at the calcaneus, and the Achilles tendon. Asymmetric lower-extremity oligoarthritis with involvement of the hips and midfoot is highly suggestive of the disease.

The anterior uveitis associated with juvenile spondyloarthropathies usually has an acute onset with photophobia, pain, and a red eye.

Gmuca S, Weiss PF. Juvenile spondyloarthritis. *Curr Opin Rheumatol.* 2015;27(4):364–372.

Table 24-4 Types of Juvenile Spondyloarthropathies

Type	Additional Systemic Manifestations	Uveitis Prevalence and Characteristics
Enthesitis-related arthritis	None	Occurs in 20% of affected children Acute, symptomatic Unilateral, but both eyes may be affected at different times
Juvenile psoriatic arthritis	Nail changes (pitting or onycholysis), dactylitis, psoriasis	Occurs in 10% of affected children Insidious and chronic anterior uveitis Usually bilateral
Juvenile ankylosing spondylitis	Involves the spine Sacroiliitis, which may be subclinical Cardiac disease rare in children	Occurs in 20%–30% of those affected Acute, symptomatic Unilateral, but both eyes may be affected at different times
Enteropathic arthritis	Crohn disease, ulcerative colitis	Occurs in 5% of those affected
Reactive arthritis	Follows an infection not involving the joints Urethritis	Occurs in 12% of those affected Acute, symptomatic Unilateral and recurrent anterior uveitis Conjunctivitis may also be present

幼年脊柱关节病

幼年脊柱关节病是一组 HLA–B27 相关疾病，25% 的患者有葡萄膜炎。男孩多于女孩，且常在青春期的早期发病。有分化的和未分化 2 种类型。分化的类型有附着点相关性关节炎、幼年强直性脊柱炎、幼年银屑病关节炎、反应性关节炎和与炎性肠病（肠病）相关的关节炎（表 24–4）。分化型的一个特征是附着点炎，即一种韧带、肌腱和关节囊附着于骨的部位的炎症。附着点炎最常见的部位是髌骨下方髌骨韧带、跟骨的跖腱膜和跟腱的止点。若有不对称下肢少关节炎并累及臀部和中足，高度提示该疾病。

幼年脊柱关节病相关的前葡萄膜炎常急性发作，伴有畏光、疼痛和红眼。

Gmuca S, Weiss PF. Juvenile spondyloarthritis. *Curr Opin Rheumatol.* 2015;27(4):364–372.

表 24–4　幼年脊柱关节病的类型

类型	其他全身表现	葡萄膜炎的患病率和特征
附着点相关性关节炎	无	20%的受累儿童发病 急性发病、有症状 单眼发病，但双眼可能在不同时间受累
幼年银屑病关节炎	指甲改变（点蚀或甲剥离）、指（趾）炎、银屑病	10%的受累儿童发病 隐匿性和慢性前葡萄膜炎 常累及双眼
幼年强直性脊柱炎	累及脊椎 骶髂关节炎呈亚临床表现 在心脏病儿童中罕见	20%~30%的受累患儿发病 急性发病，有症状 单眼发病，但双眼可能在不同的时间受到影响
肠病性关节炎	Crohn病，溃疡性结肠炎	5%的受累患儿发病
反应性关节炎	感染后不累及关节 尿道炎	12%的受累患儿发病 急性发病，有症状 单眼发病和复发性前葡萄膜炎 也有结膜炎

Tubulointerstitial Nephritis and Uveitis Syndrome

Tubulointerstitial nephritis and uveitis (TINU) syndrome is kidney disease associated with chronic or recurrent anterior uveitis in adolescents. The median age at onset is 15 years. The renal disease is characterized by low-grade fever, fatigue, pallor, and weight loss. Elevated levels of β_2-microglobulin are usually present in the urine. The uveitis is usually bilateral and may occur before, simultaneously with, or after the renal disease. The prognosis is generally good, but long-term follow-up is required because the inflammation may recur.

Kawasaki Disease

Kawasaki disease, also known as *mucocutaneous lymph node syndrome*, is a primary vasculitis mediated by immunoglobulin (Ig) A affecting children younger than 5 years. Abnormalities include fever, conjunctival injection, mucous membrane changes, extremity changes involving the skin, rash, and cervical lymphadenopathy. The most significant complication of Kawasaki disease is coronary artery aneurysm, which occurs in 15%–25% of untreated children. Treatment with aspirin and intravenous IgG reduces the incidence of coronary artery aneurysm formation. After conjunctivitis, a generally self-limited anterior uveitis during the acute phase of the illness is the second most common ocular finding, occurring in approximately 10% of cases.

Other Causes of Anterior Uveitis

Many cases of anterior uveitis are idiopathic or are caused by trauma. Other causes include a variety of infectious and noninfectious diseases (see Table 24-1).

Intermediate Uveitis

The term *intermediate uveitis* is an anatomically based description of the primary site of the ocular inflammation. The inflammation is localized to the vitreous base overlying the ciliary body, pars plana, and peripheral retina, as well as the anterior vitreous (Fig 24-2). Intermediate uveitis accounts for 12%–28% of uveitis cases in the pediatric age group. In children, it may occur with various conditions, including sarcoidosis, syphilis, Lyme disease, multiple sclerosis, and tuberculosis. Idiopathic disease, known as *pars planitis*, accounts for 85%–90% of cases.

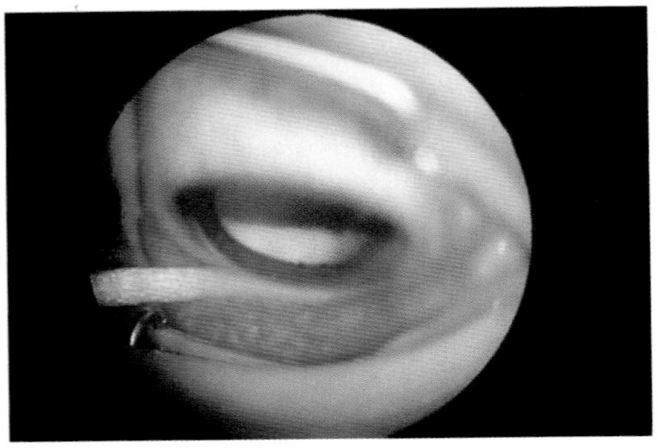

Figure 24-2 Intermediate uveitis with inferior snowbank formation (inflammatory exudative accumulation on the inferior pars plana ["snow bank"]), right eye.

肾小管间质性肾炎和葡萄膜炎综合征

肾小管间质性肾炎和葡萄膜炎（TINU）综合征是一种肾病，伴有青春期慢性或复发性前葡萄膜炎。平均发病年龄为 15 岁。肾病表现为低热、疲劳、苍白和体重减轻。尿中 β_2- 微球蛋白水平升高。葡萄膜炎为双眼，可能发生在肾病之前、同时或之后。预后良好，但炎症可能复发，需要长期随访。

Kawasaki 病（川崎病）

Kawasaki 病（川崎病），也称为*皮肤黏膜淋巴结综合征*，是一种免疫球蛋白（Ig）A 介导的原发性血管炎，累及 5 岁以下的儿童。异常症状有发热、结膜充血、口腔黏膜改变、肢端皮肤变化如皮疹，和颈淋巴结病。Kawasaki 病（川崎病）的主要并发症是冠状动脉瘤，发生于 15% ~ 25%的未治疗儿童。阿司匹林和静脉注射 IgG 治疗可降低冠状动脉瘤形成的发生率。除结膜炎外，第 2 种最常见的眼病是自限性前葡萄膜炎，急性期出现，发生率约为 10%。

前葡萄膜炎的其他病因

许多前葡萄膜炎是特发性的或是由外伤引起的，其他原因包括各种传染病和非传染病（见表 24–1）。

中间葡萄膜炎

*中间葡萄膜炎*一词是描述眼部炎症主要受累部位的解剖学术语。炎症局限于玻璃体基底部，包括睫状体、扁平部、周边视网膜以及前玻璃体（图 24–2）。中间葡萄膜炎占儿童年龄组葡萄膜炎的 12% ~ 28%，可出现在多种疾病中，包括结节病、梅毒、Lyme 病、多发性硬化和肺结核。特发性疾病称为*睫状体扁平部炎*，占 85% ~ 90%。

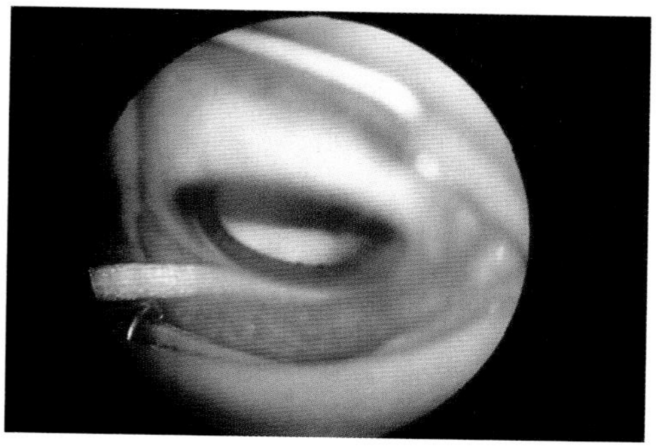

图 24–2　中间葡萄膜炎伴有下方的雪堤形成［炎症渗出物积聚在下方睫状体扁平部（“雪堤”）］，右眼。

Posterior Uveitis

Posterior uveitis is defined as intraocular inflammation primarily involving the choroid; often, there is also retinal involvement.

Toxoplasmosis

Toxoplasmosis is the most common cause of posterior uveitis in children. It is discussed in Chapter 28.

Toxocariasis

Ocular toxocariasis is caused by the nematode larvae of a common intestinal parasite of dogs (*Toxocara canis*) or cats (*Toxocara cati*). This disease, contracted through ingestion of ascarid ova in soil contaminated by dog or cat feces, primarily affects children. *Visceral larva migrans (VLM)* is an acute systemic infection produced by these organisms; it commonly occurs at approximately age 2 years. If symptomatic, it is associated with fever, cough, rashes, malaise, and anorexia. Laboratory testing reveals eosinophilia. VLM and ocular toxocariasis, for unknown reasons, seldom occur in the same patient.

Ocular toxocariasis is usually unilateral and is not associated with systemic illness or an elevated eosinophil count. The average age at onset is 11.5 years. The 3 major retinal forms of the disease include posterior pole granuloma, peripheral granuloma with macular traction (Fig 24-3), and endophthalmitis. There is often little external evidence of inflammation. Patients may present with leukocoria, strabismus, or decreased vision. These are also common presenting signs and symptoms of retinoblastoma, which must be differentiated from ocular toxocariasis. Because elevated *Toxocara* titers may be found in a significant percentage of children, a positive result on tests such as the enzyme-linked immunosorbent assay does not rule out other possibilities, including retinoblastoma.

Treatment includes observation of peripheral lesions, periocular or systemic steroids for posterior lesions and endophthalmitis, or surgical intervention to address retinal traction, cataract, glaucoma, or cyclitic membranes. Systemic anthelmintics are not useful in treating ocular toxocariasis because the organism may already be dead or its death can produce significant inflammation.

Woodhall D, Starr MC, Montgomery SP, et al. Ocular toxocariasis: epidemiologic, anatomic, and therapeutic variations based on a survey of ophthalmic subspecialists. *Ophthalmology*. 2012;119(6):1211–1217.

Other Causes of Posterior Uveitis

Other causes of posterior uveitis are listed in Table 24-1.

后葡萄膜炎

*后葡萄膜炎*指主要累及脉络膜的眼内炎症，常有视网膜受累。

弓形虫病

弓形虫病是儿童后葡萄膜炎的最常见原因，详情见第 28 章。

弓蛔虫病

眼部弓蛔虫病是由线虫幼虫引起的，常见于狗（*犬弓蛔虫*）或猫（*猫弓蛔虫*）的肠道寄生虫。此病是摄入了被狗或猫粪便污染的土壤中蛔虫卵而感染的，主要累及儿童。*内脏幼虫移行症（VLM）*是由线虫幼虫引起的急性全身感染，常发生在 2 岁左右。症状有发烧、咳嗽、皮疹、不适和厌食。实验室试验显示嗜酸性粒细胞增多。内脏幼虫移行症（VLM）和眼部弓蛔虫病很少发生于同一患儿，原因不明。

眼部弓蛔虫病通常是单眼的，与全身性疾病或嗜酸性粒细胞计数升高无关。平均发病年龄为 11.5 岁。主要有 3 种视网膜病变，有后极肉芽肿、周边肉芽肿伴黄斑牵引（图 24–3）和眼内炎。外眼很少有炎症表现。患儿可出现白瞳症、斜视或视力下降，这些也是视网膜母细胞瘤的常见症状和体征，需与眼弓蛔虫病相鉴别。因为许多儿童的*弓蛔虫*滴度升高，阳性结果，如酶联免疫吸附试验，并不排除其他疾病的可能性，包括视网膜母细胞瘤。

治疗包括观察视网膜周边病变、眼周或全身类固醇治疗后的极部病变和眼内炎，或手术干预，以解除视网膜牵拉、白内障、青光眼或睫状体膜炎。全身驱虫剂治疗眼部弓蛔虫病无效的，因为线虫幼虫可能已经死亡，或其死亡可以引发严重炎症。

Woodhall D, Starr MC, Montgomery SP, et al. Ocular toxocariasis: epidemiologic, anatomic, and therapeutic variations based on a survey of ophthalmic subspecialists. *Ophthalmology*. 2012;119(6):1211–1217.

后葡萄膜炎的其他病因

后葡萄膜炎的其他病因被列举在表 24–1 中。

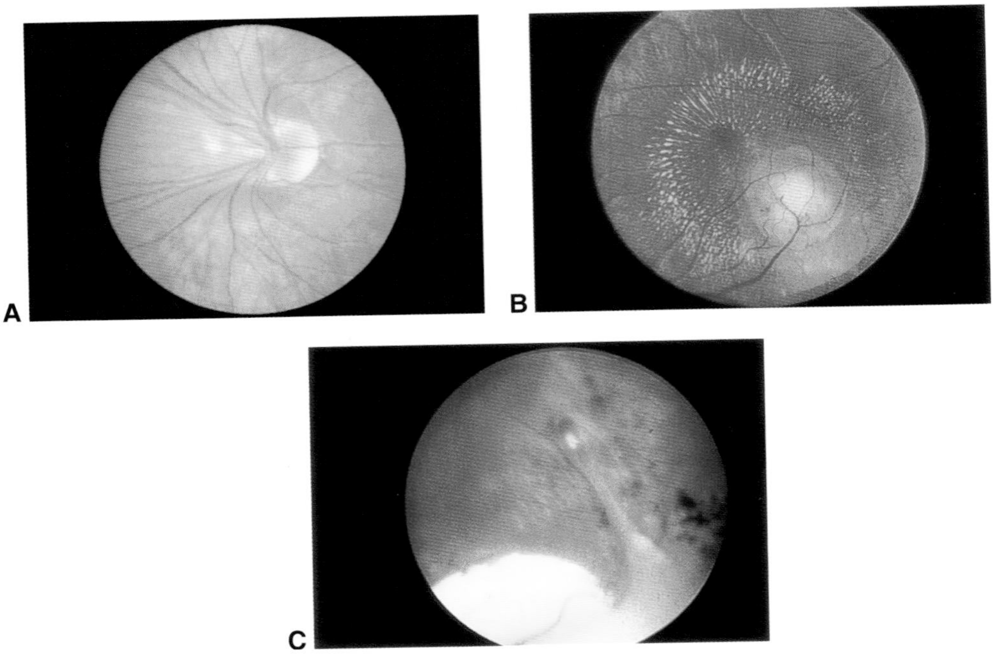

Figure 24-3 Toxocariasis. **A,** Distortion of posterior pole vessels, right eye. **B,** Fundus photograph showing macular granuloma. **C,** Fundus photograph of peripheral granuloma.

Panuveitis

In panuveitis, inflammation is diffuse without a predominant site. Inflammation is observed in the anterior chamber, vitreous, and choroid.

Sarcoidosis

Sarcoidosis may present in 2 distinct forms in children. In young patients (<5 years), lung disease is rare, and sarcoidosis is more often characterized by the triad of uveitis, granulomatous arthritis, and rash. Early-onset sarcoidosis is considered a *pediatric granulomatous arthritis* and is phenotypically and genetically similar to familial juvenile systemic granulomatosis (discussed in the following section). Older children (8–15 years) with sarcoidosis have the pulmonary abnormalities and lymph node findings more commonly associated with the adult form of the disease and are also at risk for uveitis. Although anterior uveitis (Fig 24-4) is the most common manifestation of ocular sarcoidosis in children, this disease can produce a panuveitis.

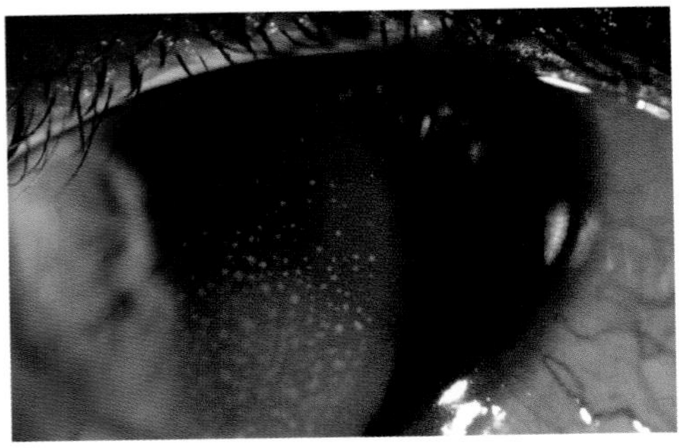

Figure 24-4 Keratic precipitates in sarcoidosis. *(Courtesy of Ken K. Nischal, MD.)*

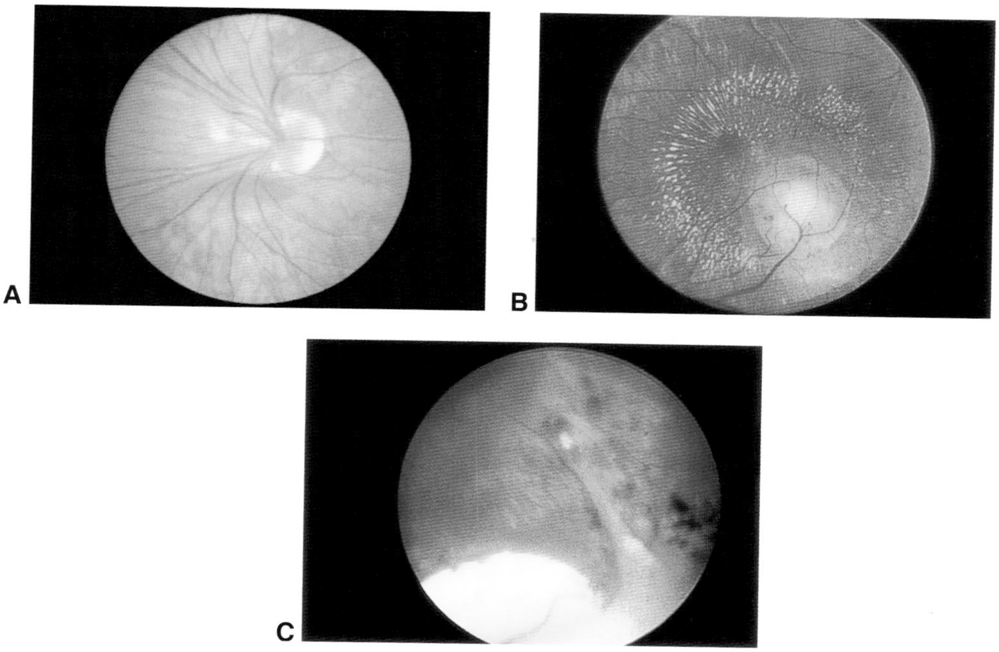

图 24–3　弓蛔虫病。**A.** 后极血管扭曲，右眼。**B.** 眼底照片显示黄斑肉芽肿。**C.** 周边肉芽肿眼底照。

全葡萄膜炎

在全葡萄膜炎中，炎症是弥漫性的，没有主要的累及部位。在前房、玻璃体和脉络膜中均可见到炎症反应。

结节病

结节病在儿童中有 2 种不同的表现形式。低龄患儿（<5 岁）的肺部疾病很少见，其结节病表现为葡萄膜炎、肉芽肿性关节炎和皮疹三联征。早发性结节病被认为是一种*儿童肉芽肿性关节炎*，其表型和遗传性与家族性幼年全身肉芽肿病相似（下一节讨论）。大龄儿童（8 ~ 15 岁）与成人表现相同，结节病有肺部异常和淋巴结肿大，也有患葡萄膜炎的风险。前葡萄膜炎（图 24–4）是儿童眼部结节病最常见的表现，但也可导致全葡萄膜炎。

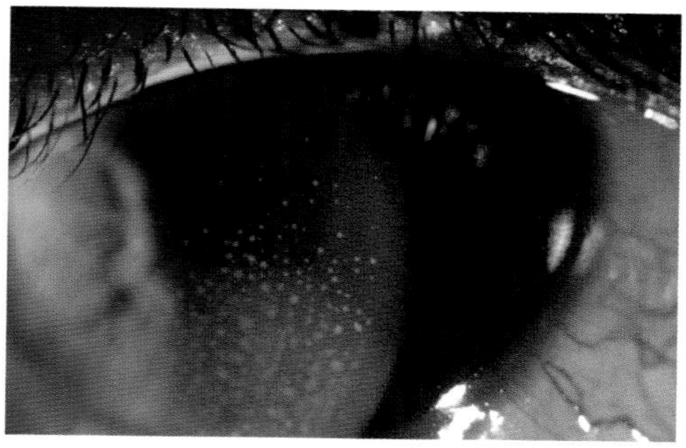

图 24–4　结节病的角膜后沉着物。*（译者注：资料来源见前页原文。）*

Diagnosis and treatment in children is similar to that in adults (see BCSC Section 9, *Uveitis and Ocular Inflammation*). However, serum angiotensin-converting enzyme levels, which may be abnormally elevated in patients with sarcoidosis, are normally higher in healthy children than in adults and thus can be misleading in diagnosis of this disease.

Familial Juvenile Systemic Granulomatosis

Familial juvenile systemic granulomatosis (*Blau syndrome*) is an autosomal dominant disease that may be identical to early-onset sarcoidosis; both are classified as *pediatric granulomatous arthritides.* In both diseases, there are mutations in the nucleotide binding oligomerization domain containing 2 gene *(NOD2)* on chromosome 16; however, in Blau syndrome, other family members are affected. Both diseases present with granulomatous arthritis, uveitis, and rash during childhood, but pulmonary involvement and lymphadenopathy are absent in Blau syndrome. Chronic panuveitis associated with multifocal choroiditis is the most common ocular presentation; in some cases, the uveitis may be limited to the anterior segment and the disease misdiagnosed as JIA. Ocular complications, including cataract, glaucoma, band keratopathy, and vision loss, are common.

Vogt-Koyanagi-Harada Syndrome

Vogt-Koyanagi-Harada syndrome is a chronic, progressive bilateral panuveitis that is associated with exudative retinal detachments and may be accompanied by meningeal irritation, auditory disturbances, and skin changes. It is rare in children, but in those affected, the rate of ocular complications such as cataract and glaucoma is higher and the visual prognosis poorer compared with that for adults. For further discussion, see BCSC Section 9, *Uveitis and Ocular Inflammation.*

Other Causes of Panuveitis

Other causes of panuveitis are listed in Table 24-1.

Masquerade Syndromes

Various conditions can simulate pediatric uveitis. Table 24-5 lists these masquerade syndromes and their diagnostic features.

Evaluation of Pediatric Uveitis

Establishing the correct diagnosis is important in managing a pediatric patient with uveitis, but some ophthalmologists defer the workup of isolated anterior uveitis unless it is recurrent or unresponsive to initial therapy. Accurate diagnosis requires a detailed history, thorough ophthalmic examination, and selected laboratory tests. An examination under anesthesia may be necessary if the child is not cooperative enough for an office evaluation. Laboratory investigations are chosen based on the suspected diagnoses (Table 24-6; see also Table 24-5).

儿童的诊断和治疗与成人相似（见 BCSC 第 9 册《*葡萄膜炎与眼部炎症*》）。结节病患儿的血清血管紧张素转换酶水平可能异常升高，但在正常情况下，健康儿童的转换酶水平高于成人，因此可能误导该疾病的诊断。

家族性幼年全身性肉芽肿病

家族性幼年全身性肉芽肿病（*Blau 综合征*）是一种常染色体显性遗传疾病，可能与早发性结节病相同，两者都被归为*儿童肉芽肿性关节炎*。在这 2 种疾病中，16 号染色体上含有 2 个基因（*NOD2*）的核苷酸结合寡聚化结构域存在突变；而在 Blau 综合征中，其他家族成员亦受累。这 2 种疾病的儿童时期，都表现为肉芽肿性关节炎、葡萄膜炎和皮疹，但 Blau 综合征中肺部不受累和无淋巴结病。慢性全葡萄膜炎合并多灶性脉络膜炎是最常见的眼部表现，有时葡萄膜炎限于前节，被误诊为幼儿特发性关节炎。眼部并发症包括白内障、青光眼、带状角膜病变和视力丧失。

Vogt-Koyanagi-Harada 综合征

Vogt-Koyanagi-Harada 综合征是一种慢性进行性双眼全葡萄膜炎，伴有渗出性视网膜脱离，可能伴有脑膜刺激征、听觉障碍和皮肤变化。儿童很少见，一旦受累，白内障和青光眼等眼部并发症的发生率较高。与成人相比，视力预后较差。相关的进一步讨论，见 BCSC 第 9 册《*葡萄膜炎与眼部炎症*》。

全葡萄膜炎的其他原因

引起全葡萄膜炎的其他原因详见表 24-1。

伪装综合征

各种条件都可以模拟小儿葡萄膜炎。表 24-5 列出了这些伪装综合征及其诊断特征。

小儿葡萄膜炎的评估

正确的诊断对治疗儿童葡萄膜炎很重要，但一些眼科医生推迟了对孤立的前葡萄膜炎的病情检查，除非病情复发或对初始的治疗没有反应。精准的诊断需要详细的病史、完整的眼科检查和选择性的实验室检查。如果患儿在门诊不能配合检查，则需要麻醉。根据疑似诊断选择实验室检查（表 24-6，另见表 24-5）。

Table 24-5 Uveitis Masquerade Syndromes in Children

Disease or Condition	Age, y	Signs of Inflammation	Examination/Diagnostic Studies
Anterior segment			
Retinoblastoma	<15	Flare, cells, pseudohypopyon	Ultrasonography, MRI
Leukemia	<15	Flare, cells, hypopyon, heterochromia, hyphema	Bone marrow biopsy, peripheral blood smear
Intraocular foreign body	Any age	Flare, cells	X-ray, CT, ultrasonography
Malignant melanoma	Any age	Flare, cells	Fluorescein angiography, ultrasonography, OCT
Juvenile xanthogranuloma	<15	Flare, cells, hyphema	Examination of skin, iris biopsy
Peripheral retinal detachment	Any age	Flare, cells	Ophthalmoscopy
Posterior segment			
Retinitis pigmentosa	Any age	Cells in vitreous, waxy disc pallor, bone-spicule pigmentary changes in midperiphery	ERG, visual fields
Systemic lymphoma	≥15	Retinal hemorrhage or exudates, vitreous cells	Node biopsy, bone marrow biopsy, physical examination
Retinoblastoma	<15	Vitreous cells, retinal exudates	Ultrasonography, MRI
Malignant melanoma	≥15	Vitreous cells	Fluorescein angiography, ultrasonography, OCT
Multiple sclerosis	≥15	Periphlebitis, pars planitis	Neurologic examination

CT = computed tomography; ERG = electroretinogram; MRI = magnetic resonance imaging; OCT = optical coherence tomography.

Treatment of Pediatric Uveitis

The goals of treatment of uveitis in children are to eliminate the inflammation of the eye before ocular complications occur and to monitor for ocular and systemic adverse effects of the treatment. It is important to note that although the presence of cells in the anterior chamber indicates active inflammation, flare (protein) may persist long after the inflammation has been successfully treated.

Infectious diseases and malignancies producing uveitis should be identified and treated appropriately. Treatment of noninfectious uveitis is discussed in the following sections.

Management of Inflammation

Anterior segment inflammation is initially treated with topical corticosteroid and mydriatic/cycloplegic agents. Because topical corticosteroids do not penetrate well into the vitreous or posterior segment, sub-Tenon injections of a corticosteroid may be useful in the treatment of intermediate or posterior uveitis. Short courses of oral corticosteroids may be used, but long-term use is usually avoided because of the potential for significant ocular and systemic adverse effects. Corticosteroid intravitreal implants containing either fluocinolone acetonide or dexamethasone have been used successfully to treat posterior uveitis in children.

表24-5　儿童葡萄膜炎伪装综合征

疾病或条件	年龄/岁	炎症表现	检查/诊断
眼前节			
视网膜母细胞瘤	<15	房闪，细胞，假性前房积脓	超声，MRI，骨髓活检
白血病	<15	房闪，细胞，前房积脓，异色症，前房积血	外周血涂片
眼内异物	任何年龄	房闪，细胞	X线，CT，超声
恶性黑色素瘤	任何年龄	房闪，细胞	荧光血管造影，超声，OCT
幼年黄色肉芽肿	<15	房闪，细胞，前房积血	检查皮肤，虹膜活检
周边视网膜脱离	任何年龄	房闪，细胞	眼底镜
眼后节			
视网膜色素变性	任何年龄	玻璃体细胞，视盘蜡样苍白，中周部骨针样色素沉着	ERG，视野
全身性淋巴瘤	≥15	视网膜出血或渗出物，玻璃体细胞	淋巴结活检，骨髓活检，体格检查
视网膜母细胞瘤	<15	玻璃体细胞，视网膜渗出物	超声，MRI
恶性黑色素瘤	≥15	玻璃体细胞	荧光血管造影，超声，OCT
多发性硬化症	≥15	静脉周围炎，睫状体扁平部炎	神经系统检查

CT =计算机断层扫描；ERG = 视网膜电图；MRI =核磁共振；OCT = 光学相干断层扫描。

儿童葡萄膜炎的治疗

儿童葡萄膜炎的治疗目标是在眼部并发症发生前消除眼部炎症，并监测治疗对眼部和全身的不良反应。值得注意的是，尽管前房细胞的存在表明有活动性炎症，前房闪辉（蛋白）可能长期存在，即使炎症已得到成功的治疗。

对引起葡萄膜炎的传染病和恶性肿瘤应予以鉴别和适当治疗。非感染性葡萄膜炎的治疗将在以下章节中讨论。

炎症处理

最初可使用局部皮质类固醇和散瞳 / 睫状肌麻痹剂治疗前节炎症。由于局部皮质类固醇不能很好地穿透玻璃体或后节，在 Tenon 囊下注射皮质类固醇可能有助于治疗中间葡萄膜炎或后葡萄膜炎。可以短期使用口服皮质类固醇，但应避免长期使用，因为可能出现明显的眼部和全身的不良反应。含有氟轻松或地塞米松的皮质类固醇玻璃体内植入物已被成功地用于治疗儿童后葡萄膜炎。

Table 24-6 Laboratory Tests and Imaging for Various Types of Uveitis

Anterior uveitis
- Antinuclear antibody (JIA)
- ACE, lysozyme (sarcoidosis)
- Chest x-ray (sarcoidosis, tuberculosis)
- Tuberculin skin test, interferon-γ release assay (tuberculosis)
- FTA-ABS (syphilis)
- Lyme serology (Lyme disease)
- Complete blood count (leukemia)
- HLA-B27 and sacroiliac joint films (enthesitis-related arthritis, ankylosing spondylitis)
- Gastrointestinal series (if ulcerative colitis or regional enteritis [Crohn disease] is suspected)
- Urinalysis, blood urea nitrogen, serum creatinine, urine β_2-microglobulin (TINU syndrome)
- Antineutrophil cytoplasmic antibody (granulomatosis with polyangiitis)

Intermediate uveitis
- ACE, lysozyme (sarcoidosis)
- Chest x-ray (sarcoidosis, tuberculosis)
- Tuberculin skin test, interferon-γ release assay (tuberculosis)
- FTA-ABS (syphilis)
- Lyme serology (Lyme disease)

Posterior uveitis and panuveitis
- Toxoplasmosis PCR, ELISA
- Toxocariasis PCR, ELISA
- ACE, lysozyme (sarcoidosis)
- Chest x-ray (sarcoidosis, tuberculosis)
- Tuberculin skin test, interferon-γ release assay (tuberculosis)
- FTA-ABS (syphilis)
- Lyme serology (Lyme disease)
- PCR, blood cultures, viral cultures, or antibody levels (if cytomegalovirus, herpes simplex, herpes zoster, rubella, measles, or *Bartonella henselae* infection is suspected)

ACE=angiotensin-converting enzyme; ELISA=enzyme-linked immunosorbent assay; FTA-ABS=fluorescent treponemal antibody absorption; HLA=human leukocyte antigen; JIA=juvenile idiopathic arthritis; PCR=polymerase chain reaction; TINU=tubulointerstitial nephritis and uveitis.

Glaucoma and cataract formation are the most serious ocular complications of any corticosteroid therapy. In general, more potent topical corticosteroids are more likely to increase intraocular pressure. Periocular injections of corticosteroids can elevate intraocular pressure for weeks to months after injection. Cataracts and glaucoma are reported adverse effects of intravitreal steroid implants. Risks of long-term systemic corticosteroid use in children include growth retardation, osteoporosis and bone fractures, cushingoid appearance, diabetes mellitus, peptic ulcers, myopathy, hypertension, altered mental status, idiopathic intracranial hypertension, and increased risk of infection. Patients may also require increased doses of corticosteroids during times of stress to avoid an addisonian crisis.

Systemic immunosuppressive therapy is beneficial in treating both uveitis and arthritis. It can sometimes reduce or eliminate the need for steroids. The therapy should be undertaken in cooperation with a pediatric specialist familiar with the use of immunosuppressive and immunomodulatory medications. In patients with JIA, immunosuppressive drugs reduce the risk of vision loss from uveitis.

表24-6　各类葡萄膜炎的实验室检查及影像学检查

前葡萄膜炎
- 抗核抗体（幼年特发性关节炎）
- 血管紧张素转化酶（ACE），溶菌酶（结节病）
- 胸部X线（结节病，肺结核）
- 结核菌素皮肤试验,干扰素-γ释放试验（肺结核）
- 免疫发光法梅毒螺旋体检测（梅毒）
- Lyme血清学（Lyme病）
- 全血细胞计数（白血病）
- HLA-B27和骶髂关节片（与附着点炎有关的关节炎，强直性脊柱炎）
- 胃肠系列［如果怀疑溃疡性结肠炎或区域性肠炎（Crohn病）］
- 尿液分析，血尿素氮，血清肌酐，尿 β_2-微球蛋白（肾小管间质性肾炎和葡萄膜炎综合征TINU 综合征）
- 抗中性粒细胞胞浆抗体（多关节炎肉芽肿病）

中间葡萄膜炎
- 血管紧张素转化酶（ACE），溶菌酶（结节病）
- 胸部X线（结节病，肺结核）
- 结核菌素皮肤试验，干扰素-γ释放试验（结核病）
- 免疫发光法梅毒螺旋体检测（梅毒）
- Lyme血清学（Lyme病）

后部葡萄膜炎和全葡萄膜炎
- 弓形虫病PCR，ELISA
- 弓蛔虫病PCR, ELISA
- ACE，溶菌酶（结节病）
- 胸部X线（结节病，肺结核）
- 结核菌素皮肤试验，干扰素-γ释放试验（结核病）
- 免疫发光法梅毒螺旋体检测（梅毒）
- Lyme血清学（Lyme病）
- PCR，血培养，病毒培养或抗体水平（怀疑巨细胞病毒、单纯疱疹、带状疱疹、风疹、麻疹或巴尔通体感染）

ACE = 血管紧张素转化酶，ELISA = 酶联免疫吸附测定，FTA-ABS =免疫发光法梅毒螺旋体检测，HLA =人类白细胞抗原，JIA =幼年特发性关节炎，PCR =聚合酶链反应，TINU =肾小管间质性肾炎和葡萄膜炎。

青光眼和白内障的形成是所有皮质类固醇治疗中最严重的眼部并发症。通常，越是有效的局部皮质类固醇，越有可能升高眼内压。眼周注射皮质类固醇后，可引起数周至数月的眼压升高。有报道称，白内障和青光眼是玻璃体内类固醇植入物的不良反应。儿童长期全身使用皮质类固醇的风险包括生长迟缓、骨质疏松和骨折、cushing 面容、糖尿病、胃溃疡、肌病、高血压、精神状态改变、特发性颅内高压和感染风险增加。有压力时，患者还需增加皮质类固醇的剂量，以避免发生 Addison 危象（急性肾上腺皮质危象）。

全身免疫抑制治疗对葡萄膜炎和关节炎都有好处，有时可减少或消除对类固醇的依赖。应用该治疗方法时应与儿科专家合作，他们熟悉免疫抑制和免疫调节药物的使用。对幼年特发性关节炎（JIA）使用免疫抑制剂，可以降低因葡萄膜炎导致的视力丧失的风险。

Methotrexate is the most common antimetabolite used to treat arthritis and uveitis in children. Less commonly used antimetabolites include azathioprine and mycophenolate mofetil. These agents inhibit nucleic acid synthesis by a variety of mechanisms. Gastrointestinal disturbance is the most common adverse effect of oral methotrexate and can be alleviated by switching to subcutaneous injections. Oral folic acid supplementation is often recommended for patients using methotrexate. Hepatic toxicity, interstitial pneumonitis, and cytopenia are rare but serious adverse effects of methotrexate use.

Biologic drugs for the treatment of uveitis are used with increasing frequency to suppress the immune system in children. The 2 classes of biologic medications are tumor necrosis factor α (TNF-α) inhibitors and cell-specific antibodies. The TNF-α inhibitors most commonly used to treat uveitis are infliximab and adalimumab, which are monoclonal IgG antibodies against TNF-α. Commonly used cell-specific antibodies include abatacept (antibody to CD80 and CD86) and rituximab (antibody to interleukin-2). Etanercept should be avoided because new-onset inflammatory eye disease (uveitis, scleritis, optic neuritis) has been associated with its use, caused by poor drug efficacy and/or adverse effect of the drug. In general, TNF-α inhibitors are used before cell-specific antibodies. TNF-α inhibitors should not be used during periods of active infection. All these biologic drugs used to treat uveitis require intravenous infusion, except for adalimumab, which can be given subcutaneously. There is concern that children and adolescents treated with TNF-α blockers may be at increased risk for malignancies; however, a recent study showed that children with JIA are at increased risk for malignancies unrelated to the use of biologic drugs.

Beukelman T, Haynes K, Curtis JR, et al; Safety Assessment of Biological Therapeutics Collaboration. Rates of malignancy associated with juvenile idiopathic arthritis and its treatment. *Arthritis Rheum.* 2012;64(4):1263–1271.

Gregory AC II, Kempen JH, Daniel E, et al; Systemic Immunosuppressive Therapy for Eye Diseases Cohort Study Research Group. Risk factors for loss of visual acuity among patients with uveitis associated with juvenile idiopathic arthritis: the Systemic Immunosuppressive Therapy for Eye Diseases Study. *Ophthalmology.* 2013;120(1):186–192.

Klotsche J, Niewerth M, Haas JP. Long-term safety of etanercept and adalimumab compared to methotrexate in patients with juvenile idiopathic arthritis (JIA). *Ann Rheum Dis.* 2016;75(5):855–861.

Reiff A, Kadayifcilar S, Özen S. Rheumatic inflammatory eye diseases of childhood. *Rheum Dis Clin North Am.* 2013;39(4):801–832.

Surgical Treatment of Complications of Uveitis

Complications of uveitis include band keratopathy, cataract, and glaucoma. Band keratopathy can be treated by removal of corneal epithelium, followed by calcium chelation with ethylenediaminetetraacetic acid (EDTA). Treatment may have to be repeated. Phototherapeutic keratectomy has also been used to treat band keratopathy.

Cataract surgery for patients with uveitis can be complicated by hypotony, glaucoma, synechiae formation, cystoid macular edema, and retinal detachment. In patients with JIA, combined lensectomy and vitrectomy seems to produce better results than cataract extraction alone. Uveitis must be aggressively treated so that it is under control both before and after surgery. Intraocular lens implantation is usually not considered in children with uveitis until after a prolonged period of quiescence.

甲氨蝶呤是治疗儿童关节炎和葡萄膜炎最常用的抗代谢物。使用较少的抗代谢物有咪唑硫嘌呤和霉酚酸酯，其通过多种机制抑制核酸合成。胃肠道紊乱是口服甲氨蝶呤最常见的不良反应，改用皮下注射则可以缓解。使用甲氨蝶呤时，建议口服补充叶酸。肝毒性、间质性肺炎和血细胞减少是甲氨蝶呤少见且严重的副作用。

越来越多的生物制剂用于治疗葡萄膜炎，以抑制儿童的免疫系统疾病。2 类生物制剂分别是是肿瘤坏死因子 α（TNF-α）抑制剂和细胞特异性抗体。最常用于治疗葡萄膜炎的 TNF-α 抑制剂是英夫利昔单抗和阿达木单抗，其针对的是 TNF-α 的单克隆 IgG 抗体。常用的细胞特异性抗体包括阿巴西普（CD80 和 CD86 的抗体）和利妥昔单抗（白细胞介素 -2 的抗体）。应避免使用依那西普（抗 TNF），新发病的炎症性眼病（葡萄膜炎、巩膜炎、视神经炎）与该药的使用有关，可能是因为该药的疗效差和（或）不良反应所致。总之，TNF-α 抑制剂的使用应先于细胞特异性抗体， 但 TNF-α 抑制剂不应在活动性感染期使用。治疗葡萄膜炎的所有生物制剂均须静脉滴注，但阿达木单抗可以皮下注射。有人担心接受 TNF-α 阻滞剂治疗的儿童和青少年可能增加患恶性肿瘤的风险。然而，最近的一项研究表明，幼年特发性关节炎（JIA）的患儿患恶性肿瘤的风险增加与使用生物制剂无关。

Beukelman T, Haynes K, Curtis JR, et al; Safety Assessment of Biological Therapeutics Collaboration. Rates of malignancy associated with juvenile idiopathic arthritis and its treatment. *Arthritis Rheum.* 2012;64(4):1263–1271.

Gregory AC II, Kempen JH, Daniel E, et al; Systemic Immunosuppressive Therapy for Eye Diseases Cohort Study Research Group. Risk factors for loss of visual acuity among patients with uveitis associated with juvenile idiopathic arthritis: the Systemic Immunosuppressive Therapy for Eye Diseases Study. *Ophthalmology.* 2013;120(1):186–192.

Klotsche J, Niewerth M, Haas JP. Long-term safety of etanercept and adalimumab compared to methotrexate in patients with juvenile idiopathic arthritis (JIA). *Ann Rheum Dis.* 2016;75(5):855–861.

Reiff A, Kadayifcilar S, Özen S. Rheumatic inflammatory eye diseases of childhood. *Rheum Dis Clin North Am.* 2013;39(4):801–832.

葡萄膜炎并发症的手术治疗

葡萄膜炎的并发症包括带状角膜病变、白内障和青光眼。带状角膜病变的治疗方法是去除角膜上皮，然后用乙二胺四乙酸（EDTA）螯合钙，需要重复治疗。治疗性激光角膜切除术也用于治疗带状角膜病变。

葡萄膜炎的白内障手术较为复杂，因为其伴有低眼压、青光眼、虹膜粘连、黄斑囊样水肿和视网膜脱离。对幼年特发性关节炎（JIA）患儿联合施行晶状体切除术和玻璃体切除术，效果好于单纯行白内障摘除术。葡萄膜炎必须积极治疗，以便在手术前、后得到控制。葡萄膜炎患儿不考虑人工晶体植入，直到葡萄膜炎静止较长一段时间后再做考虑。

Glaucoma surgery may become necessary in children with uveitis. Many techniques have been used, and long-term success rates vary. Standard trabeculectomy is associated with a high rate of failure due to scarring. Goniotomy or trabeculotomy is effective in many children and can be the initial surgery if the anterior chamber angle is visible. Tube shunts can be used when goniotomy fails or if the angle is closed.

Bohnsack BL, Freedman SF. Surgical outcomes in childhood uveitic glaucoma. *Am J Ophthalmol.* 2013;155(1):134–142.

葡萄膜炎患儿可能需要行青光眼手术。已有许多可用技术，远期成功率各不相同。标准小梁切除术的失败率高，这与瘢痕形成有关。房角切开术或小梁切开术对许多儿童有效，如果可以看到前房角，则可以作为首选手术。当房角切开术失败或房角关闭时，可以使用引流管。

Bohnsack BL, Freedman SF. Surgical outcomes in childhood uveitic glaucoma. *Am J Ophthalmol.* 2013;155(1):134–142.

（翻译 陈晓航 袁立飞 // 审校 刘陇黔 石一宁 蒋宁 // 章节审校 石广礼）

CHAPTER 25

Disorders of the Retina and Vitreous

This chapter includes related videos, which can be accessed by scanning the QR codes provided in the text or going to www. aao. org/ bcscvideo_ section06.

This chapter focuses on retinal diseases that are most often diagnosed in the first 2 decades of life. These include retinopathy of prematurity, Leber congenital amaurosis, and retinoblastoma. Many of the topics covered in this chapter are also discussed in BCSC Section 12, *Retina and Vitreous*. See BCSC Section 4, *Ophthalmic Pathology and Intraocular Tumors*, for detailed discussion of tumors.

Congenital and Developmental Abnormalities

PersistentFetal Vasculature

Persistentfetal vasculature is covered in Chapter 23.

Retinopathy of Prematurity

Retinopathy of prematurity (ROP) is a vasoproliferative retinal disorder unique to premature infants. First described in the 1950s, ROP is a leading cause of childhood blindness in the United States, second only to cerebral visual impairment.

Pathophysiology

Retinal vascularization begins during week 16 of gestation. Mesenchymal tissue (the source of retinal vessels) grows centrifugally from the optic disc, reaching the nasal ora serrata by 36 weeks' gestation and the temporal ora serrata by 40 weeks' gestation. ROP results from abnormal growth of these retinal blood vessels in premature infants because of a complex interaction between vascular endothelial growth factor (VEGF) and insulin-like growth factor I (IGF-I). The pathophysiology of ROP is currently thought of as a 2-phase process and is outlined in Table 25-1.

Classification

The International Classification of Retinopathy of Prematurity (ICROP) describes the disease by location (zone), stage, and extent (Table 25-2; Figs 25-1 through 25-5). Higher stage numbers and lower zone numbers indicate more severe ROP.

第 25 章

视网膜玻璃体疾病

本章所包含的相关视频，可通过扫描文中的二维码或访问网站 www.aao.org/bcscvideo_section06 观看。

本章重点介绍 20 岁前诊断的视网膜疾病，包括早产儿视网膜病变、Leber 先天性黑矇和视网膜母细胞瘤。本章涉及的许多内容在 BCSC 第 12 册《*视网膜与玻璃体*》中也有讨论。肿瘤相关内容详见 BCSC 第 4 册《*眼病理学与眼内肿瘤*》。

先天性和发育性异常

永存 / 永久性胎儿血管

第 23 章包含永存性胎儿血管相关内容。

早产儿视网膜病变

早产儿视网膜病变（ROP）是一种特发于早产儿的血管增生性视网膜病变。早产儿视网膜病变（ROP）早在 20 世纪 50 年代就被提出，是美国儿童失明的主要原因之一，仅次于中枢性视觉损伤。

病理生理学

视网膜血管化始于妊娠第 16 周。间充质组织（视网膜血管的来源）从视盘处离心式生长，在妊娠 36 周时到达鼻侧锯齿缘，在妊娠 40 周时到达颞侧锯齿缘。在血管内皮生长因子（VEGF）和胰岛素样生长因子 -I（IGF-I）之间复杂的相互作用下，早产儿的这些视网膜血管异常生长，导致早产儿视网膜病变（ROP）。目前认为，早产儿视网膜病变（ROP）的病理生理学机制经历了 2 个阶段，详见表 25-1。

分类

早产儿视网膜病变国际分类（ICROP）按位置（区域）、分期和范围对该疾病进行描述（表 25-2；图 25-1 至 25-5）。分期越高、位置分区越低，提示早产儿视网膜病变病情越严重。

Table 25-1 Interaction Between VEGF and IGF-I in Development of ROP

Phase I

Occurs at 22–30 weeks' gestational age
Retina is hyperoxic (relative to intrauterine oxygen levels)
VEGF levels are low
Retinal blood vessels stop growing; this arrested growth is
- worsened by high oxygen levels
- worsened by low levels of IGF-I
- correlated with poor weight gain

Phase II

Occurs at 31–44 weeks' gestational age
Avascular retina is hypoxic
VEGF levels rise (due to the hypoxic avascular retina)
Neovascularization occurs

Treatment of ROP

Laser therapy destroys hypoxic avascular retina, so VEGF levels fall
Bevacizumab inhibits VEGF

IGF-I = insulin-like growth factor I; ROP = retinopathy of prematurity; VEGF = vascular endothelial growth factor.

Table 25-2 International Classification of Retinopathy of Prematurity

Location: zones II and III based on convention rather than strict anatomy (see Fig 25-1)
Zone I (posterior pole): a circle centered on the optic disc with a radius equal to twice the distance from the center of the disc to the macula. Clinically, the temporal edge of zone I is visible with a 25 or 28 D lens, with the other edge of the field of view centered on the nasal disc margin
Zone II: a circle centered on the optic disc with a radius equal to the distance from the center of the optic disc to the nasal ora serrata
Zone III: residual crescent anterior to zone II

Extent: specified as hours of the clock as observer looks at each eye

Stages

Stage 0: immature vascularization, no ROP
Stage 1: presence of a demarcation line between vascularized retina posteriorly and avascular retina anteriorly (see Fig 25-2)
Stage 2: presence of a ridge with height and width, with or without small tufts of fibrovascular proliferation ("popcorn") (see Fig 25-3)
Stage 3: ridge with extraretinal fibrovascular proliferation (see Fig 25-4)
- mild fibrovascular proliferation
- moderate fibrovascular proliferation
- severe fibrovascular proliferation

Stage 4: subtotal retinal detachment (see Fig 25-5)
A. extrafoveal retinal detachment
B. retinal detachment including fovea
Stage 5: total retinal detachment; open or closed funnel

Plus disease: venous dilatation and arteriolar tortuosity present in posterior pole retinal vessels in at least 2 quadrants of the retina; standard photograph used to define the minimum amount of vascular abnormalities necessary to make the diagnosis; plus symbol (+) added to ROP stage denotes presence of plus disease (eg, stage 3 + ROP)

Pre–plus disease: venous dilatation and arteriolar tortuosity in the posterior pole but not as severe as the vascular abnormalities seen in plus disease

Aggressive posterior ROP: zone I or posterior zone II ROP associated with plus disease involving all 4 quadrants of the posterior pole retinal vessels, shunt vessels, and flat neovascularization at the junction between vascularized and avascular retina. Without treatment, typically progresses quickly to stage 4 or 5 ROP. Was formerly known as *Rush disease*

D = diopter.

Information from International Committee for the Classification of Retinopathy of Prematurity. The International Classification of Retinopathy of Prematurity revisited. *Arch Ophthalmol.* 2005;123(7):991–999.

表25-1　早产儿视网膜病变（ROP）形成过程中VEGF和IGF-I的相互作用

阶段I

22～30 周胎龄时发生
视网膜含氧量高（相对于子宫内含氧水平）
VEGF水平低
视网膜血管停止生长，这种生长受阻
- 受高氧含量而恶化
- 受低水平IGF-I而恶化
- 与体重增长缓慢相关

阶段II

31～44周胎龄时发生
无血管区视网膜含氧量低
VEGF水平升高(由含氧量低的无血管区视网膜所致）
新生血管形成

ROP的治疗

激光治疗破坏含氧量低的无血管区视网膜，故VEGF水平下降
贝伐单抗抑制VEGF

IGF-I：胰岛素样生长因子-I；ROP：早产儿视网膜病变；VEGF：血管内皮生长因子。

表25-2　早产儿视网膜病变的国际分类

区域：II区和III区的划分基于惯例而非严格的解剖学特征（详见图25-1）

I区（后极部）：以视盘为中心，以视盘中心到黄斑中心凹距离的2倍为半径的圆形区域。临床上用25D或28D透镜可观察到I区的颞侧缘，而视野的另一边为鼻侧盘缘

II区：以视盘为中心，以视盘中心到鼻侧锯齿缘的距离为半径的圆形区域

III区：II区之外的新月形区域

范围：当检查者观察每只眼睛时，以时钟的钟点表示

分期：

0期：视网膜血管化未成熟，无ROP病变

1期：后方有血管区和前方无血管区视网膜之间出现明显的分界线（详见图25-2）

2期：出现一定高度和宽度的嵴，有或无小簇纤维血管增生（“爆米花”）（详见图25-3）

3期：嵴形成并伴有视网膜外纤维血管增生（详见图25-4）
- 轻度纤维血管增生
- 中度纤维血管增生
- 重度纤维血管增生

4期：部分视网膜脱离（详见图25-5）
A. 未累及中心凹的视网膜脱离
B. 累及中心凹的视网膜脱离

5期：全视网膜脱离；开或闭的漏斗状

附加病变：后极部视网膜血管中的静脉扩张和小动脉迂曲，至少2个象限；诊断时采用标准化照片，确定血管异常最小量；ROP分期后加上加号（+）表示存在附加病变（如3期+ ROP）

前附加病变：后极部静脉扩张和小动脉迂曲，但血管异常没有附加病变的严重

急性进展性后极部ROP：ROP I区或II区后极部，附加病变累及后极部4个象限的视网膜血管、分流血管、血管化和无血管化视网膜交界处的平坦新生血管形成。如果不进行治疗，会快速进入ROP 4期或5期。曾被称为*Rush病*

D = 屈光度。

（译者注：资料来源见前页原文。）

BOOST-II Australia and United Kingdom Collaborative Groups; Tarnow-Mordi W, Stenson B, Kirby A, et al. Outcomes of two trials of oxygen-saturation targets in preterm infants. *N Engl J Med*. 2016;374(8):749–760.

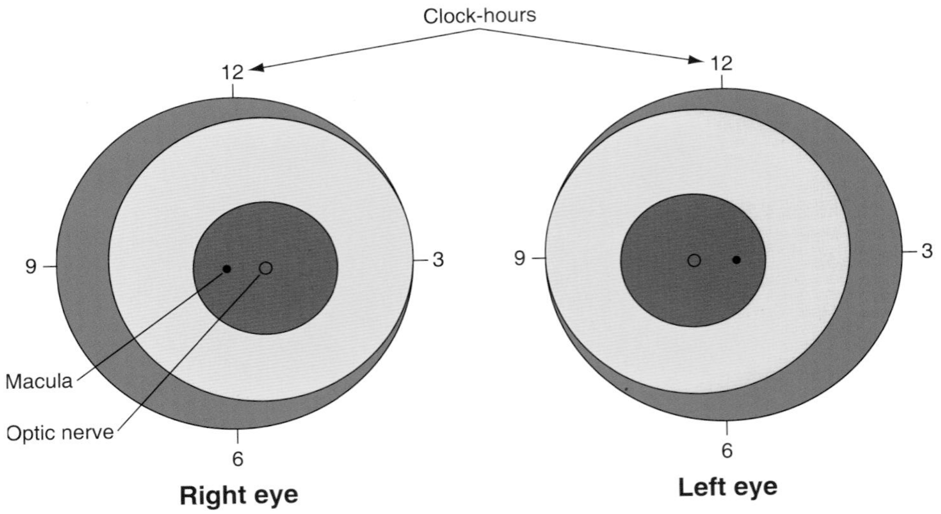

Figure 25-1 Schematic of the retina of the right and left eyes, showing the area of zones I *(red)*, II *(yellow)*, and III *(green)*, which are used to describe the location of retinopathy of prematurity (ROP). The extent of ROP is specified as hours of the clock.

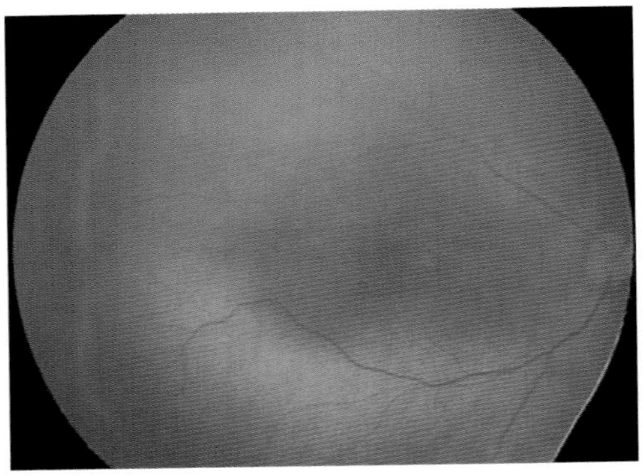

Figure 25-2 Stage 1 ROP. The demarcation line has no height. *(Courtesy of Daniel Weaver, MD.)*

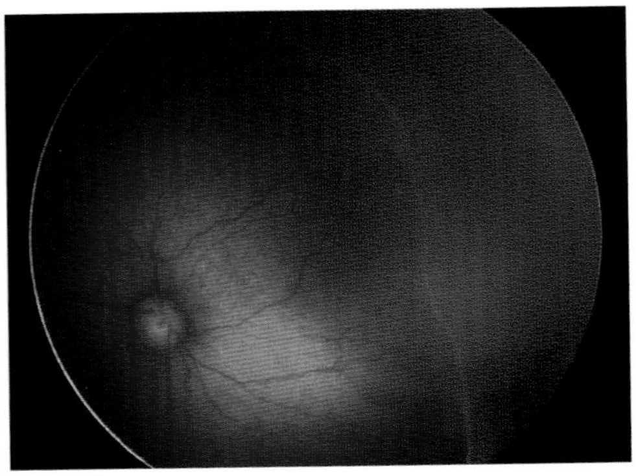

Figure 25-3 Stage 2 ROP. The demarcation line has height and width, creating a ridge. *(Courtesy of Daniel Weaver, MD.)*

BOOST-II Australia and United Kingdom Collaborative Groups; Tarnow-Mordi W, Stenson B, Kirby A, et al. Outcomes of two trials of oxygen-saturation targets in preterm infants. *N Engl J Med*. 2016;374(8):749–760.

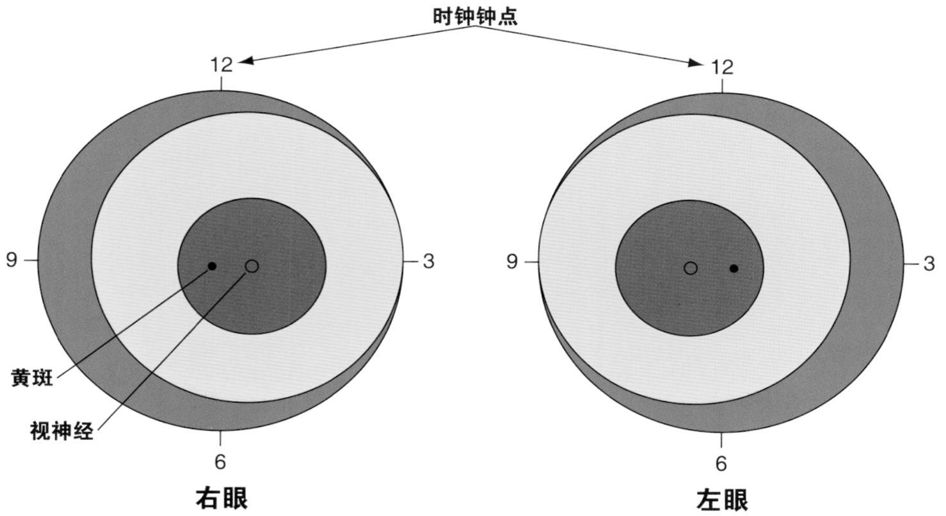

图 25-1　用于描述早产儿视网膜病变区域的双眼视网膜分区示意图：I 区（*红色*）、II 区（*黄色*）和 III 区（*绿色*）。早产儿视网膜病变的范围用时钟的钟点表示。

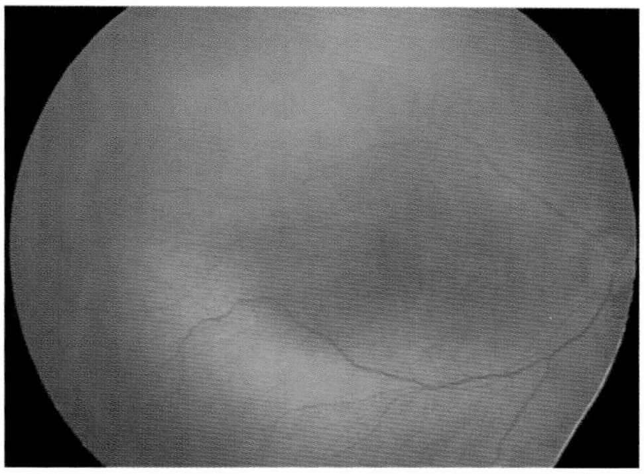

图 25-2　早产儿视网膜病变 1 期。分界线没有隆起。*（译者注：资料来源见前页原文。）*

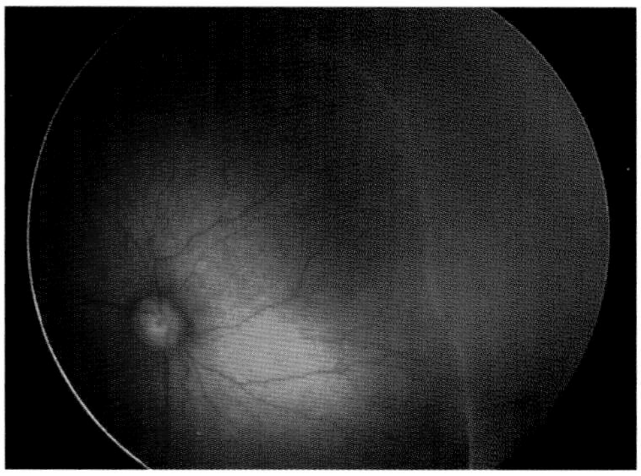

图 25-3　早产儿视网膜病变 2 期。分界线隆起且较宽，形成嵴。*（译者注：资料来源见前页原文。）*

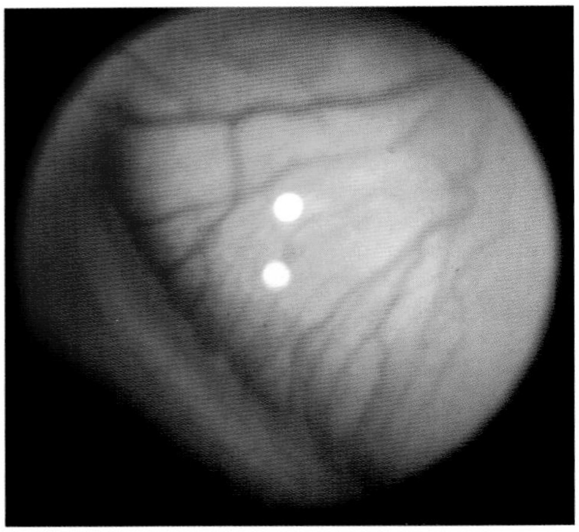

Figure 25-4 Stage 3 ROP. Ridge with extraretinal fibrovascular proliferation. *(Reproduced with permission from Lueder GT. Pediatric Practice Ophthalmology. New York: McGraw-Hill; 2011:232.)*

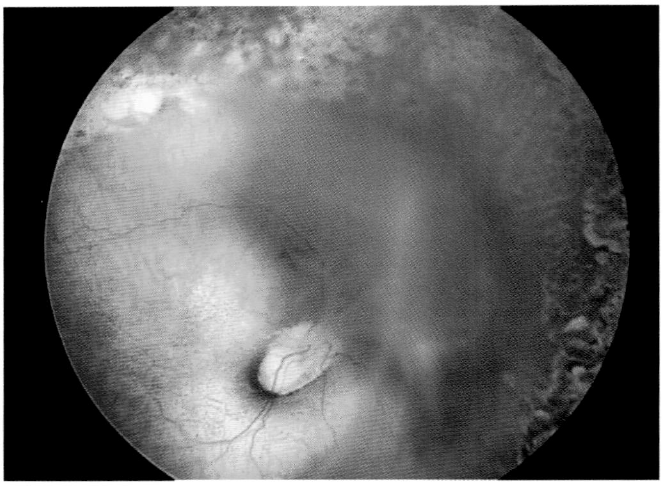

Figure 25-5 Subtotal extrafoveal retinal detachment in the right eye of a patient with stage 4A ROP treated with laser. *(Courtesy of Robert W. Hered, MD.)*

Plus disease refers to marked arteriolar tortuosity and venous engorgement of the posterior pole vasculature and is diagnosed by comparison with a standard photograph. It implies vascular shunting through the new vessels and signifies severe disease (Fig 25-6). *Pre–plus disease* refers to dilatation and tortuosity that are abnormal but less than that seen in the standard photograph (Fig 25-7).

Aggressive posterior ROP (AP-ROP; formerly known as *Rush disease*) is a severe form of ROP defined as zone I or posterior zone II disease, associated with plus disease involving all 4 quadrants of the posterior pole retinal vessels, shunt vessels, and flat neovascularization at the junction between vascularized and avascular retina. Without treatment, AP-ROP typically progresses quickly to stage 4 or 5 ROP (Fig 25-8).

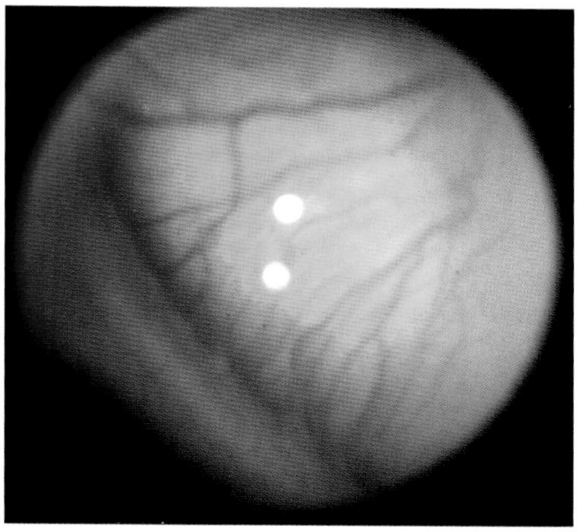

图 25-4　早产儿视网膜病变 3 期。形成嵴并伴有视网膜外纤维血管增生。*（译者注：资料来源见前页原文。）*

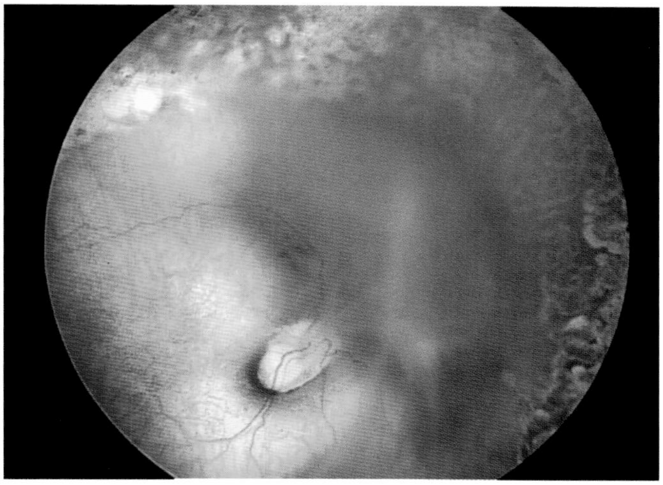

图 25-5　经激光治疗的右眼 4A 期早产儿视网膜病变，部分视网膜脱离，未累及中心凹。*（译者注：资料来源见前页原文。）*

*附加病变*指后极部出现明显的小动脉迂曲和静脉扩张，采用标准化照片比较诊断。这提示有新生血管分流，病情较严重（图 25-6）。*前附加病变*指标准化照片仅显示轻微的血管异常扩张和迂曲（图 25-7）。

进行性后极部早产儿视网膜病变（AP-ROP，曾被称为 *Rush 病变*）是一种发生在 I 区或 II 区后部的严重早产儿视网膜病变（ROP），伴有附加病变累及后极部 4 个象限的视网膜血管、分流血管、血管化和无血管化视网膜交界处的平坦新生血管形成。如不治疗，进行性后极部早产儿视网膜病变（AP-ROP）会快速进入早产儿视网膜病变（ROP）4 期或 5 期（图 25-8）。

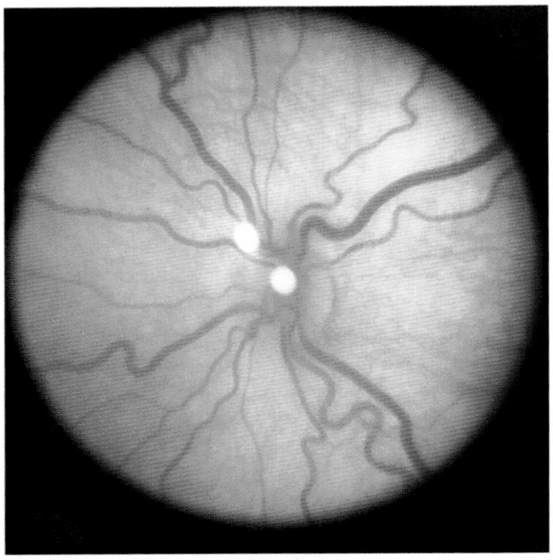

Figure 25-6 Plus disease. *(Reproduced with permission from Lueder GT. Pediatric Practice Ophthalmology. New York: McGraw-Hill; 2011:231.)*

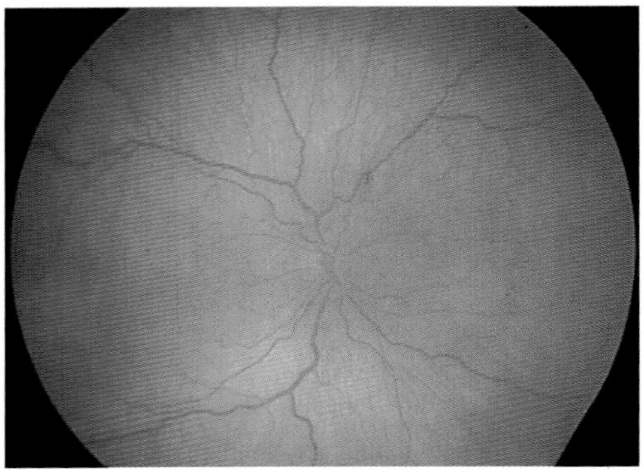

Figure 25-7 Pre–plus disease. *(Courtesy of Daniel Weaver, MD.)*

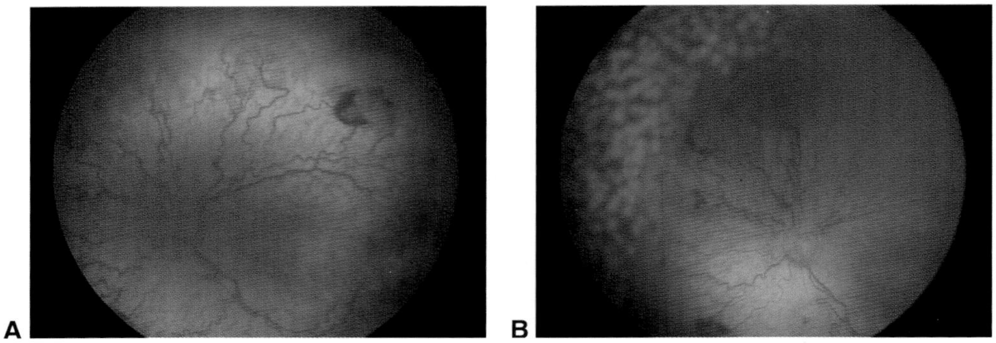

Figure 25-8 Aggressive posterior ROP, left eye, prior to treatment **(A)** and shortly after laser treatment **(B).** *(Courtesy of Robert W. Hered, MD.)*

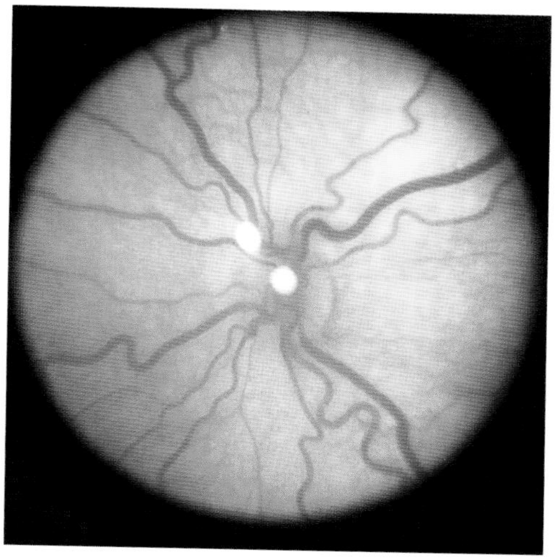

图 25-6　附加病变。*（译者注：资料来源见前页原文。）*

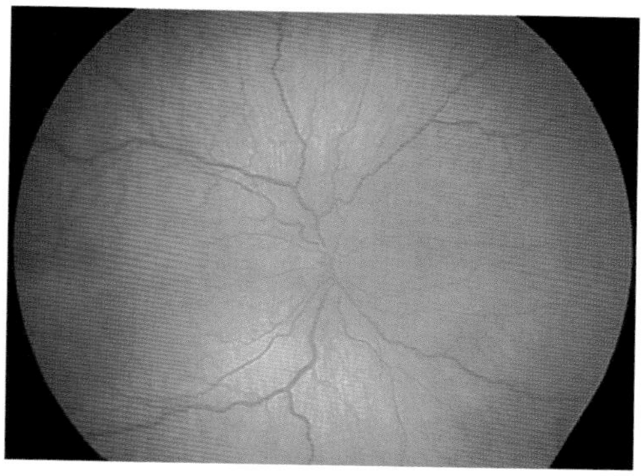

图 25-7　前附加病变。*（译者注：资料来源见前页原文。）*

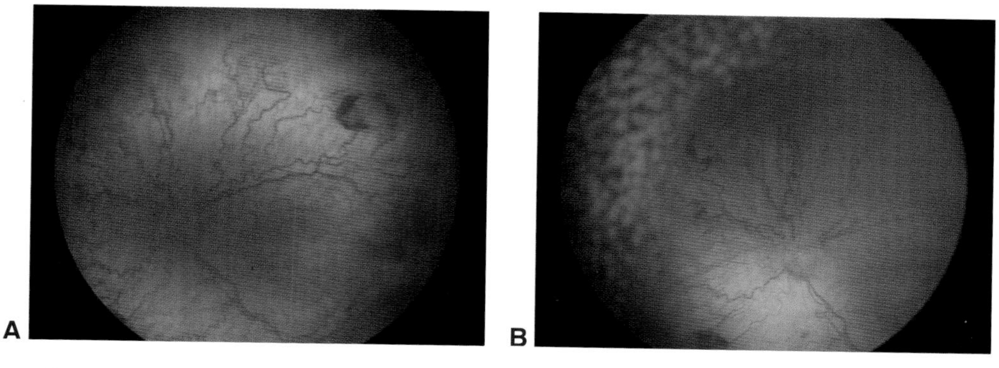

图 25-8　进行性 / 急进性后极部早产儿视网膜病变，左眼，治疗前（**A**）和激光治疗后（**B**）。*（译者注：资料来源见前页原文。）*

Table 25-3 ETROP Classification of ROP

Type 1	
	Zone I, any stage ROP with plus disease
	Zone I, stage 3 ROP without plus disease
	Zone II, stage 2 or 3 ROP with plus disease
Type 2	
	Zone I, stage 1 or 2 ROP without plus disease
	Zone II, stage 3 ROP without plus disease

ETROP = Early Treatment for Retinopathy of Prematurity.

Modified from Wallace DK. Retinopathy of prematurity. *Focal Points: Clinical Modules for Ophthalmologists.* San Francisco: American Academy of Ophthalmology; 2008, module 12:p 4.

The Cryotherapy for Retinopathy of Prematurity (CRYO-ROP) trial defined *threshold* disease as 5 contiguous or 8 total clock-hours of stage 3 ROP in zone I or II in the presence of plus disease. The Early Treatment for Retinopathy of Prematurity (ETROP) trial defined *prethreshold disease* as all zone I and zone II ROP changes that do not meet threshold treatment criteria, except for zone II stage 1 and zone II stage 2 without plus disease. ETROP further divided prethreshold ROP into *type 1* and *type 2* disease to delineate which babies would benefit from treatment before the development of threshold disease (Table 25-3).

International Committee for the Classification of Retinopathy of Prematurity. The International Classification of Retinopathy of Prematurity revisited. *Arch Ophthalmol.* 2005;123(7):991–999.

Risk factors for development of ROP

Premature birth (≤30 weeks' gestational age) and low birth weight (≤1500 g) are the most significant risk factors for development of ROP. Excessive administration of supplementaloxygen during the early postnatal period is also a risk factor for ROP development. Despite decades of research, however, the ideal amount of oxygen required by a premature infant remains unknown. Low target ranges of oxygen saturation have been associated with an increased risk of death and disability. Low levels of serum IGF-I are associated with poor postnatal weight gain and more severe ROP. Numerous algorithms using postnatal weight gain to identify infants at risk for type 1 ROP have been developed and are under investigation. African American preterm infants are at lower risk for needing ROP treatment.

Saugstad OD, Aune D. Optimal oxygenation of extremely low birth weight infants: a metaanalysis and systematic review of the oxygen saturation target studies. *Neonatology.* 2014;105(1):55–63.

Screening and diagnosis

Current guidelines from the American Academy of Pediatrics, American Academy of Ophthalmology, and American Association for Pediatric Ophthalmology and Strabismus recommend that infants with gestational age of 30 weeks or less, birth weight of 1500 g or less, or a complicated clinical course be screened for ROP. The first examination should be performed at 4 weeks' chronologic (postnatal) age or at a corrected gestational age of 31 weeks, whichever is later (but not later than 6 weeks' chronologic age). Current screening recommendations can be found on the website of the American Academy of Pediatrics (http:// pediatrics. aappublications. org/content/131/1/189). In developing countries, ROP occurs in infants at an older gestational age and with a higher birth weight compared with infants in the United States. This suggests that screening criteria for ROP do not apply globally and should be modified in other regions of the world.

表25-3 早产儿视网膜病变ETROP分类

1型
I区，伴有附加病变的任何分期ROP
I区，不伴附加病变的ROP 3期
II区，伴有附加病变的ROP 2期或3期
2型
I区，不伴附加病变的ROP 1期或2期
II区，不伴附加病变的ROP 3期

ETROP：=ROP早期治疗试验。

（译者注：资料来源见前页原文。）

早产儿视网膜病变的冷冻疗法（CRYO-ROP）试验将*阈值病变*定义为附加病变，合并了I区或II区中连续5个钟点或共计8个钟点的ROP 3期病变。早产儿视网膜病变的早期治疗（ETROP）试验将*阈前病变*定义为不符合阈值治疗标准的所有I区和II区ROP变化，除外II区1期不伴附加病变和II区2期ROP病变。ETROP进一步将阈前早产儿视网膜病变（ROP）分为*1型*和*2型*，以划分出可在阈值病变形成前治疗的婴儿，使其受益（表25-3）。

International Committee for the Classification of Retinopathy of Prematurity. The International Classification of Retinopathy of Prematurity revisited. *Arch Ophthalmol.* 2005;123(7):991–999.

早产儿视网膜病变（ROP）的危险因素

早产儿（胎龄≤30周）和低出生体重儿（≤1500g）是发生早产儿视网膜病变（ROP）最重要的危险因素。出生后早期过量吸氧也是早产儿视网膜病变（ROP）发展的危险因素。尽管进行了数十年的研究，早产儿所需的理想氧气量仍未知。低目标范围/流量的氧饱和度与早产儿死亡和残疾风险增加有关。低水平的血清IGF-I与生后体重增长缓慢和严重的早产儿视网膜病变（ROP）有关。正在研发通过计算产后体重增加来确定1型早产儿视网膜病变（ROP）风险婴儿。非裔美国早产儿较少需要进行早产儿视网膜病变（ROP）的治疗。

Saugstad OD, Aune D. Optimal oxygenation of extremely low birth weight infants: a metaanalysis and systematic review of the oxygen saturation target studies. *Neonatology.* 2014;105(1):55–63.

筛查和诊断

美国儿科学会、美国眼科学会和美国小儿眼科与斜视学会的现行指南建议，胎龄30周及以下、出生体重不超过1500克或产程不顺利的婴儿应进行筛查，第一次检查应在出生后4周龄，或矫正胎龄31周，以后者为准（但不晚于出生后6周龄）。最新的筛查建议可登录美国儿科学会的网站（http://pediatrics.aappublications.org/content/131/1/189）查看。与美国婴儿相比，发展中国家的早产儿视网膜病变（ROP）发生在胎龄较大且出生体重较重的婴儿，提示早产儿视网膜病变（ROP）的筛查标准不适用于全球，在世界其他地区使用时需进行修改。

ROP examinations are performed after pharmacologic dilation of the pupils. Combination eyedrops of relatively low concentration (cyclopentolate 0.2% and phenylephrine 1%) are typically used. Sterile instruments should be used to examine the infant. A nurse should be present for examinations in the neonatal intensive care unit because an infant may experience apnea and bradycardia during examination. If an examination must be postponed, the postponement and medical reason should be documented in the patient's medical record. Suggested intervals for follow-up ophthalmic examinations for ROP without plus disease are given in Table 25-4; discontinuation of screening examinations is summarized in Table 25-5. Most ROP regresses spontaneously via involution.

Table 25-4 Recommended Intervals of Follow-up Eye Examinations for ROPWithout Plus Disease

1 Week or Less
- Immature vascularization: zone I or posterior zone II
- Stage 1 or 2 ROP: zone I
- Stage 3 ROP: zone II
- Presence or suspected presence of aggressive posterior ROP

1 to 2 Weeks
- Immature vascularization: posterior zone II
- Stage 2 ROP: zone II
- Unequivocally regressing ROP: zone I

2 Weeks
- Stage 1 ROP: zone II
- Immature vascularization: zone II
- Unequivocally regressing ROP: zone II

2 to 3 Weeks
- Stage 1 or 2 ROP: zone III
- Regressing ROP: zone III

Information from Fierson WM; American Academy of Pediatrics Section on Ophthalmology; American Academy of Ophthalmology; American Association for Pediatric Ophthalmology and Strabismus; American Association of Certified Orthoptists. Screening examination of premature infants for retinopathy of prematurity. *Pediatrics.* 2013;131(1):189–195.

Table 25-5 Criteria for Discontinuation of ROP Screening Examinations[a]

- Fully vascularized retina
- Zone III vascularization without previous zone I or II ROP
- Lack of development of prethreshold or worse ROP by 50 weeks' postmenstrual age
- Regression of ROP in zone III without abnormal vascular tissue capable of reactivation in zone II or III

[a] May consider discontinuation if any of the criteria are met. Applies to infants who did not require treatment.

Adapted from Shulman JP, Hobbs R, Hartnett ME. Retinopathy of prematurity: evolving concepts in diagnosis and management. *Focal Points: Clinical Modules for Ophthalmologists.* San Francisco: American Academy of Ophthalmology; 2015, module 1.

Diagnosis of ROP via digital retinal photography and telemedicine is under investigation. It is currently being used in developing countries and areas where ophthalmologists are not available to perform ROP examinations.

Fierson WM; American Academy of Pediatrics Section on Ophthalmology; American Academy of Ophthalmology; American Association for Pediatric Ophthalmology and Strabismus; American Association of Certified Orthoptists. Screening examination of premature infants for retinopathy of prematurity. *Pediatrics.* 2013;131(1):189–195.

早产儿视网膜病变（ROP）检查应在药物性散瞳后进行。常使用浓度相对较低的复合滴眼液（0.2%环喷托酯和1%苯肾上腺素）、无菌器械检查婴儿。应在新生儿重症监护室和护士陪同下进行检查，因为检查期间婴儿可能会出现呼吸暂停和心动过缓。如果需推迟检查，应将延期和医疗原因记录在患儿的病历中。表 25-4 给出了无附加病变的早产儿视网膜病变（ROP）进行眼科随访检查的推荐时间间隔，表 25-5 汇总了筛查终止时间。多数早产儿视网膜病变（ROP）病变逐步退化、自行消退。

表25-4　无附加病变ROP推荐眼科检查随访时间间隔

1 周及以内
- 未成熟血管化：I区或II区后极部
- 1期或2期ROP：I区
- 3期ROP：II区
- 存在或可疑存在进行性后极部ROP

1 ~ 2周
- 未成熟血管化：II区后极部
- 2期ROP：II区
- 病变明确退化的ROP：I区

2周
- 1期ROP：II区
- 未成熟血管化：II区
- 病变明确退化的ROP：II区

2 ~ 3周
- 1期或2期ROP：III区
- 病变退化的ROP：III区

（译者注：资料来源见前页原文。）

表25-5　终止ROP筛查标准[a]

- 视网膜完全血管化
- III区血管化，且既往无I区或II区ROP
- 当矫正胎龄达50周时仍未发生阈值前病变或更严重的ROP
- III区中病变退化的ROP，且在II区或III区中无恢复活性的异常血管组织

[a]如果满足任何标准，可考虑停止随访筛查。适用于不需要治疗的婴儿。

（译者注：资料来源见前页原文。）

正在研发通过数字视网膜摄影和远程医疗途径诊断早产儿视网膜病变（ROP）的技术，目前该技术正应用于眼科医生无法进行早产儿视网膜病变（ROP）检查的发展中国家和地区。

Fierson WM; American Academy of Pediatrics Section on Ophthalmology; American Academy of Ophthalmology; American Association for Pediatric Ophthalmology and Strabismus; American Association of Certified Orthoptists. Screening examination of premature infants for retinopathy of prematurity. *Pediatrics.* 2013;131(1):189–195.

Vinekar A, Jayadev C, Mangalesh S, Shetty B, Vidyasagar D. Role of tele-medicine in retinopathy of prematurity screening in rural outreach centers in India—a report of 20,214 imaging sessions in the KIDROP program. *Semin Fetal Neonatal Med.* 2015;20(5):335–345.

Treatment

Approximately 10% of infants examined for ROP require treatment. Several multicenter ROP trials have been influential in guiding treatment of the disease. The initial ROP treatment study, CRYO-ROP, recommended treatment with cryotherapy when the disease reached a certain level of severity, termed *threshold*. Current treatment guidelines are based on results of the ETROP trial (see Table 25-3 for ETROP classification), which found that earlier treatment in prethreshold eyes classified as type 1 resulted in better structural and visual outcomes than did conventional treatment. Panretinal laser photocoagulation is performed to ablate the peripheral avascular retina (Fig 25-9). Current guidelines strongly recommend treatment for any eye with type 1 ROP. Eyes with type 2 ROP should be closely observed for progression to type 1 disease (Videos 25-1 through 25-4 show ROP progression and response to laser treatment).

VIDEO 25-1 Stage 3 retinopathy of prematurity.

Courtesy of Leslie D. MacKeen, BSc, and Anna L. Ells, MD, FRCS(C). Dynamic documentation of the evolution of retinopathy of prematurity in video format. J AAPOS. 2008;12(4):349–351.

Access all Section 6 videos at www.aao.org/bcscvideo section06.

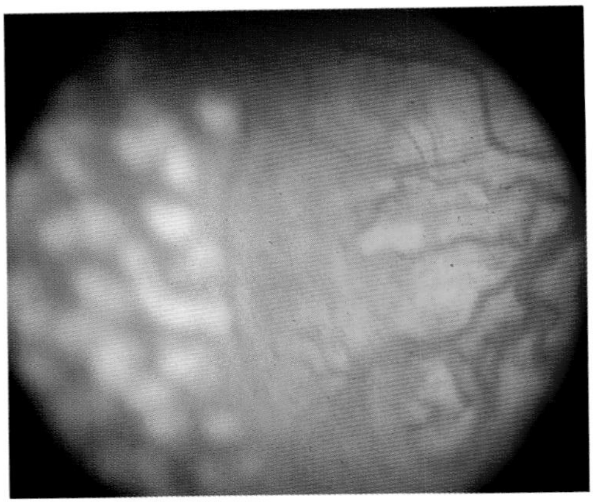

Figure 25-9 Laser photocoagulation applied anterior to avascular retina. Laser treatment should not be applied directly to the ridge. Note the thick band of neovascularization and plus disease. *(Courtesy of Philip J. Ferrone, MD.)*

VIDEO 25-2 Aggressive posterior retinopathy of prematurity with laser treatment.

Courtesy of Leslie D. MacKeen, BSc, and Anna L. Ells, MD, FRCS(C).

Dynamic documentation of the evolution of retinopathy of prematurity in video format.

J AAPOS. 2008;12(4):349–351.

VIDEO 25-3 Retinopathy of prematurity—the movie, 2.

Courtesy of Anna L. Ells, MD, FRCS(C), and Leslie D. MacKeen, BSc.

Retinopathy of prematurity—the movie. J AAPOS. 2004;8(4):389.

Vinekar A, Jayadev C, Mangalesh S, Shetty B, Vidyasagar D. Role of tele-medicine in retinopathy of prematurity screening in rural outreach centers in India—a report of 20,214 imaging sessions in the KIDROP program. *Semin Fetal Neonatal Med.* 2015;20(5):335–345.

治疗

接受 ROP 检查的婴儿中，约有 10% 需要治疗。一些多中心早产儿视网膜病变（ROP）试验在指导疾病治疗方面具有重要影响。初始的 ROP 治疗研究，早产儿视网膜病变的冷冻疗法 CRYO-ROP 试验建议在疾病达到一定的严重程度，即达到*阈值*时，应使用冷冻疗法进行治疗。目前的治疗指南是基于早产儿视网膜病变的早期治疗 ETROP 试验的结果（ETROP 分类参见表 25-3）。该研究发现，当患眼为 1 型阈值前病变时进行早期治疗，比常规治疗在结构和视功能上预后更好。可进行全视网膜激光光凝术，以消除周边视网膜无血管区（图 25-9）。目前的指南强烈建议对 1 型早产儿视网膜病变（ROP）患者进行治疗。应密切观察 2 型早产儿视网膜病变（ROP）患者的情况，预防其发展为 1 型早产儿视网膜病变（ROP）[视频 25-1 至 25-4 显示早产儿视网膜病变（ROP）的进展和对激光治疗的反应]。

视频 25-1　ROP 3期。*（译者注：资料来源见前页原文。）*
可登陆网站www.aao.org/bcscvideo_section06观看第6册中的所有视频。

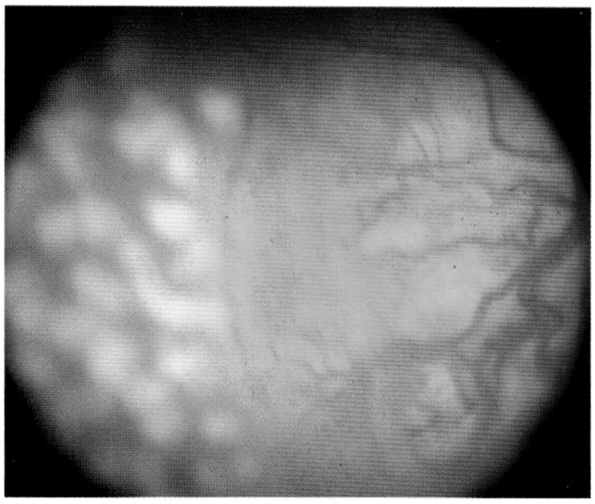

图 25-9　激光光凝术应用于嵴前视网膜无血管区。激光治疗不应直接用于视网膜嵴。注意新血管形成的厚带区域和附加疾病。*（译者注：资料来源见前页原文。）*

视频 25-2　激光治疗急性进展性后极部早产儿视网膜病变。
（译者注：资料来源见前页原文。）

视频 25-3　早产儿视网膜病变——短片2。
（译者注：资料来源见前页原文。）

VIDEO 25-4 Retinopathy of prematurity—the movie, 7.
Courtesy of Anna L. Ells, MD, FRCS(C), and Leslie D. MacKeen, BSc.
Retinopathy of prematurity—the movie. J AAPOS. 2004;8(4):389.

AP - ROP typically occurs in zone I or posterior zone II, progresses rapidly, is often difficult to treat, and has a poor prognosis (see Table 25-2 and Fig 25-8). Another characteristic of AP- ROP is that it does not progress in the typical fashion (ie, through stages 1, 2, and 3), and stage 3 can often appear as flat neovascularization.

The most recent treatment option for type 1 ROP is intravitreal injection of anti-VEGF agents bevacizumab and ranibizumab. The initial study of anti-VEGF agents for treatment of ROP, and the most influential, was Bevacizumab Eliminates the Angiogenic Threat of Retinopathy of Prematurity (BEAT-ROP), which found a significant benefit to structural outcome for zone I eyes that received intravitreal bevacizumab monotherapy compared with those that received laser treatment. Subsequent publications have documented that ROP may recur months after treatment with anti-VEGF agents; thus, prolonged surveillance and re-treatment may be necessary after intravitreal anti-VEGF injections. Anti-VEGF treatment should not be administered to infants who are unlikely to return for frequent follow-up examinations after they are discharged from the hospital.

There is concern that antiangiogenic drugs' effects on the developing vasculature in other areas of the body may lead to adverse developmental outcomes. Abnormalities of retinal vasculature have been documented by fluorescein angiography years after anti-VEGF treatment. Further study is necessary to determine the long-term ocular and systemic effects of anti-VEGF agents used to treat ROP.

Early Treatment for Retinopathy of Prematurity Cooperative Group. Revised indications for the treatment of retinopathy of prematurity: results of the Early Treatment for Retinopathy of Prematurity randomized trial. *Arch Ophthalmol.* 2003;121(12):1684–1694.

Early Treatment for Retinopathy of Prematurity Cooperative Group; Good WV, Hardy RJ, Dobson V, et al. Final visual acuity results in the Early Treatment for Retinopathy of Prematurity study. *Arch Ophthalmol.* 2010;128(6):663–671.

Lepore D, Quinn GE, Molle F, et al. Intravitreal bevacizumab versus laser treatment in type 1 retinopathy of prematurity: report on fluorescein angiographic findings. *Ophthalmology*. 2014;121(11):2212–2219.

Mintz-Hittner HA, Kennedy KA, Chuang AZ; BEAT-ROP Cooperative Group. Efficacy of intravitreal bevacizumab for stage 3+ retinopathy of prematurity. *N Engl J Med.* 2011;364(7):603–615.

Morin J, Luu TM, Superstein R, et al; Canadian Neonatal Network and the Canadian Neonatal Follow-Up Network Investigators. Neurodevelopmental outcomes following bevacizumab injections for retinopathy of prematurity. *Pediatrics*. 2016;137(4). pii: e20153218.

Sequelae and complications

One of the most common sequelae of significant ROP, whether treated or spontaneously regressed, is myopia, which may be severe. Also, premature infants with ROP, especially those who required treatment, are at higher risk for strabismus and amblyopia. Another recognized risk is glaucoma from crowding of the anterior chamber angle.

视频 25-4　早产儿视网膜病变——短片7。
（译者注：资料来源见前页原文。）

急进性 / 进行性后极部早产儿视网膜病变（AP-ROP）通常发生在 I 区或 II 区后部，进展迅速、治疗困难、预后不良（见表 25-2 和图 25-8）。其另一个特征是不遵循常规的早产儿视网膜病变（ROP）发展规律（即 1 期向 2 期和 3 期逐渐发展），且 3 期可表现为扁平的新生血管形成。

1 型 ROP 的最新治疗选择是向玻璃体腔内注射抗 VEGF 试剂贝伐单抗和雷珠单抗。贝伐单抗消除早产儿视网膜病变血管生成风险（BEAT-ROP）是最早也最具影响力的探索抗 VEGF 药物治疗 ROP 的研究。该研究发现，与激光治疗相比，I 区 ROP 接受玻璃体腔内注射贝伐单抗单药治疗，更有助于改善结构预后。随后的研究结果显示，ROP 可能在用抗 VEGF 药物治疗后数月复发，因此，玻璃体腔内抗 VEGF 注射治疗后可能需要长时间的随访监测和再治疗。对于出院后不能随访监测的婴儿，不应给予抗 VEGF 治疗。

人们担心抗血管生成药物会对身体其他部位发育中的血管系统有影响，导致发育不良。在抗 VEGF 治疗数年后，荧光素血管造影仍发现视网膜血管系统的异常。治疗 ROP 的抗 VEGF 药物对于眼部和全身的长期影响尚需进一步研究。

Early Treatment for Retinopathy of Prematurity Cooperative Group. Revised indications for the treatment of retinopathy of prematurity: results of the Early Treatment for Retinopathy of Prematurity randomized trial. *Arch Ophthalmol.* 2003;121(12):1684–1694.

Early Treatment for Retinopathy of Prematurity Cooperative Group; Good WV, Hardy RJ, Dobson V, et al. Final visual acuity results in the Early Treatment for Retinopathy of Prematurity study. *Arch Ophthalmol.* 2010;128(6):663–671.

Lepore D, Quinn GE, Molle F, et al. Intravitreal bevacizumab versus laser treatment in type 1 retinopathy of prematurity: report on fluorescein angiographic findings. *Ophthalmology.* 2014;121(11):2212–2219.

Mintz-Hittner HA, Kennedy KA, Chuang AZ; BEAT-ROP Cooperative Group. Efficacy of intravitreal bevacizumab for stage 3+ retinopathy of prematurity. *N Engl J Med.* 2011;364(7):603–615.

Morin J, Luu TM, Superstein R, et al; Canadian Neonatal Network and the Canadian Neonatal Follow-Up Network Investigators. Neurodevelopmental outcomes following bevacizumab injections for retinopathy of prematurity. *Pediatrics.* 2016;137(4). pii: e20153218.

后遗症和并发症

无论是治疗的，还是自发退化的 ROP，最常见的后遗症是近视，甚至是高度近视。此外，ROP 的早产儿，特别是治疗的婴儿，患斜视和弱视的风险很高。另一个公认的风险是前房角狭窄所致的青光眼。

Various sequelae due to ROP involution may be noted in the retina and its vasculature, including latticelike degeneration, failure of peripheral vascularization, and tortuous vessels. Dragging of the macula can occur, giving rise to pseudoexotropia as a result of a large positive angle kappa (Figs 25-10, 25-11) (see Chapter 7 for a discussion of angle kappa). Eyes that have undergone treatment may also experience late retinal detachments at the border between treated and untreated retina. A child who has had ROP thus requires periodic ophthalmic examinations beyond the newborn period. Late changes associated with stage 5 ROP include cataract, glaucoma, and phthisis bulbi.

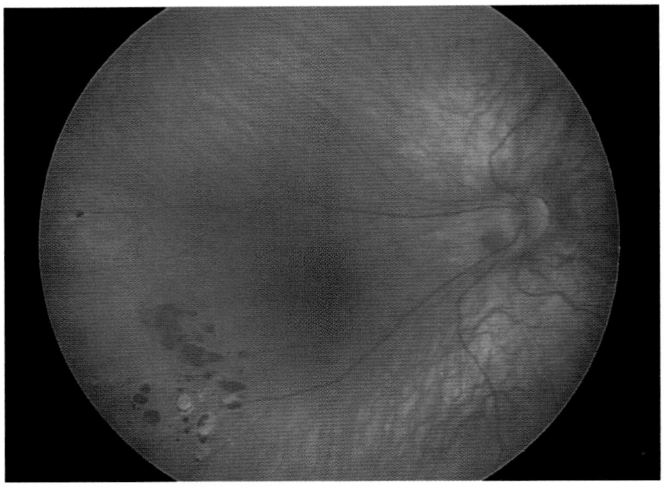

Figure 25-10 Posterior pole traction and dragging of the macula (right eye), a sequela of ROP. *(Courtesy of Robert W. Hered, MD.)*

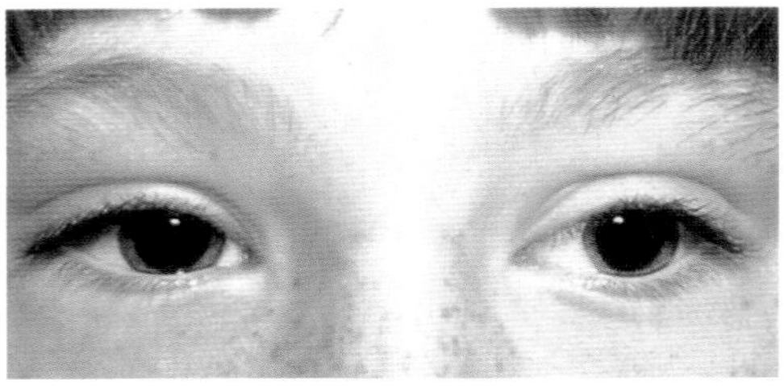

Figure 25-11 Pseudoexotropia in a fixating left eye in ROP. The patient has a positive angle kappa as a result of macular dragging.

When laser treatment, cryotherapy, or intravitreal bevacizumab monotherapy has not prevented the progression of ROP to stage 4 or 5 (retinal detachment), scleral buckling and vitrectomy may be indicated. Anatomical success varies depending on many factors, but visual acuity results have been disappointing, particularly with stage 5 eyes.

Unfortunately, even with the current guidelines for screening and treatment, approximately 400–600 babies become legally blind because of ROP each year in the United States. Poor ROP outcomes may be perceived as medical malpractice and therefore pose a risk for litigation by patients or their families. The Ophthalmic Mutual Insurance Company (www.omic.com) offers numerous tools to help ophthalmologists limit their liability risk.

Repka MX, Tung B, Good WV, Capone A Jr, Shapiro MJ. Outcome of eyes developing Retinal detachment during the Early Treatment for Retinopathy of Prematurity study. *Arch Ophthalmol.* 2011;129(9):1175–1179.

在视网膜及其血管系统中，可见到 ROP 退化引起的各种后遗症，包括格子变性、周边部血管未形成和血管扭曲。黄斑牵拉产生假性外斜视，系大角度的正 kappa 角所致（图 25-10，图 25-11）（关于 kappa 角的讨论详见第 7 章）。治疗眼可发生迟发性视网膜脱离，发生在治疗和未治疗的视网膜交界处。因此，ROP 儿童在出生后需要定期进行眼科检查。与 ROP 5 期相关的晚期病变包括白内障、青光眼和眼球萎缩。

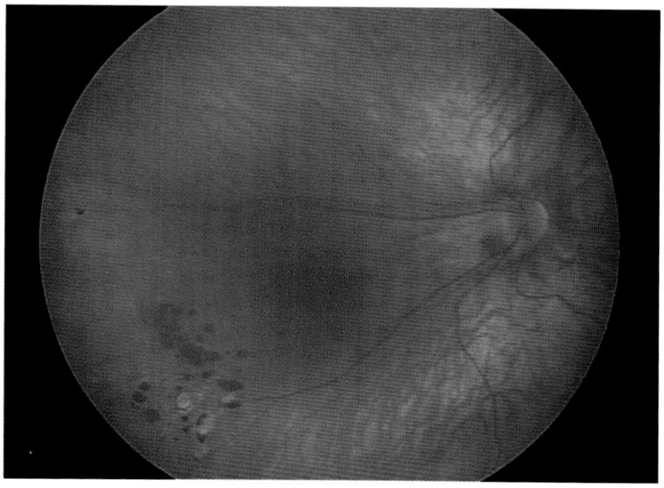

图 25-10　早产儿视网膜病变后遗症：后极部牵拉和黄斑牵拉（右眼）。*（译者注：资料来源见前页原文。）*

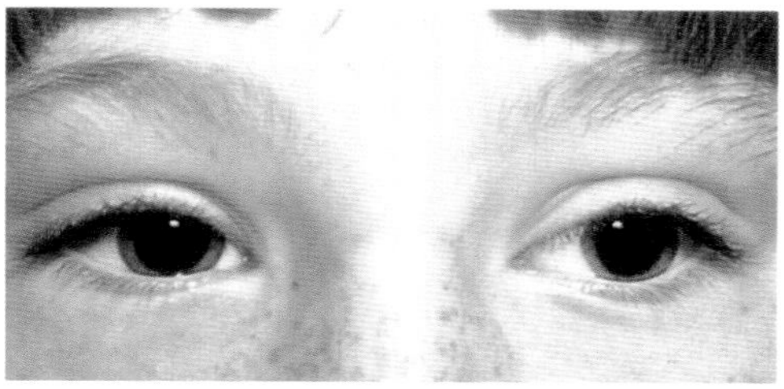

图 25-11　ROP 患者左眼假性外斜视。由于黄斑牵拉导致正 kappa 角。

当激光治疗、冷冻治疗或玻璃体腔内注射贝伐单抗都不能阻止早产儿视网膜病变（ROP）进展到 4 期或 5 期（视网膜脱离）时，可考虑巩膜环扎术和玻璃体切除术。解剖成功取决于许多因素，但视力预后较差，特别是 5 期患儿。

不幸的是，即便应用目前的筛查和治疗指南，美国每年仍有 400 ~ 600 名婴儿因早产儿视网膜病变而失明。不良的 ROP 预后可能会被视为医疗事故，因此有被患者或其家庭起诉的风险。眼科互助保险公司（www.omic.com）提供了多种方法，帮助眼科医生降低责任风险。

Repka MX, Tung B, Good WV, Capone A Jr, Shapiro MJ. Outcome of eyes developing Retinal detachment during the Early Treatment for Retinopathy of Prematurity study. *Arch Ophthalmol.* 2011;129(9):1175–1179.

Hereditary Retinal Disease

Nystagmus is the most common presenting sign of hereditary retinal disease. The onset of nystagmus typically occurs between 8 and 12 weeks of age and indicates limited visual potential if the cause is retinal disease (see Chapter 13). In infantile nystagmus caused by certain forms of Leber congenital amaurosis, achromatopsia, or X-linked congenital stationary night blindness, the retinal appearance can be normal.

Nystagmus does not develop in all patients with hereditary retinal disease; for example, it may not develop in those with less severe retinal damage. Poor visual function or failed vision screening may be the presenting abnormality in older children with retinal disease. The paradoxical pupillary response (pupils that initially constrict in the dark rather than dilate) is common in hereditary retinal dystrophies (Table 25-6).

Tests utilized to evaluate a patient with a possible hereditary retinal disorder include electroretinography (ERG), electro-oculography (EOG), and optical coherence tomography (OCT), as well as color vision, visual field, and dark adaptation tests. Sedation or general anesthesia may be required in order to perform ERG or OCT in young children. Because significant retinal maturation occurs during the first few years of life, an ERG can appear subnormal in a healthy infant. To obtain more reliable results, ERG is performed after 6–10 months of age. Repeated ERG testing may be necessary to confirm abnormalities of phototransduction.

Table 25-6 Differential Diagnosis of Paradoxical Pupils

Achromatopsia (complete, incomplete, or blue-cone monochromatism)
Albinism
Best disease
Congenital stationary night blindness
Leber congenital amaurosis
Optic nerve hypoplasia
Retinitis pigmentosa

Hereditary retinal diseases with onset late in childhood are much like those in adulthood and are not covered here. See BCSC Section 12, *Retina and Vitreous.*

Leber congenital amaurosis

Leber congenital amaurosis (LCA) is a group of hereditary (usually autosomal recessive) retinal dystrophies that affect both rod and cone photoreceptors. LCA is characterized by severe vision loss in infancy, nystagmus, poorly reactive pupils, and an extinguished ERG. Visual acuity typically ranges from 20/200 to bare light perception, but in some patients is not very low.

Ophthalmoscopic appearance varies greatly, depending on the genotype. It ranges from a normal appearance, particularly in infancy; to pigment clumping in the retinal pigment epithelium (RPE); to resemblance of classic retinitis pigmentosa, with bone spicules, attenuation of arterioles, and disc pallor. Other reported but less common fundus findings include extensive chorioretinal atrophy, macular coloboma, white dots (similar to those seen in retinitis punctata albescens), and marbleized retinal appearance (Fig 25-12). Histologic examination shows diffuse absence of photoreceptors.

Additional ocular manifestations include the oculodigital reflex (rubbing or poking the eye), photoaversion, cataracts, keratoconus, and keratoglobus. High refractive errors, usually high hyperopia, are common.

遗传性视网膜疾病

眼球震颤是遗传性视网膜疾病的最常见表现。眼球震颤常发生在出生后 8 ～ 12 周，如果是视网膜疾病所致，提示视觉发育受限（见第 13 章）。如果婴儿眼球震颤是由某一类型的 Leber 先天性黑矇、色盲或 X 连锁先天性静止性夜盲症引起的，视网膜外观可能正常。

并非所有遗传性视网膜疾病患儿都会出现眼球震颤，如视网膜病变较轻时，不会出现眼球震颤。大龄儿童有视力低下或无法进行视力筛查时，可有视网膜疾病的异常表现。矛盾性瞳孔反应（瞳孔在黑暗中最初表现为收缩而不是扩张）在遗传性视网膜营养不良中很常见（表 25–6）。

评估患者是否患有遗传性视网膜疾病的检查有视网膜电图（ERG）、眼电图（EOG）和光学相干断层扫描（OCT），以及色觉、视野和暗适应。幼儿进行视网膜电图 ERG 或光学相干断层扫描 OCT 检查时，需使用镇静剂或进行全身麻醉。因为在出生后几年内，视网膜逐步发育成熟，所以健康婴儿的视网膜电图 ERG 可能会出现异常。为了获得更可靠的结果，常在 6 ～ 10 个月龄后进行视网膜电图 ERG 检查。确定是否有光传导异常需重复检测视网膜电图（ERG）。

表25–6　矛盾性瞳孔反应的鉴别诊断

色盲（完全性、不完全性、蓝色色盲）
白化病
Best病
先天性静止性夜盲
Leber先天性黑矇
视神经发育不全
视网膜色素变性

大龄儿童迟发性遗传性视网膜疾病与成年人的表现相似，本节不赘述。见 BCSC 第 12 册《*视网膜与玻璃体*》。

Leber 先天性黑矇

Leber 先天性黑矇（LCA）是一组遗传性（多为常染色体隐性遗传）视网膜营养不良疾病，影响视锥和视杆细胞。Leber 先天性黑矇（LCA）的特点是婴儿期视力严重丧失、眼球震颤、瞳孔反射差和熄灭性视网膜电图 ERG。视力在微弱光感至 20/200 之间，但有的患儿视力并不差。

基因型不同，其眼底表现差别很大，眼底可正常（特别是婴儿期），也可表现为视网膜色素上皮层（RPE）色素沉着，类似于典型视网膜色素变性的骨针状色素沉着、视网膜小动脉血管狭窄和视盘苍白。有报告称，个别病例眼底表现呈广泛的脉络膜视网膜萎缩、黄斑缺损、视网膜白点（类似于白点状视网膜炎 / 病变）和大理石样的视网膜外观（图 25–12）。组织学检查显示视网膜光感受器弥漫性缺失。

其他眼部表现有眼手指反射（揉眼或按压眼球）、畏光、白内障、圆锥角膜和球形角膜。常见高度屈光不正，特别是高度远视。

LCA-like phenotypes can be found in a number of systemic diseases, including peroxisomal disorders (Zellweger [cerebrohepatorenal] syndrome, neonatal adrenoleukodystrophy, and infantile Refsum disease) and the ciliopathies (Alström syndrome, Joubert syndrome, Senior-Løken syndrome, and Bardet-Biedl syndrome). The ciliopathies are a group of genetic disorders in which the structure and/or function of the cilia is affected, manifesting in cerebral anomalies and renal and retinal disease. Retinal involvement is common because the junction between inner and outer segments of the photoreceptor cell is modified nonmotile cilium (see Chapter 28). Thus, ophthalmologists should be aware that an LCA-like phenotype may be the first sign of an undiagnosed systemic disease.

Diagnosis An ERG is typically used to diagnose LCA. However, in a child with an obvious phenotype (oculodigital reflex, severely decreased vision at birth, and pigmentary retinopathy), ERG is not always necessary. genetic testing is important and can be used to confirm the diagnosis, distinguish LCA from other retinal diseases, predict prognosis, and help with family planning. Molecular diagnosis of LCA is hindered by the fact that the disease is heterogeneous. At least 20 different genetic mutations are known to cause LCA; the most frequent involve *CEP290* (15%), *GUCY2D* (12%), and *CRB1* (10%), as well as *RPE65* (6%).

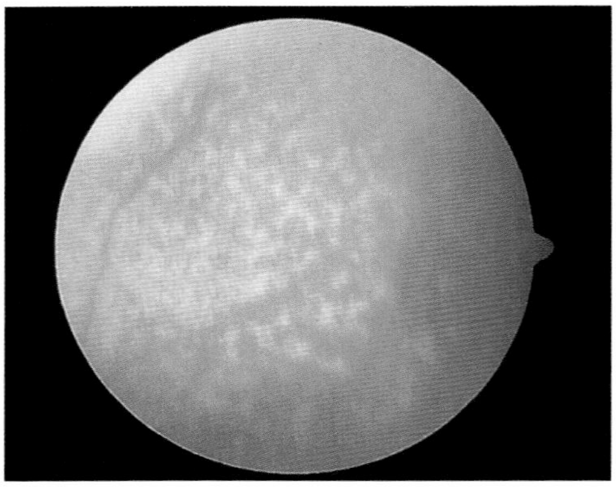

Figure 25-11 Leber congenital amaurosis with marbleized fundus.

Treatment Gene therapy is available for biallelic *RPE65* disease. Studies have demonstrated improvement in subjective and objective vision after subretinal injections of the gene promoter attached to an adenovirus viral particle, but it is unclear whether these results will be sustainable. Results seem most promising in young children.

Alkharashi M, Fulton AB. Available evidence on Leber congenital amaurosis and gene therapy. *Semin Ophthalmol.* 2017;32(1):14–21.

Weleber RG, Pennesi ME, Wilson DJ, et al. Results at 2 years after gene therapy for RPE65-deficient Leber congenital amaurosis and severe early-childhood-onset retinal dystrophy. *Ophthalmology.* 2016;123(7):1606–1620.

Achromatopsia

Complete achromatopsia, also known as *rod monochromatism*, is an autosomal recessive congenital disorder of the cone photoreceptors in which patients have no color vision, poor central vision, nystagmus, and photophobia. These patients see the world in shades of gray. Hemeralopia, the inability to see clearly in bright light, occurs in these patients.

许多全身性疾病中可见到类似 Leber 先天性黑矇（LCA）表型，如过氧化物酶病[Zellweger（脑肝肾）综合征、新生儿肾上腺脑白质营养不良和婴儿 Refsum 病]和纤毛病（Alström 综合征、Joubert 综合征、Senior - Løken 综合征和 Bardet–Biedl 综合征）。纤毛病是一组遗传性疾病，纤毛的结构和/或功能受到影响，表现为大脑异常和肾脏及视网膜疾病。纤毛病常累及视网膜，因为光感受器细胞内节和外节之间的连接处是修饰过的非运动性纤毛（见第 28 章），所以，眼科医师应认识到，类 Leber 先天性黑矇（LCA）表型眼部表现可能是全身性疾病确诊前的第一个征兆。

诊断　视网膜电图（ERG）常用于 Leber 先天性黑矇（LCA）的诊断。但对有典型表型的儿童（眼手指反射、出生时视力严重下降和色素性视网膜病变），不需进行视网膜电图（ERG）检测。基因检测很重要，可用于确诊此病、与其他视网膜疾病相鉴别、评估预后、帮助计划生育。而此病的异质性阻碍了 Leber 先天性黑矇（LCA）的分子学诊断。已知至少有 20 种不同的基因突变会导致 Leber 先天性黑矇（LCA），最常见的基因有 *CEP290*（15%）、*GUCY2D*（12%）和 *CRB1*（10%），以及 *RPE65*（6%）。

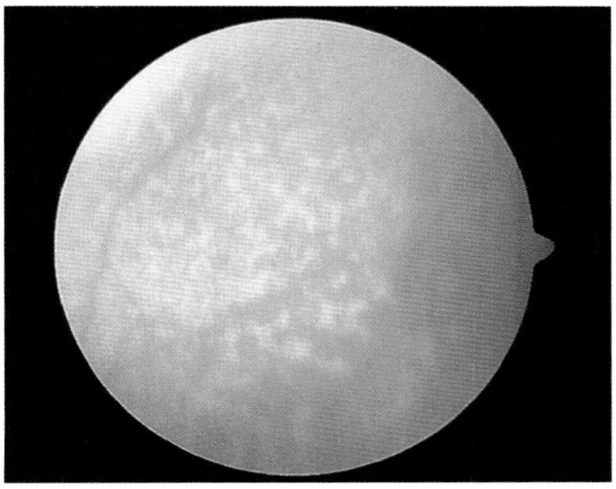

图 25–12　Leber 先天性黑矇，大理石样眼底。

治疗　基因疗法可用于等位基因 *RPE65* 病。研究表明，将与腺病毒颗粒相连的基因启动子注入视网膜下，患儿的主观视力和客观视力都有提高，但不清楚能持续多久。这一结果有望用于幼儿的治疗。

Alkharashi M, Fulton AB. Available evidence on Leber congenital amaurosis and gene therapy. *Semin Ophthalmol*. 2017;32(1):14–21.

Weleber RG, Pennesi ME, Wilson DJ, et al. Results at 2 years after gene therapy for RPE65-deficient Leber congenital amaurosis and severe early-childhood-onset retinal dystrophy. *Ophthalmology*. 2016;123(7):1606–1620.

全色盲

完全性色盲，又称*杆体全/单色盲*，是一种先天性锥体光感受器病，常染色体隐性遗传，患儿没有色觉、中心视力差、眼球震颤和畏光，看到的是灰色的世界。患儿有昼盲症，即在强光下看不清楚。

Findings on retinal examination are usually normal, with the possible exception of a poor or absent foveal reflex. Although achromatopsia was initially thought to be a stationary disorder, results of recent studies have shown deterioration of visual acuity, macular appearance, and cone function on ERG.

Diagnosis Results of color vision testing are markedly abnormal. The ERG is subnormal, showing extinguished cone or photopic responses but normal or nearly normal rod responses. Several recessive gene mutations have been identified as the cause of achromatopsia, including mutations in *CNGA3*, *CNGB3* (most common), *GNAT2*, *PDE6C*, and *PDE6H*.

Other cone dystrophies causing early-onset visual impairment and nystagmus include *incomplete achromatopsia*, which is an autosomal recessive condition, and *blue-cone monochromatism*, which is an X-linked disorder. In both disorders, patients usually have better vision than do those with complete achromatopsia. In incomplete achromatopsia,some residual cone function is observed on ERG testing. In blue-cone monochromatism, the blue (short-wavelength) cones show normal function on specialized ERG testing, but the photopic response is usually extinguished.

Treatment Glasses with dark lenses or red lenses that exclude short wavelengths may help. Gene therapy has been used in animal models.

Congenital stationary night blindness

Congenital stationary night blindness (CSNB) refers to a group of nonprogressive retinal disorders characterized predominantly by abnormal function of the rod system. The condition may be X-linked (the most common form), autosomal recessive, or autosomal dominant.

Children with CSNB, especially the autosomal recessive and X-linked forms, usually present in early infancy with nystagmus and a normal fundus appearance. These forms are often also associated with myopia and decreased visual acuity of roughly 20/200. However, the range of vision in these patients is wide, and occasionally, patients have normal vision. The retina usually appears normal, but the optic nerve may show myopic tilt and temporal pallor.

Diagnosis An ERG or genetic testing is necessary for diagnosis. The most common ERG pattern seen in CSNB is the "negative" dark-adapted ERG: a large a-wave and a reducedamplitude (negative) b-wave. Dark adaptation is abnormal in all patients with CSNB. Infants with CSNB may have a flat ERG until approximately 6 months of age, when it converts to the classic negative configuration.

Treatment Bright illumination should be used for visual tasks and refractive errors corrected.

Foveal hypoplasia

Foveal hypoplasia, or incomplete development of the fovea, is another cause of nystagmus in early infancy. Although this condition is most often associated with albinism or aniridia, it may also be isolated or familial and may be related to a defect in the *PAX6* gene. On ophthalmoscopic examination, the foveal reflex is poor or absent, and the macula exhibits hypoplasia to varying degrees, which can also be seen in patients with complete achromatopsia.

Al-Saleh AA, Hellani A, Abu-Amero KK. Isolated foveal hypoplasia: report of a new case and detailed genetic investigation. *Int Ophthalmol.* 2011;31(2):117–120.

Diagnosis Fundus examination showing foveal hypoplasia is diagnostic. OCT may be useful.

视网膜检查正常，仅中心凹反光较弱或消失。全色盲最初被视为静止性疾病，但近期的研究结果提示，视力、黄斑外观以及视网膜电图（ERG）锥体功能均呈现恶化。

诊断　色觉检查有明显异常。视网膜电图（ERG）低于正常，呈锥体/视锥反应或明反应熄灭，而杆体/视杆反应正常或接近正常。几种隐性基因突变可引起全色盲，包括*CNGA3*、*CNGB3*（最常见）、*GNAT2*、*PDE6C* 和 *PDE6H*。

导致早期出现视力损害和眼球震颤的其他锥体营养不良，包括*不完全性全色盲*（常染色体隐性）和*蓝锥体单色盲*（X 连锁遗传），患者的视力比完全性全色盲好。不完全性全色盲患者的视网膜电图（ERG）检测，尚残存部分视锥功能。蓝锥体单色盲中，特殊 ERG 检测时，蓝锥体（短波长）功能正常，但明反应熄灭。

治疗　滤除短波长的深色镜片或红色镜片对治疗有帮助。基因疗法已用于动物模型。

先天性静止型夜盲

先天性静止型夜盲（CSNB）是一组以杆体细胞功能异常为主要特征的非进行性视网膜病。遗传方式有 X- 连锁遗传（最常见）、常染色体隐性遗传或常染色体显性遗传。

先天性静止型夜盲（CSNB），特别是常染色体隐性遗传和 X- 连锁遗传，常在婴儿早期出现眼球震颤，而眼底正常。此类型常伴近视和视力低下（约 20/200）。但患者的视力变化较大，偶有视力正常。视网膜外观正常，视盘呈近视性倾斜和颞侧视盘苍白。

诊断　视网膜电图（ERG）或基因检测是诊断必需的。视网膜电图（ERG）表现为“负性”的暗适应 ERG：一个大的 a 波和低振幅（负波性）b 波。所有先天性静止型夜盲（CSNB）的暗适应异常。先天性静止型夜盲（CSNB）婴儿在 6 个月龄前 ERG 平坦，之后转变为典型的负波。

治疗　用眼时应给以明亮照明，并矫正屈光不正。

黄斑中心凹发育不全

黄斑中心凹发育不全，或者说黄斑中心凹不完全发育，是婴儿早期眼球震颤的另一个原因。尽管此病伴白化病或无虹膜，但可能是散发/孤立的或家族性的，与 *PAX6* 基因缺陷有关。眼底镜检查可见，黄斑中心凹反光差或消失，黄斑区表现为不同程度的发育不全，也见于完全性全色盲。

Al-Saleh AA, Hellani A, Abu-Amero KK. Isolated foveal hypoplasia: report of a new case and detailed genetic investigation. *Int Ophthalmol*. 2011;31(2):117–120.

诊断　眼底镜检查显示黄斑中心凹发育不全即可诊断。OCT 可帮助诊断。

Treatment No treatment is currently available.

Aicardi syndrome

Aicardi syndrome is a presumed X-linked autosomal dominant disorder characterized by the clinical triad of widespread round or oval depigmented chorioretinal lacunae (Fig 25-13), infantile spasms, and agenesis of the corpus callosum. Chorioretinal lacunae have been shown to occur in 88% of patients; optic nerve abnormalities, in 81%. Colobomas,Persistent pupillary membranes, and microphthalmia may also occur. Aicardi syndrome is typically lethal in males.

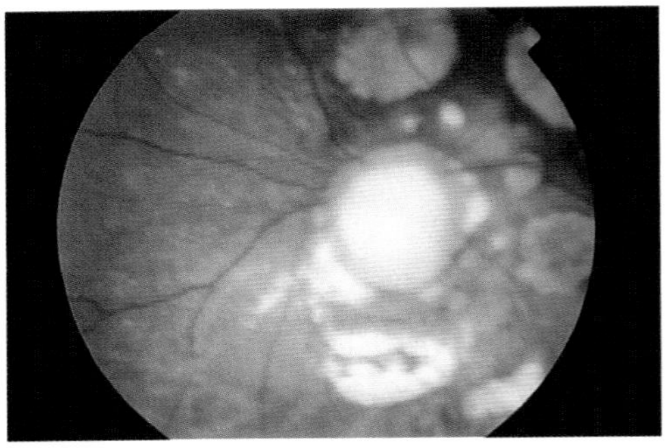

Figure 25-13 Aicardi syndrome. Fundus photograph showing optic disc coloboma and chorioretinal lacunae.

Fruhman G, Eble TN, Gambhir N, Sutton VR, Van den Veyver IB, Lewis RA. Ophthalmologic findings in Aicardi syndrome. *J AAPOS.* 2012;16(3):238–241.

Diagnosis The clinical picture provides the foundation for diagnosis.

Treatment No treatment is currently available.

Hereditary Macular Dystrophies

Macular abnormalities are seen in a number of hereditary disorders. The abnormality can be associated with a hereditary systemic disease (eg, the cherry-red spot in GM_2 gangliosidosis type I) or can reflect a primary retinal disorder, such as Stargardt disease or Best disease. Only primary retinal disorders are discussed here.

Stargardt disease

Stargardt disease (juvenile macular degeneration) is the most common hereditary macular dystrophy. Inheritance is usually autosomal recessive; in rare cases, it is autosomal dominant. Most cases are caused by mutations in the retina-specific adenosine triphosphate–binding transporter gene *(ABCA4)*. Children with Stargardt disease usually present between ages 8 and 15 years with a decrease in vision, photophobia, or color vision abnormalities. The condition is bilateral, symmetric, and progressive; visual acuity levels off at approximately 20/50–20/200.

治疗　目前尚无有效治疗方法。

Aicardi 综合征

Aicardi 综合征是一种 X- 连锁和常染色体显性遗传疾病，临床三联征有广泛的圆形或椭圆形色素脱失性脉络膜视网膜腔（图 25-13）、婴儿痉挛症和胼胝体发育不全。88% 出现脉络膜视网膜腔，81% 出现视神经异常，也可能出现脉络膜视网膜缺损、永久性瞳孔残膜和小眼球。男性 Aicardi 综合征常是致命的。

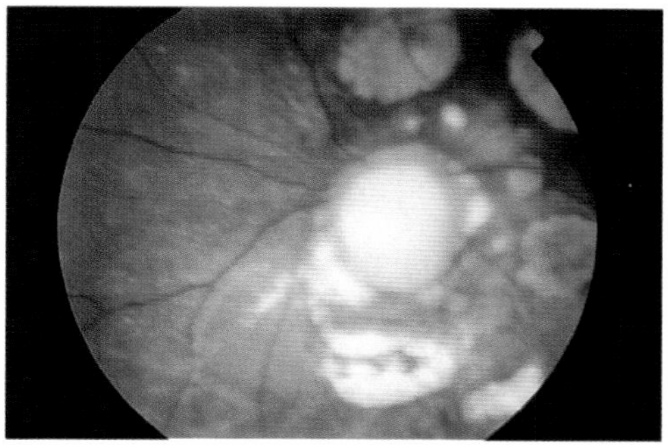

图 25-13　Aicardi 综合征。眼底照片显示视盘缺损和脉络膜视网膜腔。

Fruhman G, Eble TN, Gambhir N, Sutton VR, Van den Veyver IB, Lewis RA. Ophthalmologic findings in Aicardi syndrome. *J AAPOS*. 2012;16(3):238–241.

诊断　临床图像是诊断的基础。

治疗　目前没有治疗手段。

遗传性黄斑营养不良

黄斑异常见于许多遗传性疾病，与全身遗传性疾病（如 GM2 导致的 I 型神经节病出现黄斑区的“樱桃红”样点）有关，也可为原发性视网膜疾病，如 Stargardt 病或 Best 病。本节只讨论原发性视网膜疾病。

Stargardt 病

Stargardt 病（青少年黄斑变性）是最常见的遗传性黄斑营养不良，多为常染色体隐性遗传，偶尔是常染色体显性遗传。大多数是视网膜特异性三磷酸腺苷结合转运体基因（*ABCA4*）突变引起的。Stargardt 病的年龄在 8 ~ 15 岁，表现为视力下降、畏光或色觉异常，常呈双眼对称性进行性，视力下降至 20/50 ~ 20/200。

Diagnosis The disease often progresses through stages. Initially, the fundus appears normal even when vision is decreased, and the condition may be misdiagnosed as functional vision loss. The first ophthalmoscopic changes observed are loss of foveal reflex, followed by development of a characteristic macular bull's-eye atrophy surrounded by round or pisciform yellowish flecks, which develop in the posterior pole at the level of the RPE. If the flecks are scattered throughout the fundus, the condition may be referred to as *fundus flavimaculatus*. Before the flecks develop, the macula often appears atrophic due to diseased RPE, inducing a peculiar light-reflecting quality resembling that of beaten bronze (Figs 25-14, 25-15).

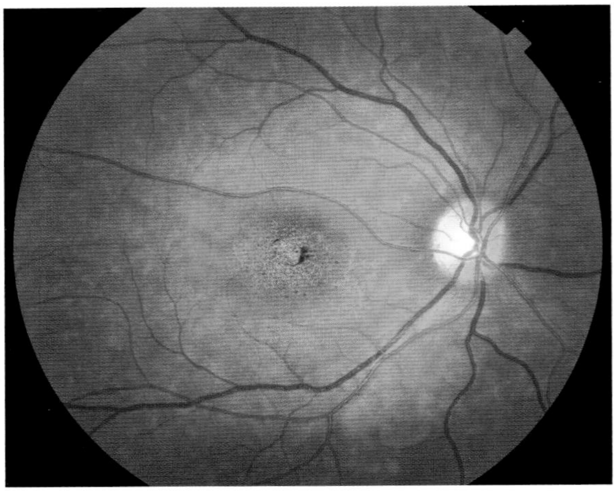

Figure 25-14 Stargardt disease. Macular atrophy, pisciform yellow-white flecks, and a beatenbronze appearance. Note the peripapillary sparing of retina. *(Courtesy of Marc T. Mathias, MD.)*

The "dark choroid" sign on fluorescein angiography is distinctive but is not present in all patients. This phenomenon is due to the accumulation of lipofuscin within the RPE, which blocks the choroidal fluorescence. Fluorescein angiography has been largely replaced by fundus autofluorescence (FAF) testing for the confirmation of Stargardt disease. FAF reveals both increased autofluorescence due to lipofuscin accumulation in the RPE and reduced autofluorescence in areas of RPE atrophy and photoreceptor loss (see Fig 25-15C, D). OCT imaging of the macula can reveal lipofuscin accumulation in the RPE and photoreceptor loss.

Results of visual field testing may be normal in the early stages of the disease. Disease progression will result in a central scotoma.

ERG results are often normal in the early stages of Stargardt disease. Stargardt disease can be associated with a progressive cone–rod dystrophy that has a much worse visual prognosis and an extinguished ERG.

Detection of *ABCA4* mutations viagenetic testing may be diagnostic.

诊断　此病的发展呈阶段性。初期，即便视力下降，眼底表现正常，此期可能被误诊为功能性视力丧失。第一个眼底变化是黄斑中心凹反光消失，随后呈特征性“牛眼”状萎缩改变，环绕圆形或豌豆状形的微黄色斑点，位于后极部的 RPE 层。如果斑点散在整个眼底，则被称为*眼底黄色斑点症*。在斑点形成之前，由于 RPE 病变，黄斑区萎缩，故呈现特有的金箔样反光，如同被捶打过的青铜片样外观（图 25–14，图 25–15）。

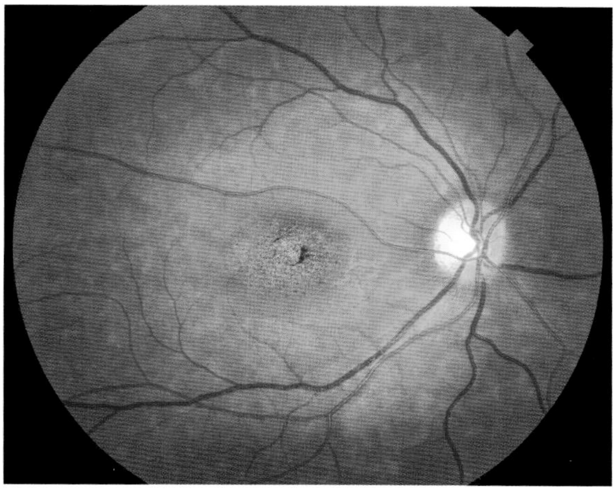

图 25–14　Stargardt 病。黄斑萎缩，豌豆状黄白色斑点，青铜片样外观。注意视乳头周围的视网膜赦免。*（译者注：资料来源见前页原文。）*

眼底荧光血管造影“脉络膜湮灭”征是特征性的，但并非所有患者都有，是视网膜色素上皮（RPE）细胞内脂褐质沉积，遮挡了脉络膜荧光。眼底自发荧光（FAF）检查可以诊断 Stargardt 病，基本取代了眼底荧光血管造影检查。眼底自发荧光（FAF）检查可发现视网膜色素上皮（RPE）中脂褐质积累导致的自发荧光增强，以及局部视网膜色素上皮 RPE 萎缩和光感受器丧失导致的自发荧光减弱（见图 25–15C, D）。黄斑的光学相干断层扫描 OCT 成像可见 RPE 中脂褐质积累和光感受器缺损。

视野检查在早期可正常，随着病情的发展，可出现中心暗点。

视网膜电图（ERG）在 Stargardt 病早期是正常的。Stargardt 病可伴有进行性视锥视杆 / 锥体杆体细胞营养不良，后者视觉预后更差，以熄灭性视网膜电图（ERG）为特征。

基因检测 *ABCA4* 基因突变可诊断。

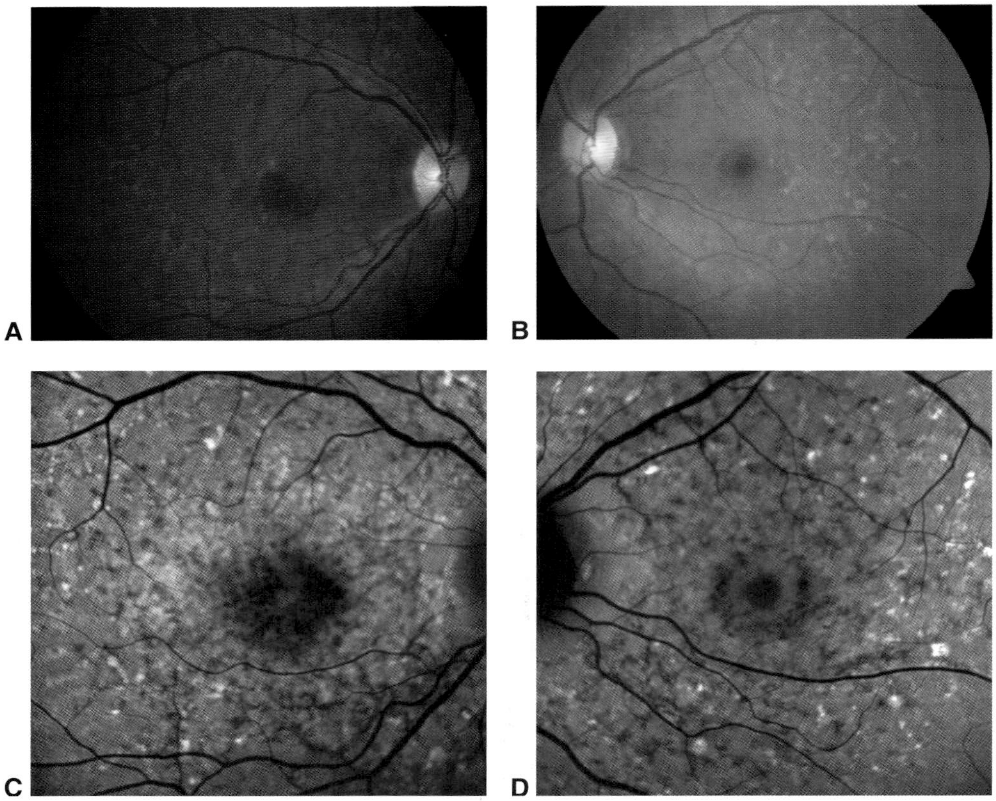

Figure 25-15 Fundus photographs from a patient with Stargardt disease. The right eye **(A)** and left eye **(B)** demonstrate classic pisciform yellow-white flecks throughout the macula, with mottling of the central retinal pigment epithelium (RPE). Corresponding right **(C)** and left **(D)** fundus autofluorescence (FAF) images reveal mottled hypo-and hyperautofluorescence with hyperautofluorescent flecks (corresponding to the pisciform flecks) and a bull's-eye maculopathy, greater in the left eye than in the right eye. *(Courtesy of Marc T. Mathias, MD.)*

Treatment Gene therapy for Stargardt disease has been used in animal models and is being studied in phase 1/2a clinical trials in humans.

Han Z, Conley SM, Naash MI. Gene therapy for Stargardt disease associated with *ABCA4* gene. *Adv Exp Med Biol.* 2014;801:719–724.

Best disease

Classic Best disease, or *juvenile-onset vitelliform macular dystrophy (VMD)*, is an autosomal dominant retinal disorder with variable penetrance and expressivity. The condition is caused by mutations in the *BEST1* gene on chromosome 11, which encodes for the protein bestrophin. Patients usually present asymptomatically in childhood with the classic retinal appearance, or later in life with decrease in vision.

Over the last decade, a rare, distinct phenotype—*autosomal dominant vitreoretinochoroidopathy (ADVIRC)*—has been recognized. ADVIRC results from exon-skipping mutation in BEST1. A separate, distinct phenotype caused by biallelic null mutations in *BEST1* also exists. The various phenotypes caused by heterozygous or biallelic mutations of *BEST1* are collectively termed *bestrophinopathies*.

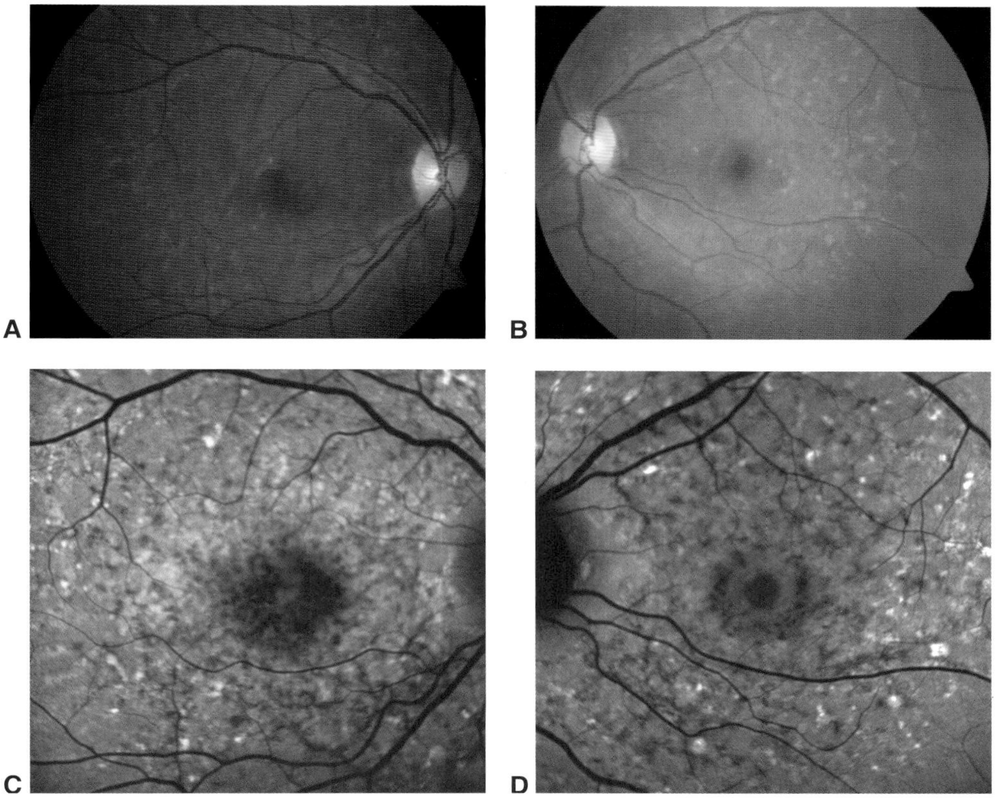

图 25-15　Stargardt 病眼底照片。右眼（**A**）和左眼（**B**）可见黄斑区典型的豌豆状黄白色斑点，中央视网膜色素上皮（RPE）斑驳样。相应的右眼（**C**）和左眼（**D**）眼底自发荧光（FAF）图像显示了斑驳的低自发荧光和高自发荧光，具有高自发荧光斑点（对应于豌豆状斑点）和“牛眼状”黄斑病变，左眼比右眼大。*（译者注：资料来源见前页原文。）*

治疗　Stargardt 病的基因疗法已经在动物模型中进行，并正在进行人的 1/2a 阶段的临床试验。

Han Z, Conley SM, Naash MI. Gene therapy for Stargardt disease associated with *ABCA4* gene. *Adv Exp Med Biol*. 2014;801:719–724.

Best 病

典型的 Best 病，或*青少年/少年发病的卵黄状黄斑营养不良*（VMD），是一种常染色体显性遗传性视网膜疾病，具有多变的外显率和表达性。其 11 号染色体的 *BEST1* 基因突变，进行 Bestrophin 蛋白编码。常在儿童时期出现典型的卵黄状视网膜外观，但无临床症状，随后视力逐步下降。

近 10 年发现一种罕见独特的表型——*常染色体显性玻璃体视网膜-脉络膜病*（ADVIRC），是 *BEST1* 基因外显子跳跃突变。*BEST1* 中的等位基因无效/无义突变则引起另一种不同的/分离的独特的表型。由 *BEST1* 杂合子或等位基因突变引起的各种表型统称为 *bestrophin 病变*。

Pasquay C, Wang LF, Lorenz B, Preising MN. Bestrophin 1—phenotypes and functional aspects in bestrophinopathies. *Ophthalmic Genet.* 2015;36(3):193–212.

Diagnosis The retina may appear normal at first, but between 4 and 10 years of age, the "egg yolk," or vitelliform, stage begins (Fig 25-16). A yellow-orange cystlike structure is seen, usually in the macula; however, the lesion may occur elsewhere, and occasionally there are multiple lesions. The lesions are usually 1.5–5.0 disc diameters in size. The egg yolk–like appearance is associated with good central vision.

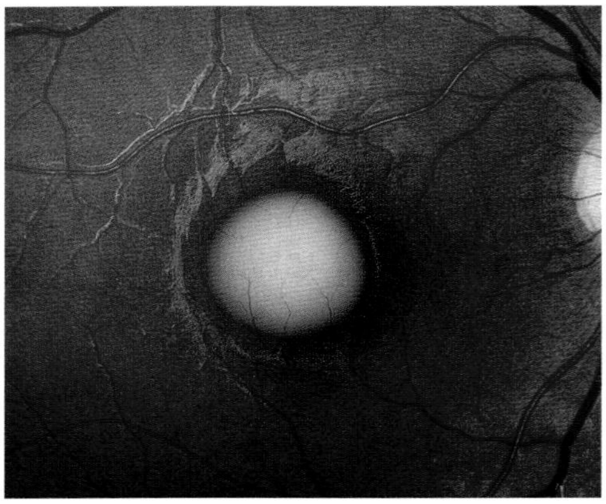

Figure 25-16 Best disease, "egg yolk" stage. *(Courtesy of Joseph Morales, CRA, COA. Cover image for Ophthalmology Retina [Sept/Oct 2017 issue].)*

With time, the cystic material may become granular, giving rise to the "scrambled egg" stage. At this stage, central vision usually remains good, with visual acuity roughly 20/30. The cyst may rupture and become partially resorbed; a pseudohypopyon may form from cystic contents. *Choroidal neovascular membranes (CNVMs)* and *pigment epithelial detachments (PEDs)* develop in 20% of patients (Fig 25-17A). Subretinal hemorrhage may occur, and visual acuity may deteriorate to 20/100 or worse. FAF reveals central macular hyperautofluorescence due to vitelliform material (Fig 25-17B). Fluorescein angiography reveals central macular hyperfluorescence due to staining of the vitelliform material as well as late leakage from a CNVM, if present (Fig 25-17C, D). Spectral-domain OCT (SD-OCT) imaging can further illustrate the central macular abnormalities (Fig 25-17E, F).

The EOG is usually abnormal in affected patients and carriers. This disorder is one of the few in which the EOG is abnormal and the ERG is normal. *BEST1* gene mutations are found in 60%–83% of affected patients. Carriers can be identified by the presence of an abnormal EOG with a normal retina or a *BEST1* gene mutation.

Meunier I, Sénéchal A, Dhaenens CM, et al. Systematic screening for *BEST1* and *PRPH2* in juvenile and adult vitelliform macular dystrophies: a rationale for molecular analysis. *Ophthalmology.* 2011;118(6):1130–1136.

Treatment No treatment is indicated unless subretinal neovascularization occurs.

Hereditary Vitreoretinopathies

Hereditary vitreoretinopathies include a broad range of disease entities. The ones discussed here characteristically present in childhood.

Pasquay C, Wang LF, Lorenz B, Preising MN. Bestrophin 1—phenotypes and functional aspects in bestrophinopathies. *Ophthalmic Genet*. 2015;36(3):193–212.

诊断　早期视网膜正常，4 ~ 10 岁开始出现“卵黄”，或卵黄形成阶段（图 25–16），黄斑处可见黄橙色的囊样结构，病变可能发生在其他部位，也有多处病变。病变大小为 1.5 ~ 5.0 视盘直径。卵黄样外观可伴有良好的中心视力。

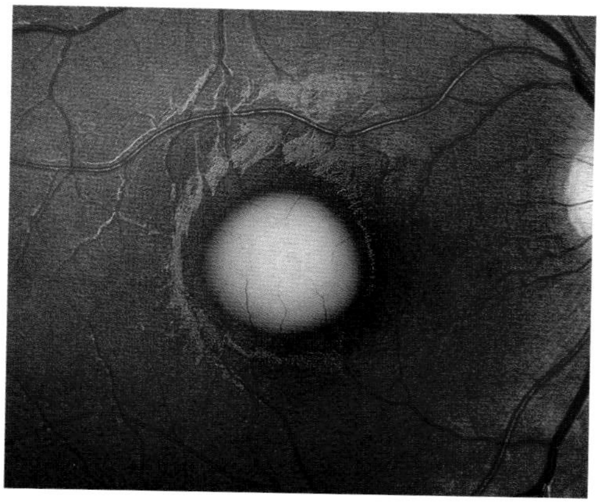

图 25–16　Best 病，“卵黄”阶段。*（译者注：资料来源见前页原文。）*

随着时间的推移，囊的物质可能变成颗粒状，从而进入“炒鸡蛋”阶段。这个阶段的中心视力保持良好，约为 20/30。囊破裂并部分吸收，囊内物质可形成假性积脓。20% 的患者出现*脉络膜新生血管膜（CNVMs）*和*色素上皮分离（PEDS）*（图 25–17A）。患者可能会出现视网膜下出血，视力下降至 20/100 或更差。眼底自发荧光 FAF 可见卵黄状物质引起的黄斑中央区高自发荧光（图 25–17B）。荧光血管造影显示卵黄状物质染色导致黄斑中央区高荧光，以及存在的脉络膜新生血管膜 CNVM 导致的晚期渗漏（图 25–17C，D）。谱域光学相干断层扫描（SD–OCT）可帮助进一步了解黄斑中央区异常（图 25–17E，F）。

患者和携带者的眼电图（EOG）常是异常的，是几种眼电图（EOG）异常而视网膜电图（ERG）正常的疾病之一。60% ~ 83% 的患者有 *BEST1* 基因突变。可通过携带者视网膜表现正常、眼电图（EOG）异常或存在 *BEST1* 基因突变进行诊断。

Meunier I, Sénéchal A, Dhaenens CM, et al. Systematic screening for *BEST1* and *PRPH2* in juvenile and adult vitelliform macular dystrophies: a rationale for molecular analysis. *Ophthalmology*. 2011;118(6):1130–1136.

治疗　未发生视网膜下新生血管，不需要治疗。

遗传性玻璃体视网膜病变

遗传性玻璃体视网膜病变包括多种疾病。本节讨论存在于儿童期的病变。

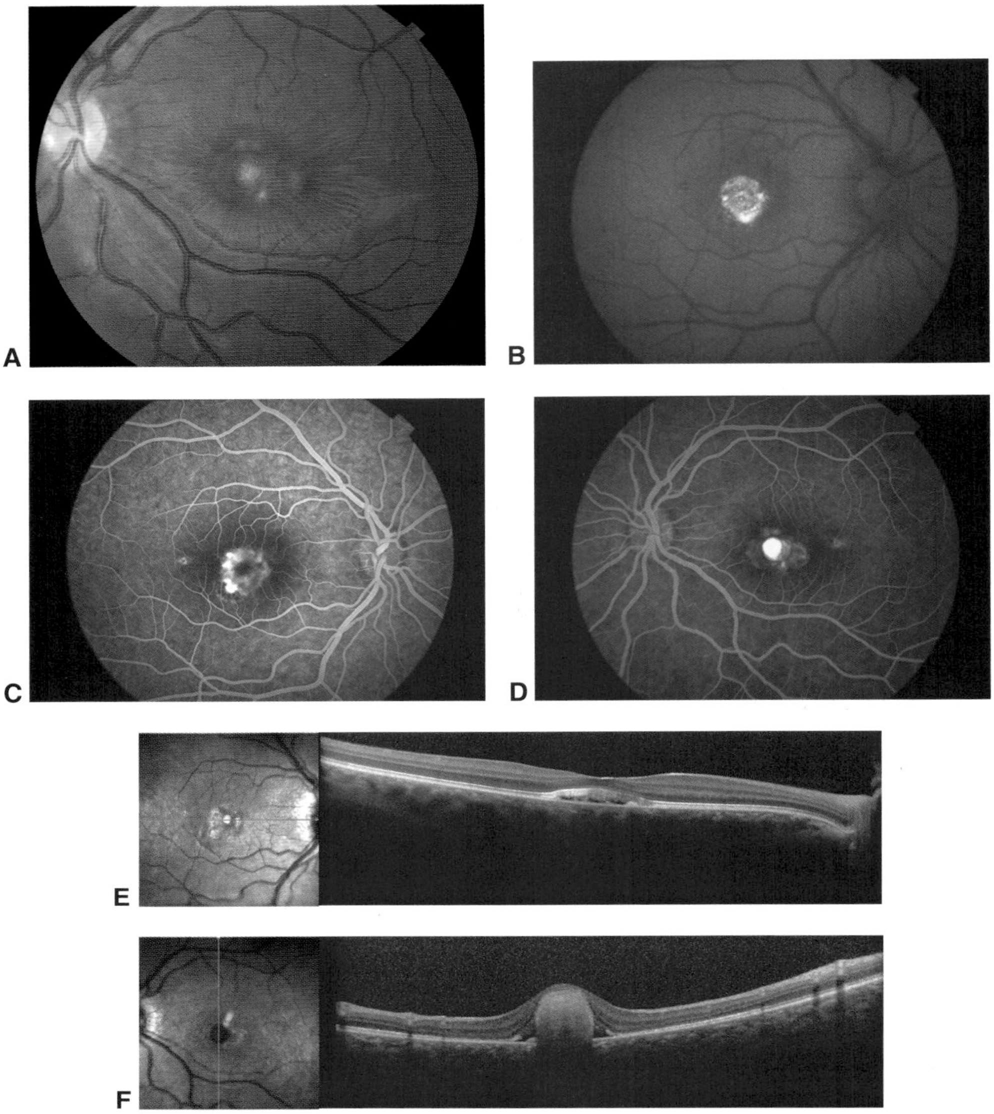

Figure 25-17 Best disease. **A,** Left eye with vitelliform lesion and central dome-shaped choroidal neovascular membrane (CNVM). **B,** Right eye with central macular hyperautofluorescence due to vitelliform material, as seen on FAF imaging. **C,** Fluorescein angiography image (right eye) reveals central macular hyperfluorescence due to staining of vitelliform material. **D,** Fluorescein angiography image (left eye) shows late central hyperfluorescence from leakage of CNVM. **E,** Spectral-domain OCT (SD-OCT) image (right eye) reveals subretinal hyperreflective material with a hyporeflective cleft corresponding to the vitelliform lesion. **F,** SD-OCT image (left eye) reveals a large subfoveal pigment epithelial detachment with subretinal hyperreflective material and subretinal fluid. *(Courtesy of Marc T. Mathias, MD.)*

Juvenile retinoschisis

Juvenile retinoschisis (splitting of the retina) is an X-linked disease caused by mutations in the *RS1* gene, which encodes for the retinal protein retinoschisin, an adhesion protein that is believed to be essential to the health of Müller cells. Affected males usually present in early childhood with decreased vision. Visual acuity varies but usually deteriorates to roughly 20/200.

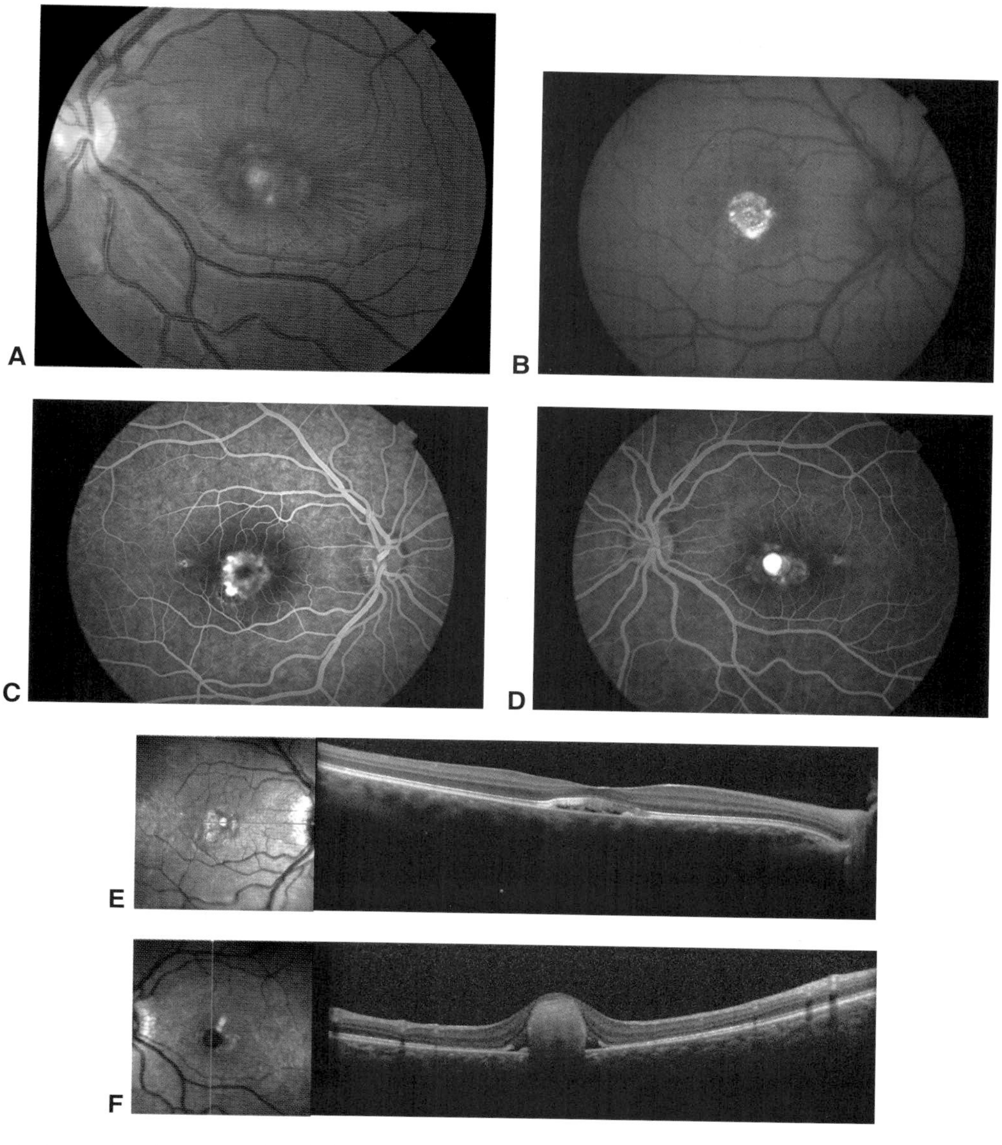

图 25-17　Best 病。**A.** 左眼卵黄状病变，中央圆形脉络膜新生血管膜（CNVM）。**B.** 自发荧光 FAF 显示，右眼卵黄状物质引起黄斑中央高自发荧光。**C.** 荧光血管造影（右眼）显示，卵黄状物质着色导致的黄斑中央区高荧光。**D.** 荧光血管造影（左眼）显示，脉络膜新生血管膜 CNVM 渗漏可导致晚期中央区高荧光。**E.** 谱域光学相干断层扫描（SD-OCT）（右眼）显示，视网膜下高反射物质，低反射裂隙相对应于卵黄样病变。**F.** 谱域光学相干断层扫描 SD-OCT（左眼）显示，较大中心凹下视网膜色素上皮脱离，视网膜下高反射物质和视网膜下液。*（译者注：资料来源见前页原文。）*

青少年视网膜劈裂

青少年视网膜劈裂（视网膜层间的分离）是一种 X- 连锁 /X- 连锁遗传病，其 *RS1* 基因突变，该基因编码视网膜蛋白 retinoschisin，是一种维持正常视网膜 Müller 细胞所需的黏附蛋白。受累男性常在儿童早期视力下降，严重程度不同，但常下降至 20/200。

Diagnosis Foveal retinoschisis is present in almost all cases; peripheral retinoschisis, in approximately 50% of patients. The fovea has a stellate or spokelike configuration that may resemble cystoid macular edema; it becomes less distinct over time. SD-OCT shows schisis spaces in the middle layers of the macula (Fig 25-18A). Vitreous veils or strands are common, and vitreal syneresis, or liquefaction, is prominent. Complications include vitreous hemorrhage and various types of retinal detachment (Figs 25-18B, 25-19). The ERG shows a reduction of the scotopic b-wave with preservation of the a-wave.

Treatment Contact sports should be avoided because the retina in affected eyes is more susceptible to trauma. Gene replacement has shown some success in mouse models. Use of carbonic anhydrase inhibitors to treat cystic macular lesions is under investigation.

Verbakel SK, van de Ven JP, Le Blanc LM, et al. Carbonic anhydrase inhibitors for the treatment of cystic macular lesions in children with X-linked juvenile retinoschisis. *Invest Ophthalmol Vis Sci.* 2016;57(13):5143–5147.

A

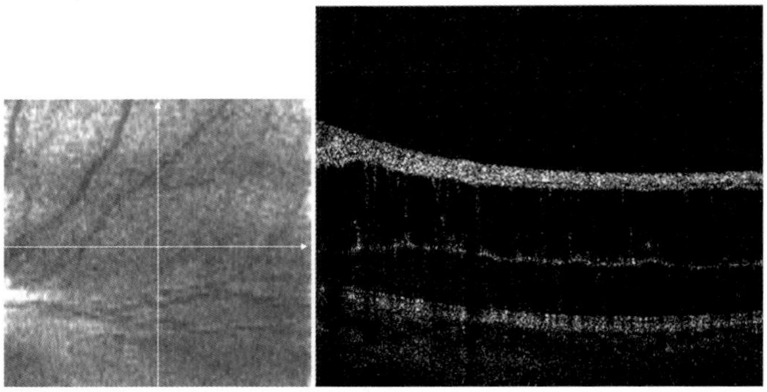

B

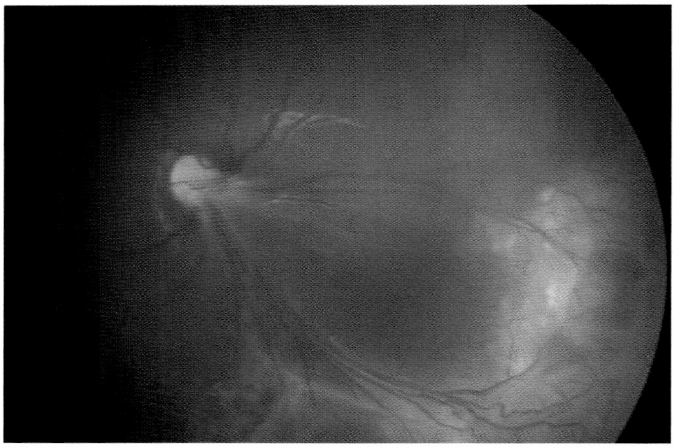

Figure 25-18 Juvenile retinoschisis. **A,** SD-OCT image shows schisis of retina. **B,** Combined tractional and rhegmatogenous retinal detachment. (*Courtesy of Scott C. Oliver, MD.*)

诊断 多存在黄斑中心凹处视网膜劈裂，50% 有周边的视网膜劈裂。黄斑中央凹呈放射状或轮辐状改变，类似黄斑囊样水肿。随着病程进展，这些改变不明显。谱域光学相干断层扫描 SD-OCT 显示黄斑中间层劈裂（图 25-18A）。常见玻璃体纱膜或条索，玻璃体脱水收缩或液化明显。并发症包括玻璃体积血和各类型的视网膜脱离（图 25-18B，图 25-19）。视网膜电图 ERG 表现为暗适应 b 波振幅明显下降，a 波振幅正常。

治疗 视网膜劈裂的视网膜易受外伤损伤，要尽量避免创击性运动。基因替换成功用于小鼠模型。碳酸酐酶抑制剂治疗黄斑囊样病变正在研究中。

Verbakel SK, van de Ven JP, Le Blanc LM, et al. Carbonic anhydrase inhibitors for the treatment of cystic macular lesions in children with X-linked juvenile retinoschisis. *Invest Ophthalmol Vis Sci.* 2016;57(13):5143–5147.

A

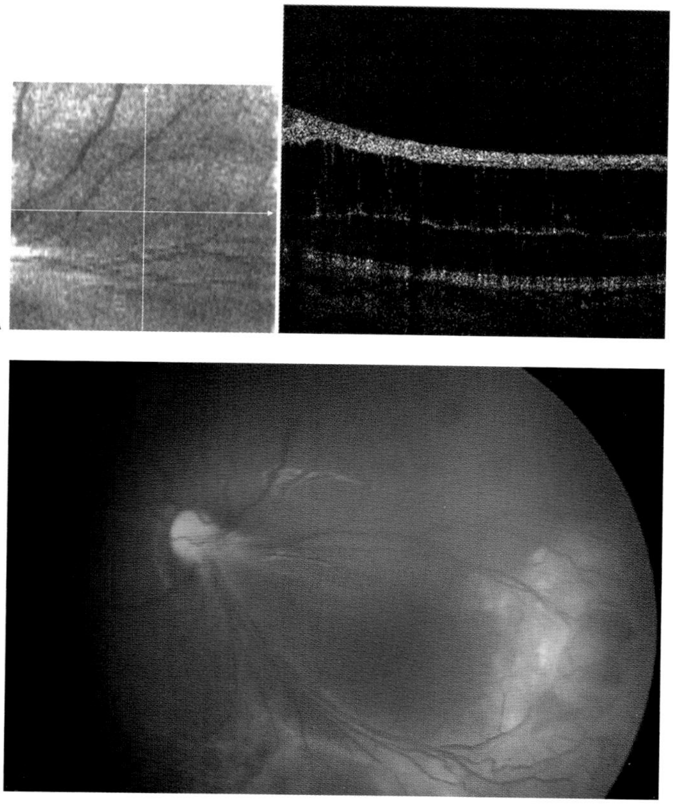

B

图 25-18 青少年视网膜劈裂。**A.** 谱域光学相干断层扫描 SD-OCT 显示视网膜劈裂。**B.** 牵拉性视网膜脱离合并孔源性视网膜脱离。*（译者注：资料来源见前页原文。）*

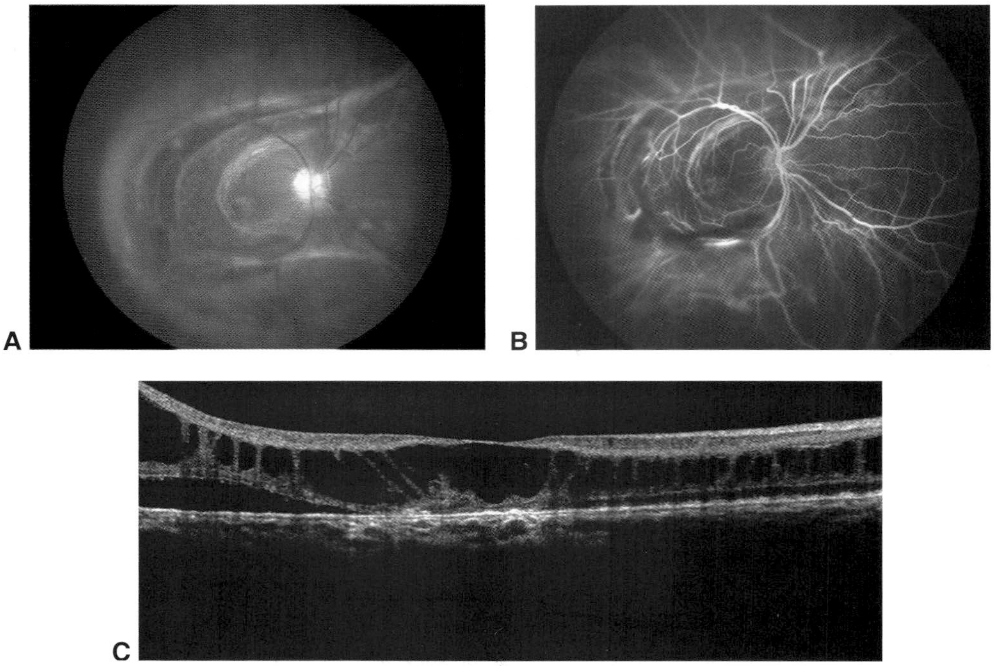

Figure 25-19 Three-year-old with juvenile retinoschisis. **A,** Central and extensive peripheral retinoschisis with mild vitreous and preretinal hemorrhage. There is a large circumferential tractional retinal detachment around the arcades, encroaching on the central macula. A retinal hole is also present. **B,** Fluorescein angiography reveals an extensive tractional detachment. **C,** Macular OCT image demonstrates retinoschisis with a tractional detachment and subretinal fluid encroaching on the fovea. *(Courtesy of Marc T. Mathias, MD.)*

Stickler syndrome

Stickler syndrome is a group of connective tissue disorders with variable phenotypic expression. The most common type of Stickler syndrome is autosomal dominant, has ocular and systemic findings, and is caused by a mutation in *COL2A1*, the gene that encodes for type II procollagen. Some mutations in the gene cause an ocular-only phenotype.

Diagnosis The diagnosis is made based on the clinical features as well as the results of genetic testing. Common ocular abnormalities include an optically empty vitreous due to vitreous liquefaction, high myopia, lattice degeneration, and proliferative vitreoretinopathy. In addition, there is a high incidence of retinal detachment secondary to retinal breaks. Anterior chamber angle anomalies, ectopia lentis, cataracts, ptosis, and strabismus are less common.

Characteristic systemic abnormalities are a flat midface, progressive hearing loss, cleft palate, Pierre Robin sequence, mitral valve prolapse, and progressive arthropathy with spondyloepiphyseal dysplasia. Although the arthropathy may not be symptomatic initially, children with Stickler syndrome often show radiographic abnormalities of the long bones and joints, and associated symptoms develop.

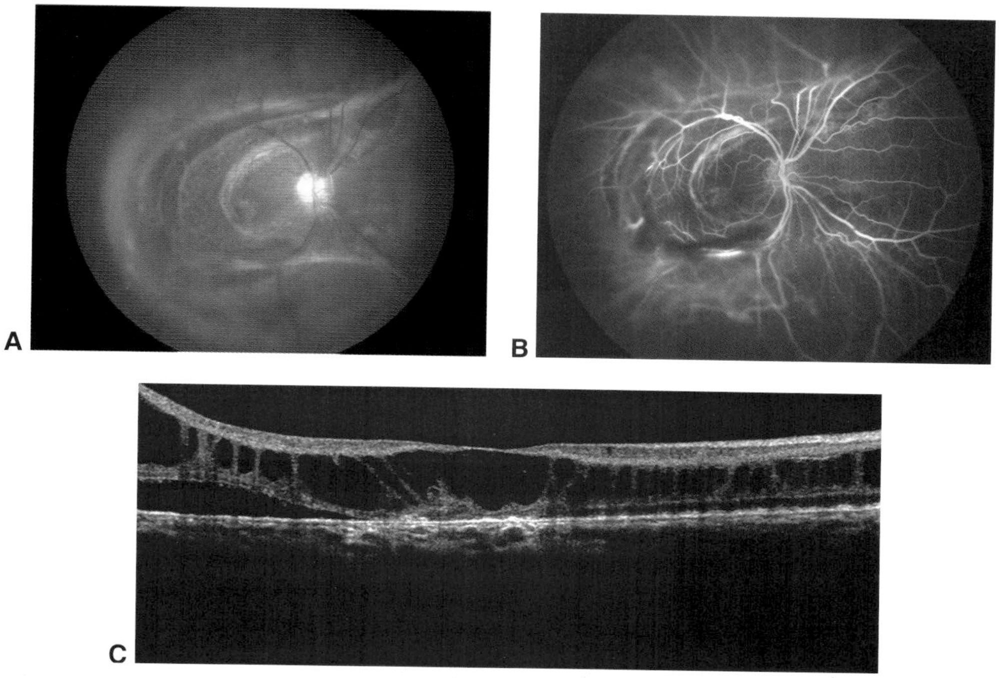

图 25-19　青少年视网膜劈裂症，3 岁。**A.** 中心和周边视网膜劈裂伴轻度玻璃体和视网膜前积血，沿血管弓存在的环形牵拉性视网膜脱离，累及中央黄斑区，并存在视网膜裂孔。**B.** 荧光血管造影显示广泛的牵拉性视网膜脱离。**C.** 黄斑光学相干断层扫描 OCT 显示视网膜劈裂，伴累及中心凹的牵拉性视网膜脱离和视网膜下积液。*（译者注：资料来源见前页原文。）*

Stickler 综合征

Stickler 综合征是一组具有多种表型的结缔组织疾病，最常见常染色体显性遗传，有眼部和全身的表现，由编码Ⅱ型原胶原的 *COL2A1* 基因突变引起。某些突变仅有眼部改变的表型。

诊断　根据临床特点和遗传检测结果即可诊断。常见的眼部表现有玻璃体液化形成的玻璃体空腔、高度近视、视网膜格子样变性和增生性玻璃体视网膜病变。此外，视网膜裂孔导致的视网膜脱离发生率较高。前房角异常、晶状体脱位、白内障、上睑下垂和斜视也偶有发生。

典型的全身性异常包括：面中部扁平、进行性听力损失、腭裂、Pierre-Robin 序列征、二尖瓣脱垂和进行性关节病伴脊柱 / 椎骨骺发育不良。最初关节病变没有症状，但 Stickler 综合征患儿常有长骨和关节的影像学异常，并出现相关症状。

Treatment The retinal detachments are often difficult to repair because these patients may have large retinal breaks posteriorly and the incidence of proliferative vitreoretinopathy is high. The incidence of vitreous loss during cataract surgery is high, as is the rate of subsequent retinal detachment. Retinal folds and breaks should be treated before cataract extraction. Prophylactic retinopexy may be appropriate in certain patients.

Fincham GS, Pasea L, Carroll C, et al. Prevention of retinal detachment in Stickler syndrome: the Cambridge prophylactic cryotherapy protocol. Ophthalmology. 2014;121(8):1588–1597.

Knobloch syndrome

Knobloch syndrome is a vitreoretinopathy caused by biallelic mutations in *COL18A1*. It is classically defined by the triad of occipital encephalocele, high myopia, and predisposition to retinal detachment.

Diagnosis The ocular phenotype is characterized by a distinct vitreoretinal degeneration—very severe RPE atrophic changes with prominent choroidal vessels (Fig 25-20A) out of proportion to the degree of myopia, macular atrophic lesions with or without a "punchedout" appearance, and white fibrillar vitreous condensations. These eyes have a strong predisposition to spontaneous retinal detachment. Smooth (cryptless) irides are universal in affected eyes (Fig 25-20B); ectopia lentis is an occasional finding. Taken together, these ocular findings are pathognomonic for biallelic *COL18A1* mutations.

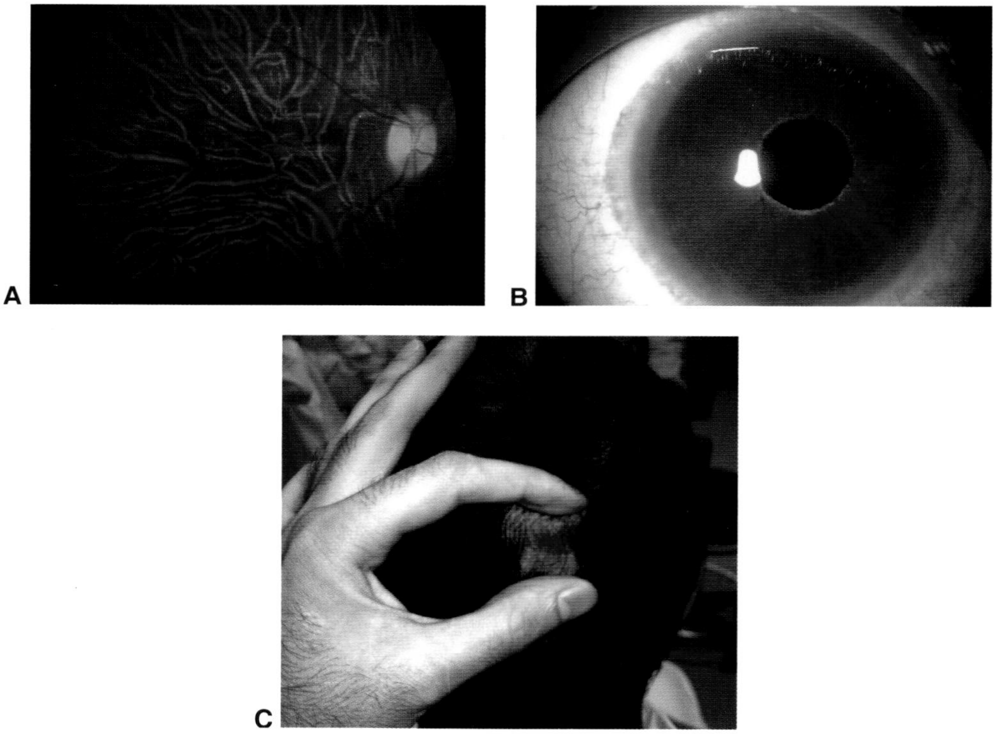

Figure 25-20 Knobloch syndrome. **A,** With severe chorioretinal atrophy. **B,** With cryptless iris. **C,** With scalp abnormality. *(Courtesy of Arif O. Khan, MD.)*

治疗 视网膜脱离复位较难，因为后极部视网膜裂孔较大、增殖性玻璃体视网膜病变发生率较高。白内障手术中玻璃体丢失的发生率很高，视网膜脱离的发生率也很高。白内障摘除前应先处理视网膜皱襞和裂孔，一些患者应行预防性视网膜加固术。

Fincham GS, Pasea L, Carroll C, et al. Prevention of retinal detachment in Stickler syndrome: the Cambridge prophylactic cryotherapy protocol. Ophthalmology. 2014;121(8):1588–1597.

Knobloch 综合征

Knobloch 综合征是玻璃体视网膜病变，由 *COL18A1* 等位基因突变引起。典型的三联征表现为枕叶脑膨出、高度近视和视网膜脱离多发。

诊断 眼部表现为特殊的玻璃体视网膜退行性病变——非常严重的视网膜色素上皮 RPE 萎缩，明显的脉络膜血管（图 25–20A）远较其近视程度严重；黄斑萎缩病变，可呈“穿孔样”外观；玻璃体浓缩的白色纤维。易自发性视网膜脱离。受累眼见光滑的（无隐窝）虹膜（图 25–20B），少见晶状体脱位。这些眼部症状是特征性等位基因 *COL18A1* 突变所致。

A B C
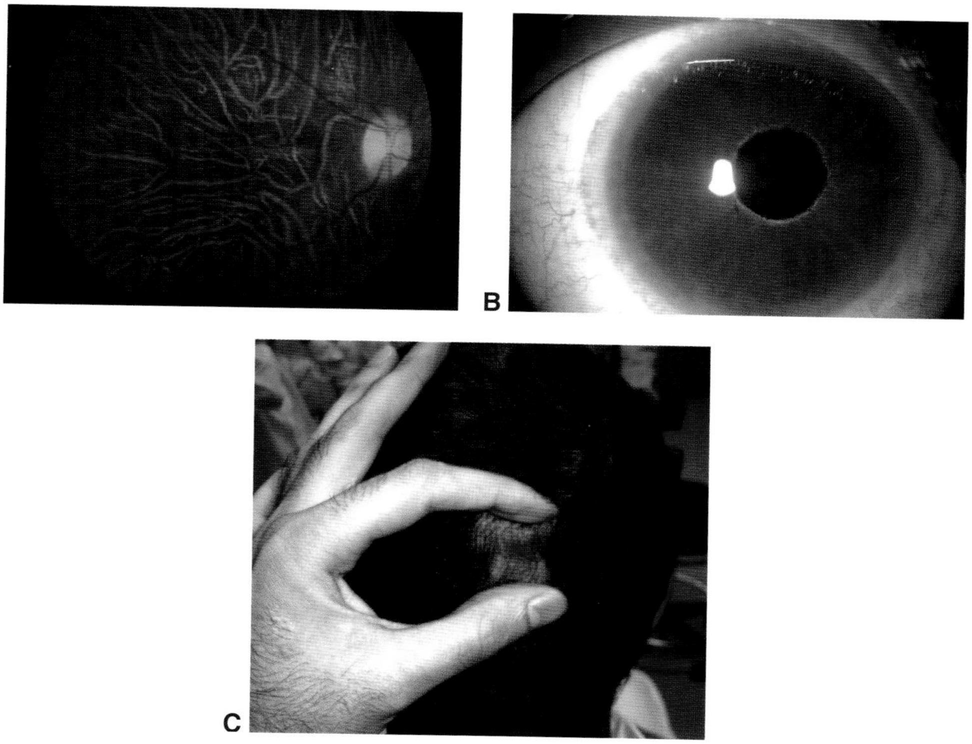

图 25–20 Knobloch 综合征。**A.** 伴有严重的脉络膜视网膜萎缩。**B.** 无隐窝虹膜。**C.** 伴有头皮异常。*（译者注：资料来源见前页原文。）*

ERG shows cone–rod dysfunction. Pigment dispersion glaucoma has been reported in 2 patients.

Systemic manifestations are variable and not always present; they include occipital abnormalities (Fig 25-20C) (ranging from scalp abnormalities to encephalocele), congenital renal malformations, developmental delay, seizures, and heterotopic gray matter.

Treatment Therapy is based on disease manifestations.

Khan AO, Aldahmesh MA, Mohamed JY, Al-Mesfer S, Alkuraya FS. The distinct ophthalmic phenotype of Knobloch syndrome in children. *Br J Ophthalmol.* 2012;96(6):890–895.

Norrie disease

Norrie disease is an X-linked recessive disorder of retinal dysplasia caused by a mutation in the *NDP* gene, which encodes for the protein norrin. Affected boys are typically born blind and have varying degrees of hearing impairment and intellectual disability.

Diagnosis The condition is characterized by a distinctive retinal appearance: a globular, severely dystrophic retina with pigmentary changes in the avascular periphery. During the first few days or weeks of life, a bilateral, yellowish retinal detachment appears, followed by a whiter mass behind the clear lens. Over time, the lenses, and later the cornea, opacify; phthisis bulbi may ensue by age 10 years or earlier. Female carriers show peripheral retinal abnormalities.

Treatment No treatment exists.

Familial exudative vitreoretinopathy

Familial exudative vitreoretinopathy (FEVR) is a disease of abnormal retinal vascularization similar to that seen in ROP (discussed earlier in the chapter). There is failure of the peripheral retina to vascularize. FEVR is typically autosomal dominant, but autosomal recessive and X-linked forms exist as well, the latter resulting from mutations in the same gene involved in Norrie disease *(NDP).*

Khan AO, Lenzner S, Bolz HJ. A family harboring homozygous *FZD4* deletion supports the existence of recessive *FZD4*-related familial exudative vitreoretinopathy. *Ophthalmic Genet.* 2017;38(4):380 –382.

Diagnosis Posterior pole findings in FEVR include retinal traction, folds, breaks, and detachment secondary to vitreous traction (Fig 25-21A). Posterior vitreous detachment and thick peripheral intraretinal and subretinal exudates may develop (Fig 25-21B). The disease is bilateral and can mimic ROP but affects infants born at full term. Fluorescein angiography shows areas of retinal nonperfusion and neovascularization (Fig 25-21C). Examination of family members is important in the diagnosis of FEVR. Affected family members can show marked variation in severity, from minimal straightening of retinal vessels and peripheral nonperfusion to total retinal detachment.

视网膜电图 ERG 显示视锥视杆 / 锥体杆体细胞功能障碍。报道称有 2 例出现色素播散性青光眼。

全身症状变化较大或缺如，有枕叶异常（图 25–20C）（有头皮异常或脑膨出）、先天性肾脏畸形、发育迟缓、癫痫和大脑灰质异位症。

治疗　治疗取决于疾病的临床表现。

Khan AO, Aldahmesh MA, Mohamed JY, Al-Mesfer S, Alkuraya FS. The distinct ophthalmic phenotype of Knobloch syndrome in children. *Br J Ophthalmol.* 2012;96(6):890–895.

Norrie 病

Norrie 病是一种 X– 连锁隐形遗传的视网膜发育不良疾病，由编码 norrin 蛋白的 *NDP* 基因突变引起。受累男孩出生时即失明，有不同程度的听力损伤和智力障碍。

诊断　视网膜独特的外观：在周边无血管区，有球形、伴色素改变的严重视网膜发育不良。出生后几天或几周内，出现双眼的黄色视网膜脱离，随后在透明晶状体后出现白色团块。随着时间的推移，晶状体、角膜依次混浊，10 岁或更早发生眼球萎缩。女性携带者表现为周边视网膜异常。

治疗　尚无有效的治疗方法。

家族性渗出性玻璃体视网膜病变

家族性渗出性玻璃体视网膜病变（FEVR）是一种视网膜血管化异常的疾病，类似于早产儿视网膜病变(见本章前节讨论)，周边视网膜未血管化。家族性渗出性玻璃体视网膜病变(FEVR)多为常染色体显性遗传，也有常染色体隐性遗传和 X – 连锁遗传。X– 连锁遗传是由 Norrie 病（*NDP*）中的同一基因突变引起的。

Khan AO, Lenzner S, Bolz HJ. A family harboring homozygous *FZD4* deletion supports the existence of recessive *FZD4*-related familial exudative vitreoretinopathy. *Ophthalmic Genet*. 2017;38(4):380 –382.

诊断　家族性渗出性玻璃体视网膜病变（FEVR）的后极部表现有视网膜牵引、皱襞 / 折、裂孔和玻璃体牵拉 / 引性视网膜脱离（图 25–21A），可形成玻璃体后脱离和周边视网膜层间、视网膜下致密渗出物（图 25–21B）。家族性渗出性玻璃体视网膜病变（FEVR）是双眼发病，与早产儿视网膜病变（ROP）表现相似，但发生在足月出生的婴儿。荧光血管造影显示，视网膜无灌注区和新生血管形成（图 25–21C）。家庭成员检查对 FEVR 的诊断很重要，患病的家庭成员有不同程度的表现：或视网膜血管略微变直，或周围无灌注区，或视网膜完全脱离。

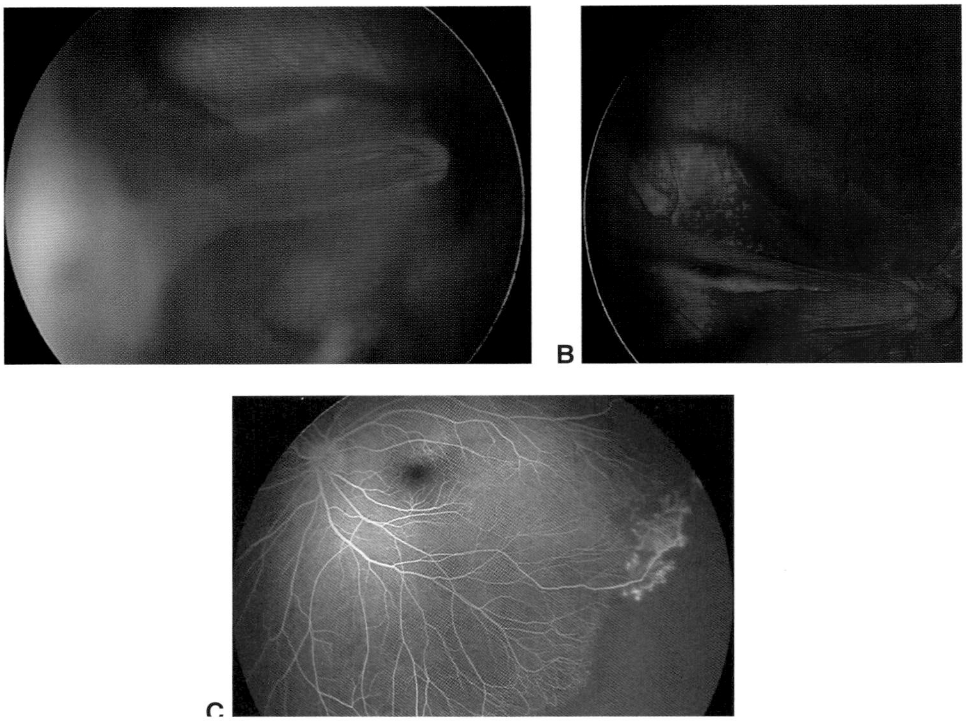

Figure 25-21 Familial exudative vitreoretinopathy. **A,** Tractional retinal detachment with a knot of anterior fibrotic tissue. **B,** Tractional detachment treated with a radially oriented sponge. Note the subretinal exudates. **C,** Fluorescein angiography image shows peripheral avascular retina and hyperfluorescence from leakage of peripheral vessels. *(Courtesy of Scott C. Oliver, MD.)*

Treatment Cryopexy, photocoagulation, vitrectomy, and cataract surgery have been used to manage patients with this disorder.

Infectious Diseases

Herpes Simplex Virus and Cytomegalovirus

Herpes simplex virus and cytomegalovirus are discussed in Chapter 28.

Human Immunodeficiency Virus

The ocular complications of HIV infection have been noted only rarely since the advent of potent antiretroviral therapy. Such complications typically occur only in children with advanced HIV infection who are severely immunocompromised. For more information, see BCSC Section 9, *Uveitis and Ocular Inflammation*, and Section 12, *Retina and Vitreous.*

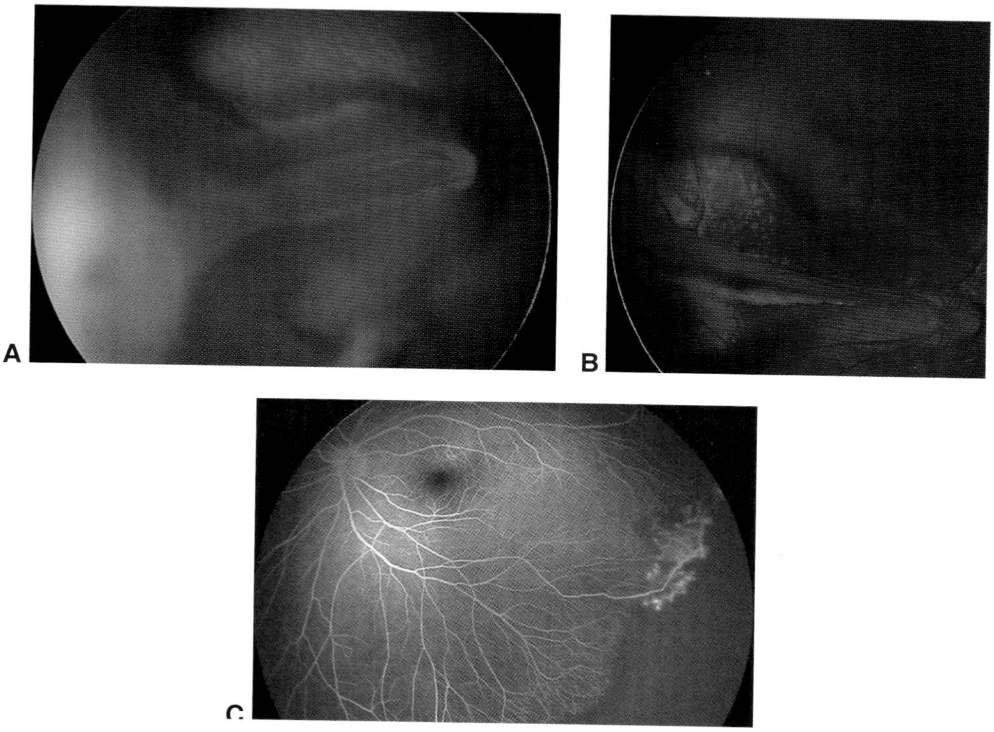

图 25-21　家族性渗出性玻璃体视网膜病变。**A.** 牵拉性视网膜脱离，伴前部纤维组织结节。**B**. 放射状硅海绵加压治疗牵拉性视网膜脱离，可见视网膜下渗出物。**C.** 荧光血管造影显示，周边无血管区视网膜和周边血管渗漏引起的高荧光。*（译者注：资料来源见前页原文。）*

治疗　冷冻治疗、视网膜激光光凝、玻璃体切除术和白内障手术可用来治疗有相应症状的患者。

感染性疾病

单纯疱疹病毒和巨细胞病毒

单纯疱疹病毒和巨细胞病毒感染在第 28 章讨论。

人类免疫缺陷病毒

自从有效的抗逆转录病毒疗法出现以来，人类免疫缺陷病毒 HIV 感染引起的眼部并发症很少发生。眼部并发症仅见于免疫功能低下的晚期人类免疫缺陷病毒 HIV 感染儿童。更多信息见 BCSC 第 9 册《*葡萄膜炎与眼部炎症*》和第 12 册《*视网膜与玻璃体*》。

Tumors

Choroidal and Retinal Pigment Epithelial Lesions

A pigmented fundus lesion in a child is usually benign. Flat choroidal nevi are common and are not a cause for concern. Malignant melanoma of the choroid is extremely rare in children. Choroidal osteoma is a benign bony tumor of the uveal tract that may occur in childhood, usually presenting with decreased vision. Diffuse hemangioma of the choroid associated with Sturge-Weber syndrome is discussed in Chapter 28. Patients with neurofibromatosis type 1 often have flat, tan-colored spots in the choroid (see Chapter 28).

Congenital hypertrophy of the retinal pigment epithelium (CHRPE) is a sharply demarcated, flat, hyperpigmented lesion that may be isolated or multifocal (Fig 25-22). Such lesions are sometimes grouped, in which case they are also called *bear tracks.*

Pigmented lesions similar to CHRPE have been associated with Gardner syndrome, an autosomal dominant condition caused by a mutation in the APC gene, located at 5q22.2. Patients with Gardner syndrome have many polyps of the colon, which carry a very high risk for malignant transformation. Affected individuals often require a colectomy in early adulthood to prevent cancer. They may also have skeletal hamartomas and various other soft-tissue tumors. The pigmented retinal lesions associated with Gardner syndrome are different from CHRPE in that they are typically multiple, bilateral, and dispersed; in addition, they often have a surrounding halo and tail of depigmentation that is oriented radially and directed toward the optic nerve (Fig 25-23).

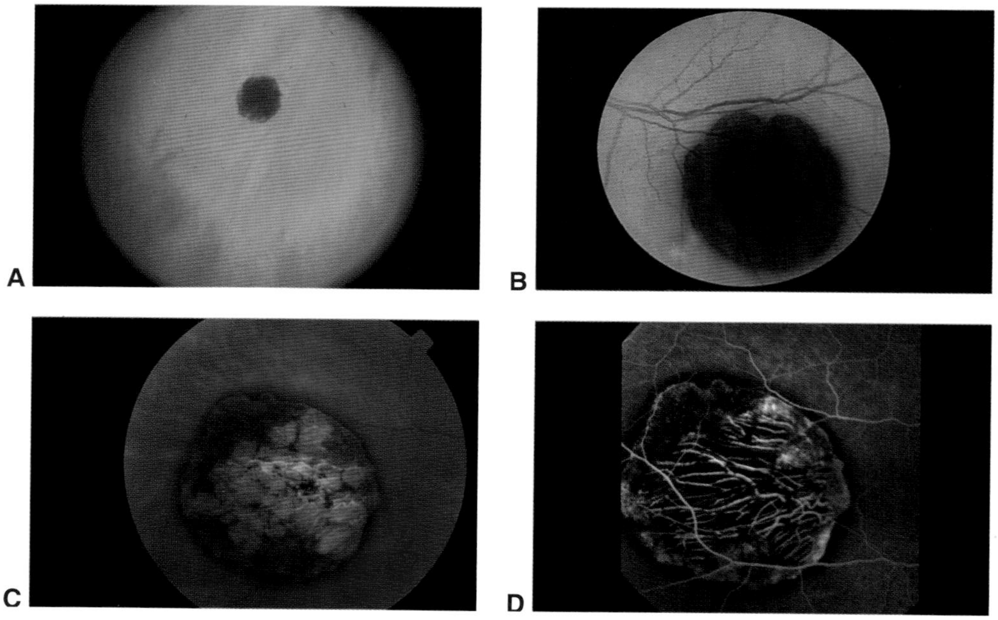

Figure 25-22 Congenital hypertrophy of the RPE (CHRPE). Examples of varying clinical appearances. **A,** Small lesion. **B,** Medium-sized lesion; note the homogeneous black color and well-defined margins of this nummular lesion. **C,** Color fundus photograph of a large lesion. **D,** Corresponding fluorescein angiogram of the large lesion. Note the loss of RPE architecture and highlighted choroidal vasculature. *(Parts A, C, and D courtesy of Timothy G. Murray, MD.)*

肿瘤

脉络膜和视网膜色素上皮病变

儿童色素沉着的眼底病变多是良性的。扁平脉络膜痣常见，不需关注。恶性脉络膜黑色素瘤在儿童中极为罕见。脉络膜骨瘤是儿童时期可能发病的良性葡萄膜骨肿瘤，表现为视力下降。与 Sturge-Weber 综合征相关的脉络膜弥漫性血管瘤在第 28 章讨论。1 型神经纤维瘤病常有脉络膜的扁平褐色斑点（见第 28 章）。

*先天性视网膜色素上皮肥大（CHRPE）*是一种边界清楚、扁平、色素沉着的病变，病灶可以是孤立的或多灶性的（图 25-22）。病灶成群出现时称为*熊脚迹*。

类似于先天性视网膜色素上皮肥大（CHRPE）的色素沉着病灶，可能与 Gardner 综合征有关。Gardner 综合征是一种常染色体显性疾病，是由位于 5q22.2 的 APC 基因突变所致。Gardner 综合征有多发结肠息肉，极易恶变。常在成年早期行结肠切除术，预防恶性肿瘤。同时可患有骨骼错构瘤和多种其他软组织肿瘤。Gardner 综合征不同于先天性视网膜色素上皮肥大（CHRPE），其视网膜色素病灶双眼多发，散在分布，且有环绕脱色素的光环和尾部，呈放射状指向视神经（图 25-23）。

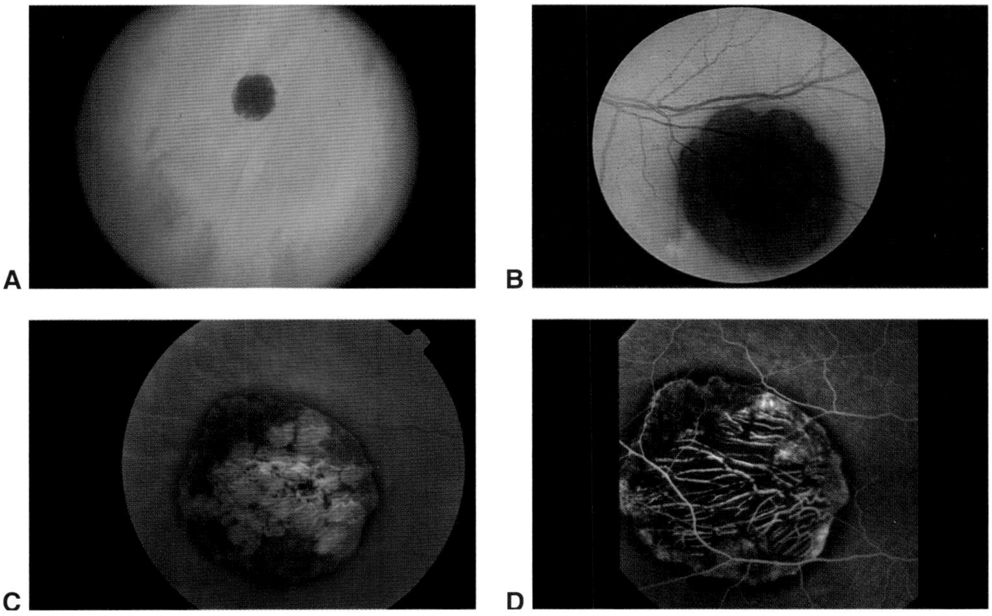

图 25-22　先天性视网膜色素上皮肥大（CHRPE）。不同临床表现病例。**A.** 小病灶。**B.** 中等病灶，可见均质黑色的、边界清楚的圆形病变。**C.** 大病灶的彩色眼底照片。**D.** 大病灶对应的荧光血管造影，可见视网膜色素上皮结构的缺失和凸显的脉络膜血管。*（译者注：资料来源见前页原文。）*

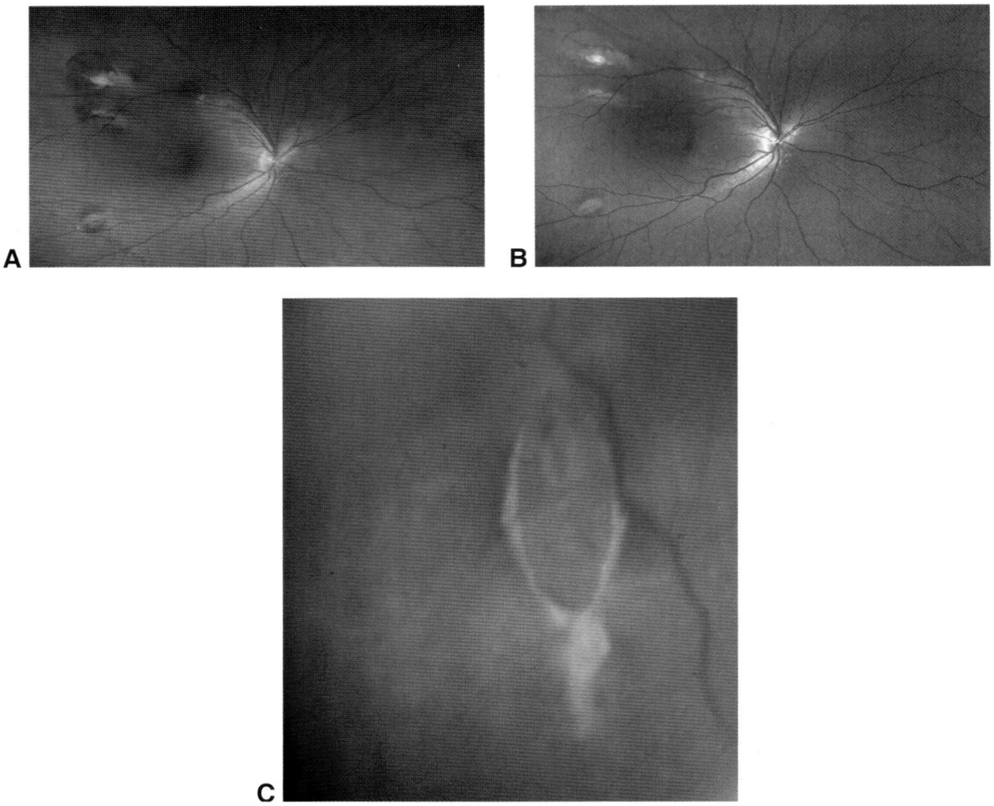

Figure 25-23 Gardner Syndrome. **A,** Ultra-wide-angle fundus photograph shows multiple pigmented retinal lesions with areas of depigmentation oriented radially to the optic nerve. **B,** FAF reveals areas of hypo-and hyperautofluorescence within pigmented lesions. **C,** Retinal lesion with a "fish-tail" configuration. *(Parts A and B courtesy of Cara E. Capitena, MD; part C courtesy of Robert W. Hered, MD.)*

Combined hamartoma of the retina and RPE is an ill-defined, elevated, variably pigmented tumor that may be juxtapapillary or located in the retinal periphery. The tumor is often minimally elevated; retinal traction and tortuous retinal vessels are often present. In peripheral tumors, dragging of the retinal vessels is a prominent feature. The tumors have a variable composition of glial tissue and RPE. This condition can be associated with neurofibromatosis (type 1 or 2), incontinentia pigmenti, X-linked retinoschisis, and facial hemangiomas. Bilateral lesions in a child should raise suspicion for neurofibromatosis type 2.

Traboulsi EI. Ocular manifestations of familial adenomatous polyposis (Gardner syndrome). *Ophthalmol Clin North Am.* 2005;18(1):163–166.

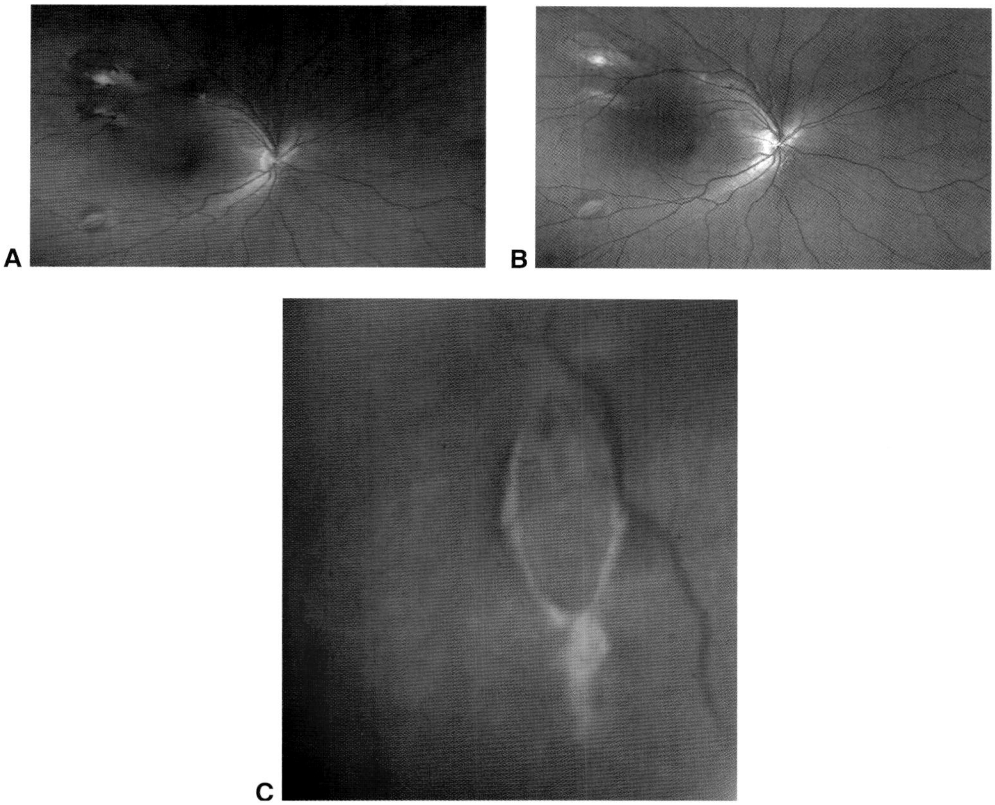

图 25-23　Gardner 综合征。**A.** 超广角眼底照相显示，多处视网膜色素沉着性病灶及放射状指向视神经的脱色素区域。**B.** 眼底自发荧光 FAF 显示色素沉着病灶内的高自发荧光区和低自发荧光区。**C.** “鱼尾样”的视网膜病灶。*（译者注：资料来源见前页原文。）*

*视网膜和色素上皮 RPE 的合并错构瘤*是一种边界不清的、隆起、形态多样的色素肿瘤，位于视乳头附近或周边视网膜。肿瘤略微隆起，牵拉视网膜和血管扭曲。周边部肿瘤的显著特征是视网膜血管的牵拉。肿瘤由不同的神经胶质组织和视网膜色素上皮 RPE 构成，可能伴神经纤维瘤病（1 型或 2 型）、色素失调 / 禁症、X- 连锁性视网膜劈裂和面部血管瘤。儿童双眼患病时，应怀疑 2 型神经纤维瘤病。

Traboulsi EI. Ocular manifestations of familial adenomatous polyposis (Gardner syndrome). *Ophthalmol Clin North Am*. 2005;18(1):163–166.

Retinoblastoma

Retinoblastoma is the most common malignant intraocular tumor of childhood and one of the most common pediatric solid tumors, with an incidence of 1:14,000–1:20,000 live births. It is equally common in both sexes and has no racial predilection. Retinoblastoma is a neuroblastic tumor and is therefore biologically similar to neuroblastoma and medulloblastoma. The tumor can be unilateral or bilateral; 30%–40% of cases are bilateral. In familial and bilateral cases, retinoblastoma is typically diagnosed during the first year of life; in sporadic unilateral cases, between 1 and 3 years of age. Approximately 90% of cases are diagnosed before 3 years of age; onset later than age 5 years is rare but can occur.

The most common initial sign is leukocoria (white pupillary reflex), which is usually first noticed by the family and described as a glow, glint, or cat's-eye appearance (Fig 25-24). The differential diagnosis of leukocoria is presented in Table 25-7. Approximately 25% of cases present with strabismus (esotropia or exotropia). Less common presen ta tions include vitreous hemorrhage, hyphema, ocular or periocular inflammation, glaucoma, proptosis, and pseudohypopyon.

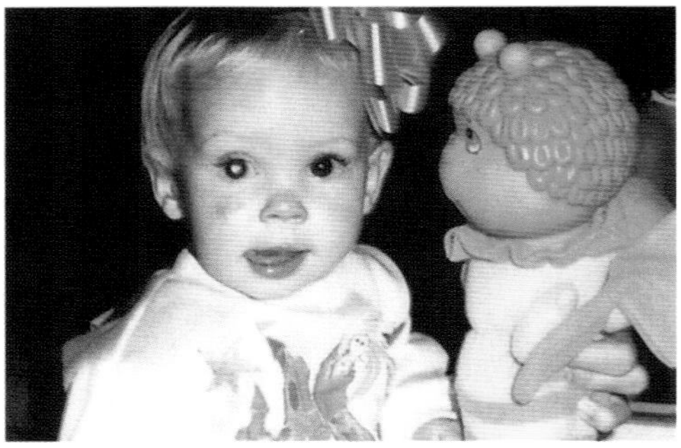

Figure 25-24 Leukocoria of the right eye, which is visible in this family photograph of a 1-year-old girl with retinoblastoma. *(Courtesy of A. Linn Murphree, MD.)*

Table 25-7 Differential Diagnosis of Leukocoria

Cataract
Coats disease
Coloboma of choroid or optic disc
Congenital retinal fold
Corneal opacity
Familial exudative vitreoretinopathy
High myopia or anisometropia
Myelinated nerve fibers
Norrie disease
Organizing vitreous hemorrhage
Persistent fetal vasculature
Photographic artifact
Retinal detachment
Retinal dysplasia
Retinoblastoma
Retinopathy of prematurity
Toxocariasis
Uveitis

视网膜母细胞瘤

视网膜母细胞瘤是儿童最常见的眼内恶性肿瘤，也是最常见的儿童实体肿瘤，发病率为 1 : 20000 ~ 1 : 14000，没有性别及种族差异。视网膜母细胞瘤是一种神经母细胞肿瘤，类似于神经母细胞瘤和髓母细胞瘤的生物学特性。肿瘤可以是单眼或双眼，30% ~ 40%是双眼发病。在家族性和双眼发病的病例中，视网膜母细胞瘤在出生后第一年被确诊，在散发单眼病例中，则在 1 ~ 3 岁被确诊。90%的病例在 3 岁之前被确诊，5 岁以后发病较罕见，但也有可能发生。

最常见的初始症状是白瞳症（白色瞳孔反光），家人首先发现，并描述其为一种发光、闪光或猫眼样外观（图 25-24）。白瞳症的鉴别诊断见表 25-7。约 25% 的病例有斜视（内斜视或外斜视）。少见的临床表现有玻璃体积血、前房积血、眼内炎或眼周炎症、青光眼、眼球突出和假性前房积脓。

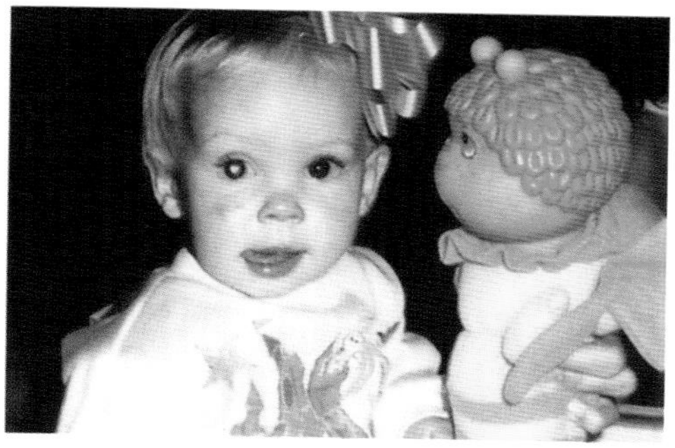

图 25-24　右眼白瞳症。患视网膜母细胞瘤的 1 岁女孩。*（译者注：资料来源见前页原文。）*

表 25-7　白瞳症的鉴别诊断

白内障
Coats病
脉络膜或视盘缺损
先天性视网膜皱襞
角膜混浊
家族性渗出性玻璃体视网膜病变
高度近视或屈光参差
有髓神经纤维
Norrie病
机化的玻璃体积血
永存/永久性胎儿血管
照相伪影
视网膜脱离
视网膜发育不良
视网膜母细胞瘤
早产儿视网膜病变
弓蛔虫病
葡萄膜炎

Diagnosis

Diagnosis of retinoblastoma is usually based on its ophthalmoscopic appearance. Intraocular retinoblastoma can exhibit a variety of growth patterns. With endophytic growth, it appears as a white to cream-colored mass that breaks through the internal limiting membrane (Fig 25-25). Endophytic retinoblastoma is sometimes associated with vitreous seeding, in which individual cells or fragments of tumor tissue become separated from the main mass, as shown in Figure 25-26. Vitreous seeds may be few and localized or so extensive that the clinical picture resembles endophthalmitis. Occasionally, malignant cells enter the anterior chamber and form a pseudohypopyon.

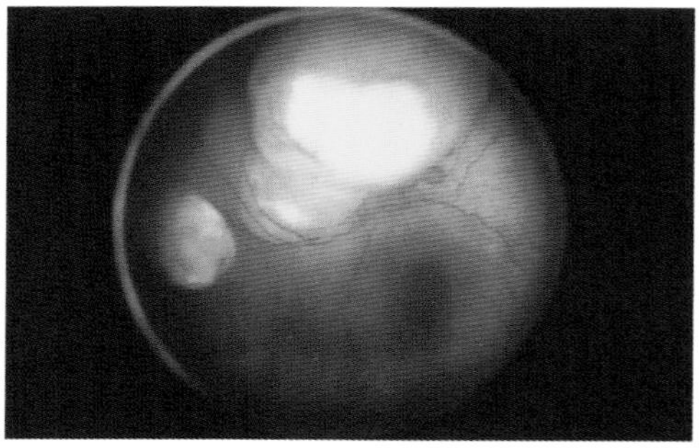

Figure 25-25 Fundus photograph showing multiple endophytic retinoblastoma lesions, left eye. *(Courtesy of A. Linn Murphree, MD.)*

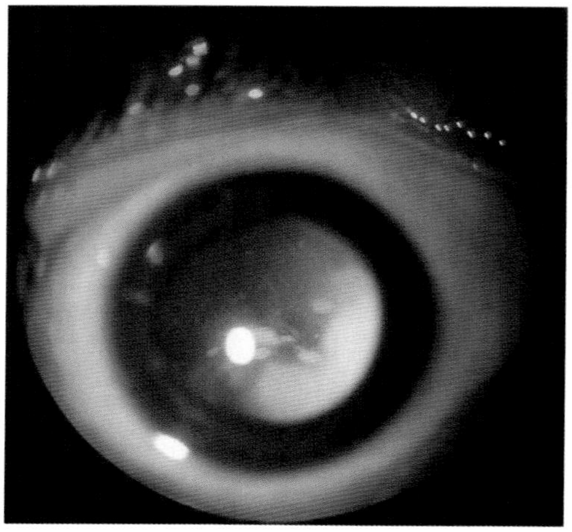

Figure 25-26 Endophytic retinoblastoma with vitreous seeding.

Exophytic tumors are usually yellow-white and occur in the subretinal space; the overlying retinal vessels are commonly larger in caliber and more tortuous (Fig 25-27). Exophytic retinoblastoma growth is often associated with subretinal fluid accumulation, which can obscure the tumor and closely mimic the appearance of an exudative retinal detachment suggestive of advanced Coats disease. Retinoblastoma cells have the potential to implant on previously uninvolved retinal tissue and grow, thereby creating an impression of multicentricity in an eye with only a single primary tumor.

诊断

视网膜母细胞瘤常依据检眼镜下表现来做出诊断。眼内视网膜母细胞瘤有多种生长模式。内生型肿瘤的生长突破内界膜时，外观呈白色或奶油色包块（图 25–25）。如图 25–26 所示，内生型视网膜母细胞瘤可伴有玻璃体腔内种植，单个细胞或肿瘤组织碎片与瘤体分离，玻璃体种植少且局限，或非常广泛，类似于眼内炎。偶见肿瘤细胞进入前房，形成假性前房积脓。

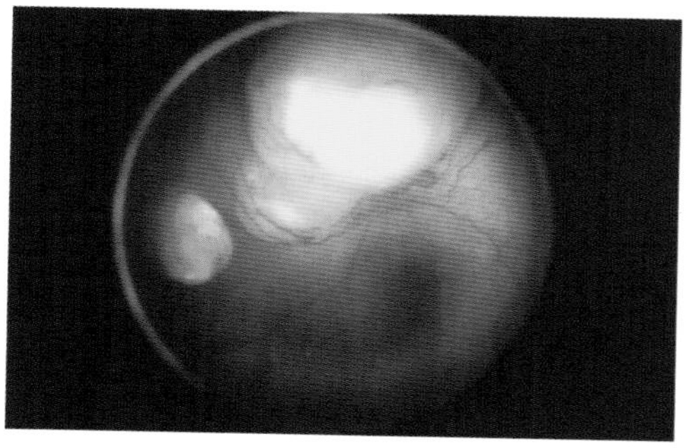

图 25–25 眼底照相显示多灶内生型视网膜母细胞瘤（左眼）。*（译者注：资料来源见前页原文。）*

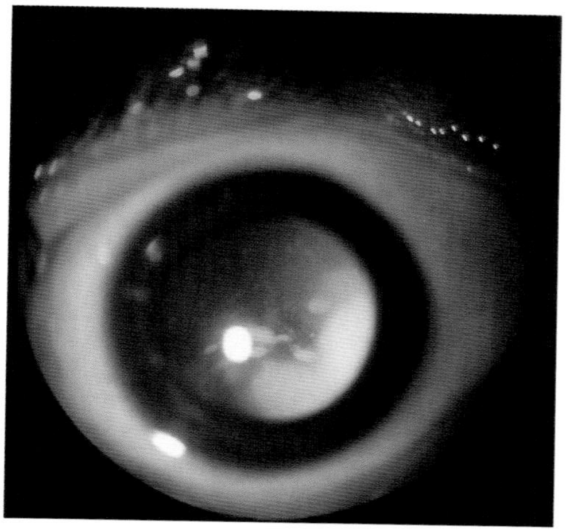

图 25–26 内生型视网膜母细胞瘤伴玻璃体种植。

外生型肿瘤常为黄白色，位于视网膜下腔。肿瘤表面视网膜血管管径粗大且扭曲（图 25–27）。外生型视网膜母细胞瘤常伴视网膜下积液，遮掩肿瘤，类似于渗出性视网膜脱离，易被误诊为晚期 Coats 病。视网膜母细胞瘤细胞可以提前植入未受累的视网膜，并生长，呈现单个原发性肿瘤的多中心病灶。

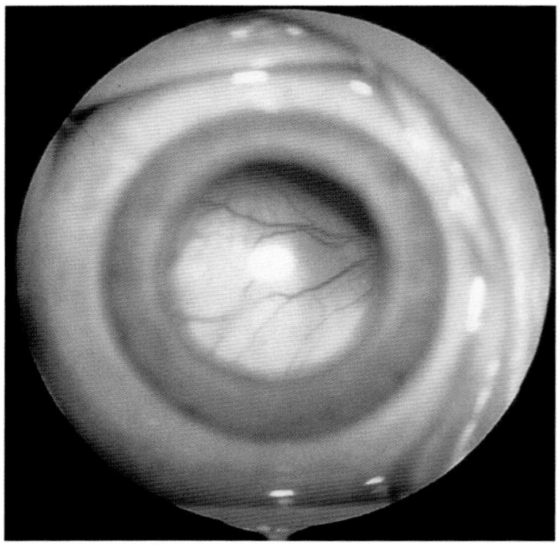

Figure 25-27 Exophytic retinoblastoma with overlying detached retina.

Large tumors often show signs of both endophytic and exophytic growth. Small retinoblastoma lesions appear as a grayish mass and are frequently confined between the internal and external limiting membranes. A third pattern, diffuse infiltrative retinoblastoma, is usually unilateral and nonhereditary. It is found in children older than 5 years. The tumor presents with conjunctival injection, anterior chamber seeds, pseudohypopyon, large clumps of vitreous cells, and retinal infiltration of tumor. Because no distinct tumor mass is present, diagnostic confusion with inflammatory conditions is common.

Spontaneous regression of retinoblastoma is possible. It can be asymptomatic, resulting in the development of a benign retinocytoma, or it can be associated with inflammation and, ultimately, phthisis bulbi. In either case, the genetic implications are the same as for an individual with an active retinoblastoma.

The most common retinal lesion simulating retinoblastoma is seen in Coats disease. The presence of crystalline material, extensive subretinal fluid, and peripheral vascular abnormalities—combined with the absence of calcium—suggests Coats disease. *Astrocytic hamartomas* and *hemangioblastomas* are benign retinal tumors that may simulate the appearance of small retinoblastomas. Both are usually associated with neuro-oculocutaneous syndromes (see Chapter 28).

Evaluation of a patient with presumed retinoblastoma requires imaging of the head and orbits, which can confirm the diagnosis and assess for extraocular extension and intracranial disease. Computed tomography is discouraged because of the possible increased risk of secondary tumors due to radiation exposure. Magnetic resonance imaging and ultrasonography are recommended. More invasive tests are reserved for atypical cases. Aspiration of ocular fluids for diagnostic testing should be performed only under the most unusual circumstances because such procedures can disseminate malignant cells. Recently, however, it was demonstrated that cell-free tumor-derived DNA may be obtained from aqueous humor.

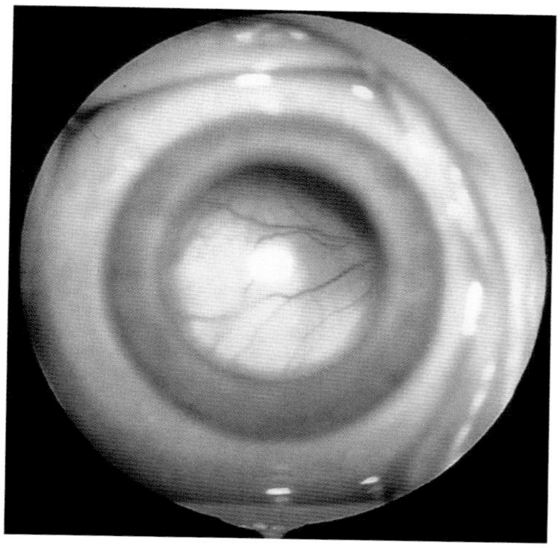

图 25-27　外生型视网膜母细胞瘤伴肿瘤表面视网膜脱离。

大的视网膜母细胞瘤常同时表现出内生型和外生型生长；小的视网膜母细胞瘤的外观呈浅灰色肿块，限制在内界膜和外界膜之间。第 3 种生长模式为弥漫浸润型视网膜母细胞瘤，为单眼和非遗传性的，常见于 5 岁以上的儿童，表现为结膜充血、前房种植、假性前房积脓、玻璃体内大团块细胞和肿瘤的视网膜浸润。因为无明显的肿块，常被误诊为眼内炎。

视网膜母细胞瘤可自行消退。它可以无症状，并发展为良性视网膜细胞瘤，或伴随炎症，最终眼球萎缩。无论是何种情况，对于每个活动性视网膜母细胞瘤而言，其遗传学意义是一样的。

Coats 病是最常见的类似视网膜母细胞瘤的视网膜病。眼底表现有结晶样物质、广泛的视网膜下液和周边血管异常，若伴钙化缺如，常提示为 Coats 病。*星形细胞错构瘤*和*血管母细胞瘤*是良性视网膜肿瘤，类似于小视网膜母细胞瘤，两者伴有神经眼皮肤综合征 / 母斑病（见第 28 章）。

疑似视网膜母细胞瘤应进行头部和眼眶影像学检查确诊并评估眼外扩散和颅内病变。不建议使用计算机断层扫描 CT 检测，因为辐射暴露可增加继发性肿瘤的风险，建议使用磁共振成像 MRI 和超声检查。对非典型病例不建议行侵入性检查，诊断性眼内穿刺仅在特殊情况下进行，因为这样的操作可致恶性肿瘤细胞扩散。最近的研究表明，房水中可获得无细胞肿瘤源性 DNA。

The characteristic histologic features of retinoblastoma include Flexner-Wintersteiner rosettes, which are usually present, and fleurettes, which are less common. Both represent limited degrees of retinal cellular differentiation. Homer Wright rosettes are also frequently present but are less specific for retinoblastoma because they are common in other neuroblastic tumors. Calcification of varying extent is usually present.

Berry JL, Xu L, Murphree AL, et al. Potential of aqueous humor as a surrogate tumor biopsy for retinoblastoma. *JAMA Ophthalmol.* 2017;135(11):1221–1230.

de Graaf P, Göricke S, Rodjan F, et al; European Retinoblastoma Imaging Collaboration. Guidelines for imaging retinoblastoma: imaging Principles and MRI standardization. *Pediatr Radiol.* 2012;42(1):2–14.

Genetics The retinoblastoma gene *(RB1)* maps to a locus within the q14 band of chromosome 13 and codes for a protein, pRB, that suppresses tumor formation. For retinoblastoma to occur, both *RB1* genes must have a mutation. Approximately 60% of retinoblastoma cases arise from somatic nonhereditary mutations of both alleles of *RB1* in a retinal cell. These mutations generally result in unifocal and unilateral tumors. In the other 40% of patients, a germline mutation in 1 of the 2 alleles of *RB1* either is inherited from an affected parent (10% of all retinoblastoma cases) or occurs spontaneously in 1 of the gametes. A second somatic mutation in a retinal cell is all that is necessary for retinoblastoma to develop; such cases are often multicentric and bilateral.

Genetic counseling for families of retinoblastoma patients is complex (Table 25-8). Both parents and all siblings should be examined. In approximately 1% of cases, a parent may be found to have an unsuspected fundus lesion that represents a spontaneously regressed retinoblastoma (retinocytoma).

Genetic testing for retinoblastoma is important for determining the risk of subsequent cancers (both retinoblastoma and other primary neoplasms) in the affected child and the risk of retinoblastoma in other family members. The probability of detecting the *RB1* gene depends on many factors, including the capabilities of the molecular diagnostic laboratory, the presence of tumor tissue, and the ability to test other affected family members.

Preimplantation genetic testing can be performed, and in vitro fertilization techniques have been used successfully to select embryos that are free from the germinal *RB1* mutation.

Dhar SU, Chintagumpala M, Noll C, Chévez-Barrios P, Paysse EA, Plon SE. Outcomes of integrating genetics in management of patients with retinoblastoma. *Arch Ophthalmol.* 2011;129(11):1428–1434.

Classification of retinoblastoma The International Classification of Retinoblastoma (ICRB; Table 25-9) is useful for predicting the success of chemoreduction and has superseded the Reese-Ellsworth classification, which was originally developed to predict globe salvage after external-beam radiotherapy. The American Joint Committee on Cancer (AJCC) also has a staging system for retinoblastoma that addresses both intraocular and extraocular disease (see BCSC Section 4, *Ophthalmic Pathology and Intraocular Tumors*).

Shields CL, Mashayekhi A, Au AK, et al. The International Classification of Retinoblastoma predicts chemoreduction success. *Ophthalmology.* 2006;113(12):2276–2280.

视网膜母细胞瘤的典型组织学特征有 Flexner–Wintersteiner 菊形团（较多见）和花状饰（较少见），两者均提示视网膜细胞分化程度有限。Homer–Wright 菊形团也常见，不是视网膜母细胞瘤特异性的，也可见于其他神经母细胞瘤中。肿瘤常存在不同程度的钙化。

Berry JL, Xu L, Murphree AL, et al. Potential of aqueous humor as a surrogate tumor biopsy for retinoblastoma. *JAMA Ophthalmol.* 2017;135(11):1221–1230.

de Graaf P, Göricke S, Rodjan F, et al; European Retinoblastoma Imaging Collaboration. Guidelines for imaging retinoblastoma: imaging Principles and MRI standardization. *Pediatr Radiol.* 2012;42(1):2–14.

遗传学　视网膜母细胞瘤基因（*RB1*）位于染色体 13q14 区，并编码抑制肿瘤形成的蛋白质 pRB。视网膜母细胞瘤的发生，是 2 个视网膜母细胞瘤基因（*RB1*）都发生突变所致。约 60% 的视网膜母细胞瘤是视网膜细胞中 *RB1* 的 2 个等位基因发生体细胞非遗传突变，这些突变导致单灶和单眼肿瘤。另 40% 是由于 *RB1* 的 2 个等位基因中的 1 个发生生殖系突变，源于受累的父母亲（占视网膜母细胞瘤的 10%），或源于其中 1 个配子的自发突变，另 1 个视网膜细胞的体细胞突变才是视网膜母细胞瘤发生所必需的。肿瘤通常是多灶性和双眼的。

视网膜母细胞瘤患者家族的遗传咨询较为复杂（表 25–8）。父母和所有兄弟姐妹都应检查，1% 的病例中可能发现父母一方有眼底病变，表现为自发性退化的视网膜母细胞瘤（视网膜细胞瘤）。

视网膜母细胞瘤的基因检测对于确定患病儿童后续肿瘤（视网膜母细胞瘤和其他原发性肿瘤）的风险，以及其他家庭成员患视网膜母细胞瘤的风险非常重要。检测出 *RB1* 基因的概率取决于许多因素，包括分子诊断实验室的检测能力、肿瘤组织的表达，以及能否检测到其他受累的家庭成员。

可进行胚胎植入前基因检测，体外受精技术可以成功选择不含 *RB1* 种系 / 生殖突变的胚胎。

Dhar SU, Chintagumpala M, Noll C, Chévez-Barrios P, Paysse EA, Plon SE. Outcomes of integrating genetics in management of patients with retinoblastoma. *Arch Ophthalmol.* 2011;129(11):1428–1434.

视网膜母细胞瘤的分类　视网膜母细胞瘤的国际分类（ICRB，表 25–9）可用于预测化学减容的疗效，并取代了 Reese–Ellsworth 分类，后者用于预测外照射放疗后的保眼球治疗效果。美国癌症联合委员会（AJCC）也有视网膜母细胞瘤分期系统，用于眼内和眼外肿瘤（见 BCSC 第 4 册《*眼病理学与眼内肿瘤*》）。

Shields CL, Mashayekhi A, Au AK, et al. The International Classification of Retinoblastoma predicts chemoreduction success. *Ophthalmology.* 2006;113(12):2276–2280.

Table 25-8 Genetic Counseling for Retinoblastoma

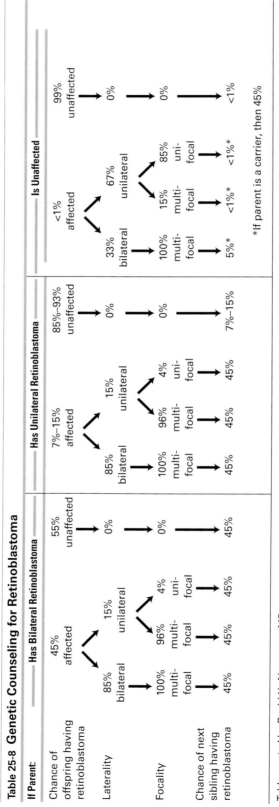

If Parent:	Has Bilateral Retinoblastoma				Has Unilateral Retinoblastoma				Is Unaffected			
Chance of offspring having retinoblastoma	45% affected			55% unaffected	7%–15% affected			85%–93% unaffected	<1% affected			99% unaffected
Laterality	85% bilateral	15% unilateral		0%	85% bilateral	15% unilateral		0%	33% bilateral	67% unilateral		0%
Focality	100% multi-focal	96% multi-focal	4% uni-focal	0%	100% multi-focal	96% multi-focal	4% uni-focal	0%	100% multi-focal	15% multi-focal	85% uni-focal	0%
Chance of next sibling having retinoblastoma	45%	45%	45%	45%	45%	45%	45%	7%–15%	5%*	<1%*	<1%*	<1%

*If parent is a carrier, then 45%

Table created by David H. Abramson, MD.

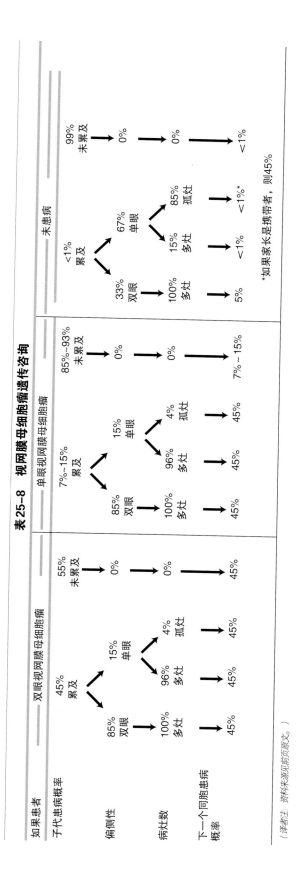

表 25-8　视网膜母细胞瘤遗传咨询

如果患者	双眼视网膜母细胞瘤				单眼视网膜母细胞瘤				未患病			
子代患病概率	45% 累及			55% 未累及	7%~15% 累及			85%~93% 未累及	<1% 累及			99% 未累及
偏侧性	85% 双眼	15% 单眼		0%	85% 双眼	15% 单眼		0%	33% 双眼	67% 单眼		0%
病灶数	100% 多灶	96% 多灶	4% 孤灶	0%	100% 多灶	96% 多灶	4% 孤灶	0%	100% 多灶	15% 多灶	85% 孤灶	0%
下一个同胞患病概率	45%	45%	45%	45%	45%	45%	45%	7% ~ 15%	5%	<1%	<1%*	<1%

*如果家长是携带者，则45%

（译者注：资料来源见前页原文。）

Table 25-9 International Classification of Retinoblastoma

Group	Features
A	Small tumors (≤3 mm) confined to the retina; >3 mm from the fovea; >1.5 mm from the optic disc
B	Tumors (>3 mm) confined to the retina in any location, with clear subretinal fluid ≤6 mm from the tumor margin
C	Localized vitreous and/or subretinal seeding (<6 mm total from tumor margin) If there is more than 1 site of subretinal or vitreous seeding, the total of these sites is <6 mm
D	Diffuse vitreous and/or subretinal seeding (≥6 mm total from tumor margin) If there is more than 1 site of subretinal or vitreous seeding, the total of these sites is ≥6 mm Subretinal fluid >6 mm from tumor margin
E	No visual potential or Presence of any of the following: • tumor in the anterior segment • tumor in or on the ciliary body • neovascular glaucoma • vitreous hemorrhage obscuring the tumor or significant hyphema • phthisical or prephthisical eye • orbital cellulitis-like presentation

Modified from Shields CL, Mashayekhi A, Au AK, et al. The International Classification of Retinoblastoma predicts chemoreduction success. *Ophthalmology.* 2006;113(12):2276–2280.

Treatment

The management of retinoblastoma has changed dramatically over the past decade and continues to evolve. Many specialists may be involved, including ocular oncologists, pediatric ophthalmologists, geneticists, genetic counselors, pediatric oncologists, and radiation oncologists. External-beam radiation is seldom used to treat intraocular retinoblastoma because of its high association with development of craniofacial deformity and secondary tumors in the field of radiation. When the likelihood of salvaging vision is low, primary enucleation of eyes with advanced unilateral retinoblastoma is often performed to avoid the adverse effects of systemic chemotherapy. To prevent extraocular spread of the tumor, the surgeon should minimize manipulation of the globe and obtain a long segment of optic nerve. Small retinoblastoma tumors can often be treated with either laser photocoagulation or cryotherapy.

Primary systemic chemotherapy (chemoreduction) followed by local therapy (consolidation) has been used to spare vision for larger tumors (Fig 25-28) and is often used in cases of bilateral retinoblastoma. Most studies of chemoreduction for retinoblastoma have used vincristine, carboplatin, and an epipodophyllotoxin. Others have added cyclosporine. Chemotherapy is rarely successful when used alone and often requires local therapy (cryotherapy, laser photocoagulation, thermotherapy, or plaque radiotherapy) as well. Adverse effects of chemoreduction treatment include low blood count, hair loss, hearing loss, renal toxicity, neurologic and cardiac disturbances, and possible increased risk for acute myelogenous leukemia.

表25-9　视网膜母细胞瘤的国际分类

分组	特点
A	局限于视网膜的小肿瘤（≤3mm）；距离中央凹>3mm；距视盘>1.5mm
B	肿瘤（> 3 mm）局限于视网膜任何部位，距肿瘤边缘≤6mm的透明视网膜下液
C	局限性玻璃体和/或视网膜下的种植灶（距离肿瘤边缘<6 mm） 如果有超过视网膜或玻璃体种植灶多于1个，全部病灶<6mm
D	弥漫性玻璃体和/或视网膜下种植（距离肿瘤边缘≥6mm） 如果视网膜下或玻璃体种植灶多于1个，全部病灶≥6mm 距肿瘤边缘>6mm的视网膜下液
E	视功能丧失或有以下任何一种情况： • 眼前节的肿瘤 • 位于睫状体内或表面的肿瘤 • 新生血管性青光眼 • 大量玻璃体出血使肿瘤变得模糊，或明显的前房出血 • 眼球痨或眼球痨前期 • 眼眶蜂窝织炎样表现

（译者注：资料来源见前页原文。）

治疗

视网膜母细胞瘤的治疗在过去的 10 年里发生了巨大变化，并且还在不断进步。许多专家参与其中，包括眼肿瘤、小儿眼科、遗传学、遗传咨询、儿童肿瘤以及放射肿瘤等专家。外放射治疗很少用于治疗眼内视网膜母细胞瘤，因为放射治疗区可能发生颅面畸形和继发性肿瘤。当视力无法挽救时，做单眼晚期视网膜母细胞瘤手术应摘除眼球，以避免全身化学治疗的副作用。为防止肿瘤的眼外扩散，手术医生应尽量减少对眼球的操作，并应截取较长的视神经。较小的视网膜母细胞瘤可用激光光凝或冷冻治疗。

首先进行全身化疗（化学减容），然后进行局部治疗（联合），用于保留较大肿瘤的治疗后视力（图 25-28），并适用于双眼视网膜母细胞瘤。视网膜母细胞瘤化学减容治疗中，多使用长春新碱、卡 / 波铂和表鬼臼毒素，还可联合使用环孢霉素。单独使用化疗无法治愈视网膜母细胞瘤，常需联合局部治疗（冷冻治疗、激光光凝、透热治疗或放射敷贴治疗）。化学减容治疗的副作用有血细胞计数下降、脱发、听力丧失、肾毒性、神经系统和心血管系统紊乱，急性髓细胞性白血病的患病风险增加。

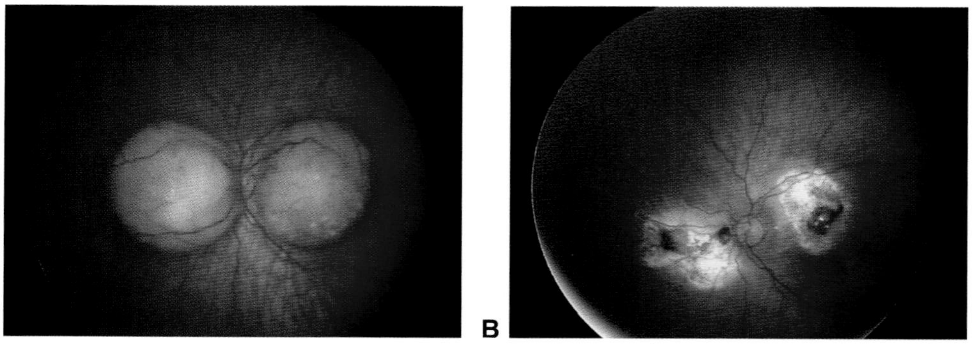

A B

Figure 25-28 **A,** Left eye of an infant with bilateral retinoblastoma; 2 tumors straddle the optic nerve. **B,** After chemoreduction and laser consolidation, the tumors are nonviable. The child's visual acuity was 20/25 at age 5 years.

Intra-arterial chemotherapy has recently been reported as an alternative to systemic chemoreduction for unilateral retinoblastoma in group B, C, D, or E eyes. Chemotherapy is delivered via cannulation of the ophthalmic artery in single or multiple sessions. Many chemotherapy agents have been used; melphalan is the most common. Overall, the results show higher rates of globe salvage in eyes treated initially and in those that did not respond to prior treatments. Systemic complications include neutropenia and metastasis. Ocular complications include vascular occlusion, blepharoptosis, cilia loss, temporary dysmotility, and periocular edema in the distribution of the supratrochlear artery. There is concern about the radiation that is delivered during the procedure, especially for patients with germline *RB1* gene mutations, who are at higher risk for malignant tumors.

Intravitreal chemotherapy has been used for refractory and recurrent vitreous seeding from retinoblastoma. Periocular injections have been used for adjuvant chemotherapy.

Treated retinoblastoma sometimes disappears altogether, but more often it persists as a calcified mass (type 1, or "cottage cheese," pattern) or a noncalcified, translucent grayish lesion (type 2, or "fish flesh," pattern), which may be difficult to distinguish from untreated tumor. Type 3 regression has elements of both types 1 and 2, and type 4 regression is a flat, atrophic scar. A child with treated retinoblastoma must be observed closely for new or recurrent tumor formation, with frequent examinations under anesthesia if necessary.

Extraocular retinoblastoma, though uncommon in the United States, is still problematic in developing countries, primarily because of delay in diagnosis. The 4 major types are optic nerve involvement, orbital invasion, central nervous system (CNS) involvement, and distant metastasis. Treatment of extraocular retinoblastoma includes intensive multimodality chemotherapy, autologous hematopoietic stem cell rescue, and external-beam radiotherapy. Long-term disease-free survival is possible if the CNS is not involved; otherwise, the prognosis is usually poor.

Patients with trilateral retinoblastoma have a primitive neuroectodermal tumor (PNET) of the pineal gland or parasellar region in addition to retinoblastoma. In patients with unilateral retinoblastoma, the risk of trilateral retinoblastoma has been less than 0.5%; in those with bilateral retinoblastoma, less than 5%–15%. However, the rate of trilateral retinoblastoma appears to be lower in patients treated with chemoreduction. Treatment usually involves a multimodal approach, and the prognosis is poor.

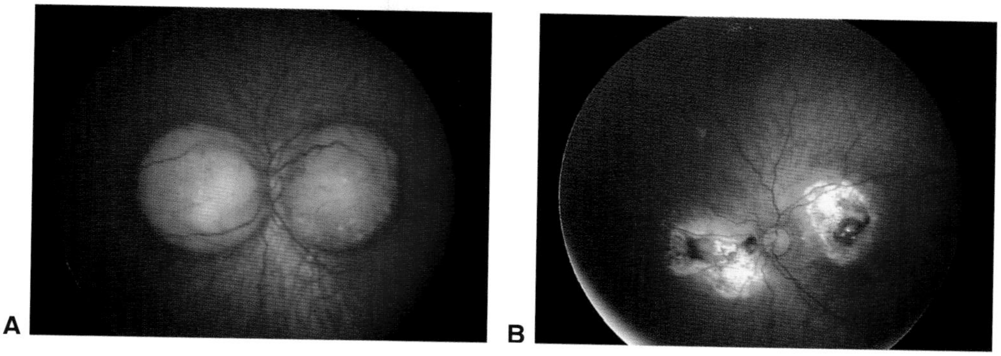

图 25-28 A. 双眼视网膜母细胞瘤，左眼，2 个肿瘤跨在视盘两侧。B. 化学减容联合激光治疗后，肿瘤失去活性，5 岁时视力为 20/25。

近期有报道使用动脉内化学治疗替代全身化学减容的方案，应用在 B、C、D 或 E 期单眼视网膜母细胞瘤。通过单次或多次眼动脉插管来进行化学治疗，已有许多化疗药物应用在动脉内化学治疗中，最常用美法仑。总体上看，与先前治疗无效后选择动脉内化疗的患者相比，首选动脉内化学治疗的眼球保留成功率更高。全身并发症有中性粒细胞减少和转移瘤，眼部并发症有血管闭塞、上睑下垂、睫毛脱落、暂时性运动障碍和滑车上动脉分布区的眼周水肿。插管化疗手术中应当要考虑辐射的影响，特别是具有较高恶性肿瘤风险的 RB1 生殖 / 胚系基因突变的患者。

玻璃体腔内化学治疗用于视网膜母细胞瘤的难治性和复发性玻璃体腔种植，眼周注射作为辅助化学治疗。

经过治疗的视网膜母细胞瘤有时会完全消失，但更多的是以钙化团块持续存在（1 型，或“松软奶酪”模式），或非钙化的半透明灰色病灶（2 型，或“鱼肉”模式），后者难以与未经治疗的肿瘤相鉴别。3 型的消退同时具有 1 型和 2 型的特点，4 型的消退呈平坦的萎缩瘢痕。治疗后的视网膜母细胞瘤的儿童需密切观察，是否有新的或复发的肿瘤，必要时可在麻醉状态下反复检查。

眼外视网膜母细胞瘤虽然在美国不常见，但在发展中国家仍是一个问题，主要是因为延误诊断。其 4 种主要类型有视神经受累、眼眶侵犯、中枢神经系统（CNS）受累和远处转移。眼外视网膜母细胞瘤的治疗有强化的多模式化学治疗、自体造血干细胞抢救和外放射治疗。如不累及中枢神经系统（CNS），患者可以长期无病生存，否则预后较差。

三侧性视网膜母细胞瘤，除视网膜母细胞瘤外，还有松果体或鞍旁原发性神经外胚层肿瘤（PNET）。单眼视网膜母细胞瘤患三侧性视网膜母细胞瘤的风险＜0.5%，双眼视网膜母细胞瘤的风险小于 5% ~ 15%。进行了化学减容治疗的患者，发生三侧性视网膜母细胞瘤的风险降低。三侧性视网膜母细胞瘤的治疗包括多种方式，但预后很差。

Abramson DH, Dunkel IJ, Brodie SE, Marr B, Gobin YP. Superselective ophthalmic artery chemotherapy as primary treatment for retinoblastoma (chemosurgery). *Ophthalmology.* 2010;117(8):1623–1629.

Shields CL, Alset AE, Say EA, Caywood E, Jabbour P, Shields JA. Retinoblastoma control with primary intra-arterial chemotherapy: outcomes before and during the intravitreal chemotherapy era. *J Pediatr Ophthalmol Strabismus.* 2016;53(5):275–284.

Monitoring Identification of *RB1* mutations is very useful in determining how frequently to monitor patients. Patients with unilateral tumors who have somatic mutations are not at risk for development of additional tumors (ocular or systemic). Patients who undergo globe salvage require frequent examinations to monitor for tumor recurrence. In these patients, examinations under anesthesia are typically performed every 4–8 weeks until age 3 years. Recurrence of retinoblastoma is common and can occur years after treatment.

In patients with germline mutations, periodic MRI of the brain is performed to screen for CNS metastases and PNET, which have poor prognoses. Results of genetic testing can also help determine whether siblings need to be monitored. If genetic testing is not available, siblings should be monitored routinely during the first 2 years of life.

Because of their risk of developing secondary malignancies, patients with germline mutations require long-term follow-up by oncologists and ophthalmologists. Nonocular tumors are common in these patients; the estimated incidence rate is 1% per year of life (eg, 10% prevalence by age 10 years, 30% by age 30 years). The incidence is higher among patients treated with external-beam radiation before 1 year of age. The most common secondary tumors (and the mean age at diagnosis) are PNET (2.7 years), sarcoma (13 years), melanoma (27 years), and carcinomas (29 years). For patients with second nonocular tumors, the risk of additional malignant tumors is even greater.

Correa ZM, Berry JL. Review of retinoblastoma. Pediatric Ophthalmology Education Center. April 28, 2016. Available at https://www. aao. org/disease-review/review-of-retinoblastoma.

Woo KI, Harbour JW. Review of 676 second primary tumors in patients with retinoblastoma: association between age at onset and tumor type. *Arch Ophthalmol.* 2010;128(7):865–870.

Acquired Disorders

Coats Disease

The classic findings in Coats disease are yellow subretinal and intraretinal lipid exudates associated with retinal vascular abnormalities—most often telangiectasia, tortuosity, aneurysmal dilatations, and retinal capillary nonperfusion. The clinical presentation varies, ranging from mild changes to total retinal detachment (Fig 25-29).

Males are affected more frequently than females, and the condition is usually, but not always, unilateral. The average age at diagnosis is 6–8 years, but the disease has also been observed in infants. The etiology of Coats disease is unknown. Associations with various gene deletions have been reported, but the disease is isolated in most cases.

Abramson DH, Dunkel IJ, Brodie SE, Marr B, Gobin YP. Superselective ophthalmic artery chemotherapy as primary treatment for retinoblastoma (chemosurgery). *Ophthalmology*. 2010;117(8):1623–1629.

Shields CL, Alset AE, Say EA, Caywood E, Jabbour P, Shields JA. Retinoblastoma control with primary intra-arterial chemotherapy: outcomes before and during the intravitreal chemotherapy era. *J Pediatr Ophthalmol Strabismus*. 2016;53(5):275–284.

监测　*RB1* 基因突变的鉴定有助于确定随访频率。体细胞基因突变的单眼肿瘤的患者没有发生其他肿瘤（眼部或全身）的风险。保留眼球治疗的患儿需频繁检查，以监测肿瘤的复发。常间隔 4 ~ 8 周行麻醉下检查，直至 3 岁。视网膜母细胞瘤的复发很常见，治疗后数年仍可复发。

生殖系突变的患者需定期进行头部磁共振成像（MRI），以筛查预后较差的中枢神经系统（CNS）转移和原发性神经外胚层肿瘤（PNET）。基因检测的结果可以帮助确定是否需要监测患者的兄弟姐妹。如果没有条件进行基因测试，其兄弟姐妹应在 2 岁前进行常规监测。

生殖系突变患者有继发恶性肿瘤的风险，需要肿瘤科和眼科医生进行长期随访。常见非眼部肿瘤，发病率每年增加 1%（如 10 岁的患病率为 10%，30 岁的患病率则为 30%），1 岁前有过外放射治疗的患者发病率更高。最常见的继发性肿瘤（和平均诊断年龄）是原发性神经外胚层肿瘤 PNET（2.7 岁）、肉瘤（13 岁）、黑色素瘤（27 岁）和癌（29 岁）。患有第 2 种非眼部肿瘤的患者，发生其他恶性肿瘤的风险会更大。

Correa ZM, Berry JL. Review of retinoblastoma. Pediatric Ophthalmology Education Center. April 28, 2016. Available at https://www. aao. org/disease-review/review-of-retinoblastoma.

Woo KI, Harbour JW. Review of 676 second primary tumors in patients with retinoblastoma: association between age at onset and tumor type. *Arch Ophthalmol*. 2010;128(7):865–870.

获得性疾病

Coats 病

Coats 病的典型表现是视网膜下和视网膜内黄色脂质渗出物，伴视网膜血管异常，后者常表现为毛细血管扩张、扭曲、动脉瘤样扩张和视网膜毛细血管无灌注。临床表现变异很大，可从轻度改变到全视网膜脱离（图 25–29）。

男性比女性更易发病，多累及单眼，平均确诊年龄为 6 ~ 8 岁，但也可见于婴儿。Coats 病的病因尚不明，已报道与多种基因缺失有关，但多数发病呈散发性。

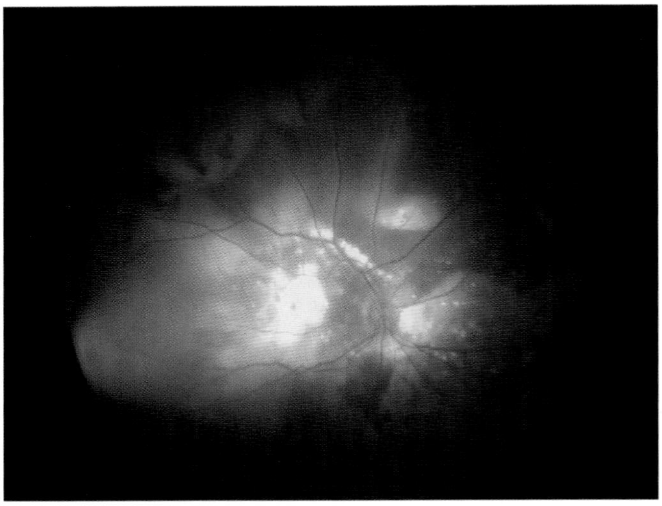

Figure 25-29 Advanced Coats disease with extensive subretinal exudation and total retinal detachment. Superior retinal macrocysts—associated with macroaneurysms and dilatated, tortuous vessels—are present. *(Courtesy of Scott C. Oliver, MD.)*

Diagnosis

The diagnosis of Coats disease requires the presence of abnormal retinal vessels, which occasionally are small and difficult to find. The subretinal exudate is thought to come from the leaking anomalous vessels. Fluorescein angiography may be helpful in identifying leakage from the telangiectatic vessels and in assessing the effectiveness of therapy (Fig 25-30). Oral fluorescein can be used in place of intravenous fluorescein in the ambulatory setting to monitor disease and avoid examination under anesthesia.

A 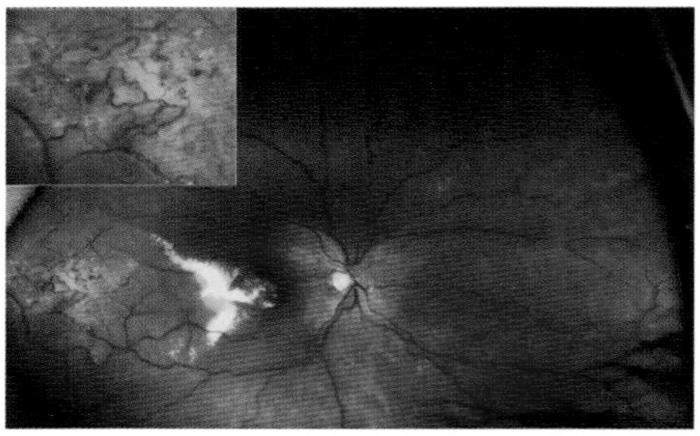 B 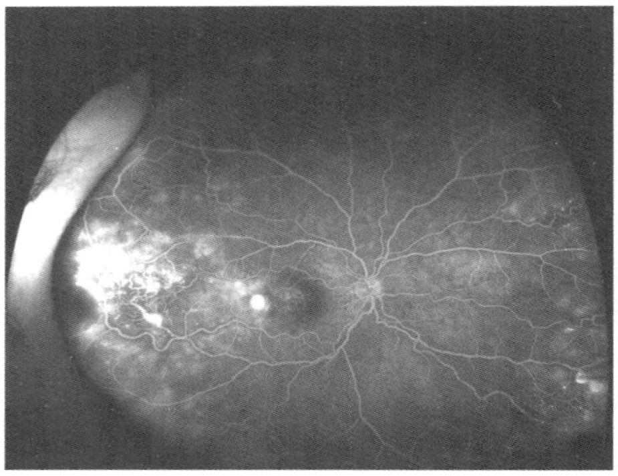

Figure 25-30 Coats disease. **A,** Ultra-wide-angle color photograph reveals foveal exudation with temporal macroaneurysms and telangiectasias. Inset shows magnification of macroaneurysms and telangiectasias. Subtle nasal telangiectasias are also present. **B,** Image obtained with oral fluorescein angiography shows extensive leakage from temporal macroaneurysms, mild leakage from temporal and nasal telangiectasias, and macular leakage with some staining. *(Courtesy of Scott C. Oliver, MD.)*

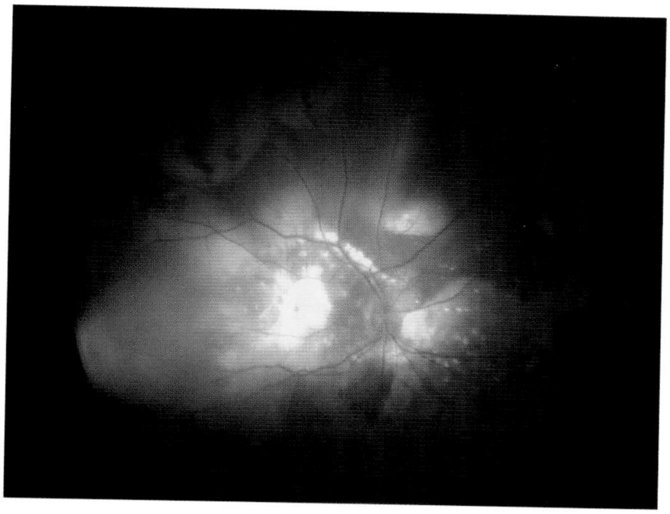

图 25-29　晚期 Coats 病伴广泛视网膜下渗出和全视网膜脱离。上方视网膜大囊肿，伴大动脉瘤和扩张扭曲的血管。*（译者注：资料来源见前页原文。）*

诊断

Coats 病的诊断需存在异常视网膜血管，偶见异常血管很小，不易被发现。视网膜下渗出源于异常血管的渗漏。荧光血管造影有助于识别这些毛细血管扩张的渗漏和评估治疗效果（图 25-30）。在便携式设备中，口服荧光剂可以代替静脉注射荧光素，监测病情，避免麻醉。

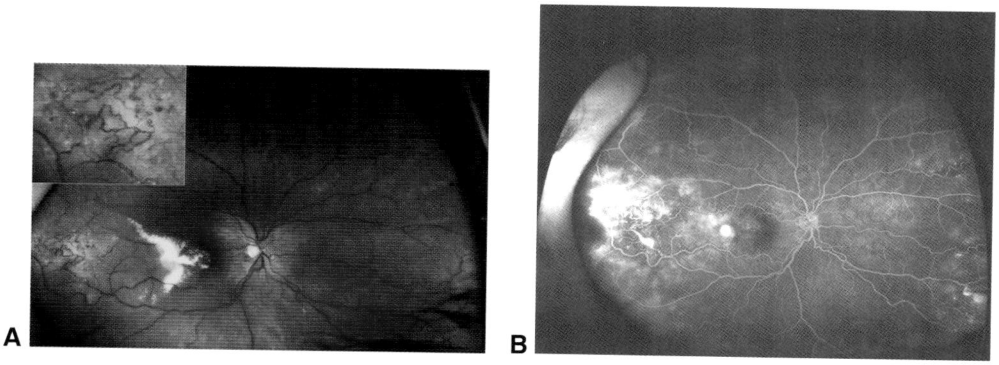

图 25-30　Costs 病。**A.** 超广角彩色照片显示，中心凹渗出伴有颞侧大动脉瘤和毛细血管扩张；小插图为大动脉瘤和毛细血管扩张的放大图像，鼻侧毛细血管略微扩张。**B.** 口服荧光血管造影显示，颞侧大动脉瘤广泛渗漏、颞侧和鼻侧扩张毛细血管轻度渗漏、黄斑渗漏和染色。*（译者注：资料来源见前页原文。）*

The differential diagnosis includes persistentfetal vasculature, ROP, toxocariasis, FEVR, Norrie disease, retinal dysplasia, endophthalmitis, leukemia, and retinoblastoma. Calcium is frequently detected by ultrasonography in retinoblastoma but is distinctly rare in Coats disease. Coats disease often presents with xanthocoria (yellow pupillary reflex), whereas retinoblastoma presents with leukocoria.

Treatment

Treatment is directed at obliterating the abnormal leaking vessels and includes cryotherapy, laser photocoagulation, vitrectomy, and silicone oil. Exudative retinal detachments and subretinal fibrosis develop in eyes with progressive disease. Once the fovea is detached and the subretinal exudate becomes or ga nized, the prognosis for restoration of central vision is poor. Use of intravitreal bevacizumab in addition to laser treatment has been reported, but one study found that this approach was associated with a higher incidence of vitreoretinal fibrosis and tractional retinal detachment.

Mulvihill A, Morris B. A population-based study of Coats disease in the United Kingdom II: investigation, treatment, and outcomes. *Eye (Lond).* 2010;24(12):1802–1807.

Ramasubramanian A, Shields CL. Bevacizumab for Coats disease with exudative retinal detachment and risk of vitreoretinal traction. *Br J Ophthalmol.* 2012;96(3):356–359.

鉴别诊断有永久性胎儿血管、早产儿视网膜病变（ROP）、弓蛔虫病、家族性渗出性玻璃体视网膜病变 FEVR、Norrie 病、视网膜发育不良、眼内炎、白血病和视网膜母细胞瘤。视网膜母细胞瘤的超声检查常见钙化回声，但 Coats 病罕见。Coats 病常表现为黄瞳症（黄色瞳孔反光），而视网膜母细胞瘤则为白瞳症。

治疗

治疗旨在消除异常渗漏血管，方法有冷冻治疗、激光光凝、玻璃体切除术和硅油填充。进展期可形成渗出性视网膜脱离和视网膜下纤维化。一旦中央凹视网膜脱离且视网膜下渗出物机化，中心视力的恢复很差。除激光治疗外，可使用玻璃体腔内注射贝伐单抗，但有研究发现这可能会导致玻璃体视网膜纤维化和牵拉性视网膜脱离发生率的增加。

Mulvihill A, Morris B. A population-based study of Coats disease in the United Kingdom II: investigation, treatment, and outcomes. *Eye (Lond)*. 2010;24(12):1802–1807.

Ramasubramanian A, Shields CL. Bevacizumab for Coats disease with exudative retinal detachment and risk of vitreoretinal traction. *Br J Ophthalmol*. 2012;96(3):356–359.

（翻译　赵晓燕　孙新成　马君鑫 // 审校　刘虎　石一宁　蒋宁 // 章节审校　石广礼）

CHAPTER 26

Optic Disc Abnormalities

This chapter includes a related video, which can be accessed by scanning the QR code provided in the text or going to www. aao. org/ bcscvideo_ section06.

Developmental Anomalies

Developmental abnormalities of the optic nerve may or may not limit vision. To maximize visual potential in a child with an optic disc (also called *optic nerve head*) abnormality, treatment of possible superimposed amblyopia should always be considered.

Optic Nerve Hypoplasia

Optic nerve hypoplasia (ONH), the most common developmental optic disc anomaly, is characterized by a decreased number of optic nerve axons. It can be unilateral, bilateral, or segmental and is often asymmetric if bilateral. The typical affected disc can be pale, gray, and relatively small with vascular tortuosity (Fig 26-1A). A yellow-to-white ring around the disc (corresponding to abnormal extension of retina over the lamina cribrosa), known as the *double ring sign*, may be present. When the double ring sign is present, the hypoplastic disc–ring complex can be mistaken for a normal-sized optic nerve with normal cup–disc ratio (Fig 26-1B, C).

Visual acuity can range from 20/20 to no light perception. The extent of papillomacular fiber involvement and any associated amblyopia determines visual acuity.

ONH is usually idiopathic and sporadic. It is more prevalent in fetal alcohol syndrome. Segmental ONH may be associated with maternal diabetes mellitus. ONH may be associated with central nervous system (CNS) abnormalities and pituitary gland dysfunction.

Septo-optic dysplasia (*de Morsier syndrome*) is the association of ONH with absence of the septum pellucidum and agenesis of the corpus callosum (Figs 26-2, 26-3). As isolated abnormalities, these neuroimaging findings are not associated with neurodevelopmental or endocrinologic problems. Cerebral hemisphere abnormalities such as schizencephaly, periventricular leukomalacia, and encephalomalacia occur in approximately 45% of patients with ONH and are associated with neurodevelopmental defects.

第 26 章

视盘异常

本章所包含的相关视频，可通过扫描文中的二维码或访问网站 www.aao.org/bcscvideo_section06 观看。

发育异常

视神经发育异常可能影响视力，也可能不影响。为了使视盘异常（又称*视神经头部*）儿童的视觉潜力得以最充分发育，应对合并的弱视进行治疗。

视神经发育不良

视神经发育不良（ONH）是最常见的发育性视盘异常，其特征是视神经轴突数量减少，呈单眼、双眼或节段的，若是双眼则常不对称。典型的受累视盘呈浅灰色，相对较小，血管弯曲（图 26–1A）。视盘围绕着黄到白的环（对应于筛板上视网膜的异常延伸），称为*双环征*。当出现双环征时，可将发育不全的盘 – 环复合体误认为是正常大小的视神经，以及伴有正常的杯 – 盘比（图 26–1B，C）。

视力从 20/20 到无光感，视力取决于乳头黄斑纤维受累程度和伴随的弱视。

视神经发育不良 ONH 常为特发和散发的，更多见于胎儿酒精综合征。节段性视神经发育不良（ONH）与母亲糖尿病有关。视神经发育不良（ONH）可伴有中枢神经系统（CNS）异常和垂体功能障碍。

*视隔发育不良（综合征）*是视神经发育不良（ONH），伴透明隔缺失和胼胝体发育不全（图 26–2，图 26–3）。孤立病变的神经影像学表现，并不伴有神经发育异常或内分泌异常。45% 的视神经发育不良（ONH）出现大脑半球异常，如脑裂畸形、脑室周围白质软化和脑软化，并伴有神经发育缺陷。

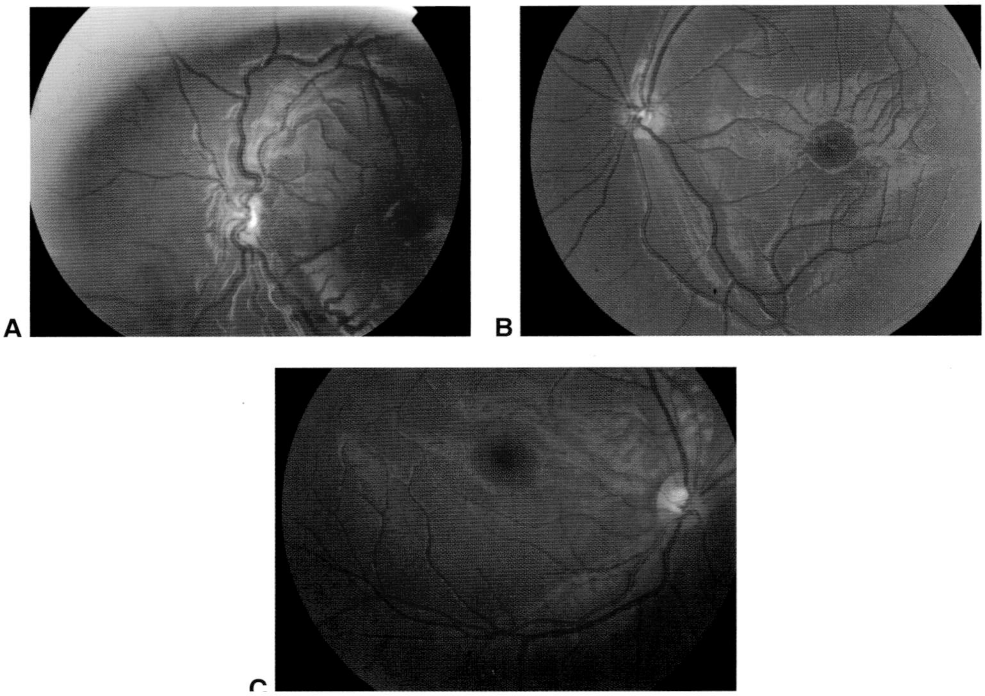

Figure 26-1 **A,** Left optic nerve hypoplasia. Note the small, pale disc with vascular tortuosity. **B,** Left optic nerve hypoplasia with the double ring sign. When viewed quickly, the hypoplastic disc–ring complex may be mistaken for a normal-sized optic nerve. **C,** The normal right optic disc of the patient shown in part B. *(Courtesy of Arif O. Khan, MD.)*

Patients with ONH can have pituitary gland abnormalities, which are important to rule out in children who present with ONH. Magnetic resonance imaging (MRI) in affected patients reveals an ectopic posterior pituitary bright spot at the upper infundibulum. This finding is associated with pituitary hormone deficiencies, including growth hormone deficiency, hypothyroidism, hyperprolactinemia, hypocortisolism, panhypopituitarism, and diabetes insipidus. A history of neonatal jaundice suggests hypothyroidism; neonatal hypoglycemia or seizures indicate possible panhypopituitarism. Patients with ONH and hypocortisolism, especially with diabetes insipidus, can have problems with thermal regulation and dehydration and must be monitored carefully during febrile illnesses.

Children with periventricular leukomalacia can have a variant of ONH that may be mistaken for glaucomatous cupping. The optic nerve has a large cup within a normal-sized optic disc secondary to transsynaptic degeneration of optic axons, a consequence of lesions in the optic radiations. This form of ONH is not associated with endocrine deficiencies.

Garcia-Filion P, Borchert M. Optic nerve hypoplasia syndrome: a review of the epidemiology and clinical associations. *Curr Treat Options Neurol.* 2013;15(1):78–89.

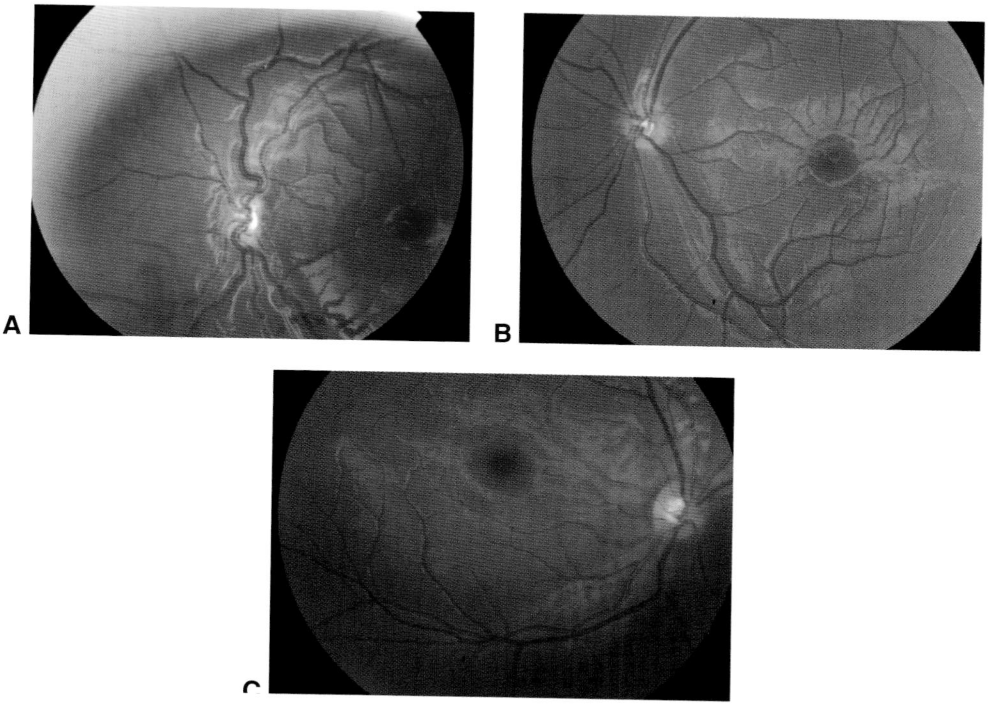

图 26–1　**A.** 左眼视神经发育不良。可见小而苍白的视盘，伴血管扭曲。**B.** 左眼视神经发育不全伴双环征。快速看时，发育不全的盘 – 环复合体可能被误认为是正常视神经。**C.**B 图的右眼正常视神经盘。*（译者注：资料来源见前页原文。）*

视神经发育不良（ONH）可有垂体异常，这是排除视神经发育不良（ONH）的重要指征。患儿磁共振成像（MRI）显示，上漏斗管有一个异位垂体后叶亮点，同时伴有垂体激素缺乏，包括生长激素缺乏、甲状腺功能减退、高催乳素血症、肾上腺皮质功能减退、全垂体功能减退和尿崩症。新生儿黄疸史提示，甲状腺功能减退，新生儿低血糖症或癫痫发作提示可能伴全垂体功能减退。患视神经发育不良（ONH）和肾上腺皮质功能减退者，特别是伴尿崩症时，可能会出现热调节问题和脱水现象，所以在发热性疾病期间需严密监测。

伴室周白质软化症的儿童有多种视神经发育不良（ONH）的表现，可能被误诊为青光眼视杯。视神经呈现在正常大小的视盘内有一个较大的视杯，继发于视神经轴突的跨突触变性，是视神经辐射损伤的结果。这种视神经发育不良（ONH）不伴有内分泌功能缺陷。

Garcia-Filion P, Borchert M. Optic nerve hypoplasia syndrome: a review of the epidemiology and clinical associations. *Curr Treat Options Neurol.* 2013;15(1):78–89.

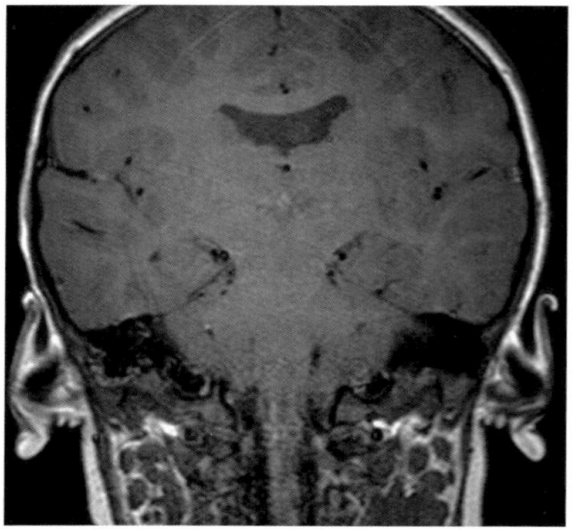

Figure 26-2 Coronal T1-weighted magnetic resonance imaging (MRI) scan of the lateral ventricles: the septum pellucidum (interventricular septum) is absent. *(Courtesy of Jane L. Weissman, MD.)*

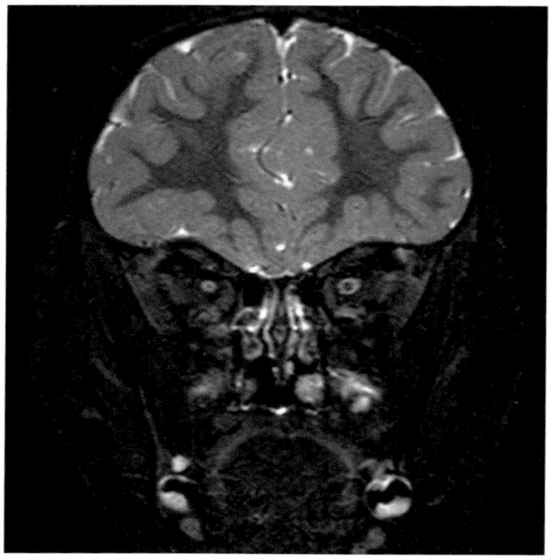

Figure 26-3 Coronal T2-weighted MRI scan of the orbits: the right optic nerve is smaller and more T2 hyperintense than the left optic nerve. *(Courtesy of Jane L. Weissman, MD.)*

Morning Glory Disc Anomaly

Morning glory disc anomaly (MGDA) is the result of abnormal development of the distal optic stalk at its junction with the primitive optic vesicle. The anomaly is typically unilateral and is more common in girls. Serous retinal detachments occur in one-third of cases.
MGDA has been associated with basal encephalocele in patients with midline abnormalities, PHACE syndrome (*p*osterior fossa malformations, *h*emangiomas, *a*rterial lesions, *c*ardiac and *e*ye anomalies), and carotid circulation abnormalities (moyamoya disease).

MGDA typically appears as a funnel-shaped excavation of the posterior fundus that incorporates an enlarged optic disc with elevated surrounding retinal pigment epithelium and an increased number of blood vessels looping at the edges of the disc (Fig 26-4). A core of white glial tissue occupies the normal position of the optic cup. This tissue may have contractile elements, as the optic cup can sometimes be seen to open and close with some periodicity.

Visual acuity ranges from 20/20 to no light perception, but it is usually 20/100 to 20/200. Because of the potential for associated CNS abnormalities, MRI and MR angiography should be considered.

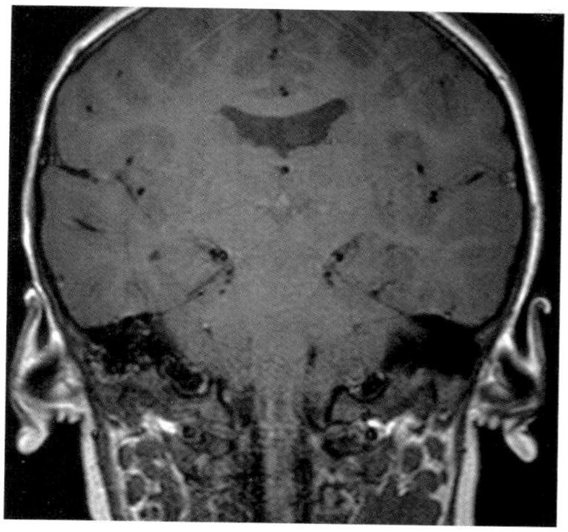

图 26–2　冠状位 T1– 加权磁共振（MRI）扫描侧脑室：透明膈（室间膈）缺如。*（译者注：资料来源见前页原文。）*

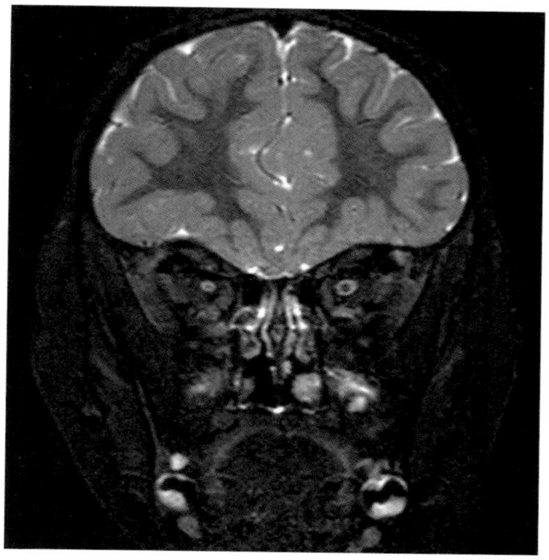

图 26–3　冠状位 T2– 加权磁共振（MRI）扫描眼眶：右眼视神经较小，且与左眼视神经相比，呈 T2 高信号。*（译者注：资料来源见前页原文。）*

牵牛花综合征

牵牛花综合征（MGDA）是远端视柄与原始视泡交界处的发育异常，常为单眼，多见于女性。1/3 病例发生浆液性视网膜脱离。

牵牛花综合征（MGDA）伴有基底脑膨出和中线异常，后者包括 PHACE 综合征（即后颅窝畸形、血管瘤、动脉病变、心脏异常和眼异常）和颈动脉循环异常（脑底异常血管网病 / 云雾病）。

牵牛花综合征（MGDA）典型表现为后级部的漏斗状深凹陷，其中有增大的视盘、环绕视盘并略增高的色素上皮和在视盘边缘增多的血管攀（图 26–4）。白色胶质组织居于视杯位置，具有收缩成分，可见视杯周期性打开和关闭。

视力从 20/20 到无光感，多为 20/200 ~ 20/100。因为多伴有中枢神经系统异常，应考虑行磁共振（MRI）和磁共振血管造影（MRA）检查。

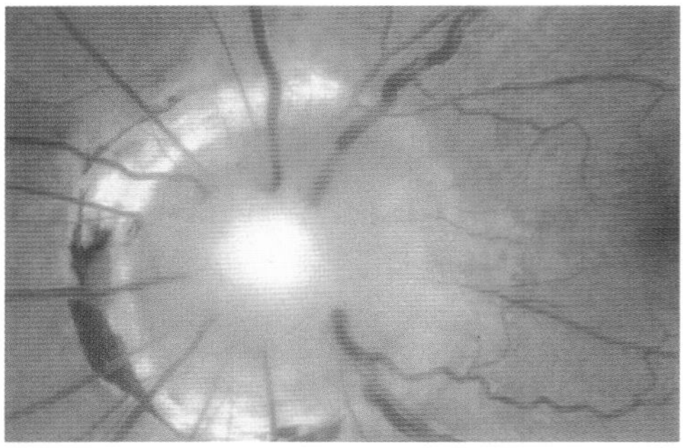

Figure 26-4 Morning glory disc anomaly, left eye.

Optic Nerve Coloboma

Optic nerve coloboma results from incomplete closure of the embryonic fissure. It can be associated with iris coloboma and adjacent or peripheral chorioretinal coloboma. Optic nerve coloboma can be unilateral or bilateral and is often asymmetric.

Typically, there is an inferonasal excavation of the optic disc that, when mild, may be confused with glaucomatous damage. More extensive defects appear as an enlargement of the peripapillary area with a deep central excavation lined by a glistening white tissue; blood vessels overlie this deep cavity (Fig 26-5). When chorioretinal coloboma is coexistent, there is a risk for retinal detachment. Visual acuity is related to involvement of the papillomacular or foveal region and is difficult to predict.

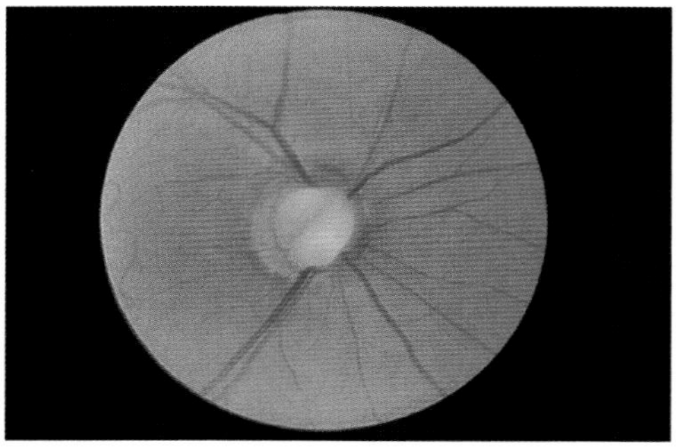

Figure 26-5 Optic nerve coloboma, right eye.

Ocular colobomas may be associated with multiple systemic abnormalities and a number of syndromes, such as the CHARGE syndrome (*c*oloboma, *h*eart defects, *c*hoanal atresia, *m*ental retardation, *g*enitourinary abnormalities, and *e*ar abnormalities).

Optic Nerve Pit

Optic nerve pit (optic hole) represents herniation of dysplastic retina into a collagen-lined pocket extending posteriorly, often into the subarachnoid space, through a defect in the lamina cribrosa. It is typically unilateral. There is an association with serous macular detachments in the second and third decades of life.

The typical appearance is a round or oval, gray, white, or yellowish depression in the inferotemporal quadrant or central portion of the disc, often covered with a gray veil of tissue and emerging cilioretinal vessels (Fig 26-6).

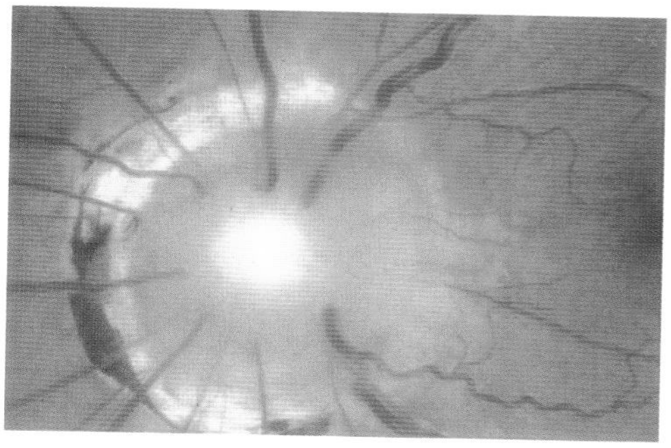

图 26–4　牵牛花综合征，左眼。

视神经缺损

视神经缺损是胚胎裂闭合不全，可伴虹膜缺损及邻近或周围脉络膜视网膜缺损。视神经缺损可以是单眼或双眼，常不对称。

典型表现为视盘鼻下方的深凹陷，轻度凹陷可能与青光眼损害混淆。广泛的缺损表现为视盘周围区域的扩大和中央深凹陷，后者内衬闪亮的白色组织，其上覆盖有血管（图 26–5）。当脉络膜视网膜缺损并存时，有视网膜脱离的风险。视力难以预测，与累及的乳头黄斑区或中央凹区有关。

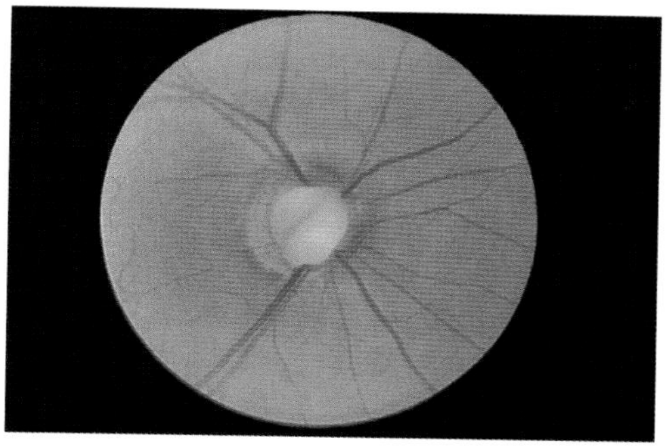

图 26–5　视神经缺损，左眼。

眼部缺损可能与多种系统性异常和多种综合征有关，如 CHARGE 综合征［即眼组织缺损（*c*oloboma）、心脏缺陷（*h*eart defects）、后鼻孔闭锁（*c*oloboma atresia）、智力发育迟缓（*m*ental retardation）、泌尿生殖系统异常（*g*enitourinary abnormalities）和耳朵异常（*e*ar abnormalities）］。

视神经小凹

视神经小凹（视孔）是指发育不良的视网膜疝通过筛板上的缺陷，进入向后延伸内衬胶原囊袋，并进入蛛网膜下腔。常是单眼，20 ~ 30 岁发生浆液性黄斑脱离。

典型的表现是颞下象限或视盘中央的圆形或椭圆形灰色、白色或黄色凹陷，常被灰色膜组织和睫网血管覆盖（图 26–6）。

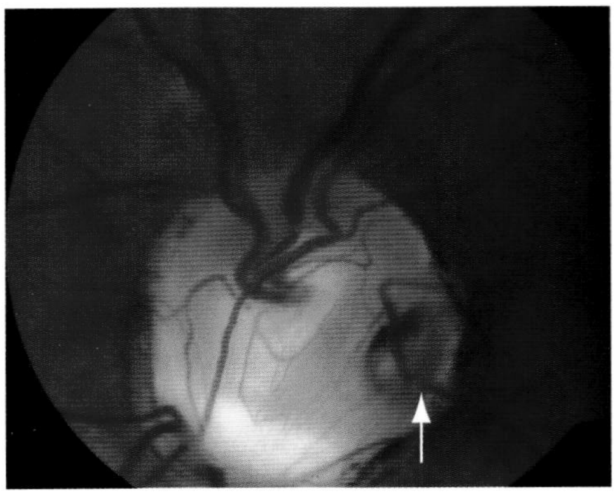

Figure 26-6 Left optic nerve with a temporal optic nerve pit (*arrow*) and a mild inferonasal disc coloboma. Cilioretinal vessels can be seen emanating from the optic nerve pit. *(Courtesy of Paul Phillips, MD.)*

Some have considered this entity to be a variant of coloboma, but it is distinct and there is no association with iris or chorioretinal coloboma.

Myelinated Retinal Nerve Fiber Layer

Myelination of the optic nerve normally stops at the lamina cribrosa. Inappropriate myelination anterior to the lamina cribrosa causes scotomata or central vision loss. Particularly when the macula is involved, myelinated retinal nerve fibers are associated with ipsilateral high myopia and resultant anisometropic amblyopia. In some cases, the macula is hypoplastic.

Clinically, myelinated nerve fibers appear as a white superficial retinal area, the frayed and feathered edges of which tend to follow the same orientation as that of the normal retinal nerve fibers (Fig 26-7). Retinal vessels that pass within the superficial layer of the nerve fibers are obscured. The myelinated fibers may occur as a single spot or as several noncontiguous patches. The most common location is along the disc margin.

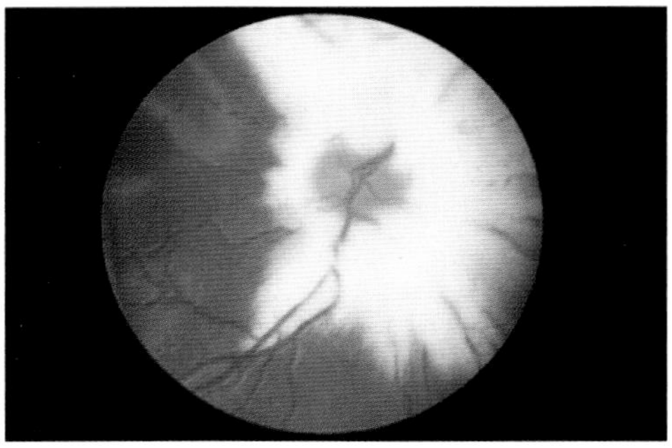

Figure 26-7 Myelinated nerve fibers of the optic nerve and retina, right eye.

Tilted Disc

In a patient with a tilted disc, often the superior pole of the optic disc appears elevated, with posterior displacement of the inferior nasal disc. Alternatively, the disc is tilted horizontally, resulting in an oval disc with an oblique long axis (Fig 26-8). Tilted disc is often associated with a scleral crescent located inferiorly or inferonasally, situs inversus, posterior ectasia of the inferior nasal fundus, and myopia and astigmatism.

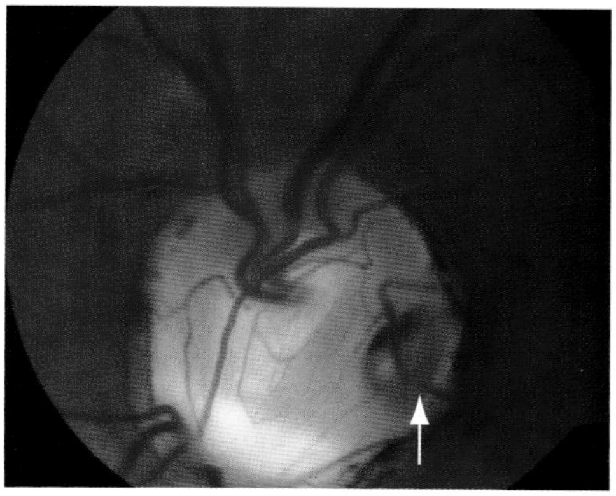

图 26–6　左眼视神经，伴颞侧视神经小凹（*箭头*）和轻度鼻下方视盘缺损。可见睫网血管从视神经小凹发出。（*译者注：资料来源见前页原文。*）

有人认为本质上这是眼缺损的一种变异，但是特殊的，不伴有虹膜或脉络膜视网膜缺损。

髓鞘神经纤维层

视神经髓鞘化在筛板处终止，筛板前的髓鞘会导致暗点或中央视力丧失，特别是累及黄斑，髓鞘神经纤维伴同侧高度近视，导致屈光参差性弱视。有时黄斑发育不良。

临床上，髓鞘神经纤维表现为视网膜浅层白色病灶、边缘不齐的羽毛状，沿正常视网膜神经纤维的方向分布（图 26–7），遮蔽经过神经纤维表层的视网膜血管。髓鞘神经纤维也可呈单个斑点或几个不接续的斑块，多见于视盘边缘。

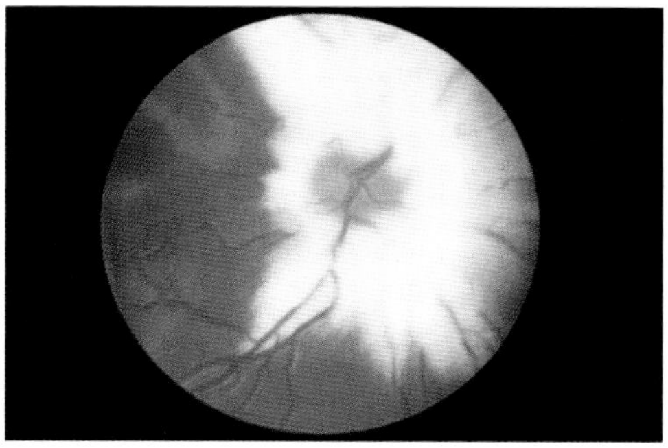

图 26–7　视神经和视网膜的髓鞘神经纤维，右眼。

视盘倾斜

视盘倾斜常表现为视盘上方常隆起、视盘鼻下方向后移位。也表现为视盘水平倾斜，呈椭圆形视盘、长轴斜行（图 26–8）。倾斜视盘常伴有巩膜弧形斑，位于下方或鼻下方，逆转 / 转位，鼻下方眼底后扩张，近视和散光。

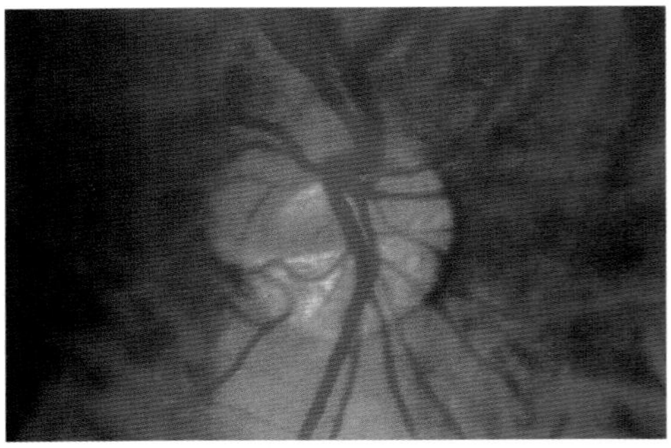

Figure 26-8 Tilted disc, right eye.

Patients may demonstrate superotemporal visual field defects, which may resolve with refractive correction. Tilted discs, myopic astigmatism, bilateral decreased vision, and visual difficulty at night suggest the possibility of X-linked congenital stationary night blindness (see Chapter 25). Acquired tilted disc and peripapillary crescent formation have been documented in children with myopic progression.

Kim TW, Kim M, Weinreb RN, et al. Optic disc changes with incipient myopia of childhood. *Ophthalmology.* 2012;119(1):21–26.

Bergmeister Papilla

A form of persistentfetal vasculature, Bergmeister papilla is a benign prepapillary glial remnant of the hyaloid artery, which is normally resorbed before birth. In some cases, a hyaloid artery remnant extends from the optic disc to the lens (typically inferonasally) and may contain blood.

Megalopapilla

Megalopapilla is an abnormally large optic disc (area $>2.5mm^2$). The commonly associated large cup can be mistaken for glaucomatous damage.

Peripapillary Staphyloma

Peripapillary staphyloma is a posterior bulging of the sclera encompassing the optic disc. White sclera encircling the disc is often visible. Vision is usually poor. The condition is usually unilateral and rarely bilateral.

Optic Nerve Aplasia

Optic nerve aplasia, a lack of optic nerve axons and retinal blood vessels, is very rare. The choroidal pattern is clearly visible. When bilateral, optic nerve aplasia is usually associated with other CNS malformations; when unilateral, it can occur with normal brain development.

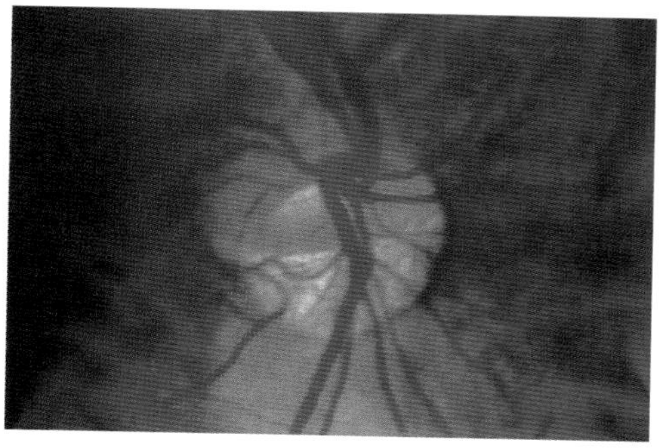

图 26-8 视盘倾斜，右眼。

患者可表现为颞上方视野缺损，可用屈光矫正。倾斜的视盘、近视性散光、双眼视力下降、夜间视力障碍均需考虑 X- 染色体的先天性静止型夜盲症（见第 25 章）。获得性倾斜视盘和乳头周弧形斑形成则为儿童进行性近视。

Kim TW, Kim M, Weinreb RN, et al. Optic disc changes with incipient myopia of childhood. *Ophthalmology*. 2012;119(1):21–26.

Bergmeister 乳头

Bergmeister 乳头是永久性胎儿血管的一种表现形式，是玻璃体动脉在视盘前的胶质残留，正常时在出生前被吸收。有时玻璃体动脉残留从视盘延伸到晶状体（常见下鼻方），并可含有血液。

巨大视盘

巨大视盘是一个异常大的视盘（面积 >2.5mm²）。伴有的大视杯常被误诊为青光眼损害。

视神经盘旁葡萄肿

视盘周围葡萄肿是巩膜的后凸包绕视盘，视盘周围常可见白色巩膜，视力较差。常单眼，少为双眼。

视神经发育不全

视神经发育不全是一种缺乏视神经轴突和视网膜血管的异常，很罕见。脉络膜结构清晰可见。双眼视神经发育不良常伴有其他中枢神经系统畸形。单眼发病时，其大脑发育正常。

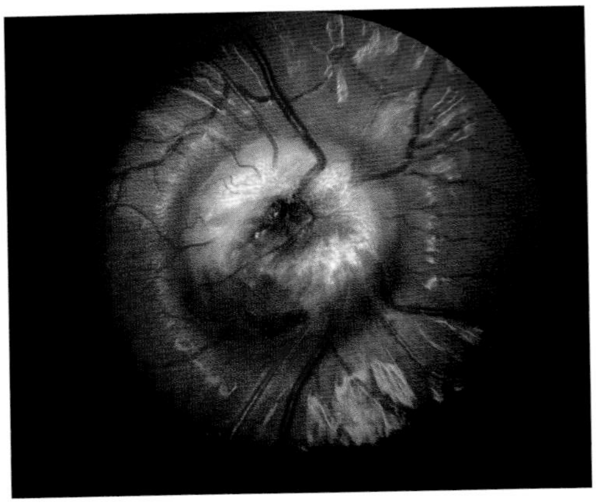

Figure 26-9 Melanocytoma of the optic disc and adjacent retina. *(Courtesy of Scott Lambert, MD.)*

Melanocytoma of the Optic Disc

Melanocytoma is a darkly pigmented tumor with little or no growth potential. It usually involves the optic disc and adjacent retina (Fig 26-9).

Optic Atrophy

Optic atrophy in children can be inherited (autosomal dominant, autosomal recessive, X-linked, or mitochondrial) or can be secondary to anterior visual pathway disease such as inflammation (optic neuritis), perinatal hypoxic–ischemic injury, hydrocephalus, or optic nerve or chiasmal tumors. Table 26-1 lists causes of acquired optic atrophy. Neuroimaging should be considered for all patients with optic atrophy of undetermined etiology because tumor or hydrocephalus is present in over 40% of these cases. Specific underlying gene defects may be inferred from coexisting systemic features (eg, Wolfram syndrome or Behr optic atrophy).

Table 26-1 Causes of Acquired Optic Atrophy in Childhood

Craniopharyngioma
Hereditary optic atrophy
Hydrocephalus
Optic nerve/chiasmal glioma
Optic neuritis
Perinatal hypoxic–ischemic injury
Postpapilledema
Retinal degenerative disease

Dominant Optic Atrophy, Kjer Type

Dominant optic atrophy is characterized by bilateral slow loss of central vision, usually before 10 years of age. It is caused by heterozygous mutations in *OPA1*. Visual acuity ranges from 20/40 to 20/100, with visual acuity rarely worse than 20/200. Visual field tests show central or cecocentral scotomata with normal peripheral isopters. Color vision testing reveals a blue dyschromatopsia. The optic disc shows a characteristic temporal wedge of pallor, often with triangular excavation (Fig 26-10).

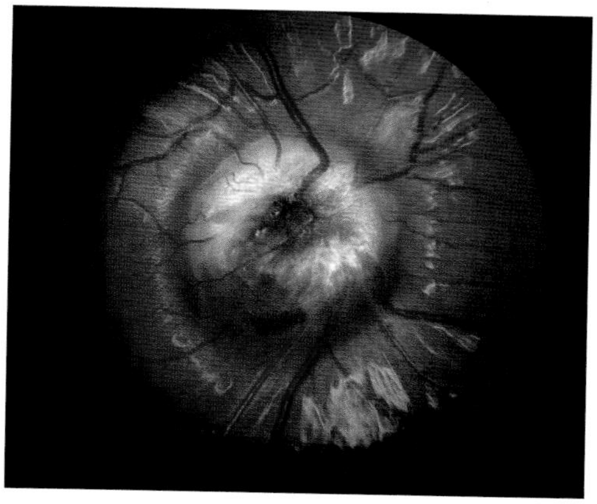

图 26–9　视盘黑素细胞瘤，视盘和周围视网膜。*（译者注：资料来源见前页原文。）*

视盘黑素细胞瘤

黑素细胞瘤是一种深色素肿瘤，几乎不生长，常累及视盘和周围视网膜（图 26–9）。

视神经萎缩

儿童的视神经萎缩可是遗传性的（常染色体显性、常染色体隐性、X– 连锁或线粒体），也可继发于前视路疾病，如炎症（视神经炎）、围产期缺氧缺血性损伤、脑积水、视神经或交叉肿瘤。表 26–1 列出了获得性视神经萎缩的原因。所有病因不明的视神经萎缩都应进行神经影像学检查，因为 40% 以上的患者有肿瘤或脑积水。特定的基因缺陷从共存的全身特征（如 Wolfram 综合征或 Behr 视神经萎缩）可以推断出来。

表 26–1　儿童期获得性视神经萎缩的原因

颅咽管瘤
遗传性视神经萎缩
脑积水
视神经/交叉的神经胶质瘤
视神经炎
围产期缺氧缺血损伤
后视神经乳头水肿
视网膜退行性疾病

显性遗传性视神经萎缩，Kjer 型

显性遗传性视神经萎缩的特征是 10 岁前双眼中央视力缓慢丧失，是 *OPA1* 杂合突变。视力 20/100 ~ 20/40，罕见＜ 20/200。视野检查显示中心或中心盲点性暗点伴正常周边等高线。色觉测试显示蓝色盲。视盘呈现一个典型的楔形颞侧苍白，呈三角形凹陷（图 26–10）。

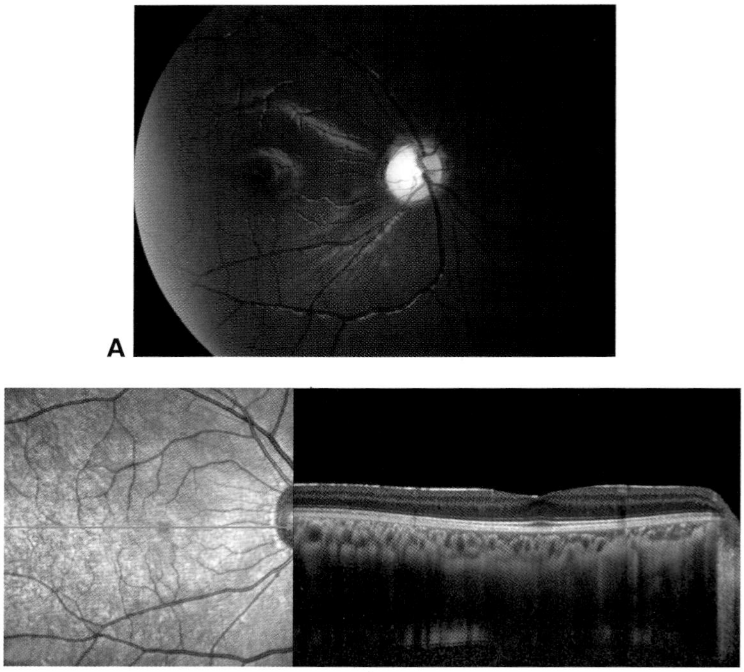

Figure 26-10 A, The optic disc, right eye, shows temporal pallor. The left eye was similar in this boy with dominant optic atrophy and confirmed heterozygous OPA1 mutation. B, Corresponding optical coherence tomography image shows a lack of nerve fiber and ganglion cell layers (left eye was similar). *(Courtesy of Arif O. Khan, MD.)*

Recessive Optic Atrophy

Recessive optic atrophy is characterized by severe bilateral vision loss before 5 years of age, often associated with nystagmus. Wolfram syndrome is optic atrophy caused by biallelic mutations in *WFS1*, with variable expressivity of hearing loss and diabetes mellitus. Similarly, Behr optic atrophy is caused by biallelic mutations in *OPA1*, with variable expressivity of neurologic findings such as ataxia, pyramidal signs, spasticity, bladder dysfunction, and intellectual disability.

Leber Hereditary Optic Neuropathy

Leber hereditary optic neuropathy is a maternally inherited (mitochondrial) disease characterized by acute or subacute bilateral loss of central vision, optic disc edema in the acute phase, acquired red-green dyschromatopsia, and central or cecocentral scotomata in otherwise healthy patients (usually males) in their second to fourth decade of life. See BCSC Section 5, *Neuro-Ophthalmology*, for further discussion.

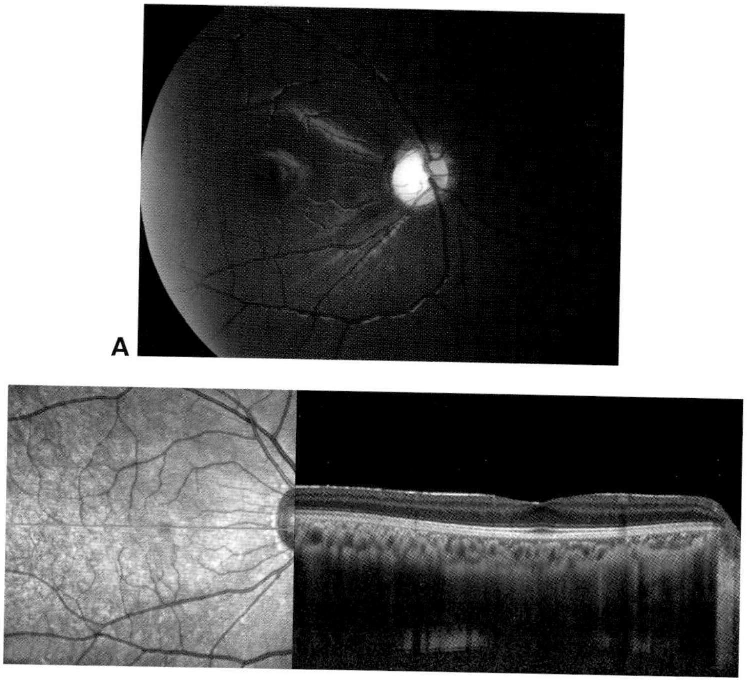

图 26-10　**A.** 视盘，右眼，显示颞部苍白。男孩的左眼改变相同，证实为 OPA1 的杂合突变的显性遗传性视神经萎缩。**B.** 相应的光学相干断层扫描图像显示，神经纤维和神经节细胞层缺失（左眼与之相同）。*（译者注：资料来源见前页原文。）*

隐性遗传性视神经萎缩

隐性遗传性视神经萎缩的特征是 5 岁前严重的双眼视力丧失，伴眼球震颤。Wolfram 综合征是 *WFS1* 双等位基因突变引起的视神经萎缩，伴多种形式的听力下降和糖尿病。同样，Behr 视神经萎缩是 *OPA1* 的双等位基因突变，表现为多种形式的神经系统异常，如共济失调、锥体征、痉挛、膀胱功能障碍和智力障碍。

Leber 遗传性视神经病变

Leber 遗传性视神经病变是一个母体遗传性（线粒体）疾病，其特征是急性或亚急性双眼中心视力丧失、急性期视盘水肿、获得性红绿色盲，或无症状患者（男性）在 20 ~ 40 岁出现中心或者中心盲点性暗点。详见 BCSC 第 5 册《*神经眼科学*》。

Optic Neuritis

Optic neuritis in childhood is often seen after systemic infections such as viral illnesses. It can also be associated with immunizations and bee stings. The cause of the postinfectious form of viral optic neuritis is unknown. It has been speculated that an autoimmune process, triggered by a previous viral infection, results in a demyelinating injury.

Optic neuritis in children, in contrast with that in adults, is more often bilateral and associated with disc edema. Vision loss can be severe. Over half of affected children have systemic symptoms, including headache, nausea, vomiting, lethargy, or malaise.

In children, optic neuritis can occur as an isolated neurologic deficit or as a component of more generalized neurologic disease, such as acute disseminated encephalomyelitis, neuromyelitis optica, or multiple sclerosis. The relationship between optic neuritis and the later development of multiple sclerosis, which is common in adults, is less clear in children. In a small subset of children with optic neuritis, signs and symptoms consistent with multiple sclerosis develop. Older age and MRI findings extrinsic to the visual system are associated with increased risk of multiple sclerosis.

Treatment of optic neuritis in children is controversial. As vision loss is often bilateral, treatment with intravenous corticosteroids should be considered in order to hasten visual recovery. The Optic Neuritis Treatment Trial did not specifically address the issue of treatment in children, so it is difficult to apply the results of this study to these patients. See also BCSC Section 5, *Neuro-Ophthalmology.*

Neuroretinitis denotes inflammatory disc edema associated with a stellate pattern of exudates in the macula (macular star; Fig 26-11). Common etiologies differ by region. In North America , a common etiology is *Bartonella henselae* infection (cat-scratch disease). Other infectious etiologies include mumps, toxocariasis, tuberculosis, and syphilis. Patients with neuroretinitis are not at risk for development of multiple sclerosis.

Children initially suspected to have optic neuritis should be reevaluated for potential emergence of macular edema, which would reclassify the diagnosis as neuroretinitis.

Waldman AT, Stull LB, Galetta SL, Balcer LJ, Liu GT. Pediatric optic neuritis and risk of multiple sclerosis: meta-analysis of observational studies. *J AAPOS.* 2011;15(5):441–446.

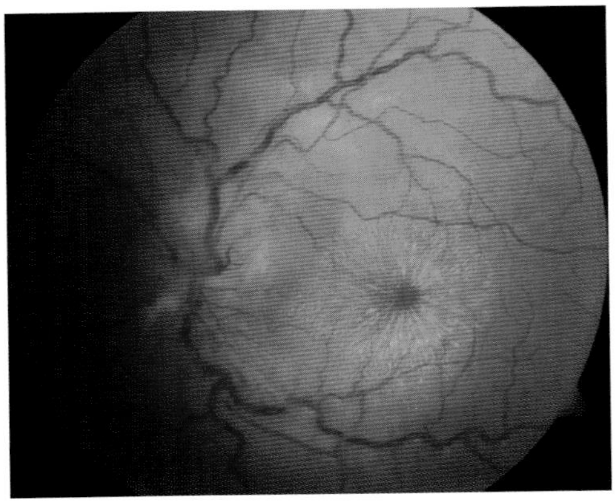

Figure 26-11 Neuroretinitis. Inflammatory optic disc edema with a macular star. *(Courtesy of Paul Phillips, MD.)*

视神经炎

儿童视神经炎常发生在全身感染后，如病毒感染，也可与免疫接种和蜜蜂叮咬有关。病毒感染后的视神经炎形成原因尚不清楚。据推测，之前的病毒感染引发自身免疫过程，导致脱髓鞘损伤。

与成人相比，儿童视神经炎常是双眼，伴视盘水肿，严重视力下降。1/2 以上的受累儿童有全身症状，包括头痛、恶心、呕吐、嗜睡或不适。

儿童中，视神经炎可表现为孤立的神经系统病变，也可为神经系统疾病的一部分，如急性播散性脑脊髓炎、视神经脊髓炎或多发性硬化症。儿童的视神经炎与多发性硬化症（多见于成人）晚期的发展关系尚不清楚。部分儿童视神经炎的进展与多发性硬化症症状和体征一致。大龄儿童和视觉系统以外的磁共振（MRI）检查异常，增加了多发性硬化的风险。

对于儿童视神经炎的治疗有争议。由于视力丧失呈双眼性的，应考虑静脉注射皮质类固醇，以加速视力康复。视神经炎治疗试验（*Neuritis Treatment Trial*）并没有明确强调儿童的治疗问题，因此很难将这项研究的结果应用于儿童患者。见 BCSC 第 5 册《*神经眼科学*》。

*视神经视网膜炎指炎*性视盘水肿，伴黄斑星状渗出（星状黄斑，图 26-11）。不同地区的病因不同。北美常见病因是*巴通体感染*（猫抓病）。其他感染原因有流行性腮腺炎、弓蛔虫病、结核和梅毒。

患视神经视网膜炎的患者不会发展为多发性硬化症。最初怀疑为视神经炎的儿童应再次评估是否存在黄斑水肿，以修正诊断为神经视网膜炎。

Waldman AT, Stull LB, Galetta SL, Balcer LJ, Liu GT. Pediatric optic neuritis and risk of multiple sclerosis: meta-analysis of observational studies. *J AAPOS*. 2011;15(5):441–446.

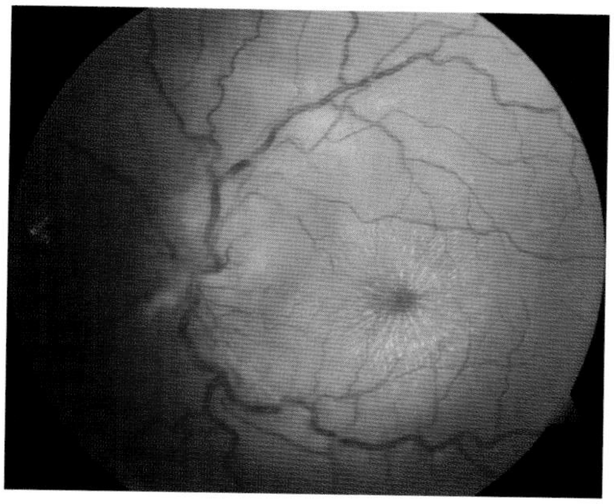

图 26–11　视神经视网膜炎。炎性视盘水肿，伴星状黄斑。*（译者注：资料来源见前页原文。）*

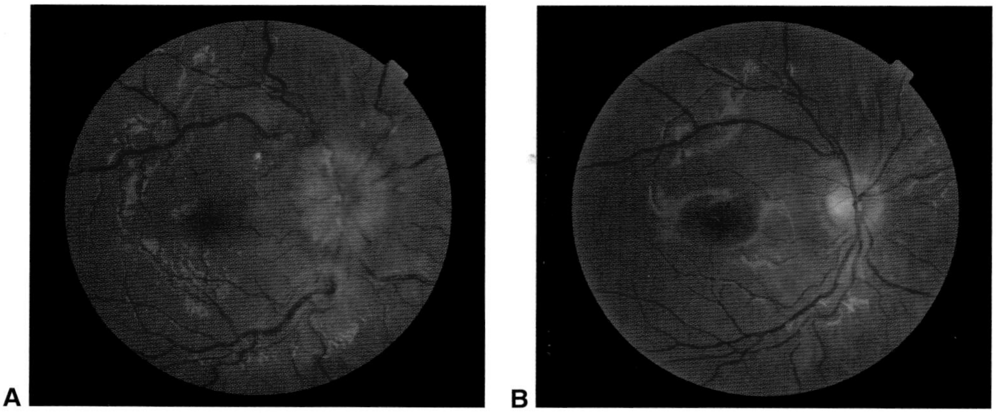

Figure 26-12 Papilledema in the right eye of a child with idiopathic intracranial hypertension before treatment **(A)** and 3 months after treatment with oral acetazolamide **(B).** Resolution in the left eye was similar. Also see Video 26-1. *(Courtesy of Robert W. Hered, MD.)*

Papilledema

Papilledema refers to optic disc edema secondary to elevated intracranial pressure (ICP) (Fig 26-12). It is typically bilateral. Initially, visual acuity, color vision, and pupillary reactions are normal. However, visual dysfunction may occur as a result of severe or chronic papilledema. Classic signs include disc hyperemia, retinal hemorrhages and exudates, and obscuration of vessels at the disc margin.

A number of conditions (eg, hydrocephalus, intracranial mass lesions, meningitis, idiopathic intracranial hypertension) can cause increased ICP in children and thus disc swelling (Table 26-2). A full evaluation, including neuroimaging possibly followed by lumbar puncture, is indicated. In infants, increased ICP results in firmness and distention of the open fontanelles. Significantly elevated pressure is usually accompanied by nausea, vomiting, and headaches. Older children may describe transient visual obscurations. Sixth nerve palsy can be a sign of elevated ICP.

Idiopathic Intracranial Hypertension

Idiopathic intracranial hypertension (IIH), or *pseudotumor cerebri*, is characterized by increased ICP with normal-sized or small ventricles on neuroimaging, and normal cerebrospinal fluid. IIH is uncommon in childhood but can occur at any age. It may be associated with viral infections, excessive vitamin A, and certain drugs (eg, tetracycline, corticosteroids, nalidixic acid, thyroid medications, and growth hormone). Magnetic resonance venography is recommended to rule out cerebral venous sinus thrombosis. In *prepubescent* children with IIH, the incidence of obesity is lower compared with that in adult IIH patients, and the male to female ratio is approximately equal. *Postpubescent* children with IIH have a clinical profile similar to that of adult IIH patients, with a higher incidence of obesity and female preponderance. Down syndrome is also associated with IIH.

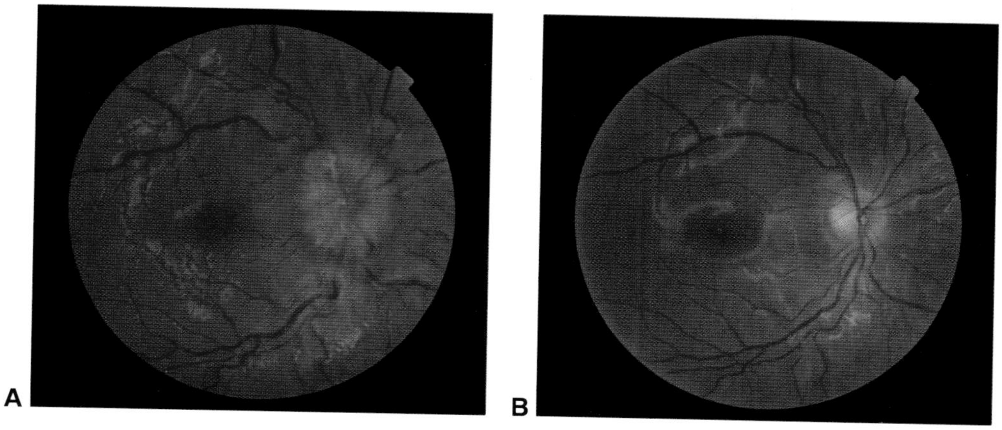

图 26–12　右眼特发性颅内高压致视乳头水肿，治疗前（**A**）和口服乙酰唑胺治疗 3 个月后（**B**）。左眼相同。见视频 26–1。*（译者注：资料来源见前页原文。）*

视乳头水肿

*视乳头水肿*指视盘水肿，继发颅内压（ICP）升高（图 26–12），常双眼发病。发病初期的视力、色觉和瞳孔反应正常。严重或慢性的视盘水肿可导致视功能障碍。临床表现为视盘充血、视网膜出血、渗出和视盘边缘血管模糊不清。

许多疾病（如脑积水、颅内肿块、脑膜炎、特发性颅内高压）可导致儿童颅内压 ICP 升高，从而导致视盘水肿（表 26–2）。全面评估，包括神经影像学检查和腰椎穿刺。婴儿的颅内压 ICP 升高会使开放的囟门僵硬和膨出。明显升高时，常伴恶心、呕吐和头痛。大龄儿童可主述有一过性视觉模糊。Ⅵ颅神经麻痹可能是颅内压 ICP 升高的特征。

特发性颅内高压

特发性颅内高压（IIH）*或脑性假瘤*，其特征是颅内压升高、神经影像学显示脑室大小正常或较小、脑脊液正常。特发性颅内高压（IIH）少见于儿童，但可以发生在任何年龄。可能与病毒感染、过量服用维生素 A 和某些药物（如四环素、皮质类固醇、萘啶酸、甲状腺药物和生长激素）有关。磁共振静脉造影用于排除脑静脉窦血栓形成。*青春期前*的儿童伴特发性颅内高压（IIH）时，肥胖的发生率低于成人特发性颅内高压（IIH）患者，男女比例相等。*青春期后*的儿童伴特发性颅内高压（IIH）时，临床特征与成人特发性颅内高压（IIH）相似，肥胖率较高，女性较多。Down 综合征也伴有特发性颅内高压（IIH）。

Table 26-2 Conditions Associated With Pediatric Optic Disc Swelling

- Papillitis
- Optic neuritis (postinfectious)
- Toxoplasmosis
- Lyme disease
- *Bartonella* infection
- Neuroretinitis
- *Toxocara* infection of disc
- Leber hereditary optic neuropathy
- Papilledema
  - Intracranial mass
  - Meningitis
  - Idiopathic intracranial hypertension
  - Dural sinus thrombosis
  - Cranial synostosis
  - Hydrocephalus
    - Chiari malformation
    - Aqueductal stenosis
    - Dandy-Walker syndrome
    - Infection
- Hypertension
- Optic nerve glioma
- Leukemic infiltrate
- Pseudopapilledema
  - Astrocytoma of optic disc (tuberous sclerosis)
  - Optic disc drusen
  - Hyperopic discs
  - Prominent disc glial tissue

Common presenting symptoms are headache, vision loss, transient visual obscurations, and diplopia. Papilledema may be noted on routine examination of an asymptomatic child. Examination frequently reveals excellent visual acuity with bilateral papilledema. Unilateral or bilateral sixth nerve palsy may be present. The patient should be monitored closely for decreased visual acuity, visual field loss, and worsening headaches. Visual field tests can be difficult to interpret in children but should be performed if possible.

Treatment of IIH begins with discontinuation of any causative medications. Medical treatment includes acetazolamide and topiramate (see Fig 26-12). Video 26-1 shows the gradual resolution (over a 3-month period) of papilledema in a child being treated for IIH. Surgical treatment options include optic nerve sheath fenestration or shunting procedures (lumbar or ventriculoperitoneal), both of which can reduce the incidence of vision loss. Shunting procedures are preferred for patients with good visual function and severe headaches unresponsive to medical management. With treatment, the visual prognosis is excellent for most patients, although vision loss can occur secondary to chronic papilledema. In most cases, spontaneous resolution occurs within 12–18 months of initial treatment. See BCSC Section 5, *Neuro-Ophthalmology,* for further discussion.

VIDEO 26-1 Gradual resolution of papilledema during treatment of idiopathic intracranial hypertension
Courtesy of Robert W. Hered, MD.
Access all Section 6 videos at www.aao.org/bcscvideo_section06.

表26-2　伴儿童视盘水肿的病变

- 视乳头炎
- 视神经炎（感染后）
- 弓形体病
- Lyme病
- *巴通体*感染
- 视神经视网膜炎
- 视盘*弓蛔虫*感染
- 遗传性视神经病变
- 视乳头水肿
    - 颅内肿物
    - 脑膜炎
    - 特发性颅内高压
    - 硬脑膜窦栓塞
    - 颅骨骨性融合
    - 脑积水
        - Chiari畸形/小脑扁桃体下疝畸形
        - 中脑导水管硬化
        - Dandy–Walker综合征
        - 感染
- 高血压
- 视神经胶质瘤
- 白血病浸润
- 假性视盘水肿
    - 视盘星形细胞瘤（结节性硬化）
    - 视盘玻璃膜疣
    - 远视眼视盘
    - 突出的视盘胶质组织

常见症状有头痛、视力下降、一过性视物模糊和复视。无症状患儿在常规体检中发现视乳头水肿。体检时视力正常，但双眼视乳头水肿，同时合并单眼或双眼Ⅵ颅神经麻痹。应密切观察患儿，是否有视力下降、视野丢失以及头痛加剧。儿童的视野检查很困难，但应尽量检测。

对于特发性颅内高压 IIH 的治疗，首先应停用任何可能诱发颅内高压的药物。药物治疗包括乙酰唑胺和托吡酯（图 26–12）。视频 26–1 示一例特发性颅内高压（IIH）儿童的视盘水肿，治疗后逐渐好转（经过 3 个月）。手术治疗包括视神经鞘开窗术或分流术（腰部或脑室腹腔分流），两者均可降低视力丧失的发生率。分流术用于视功能良好但头痛严重，且对药物治疗无反应的患者。大多数病人治疗后，视力预后较好，但视力下降也可继发于慢性视盘水肿。大多数患者在初次治疗的 12 ~ 18 个月内可自愈。详见 BCSC 第 5 册《*神经眼科学*》。

视频26–1　特发性颅内高压治疗中视盘水肿逐渐减轻的过程。*（译者注：资料来源见前页原文。）*
可登陆网站www.aao.org/bcscvideo_section06观看第6册中的所有视频。

Pseudopapilledema

Pseudopapilledema refers to any elevated anomaly of the optic disc that resembles papilledema (see Table 26-2). Conditions that are frequently confused with papilledema in children include disc drusen, hyperopic discs, and prominent disc glial tissue. Pseudopapilledema can be differentiated from true papilledema by the absence of disc hyperemia and retinal hemorrhages and exudates, and by the lack of obscuration of vessels at the disc margin (Fig 26-13). Pseudopapilledema can be associated with anomalous branching of the large peripapillary retinal vessels. However, clinical examination findings can be ambiguous.

Most children with pseudopapilledema do not have other related ophthalmic or systemic abnormalities. However, pseudopapilledema is associated with retinal dystrophy, Down syndrome, and Alagille syndrome. Down syndrome is associated with IIH as well; thus, an elevated optic disc in a child with Down syndrome should not be assumed to be benign. If clinical symptoms and signs of elevated ICP (headaches, sixth nerve palsy, true papilledema) are present, neuroimaging followed by lumbar puncture should be obtained.

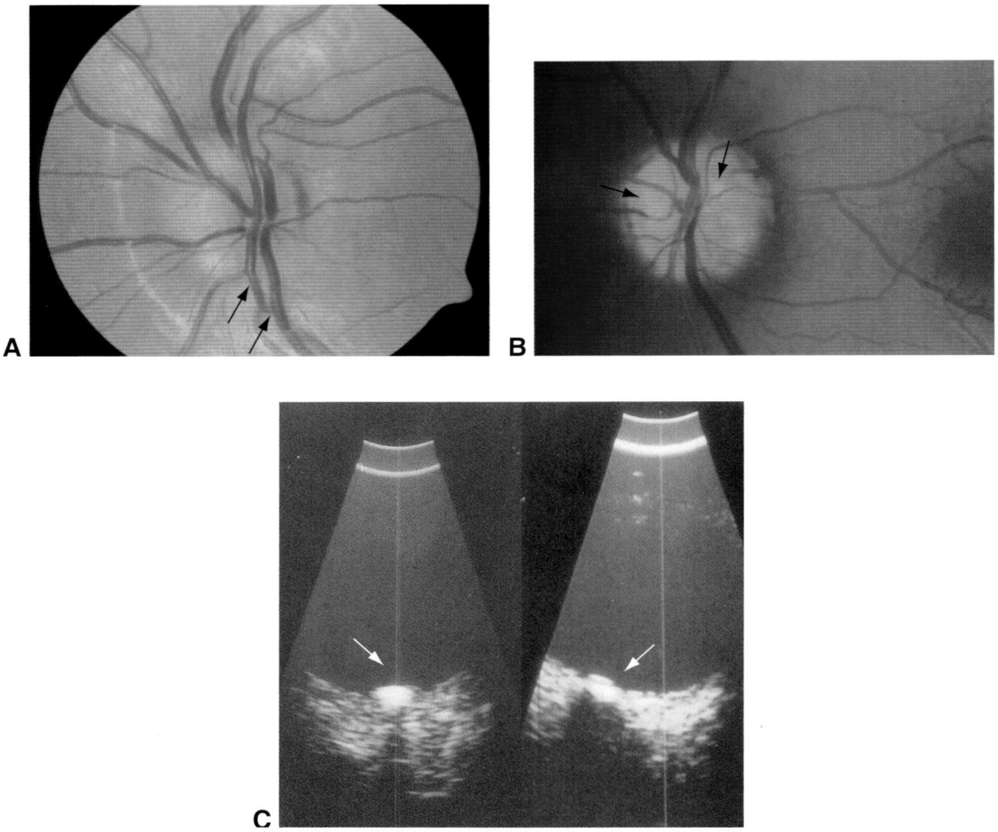

Figure 26-13 **A,** Pseudopapilledema. There is anomalous branching (*arrows*) of the large retinal vessels without disc hyperemia, retinal hemorrhages, or exudates. **B,** Optic disc drusen seen as refractile opacities on the disc surface *(arrows)*. **C,** Ultrasonographic image shows a bright spot in the optic disc *(arrows)*, consistent with drusen. *(Parts A and B courtesy of Paul Phillips, MD; part C courtesy of Edward G. Buckley, MD.)*

假性视乳头水肿

*假性视乳头水肿*是指类似于视乳头水肿的任何形式的视盘异常隆起（表 26-2）。易与儿童视乳头水肿混淆的病变有视盘玻璃膜疣、远视眼的视盘和突出的视盘胶质组织。与真性视乳头水肿的鉴别点在于，假性视乳头水肿没有视盘充血、视网膜出血和渗出、视盘边缘血管模糊（图 26-13）。假性视乳头水肿可合并视盘周围视网膜大血管的异常分支，但是临床检查中很难区别。

多数假性视乳头水肿的儿童不合并眼部及全身异常，但可伴有视网膜营养不良、Down 综合征和 Alagille 综合征。Down 综合征可伴特发性颅内高压 IIH，所以 Down 综合征患儿的颅内压 ICP 升高被视为良性改变。若临床出现颅内压 ICP 升高的症状和体征（头痛、Ⅵ颅神经麻痹、真性视乳头水肿），需行神经影像学检查和腰椎穿刺。

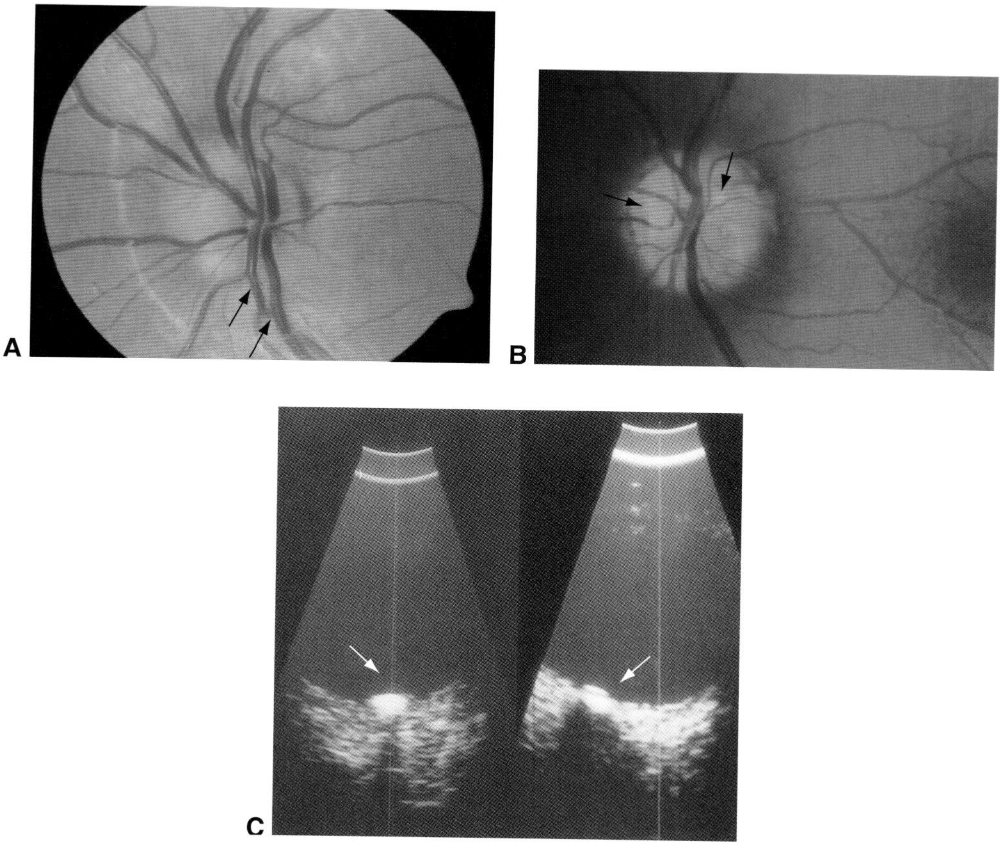

图 26-13　A. 假性视乳头水肿。可见视网膜大血管的异常分支（*箭头*），无视盘充血、视网膜出血或渗出。**B.** 视盘玻璃膜疣，可见视盘表面折射性混浊（*箭头*）。**C.** 超声显示视盘内的亮点（*箭头*），与玻璃膜疣一致。
（译者注：资料来源见前页原文。）

Drusen

Intrapapillary drusen, the most common cause of pseudopapilledema in children, can appear within the first or second decade of life (Fig 26-14; see also Fig 26-13B). Drusen are frequently inherited (autosomal dominant); thus, examination of the parents is helpful when drusen are suspected in children.

Clinically, the elevated disc does not obscure the retinal arterioles lying anteriorly and often has an irregular border suggesting the presence of drusen beneath the surface. There is no dilatation of the papillary network, and superficial retinal hemorrhages and exudates are absent. Peripapillary subretinal hemorrhages and subretinal neovascular membranes rarely occur. When drusen are not buried, they appear as shiny refractile bodies visible on the disc surface, with a gray-yellow translucent appearance. Visual field defects are frequently associated; inferior nasal field defects are common. Concentric narrowing, an arcuate scotoma, and central defects can also occur. These defects can be slowly progressive. Visual acuity is rarely affected.

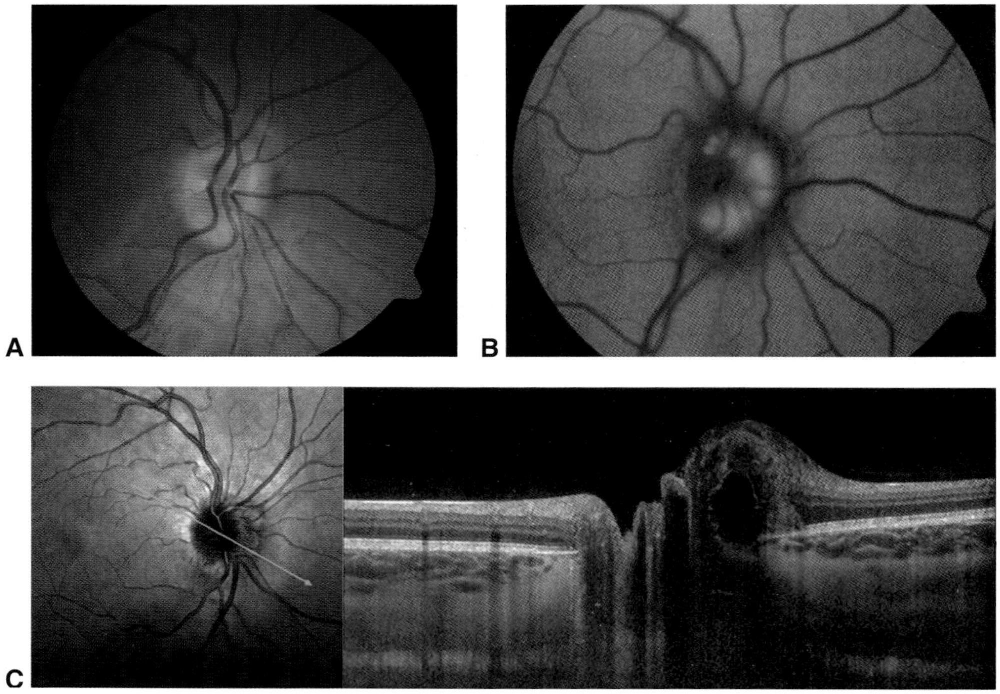

Figure 26-14 **A,** Superficial optic disc drusen, right eye. **B,** Appearance with autofluorescence. **C,** Optical coherence tomography image from a different child with drusen reveals the typical "lumpy bumpy" appearance. *(Courtesy of Wayne T. Cornblath, MD.)*

In some patients, fundus evaluation can identify drusen as the cause of the swollen disc appearance. In others, B-scan ultrasonography can be helpful in detecting bright calcific reflections at the optic disc (see Fig 26-13C). Autofluorescence imaging and optical coherence tomography can also be useful (see Fig 26-14).

Most children with optic disc drusen do not have other related ophthalmic or systemic abnormalities. However, children with retinal dystrophy or pseudoxanthoma elasticum have a higher incidence of optic disc drusen compared with the general population.

玻璃膜疣

视乳头内的玻璃膜疣，是儿童假性视盘水肿最常见的原因，见于 10 ~ 20 岁（图 26-14，图 26-13B），有遗传性（常染色体显性遗传）。当怀疑患儿有玻璃膜疣时，对其父母的检查有助于诊断。

临床上，隆起的视盘不会使位于其表面的视网膜小动脉边界模糊，且视盘边缘不规则提示下面存在玻璃膜疣。没有视乳头毛细血管网的扩张、视网膜出血和渗出，也罕见视盘周围视网膜下出血和视网膜下新生血管膜。如果玻璃膜疣没有包埋，常可见视盘表面的闪光折射小体，呈灰黄色的半透明外观。伴视野缺损。常见鼻下方视野缺损。向心性缩小、弧形暗点和中心缺损也常见。视野的缺损进展缓慢，视力不受影响。

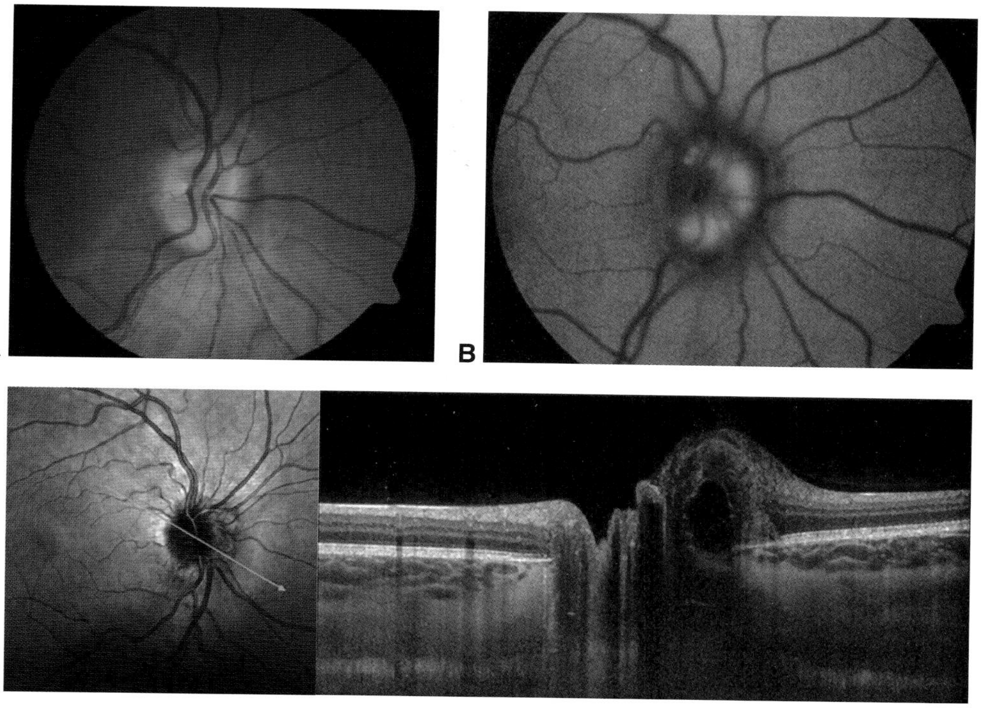

A B C

图 26-14 **A.** 视盘表面的玻璃膜疣，右眼。**B.** 自发荧光。**C.** 另一患儿的光学相干断层扫描 OCT，玻璃膜疣呈典型的凹凸不平外观。*（译者注：资料来源见前页原文。）*

一些患者的眼底见玻璃膜疣，导致视盘水肿。一些患者的 B 超检测可见视盘高密度钙化斑（图 26-13C）。自发荧光和光学相干断层扫描也有助于观察（图 26-14）。

大多数视盘玻璃膜疣的儿童不合并其他眼部及全身异常。总体来看，合并视网膜营养不良或者弹性假黄色瘤的儿童，视盘玻璃膜疣的发生率较高。

（翻译 张宁 赵方宇 // 审校 刘陇黔 石一宁 蒋宁 // 章节审校 石广礼）

CHAPTER 27

Ocular Trauma in Childhood

Special Considerations in the Management of Pediatric Ocular Trauma

Trauma is one of the most important causes of ocular morbidity in childhood. The management of eye trauma in very young patients requires special consideration of issues common in or unique to this patient population. One issue is the evaluation and treatment of accidental or nonaccidental trauma despite inadequate patient cooperation or an unreliable history. If the physician uses force to examine the child's eye, there is a risk of exacerbating the damage caused by penetrating wounds or blunt impact. When preliminary assessment indicates that prompt surgical treatment may be necessary, it is appropriate to defer detailed physical examination of the eye until the patient is in the operating room and under general anesthesia.

Another issue is the potential for the injury to cause amblyopia. In children younger than 5–7 years, deprivation amblyopia associated with traumatic cataract or other media opacity can cause severe, long-term reduction of vision even after appropriate management of the original physical damage. Minimizing the interval between the injury and the restoration of optimal media clarity and optics, including adequate aphakic refractive correction, is thus a high priority. Monocular occlusion following injury should be kept to a minimum; the expected benefit from an occlusive dressing must be weighed against the risk of disturbing binocular function or inducing amblyopia in a very young child.

Accidental Trauma

In younger children, most accidental ocular trauma occurs during casual play with other children. Older children and adolescents are most likely to be injured while participating in sports. Fireworks, BB guns, and various projectiles are less frequent causes of pediatric ocular trauma, but they are likely to cause severe injuries. The incidence of severe eye injury is particularly high in children aged 11–15 years compared with that in other age groups. Injured boys outnumber girls by a factor of 3 or 4 to 1.

Most serious childhood eye injuries could, in principle, be prevented by appropriate adult supervision and by regular use of protective eyewear during sports activities. These measures are particularly important for the child who already has monocular vision loss.

American Academy of Pediatrics, Committee on Sports Medicine and Fitness; American Academy of Ophthalmology, Eye Health and Public Information Task Force. Protective eyewear for young athletes. *Ophthalmology*. 2004;111(3):600–603.

第 27 章

儿童眼外伤

儿童眼外伤处理的特殊考虑

外伤是儿童时期最重要的眼病之一。处理幼儿的眼外伤时，需要特别注意其与一般人群的共同之处及特殊之处。其中的主要原因之一是，需在患儿难以配合，且病史叙述不可靠的情况下，对意外与人为外伤进行评估与处理。如果强行检查患儿的伤眼，则可能增加穿通伤或钝挫伤进一步恶化的风险。若经初步评估，患儿需立即手术处理，则应在手术室全身麻醉状态下，对伤眼进行详细检查。

另一个因素是，外伤本身可能导致弱视。对于年龄小于 5 ~ 7 岁的儿童，即使外伤经过了适当的处理，但外伤性白内障或其他屈光间质混浊所导致的形觉剥夺性弱视，仍然可造成长期严重的视力减退。因此，首要考虑最大限度地缩短外伤与恢复屈光介质的光学透明性的间隔时间，包括无晶状体眼的屈光矫正。尽量减少儿童外伤后的单眼遮盖，需权衡遮盖单眼的益处和其对幼儿双眼视功能的干扰及引发弱视的风险。

意外伤

大多数幼儿眼的意外伤是与同伴玩耍时偶然发生的，青少年多发生在体育活动中。烟花炮竹、BB 枪及其他射弹物引起的眼外伤，儿童少见，但所致的外伤较严重。11~15 岁儿童的严重眼外伤发生率较高，外伤男孩高于女孩，比例为 3∶1 ~ 4∶1。

原则上，若监护人看护得当，或在运动中常规使用护目镜，大多数严重的儿童眼外伤是可以避免的。恰当的防护措施对于独眼的儿童更为重要。

American Academy of Pediatrics, Committee on Sports Medicine and Fitness; American Academy of Ophthalmology, Eye Health and Public Information Task Force. Protective eyewear for young athletes. *Ophthalmology*. 2004;111(3):600–603.

Corneal Abrasion

Corneal abrasion is one of the most common ocular injuries in children and adults. Disruption of the corneal epithelium is usually associated with immediate pain, foreign-body sensation, tearing, and discomfort with blinking. Topical cycloplegic drops and antibiotic ointment may help reduce discomfort and the risk of infection, respectively. Traumatic corneal epithelial defects usually heal within 1–2 days. A pressure patch to keep the eyelids closed is not necessary for most abrasions. Many children find the patch uncomfortable, and patching does not reduce the time required for the abrasion to heal.

Thermal Injury

Cigarette burns of the cornea are the most common thermal injuries to the ocular surface in childhood. Usually, these occur in toddlers and are accidental, not manifestations of abuse. The burns usually result from the child running into a cigarette held at eye level by an adult. Despite the alarming initial white appearance of coagulated corneal epithelium, cigarette burns typically heal in a few days and without scarring. Treatment is the same as treatment of corneal abrasions (discussed in the previous section).

Chemical Injury

Chemical burns in childhood are generally caused by organic solvents or soaps in house hold cleaning agents. Even burns involving almost total loss of corneal epithelium are likely to heal in a week or less with or without patching. Acid and alkali burns in children, as in adults, can be much more serious. The initial and most important step in management of all chemical injuries is immediate copious irrigation and meticulous removal of any particulate matter from the conjunctival fornices. See BCSC Section 8, *External Disease and Cornea*, for additional discussion.

Corneal Foreign Body

Corneal foreign bodies in children can sometimes be dislodged with a forceful stream of irrigating solution. After topical anesthetic is applied, a cotton swab or blunt spatula can often be used to remove the corneal foreign body, with or without a slit lamp; use of sharp instruments should be avoided. If these methods are unsuccessful, the child may require sedation or general anesthesia to facilitate removal of the foreign body.

Penetrating or Perforating Injury

Unless an adult has witnessed the traumatic incident, the history cannot be relied upon to exclude the possibility of penetrating injury to the globe. The anterior segment and fundus must be thoroughly inspected. An examination under anesthesia may be necessary when a penetrating injury is suspected. An area of subconjunctival hemorrhage or chemosis or a small break in the skin of the eyelid may be the only surface manifestation of scleral perforation by a sharp-pointed object, such as a pencil or scissors blade (Fig 27-1). Distortion of the pupil may be the most evident sign of a small corneal or limbal perforation. Imaging should be considered if there is any reason to suspect an intraocular or orbital foreign body.

角膜擦伤

无论是儿童还是成年人，角膜的擦伤都是眼外伤中最常见的。角膜上皮的损伤表现为伤后即刻疼痛、异物感、流泪及不适性眨眼。局部应用睫状肌麻痹剂及抗生素眼膏，可分别缓解不适症状，降低感染风险。外伤性角膜上皮缺损 1 ~ 2d 即可痊愈，多不需使用加压包眼以使眼睑闭合，因为包眼使许多儿童感觉不适，且不能缩短上皮愈合时间。

热烧伤

角膜的烟头烧伤是最常见的儿童眼表热烧伤，常意外发生于学步幼儿，并不一定是虐童的表现，主要是由于幼儿跑向手持香烟的成人，而香烟的高度恰好在儿童眼球水平位置。烧伤后立即会出现角膜上皮白色的热烧伤凝固病灶，但香烟的烧伤数天即可愈合，不留瘢痕。治疗与角膜擦伤相同（见前一节所述）。

化学伤

儿童化学伤常由家用清洁剂的有机溶剂或肥皂引起，常致角膜上皮全层剥脱，无论是否包眼，1 周内可愈合。与成人一样，儿童酸碱烧伤较为严重。处理所有的化学伤的第一步，也是最重要的一步，就是立即用大量的水冲洗，仔细清除结膜囊穹隆部所有的颗粒异物。详见 BCSC 第 8 册《*外眼疾病与角膜*》。

角膜异物

儿童角膜异物有时可用加压冲洗来清除。局部麻醉后，在裂隙灯下或裸眼情况下，用棉签或钝刮铲清除异物。避免使用锐器。若上述方法不能奏效，则应在镇静或全身麻醉下清除。

穿通伤或贯通伤

除非成人亲眼目睹了外伤经过，否则不能依据其病史描述来排除眼球穿通伤的可能。需彻底检查眼前节及眼底。若怀疑为穿通伤，需在麻醉下检查。结膜下出血、结膜水肿或眼睑皮肤上的小伤口，都可能是锐器致巩膜穿通伤的表现，如铅笔或剪刀（图 27-1）。瞳孔变形是小的角膜或角膜缘穿通伤的直接证据。怀疑眼内或眶内异物时，需进行影像学检查。

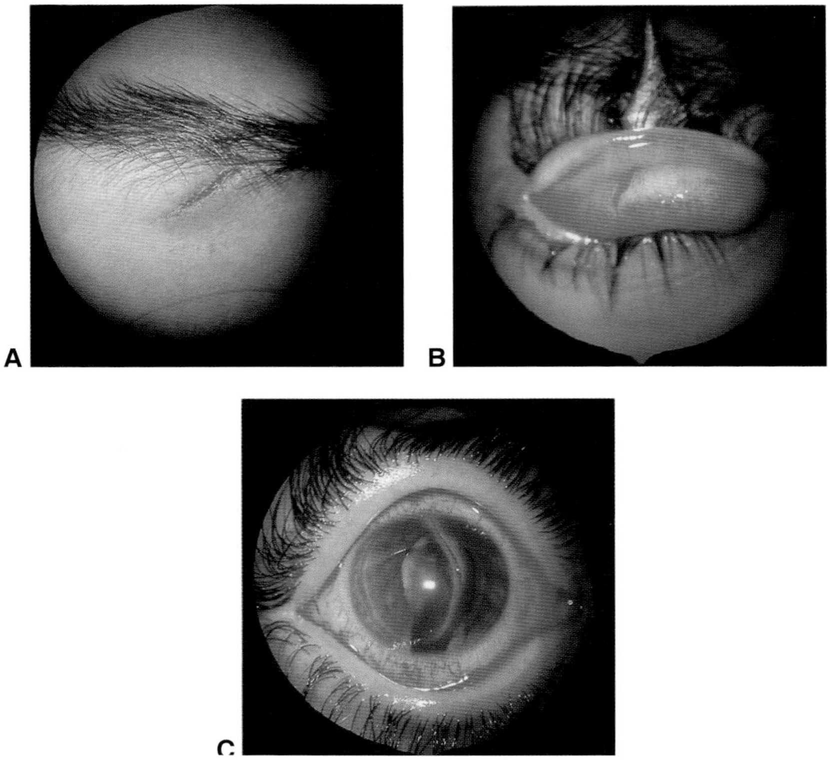

Figure 27-1 **A,** Small skin entry wound, right brow region, in a 7-year-old boy. The wound was created by a thrown dart. **B,** Conjunctival exit wound indicates complete perforation of the eyelid. **C,** Extensive injury to the anterior segment of the same eye.

Corneoscleral lacerations in children are repaired using the same Principles employed for these repairs in adults (see BCSC Section 8, *External Disease and Cornea*). Corneal wounds heal relatively rapidly in very young patients; sutures should be removed correspondingly earlier. Small conjunctival lacerations are often self-sealing.

After a penetrating injury to the cornea, fibrin clots may form quickly in the anterior chamber of a child's eye, and these can simulate the appearance of fluffy cataractous lens cortex. To avoid rendering the eye aphakic unnecessarily (and thereby compromising vision rehabilitation), the clinician should not remove the lens as part of primary wound repair unless absolutely certain that the anterior capsule has been ruptured. Even if lens cortex is exposed, postponing cataract surgery for 1–2 weeks, until severe posttraumaticinflammation has resolved, may result in a smoother postoperative recovery and reduced risk of complications without significantly worsening the visual prognosis. See also BCSC Section 11, *Lens and Cataract*.

Full-thickness eyelid lacerations, especially those involving a canaliculus, should be repaired meticulously; sedation or general anesthesia may be required, even in older children. Working near the eyes with sharp instruments and draping the face to create a sterile field are likely to frighten an awake child and add to the difficulty of the repair. Clearly superficial wounds can be repaired in the emergency department. For superficial wounds, use of an absorbable suture is acceptable if the physician wishes to avoid the need to remove nonabsorbable sutures.

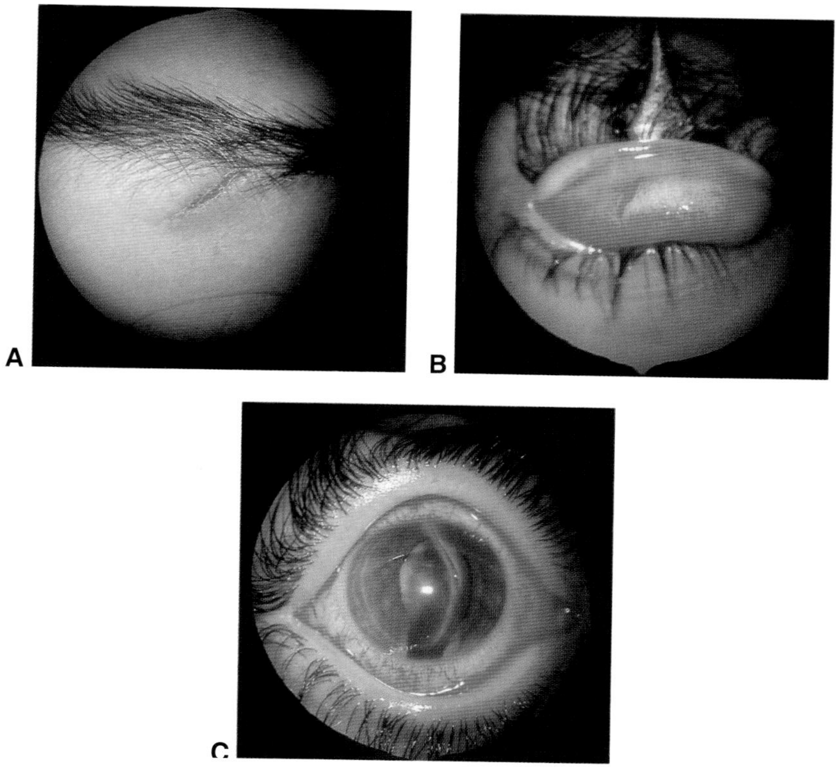

图 27–1　**A.**7 岁男孩右眉弓小的皮肤伤口，飞镖所致。**B.** 睑结膜面的外伤口，系眼睑全层贯通伤。**C.** 同一眼眼前节大范围损伤。

儿童角巩膜裂伤的修复原则与成人的相同（详见 BCSC 第 8 册《*外眼疾病与角膜*》）。幼儿的角膜伤口愈合较快，缝线可较早拆除。小的结膜裂伤可自愈。

儿童角膜穿通伤后，前房可迅速形成纤维蛋白渗出，呈松软的白内障皮质样外观。为了避免不必要的晶状体摘除（并且影响视觉康复），医生不应在一期修复伤口时摘除晶状体，除非十分明确晶状体前囊已经破裂。即使晶状体皮质已暴露，也应推迟白内障手术 1 ~ 2 周，待伤后炎症反应基本消退后进行，这样术后恢复较为平稳，并发症的风险相应降低，对视功能恢复的影响也较小。详见 BCSC 第 11 册《*晶状体与白内障*》。

全层眼睑裂伤，特别是累及泪小管断裂，应仔细修复，即使是大龄儿童，也应给予镇静和全身麻醉。在眼周围使用锐器、无菌操作遮盖面部，都会使清醒的儿童非常恐惧，从而增加手术修复的难度。单纯面部表皮外伤也可在急诊室修复。为避免拆除不可吸收缝线，建议用可吸收缝线。

Blunt Injury

Hyphema

As with all forms of pediatric trauma, the precise occurrence that led to the hyphema may be difficult to determine. The possibility of abuse must be considered, as must the possibility of a nontraumatic etiology: retinoblastoma, juvenile xanthogranuloma of the iris, and bleeding diathesis resulting from leukemia or other blood dyscrasia are relatively rare but important causes of spontaneous hyphema during the early years of life. When the findings are suspicious and the iris and fundus cannot be adequately seen, ultrasonography or magnetic resonance imaging should be performed to rule out intraocular tumor. If a bleeding disorder is suspected, a complete blood count and coagulation studies should be performed.

Intraocular pressure (IOP), an important factor in therapeutic decision making for patients with traumatic hyphema, is often difficult to monitor in the pediatric patient. The risks of inaccurate measurements and of further traumatizing the injured eye may outweigh the potential value of obtaining measurements in uncooperative children. With small hyphemas (Fig 27-2), concern about pressure is greatest in patients with sickle cell trait or disease. Sickling may develop in the anterior chamber, elevating IOP and retarding resorption of blood, or in the retinal circulation, causing vascular occlusion. All African American children with traumatic hyphema require sickle cell screening to evaluate for these conditions.

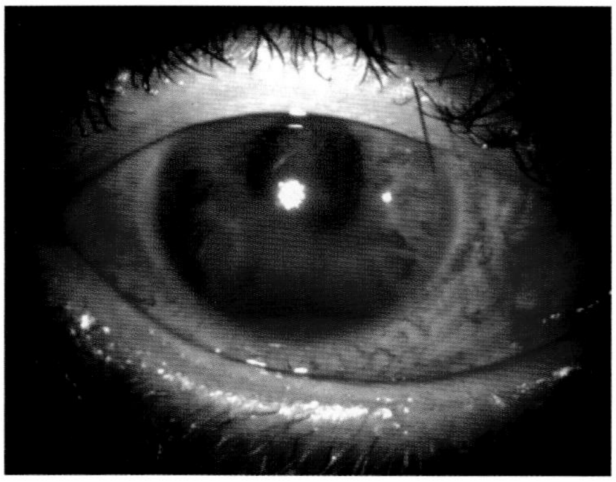

Figure 27-2 Small hyphema. Note the layering of blood inferiorly. *(Courtesy of Edward L. Raab, MD.)*

As in adults, medical management of hyphema in children remains controversial. Care must be taken to minimize the risk of rebleeding, which usually occurs between 3 and 7 days postinjury as a result of clot lysis and retraction. Outpatient management with activity restriction and close follow-up is generally accepted. However, if parental cooperation is questionable or if the patient has sickle trait, hospitalization for several days after injury, when the risk of rebleeding is greatest, remains justifiable. Many ophthalmologists routinely use cycloplegic and corticosteroid drops to facilitate fundus examination, improve comfort, and reduce the risk of inflammatory complications and rebleeding. The value of these topical agents is unproven, and some clinicians prefer to use them selectively for control of pain or obvious inflammation, or to avoid them altogether to minimize manipulation of the eye. Pressure-lowering medication is appropriate for eyes known or strongly suspected to have elevated IOP. Aspirin-containing compounds and nonsteroidal anti-inflammatory drugs can increase the risk of rebleeding and should be avoided.

钝挫伤

前房积血

与所有的小儿外伤一样，前房积血的原因很难确定。虐童是非外伤性病因之一，还有视网膜母细胞瘤、幼年虹膜黄色肉芽肿，而白血病或其他血液系统恶液质所致的出血倾向相对少见，但却是幼年时期自发性前房出血的重要原因。当高度怀疑这些非创伤性因素，且虹膜和眼底观察不清时，应行超声和磁共振检查，以排除眼内肿瘤。若怀疑为出血性疾病时，应检测血细胞计数及凝血相关指标。

眼压 IOP 是决定外伤性前房积血治疗方案的重要因素之一，但儿童很难检测。对于不配合的患儿施行眼压测量，可能会带来眼压评估不准确以及进一步损伤患眼的风险。镰刀型细胞贫血症的患儿伴少量的前房积血（图 27–2）时，应重视测量眼压。血细胞的镰状变形可在前房形成，使眼压升高、积血吸收延缓，或在视网膜血管内阻塞血管。所有非裔美国儿童发生外伤性前房积血后，需行镰状细胞的筛查进行评估。

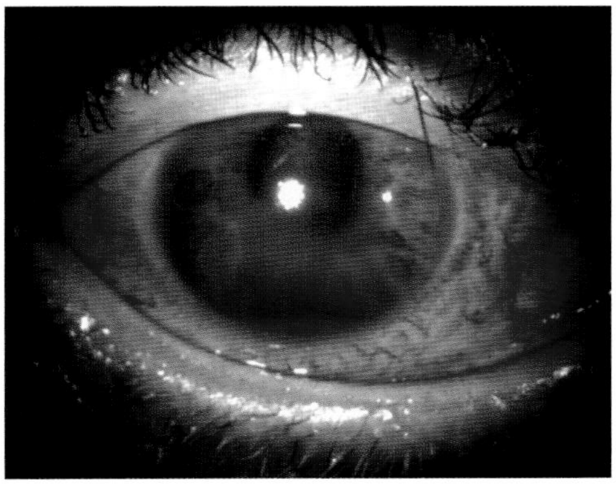

图 27–2　少量前房积血。下方可见积血液平面。*（译者注：资料来源见前页原文。）*

同成人一样，儿童前房积血的药物治疗存在争议。需加强护理以防再出血，血凝块常在伤后 3~7 天溶解收缩。门诊患儿伤后需限制活动，密切随诊。如果家长不能配合，或有镰刀细胞遗传性状，再出血风险较高的患儿应住院观察治疗。许多眼科医生常规使用睫状肌麻痹剂和糖皮质激素眼液，以协助眼底检查，改善舒适度，减少炎症所致的并发症和再出血的风险。这些局部药物的效果尚不确定，有的医生选择性地应用药物，以减轻患儿疼痛或炎症反应，或不用药物，以减少对伤眼过多干扰。若存在眼压升高或高度怀疑时，需使用降眼压药物。含阿司匹林的复合制剂和非甾体抗炎药可增加再出血的风险，应避免使用。

Many treatments have been proposed to prevent rebleeding in traumatic hyphema, although none is universally accepted. See Chapter 14 in BCSC Section 8, *External Disease and Cornea*, for a discussion of treatment considerations for traumatic hyphema.

The difficulty of detecting early corneal blood staining in a child and the risk that staining may cause severe deprivation amblyopia, coupled with the problems of accurately measuring IOP, justify early surgical intervention whenever a total hyphema persists for 4–5 days. In children with sickle cell trait or disease, it may be necessary to perform surgery even earlier if elevated pressures (>25 mm Hg for over 24 hours) occur.

Late glaucoma is a potential complication of traumatic hyphema in children, as in adults, and may occur with no symptoms. Gonioscopy can be performed after the eye has healed and the child is able to cooperate. Annual follow-up should be continued in children with a history of traumatic hyphema, in light of the potential late complications of cataract, retinal detachment, and glaucoma.

Orbital Fractures

Orbital floor fractures

Blunt facial trauma is the usual cause of orbital floor fractures. The term *blowout fracture* is used when the rim remains intact. Orbital floor fracture is thought to be due to either of the following: an acute increase in intraorbital pressure, which occurs when a direct impact occludes the orbital entrance; or compression of the rim, which results in buckling of the floor. Orbital floor fracture can be part of more extensive fractures of the orbit and midface. In some cases, the mechanism causing floor fractures extends to include the medial wall as well.

Periorbital ecchymosis and diplopia are common in the immediate posttrauma period. Injury to the inferior rectus muscle or to its nerve, with resultant weakness, may be caused by hemorrhage or ischemia, in addition to restriction. This injury can occur either at the time of the fracture or during its repair. Injury to the inferior rectus muscle can manifest as either limited elevation or depression. Hypoesthesia in the cutaneous distribution of the infraorbital nerve can also occur.

In a patient with limited elevation, a positive forced duction test indicates the presence of restriction. Bradycardia, heart block, nausea, or syncope can occur as a vagal response to entrapment. When the entrapment involves the more anterior portion of the orbital floor or when there is associated injury to the inferior rectus muscle or its nerve, there can also be limited depression. Reduced saccadic velocity and force generation on attempted downgaze suggest weak muscle action. Orbital computed tomography and high-resolution, multipositional magnetic resonance imaging are useful for revealing the presence and extent of the injury.

A special presentation, the *white-eyed blowout fracture*, is characterized by marked restriction (in both directions) of vertical ocular motility despite minimal signs of softtissue injury. This restriction is due to entrapment of the inferior rectus muscle or orbital tissue either beneath a trapdoor fracture or, unique to children, in a linear opening caused by flexion deformity of the floor. In this condition, early surgery, rather than observation, is required in order to minimize permanent muscle and nerve damage.

Wei LA, Durairaj VD. Pediatric orbital floor fractures. *J AAPOS*. 2011;15(2):173–180.

多种治疗方案可防止外伤性前房积血的再出血，但尚未统一。详见 BCSC 第 8 册《外眼疾病与角膜》，第 14 章中外伤性前房积血的治疗。

儿童角膜血染早期很难发现，血染可导致严重的形觉剥夺性弱视，同时很难精确测量眼压 IOP，这些都提示一旦全前房积血持续达 4 ~ 5d，应尽早手术干预。镰刀型细胞遗传性状或病变的患儿，若眼压升高（ > 25mmHg，持续 24h），应更早施行手术。

与成人一样，儿童外伤性前房积血后晚期可发生迟发性青光眼，且无症状。在伤眼治愈，且患儿能够配合的情况下，可行前房角镜检查。因为存在远期并发症的风险，如白内障、视网膜脱离和青光眼，外伤性前房积血病史的患儿需每年随诊观察。

眼眶骨折

眶下壁骨折

钝性面部外伤多引起眶下壁骨折。*爆裂性骨折*常用于眶缘完整的骨折。眶下壁骨折或是直接堵塞眼眶入口引起的眶内压急剧升高，或是对眶缘的挤压致眶下壁的弯曲。眶下壁骨折也可能是广泛的眼眶和面中部骨折的一部分，有时可能是眶内壁骨折的延伸。

眶周淤血和复视伤后立即出现。外伤性出血或缺血以及运动受限，导致下直肌或其支配神经的损伤，导致肌力减弱。这种情况可发生于受伤骨折时，也可发生于手术修复过程中。下直肌损伤可表现为上转受限或下转。若损伤眶下神经则可出现其支配区域的感觉迟钝。

上转受限时，被动牵拉试验阳性提示限制因素的存在。下直肌嵌顿引起的迷走反射，可出现心动过缓、心脏骤停、恶心，甚至晕厥。嵌顿位于眶下壁前的部分骨折，或同时合并下直肌或其支配神经的损伤，也可出现下转受限。扫视速度的降低和下方注视的力量减弱，均提示肌肉力量的减弱。眼眶计算机断层扫描、高分辨多方位磁共振影像有助于明确骨折位置和损伤范围。

*白眼爆裂性骨折*是一种特殊的临床表现，即垂直运动（上下 2 个方向）明显受限，仅伴轻微的软组织损伤，这是由于下直肌或眶组织嵌顿到骨折下陷口内，或儿童特有的由眶下壁挤压变形，嵌顿到线状骨折缝内。这种情况不需要观察，应早期手术，以减小肌肉和神经的永久性损伤。

Wei LA, Durairaj VD. Pediatric orbital floor fractures. *J AAPOS*. 2011;15(2):173–180.

Management There are several approaches to the management of orbital floor fractures. Some clinicians advocate surgical exploration in all cases, irrespective of the results of forced duction testing. The justification for this approach is that, especially with large bony defects, progressive herniation of orbital contents into the adjacent maxillary sinus can occur, resulting in disfiguring enophthalmos. Others recommend waiting for a few days to 2 weeks to allow periorbital ecchymosis to subside. For these surgeons, the main indication to operate is evidence of restriction with unresolved diplopia in primary position. Diplopia immediately after the injury is common and is not necessarily an indication for urgent intervention. Management of persistentdiplopia is covered in Chapter 11.

Orbital roof fractures

Though rare in older patients, orbital roof fractures are common in children younger than 10 years. Isolated roof fractures typically result from impact to the brow region in a fall, often from a height of only a few feet. The principal external manifestation is upper eyelid hematoma (Fig 27-3). These fractures often heal without treatment.

For further discussion of diagnosis and management of orbital trauma, see BCSC Section 7, *Oculofacial Plastic and Orbital Surgery.*

A 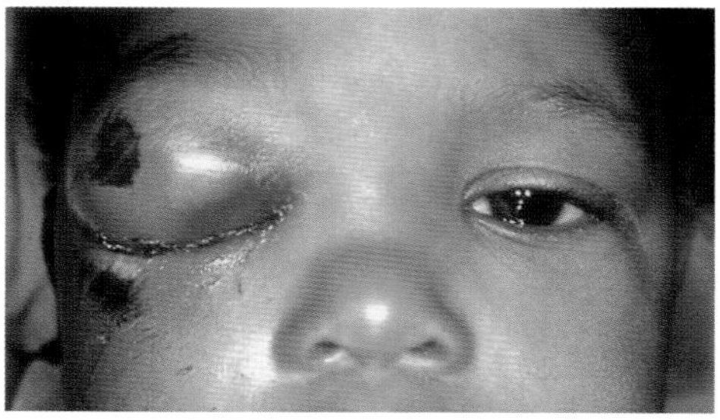 B 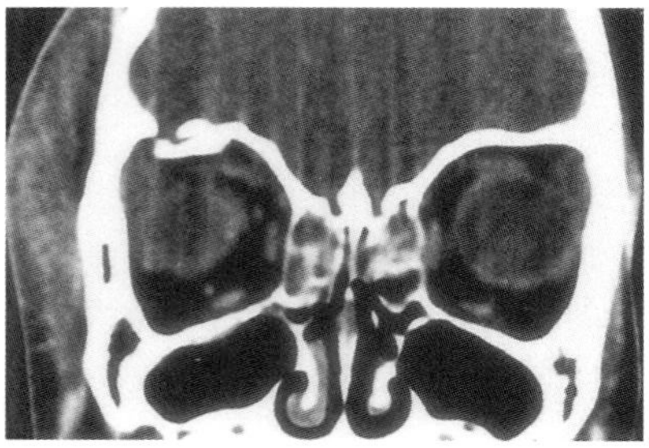

Figure 27-3 Orbital roof fracture in a child, resulting from direct impact to the brow region in a fall. **A,** Marked right upper eyelid swelling from a hematoma originating in the superior orbit, adjacent to a linear fracture. **B,** Coronal computed tomography shows a bone fragment displaced into the right orbit.

Traumatic Optic Neuropathy

The optic nerve may be damaged by trauma to the head, orbit, or globe. Vision loss is usually immediate and severe with a relative afferent pupillary defect present. Initially, the optic nerve appears normal, but it becomes atrophic within 1–2 months of injury. Management is controversial and may include high-dose intravenous steroids and optic canal decompression.

For further discussion of diagnosis and management of traumatic optic neuropathy, see BCSC Section 5, *Neuro-Ophthalmology.*

治疗　眶下壁骨折有多种处理方式。有的医生建议，无论牵拉试验结果如何，所有患者均应手术探查。因为当伴有大面积骨缺损时，眶内容物会渐渐疝入邻近的上颌窦，导致眼球内陷，影响外观。其他医生则建议观察数天到 2 周，待眶周淤血消退。其手术指征是运动受限制，第一眼位复视无法恢复，因为伤后即刻出现的复视很常见，并不是急诊干预的指征。持续性复视的治疗见第 11 章。

眶上壁骨折

眶上壁骨折在大龄儿童不常见，但常见于 10 岁以下的儿童。孤立的眶上壁骨折常见于跌落时撞击到眉区，且常仅仅是从数英尺高度跌落。主要表现是上眼睑血肿（图 27–3）。这种骨折常可自愈。

眼眶外伤的进一步诊断和治疗，见 BCSC 第 7 册《*眼面部整形与眼眶手术*》。

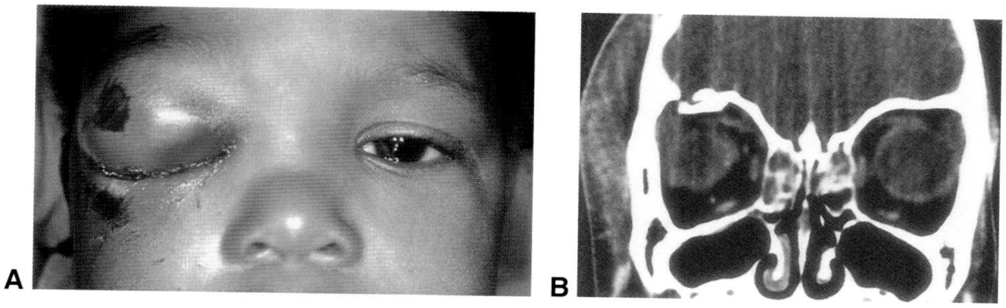

图 27–3　儿童眶上壁骨折，跌落时直接撞击眉区。**A.** 明显的右上睑血肿肿胀，源于线性骨折附近的眶上壁。**B.** 冠状计算机断层扫描 CT 显示骨折片向右眼眶移位。

外伤性视神经病变

视神经可因头部、眼眶或眼球的外伤而受损，常伴当即严重的视力下降、相对性瞳孔传入障碍。最初视神经外观正常，伤后 1 ～ 2 个月萎缩。治疗方法尚有争议，包括静脉使用大剂量类固醇和视神经管减压。

外伤性视神经病变诊断和治疗的更多内容，见 BCSC 第 5 册《*神经眼科学*》。

Nonaccidental Trauma

Although most eye injuries in childhood are accidental or innocently caused by other children, a significant number of them result from physical abuse by adults. The terms used for intentional physical abuse of a child include *nonaccidental trauma and child abuse*. Child abuse includes emotional abuse, sexual abuse, and neglect as well as physical abuse. It is a pervasive problem, with an estimated 750,000 cases per year in the United States.

A reliable history is often difficult to obtain when nonaccidental trauma has occurred. Suspicion of nonaccidental trauma should be aroused when repeated accounts of the circumstances of injury or histories obtained from different individuals are inconsistent or when the events described do not correlate with the injuries (eg, bruises on multiple aspects of the head after "a fall") or with the child's developmental level (eg, a 1-month-old "rolling off a bed" or a 4-month-old "climbing out of a high chair").

Any physician who suspects child abuse is required by law in every US state and Canadian province to report the incident to a designated governmental agency. Once this obligation has been discharged, full investigation of the situation by appropriate specialists and authorities is usually performed. Physicians should be familiar with the regulations in their own country. If possible, ocular abnormalities should be documented photographically or with a detailed drawing to use as evidence in court.

Abusive Head Trauma

A unique complex of ocular, intracranial, and sometimes other injuries occurs in infants who have been abused by violent shaking. This is recognized as one of the most important manifestations of child abuse. Although the term *shaken baby syndrome* is still occasionally used, it has largely been replaced with the terms *abusive head trauma (AHT)* and *inflicted childhood neurotrauma* because these infants may sustain impact injury as well as shaking injury involving the head.

Patients with AHT are usually younger than 5 years and most often younger than 12 months. When a reliable history is available, it typically involves a parent or other caregiver who shook an inconsolable crying baby in anger or frustration. Often, however, the only information provided is that the child's mental status deteriorated or that a seizure or respiratory difficulty developed. The involved caregiver may relate that an episode of relatively minor trauma occurred, such as a fall from a bed. Even without a supporting history, the diagnosis of AHT can still be made with confidence on the basis of characteristic clinical findings. It must be kept in mind, however, that answers to important questions concerning the timing and circumstances of injury and the identity of the perpetrator frequently cannot be inferred from medical evidence alone.

Intracranial injury in AHT frequently includes subdural hematoma (typically bilateral over the cerebral convexities or in the interhemispheric fissure) and subarachnoid hemorrhage. Displacement of the brain in relation to the skull and dura mater ruptures bridging vessels, and compression against the cranial bones produces further damage. Neuroimaging may also show intracranial edema, ischemia, or contusion in the acute stage and atrophy in later stages. These findings are thought to result from repetitive, abrupt accelerationdeceleration of the child's head as it whiplashes back and forth during the shaking episode. Some authorities, citing the frequency with which patients with AHT also show evidence of having received blows to the head, think that impact is an essential component, although in many cases no sign of impact is found.

人为外伤

大多数儿童眼外伤是由于意外或其他儿童无意中造成的，但很大一部分是成人对儿童的虐待造成的。用于儿童有意身体虐待的术语包括*人为外伤*和*儿童虐待*。儿童虐待包括情感虐待、性虐待、忽视以及身体虐待。这是一个很普遍的问题，据估计，美国每年发生 750000 起儿童虐待事件。

当发生人为外伤时，很难获得可靠的病史。当重复询问受伤情况或病史时，不同的人描述不一致，或所描述的与受伤不符（如“摔倒”后头部多处淤伤），或与儿童发育水平不符（如 1 个月龄婴儿“滚落坠床”或 4 个月龄婴儿“爬出高椅”），都应怀疑为人为外伤。

根据美国每一个州和加拿大每一个省的法律，医生怀疑发生儿童虐待时，应向指定的政府机构报告。接到报告后，相关的专家和当局应对该情况进行全面调查。医生应熟悉所在国的法规。如有可能，应采用照片或详细地画图记录眼部异常，以便在法庭上作为证据。

虐待性头部外伤

被剧烈摇晃虐待的婴儿发生眼部、颅内以及其他特有的复合性伤，是虐待儿童的最重要表现之一。虽然*摇晃婴儿综合征*一词被偶尔使用，但它已经被*虐待性头部外伤（AHT）*和*获得性儿童神经损伤*所替代，因为这些婴儿可能会遭受头部撞击伤和摇晃伤。

虐待性头部外伤（AHT）患儿多小于 5 岁，最常见小于 12 个月龄。由可靠的病史得知，父母或其他看护者在愤怒或沮丧时会摇晃哭闹不止的婴儿。但常常可获得的唯一信息是，儿童的精神状况差、有癫痫或呼吸困难。看护者可能会提及曾发生过轻微外伤（如坠床）。即使没有病史支持，根据典型的临床表现即可诊断虐待性头部外伤（AHT）。但需注意，外伤时间和受伤的状态，以及施暴者身份常不能仅仅从医学证据中推断出来。

虐待性头部外伤（AHT）的颅内损伤有硬膜下血肿（双侧大脑凸面或半球间裂 / 纵裂）和蛛网膜下腔出血。脑与颅骨和硬脑膜的相对移位，撕裂桥接血管，脑向颅骨的挤压产生进一步的损伤。神经影像学检查显示，颅内水肿、缺血，或急性期脑挫伤、晚期脑萎缩，是在摇晃过程中，儿童头部反复突然加速 – 减速，类似于来回鞭打脑组织所致。一些专家参考了虐待性头部外伤（AHT）患儿头部遭受撞击的频率，证实为头部受到撞击，他们认为撞击是重要原因，即使在许多病例中并没有发现撞击的迹象。

Ocular involvement

The most common ocular manifestation of AHT, present in approximately 80% of cases, is retinal hemorrhage. These hemorrhages can be seen in all layers of the retina and may be unilateral or bilateral. They are found most commonly in the posterior pole but often extend to the periphery (Fig 27-4). Vitreous hemorrhage may also develop, usually as a secondary phenomenon resulting from migration of blood from a preretinal hemorrhage into the vitreous. Occasionally, the vitreous becomes almost completely opacified by dispersed hemorrhage within a few days of injury. Retinal hemorrhages in shaken infants cannot be dated with precision and usually resolve over a period of weeks to months. Vitrectomy should be considered if there is a risk of amblyopia due to persistentvitreous hemorrhage.

Some eyes show evidence of retinal tissue disruption in addition to hemorrhage. Fullthickness perimacular folds in the neurosensory retina, typically with circumferential orientation around the macula that creates a craterlike appearance, are highly characteristic.

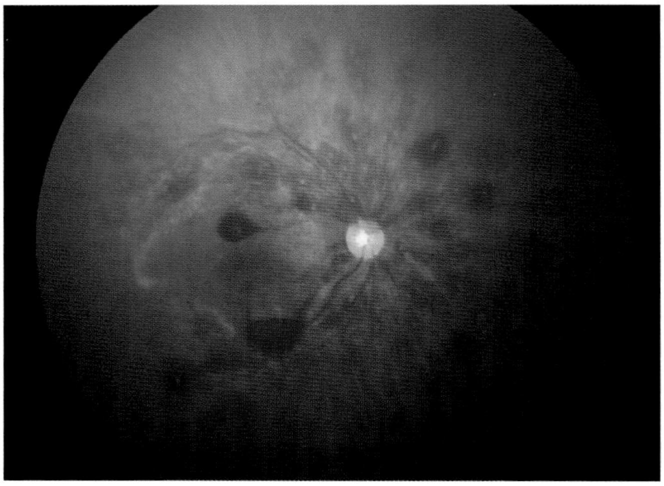

Figure 27-4 Extensive retinal hemorrhages in a 4-month-old infant suspected to have been violently shaken. *(Courtesy of Sophia Ying Fang, MD.)*

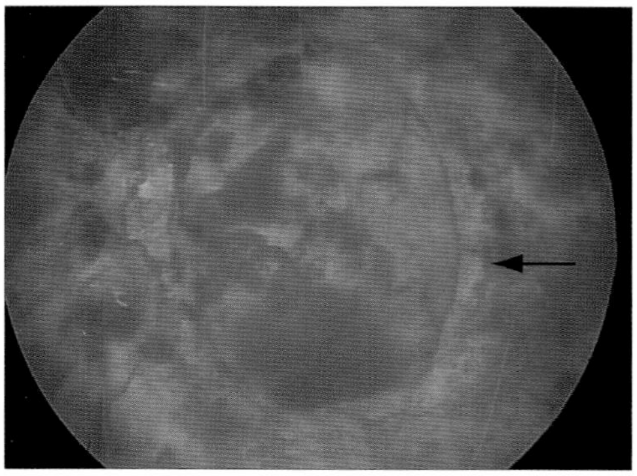

Figure 27-5 Traumatic retinoschisis with perimacular folds *(arrow)*. *(Courtesy of Ken K. Nischal, MD.)*

眼部受累

虐待性头部外伤（AHT）最常见的眼部表现是视网膜出血，约占 80%，可见于视网膜全层，单眼或双眼。最常见于后极部，但常累及周边部（图 27–4）。也可见玻璃体积血，继发于视网膜前出血扩散到玻璃体。偶见受伤后几天内出血扩散，玻璃体混浊。被摇晃婴儿的视网膜出血无法确定具体日期，需要几周到几个月才能被吸收。如果玻璃体积血持续存在，并有导致弱视的风险，应考虑玻璃体切除术。

除出血外，某些病例还有视网膜组织破裂。黄斑周视网膜神经感觉层全层皱襞具有特征性表现，即环绕黄斑的环形方向呈陨石坑样外观。

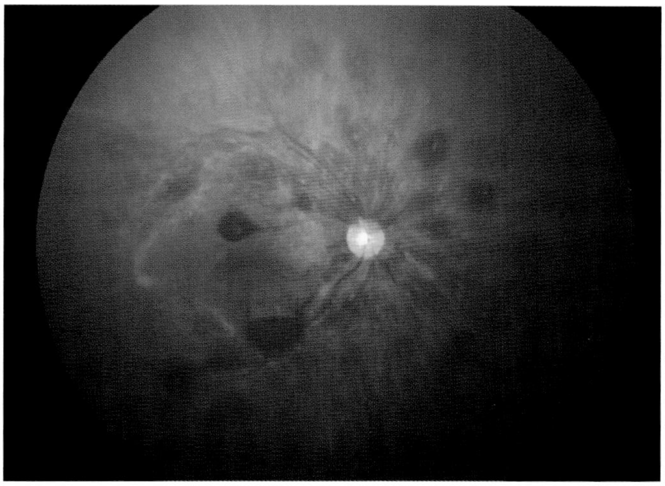

图 27–4　广泛的视网膜出血，4 月龄婴儿，怀疑被剧烈摇晃。*（译者注：资料来源见前页原文。）*

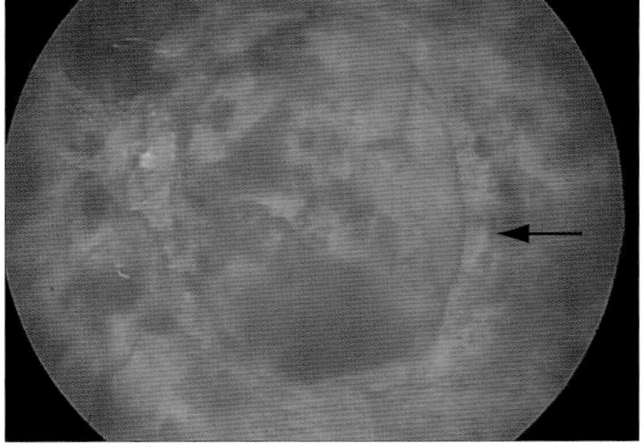

图 27–5　外伤性视网膜劈裂，伴黄斑周皱襞*（箭头）*。*（译者注：资料来源见前页原文。）*

Splitting of the retina (traumatic retinoschisis), either deep to the nerve fiber layer or superficial (involving only the internal limiting membrane), may create cavities of considerable extent that are partially filled with blood, also usually in the macular region (Fig 27-5). Full-thickness retinal breaks and detachment are rare. Retinal folds usually flatten out within a few weeks of injury, but schisis cavities can persist indefinitely.

A striking feature of AHT is the typical lack of external evidence of trauma. The ocular adnexa and anterior segment may appear entirely normal. Occasionally, the trunk or extremities show bruises representing the imprint of the perpetrator's hands. In a minority of cases, broken ribs or characteristic metaphyseal fractures of the long bones result from forces generated during shaking. It must be kept in mind, however, that these patients may have been subjected to other forms of abuse.

When extensive retinal hemorrhage accompanied by perimacular folds and schisis cavities is found in association with intracranial hemorrhage or other evidence of trauma to the brain in an infant, AHT can usually be diagnosed with confidence regardless of other circumstances. Severe accidental head trauma (eg, sustained in a fall from a second-story level or in a motor vehicle collision) is not frequently accompanied by retinal hemorrhage, and hemorrhage is not extensive when present. Retinal hemorrhage is rare and has never been documented to be extensive following cardiopulmonary resuscitation by trained personnel. Severe, fatal, acute head-crush injury rarely causes hemorrhagic retinopathy with perimacular folds, which can be differentiated from AHT by the associated injuries.

Extensive retinal hemorrhage without other ocular findings strongly suggests that intracranial injury has been caused by AHT, but alternative possibilities such as a coagulation disorder must be considered as well. Retinal hemorrhages resulting from birth trauma are common in newborns, but they seldom persist beyond the age of 1 month. Other possible causes of retinal hemorrhage in children include anemia, hypertension, acutely increased intracranial pressure, leukemia, meningitis, glutaricaciduria, and retinopathy of prematurity.

American Academy of Ophthalmology, Hoskins Center. Clinical Statement. *Abusive Head Trauma/Shaken Baby Syndrome—2015*. San Francisco: American Academy of Ophthalmology; 2015. Available at https://www.aao.org/clinical-statement/abusive-head-traumashaken-baby-syndrome.

Christian CW, Block R; Committee on Child Abuse and Neglect; American Academy of Pediatrics. Abusive head trauma in infants and children. *Pediatrics*. 2009;123(5): 1409–1411.

Maguire SA, Watts PO, Shaw AD, et al. Retinal haemorrhages and related findings in abusive and nonabusive head trauma: a systematic review. *Eye (Lond)*. 2013;27(1):28–36.

Prognosis

In one large study, 29% of children with AHT died of their injuries. Poor visual and pupillary responses were correlated with a higher risk of mortality. Survivors often had permanent impairment ranging from mild learning disability and motor disturbances to severe cognitive impairment and quadriparesis. The most common cause of vision loss is cortical injury followed by optic atrophy. Dense vitreous hemorrhage, usually associated with deep traumatic retinoschisis, carries a poor prognosis for both vision and life.

Kivlin JD, Simons KB, Lazoritz S, Ruttum MS. Shaken baby syndrome. *Ophthalmology*. 2000;107(7):1246–1254.

视网膜劈裂（外伤性视网膜劈裂），可能深达神经纤维层或仅累及表面（内界膜），可产生较大范围的腔隙，部分充填血液，常见于黄斑区（图 27-5）。全层裂孔和视网膜脱离罕见。视网膜皱襞在损伤后几周内变平，但劈裂腔可持续存在。

虐待性头部外伤（AHT）的一个显著特点是缺乏外伤的外部证据。眼附属器和眼前节可能完全正常。偶见躯干或四肢出现淤伤，呈现施暴者手印。在少数情况下，摇晃过程中产生的力可导致肋骨骨折或特征性长骨干骺端骨折。需注意，这些患儿可能遭受过其他形式的虐待。

如果发现婴儿广泛性视网膜出血，伴黄斑周皱襞和劈裂腔，同时伴颅内出血或其他脑损伤，无论其他情况如何，可确诊虐待性头部外伤（AHT）。严重的意外头部创伤（如从二楼跌落或机动车碰撞）少见视网膜出血，即使有出血，范围也较小。训练有素的人员进行心肺复苏后，罕见视网膜出血，且未见报道。严重致命的急性头部挤压伤罕见伴黄斑周褶皱的出血性视网膜病变，可通过相关损伤与虐待性头部外伤（AHT）进行鉴别。

不伴其他眼部表现的广泛性视网膜出血强烈提示颅内损伤，由虐待性头部外伤（AHT）所致。还应考虑凝血障碍。新生儿产伤导致的视网膜出血较为常见，但很少持续 1 个月。其他儿童视网膜出血的可能原因包括贫血、高血压、急性颅内压升高、白血病、脑膜炎、戊二酸尿症和早产儿视网膜病变。

American Academy of Ophthalmology, Hoskins Center. Clinical Statement. *Abusive Head Trauma/Shaken Baby Syndrome—2015*. San Francisco: American Academy of Ophthalmology; 2015. Available at https://www.aao.org/clinical-statement/abusive-head-traumashaken-baby-syndrome.

Christian CW, Block R; Committee on Child Abuse and Neglect; American Academy of Pediatrics. Abusive head trauma in infants and children. *Pediatrics*. 2009;123(5): 1409–1411.

Maguire SA, Watts PO, Shaw AD, et al. Retinal haemorrhages and related findings in abusive and nonabusive head trauma: a systematic review. *Eye (Lond)*. 2013;27(1):28–36.

预后

在一项大型研究中，29% 的虐待性头部外伤（AHT）儿童死亡，视力较差和瞳孔反应迟钝预示死亡率更高。幸存者多伴有永久性损伤，可从轻度学习障碍和运动障碍，到严重认知障碍和四肢瘫痪。视力丧失最常见的原因是皮质损伤，其次是视神经萎缩。致密玻璃体积血常与严重外伤性视网膜劈裂有关，患儿视力和生活均预后不良。

Kivlin JD, Simons KB, Lazoritz S, Ruttum MS. Shaken baby syndrome. *Ophthalmology*. 2000;107(7):1246–1254.

Ocular Injury Secondary to Nonaccidental Trauma

The presenting sign of child abuse involves the eye in approximately 5% of cases. Blunt trauma inflicted with fin gers, fists, or implements such as belts or straps is the usual mechanism of nonaccidental injury to the ocular adnexa or anterior segment. Periorbital ecchymosis, subconjunctival hemorrhage, and hyphema should raise suspicion of recent abuse if the explanation provided is implausible (see the section "Hyphema" earlier in this chapter). Cataract and lens dislocation may be a sign of repeated injury or trauma inflicted earlier. Child abuse should also be suspected with rhegmatogenous retinal detachment in a child without a history of injury or an apparent predisposing factor, such as high myopia.

继发于人为外伤的眼部损伤

儿童受虐待的症状中，约 5% 表现在眼部。手指、拳头或皮带、带子等工具造成的钝挫伤，是眼附属器或眼前节人为外伤的常见原因。有眶周淤斑、结膜下出血和前房积血症状时，如果提供的解释不合情理（参见本章“前房积血”一节），应怀疑近期有儿童虐待。白内障和晶状体脱位可能是反复受伤或创伤的早期体征。儿童孔源性视网膜脱离，若没有外伤史或易患因素（高度近视），也应怀疑为儿童虐待。

（翻译 赵方宇 朱晓鹃 // 审校 刘陇黔 石一宁 蒋宁 // 章节审校 石广礼）

CHAPTER 28

Ocular Manifestations of Systemic Disease

This chapter focuses on select systemic disorders with multiple types of ocular involvement. Systemic disorders with 1 primary ocular abnormality are discussed in other chapters in this volume. Often, the ophthalmologist can help to make the correct systemic diagnosis.

Diseases due to Chromosomal Abnormalities

Abnormalities in chromosomal number (aneuploidy: trisomy or monosomy), structure (duplications, deletions, translocations, inversions, or rings), or type (autosomal or sex chromosome) occur in approximately 1 in 150 live births. Table 28-1 lists select chromosomal abnormalities commonly associated with ocular findings. Also see BCSC Section 2, *Fundamentals and Principles of Ophthalmology*, Chapter 6.

Inborn Errors of Metabolism

Inborn errors of metabolism are estimated to occur in 1 in 1400 births and are typically caused by biallelic mutations. Ocular findings can result from direct toxicity of abnormal metabolic products, accumulation of abnormal (or normal) metabolites, errors of synthetic pathways, or deficient production of energy. The age at onset of ocular manifestations of inborn errors of metabolism varies. Table 28-2 summarizes the common ophthalmic manifestations of select conditions. Also see Chapter 21. Following are examples of ocular structural abnormalities secondary to metabolic disorders:

- Corneal clouding or deposits: certain mucopolysaccharidoses (Fig 28-1), cystinosis (Fig 28-2), Schnyder corneal dystrophy (Fig 28-3)
- Corneal pseudodendritic ulcerations: tyrosinemia
- Cataracts: diabetes mellitus, galactosemia, Smith-Lemli-Opitz syndrome, cerebrotendinous xanthomatosis (Fig 28-4)
- Lens luxation or subluxation: homocystinuria (Fig 28-5)
- Retinal degeneration: peroxisomal disorders (Zellweger syndrome, Refsum disease), lysosomal disorders (eg, neuronal ceroid lipofuscinosis), mitochondrial disorders (eg, Kearns-Sayre syndrome [Fig 28-6])

第 28 章

全身性疾病的眼部表现

本章着重介绍具有多种眼部表现的全身性疾病。在本书的其他章节中讨论了全身性疾病伴 1 种原发性眼部异常。通常，眼科医生可帮助做出正确的全身疾病诊断。

染色体异常导致的疾病

1/150 的活产儿可发生染色体异常，有数目异常（非整倍体，如三倍体或单倍体）、结构异常（复制、缺失、易位、倒位或成环）或类型异常（常染色体或性染色体）。表 28-1 列出了伴眼部表现的染色体异常。见 BCSC 第 2 册《*眼科学基础与原理*》第 6 章。

先天性代谢缺陷

据估计，每 1400 名新生儿中就有 1 名患有先天性代谢缺陷，是等位基因突变所致。异常代谢产物的直接毒性、异常（或正常）代谢产物的蓄积、合成途径的异常或能量生产不足均导致眼部表现。先天性代谢缺陷眼部表现的发病年龄各不相同。表 28-2 总结了一些疾病的常见眼部表现。详见第 21 章。以下举例说明继发于代谢性疾病的眼部器质性异常：

- 角膜混浊或沉积物：某些类型黏多糖贮积症（图 28-1）、胱氨酸贮积症（图 28-2）、Schnyder 角膜营养不良（图 28-3）
- 角膜假性树突溃疡：酪氨酸血症
- 白内障：糖尿病、半乳糖血症、Smith-Lemli-Opitz 综合征、脑腱黄瘤病（图 28-4）
- 晶状体脱位或半脱位：同型胱氨酸尿症（图 28-5）
- 视网膜变性：过氧化物酶体疾病（Zellweger 综合征、Refsum 病）、溶酶体疾病（如神经元蜡样脂褐质沉积症）、线粒体疾病［如 Kearns-Sayre 综合征（图 28-6）］

Table 28-1 Common Chromosomal Abnormalities With Ocular Associations

Chromosomal Abnormality	Associated Ocular Findings
Trisomy 13, Patau syndrome	*More common:* microphthalmia, coloboma, retinal dysplasia with frequent islands of intraocular cartilage *Less common:* cataract, corneal opacification, cyclopia, persistent fetal vasculature, shallow supraorbital ridges, upward-slanting palpebral fissures, absent eyebrows, hypotelorism, hypertelorism, anophthalmia, glaucoma
Trisomy 18, Edwards syndrome	*More common:* short palpebral fissures, hypertelorism, epicanthus, hypoplastic supraorbital ridge *Less common:* cataract, microcornea, corneal opacification, congenital glaucoma, retinal depigmentation, colobomatous microphthalmia, cyclopia
Trisomy 21, Down syndrome (most common trisomy)	*More common:* epicanthus with upward-slanting palpebral fissures, blepharitis, Brushfield spots, congenital or acquired cataract, myopia, congenital nasolacrimal duct obstruction and difficulty with probings, ectropion, strabismus, hypoaccommodation, nystagmus, increased number of vessels at optic disc margin *Less common:* infantile glaucoma, keratoconus
Deletion 4p, Wolf-Hirschhorn syndrome	*More common:* colobomatous microphthalmia, epicanthus, downward-slanting palpebral fissures, hypertelorism, strabismus, ptosis, corneal opacification (Peters anomaly) *Less common:* anterior segment anomalies, cataract
Deletion 5p, cri-du-chat syndrome	*More common:* upward- or downward-slanting palpebral fissures, hypotelorism or hypertelorism, epicanthus, strabismus *Less common:* ptosis, decreased tear production, myopia, cataract, glaucoma, tortuous retinal vessels, foveal hypoplasia, optic atrophy, colobomatous microphthalmia
Deletion 18p	*More common:* hypertelorism, ptosis, epicanthus, and strabismus *Less common:* cataracts, retinal dysplasia, colobomatous microphthalmia, synophthalmia/cyclopia
Deletion 18q	*More common:* epicanthus, hypertelorism, downward-slanting palpebral fissures, strabismus, dysplastic or atrophic optic nerve, nystagmus *Less common:* corneal abnormalities, cataracts, blue sclera, myopia, colobomatous microphthalmia
Monosomy X, Turner syndrome	*More common:* strabismus, ptosis *Less common:* cataracts, refractive errors, corneal scars, blue sclera Incidence of color blindness similar to that in unaffected males

表28-1　常见的眼部相关染色体异常

染色体异常	相关的眼部表现
13三体，Patau综合征	*常见:* 小眼球、眼缺损、视网膜发育不良伴眼内软骨岛 *少见:* 白内障、角膜混浊、独眼、永久性胎儿血管、浅眶上嵴、睑裂向上倾斜、眉毛缺失、眼距过窄、眼距过宽、眼缺如、青光眼
18三体，Edwards综合征	*常见:* 短睑裂、眼距过宽、内眦赘皮、眶上嵴发育不全 *少见:* 白内障、小角膜、角膜混浊、先天性青光眼、视网膜色素脱失、缺损性小眼球、独眼
21三体，Down综合征（最常见三体）	*常见:* 内眦赘皮伴睑裂向上倾斜、睑缘炎、Brushfield斑、先天性或获得性白内障、近视、先天性鼻泪管阻塞且探查困难、睑外翻、斜视、调节不足、眼球震颤、视盘边缘血管数量增加 *少见:* 婴幼儿型青光眼、圆锥角膜
4p缺失，Wolf-Hirschhorn综合征	*常见:* 缺损性小眼球、内眦赘皮、睑裂向下倾斜、眼距过宽、斜视、上睑下垂、角膜混浊（Peter异常） *少见:* 眼前节异常、白内障
5p缺失，cri-du-chat综合征	*常见:* 睑裂向上或向下倾斜、眼距过窄或过宽、内眦赘皮、斜视 *少见:* 上睑下垂、泪液分泌减少、近视、白内障、青光眼、视网膜血管迂曲、中心凹发育不良、视神经萎缩、缺损性小眼球
18p缺失	*常见:* 眼距过宽、上睑下垂、内眦赘皮、斜视 *少见:* 白内障、视网膜发育不良、缺损性小眼球、并眼/独眼
18q缺失	*常见:* 内眦赘皮、眼距过宽、睑裂向下倾斜、斜视、视神经发育不良或萎缩、眼球震颤 *少见:* 角膜异常、白内障、蓝色巩膜、近视、缺损性小眼球
X单体，Turner综合征	*常见:* 斜视、上睑下垂 *少见:* 白内障、屈光不正、角膜瘢痕、蓝色巩膜 色盲的发病率与未患病男性相似

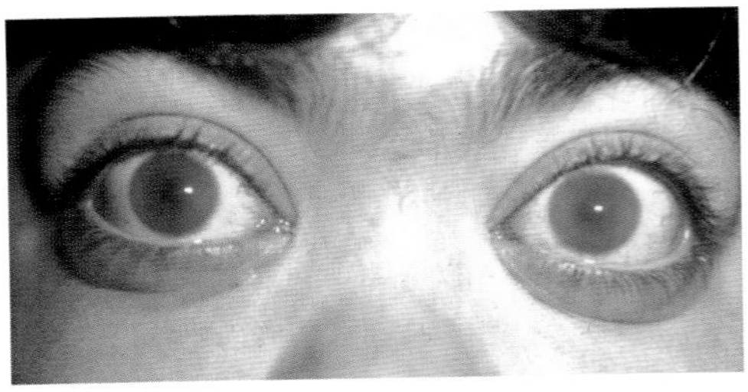

Figure 28-1 Bilateral corneal clouding in mucopolysaccharidosis VI. *(Courtesy of Edward L. Raab, MD.)*

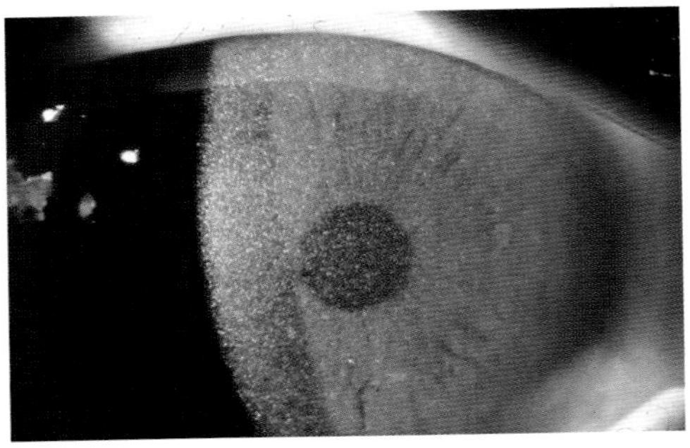

Figure 28-2 Cystinosis with corneal involvement. *(Courtesy of Gregg T. Lueder, MD.)*

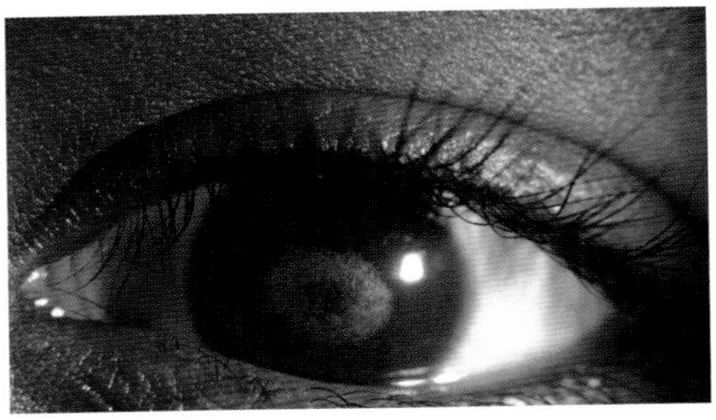

Figure 28-3 Corneal crystals in a girl with Schnyder corneal dystrophy. *(Courtesy of Arif O. Khan, MD.)*

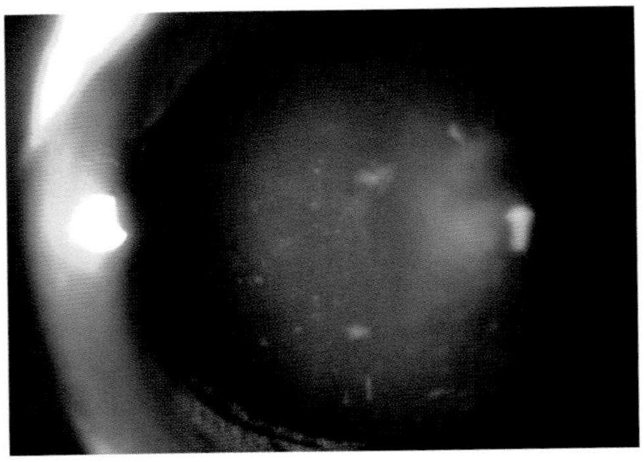

Figure 28-4 Fleck opacities and posterior capsular cataract secondary to cerebrotendinous xanthomatosis in the right eye of a boy. The patient had a history of intractable infantile diarrhea. *(Modified with permission from Khan AO, Aldahmesh MA, Mohamed JY, Alkuraya FS. Juvenile cataract morphology in 3 siblings not yet diagnosed with cerebrotendinous xanthomatosis.* Ophthalmology. *2013;120(5):956–960.)*

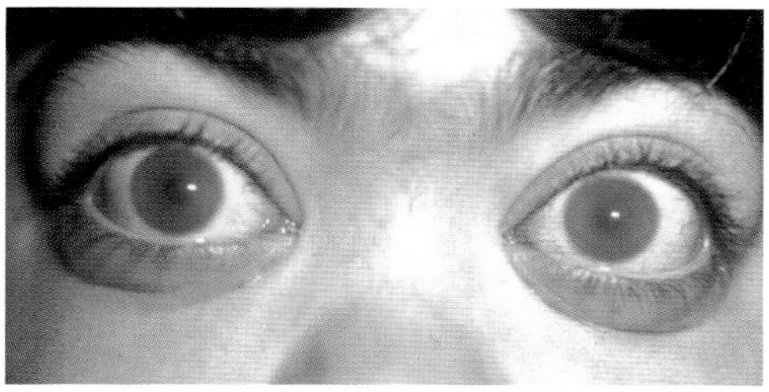

图 28–1　双眼角膜混浊，患黏多糖贮积症 VI 型。*（译者注：资料来源见前页原文。）*

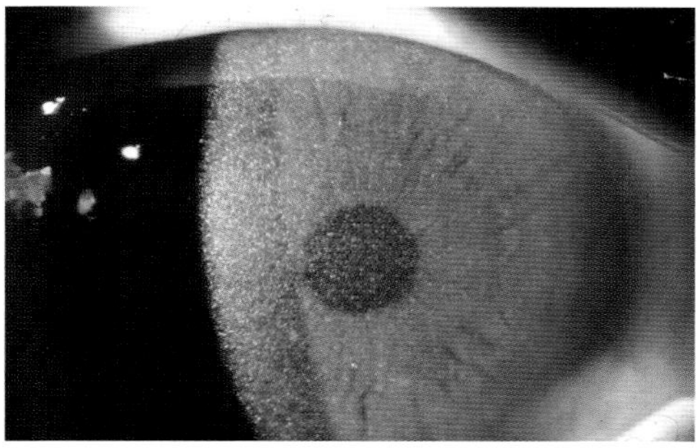

图 28–2　胱氨酸贮积症，累及角膜。*（译者注：资料来源见前页原文。）*

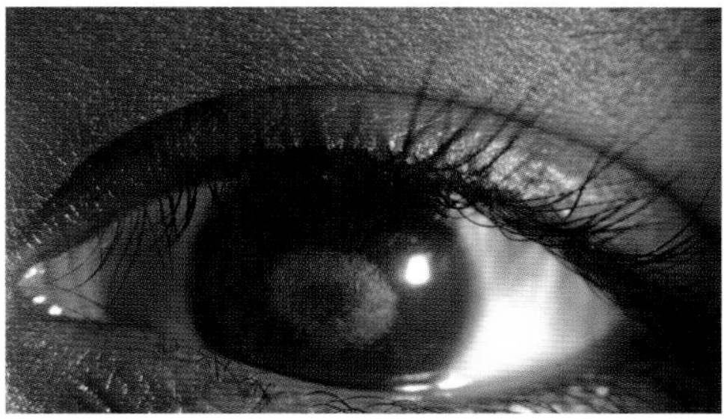

图 28–3　Schnyder 角膜营养不良伴角膜结晶，女性。*（译者注：资料来源见前页原文。）*

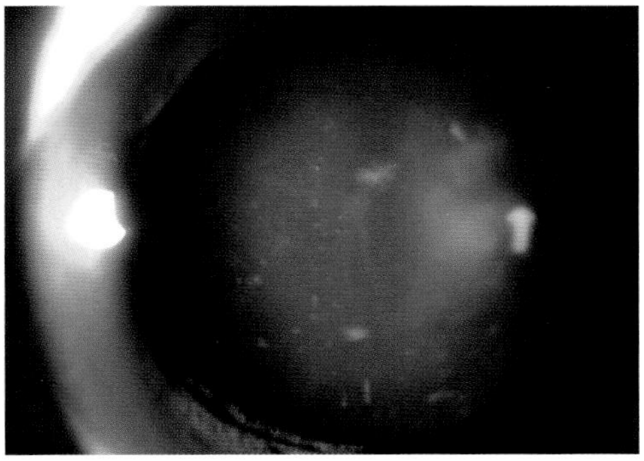

图 28–4　晶状体斑点混浊和后囊型白内障，继发于脑腱黄瘤病，男孩，右眼。患儿有顽固性婴儿腹泻病史。*（译者注：资料来源见前页原文。）*

Table 28-2 Ocular Findings in Mucopolysaccharidoses, Mucolipidoses, Lipidoses, Gangliosidoses, and Miscellaneous Disorders

Disease (code)*	Enzyme Deficiency	Corneal Clouding	Motility Disorders	Cherry-Red Spot	Retinal Dystrophy	Optic Atrophy	Other	Inheritance
Mucopolysaccharidosis (MPS) syndromes								
MPS IH (Hurler) (607014)	α-L-Iduronidase	+++	–	–	+++	+	Glaucoma; plus papilledema (IH only)	AR
MPS IS (Scheie) (607016)								
MPS II (Hunter) (309900)	Iduronate-2-sulfatase	–	–	–	++	+	–	XR
MPS III (Sanfilippo)	A: Heparan *N*-sulfatase	–	–	–	++	Rare	Late blindness	AR
A (252900)	B: α-*N*-Acetyl-glucosaminidase							
B (252920)	C: Acetyl-CoA:α-glucosaminide *N*-acetyltransferase							
C (252930)								
D (252940)	D: *N*-Acetylglucosamine-6-sulfatase							
MPS IV (Morquio)	A: *N*-Acetyl-galactosamine-6-sulfatase	++	–	–	Rare	Rare	–	A: AR
A (253200)								
B (253010)	B: β-Galactosidase							B: AR
MPS VI (Maroteaux-Lamy) (253200)	Arylsulfatase B	++	–	–	–	+	Papilledema, glaucoma	AR
MPS VII (Sly) (253220)	β-Glucuronidase	+	–	–	–	–	–	AR
Mucolipidoses								
Type I (256550)	Neuraminidase	–	+	+	+	–	Hearing loss	AR
Sialidosis (glycoproteinosis)								
"Cherry-red spot myoclonus syndrome"								
Type II (252500) (I-cell disease)	Multiple lysosomal enzymes	++	–	–	–	–	Hurler-like	AR
Type III (252600) (pseudo-Hurler polydystrophy)	Multiple lysosomal enzymes	+++	–		–	–	Hurler-like puffy eyelids	AR
Type IV (252650)	Mucolipin-1 defect	+++	–	–	++	+	Photophobia	AR
Gangliosidosis								
Lipidoses								
Niemann-Pick disease (257220)	Sphingomyelinase	+	Nystagmus	+	–	+	Eventual vision loss	AR
Fabry disease (301500)	α-Galactosidase A	Whorl-like	–	–	–	–	Angiokeratoma, spokelike cataract, aneurysmal conjunctival vessels	XR
Gaucher disease	Acid β-glucosidase	–	Paralytic strabismus, looped saccades	–	+	–	Pinguecula, conjunctival pigmentation	AR
Type I (230800)								
Type II (230900)								
Type III (231005)								
Metachromatic leukodystrophy (250100)	Arylsulfatase A	–	Nystagmus	+	–	+	Blindness, decreased pupil reaction	AR
Krabbe disease (245200)	Galactosylceramidase	–	Nystagmus	Rare	–	+	Cortical blindness	AR
Fucosidosis (230000)	α-L-Fucosidase	–	–	–	+	–	Hurler-like features, angiokeratoma, tortuous conjunctival vessels	AR

表28-2　黏多糖贮积症、黏脂质贮积症、脂贮积症、神经节苷脂病和其他疾病的眼部表现

疾病（编号）*	酶缺陷	角膜混浊	运动障碍	樱桃红斑	视网膜发育不良	视神经萎缩	其他	遗传
黏多糖贮积症(MPS)综合征								
MPS IH 型(Hurler)(607014)	α-L-艾杜糖醛酸酶	+++	-	-	++++	+	青光眼；合并视盘水肿（仅见于IH型）	AR
MPS IS型(Scheie)(607016)								
MPS II型(Hunter)(309900)	艾杜糖醛酸-2-硫酸酯酶	-	-	-	++	+	-	XR
MPS III型(Sanfilippo)	A：乙酰肝素-*N*-硫酸酯酶	-	-	-	++	罕见	迟发性盲	AR
A (252900)	B：α-*N*-乙酰-氨基葡萄糖苷酶							
B (252920)	C：乙酰-辅酶Aα-氨基葡萄糖苷							
C (252930)	*N*-乙酰转移酶							
D (252940)	D：*N*-乙酰葡糖胺-6-硫酸酯酶							
MPS IV型(Morquio)	A：*N*-乙酰葡糖胺-6-硫酸酯酶	++	-	-	罕见	罕见	-	A: AR
A (253200)								
B (253010)	B：β-半乳糖苷酶							B: AR
MPS VI型(Maroteaus-Lamy)(253200)	芳香基硫酸酯酶B	++	-	-	-	+	视盘水肿、青光眼	AR
MPS VII型(Sly)(253220)	β-葡萄糖醛酸酶	+	-	-	-	-	-	AR
黏脂质贮积症								
I型(256550)	神经氨酸苷酶	-	+	+	+	-	听力丧失	AR
唾液酸贮积症（糖蛋白贮积病）								
“樱桃红斑肌痉挛综合征”								
II型(252500)（I细胞病）	多种溶酶体酶	++	-	-	-	-	Hurler样	AR
III型(252600)（假性-Hurler多种营养不良症）	多种溶酶体酶	+++	-		-	-	Hurler样眼睑肿胀	AR
IV型(252650)	黏脂蛋白-1 缺陷	+++	-	-	++	+	畏光	AR
神经节苷脂贮积症								
脂贮积症								
Niemann-Pick病（257220）	神经鞘磷脂酶	+	眼球震颤	+	-	+	最终视力损失	AR
Fabry病（301500）	α-半乳糖苷酶 A	Whorl样	-	-	-	-	血管角皮瘤，辐辏状白内障，血管动脉瘤	XR
Gaucher病	酸性β-葡萄糖苷酶	-	麻痹性斜视，环形扫视	-	+	-	睑裂斑，结膜色素沉着	AR
I型(230800)								
II型(230900)								
III型(231005)								
异染性脑白质营养不良（250100）	芳香基硫酸酯酶A	-	眼球震颤	+	-	+	盲，瞳孔反射减弱	AR
Krabbe病（245200）	半乳糖神经酰胺酶	-	眼球震颤	罕见	-	+	皮质盲	AR
岩藻糖苷贮积症	α-L-岩藻糖苷酶	-	-	-	+	-	Hurler样改变，血管角皮瘤，结膜血管迂曲	AR

Disease (code)*	Enzyme Deficiency	Conjunctival Tortuosity	Corneal Clouding	Motility Disorders	Cherry-Red Spot	Retinal Dystrophy	Optic Atrophy	High Myopia	Blindness	Inheritance
Gangliosidoses										
Generalized (GM_1) gangliosidoses										
Type I (230500)	β-Galactosidase-1	+	±	ET, nystagmus	50% of patients	–	+	+	+	AR
Type II (230600) (juvenile GM_1, Derry disease)	β-Galactosidase-1	–	–	ET, nystagmus	–	+	±	–	Late	AR
Type III (230650) (adult GM_1)	β-Galactosidase-1	±	Rare	–	–	–	–	–	–	AR
GM_2 gangliosidoses										
Tay-Sachs disease (272800)										
Type I (classic infantile)	Hexosaminidase A	–	–	Nystagmus, ophthalmoplegia	+	–	+	–	+	AR
B1 variant (late infantile)	HEXA defect									AR
Type III (juvenile subacute)	Hexosaminidase A or B		+	Strabismus	+	+	+		+	AR
Chronic adult	HEXA defect			Ocular motor defects						AR
Type II (268800) (Sandhoff disease)	Hexosaminidase A and B	–	Rare	ET	+	–	±	–	+	AR
Type AB, Hexosaminidase activator deficiency	Activator deficiency			Strabismus	+	+	+		Late	AR

Disease (code)*	Enzyme Deficiency	Corneal Clouding	Motility Disorders	Cherry-Red Spot	Retinal Dystrophy	Optic Atrophy	Other	Inheritance
Miscellaneous disorders								
Galactosialidosis (256540)	β-Galactosidase, neuraminidase	+	–	+	–	+	Dwarfism, seizures, coarse facies	AR
Neuronal ceroid lipofuscinosis								
CLN1 Infantile Hagberg-Santavuori disease (256730)	Palmitoyl-protein thioesterase 1 (PPT-1)	–	+	Macular	+	+*	Blindness	AR
CLN2 Late infantile Hagberg-Santavuori (204500)	PPT-1	–	+	Bull's eye	+	+	Blindness	AR
CLN3 Juvenile Batten, Spielmeyer-Vogt disease (204200)	Unknown	–	+	Bull's eye	+	+	Blindness	AR
CLN4 Adult Kufs disease (204300)	Unknown	–	–	–	–	–		AR
Cystinosis (219800)	Unknown	Crystals	–	–	++	–	Conjunctival crystals, renal problems	AR
Galactosemia (230400)	Gal-1-PO_4 uridyl transferase	–	–	–	–	–	Cataracts if not treated	AR
Mannosidosis (248500)	α-Mannosidase	++	–	–	+	Pallor, blurred margin	Hurler-like, spokelike cataract	AR
Homocystinuria (236200)	Cystathionine β-synthase	–	–	–	+	–	Dislocated lens, cataract	AR
Refsum disease (266500)	Phytanic acid α-hydroxylase	–	–	–	++	–	Cataract, night blindness	AR

* Code numbers refer to the system developed by Victor McKusick and colleagues (McKusick VA, Francomano CA, Antonarakis SE. *Mendelian Inheritance in Man: Catalogs of Autosomal Dominant, Autosomal Recessive, and X-Linked Phenotypes.* 10th ed. Baltimore: The Johns Hopkins University Press; 1992). Table updates from Online Mendelian Inheritance in Man (www.ncbi.nlm.nih.gov/omim).
Plus (+) and minus (–) signs indicate the relative likelihood of occurrence of ocular findings in these systemic disorders. AR = autosomal recessive; ET = constant esotropia; XR = X-linked recessive.

疾病（编号）*	酶缺陷	结膜迂曲	角膜混浊	运动障碍	樱桃红斑	视网膜发育不良	视神经萎缩	高度近视	盲	遗传
神经节苷脂贮积症										
广泛（GM_1）神经节苷脂贮积症										
I型(230500)	β-半乳糖苷酶-1	+	±	ET，眼球震颤	50%患者	-	+	+	+	AR
II型(230600)（青少年GM1，Derry病）	β-半乳糖苷酶-1	-	-	ET，眼球震颤	-	+	±	-	迟发	AR
III型(230650)（成人GM1）	β-半乳糖苷酶-1	±	罕见	-	-	-	-	-	-	AR
GM_2神经节苷脂贮积症										
Tay-Sachs病（272800）										
I型（典型婴儿型）	氨基己糖苷酶A	-	-	眼球震颤，眼肌麻痹	+	-	+	-	+	AR
B1变异（迟发婴儿型）	HEXA缺陷									AR
III型（青少年亚急性）	氨基己糖苷酶A或B		+	斜视	+	+	+			AR
成年慢性	HEXA缺陷			眼运动缺陷					+	AR
II型（268800）（Sandhoff病）	氨基己糖苷酶A和B	-	罕见	ET	+	-	±	-	+	AR
AB型，氨基己糖苷酶激活物缺陷	激活物缺陷			斜视	+	+	+		迟发	AR

疾病（编号）*	酶缺陷	角膜混浊	运动障碍	樱桃红斑	视网膜发育不良	视神经萎缩	其他	遗传
其他疾病								
半乳糖苷唾液酸贮积症（256540）	β-半乳糖苷酶, 神经氨酸酶	+	-	+	-	+	侏儒症，癫痫发作，面容粗犷	AR
神经元蜡样质脂褐质贮积症								
CLN1婴儿型Hagberg-Santavuori病（256730）	棕榈酰-蛋白硫酯酶1（PPT-1）	-	+	黄斑	+	+	盲	AR
CLN2迟发婴儿型Hagberg-Santavuori（204500）	PPT-1	-	+	牛眼	+	+	盲	AR
CLN3青少年型Spielmeyer-Vogt病（204200）	未知	-	+	牛眼	+	+	盲	AR
CLN4成人Kufs病（204300）	未知	-	-	-	-	-		AR
胱氨酸贮积症（219800）	未知	结晶	-	-	++	-	结膜结晶，肾脏疾病	AR
半乳糖血症（230400）	半乳糖-1-PO_4尿苷转移酶	-	-	-	-	-	不治疗，则白内障	AR
甘露糖苷贮积症（248500）	α-甘露糖苷酶	++	-	-	+	苍白，边缘模糊	Hurler样，辐辏状白内障	AR
同型胱氨酸尿症（236200）	胱硫醚β-合成酶	-	-	-	+	-	晶体脱位，白内障	AR
Refsum病（266500）	植烷酸α-羟化酶	-	-	-	++	-	白内障，夜盲	AR

*编码系统开发人员ViktorMckusick and collegues (McKusick VA，Francomano CA，Antonarakis SE。*孟德尔遗传基因：染色体组，常染色体组隐性和X连锁表型*。第十版。巴尔的摩：约翰霍普金斯大学出版社；1992年)。人类孟德尔遗传学的最新表格(www.ncbi.nlm.nih.gov/omim)。加号(+)和减号(－)表示在这些系统性疾病中出现眼部表现的相对可能性。AR=常染色体隐性遗传；ET：恒定内斜视；XR=X连锁隐性。

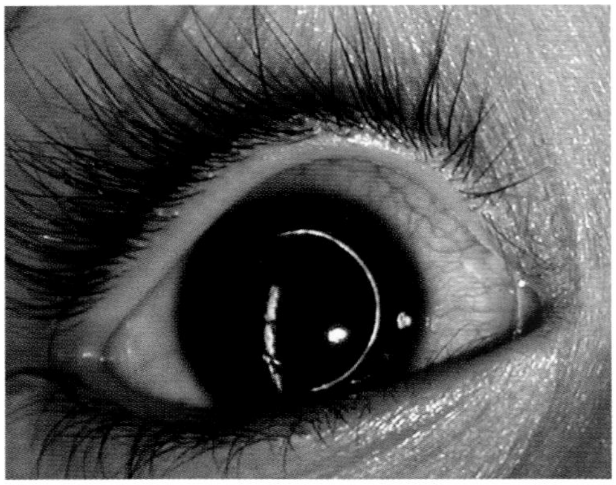

Figure 28-5 Lens luxation into the anterior chamber and acute glaucoma as the presenting sign of homocystinuria in a boy. *(Courtesy of Arif O. Khan, MD.)*

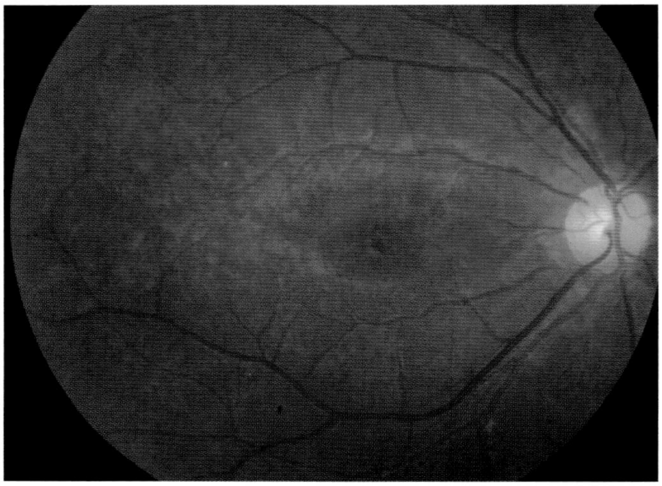

Figure 28-6 Juvenile retinal dystrophy in a boy with recent slow development of ptosis and ophthalmoplegia, which led to the diagnosis of Kearns-Sayre syndrome. *(Courtesy of Arif O. Khan, MD.)*

- Central macular cherry-red spot: GM2 gangliosidosis type I (Tay-Sachs disease) and type II (Sandhoff disease), Niemann-Pick disease. The cherry-red spot disappears over time as the intumescent ganglion cells die and optic atrophy develops. Therefore, the absence of a cherry-red spot should not be used to rule out a diagnosis, especially in older children.

In some disorders, early metabolic control greatly decreases the risk of ocular and systemic sequelae. Therefore, early recognition of metabolic disorders and timely referral to a geneticist are essential. The ophthalmologist can play a key role in the early identification of certain treatable metabolic disorders, examples of which are galactosemia, classic homocystinuria (Chapter 23), cystinosis (Chapter 21), certain mucopolysaccharidoses, and cerebrotendinous xanthomatosis (Chapter 23).

Poll-The BT, Maillette de Buy Wenniger-Prick CJ. The eye in metabolic diseases: clues to diagnosis. *Eur J Paediatr Neurol.* 2011;15(3):197–204.

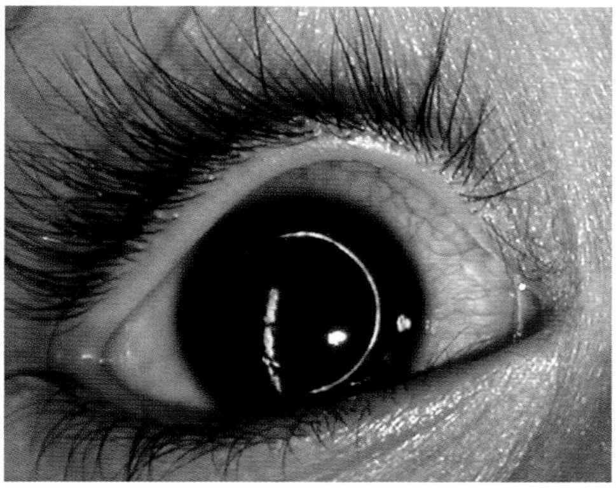

图 28-5 晶状体脱位进入前房和急性青光眼，同型胱氨酸尿症，男孩。*（译者注：资料来源见前页原文。）*

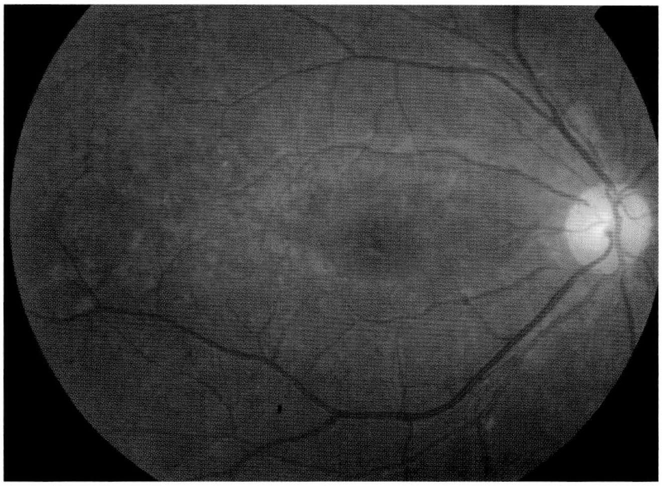

图 28-6 青少年视网膜发育不良，男孩，近期逐渐形成上睑下垂和眼肌麻痹，随后确诊为 Kearns-Sayre 综合征。*（译者注：资料来源见前页原文。）*

- 黄斑中央樱桃红斑：GM2 神经节苷脂沉积症 Ⅰ 型（Tay-Sachs 病）和 Ⅱ 型（Sandhoff 病），Niemann-Pick 病。随着肿大的神经节细胞死亡和视神经萎缩，樱桃红斑会消失。因此，樱桃红斑缺如时，不能排除诊断，特别是大龄儿童。

对一些疾病进行早期代谢控制，可大大降低眼部和全身后遗症的风险。因此，早期发现代谢性疾病，及时转诊至遗传学家非常重要。在早期发现一些可治疗的代谢性疾病中，眼科医生发挥着关键的作用，如半乳糖血症、同型胱氨酸尿症（第 23 章）、胱氨酸贮积症（第 21 章）、某些黏多糖贮积症和脑腱黄瘤病（第 23 章）。

Poll-The BT, Maillette de Buy Wenniger-Prick CJ. The eye in metabolic diseases: clues to diagnosis. *Eur J Paediatr Neurol.* 2011;15(3):197–204.

Familial Oculorenal Syndromes

Lowe Syndrome

Lowe (oculocerebrorenal) syndrome is due to hemizygous *OCRL* mutation and is characterized by both bilateral congenital cataract and glaucoma. Pupils are typically miotic. The lenses are small and thick and may exhibit posterior lenticonus. In carrier mothers, they show radially oriented punctate snowflake opacities. Systemic findings include congenital hypotonia, cognitive impairment, and infantile renal tubulopathy (Fanconi type) with resultant aminoaciduria, metabolic acidosis, proteinuria, and rickets.

Alport Syndrome

Alport syndrome shows different inheritance patterns, but X-linked inheritance is the most common. Ocular findings include anterior lenticonus or anterior subcapsular cataract, posterior polymorphous corneal dystrophy, and fleck retinopathy. Alport syndrome is a basement membrane disease that can include progressive renal failure and deafness.

Ciliopathies

Ciliopathies are disorders of organ-specific or systemic cilia dysfunction. Nonmotile cilia have a variety of specialized functions, such as cell signaling, detection of chemical gradients, and intracellular transport. Retinal involvement is frequent in ciliopathies because the junction between inner and outer segments of the photoreceptor cell is a modified nonmotile cilium. When a child has a retinopathy secondary to a systemic ciliopathy, the most common later organ dysfunction is renal. The possibility of systemic ciliopathy should be considered in all children with early-onset retinal dystrophy.

Systemic ciliopathies include Senior-Løken syndrome (retinopathy, later renal dysfunction), Bardet-Biedl syndrome (retinopathy, polydactyly [Fig 28-7], obesity, later renal dysfunction), Alström syndrome (retinopathy, cardiomyopathy, obesity, later renal dysfunction), and Joubert syndrome (retinopathy, oculomotor apraxia, developmental delay, characteristic magnetic resonance imaging [MRI] findings [Fig 28-8], later renal dysfunction).

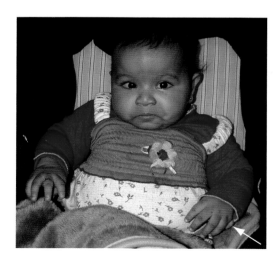

Figure 28-7 This infant with nystagmus related to retinal dystrophy also had polydactyly *(arrow)*, which led to the diagnosis of Bardet-Biedl syndrome. Systemic features such as renal impairment emerge in later childhood. *(Courtesy of Arif O. Khan, MD.)*

家族性眼肾综合征

Lowe 综合征

Lowe（眼脑肾）综合征由半合子 *OCRL* 基因突变导致，特征是双眼先天性白内障和青光眼，瞳孔缩小，晶状体小而厚、形成后圆锥形晶状体。基因携带者（母亲）的晶状体见放射状点状雪花混浊。全身性表现有先天性张力减退、认知障碍，以及婴儿肾小管病变（Fanconi 型）伴氨基酸尿症、代谢性酸中毒、蛋白尿和佝偻病。

Alport 综合征

Alport 综合征有不同的遗传模式，但最常见的遗传方式是伴 X- 染色体遗传。眼部症状主要包括前圆锥形晶状体或前囊下白内障，后部多形性角膜营养不良和斑点状视网膜病变。Alport 综合征是一种基底膜疾病，可伴进行性肾衰竭和耳聋。

纤毛病

纤毛病是指器官特异性疾病或全身纤毛功能障碍。非运动纤毛具有多种特殊的功能，如细胞信号传导，化学梯度探测和细胞内运输。纤毛病常累及视网膜，因为光感受器细胞内节和外节间的连接是修饰的非运动纤毛。当儿童继发全身性纤毛病，发生视网膜病变时，常发生晚期肾功能不全。患有早发性视网膜营养不良的所有儿童，都应考虑全身性纤毛病的可能性。

全身性纤毛病包括 Senior–Løken 综合征（视网膜病变、晚期肾功能不全），Bardet–Biedl 综合征［视网膜病变、多指畸形（图 28–7）、肥胖、晚期肾功能不全］，Alström 综合征（视网膜病变、心肌病、肥胖、晚期肾功能不全）和 Joubert 综合征［视网膜病变、动眼失用症 / 动眼神经麻痹，发育迟缓、特征性磁共振成像（MRI）（图 28–8）、晚期肾功能不全］。

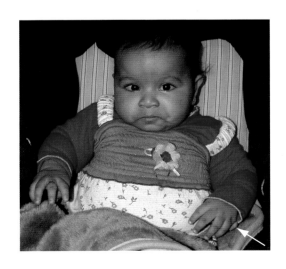

图 28–7　患儿眼球震颤，与视网膜营养不良有关，以及多指畸形（*箭头*），确诊为 Bardet–Biedl 综合征。儿童晚期出现全身性症状，如肾功能损害。*（译者注：资料来源见前页原文。）*

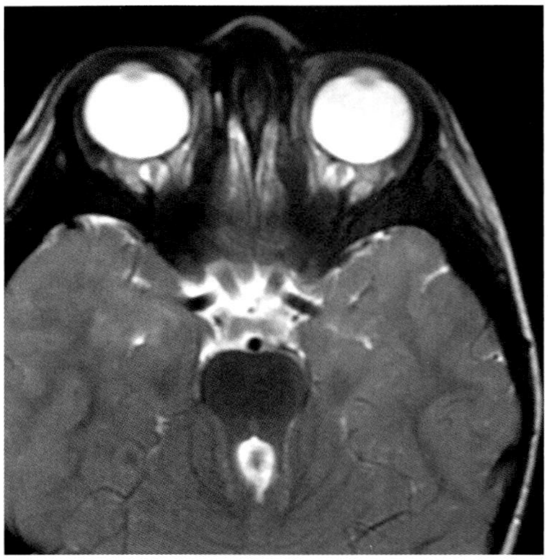

Figure 28-8 Magnetic resonance (MR) image showing the classic "molar tooth" sign in a 2-year-old girl, confirming the diagnosis of Joubert syndrome. The patient presented with developmental delay, retinal dystrophy, and oculomotor apraxia. *(Courtesy of Arif O. Khan, MD.)*

Neuro-Oculocutaneous Syndromes

Neuro-oculocutaneous syndromes (phakomatoses) are characterized by systemic hamartomas of the eye, central nervous system (CNS), and skin. Diagnosis is clinical, according to the latest published consensus criteria. Ocular involvement is frequent and can help confirm the specific diagnosis. An overview of these conditions is provided in Table 28-3.

Neurofibromatosis Type 1

Neurofibromatosis type 1 (NF1) is characterized by multiple melanocytic and neuroglial lesions. See Table 28-3 for a list of common features.

Melanocytic lesions

Café-au-lait spots, the most common cutaneous expression of NF1, are uniformly hyperpigmented macules of varying size (Fig 28-9). Some are usually present at birth; the number and size increase during the first decade of life. Unaffected individuals may have 1–3 café-au-lait spots, but greater numbers are rare except in association with NF1. Melanocytic lesions of the uveal tract are also common.

Lisch nodules are small (usually <1 mm), sharply demarcated, dome-shaped excrescences of the iris (Fig 28-10). Lisch nodules most often develop between ages 5 and 10 years and are present in nearly all adults with NF1. Multiple flat choroidal lesions 1–2 times the size of the optic disc are common. These lesions are difficult to visualize by conventional fundus examination, but near-infrared reflectance imaging has a high sensitivity for detection. Melanocytic lesions in NF1 do not affect vision.

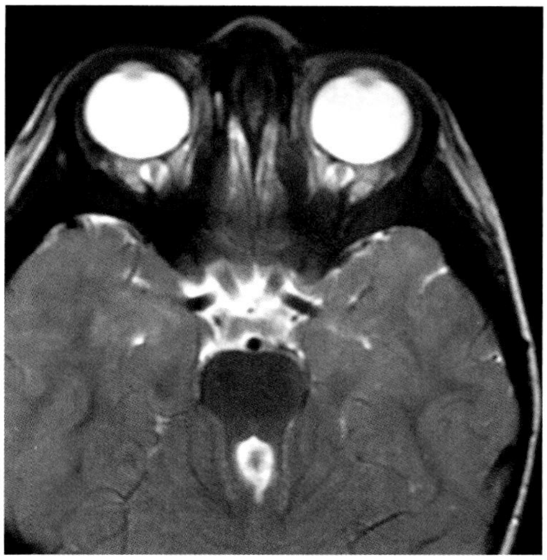

图 28-8 磁共振（MR）图像显示"臼齿"征象，2 岁女孩，确诊为 Joubert 综合征。患儿伴发育迟缓、视网膜营养不良和动眼失用症。*（译者注：资料来源见前页原文。）*

神经 – 眼皮肤综合征

神经 – 眼皮肤综合征（斑痣性错构瘤病；母斑病）的典型特征是眼部、中枢神经系统（CNS）和皮肤的全身性错构瘤。根据最新公布的共识标准，诊断主要依据临床表现。眼部受累常可以帮助明确诊断。表 28-3 对诊断分类进行了汇总。

神经纤维瘤病 1 型

神经纤维瘤病 1 型（NF1）的典型特征在于多发性黑色素细胞病变和神经胶质细胞病变。表 28-3 列出了其常见症状。

黑色素细胞病变

*皮肤的咖啡牛奶斑*是神经纤维瘤病 1 型（NF1）最常见的皮肤症状，呈大小不同的均匀色素沉着斑点（图 28-9）。有时出生即有，10 岁前其数量和大小逐渐增加。无病的儿童也可能有皮肤的咖啡牛奶斑，但不伴有神经纤维瘤病 1 型（NF1）时斑点数很少。常见葡萄膜黑色素细胞病变。

*Lisch 结节*很小（<1 mm），边界清晰，在虹膜上呈圆形隆起物（图 28-10）。Lisch 结节最常见于 5 ~ 10 岁患儿和所有成年神经纤维瘤病 1 型（NF1）患者。多发性扁平脉络膜病变，有 1 ~ 2 个视盘大小。常规眼底检查很难观察到，但近红外反射成像具有较高的检测灵敏度，可以检测出这些病变。神经纤维瘤病 1 型（NF1）的黑色素细胞病变不影响视力。

Table 28-3 Overview and Select Key Features of Neuro-Oculocutaneous Syndromes

Disease	Gene Symbol/ Chromosome Location	Inheritance Pattern	Ocular Features	Cutaneous Features	CNS and Other Systemic Features	Incidence and Comments
Neurofibromatosis type 1 (von Recklinghausen disease)	*NF1* (17q11.2); tumor suppressor	AD	Eyelid neurofibroma, glaucoma, Lisch nodules, optic pathway glioma	Café-au-lait spots, neurofibromas	Sphenoid dysplasia, other tumors	1/3500 New mutations common; variable expressivity common
Neurofibromatosis type 2	*NF2* (22q12); tumor suppressor	AD	Cataract, retinal combined hamartoma, epiretinal membrane	Café-au-lait spots	Acoustic neuromas, spinal cord tumors	1/33,000 New mutations common
Tuberous sclerosis (Bourneville disease)	*TSC1* (9q34), *TSC2* (16p13.3); tumor suppressor	AD	Retinal astrocytic hamartomas	Angiofibromas, hypopigmented macules, subungual fibromas	Seizures, cognitive impairment, renal cell carcinoma, cardiac rhabdomyoma	1/10000 New mutations very common
von Hippel–Lindau disease (retinal angiomatosis)	*VHL* (3p26-p25); tumor suppressor	AD	Retinal capillary hemangioblastoma	—	Hemangioblastoma, renal cell carcinoma, pheochromocytoma	1/36000 High penetrance; benign and malignant tumors

(Continued)

表28-3　神经-眼皮综合征的主要特征概述

疾病	基因符号/染色体位置	遗传方式	眼部特征	皮肤特征	中枢和其他全身特征	发病率和评价
1型神经纤维瘤（von Recklinghausen病）	*NF1 (17q11.2);* 肿瘤抑制因子	AD	眼睑神经纤维瘤，青光眼，Lisch结节视神经胶质瘤	牛奶咖啡斑，神经纤维瘤	蝶窦发育不良，其他肿瘤	1/35000 常见新突变，症状多样
2型神经纤维瘤	*NF2 (22q12);* 肿瘤抑制因子	AD	白内障，视网膜复合错构瘤，视网膜前膜	牛奶咖啡斑	听神经瘤，脊髓肿瘤	1/330000 常见新突变
结节性硬化症(Bourneville病)	*TSC2 (16p13.3);* 肿瘤抑制因子	AD	视网膜星形细胞错构瘤	血管纤维瘤，色素减退斑，甲下肌瘤	癫痫发作，认知障碍，肾细胞癌，心脏横纹肌瘤	1/100000 很常见新突变
von Hippel-Lindau病（视网膜病变血管瘤病）	*(3p26 - p25);* 肿瘤抑制因子	AD	视网膜毛细血管母细胞瘤	—	血管母细胞瘤，肾细胞癌，嗜铬细胞瘤	1/360000 高外显率；良性和恶性肿瘤

接续表

Table 28-3 *(continued)*

Disease	Gene Symbol/ Chromosome Location	Inheritance Pattern	Ocular Features	Cutaneous Features	CNS and Other Systemic Features	Incidence and Comments
Sturge-Weber syndrome (encephalofacial angiomatosis)	*GNAQ* (9q21)	Somatic mosaicism	Diffuse choroidal cavernous angioma, glaucoma	Nevus flammeus	Meningeal angiomas, seizures	1/50000 Nevus flammeus alone not pathognomonic
Ataxia-telangiectasia (Louis-Bar syndrome)	*ATM* (11q22.3)	AR	Saccadic initiation failure, conjunctival telangiectasias	Telangiectasias	Cerebellar dysfunction, immunodeficiency, malignancy	1/40000 *ATM* is regulator of tumor-suppressor genes and DNA repair
Incontinentia pigmenti (Bloch-Sulzberger syndrome)	*IKBKG* (Xq28)	X-linked dominant	Retinal vasculopathy	Vesicles with evolution to hyperpigmented lesions	Seizures, cognitive impairment	Evolution of skin lesions can occur in utero
Wyburn-Mason syndrome	Nonhereditary	Sporadic	Retinal racemose angioma	If present, lesions are on face	Intracranial AVMs with bleeding as sequelae	Isolated finding more common than syndrome
Klippel-Trénaunay-Weber syndrome	Nonhereditary	Sporadic	Glaucoma	Nevus flammeus similar to that in Sturge-Weber syndrome	—	Extremity with vascular nevus, varicosities, hypertrophy of bone and soft tissue, AVM

AD = autosomal dominant; AR = autosomal recessive; AVM = arteriovenous malformation; CNS = central nervous system.

续上表

疾病	基因符号/染色体位置	遗传方式	眼部特征	皮肤特征	中枢和其他全身特征	发病率和评价
Sturge-Weber综合征（脑面血管瘤病）	*GNAQ* (9q21)	体细胞嵌合体	弥漫性脉络膜海绵状血管瘤，青光眼	火焰痣	脑膜血管瘤，癫痫	1/50000 单纯火焰痣并无特异性
共济失调毛细血管扩张(Louis-Bar综合征）	*ATM* (11q22.3)	AR	扫视启动失能，结膜毛细血管扩张	毛细血管扩张	小脑功能障碍，免疫缺陷，恶性肿瘤	1/40000 ATM是肿瘤抑制基因和DNA修复的调节因子
色素失调症(Bloch-Sulzberger综合征)	*IKBKG* (Xq28)	X连锁显性	视网膜血管病变	囊泡演变为色素沉着病变	癫痫，认知障碍	子宫内膜发生皮肤病变
Wyburn-Mason综合征	非遗传	散发	视网膜蔓状血管瘤	如果发病，则面部有症状	颅内AVM伴有出血后遗症	单独出现的情况比综合征更常见
Klippel-Trénaunay-Weber 综合征	非遗传	散发	青光眼	类似于Sturge-Weber综合征的火焰痣	—	四肢血管痣，静脉曲张，骨和软组织肥大，动静脉血管畸形

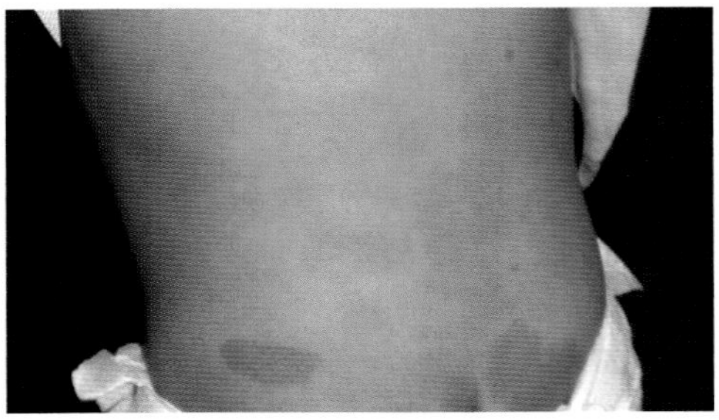

Figure 28-9 Multiple café-au-lait spots in an infant with unilateral glaucoma; neurofibromatosis type 1 (NF1) was ultimately diagnosed. *(Courtesy of Arif O. Khan, MD.)*

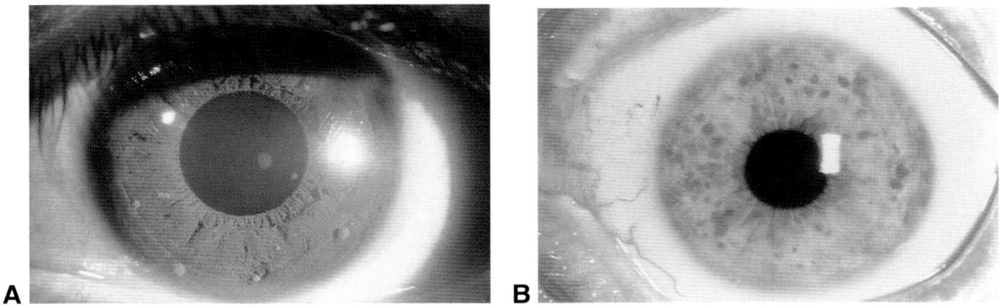

Figure 28-10 Lisch nodules of the iris in 2 patients with NF1. The brown iris has lighter-colored Lisch nodules **(A),** whereas the blue iris has darker-colored nodules **(B).**

Neuroglial lesions

Nodular cutaneous and *subcutaneous neurofibromas*, or *fibroma molluscum*, are by far the most common lesions of neuroglial origin. They typically develop in late childhood.

Plexiform neurofibromas are seen in approximately 30% of cases. These are extensive, soft subcutaneous swellings with indistinct margins, often with hyperpigmentation or hypertrichosis of the overlying skin. Hypertrophy of underlying soft tissue and bone (regional gigantism) is often present. Plexiform neurofibromas develop earlier than nodular lesions, are frequently evident in infancy or childhood, and may cause severe disfigurement and functional impairment. Approximately 10% involve the face, commonly the upper eyelid and orbit (Fig 28-11). Greater involvement of the upper eyelid's temporal portion results in an S-shaped configuration. Tumor bulk may cause complete ptosis. Glaucoma in the ipsilateral eye is found in up to 50% of cases.

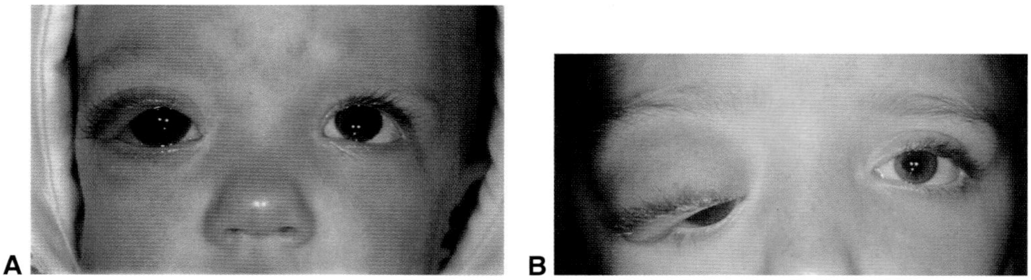

Figure 28-11 Plexiform neurofibroma involving the right upper eyelid, associated with ipsilateral buphthalmos, in a girl with NF1. **A,** Age 8 months. **B,** Age 8 years.

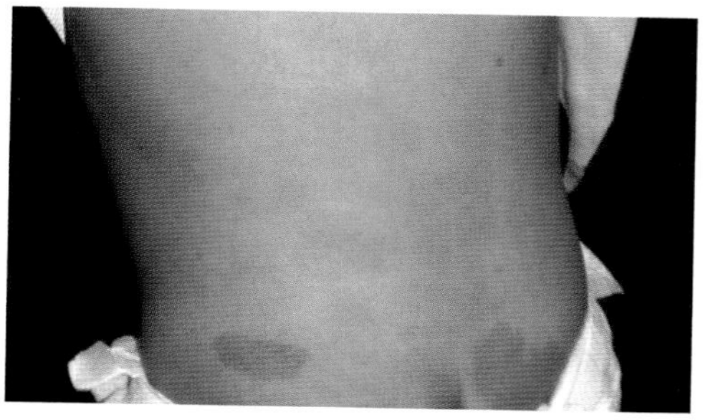

图 28–9　婴儿有多个皮肤的咖啡牛奶斑，伴单眼青光眼，诊断为神经纤维瘤病 1 型（NF1）。*（译者注：资料来源见前页原文。）*

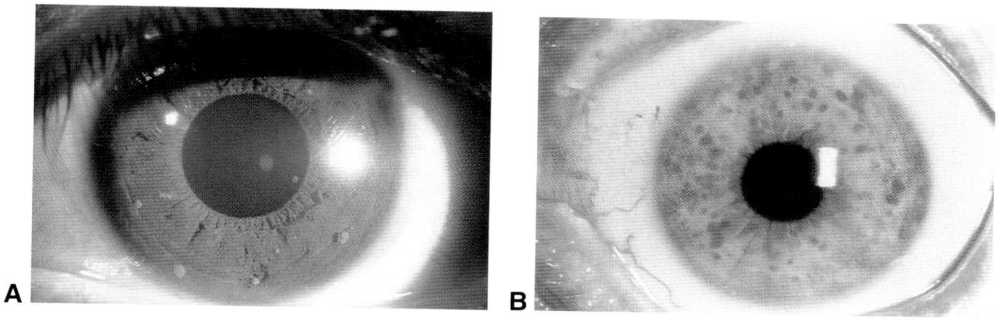

图 28–10　2 例神经纤维瘤病 1 型（NF1）虹膜上的 Lisch 结节。棕色虹膜呈浅色的 Lisch 结节（**A**），而蓝色虹膜呈深色的结节（**B**）。

神经胶质病变

*结节性皮肤*和*皮下神经纤维瘤*，或*软疣性纤维瘤*是最常见的源于神经胶质病变，常发生于大龄儿童。

*丛状神经纤维瘤*约占 30%，表现为广泛柔软的皮下水肿，边界不清，皮肤常被覆色素沉着或多毛，其下伴软组织和骨骼肥大（区域性巨形化）。丛状神经纤维瘤的发生早于结节性病变，可见于婴儿期或儿童期，引起严重的畸形和功能损害，10% 累及面部，常是上眼睑和眼眶（图 28–11）。上眼睑颞侧受累程度较重，呈现 S 形。大包块可致完全上睑下垂。同侧眼发生青光眼高达 50%。

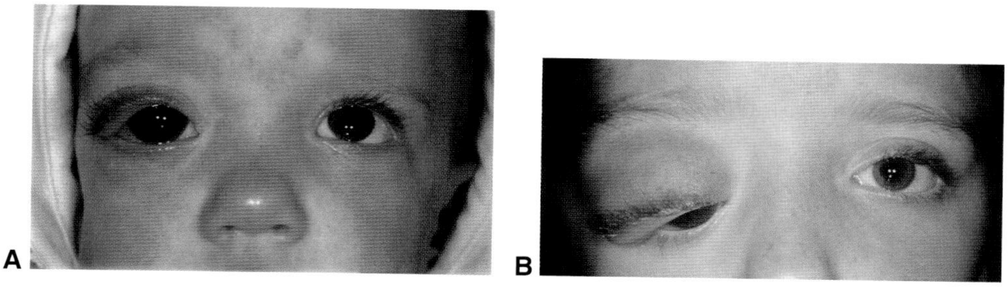

图 28–11　丛状神经纤维瘤累及右上睑，伴同侧牛眼，神经纤维瘤病 1 型 NF1，女孩。**A.** 8 月龄。**B.** 8 岁。

Complete excision of an eyelid plexiform neurofibroma is generally not possible. Treatment is directed toward the relief of specific symptoms. Surgical debulking and frontalis suspension procedures can reduce ptosis sufficiently to allow binocular vision. Clinical trials examining use of biologic agents to treat these lesions are under way.

Optic pathway glioma is a low-grade pilocytic astrocytoma involving the optic nerve, chiasm, or both. It is present in approximately 15% of affected patients and is symptomatic in 1%–5% (almost always before age 10 years, after a period of brief rapid enlargement). The efficacy of treatment (ie, chemotherapy, radiation) is unclear because of the condition's highly variable natural history, including relative stability after rapid growth and spontaneous improvement in a few cases. MRI usually shows cylindrical or fusiform enlargement (Fig 28-12), often with exaggerated sinuousness or kinking, creating an appearance of discontinuity or localized constriction on axial images. In addition to causing bilateral vision loss, tumors involving primarily the chiasm may result in significant morbidity, including hydrocephalus and hypothalamic dysfunction. Chiasmal glioma in patients with NF1 carries a better prognosis than in individuals without NF1.

Other less common neuroglial abnormalities include spinal and gastrointestinal neurofibromas, pheochromocytomas, prominence of corneal nerves (≤20%), localized orbital neurofibromas, and retinal hamartomas.

Jakacki RI, Dombi E, Potter DM, et al. Phase I trial of pegylated interferon-α-2b in young patients with plexiform neurofibromas. *Neurology*. 2011;76(3):265–272.

Other manifestations

Additional manifestations include various benign tumors that involve the skin or the eye (eg, juvenile xanthogranuloma, retinal capillary hemangioma), several forms of malignancy (leukemia, rhabdomyosarcoma, pheochromocytoma, Wilms tumor), bony defects such as scoliosis, pseudarthrosis of the tibia, and hypoplasia of the sphenoid bone (which may cause ocular pulsation). Sphenoid dysplasia may be associated with neurofibromas in the ipsilateral superficial temporal fossa as well as in the deep orbit. Several ill-defined abnormalities of the CNS (macrocephaly, aqueductal stenosis, seizures, and developmental delay) are also seen with greater frequency in patients with NF1. The diagnosis of NF1 should be considered in any child who presents with unilateral glaucoma.

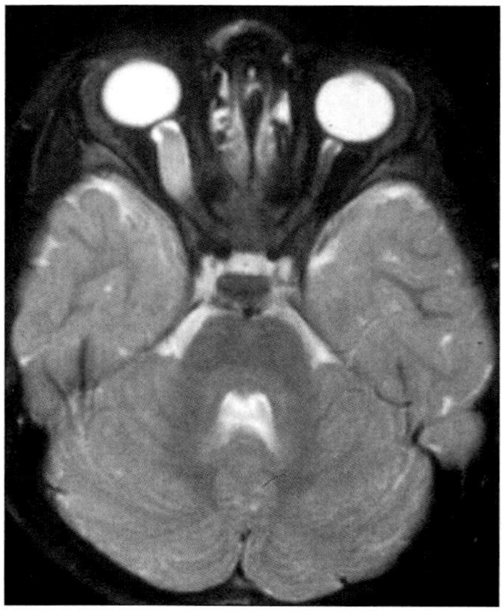

Figure 28-12 Axial MR image of a right optic pathway glioma in a child with NF1. *(Courtesy of Ken K. Nischal, MD.)*

眼睑丛状神经纤维瘤无法完全切除。治疗的目的是缓解某些症状。肿块削体切除术和额部悬吊手术可以减轻上睑下垂，有助于建立双眼视觉。采用生物制剂治疗这些病变的临床试验正在进行中。

*视路神经胶质瘤*是一种低分化毛细胞型星形细胞瘤，视神经、视交叉受累或同时受累。患者中约 15% 存在病灶，1% ~ 5% 有症状（10 岁前，短时间快速增大）。治疗效果（如化学治疗、放射治疗）尚不清楚，因为自然病程变化很大，如快速生长后的相对稳定性、少数病例的自发性改善。磁共振（MRI）显示，病灶呈圆柱形或梭形扩大（图 28-12），常有过度的弯曲或扭结，在轴向图像上显示不连续或局部收缩的外观。除了导致双眼视力丧失外，累及视交叉的肿瘤可导致严重的并发症，包括脑积水和下丘脑功能障碍。与没有神经纤维瘤病 1 型（NF1）的相比，交叉神经胶质瘤伴神经纤维瘤病 1 型（NF1）的预后更好。

其他少见的神经胶质细胞异常，包括脊髓和胃肠道神经纤维瘤、嗜铬细胞瘤、角膜神经突出（≤ 20%）、局限性眼眶神经纤维瘤和视网膜错构瘤。

Jakacki RI, Dombi E, Potter DM, et al. Phase I trial of pegylated interferon-α-2b in young patients with plexiform neurofibromas. *Neurology*. 2011;76(3):265–272.

其他表现形式

其他表现有累及皮肤或眼睛的各种良性肿瘤（如青少年黄色肉芽肿、视网膜毛细血管瘤），几种恶性肿瘤（白血病、横纹肌肉瘤、嗜铬细胞瘤、Wilms 肿瘤）、骨缺陷，如骨脊柱侧弯、胫骨假关节和蝶骨发育不全（可致眼球搏动）。蝶窦发育不良时，可伴同侧颞浅窝以及深部眼眶的神经纤维瘤。在神经纤维瘤病 1 型（NF1）患者中也伴有中枢神经系统（CNS）异常（巨头畸形、中脑导水管硬化、癫痫和发育迟缓）。患有单眼青光眼的儿童都应考虑神经纤维瘤病 1 型（NF1）的诊断。

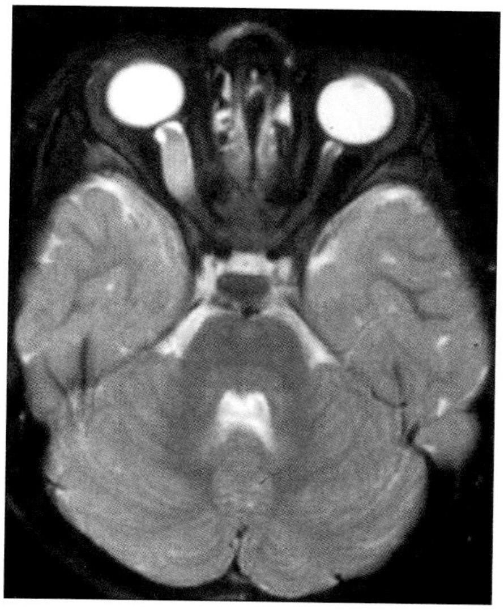

图 28-12　右侧视神经胶质瘤的轴向磁共振图像，神经纤维瘤病 1 型（NF1）患儿。*（译者注：资料来源见前页原文。）*

An appropriate interval for periodic ophthalmic reassessment in childhood is 1–2 years, unless a specific abnormality requires closer observation.

Fisher MJ, Loguidice M, Gutmann DH, et al. Visual outcomes in children with neurofibromatosis type 1–associated optic pathway glioma following chemotherapy: a multicenter retrospective analysis. *Neuro Oncol.* 2012;14(6):790–797.

Kalamarides M, Acosta MT, Babovic-Vuksanovic D, et al. Neurofibromatosis 2011: a report of the Children's Tumor Foundation annual meeting. *Acta Neuropathol.* 2012;123(3):369–380.

Neurofibromatosis Type 2

Neurofibromatosis type 2 (NF2) is diagnosed clinically by the presence of bilateral acoustic neuromas (eighth cranial nerve tumors) or by a first-degree relative with NF2 and presence of a unilateral acoustic neuroma, neurofibroma, meningioma, schwannoma, glioma, or early-onset posterior subcapsular cataract. Patients typically present in their teens or early adulthood with signs or symptoms related to the eighth nerve tumor(s), including decreased hearing or tinnitus. The most characteristic ocular finding in NF2 is lens opacity, especially posterior subcapsular cataract or wedge-shaped cortical cataracts. Up to 80% of patients have epiretinal membranes or combined hamartomas of the retina and retinal pigment epithelium (RPE). Lisch nodules of the iris can occur in NF2 but are infrequent. Salient features are summarized in Table 28-3.

Tuberous Sclerosis

Tuberous sclerosis (TS) is characterized by benign tumor growth in multiple organs, predominantly the skin, brain, heart, kidney, and eye. Prominent extraocular features are summarized in Table 28-4, with examples shown in Figures 28-13 and 28-14. The classic *Vogt triad* of clinical findings is cognitive impairment, seizures, and facial angiofibromas. The facial angiofibromas are not usually present in young children, but hypomelanotic macules ("ash-leaf spots") are.

The most frequent and characteristic ocular manifestation of TS is retinal phakoma, frequently termed *astrocytic hamartoma* (Fig 28-15). Pathologically, this growth arises from the innermost layer of the retina and is composed of nerve fibers and relatively undifferentiated cells that appear to be of glial origin. Phakomas are usually found near the posterior pole and involve the retina, the optic disc, or both. They vary in size from approximately half to twice the diameter of the disc. Vision is rarely affected.

Retinal phakomas have 3 distinct appearances. The first is typically found in very young children; these phakomas are relatively flat with a smooth surface, indistinct margins, and a gray-white color that makes them difficult to detect. The second is a sharply demarcated, elevated, yellow-white, calcified lesion with an irregular surface that has been compared to that of a mulberry. These lesions are more often found in older patients, on or adjacent to the optic disc. The third type is a transitional lesion that combines features of the first 2.

儿童进行定期眼科检查的时间间隔为 1 ～ 2 年，特殊异常需密切观察。

Fisher MJ, Loguidice M, Gutmann DH, et al. Visual outcomes in children with neurofibromatosis type 1–associated optic pathway glioma following chemotherapy: a multicenter retrospective analysis. *Neuro Oncol.* 2012;14(6):790–797.

Kalamarides M, Acosta MT, Babovic-Vuksanovic D, et al. Neurofibromatosis 2011: a report of the Children's Tumor Foundation annual meeting. *Acta Neuropathol.* 2012;123(3):369–380.

神经纤维瘤病 2 型

神经纤维瘤病 2 型（NF2）的确诊依据是，有双侧听神经瘤（Ⅷ颅神经瘤），或一级亲属患神经纤维瘤病 2 型（NF2），或有单侧听神经瘤、神经纤维瘤、脑膜瘤、神经鞘瘤、神经胶质瘤，或早发性后囊下白内障。患者常在青少年或成年早期，出现Ⅷ颅神经肿瘤的体征或症状，包括听力下降或耳鸣。NF2 中最典型的眼部症状是晶状体混浊，特别是后囊下白内障或楔形皮质白内障。80%有视网膜前膜，或伴有视网膜及色素上皮（RPE）错构瘤。虹膜 Lisch 结节可见于神经纤维瘤病 2 型（NF2），但不常见。表 28–3 汇总了其主要特征。

结节性硬化症

结节性硬化症（TS）的特征是良性肿瘤，侵犯多个器官，主要是皮肤、脑、心脏、肾脏和眼睛。表 28–4 汇总了主要的眼外特征，图 28–13 和图 28–14 为病例。临床的经典 *Vogt 三联征*是认知障碍、癫痫和面部血管纤维瘤。幼儿的面部血管纤维瘤少见，但常见脱色素斑（“灰叶斑”）。

结节性硬化症（TS）眼部最常见的特征性表现是视网膜斑痣性错构瘤病，常称为*星形细胞错构瘤*（图 28–15）。病理学上源于视网膜的最内层，由神经纤维和相对未分化的细胞组成，这些细胞源于神经胶质。视网膜斑痣性错构瘤病常位于后极部，视网膜、视盘受累或两者同时累及，其病灶大小为 1/2 ～ 2 个视盘直径。视力少有影响。

视网膜斑痣性错构瘤病有 3 种不同的表现。第 1 种见于幼儿，斑痣性错构瘤相对平坦，表面光滑，边缘模糊以及灰白色，不易被发现。第 2 种边界清晰、隆起，为黄白色，有钙化的病变，其表面不规则，似桑树表面，多见于大龄患者，位于视盘上或视盘附近。第 3 种是过渡性病变，兼有前 2 种表现。

Table 28-4 Extraocular Features in Tuberous Sclerosis

Feature	Characteristic
Ash-leaf spot	Sharply demarcated, hypopigmented skin lesion Visibility increased by ultraviolet light Onset during infancy
Adenoma sebaceum	Facial angiofibromas Occurrence in three-quarters of patients Can be mistaken for acne Onset during childhood
Subungual fibroma	Most common but can be periungual
Shagreen patch	Typically located in lumbosacral area Onset after puberty
Seizures	Periventricular or basal ganglia calcification (representing benign astrocytomas) Tuberous malformations of the cortex Cognitive impairment in 50% of patients
Other tumors	Cardiac rhabdomyomas Bone and kidney lesions

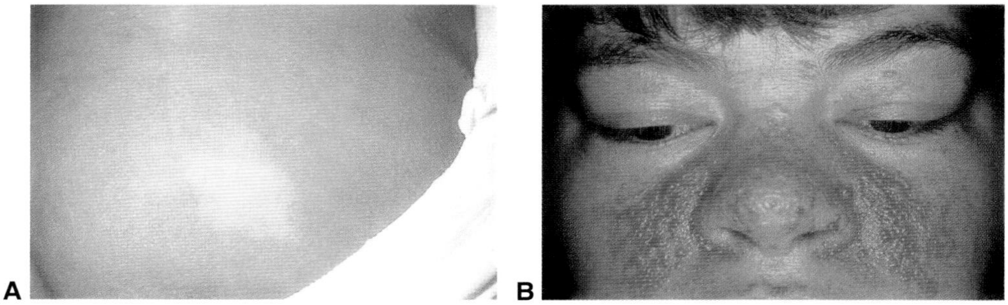

Figure 28-13 Cutaneous lesions of tuberous sclerosis. **A,** Hypomelanotic macule (ash-leaf spot). **B,** Adenoma sebaceum of the face.

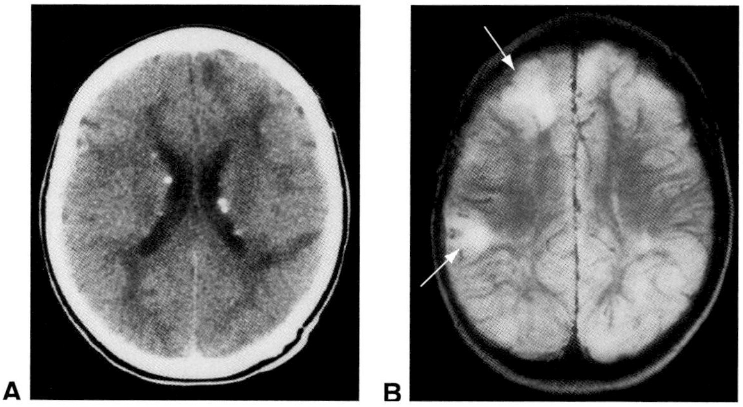

Figure 28-14 Brain lesions of tuberous sclerosis. **A,** Axial computed tomography image showing small periventricular calcifications. **B,** Axial T2-weighted MR image demonstrating tuberous malformations *(arrows)*.

表28-4　结节性硬化症的眼外特征

特征	特点
灰叶斑	边界明显，色素脱失的皮肤病变 紫外线照射其可见度增加 婴儿期发病
脂腺腺瘤	面部血管纤维瘤 3/4患者发病 误诊为粉刺 儿童期发病
甲下纤维瘤	最常见，也可在甲周
鲨鱼斑	常位于腰骶部 青春期后发病
癫痫	脑室周围或基底神经节钙化 （代表良性星形细胞瘤） 皮质结节性畸形 50%认知障碍
其他肿瘤	心脏横纹肌瘤 骨和肾脏病变

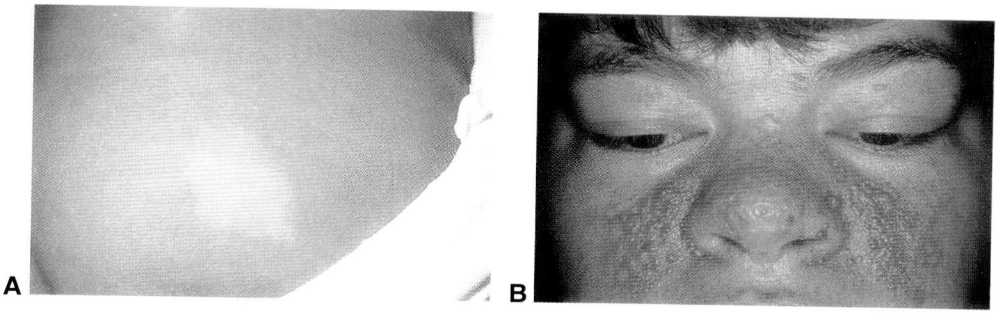

图 28-13　结节性硬化症的皮肤病变。**A.** 色素脱失斑（灰叶病）。**B.** 面部皮脂腺腺瘤。

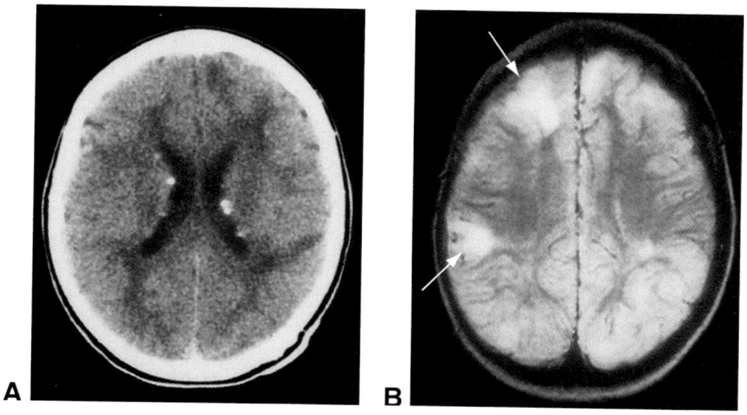

图 28-14　结节性硬化症的脑部病变。**A.** 轴向计算机断层扫描图像显示，微小脑室周围钙化灶。**B.** 轴向 T2 加权磁共振（MR）图像显示，结节畸形（*箭头*）。

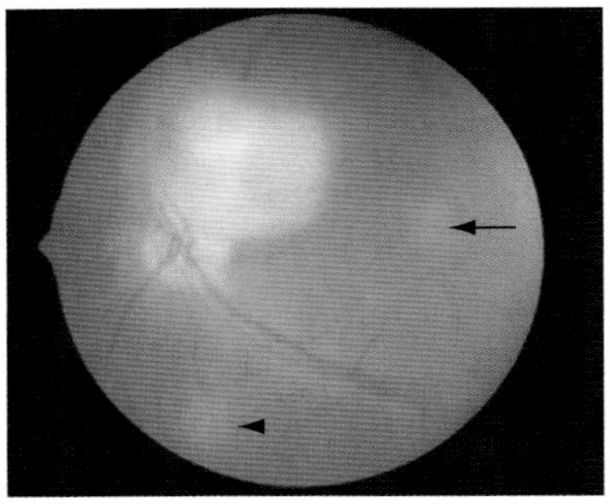

Figure 28-15 Fundus lesions of tuberous sclerosis, left eye. In addition to the large phakoma partially overlying the optic disc, a small hypopigmented lesion *(arrow)* appears in the temporal macula, and a barely visible second phakoma *(arrowhead)* partially obscures a retinal blood vessel near the edge of the photograph, directly below the disc. The lesions of tuberous sclerosis can vary considerably in their opaqueness and visibility.

Phakomas are present in 30%–50% of patients with TS. One to several phakomas may be found in a single eye, and 40% of cases are bilateral. There is no evidence that the number of lesions increases with age, but individual tumors have been documented to grow over time. Phakomas are not pathognomonic of TS; they occur occasionally in association with neurofibromatosis and in the eyes of unaffected persons. Retinal lesions are more common in individuals with mutations in the *TSC2* gene. Hypopigmented lesions analogous to ash-leaf spots are occasionally seen in the iris or choroid.

Management of TS patients by the ophthalmologist includes monitoring of vision and ocular lesions. Difficult-to-control seizures respond to vigabatrin: up to 95% of patients experience significant reduction of seizures. However, patients treated with vigabatrin are at risk for ocular complications, which may be difficult or impossible to monitor in patients with TS.

Aronow ME, Nakagawa JA, Gupta A, Traboulsi EI, Singh AD. Tuberous sclerosis complex: genotype/phenotype correlation of retinal findings. *Ophthalmology.* 2012;119(9):1917–1923.

Von Hippel–Lindau Disease

The retinal lesions seen in von Hippel–Lindau disease (VHL; angiomatosis of the retina and cerebellum) and originally described by von Hippel are capillary hemangioblastomas. These lesions usually become visible ophthalmoscopically between ages 10 and 35 years, with an average age at onset of 25 years. Retinal capillary hemangioblastomas are found in up to 85% of patients with the *VHL* mutation. Multiple tumors are present in the same eye in about one-third of cases and bilaterally in as many as one-half of cases. Tumors typically occur in the peripheral fundus, but lesions adjacent to the optic disc have been described. Prominent extraocular features of VHL are summarized in Table 28-5.

The hallmark of the mature tumor is a pair of markedly dilated vessels (artery and vein) running between the lesion and the optic disc, indicating significant arteriovenous shunting (Fig 28-16). Characteristic paired or twin retinal vessels of normal caliber may be present before the tumor becomes visible.

Histologically, retinal capillary hemangioblastomas consist of relatively well-formed capillaries; however, fluorescein angiography shows that these vessels are leaky. Transudation of fluid into the subretinal space causes lipid accumulation, retinal detachment, and consequent vision loss.

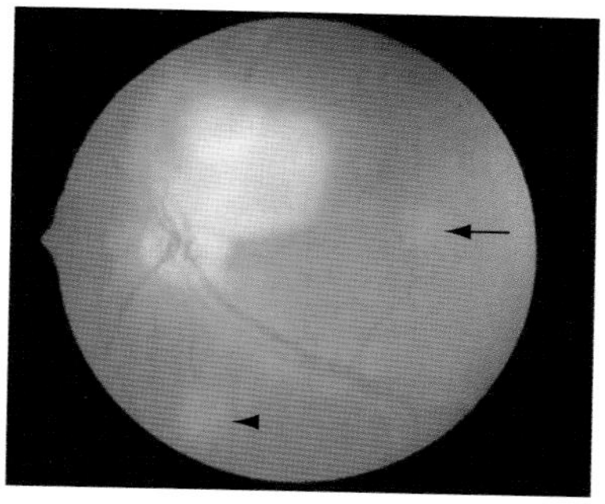

图 28-15　结节性硬化症的眼底病变，左眼。除了部分覆盖在视盘上大的错构瘤外，黄斑颞侧有 1 个小的脱色素病灶（*箭头*），以及位于视盘正下方、靠近照片边缘的隐现的第 2 个微小瘤体（*箭头*），其部分遮挡了视网膜血管。结节性硬化症病变的不透明性和可见性差异很大。

30% ~ 50%的结节性硬化症（TS）患者有斑痣性错构瘤，单眼内可见 1 到数个，40%的患者是双眼的。没有证据表明病变的数量会随着年龄的增长而增加，但单个肿瘤会随着时间而增大。斑痣性错构瘤不是结节性硬化症（TS）的典型特征，偶见于神经纤维瘤病和未患病眼中。视网膜病变常见于 *TSC2* 基因突变患者，虹膜或脉络膜偶见于类似灰叶斑的脱色素病灶。

对结节性硬化症（TS）患者，眼科医生需监测其视力和眼部病变。氨己烯酸对难以控制的癫痫发作有效， 95% 的患者癫痫发作明显减少，但有发生眼部并发症的风险，很难对结节性硬化症（TS）患者进行监测。

Aronow ME, Nakagawa JA, Gupta A, Traboulsi EI, Singh AD. Tuberous sclerosis complex: genotype/phenotype correlation of retinal findings. *Ophthalmology*. 2012;119(9):1917–1923.

Von Hippel-Lindau 病

在 von Hippel-Lindau 病（VHL，视网膜和小脑的血管瘤病）中可观察到视网膜病变，最初 von Hippel 描述为毛细血管母细胞瘤。在检眼镜下，可见病灶，发病年龄为 10 ~ 35 岁，平均年龄 25 岁。85% 视网膜毛细血管母细胞瘤患者有 *VHL* 突变。1/3 患者的单眼中有多发肿瘤，1/2 患者双眼有肿瘤。肿瘤常位于周边眼底，也有与视盘相邻的病灶。表 28-5 总结了 von Hippel-Lindau 病（VHL）的典型眼外症状。

成熟肿瘤的标志，是在病变和视盘之间存在 1 对明显扩张的血管（动脉和静脉），提示动静脉分流（图 28-16）。肿瘤明显可见前，有可能存在着 1 对正常直径的视网膜血管。

组织学上，视网膜毛细血管母细胞瘤由形态较好的毛细血管组成，但荧光血管造影显示这些血管有渗漏。液体进入视网膜下间隙会导致脂质积聚、视网膜脱离和最终视力丧失。

Table 28-5 Extraocular Features in von Hippel–Lindau Disease

Feature	Characteristic
Brain hemangioblastomas	Usually located in cerebellum Exudation from thin tumor vessel walls causes significant fluid accumulations
Cysts and tumors	Potential for cyst or tumor development in kidneys (renal cell carcinoma), pancreas, liver, epididymis, and adrenal glands (pheochromocytoma)
Rare skin lesions	Café-au-lait spots and port-wine stains (nevus flammeus) seen occasionally
Shagreen patch	Typically located in lumbosacral area Onset after puberty
Seizures	Periventricular or basal ganglia calcification (representing benign astrocytomas) Tuberous malformations of the cortex Cognitive impairment in 50% of patients
Other tumors	Cardiac rhabdomyomas Bone and kidney lesions

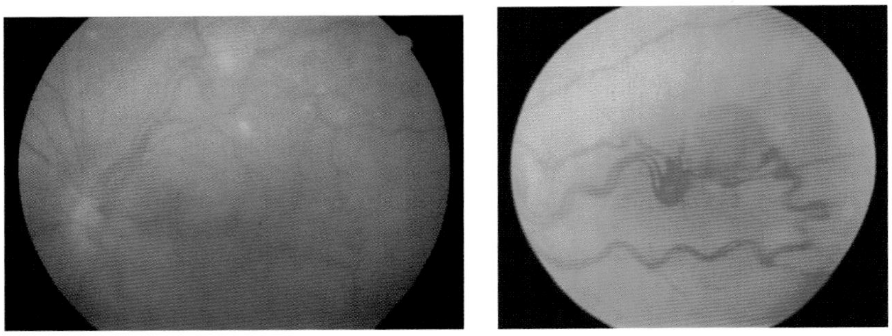

Figure 28-16 Retinal angiomatosis, left eye, in a patient with von Hippel–Lindau disease.

Retinal capillary hemangioblastomas can be effectively treated with cryotherapy or laser photocoagulation in two-thirds of cases or more, particularly when the lesions are still small. Antiangiogenic therapy has also shown potential. Early diagnosis increases the likelihood of successful treatment. The ocular lesions of VHL are asymptomatic prior to retinal detachment. Therefore, children at risk for the disease should undergo periodic ophthalmologic evaluation beginning at approximately age 5 years.

Early diagnosis of systemic tumors can significantly reduce morbidity and mortality. Molecular genetic testing has been suggested for patients with early-onset (<30 years) cerebellar hemangioblastoma, early-onset retinal capillary hemangioblastoma, or familial clear cell renal carcinoma.

Maher ER, Neumann HP, Richard S. Von Hippel–Lindau disease: a clinical and scientific review. *Eur J Hum Genet.* 2011;19(6):617–623.

Toy BC, Agrón E, Nigam D, Chew EY, Wong WT. Longitudinal analysis of retinal hemangioblastomatosis and visual function in ocular von Hippel–Lindau disease. *Ophthalmology.* 2012;119(12):2622–2630.

表28-5　von Hippel-Lindau病的眼外特征

特征	特点
脑血管母细胞瘤	常位于小脑 薄的肿瘤细胞壁的渗出导致明显的液体聚积
囊肿和肿瘤	肾脏（肾细胞癌）、胰腺、肝脏、附睾和肾上腺（嗜铬细胞瘤）有发展成囊肿或肿瘤的可能性
罕见的皮肤病变	偶见皮肤的咖啡牛奶斑和葡萄酒色斑（鲜红斑痣）
鲨鱼斑	常位于腰骶部 青春期后发病
癫痫	脑室周围或基底神经节钙化（代表良性星形细胞瘤） 皮质结节状畸形 50%存在认知障碍
其他肿瘤	心脏横纹肌瘤 骨和肾脏病变

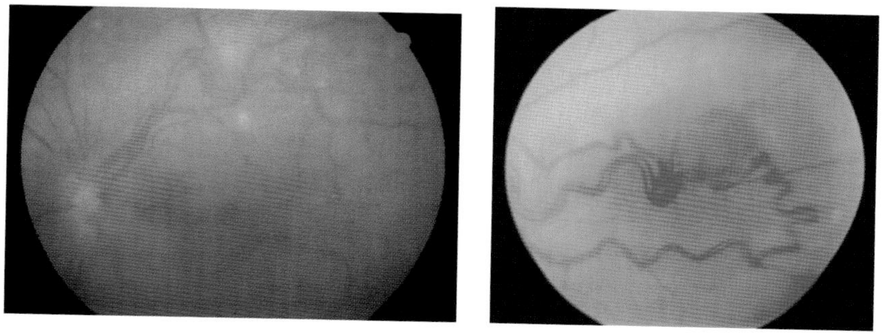

图 28-16　视网膜血管瘤病，左眼，患有 von Hippel-Lindau 病。

2/3 的视网膜毛细血管母细胞瘤可用冷冻疗法和激光光凝治疗，特别是较小的病灶。抗血管生成疗法也有效。早期诊断可提高治疗的成功率。视网膜脱离前，von Hippel-Lindau 病（VHL）无眼部症状。因此，患有该病的儿童应从 5 岁开始定期进行眼科检查，以评估风险。

全身肿瘤的早期诊断可以明显降低发病率和死亡率。对早发（<30 岁）小脑血管母细胞瘤、早发性视网膜毛细血管母细胞瘤或家族性透明细胞肾癌的患者，建议进行分子遗传学检测。

Maher ER, Neumann HP, Richard S. Von Hippel-Lindau disease: a clinical and scientific review. *Eur J Hum Genet*. 2011;19(6):617–623.

Toy BC, Agrón E, Nigam D, Chew EY, Wong WT. Longitudinal analysis of retinal hemangioblastomatosis and visual function in ocular von Hippel-Lindau disease. *Ophthalmology*. 2012;119(12):2622–2630.

Sturge-Weber Syndrome

Sturge-Weber syndrome (SWS; encephalofacial angiomatosis) consists of a facial cutaneous vascular malformation (port-wine stain) with ipsilateral leptomeningeal vascular malformation. Extraocular features are summarized in Table 28-6, with examples shown in Figures 28-17 and 28-18.

Any portion of the ocular circulation may be anomalous in SWS. When the skin lesion involves the eyelids, increased conjunctival vascularity commonly produces a pinkish discoloration. An abnormal plexus of episcleral vessels is often present.

The retina sometimes shows tortuous vessels and arteriovenous communications. Choroidal hemangioma is the most significant retinal anomaly associated with SWS. The tumor is composed of well-formed choroidal vessels, which give the fundus a uniform deep-red color that has been compared to that of tomato ketchup (Fig 28-19). Sometimes only the posterior pole is involved; in other cases, the entire fundus is affected. Choroidal hemangiomas are usually asymptomatic in childhood. During adolescence or adulthood, the choroid sometimes becomes markedly thickened. Degeneration or detachment of the overlying retina may follow. No treatment has been proven to prevent or reverse such deterioration, but scattered application of laser photocoagulation may help.

Glaucoma is the most common and most serious ocular complication. It has been reported to occur in up to approximately 70% of patients with SWS. Causes of elevated intraocular pressure (IOP) include elevated episcleral venous pressure, hyperemia of the ciliary body with hypersecretion of aqueous, and developmental anomaly of the anterior chamber angle. Involvement of the skin of the upper eyelid, choroidal hemangioma, iris heterochromia, and episcleral hemangioma increase the likelihood of glaucoma. Onset of glaucoma can be at birth or later in childhood.

Table 28-6 Extraocular Features in Sturge-Weber Syndrome

Feature	Characteristics
Port-wine stain	Congenital facial cutaneous vascular malformation (dilatation of the deep dermal plexus) Hemifacial lesion, typically unilateral
Leptomeningeal vascular malformation	Ipsilateral to port-wine stain Potentially associated with cerebral calcification (occipital, parietal, temporal, and occasionally frontal lobe), seizures, focal neurologic defect, and highly variable cognitive impairment

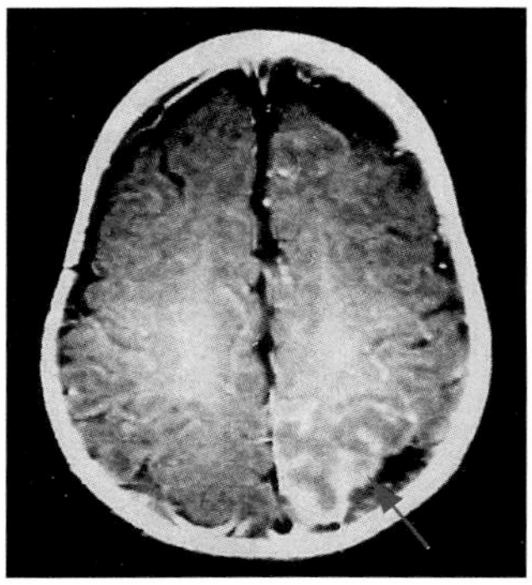

Figure 28-17 Axial gadolinium-enhanced T1-weighted MR image shows vascular malformation with underlying cortical atrophy *(arrow)* in the left occipital lobe of a 4-month-old girl with Sturge-Weber syndrome.

Sturge-Weber 综合征

Sturge-Weber 综合征（SWS；脑 - 面血管瘤病）包括面部皮肤血管畸形（葡萄酒色斑）和同侧软脑膜血管畸形。该综合征的外眼特征见表 28-6，例图见图 28-17 和图 28-18。

Sturge-Weber 综合征（SWS）的任何眼循环都可能出现异常。当皮肤病变累及眼睑时，增加的结膜血管呈粉红色，表层巩膜出现异常血管丛。

视网膜有时可见迂曲血管和动静脉瘘。脉络膜血管瘤是 Sturge-Weber 综合征（SWS）主要的视网膜异常。血管瘤由发育良好的脉络膜血管组成，眼底呈均匀的深红色，如同番茄酱（图 28-19）。有时病变仅累及后极部，有时整个眼底都会受到影响。脉络膜血管瘤在儿童时期没有症状，在青春期或成年后脉络膜显著增厚。随后被覆的视网膜发生退行性病变或脱离。尚无防止或逆转病变的有效治疗，弥散激光光凝有所帮助。

青光眼是 Sturge-Weber 综合征（SWS）最常见、最严重的眼部并发症，约 70% 的 Sturge-Weber 综合征（SWS）发生青光眼。眼内压（IOP）升高的原因有表层巩膜静脉压升高、睫状体充血伴房水过量分泌、前房角发育异常。累及上眼睑的病变、脉络膜血管瘤、虹膜异色症和表层巩膜血管瘤均会增加患青光眼的风险。青光眼可在出生时或童年期发病。

表28-6　Sturge-Weber综合征的眼外特征

特征	特点
葡萄酒色斑	先天性面部皮肤血管畸形（深部真皮血管丛扩张） 半侧颜面部病变，典型的为单侧
软脑膜血管畸形	同侧葡萄酒色斑 伴脑钙化（枕叶，顶叶，颞叶，偶见额叶），癫痫，局灶性神经系统缺陷和多种认知障碍

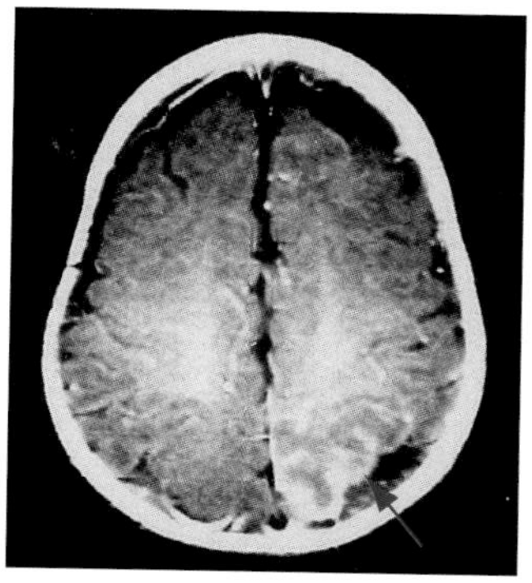

图 28-17　Sturge-Weber 综合征，4 月龄女婴，轴向钆增强 T1 加权磁共振影像（MRI），显示左侧枕叶血管畸形，伴其下方皮质萎缩*（箭头）*。

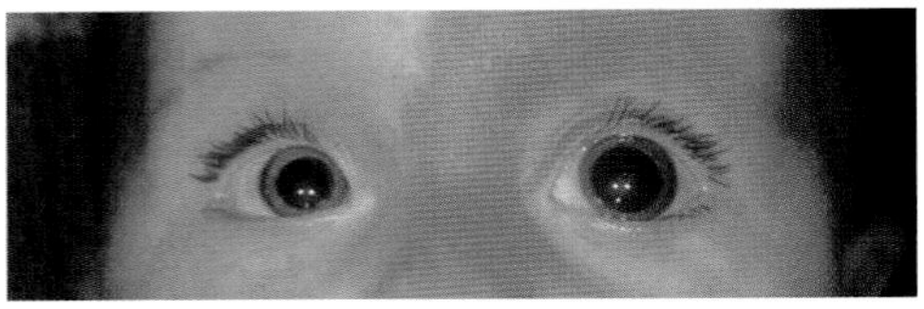

Figure 28-18 Facial port-wine stain involving the left eyelids, associated with ipsilateral buphthalmos, in an infant girl with Sturge-Weber syndrome and glaucoma.

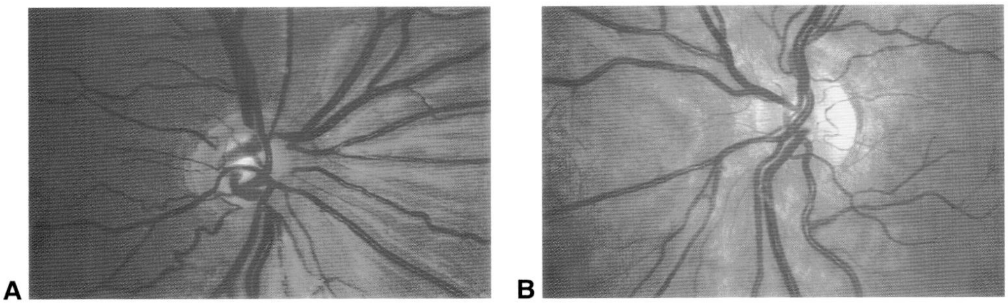

Figure 28-19 Fundus appearance in an adolescent boy with Sturge-Weber syndrome. Note the glaucomatous disc cupping and deeper red color of surrounding choroid, right eye **(A),** compared with the healthy fellow eye **(B).**

SWS glaucoma is difficult to treat. Initial therapy with topical eyedrops can be effective, especially in cases of later onset. Surgery is indicated in early-onset cases and when medical treatment is inadequate. Adequate long-term control of IOP can frequently be achieved, but multiple operations are typically necessary. A particular risk of glaucoma surgery in SWS is intraoperative or postoperative exudation or hemorrhage from anomalous choroidal vessels; this complication is caused by rapid ocular decompression. The surgeon must exercise special care with implanted glaucoma drainage devices to prevent excessive early postoperative hypotony. Postsurgical accumulation of choroidal or subretinal fluid may be dramatic, but spontaneous resorption usually occurs within 1–2 weeks.

Angle surgery (goniotomy and trabeculotomy) has been used successfully in some patients with SWS. Treatment of affected skin with a pulsed dye laser has been shown to reduce vascularity, considerably improving appearance without causing significant damage to dermal tissue.

Khaier A, Nischal KK, Espinosa M, Manoj B. Periocular port wine stain: the Great Ormond Street Hospital experience. *Ophthalmology*. 2011;118(11):2274–2278.e1.

Ataxia-Telangiectasia

Ataxia-telangiectasia (AT; Louis-Bar Syndrome) involves primarily the cerebellum, ocular surface, skin, and immune system. Extraocular features are summarized in Table 28-7.

Ocular motor abnormalities are found in many patients with AT and are frequently among the earliest manifestations. Characteristically, there is poor initiation of saccades with preservation of vestibular-ocular movements, as in congenital ocular motor apraxia. Head thrusts are used to compensate for saccades. Strabismus and nystagmus may also be present.

Telangiectasia of the conjunctiva occurs in 91% of patients and develops between the ages of 3 and 5 years. Involvement is initially interpalpebral but away from the limbus (Fig 28-20); it eventually becomes generalized. Similar vessel changes can appear in the skin of the eyelids and other sun-exposed areas.

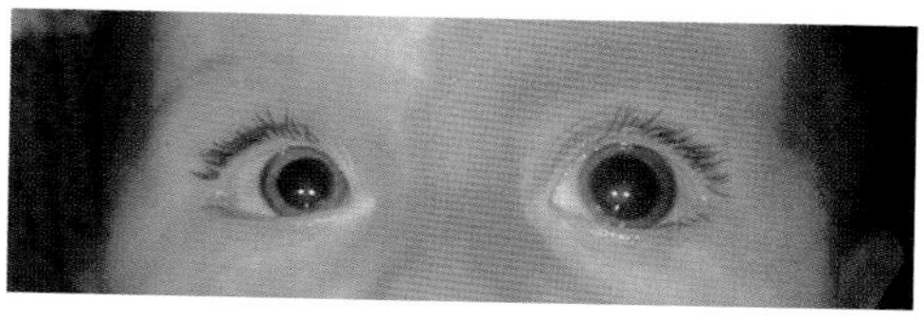

图 28-18　Sturge-Weber 综合征合并青光眼，女婴，葡萄酒色斑累及左眼睑，伴同侧牛眼。

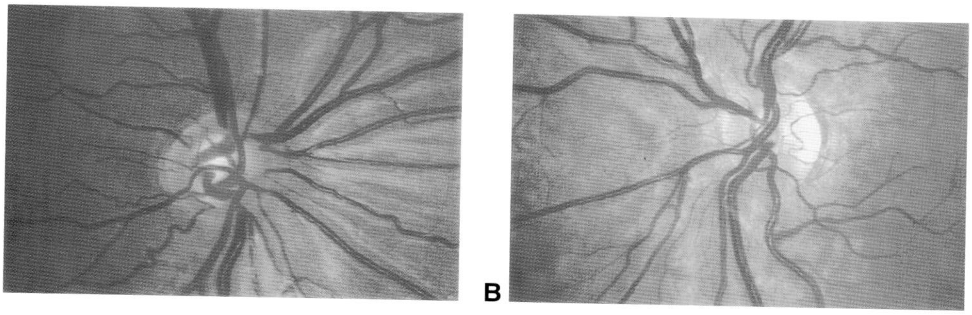

图 28-19　Sturge-Weber 综合征眼底，青春期男孩，右眼青光眼视杯及周围脉络膜深红色（**A**），与健眼比较（**B**）。

Sturge-Weber 综合征（SWS）性青光眼不易治疗。初期使用局部滴眼液可能有效，特别是发病较晚者。手术适用于早发病例和药物治疗效果不佳者，可以长期良好地控制眼压，但需多次手术。Sturge-Weber 综合征（SWS）性青光眼手术的特殊风险，是术中或术后异常脉络膜血管的渗出或出血，系眼压下降过快所致。手术医生必须特别谨慎地植入青光眼引流装置，以防术后早期眼压过度降低。术后可能有大量脉络膜或视网膜下积液，但常在 1 ~ 2 周内自发性吸收。

房角手术（前房角切开术和小梁切开术）已成功用于 Sturge-Weber 综合征（SWS）。脉冲染料激光治疗受累皮肤，可以降低血管密度，明显改善其外观，而不会对皮肤组织造成明显损害。

Khaier A, Nischal KK, Espinosa M, Manoj B. Periocular port wine stain: the Great Ormond Street Hospital experience. *Ophthalmology*. 2011;118(11):2274–2278.e1.

毛细血管扩张性共济失调

毛细血管扩张性共济失调（AT; Louis-Bar 综合征）主要累及小脑、眼表、皮肤和免疫系统。表 28-7 汇总了外眼特征。

眼球运动异常是毛细血管扩张性共济失调（AT）最早的临床表现之一，典型的特征是前庭眼反射运动正常，但眼球扫视运动的启动功能差，与先天性动眼失用症 / 眼球运动不同。患者常通过甩头来补偿扫视运动。该病也可并发斜视和眼球震颤。

91% 发生结膜毛细血管扩张，且 3 ~ 5 岁间持续发展。最初累及睑裂区，但远离角膜缘（图 28-20），最后广泛分布。类似的血管变化可出现在眼睑和其他暴露于阳光的皮肤。

Table 28-7 Extraocular Features in Ataxia-Telangiectasia

Feature	Characteristics
Neurologic findings	Truncal ataxia usually noted during second year of life Subsequent development of dysarthria, dystonia, and choreoathetosis Progressive deterioration of motor function, leading to serious disability by age 10 years Intellectual disability and microcephaly in some patients
Immunologic findings	Defective T-cell function is usually associated with hypoplasia of the thymus and decreased levels of circulating immunoglobulin Recurrent respiratory tract infections (frequent cause of mortality) Increased susceptibility to malignancy (frequent cause of mortality)
Oncologic findings	Greatly increased sensitivity to the tissue-damaging adverse effects of therapeutic radiation and many chemotherapeutic agents Increased risk of malignancy and radiation damage can also occur in heterozygous carriers
Shagreen patch	Typically located in lumbosacral area Onset after puberty

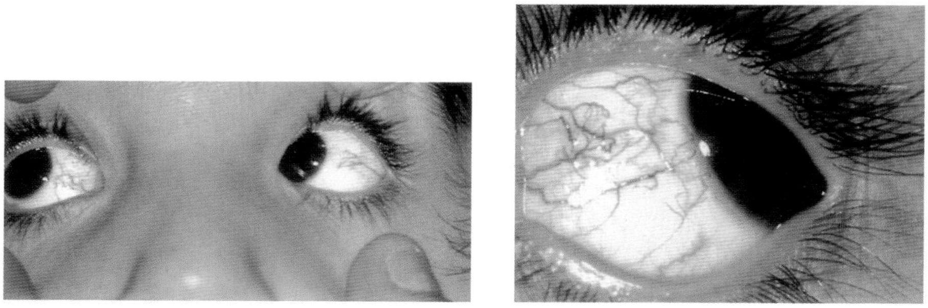

Figure 28-20 Abnormally dilated and tortuous interpalpebral conjunctival vessels in a child with ataxia-telangiectasia, seen only in the interpalpebral fissure.

Individuals with AT are much more sensitive to the tissue-damaging adverse effects of therapeutic radiation and many chemotherapeutic agents. Defective T-cell function in patients with AT is usually associated with hypoplasia of the thymus and decreased levels of circulating immunoglobulin. Recurrent respiratory tract infections and increased susceptibility to malignant tumors are frequent causes of mortality.

Incontinentia Pigmenti

Incontinentia pigmenti (IP; Bloch-Sulzberger syndrome) affects the skin, brain, and eyes. Extraocular features are summarized in Table 28-8, with examples of skin lesions shown in Figure 28-21. The condition has an X-linked dominant inheritance pattern, with a presumed lethal effect on the hemizygous male fetus.

表28-7　毛细血管扩张性共济失调的眼外特征

特征	特点
神经系统	躯干共济失调常在出生后第2年被发现 后续发展为构音障碍，肌张力障碍和舞蹈手足徐动症 运动功能逐渐恶化，10岁时发展为严重残疾 部分患者智力障碍和畸形
免疫系统	T细胞缺陷功能通常与胸腺发育不全和循环免疫球蛋白水平降低有关 反复呼吸道感染（死亡的常见原因） 对恶性肿瘤的易感性升高（死亡的常见原因）
肿瘤学	对治疗性放射和许多化学治疗剂的组织损害性副作用的敏感性显著增加 杂合子携带者发生恶性肿瘤和放射性损伤的风险增加
鲨鱼斑	典型位于骶髂区 青春期发病

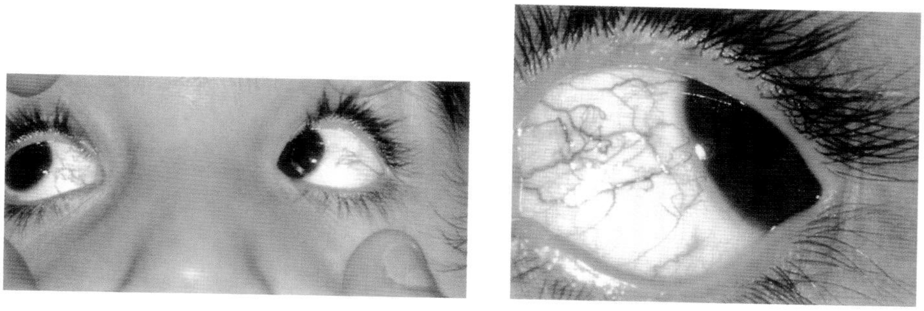

图 28-20　患有毛细血管扩张性共济失调的儿童，睑结膜血管异常扩张和迂曲，仅见于睑裂区。

毛细血管扩张性共济失调（AT）对放射治疗和化学治疗造成的组织损伤副作用较敏感。患者 T 细胞功能缺陷常伴胸腺发育不良和循环免疫球蛋白水平降低。反复的呼吸道感染和对恶性肿瘤的易感性是常见的死亡原因。

色素失调症

色素失调症（IP，Bloch-Sulzberger 综合征）累及皮肤、大脑和眼，其外眼特征汇总见表 28-8，皮肤病变见图 28-21。该病症具有 X- 连锁显性遗传模式，半合子男性胎儿可能致死。

Table 28-8 Extraocular Features in Incontinentia Pigmenti

Feature	Characteristics
Dermatologic findings	Usually normal skin appearance at birth Development of erythema and bullae during the first few days of life, usually on the extremities (see Fig 28-21A) Persistence of lesions for weeks to months When healed, appearance of lesions as clusters of small, hyperpigmented macules in a characteristic "splashed paint" distribution (see Fig 28-21B), most prominently on the trunk
Neurologic findings	Microcephaly, hydrocephalus, seizures, and varying degrees of cognitive impairment in one-third of patients
Dental findings	Missing and malformed teeth in roughly two-thirds of cases
Other findings	Scoliosis, skull deformities, cleft palate, and dwarfism, among other findings, occur less commonly

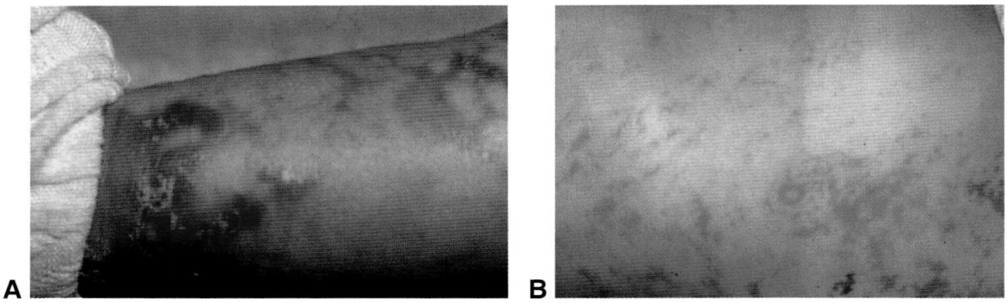

Figure 28-21 Pigmented skin lesions of incontinentia pigmenti. **A,** Bullous lesions. **B,** Hyperpigmented macules. *(Courtesy of Edward L. Raab, MD.)*

Ocular involvement occurs in 35%–77% of cases and tends to be unilateral or very asymmetric if bilateral, typically in the form of proliferative retinal vasculopathy that closely resembles retinopathy of prematurity. At birth, the only detectable abnormality may be incomplete peripheral retinal vascularization. Abnormal arteriovenous connections,microvascular abnormalities, and neovascular membranes develop at or near the junction of the vascular and avascular retina (Fig 28-22). Rapid progression sometimes leads to total retinal detachment and retrolental membrane formation within the first few months of life. Microphthalmia, cataract, glaucoma, optic atrophy, strabismus, and nystagmus may occur, usually secondary to end-stage retinopathy.

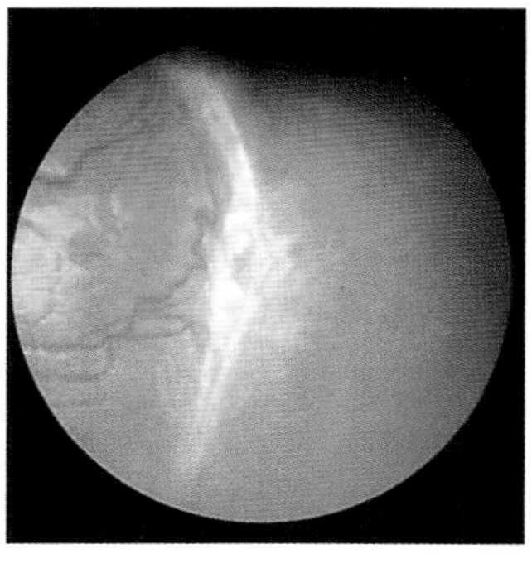

Figure 28-22 Vascular abnormalities of the temporal retina, right eye, in a 2-year-old with incontinentia pigmenti. Note the avascularity peripheral to the circumferential white vasoproliferative lesion, which showed profuse leakage on fluorescein angiography.

表28-8　色素失调症的眼外表现

特征	特点
皮肤科	出生时皮肤外观正常 出生最初几天出现红斑和大疱，常在四肢（见图28-21A） 病变持续数周到数月 愈合后，病变的外观就像一簇小的色素沉着的斑点状物质分布在一个特征性的“泼漆”图中（见图28-21B），主要位于躯干上
神经系统	1/3存在小头畸形、脑积水、癫痫以及不同程度的认知障碍
牙科	2/3存在牙缺失或畸形
其他结果	少见脊柱侧凸、颅骨畸形、腭裂和侏儒症

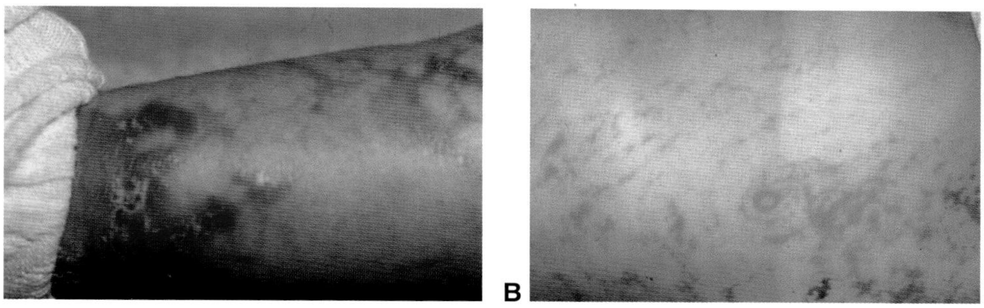

A　B

图 28-21　色素失调症患者的色素性皮肤病变。**A.** 大疱性病变。**B.** 色素沉着斑。*（译者注：资料来源见前页原文。）*

35% ~ 77% 的病例眼部受累，单眼发病，双眼时极不对称，表现为增殖性视网膜血管病变，与早产儿视网膜病变相似。出生时唯一的异常是周边视网膜不完全血管化。异常的动静脉吻合、微血管畸形、视网膜血管与无血管交界区的新生血管膜（图 28-22）。病情的快速发展导致在出生后最初几个月内，完全视网膜脱离和晶状体后膜形成。视网膜病变晚期可见小眼畸形、白内障、青光眼、视神经萎缩、斜视和眼球震颤。

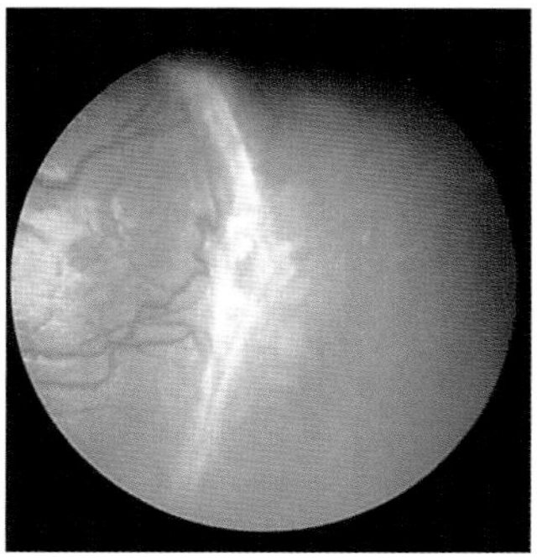

图 28-22　颞侧视网膜血管异常，右眼，2 岁的色素失调症患者。可见围绕白色血管增生性病变的无血管区，荧光血管造影见大量渗漏。

Sequential retinal evaluations for the first 1–2 years of life are necessary to identify eyes that require treatment. The retinopathy of IP has been managed by photocoagulation or cryotherapy with varying degrees of success. Treatment is usually applied primarily to the avascular peripheral retina, as in the management of retinopathy of prematurity.

O'Doherty M, Mc Creery K, Green AJ, Tuwir I, Brosnahan D. Incontinentia pigmenti—ophthalmological observation of a series of cases and review of the literature. *Br J Ophthalmol.* 2011;95(1):11–16.

Wyburn-Mason Syndrome

Wyburn-Mason syndrome (racemose angioma) is a nonhereditary arteriovenous malformation of the eye and brain. Extraocular features are summarized in Table 28-9.

Ocular manifestations are unilateral and congenital, and they may progress during childhood. The typical lesion consists of markedly dilated and tortuous vessels that shunt blood directly from arteries to veins (Fig 28-23). These vessels do not leak fluid. Vision ranges from normal to markedly reduced. Intraocular hemorrhage and secondary neovascular glaucoma are possible complications. More than half of affected eyes are blind, and an additional one-quarter have severe visual impairment.

Table 28-9 Extraocular Features in Wyburn-Mason Syndrome

Feature	Characteristics
Dermatologic findings	Maxillofacial or cutaneous facial AVM
Neurologic findings	AVM, especially in midbrain Frequent source of hemorrhage May result in seizures, mental changes, hemiparesis, and papilledema

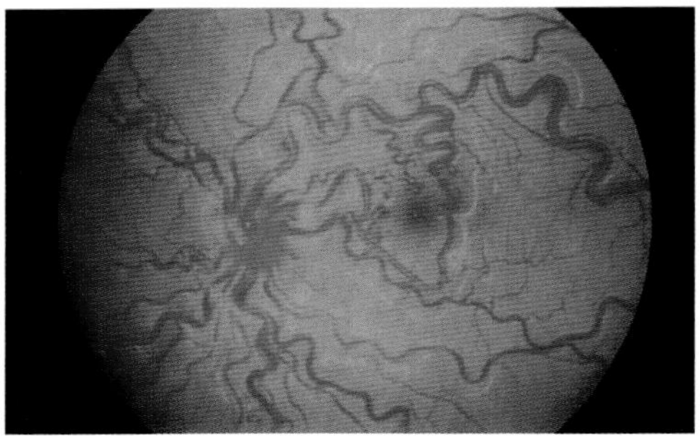

Figure 28-23 Wyburn-Mason syndrome, or racemose angioma of the retina, left eye.

No treatment is indicated for primary lesions. Treatment may be considered for associated complications, such as scatter photocoagulation for ischemic venous occlusive disease, vitrectomy for nonclearing vitreous hemorrhage, and cyclodestructive treatment for neovascular glaucoma.

需在出生后的第 1~2 年进行连续的视网膜评估，判定眼部的治疗。色素失调症 IP 的视网膜病变可进行光凝或冷冻治疗，这 2 种方法可达到不同程度的效果。与早产儿视网膜病变的治疗一样，主要是对周边无血管视网膜进行治疗。

O'Doherty M, Mc Creery K, Green AJ, Tuwir I, Brosnahan D. Incontinentia pigmenti—ophthalmological observation of a series of cases and review of the literature. *Br J Ophthalmol.* 2011;95(1):11-16.

Wyburn-Mason 综合征

Wyburn-Mason 综合征（葡萄状血管瘤）是一种非遗传性的眼部和大脑的动静脉畸形。外眼特征汇总见表 28-9。

该疾病眼部表现是单侧和先天性的，病变可能在童年时期持续发展。典型的病变为明显扩张和迂曲的血管将血液直接从动脉分流到静脉（图 28-23），这些血管不会发生渗漏。患者的视力范围为从正常视力到显著低于正常视力。该疾病可能的并发症包括眼内出血和继发性新生血管性青光眼。1/2 受累眼睛失明，另外 1/4 的人有严重的视力障碍。

表28-9　Wyburn-Mason综合征的外眼特征

特征	特点
皮肤科	颌面部或皮肤面部动静脉畸形AVM
神经系统	动静脉畸形（AVM），特别在中脑 频繁出血的原因 导致癫痫、精神症状、偏瘫和视乳头水肿

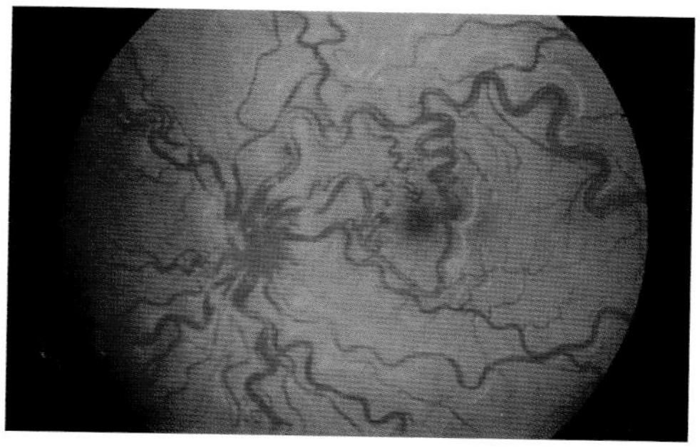

图 28-23　Wyburn-Mason 综合征，或视网膜葡萄状血管瘤，左眼。

没有适用于该疾病原发病灶的治疗措施。可考虑治疗相关并发症，例如适用于缺血性静脉闭塞性疾病的散射光凝固治疗、非清除性玻璃体出血的玻璃体切除术和新生血管性青光眼的环形破坏性治疗。

Klippel-Trénaunay Syndrome

Klippel-Trénaunay syndrome (KTS) is a neuro-oculocutaneous disorder consisting of a vascular nevus involving an extremity, varicosities of that extremity, and hypertrophy of bone and soft tissue. When arteriovenous malformation is also present, the disease is called *Klippel-Trénaunay-Weber syndrome*. Occurrence of KTS is sporadic and the etiology is unknown. Ophthalmic findings include vascular anomalies of the orbit, iris, retina, choroid, and optic nerve, as well as optic nerve and chiasmal gliomas. There is also a risk of glaucoma.

KTS is a complex syndrome with no single treatment protocol. Treatment is individualized to the patient. At present, many of the symptoms may be treated, but there is no cure for this syndrome.

Albinism

Albinism is a group of conditions that involve the synthesis of melanin in the skin and eye *(oculocutaneous albinism [OCA])* or the eye alone *(ocular albinism [OA])*.

Diagnosis

The major ophthalmic findings in all types of OCA and OA are iris transillumination from decreased pigmentation, foveal aplasia or hypoplasia, and a characteristic deficit of pigment in the retina, especially peripheral to the posterior pole (Fig 28-24A, B). Nystagmus, photophobia, high refractive errors, and reduced central visual acuity are often present, and visual acuity ranges from 20/25 to 20/200. If a child has significant foveal hypoplasia, nystagmus will begin at 2–3 months of age. The severity of the visual impairment tends to be proportional to the degree of nystagmus and foveal hypoplasia. Optical coherence tomography has demonstrated that the size of the photoreceptor outer segment is the strongest predictor of visual acuity. An abnormally large number of crossed fibers appear in the optic chiasm of patients and animals with albinism, precluding stereopsis and often inducing strabismus. Asymmetric visual evoked potentials are often seen in affected patients and may be helpful in diagnosis.

There are 4 major types of OCA, all of which exhibit various degrees of skin and hair pigmentation (Fig 28-24C). They are autosomal recessive and are caused by different gene mutations (Table 28-10).

Ocular albinism (OA1), also called *Nettleship-Falls ocular albinism*, is usually caused by a mutation in the *GPR143* gene on the X chromosome. This gene controls melanosome number and size; the mutation results in macromelanosomes, which may be revealed by skin biopsy. Affected individuals appear to have decreased pigment in the eyes but not the skin. Patches of decreased pigment in the fundus and iris transillumination are apparent in many female carriers.

Klippel-Trénaunay 综合征

Klippel–Trénaunay 综合征（KTS）是一种神经 – 眼皮肤疾病，包括累及四肢的血管痣、受累肢体静脉曲张、骨和软组织肥大。当同时存在动静脉畸形时，称为 *Klippel–Trénaunay–Weber 综合征*。Klippel–Trénaunay 综合征（KTS）散在发生，病因不明。眼科检查有眼眶、虹膜、视网膜、脉络膜和视神经血管异常，以及视神经和视交叉神经胶质瘤，还有患青光眼的风险。

Klippel–Trénaunay 综合征（KTS）是一种复杂的综合征，没有单一的治疗方案。治疗时针对患者进行个体化治疗。目前可以对症治疗，但无法治愈。

白化病

白化病是一组影响皮肤及眼部［*眼皮肤白化病*（*OCA*）］或仅影响眼部［*眼白化病*（*OA*）］的黑色素合成异常。

诊断

所有类型的眼皮肤白化病（OCA）和眼白化病（OA）的主要眼部表现为色素减少所致的虹膜透光、黄斑中心凹发育不全，以及特征性视网膜色素缺失，特别是从周边向后极部（图 28–24A、B）发展。常有眼球震颤、畏光、高度屈光不正，中心视力降低，为 20/200 ~ 20/25。如果有严重的黄斑中心凹发育不全，出生后 2~3 个月发生眼球震颤，视力损害的严重程度与眼球震颤和黄斑中心凹发育不全的程度成比例。光学相干断层扫描显示，感光器外节的大小可预测视力。白化病患者和动物的视交叉可出现大量异常交叉纤维，阻碍立体视形成，常引发斜视。患者常见不对称的视觉诱发电位，有助于诊断。

眼皮肤白化病（OCA）主要有 4 种类型，表现出不同的皮肤和毛发色素程度（图 28–24C），是常染色体隐性遗传，由不同的基因突变引起（表 28–10）。

眼白化病（OA1），也称为 *Nettleship–Falls* 眼白化病，常由 X 染色体 *GPR143* 基因突变引起。该基因控制黑色素体的数量和大小，其突变产生巨黑色素体，皮肤活检可检出。患者外观上表现为眼内的色素减少，但皮肤色素并没有减少。眼底色素脱失性斑块和虹膜透照现象在许多女性携带者中较为明显。

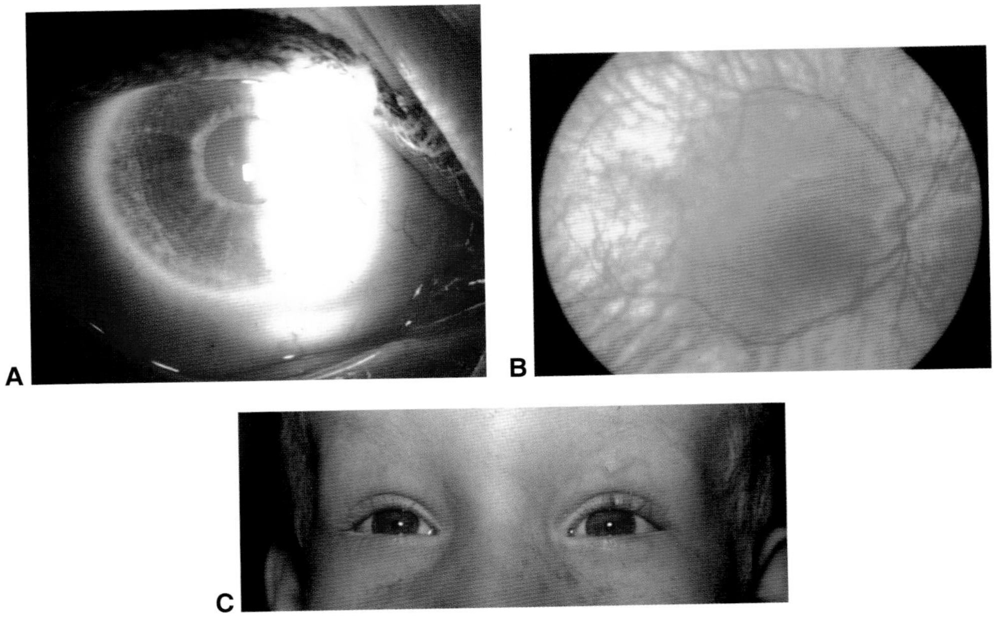

Figure 28-24 **A,** Transillumination of iris in albinism, right eye. **B,** Fundus in albinism, right eye, demonstrating complete lack of pigment and macular hypoplasia. **C,** Child with oculocutaneous albinism type 2. Note the white hair, eyebrows, and lashes and light-colored irides and freckles. (*Parts A and C courtesy of Edward L. Raab, MD.*)

Albinism can be part of a broader syndrome, such as Hermansky-Pudlak syndrome or Chédiak-Higashi syndrome, both of which are autosomal recessive. *Hermansky-Pudlak syndrome* occurs with higher frequency in Puerto Rico and consanguineous populations and is characterized by pulmonary interstitial fibrosis and bleeding abnormalities. *Chédiak-Higashi syndrome* is a rare condition characterized by increased susceptibility to bacterial infections. Whenever albinism is diagnosed in a child, the clinician should inquire whether the patient has bleeding or bruising tendencies or experiences frequent infections.

Khan AO, Tamimi M, Lenzner S, Bolz HJ. Hermansky-Pudlak syndrome genes are frequently mutated in patients with albinism from the Arabian Peninsula. *Clin Genet.* 2016;90(1):96–98.

Mohammad S, Gottlob I, Kumar A, et al. The functional significance of foveal abnormalities in albinism measured using spectral-domain optical coherence tomography. *Ophthalmology.* 2011;118(8):1645–1652.

Treatment

Significant refractive errors are treated with prescription glasses. Strabismus surgery is performed when appropriate. Tinted glasses may be used for patients with photophobia. Patients with OCA are at risk for skin cancer and should be counseled about limiting sun exposure.

Levin AV, Stroh E. Albinism for the busy clinician. *J AAPOS.* 2011;15(1):59–66.

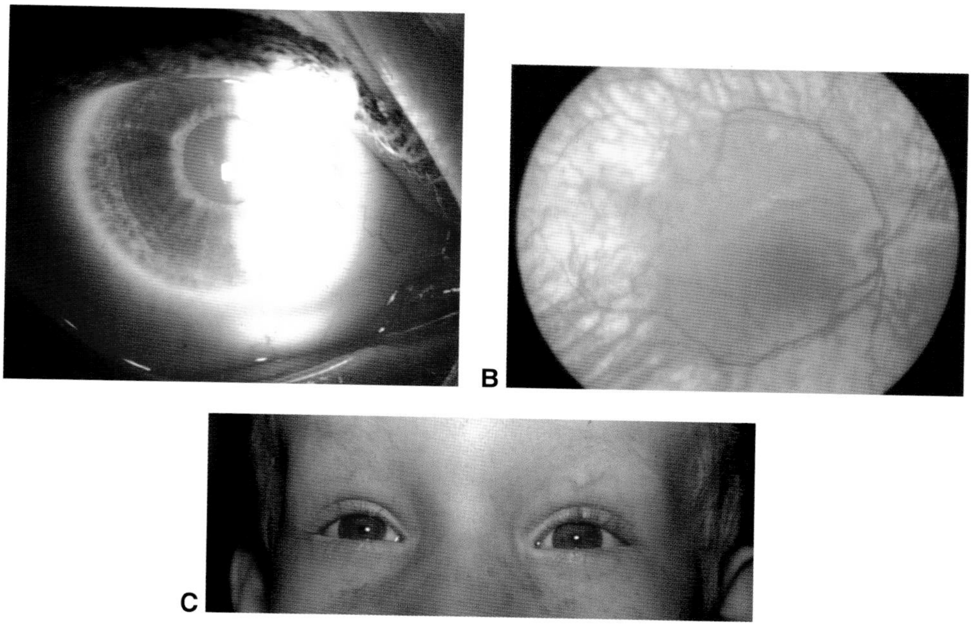

图 28-24　A. 透照法观察白化病患者的虹膜，右眼。**B.** 白化病患者的眼底，右眼，显示色素完全缺乏 / 黄斑发育不全。**C.** 眼皮肤白化病 2 型的患儿，头发、眉毛和睫毛白色，以及浅色的虹膜和雀斑。*（译者注：资料来源见前页原文。）*

白化病可能是更广泛的综合征的一部分，如 Hermansky–Pudlak 综合征，或 Chédiak–Higashi 综合征，两者都是常染色体隐性遗传。*Hermansky–Pudlak 综合征*在波多黎各和近亲群体中发生率较高，其特征是肺间质纤维化和出血异常。*Chédiak–Higashi 综合征*是一种罕见疾病，其特征是对细菌感染的易感性增加。诊断儿童白化病时，医生应询问是否有出血、淤血倾向或经常感染。

Khan AO, Tamimi M, Lenzner S, Bolz HJ. Hermansky-Pudlak syndrome genes are frequently mutated in patients with albinism from the Arabian Peninsula. *Clin Genet*. 2016;90(1):96–98.

Mohammad S, Gottlob I, Kumar A, et al. The functional significance of foveal abnormalities in albinism measured using spectral-domain optical coherence tomography. *Ophthalmology*. 2011;118(8):1645–1652.

治疗

明显的屈光不正可配镜矫正，适当时可行斜视手术。畏光可用染色眼镜。眼白化病（OCA）有患皮肤癌的风险，建议减少阳光暴露。

Levin AV, Stroh E. Albinism for the busy clinician. *J AAPOS*. 2011;15(1):59–66.

Table 28-10 Classification of Major Types of Oculocutaneous Albinism (OCA)

Type of OCA	Defective Gene	Locus	Associated Findings
OCA1A	Tyrosinase gene *(TYR)*	11q14–q21	White skin and hair; no tyrosinase; poorest vision
OCA1B	Tyrosinase gene *(TYR)*	11q14–q21	"Yellow variant"; some tyrosinase activity
OCA minimal pigment (MP)	Tyrosinase gene *(TYR)*	11q14–q21	Some tyrosinase activity
OCA temperature-sensitive	Tyrosinase gene *(TYR)*	11q14–q21	Tyrosine function in cooler areas of body only
OCA2	*OCA2* gene	15q11.2–q12	Most prevalent worldwide; seen frequently in African Americans
OCA3	Tyrosinase-related protein 1 gene *(TYRP1)*	9p23	"Red rufous" type; reddish hair; seen in persons of African descent; mild visual abnormalities
OCA4	Membrane-associated transporter protein gene *(MATP)*	5p13.3	Common in Japanese population

Diabetes Mellitus

Type 1, or insulin-dependent, diabetes mellitus was formerly called *juvenile-onset diabetes mellitus*. The prevalence of retinopathy in this condition is directly proportional to the duration of diabetes mellitus after puberty. Poor glucose control can cause cataract. Retinopathy rarely occurs less than 15 years after the onset of diabetes mellitus. Proliferative diabetic retinopathy is rare in pediatric cases (see BCSC Section 12, *Retina and Vitreous*). Diabetes mellitus, especially in young children, may be part of *DIDMOAD syndrome* (*d*iabetes *i*nsipidus, *d*iabetes *m*ellitus, *o*ptic *a*trophy, and *d*eafness). This condition, which is also known as *Wolfram syndrome*, is associated with congenital cataracts as well. BCSC Section 1, *Update on General Medicine*, discusses diabetes mellitus in greater detail.

To screen for diabetic retinopathy, the American Academy of Ophthalmology recommends annual ophthalmic examinations beginning 5 years after the onset of type 1 diabetes mellitus.

Treatment is discussed in BCSC Section 12, *Retina and Vitreous*.

American Academy of Ophthalmology Retina/Vitreous Panel. Preferred Practice Pattern Guidelines. *Diabetic Retinopathy*. San Francisco, CA: American Academy of Ophthalmology; 2017. Available at www.aao.org/ppp.

Intrauterine or Perinatal Infection

Maternally transmitted congenital infections cause ocular damage through one or more of the following means: direct action of the infecting agent, which damages tissue; a teratogenic effect, which causes malformation; or delayed reactivation of the agent after birth, which damages developed tissue by direct action or inflammation.

Most perinatal disorders have a broad spectrum of clinical presentation, ranging from silent disease to life-threatening tissue and organ damage. Common, classic types of congenital infections are represented in the mnemonic *TORCH*: *t*oxoplasmosis, *r*ubella, *c*ytomegalovirus, and *h*erpesviruses.

表28-10　眼皮肤白化病的主要类型分类

类型	缺陷基因	位点	临床表现
OCA1A	*酪氨酸酶基因(TYR)*	11q14-q21	白色皮肤和头发，酪氨酸酶缺乏
OCA1B	*酪氨酸酶基因(TYR)*	11q14-q21	“黄色变异”，酪氨酸酶有一定活性
OCA 少色素(MP)	*酪氨酸酶基因(TYR)*	11q14-q21	酪氨酸酶有一定活性
OCA 温度敏感的	*酪氨酸酶基因(TYR)*	11q14-q21	仅在体温较低部位有酪氨酸功能
OCA2	*OCA2基因*	15q11.2-q12	最常见，非裔美国人
OCA3	*酪氨酸酶相关蛋白1基因(TYRP1)*	9p23	“暗红色”型，红发，见于非洲后裔，轻度视觉异常
OCA4	*膜相关运输蛋白基因(MATP)*	5p13.3	常见于日本人

糖尿病

1 型或胰岛素依赖型糖尿病以前被称为*青少年型糖尿病*。其视网膜病变的患病率与青春期后数字糖尿病的持续时间成正比。血糖控制不良可引发白内障。视网膜病变很少发生在糖尿病发病的 15 年内。增生性糖尿病视网膜病变儿童少见（见 BCSC 第 12 册《*视网膜与玻璃体*》）。糖尿病，特别是幼儿，可能是 *DIDMOAD 综合征*［尿崩症（*d*iabetes *i*nsipidus），糖尿病（*d*iabetes *m*ellitus），视神经萎缩（optic *a*trophy）和耳聋（*d*eafness）］的一部分，也称为 *Wolfram 综合征*，伴有先天性白内障。BCSC 第 1 册《*医学最新进展*》详细探讨了糖尿病。

为了筛查糖尿病视网膜病变，美国眼科学会建议 1 型糖尿病发病 5 年后开始进行年度眼科检查。

治疗见 BCSC 第 12 册《*视网膜与玻璃体*》。

American Academy of Ophthalmology Retina/Vitreous Panel. Preferred Practice Pattern Guidelines. *Diabetic Retinopathy*. San Francisco, CA: American Academy of Ophthalmology; 2017. Available at www.aao.org/ppp.

宫内或围产期感染

母亲传播性先天性感染通过多个路径引起眼部损伤，感染的直接组织损害、致畸效应导致畸形、出生后微生物活性延迟激活，直接损伤或感染已发育组织。

多数围产期病变临床表现累及多方面，从静止性疾病到终生威胁组织和器官。常见的先天性感染可简写为 *TORCH*，即弓形体病（*t*oxoplasmosis）、风疹（*r*ubella）、巨细胞病毒感染（*c*ytomegalovirus）和疱疹病毒（*h*erpesviruses）。

Toxoplasmosis

Systemic infection in humans by the obligate intracellular parasite *Toxoplasma gondii* is common and usually goes undiagnosed. Felines are the definitive host. Signs and symptoms may include fever, lymphadenopathy, and sore throat. The percentage of antibody titer–positive persons in the United States increases with age (younger than 5 years, 5%; older than 80 years, 60%).

The incidence of congenital toxoplasmosis ranges from 1 to 10 per 10,000 live births. Toxoplasmosis can be acquired congenitally via transplacental transmission from an infected mother to the fetus. Congenital infection can result in retinitis, hepatosplenomegaly, intracranial calcifications, microcephaly, and developmental delay.

Ocular manifestations besides retinitis include choroiditis, iritis, and anterior uveitis (Fig 28-25). The area of active retinal inflammation is usually thickened and cream colored with an overlying vitritis, frequently in the macula. This area may be at the edge of an old, flat, atrophic scar (a so-called satellite lesion). Previously, apparently acquired *Toxoplasma* retinitis was thought to represent reactivation of a congenital infection; however, recent evidence suggests that most of these patients are infected postnatally. Diagnosis is primarily clinical.

Ocular toxoplasmosis does not require treatment unless it threatens vision. Systemic treatment involves the use of one or more antimicrobial drugs with or without oral corticosteroids. Commonly used antimicrobial agents are pyrimethamine and sulfadiazine. Corticosteroids should typically be used with antimicrobial coverage. Intravitreal injection of clindamycin and dexamethasone has been reported as a possible alternative treatment.

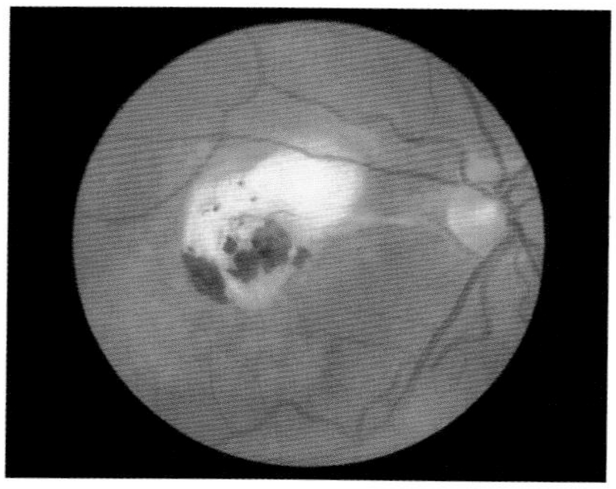

Figure 28-25 Toxoplasmosis chorioretinitis, right eye.

Further details regarding diagnosis and management can be found in BCSC Section 9, *Uveitis and Ocular Inflammation*.

Rubella

Congenital rubella (German measles) syndrome is a well-defined combination of ocular, otologic, and cardiac abnormalities, accompanied by microcephaly and variable developmental delay. The incidence has decreased markedly in North America since widespread vaccination of children was instituted in the late 1960s; however, rubella remains a cause of infant morbidity and mortality in less-developed countries.

弓形体病

由绝对细胞内寄生虫*弓形虫*引起的人全身性感染很常见，多数未予诊断，猫科动物是其终宿主。临床症状和体征有发烧、淋巴结肿大和咽喉痛。在美国，抗体滴度阳性的百分比随着年龄的增长而增加（小于 5 岁为 5%，大于 80 岁为 60%）。

先天性弓形虫病的发病率为每 10000 例活产中有 1 ~ 10 例。先天获得性的弓形虫病，由感染的母亲经胎盘传播到胎儿。先天性感染可导致视网膜炎、肝脾肿大、颅内钙化、小头畸形和发育迟缓。

除视网膜炎外，眼部表现还有脉络膜炎、虹膜炎和前葡萄膜炎（图 28–25）。活动性视网膜炎病灶区增厚，呈奶油色，其表面玻璃体炎，常位于黄斑，毗邻陈旧的扁平萎缩性瘢痕（称为卫星病变）。曾认为获得性*弓形虫*视网膜炎是先天性感染的再激活，而最近有证据表明，其大多数是出生后感染的。主要通过临床来诊断。

眼部弓形虫病未危及视力时，不需要治疗。全身治疗包括使用一种或多种抗微生物药物，加或不加口服皮质类固醇。常用的抗微生物剂是乙胺嘧啶和磺胺嘧啶。皮质类固醇常与抗菌药物一起使用。有报道称，玻璃体内注射克林霉素和地塞米松是一种可能的替代治疗方法。

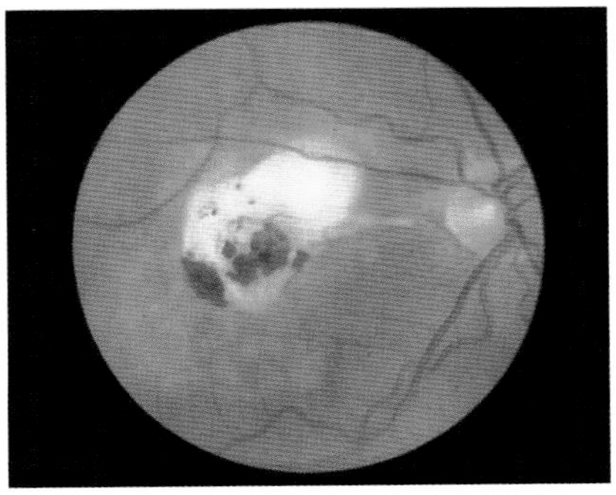

图 28–25　弓形虫病性脉络膜视网膜炎，右眼。

有关的诊断及处理见 BCSC 第 9 册《*葡萄膜炎与眼部炎症*》。

风疹

先天性风疹（德国麻疹）综合征是已明确定义为眼部、耳部和心脏异常，伴有小头畸形和多种表现的发育迟缓。自从 20 世纪 60 年代末实施广泛接种儿童疫苗以来，北美的发病率明显下降，而风疹仍是欠发达国家婴儿发病和死亡的原因之一。

Ocular abnormalities include a peculiar nuclear cataract that is sometimes floating in a liquefied lens cortex, glaucoma, microphthalmia, and retinal abnormalities that vary from a subtle salt-and-pepper retinopathy (most common finding; Fig 28-26) to pseudoretinitis pigmentosa. Diagnosis is based on this characteristic clinical picture and is supported by results of serologic testing. The virus itself can be isolated from pharyngeal swabs and from the lens contents at the time of cataract surgery.

Lensectomy is usually required for cataracts. Infected eyes are prone to postoperative inflammation and subsequent secondary membrane formation. Thus, topical steroids and mydriatics should be used aggressively. In adults, rubella virus infection has been identified as a probable cause of Fuchs heterochromic uveitis.

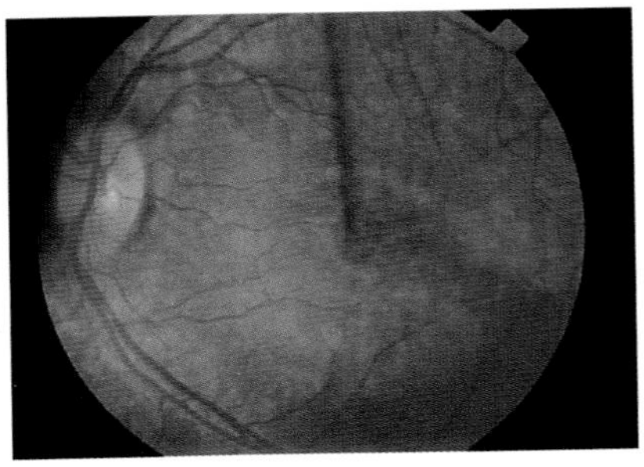

Figure 28-26 Fundus photograph from a 6-year-old patient with rubella syndrome (electroretinography results were normal).

Cytomegalovirus

Cytomegalovirus (CMV), a member of the herpesvirus family, is a ubiquitous virus that can cause a wide range of infection, from asymptomatic acquired infection in immunocompetent individuals to severe infections in newborn infants and immunocompromised patients. Over 80% of adults in developed countries have antibodies to the virus.

Congenital infection with CMV is the most common congenital infection in humans; it occurs in approximately 1% of infants. Clinically apparent disease is present in 10%–15% of infected neonates, and 20%–30% of these cases are fatal. Transmission to the fetus or newborn can occur transplacentally, from contact with an infected birth canal during delivery, or from ingestion of infected breast milk or maternal secretions. Congenital CMV disease is characterized by fever, jaundice, hematologic abnormalities, deafness, microcephaly, and periventricular calcifications.

Ophthalmic manifestations of congenital CMV infection occur primarily in infants with systemic symptoms and include retinochoroiditis (Fig 28-27), optic nerve anomalies, microphthalmia, cataract, and uveitis. The retinochoroiditis usually presents with bilateral focal involvement consisting of areas of RPE atrophy and whitish opacities mixed with retinal hemorrhages. The retinitis can be progressive, or it may present as a quiescent CMV chorioretinal scar that is difficult to differentiate from the scar seen in toxoplasmosis. CMV retinitis can be acquired in children who are immunocompromised (most frequently by infection with HIV or AIDS or following organ transplantation or chemotherapy). The retinitis is a diffuse retinal necrosis with areas of retinal thickening and whitening, hemorrhages, and venous sheathing. Vitritis may also be present.

Diagnosis is based on the clinical presentation in acquired disease and is supplemented by serologic testing for antibodies to CMV in congenital infection. In infected infants, the virus can be recovered from bodily secretions.

Infants with severe systemic or sight-threatening disease are usually treated with ganciclovir. Medications that are available for treatment of older immunocompromised children include ganciclovir, valganciclovir, foscarnet, cidofovir, and fomivirsen.

该疾病的眼部异常包括特有的核性白内障（有时可漂浮在液化晶状体皮质中）、青光眼、小眼球和多种视网膜异常，如细微的椒盐样视网膜病变（最常见的检查结果；图 28–26），或色素性假性视网膜炎。根据特征性临床表现和血清学检测即可诊断。病毒本身可以从咽拭子和白内障手术时晶状体成分中分离出来。

白内障患者常需行晶状体切除术。感染眼易发生术后炎症，形成继发性膜，因此，应大量使用局部类固醇药物和散瞳剂。已确定成人 Fuchs 异色性葡萄膜炎的可能原因是风疹病毒感染。

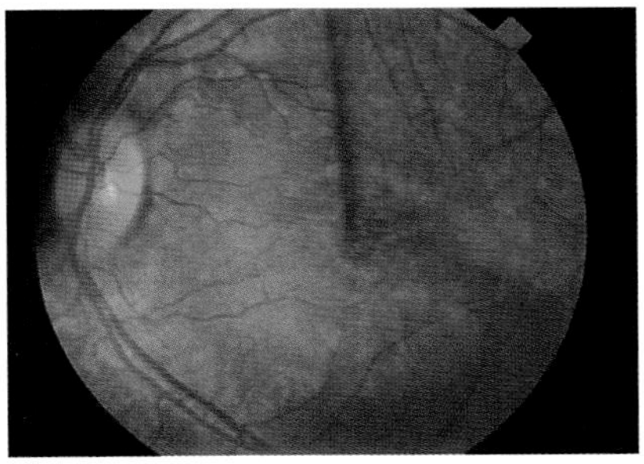

图 28–26　6 岁风疹综合征患者的眼底照片（视网膜电图检查结果正常）。

巨细胞病毒

巨细胞病毒（CMV）属于疱疹病毒家族，普遍存在于自然界，并能引起从免疫功能正常的无症状获得性感染，到新生儿和免疫功能低下患者的严重感染。超过 80% 的发达国家成人有巨细胞病毒抗体。

先天性巨细胞病毒（CMV）感染是人类最常见的先天性感染，约占婴儿的 1%。10% ~ 15% 的感染新生儿有明显的临床症状，其中 20% ~ 30% 致死。胎儿或新生儿可经胎盘、感染的产道或摄入感染的母乳、母体分泌物而感染。先天性巨细胞病毒（CMV）病的特点为发热、黄疸、血液异常、耳聋、小头畸形和心室周围钙化。

巨细胞病毒（CMV）感染的有全身症状的婴儿，出现眼部症状，包括视网膜脉络膜炎（图 28–27）、视神经异常、小眼畸形、白内障和葡萄膜炎。视网膜脉络膜炎常表现为双眼、局灶性病变，包括视网膜色素上皮（RPE）萎缩、白色混浊病灶伴有视网膜出血。视网膜炎可呈进行性，也可表现为静止的巨细胞病毒（CMV）脉络膜视网膜瘢痕，难与弓形体病的瘢痕鉴别。巨细胞病毒（CMV）性视网膜炎可发生于免疫功能低下的儿童［最常见的是人类免疫缺陷病毒（HIV）感染，或获得性免疫缺乏综合征（AIDS），或在器官移植或化学治疗后］。视网膜炎是一种弥漫性视网膜坏死，伴有视网膜增厚、变白、出血和静脉鞘。可伴有玻璃体炎。

获得性巨细胞病毒（CMV）感染的诊断以临床表现为主，先天性感染的诊断需辅助巨细胞病毒抗体的血清学检测，感染婴儿的病毒可以从身体分泌物中得到。

患有严重全身性或危及视力疾病的婴儿使用更昔洛韦进行治疗。用于治疗免疫功能受损的大龄儿童的药物有更昔洛韦、缬更昔洛韦、膦甲酸、西多福韦和福米韦生。

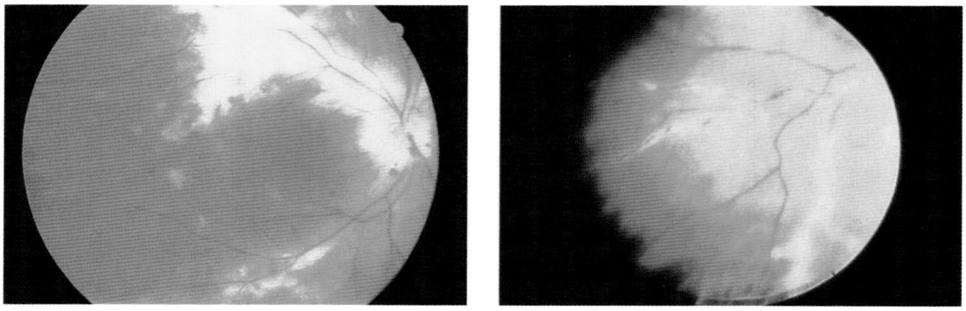

Figure 28-27 Active cytomegalovirus retinochoroiditis in a premature infant, right eye.

Herpes Simplex Virus

Herpes simplex virus (HSV) is a member of the herpesvirus family, which includes 2 types of simplex virus (HSV-1 and HSV-2), herpes zoster, Epstein-Barr virus, and CMV. Neonatal HSV infection occurs in 1 in 3000 to 20,000 births and is usually secondary to HSV-2. HSV-1 typically affects the eyes, skin, and mouth region and is transmitted by close personal contact. HSV-2 is typically associated with genital infection through venereal transmission.

Congenital HSV infection is usually acquired during passage through an infected birth canal. The neonatal infection is confined to the CNS, skin, oral cavity, and eyes in onethird of cases. It commonly manifests with vesicular skin lesions, ulcerative mouth sores, and keratoconjunctivitis. Disseminated disease occurs in two-thirds of cases and can involve the liver, adrenal glands, and lungs. Eye involvement in congenital infection can include conjunctivitis, keratitis, retinochoroiditis, and cataracts. Keratitis can be epithelial or stromal. Retinal involvement can be severe and may include massive exudates and retinal necrosis.

Affected infants are treated with systemic acyclovir. The mortality rate from disseminated disease is significant, and survivors usually have permanent ocular and CNS impairment.

Marquez L, Levy ML, Munoz FM, Palazzi DL. A report of three cases and review of intrauterine herpes simplex virus infection. *Pediatr Infect Dis J.* 2011;30(2):153–157.

Syphilis

Syphilis is caused by the spirochete *Treponema pallidum*, and sexual contact is the usual route of transmission. Fetal infection occurs following maternal spirochetemia. The longer the mother has had syphilis, the lower is the risk of transmitting the disease to her child. If a mother has contracted primary or secondary disease, approximately half of her offspring will be infected. In cases of untreated late maternal syphilis, approximately 70% of infants are healthy. The incidence of congenital syphilis in the United States is 15.7 cases per 100,000 live births.

Signs and symptoms of congenital syphilis include unexplained premature birth, large placenta, persistentrhinitis, intractable rash, unexplained jaundice, hepatosplenomegaly, pneumonia, anemia, generalized lymphadenopathy, and metaphyseal abnormalities or periostitis on radiographs. Congenitally acquired infection can lead to neonatal death. Early eye involvement in congenital syphilis is rare.

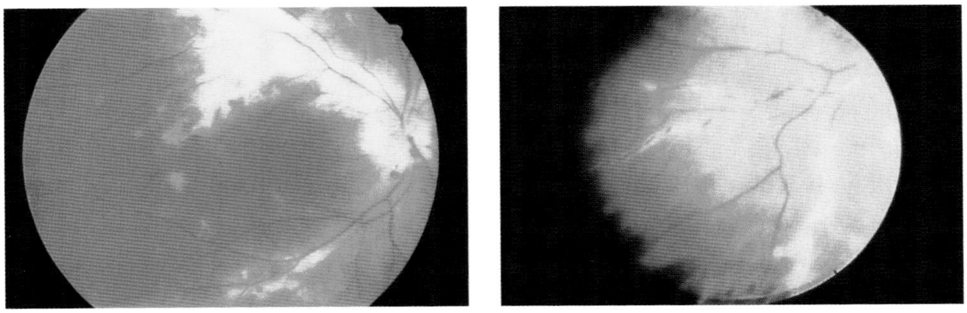

图 28–27　活动性巨细胞病毒性视网膜脉络膜炎，早产儿，右眼。

单纯疱疹病毒

单纯疱疹病毒（HSV）是疱疹病毒家族中的一员，包括 2 种类型的单纯疱疹病毒（HSV–1 和 HSV–2）、带状疱疹病毒、EB 病毒和巨细胞病毒（CMV）。新生儿单纯疱疹病毒（HSV）感染发生率为 1/20000 ~ 1/3000，常继发于单纯疱疹病毒 HSV–2。单纯疱疹病毒 HSV–1 常累及眼睛、皮肤和口腔，并通过亲密接触传播。单纯疱疹病毒 HSV–2 与生殖器感染有关，通过性传播。

先天性单纯疱疹病毒（HSV）经产道感染。1/3 的新生儿感染局限于中枢神经系统（CNS）、皮肤、口腔和眼睛。常表现为水泡性皮肤病变、溃疡性口疮和角膜结膜炎。2/3 为播散性疾病，累及肝脏、肾上腺和肺。先天性感染的累及眼部，可导致结膜炎、角膜炎、视网膜脉络膜炎和白内障，角膜炎可为上皮性或基质性，受累视网膜可能很严重，如大量渗出和视网膜坏死。

受感染的婴儿可全身使用阿昔洛韦。播散性感染的死亡率较高，幸存者留有永久性眼部和中枢神经系统（CNS）损伤。

Marquez L, Levy ML, Munoz FM, Palazzi DL. A report of three cases and review of intrauterine herpes simplex virus infection. *Pediatr Infect Dis J*. 2011;30(2):153–157.

梅毒

梅毒的病原体为*梅毒螺旋体*，通过性接触传播。胎儿感染继发于母体螺旋体血症。母亲感染梅毒的时间越长，传染给孩子的风险越低。如果母亲有原发性或继发性感染，其后代约 1/2 感染。未经治疗的晚期母体梅毒感染中，约 70% 的婴儿是健康的。在美国，先天性梅毒的发病率为每 10 万名活产婴儿中有 15.7 例。

先天性梅毒的症状和体征有：不明原因早产、大胎盘、持续性鼻炎、顽固性皮疹、不明原因的黄疸、肝脾肿大、肺炎、贫血、全身性淋巴结病，以及影像学上的干骺端异常或骨膜炎。先天获得性感染可导致新生儿死亡。先天性梅毒的早期眼部感染罕见。

In some infants, chorioretinitis appears as a salt-and-pepper granularity of the fundus. Pseudoretinitis pigmentosa may follow. In rare cases, anterior uveitis, glaucoma, or both may develop. In other cases, signs and symptoms may not appear until late childhood or adolescence. Widely spaced, peg-shaped teeth; eighth nerve deafness; and interstitial keratitis constitute the *Hutchinson triad.* Other manifestations include saddle nose, short maxilla, and linear scars around body orifices. Bilateral interstitial keratitis, the classic ophthalmic finding in older children and adults, occurs in approximately 10% of patients.

A diagnosis of congenital syphilis is confirmed by identification of T pallidum by dark-field microscopy or fluorescent antibody testing. The detection of specific immunoglobulin M is currently the most sensitive serologic method.

Congenital syphilis in neonates is treated with intravenous aqueous crystalline penicillin G. Serologic tests are repeated at 2 to 4, 6, and 12 months after the conclusion of treatment, or until results become nonreactive or the titer has decreased fourfold. Persistent positive titers or a positive cerebrospinal fluid VDRL test result at 6 months should prompt retreatment.

Also see BCSC Section 9, *Uveitis and Ocular Inflammation.*

Centers for Disease Control and Prevention. 2016 sexually transmitted diseases surveillance: syphilis. Available at https://www.cdc.gov/std/stats16/default.htm.Accessed March 7, 2018.

Lymphocytic Choriomeningitis

Lymphocytic choriomeningitis virus (LCMV) is an arenavirus that is transmitted by exposure to infected rodents (including house and laboratory mice and pet hamsters). Infants with congenital LCMV infection present with CNS abnormalities, including hydrocephaly, microcephaly, intracranial calcifications, and cognitive impairment. Chorioretinal scars, which may involve the entire macula, may occur without neurologic abnormalities. The appearance of these scars is similar to that of scars seen in patients with toxoplasmosis, CMV infection, and Aicardi syndrome. The diagnosis of LCMV infection should be considered in infants with chorioretinal scars when results of tests for these more common etiologies are negative. Elevated LCMV antibody titers establish the diagnosis. No specific treatment is available apart from exposure prevention.

Zika Virus

Zika virus is a flavivirus transmitted by the *Aedes aegypti* mosquito. It has recently been associated with congenital microcephaly and chorioretinal lesions. In a series of 29 infants in Brazil with presumed intrauterine Zika virus infection, ocular abnormalities were present in 10 infants (35%) and were bilateral in 7 infants. The characteristic lesions included posterior pole pigmentary clumping and areas of circumscribed chorioretinal atrophy. In addition, 1 baby showed iris colobomas and lens subluxation. Cerebral visual impairment is common.

de Paula Freitas B, de Oliveira Dias JR, Prazeres J, et al. Ocular findings in infants with microcephaly associated with presumed Zika virus congenital infection in Salvador, Brazil. *JAMA Ophthalmol.* 2016;134(5):529–535.

一些婴儿的脉络膜视网膜炎，眼底表现为椒盐样颗粒，随后呈假性视网膜色素病变。在极少数情况下，可出现前葡萄膜炎、青光眼，或两者同时发生。有时眼部症状和体征出现在大龄儿童或青春期。宽间距钉状牙齿 / 锯齿形牙、Ⅷ颅神经耳聋、间质性角膜炎构成 *Hutchinson 三联征*。其他表现包括鞍状鼻、短上颌骨和线状疤痕 / 体腔周围有线状疤痕。双眼间质性角膜炎是大龄儿童和成人的典型表现，约 10% 发病。

先天性梅毒的诊断是通过暗视野显微镜或荧光抗体试验来识别*梅毒螺旋体*。特异性免疫球蛋白 M 的检测是目前最敏感的血清学检测。

新生儿先天性梅毒的治疗为静脉注射青霉素 G。在治疗结束后的 2 ~ 4 个月、6 个月和 12 个月复查血清学检查，或直到结果为无反应或滴度下降 4 倍。6 个月时滴度呈持续阳性，或脑脊液 VDRL 检测结果阳性，应立即进行再治疗。

见 BCSC 第 9 册《*葡萄膜炎与眼部炎症*》。

Centers for Disease Control and Prevention. 2016 sexually transmitted diseases surveillance: syphilis. Available at https://www.cdc.gov/std/stats16/default.htm.Accessed March 7, 2018.

淋巴细胞性脉络丛脑膜炎

淋巴细胞脉络丛脑膜炎病毒(LCMV)是一种沙粒病毒，通过暴露给感染的啮齿动物(包括家鼠、实验室小鼠和宠物仓鼠）而传播。先天性淋巴细胞脉络丛脑膜炎病毒（LCMV）感染表现为中枢神经系统（CNS）异常，包括水肿、小头畸形、颅内钙化和认知功能障碍。脉络膜视网膜瘢痕可累及整个黄斑，可不伴有神经异常，这些疤痕的外观与弓形体 / 虫病、巨细胞病毒（CMV）感染和 Aicardi 综合征患者的疤痕相似。当对常见病因的检测结果为阴性时，有脉络膜视网膜瘢痕的婴儿应考虑诊断淋巴细胞脉络丛脑膜炎病毒（LCMV）感染。淋巴细胞脉络丛脑膜炎病毒（LCMV）抗体滴度提高可确诊。除防止暴露接触外，尚无治疗方法。

Zika 病毒

Zika 病毒是一种由*埃及伊*蚊传播的黄病毒。最近发现，与先天性小头畸形和脉络膜视网膜病变有关。在宫内 Zika 病毒感染的 29 名巴西婴儿中，10 人(35%)有眼部异常，其中 7 人为双眼。病变包括后极部色素沉着和局限性脉络膜视网膜萎缩。有 1 例表现为虹膜缺损和晶状体半脱位。该病常伴有大脑视觉功能损伤。

de Paula Freitas B, de Oliveira Dias JR, Prazeres J, et al. Ocular findings in infants with microcephaly associated with presumed Zika virus congenital infection in Salvador, Brazil. *JAMA Ophthalmol.* 2016;134(5):529–535.

Malignant Disease

Leukemia

Leukemia in childhood is acute in 95% of cases and is more often lymphocytic than myelocytic. Acute lymphoblastic leukemia is the most common malignant disease of childhood and is responsible for 30% of all cancer cases; there are 4000 new cases per year in the United States. Although the most common ocular manifestation of leukemia is leukemic retinopathy, all ocular structures can be affected. Ocular involvement is highly correlated with CNS involvement.

Leukemic infiltrates in the anterior segment may lead to heterochromia iridis, a change in the architecture of the iris, frank iris infiltrates, spontaneous hyphemas, leukemic cells in the anterior chamber, and pseudohypopyon. Keratic precipitates may be seen, and glaucoma develops in some affected eyes from tumor cells clogging the trabecular meshwork. Anterior chamber paracentesis for cytologic studies may be diagnostic in cases involving the anterior segment. Systemic chemotherapy, local radiation therapy, and topical steroids may be effective for anterior segment complications. Leukemic involvement of the iris may be confused with juvenile xanthogranuloma.

The most common ocular findings are retinal hemorrhages, especially flame-shaped lesions in the nerve fiber layer. They involve the posterior fundus and correlate with other aspects of the disease, such as anemia, thrombocytopenia, and coagulation abnormalities. The hemorrhages may have white centers. Retinal hemorrhages in leukemia can resemble those associated with abusive head trauma (see Chapter 27), and they have been reported as the first manifestation of leukemia. Other forms of retinal involvement include localized perivascular infiltrations, microinfarction, and discrete tumor infiltrations. Histologically, the choroid is the most frequently affected ocular tissue, but choroidal involvement is usually not apparent clinically.

Optic nerve involvement occurs if the disc has been infiltrated by leukemic cells (Fig 28-28), which may cause loss of central vision. Translucent swelling of the disc obscures the normal landmarks; with florid involvement, only a white mass is visible in the region of the disc. The presence of disc edema and loss of central vision in a child with leukemia should be considered a medical emergency because permanent loss of central vision is imminent. Such patients should undergo radiation therapy as soon as possible.

Neuroblastoma

Neuroblastoma is one of the most common childhood cancers and is the most frequent source of childhood orbital metastasis (89% of cases). It usually originates in either the adrenal gland or the sympathetic ganglion chain in the retroperitoneum or mediastinum. Approximately 20% of all patients with neuroblastoma show clinical evidence of orbital involvement, which is sometimes the initial manifestation of the tumor.

The mean age at diagnosis of patients with metastatic orbital neuroblastoma is approximately 2 years; 90% are diagnosed by 5 years of age. Unilateral or bilateral proptosis and eyelid ecchymosis are the classic presentations (Fig 28-29). Systemic signs and symptoms may include abdominal fullness and pain, venous obstruction and edema, hypertension caused by renal vascular compromise, and bone pain. Urinalysis for catecholamines is positive in 90%–95% of cases.

恶性疾病

白血病

95% 的儿童白血病是急性的，且淋巴细胞性白血病比髓细胞性白血病更常见。急性淋巴母细胞白血病是儿童最常见的恶性疾病，占所有癌症病例的 30%，美国每年有 4000 例新增病例。白血病最常见的眼部表现是白血病视网膜病变，但可累及所有眼部结构。眼球受累与中枢神经系统（CNS）受累高度相关。

白血病前节浸润可导致虹膜异色、虹膜结构改变、明显的虹膜浸润、自发性前房积血、前房白血病细胞和假性前房积脓。可见角膜后沉淀物因肿瘤细胞阻塞小梁网而导致青光眼。累及前节时，可行前房穿刺术，用于细胞学分析具有诊断价值。全身化学治疗、局部放射治疗和局部类固醇治疗，对前节并发症有效。白血病累及虹膜时，可与青少年黄色肉芽肿混淆。

最常见的眼部表现为视网膜出血，特别是神经纤维层的火焰状病变，累及后极部，与病情相关，如贫血、血小板减少和凝血异常。出血有白色中心。白血病的视网膜出血与虐待性头部创伤的出血类似（见第 27 章），是白血病的第一个表现。其他视网膜表现有局部血管周围浸润、微梗死和播散性肿瘤浸润。组织学上，脉络膜是最易累及的眼组织，但脉络膜的临床表现不明显。

一旦视盘有白血病细胞浸润，即视神经受累（图 28–28），导致中心视力丧失。视盘的半透明水肿遮盖了视盘的正常标志，仅见白色肿块。白血病儿童出现视盘水肿和中心视力丧失应急诊治疗，因为其可导致永久性视力丧失，应尽快进行放射治疗。

神经母细胞瘤

神经母细胞瘤是儿童最常见的癌症之一，也是儿童眼眶转移最常见的来源（89% 的病例）。常起源于腹膜后或纵隔的肾上腺或交感神经节链。20% 的神经母细胞瘤表现出眼眶受累，有时是肿瘤的最初表现。

转移性眼眶神经母细胞瘤的平均诊断年龄为 2 岁，90% 在 5 岁前确诊。典型的表现是单眼或双眼眼球突出和眼睑淤血（图 28–29）。全身症状和体征有腹胀和疼痛、静脉阻塞和水肿、肾血管损害引起的高血压和骨痛。尿液中儿茶酚胺的阳性率为 90% ~ 95%。

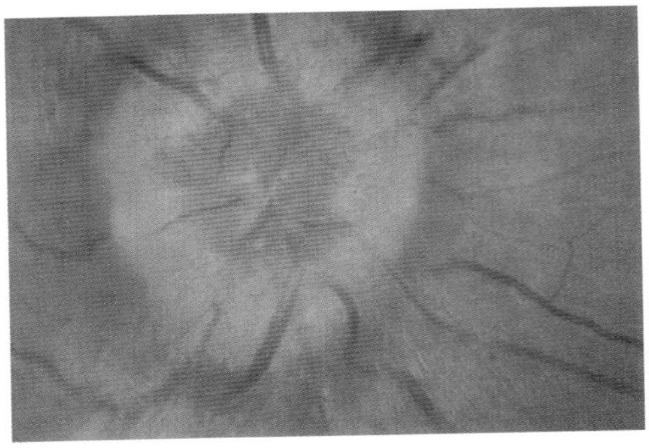

Figure 28-28 Leukemic infiltration of the optic nerve.

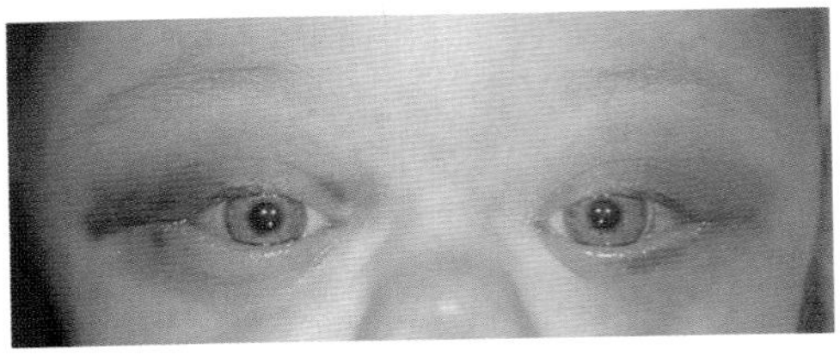

Figure 28-29 Bilateral orbital metastasis from neuroblastoma in a 2-year-old girl, presenting with periorbital ecchymosis.

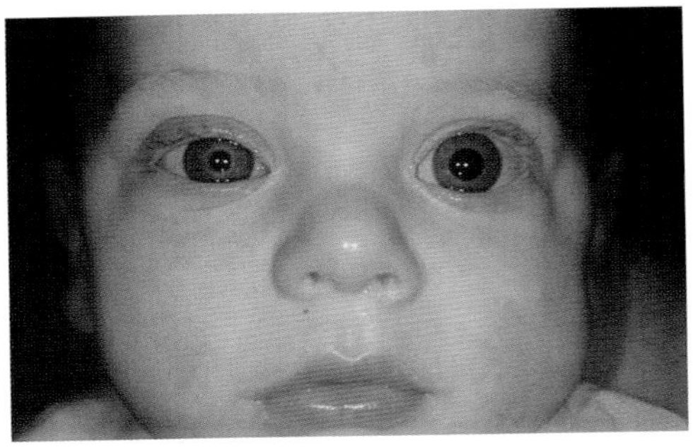

Figure 28-30 Right Horner syndrome, the presenting sign of localized intrathoracic neuroblastoma in a 6-month-old boy.

Opsoclonus, characterized by rapid, multidirectional saccadic eye movements, is a paraneoplastic syndrome that is associated with neuroblastoma and is not related to orbital involvement. It is associated with a good prognosis for survival, but neurologic deficits may persist. Horner syndrome can occur as a result of a primary cervical or apical thoracic neuroblastoma that involves the sympathetic chain (Fig 28-30).

Treatment modalities include surgery, chemotherapy, and radiation therapy. Neuroblastoma that presents in a child younger than 1 year has a more favorable prognosis than that in older children. Approximately 10% of neuroblastomas undergo spontaneous regression.

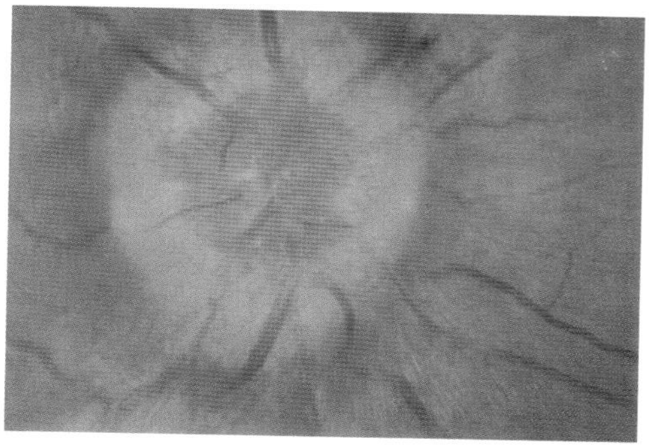

图 28–28 视神经白血病浸润。

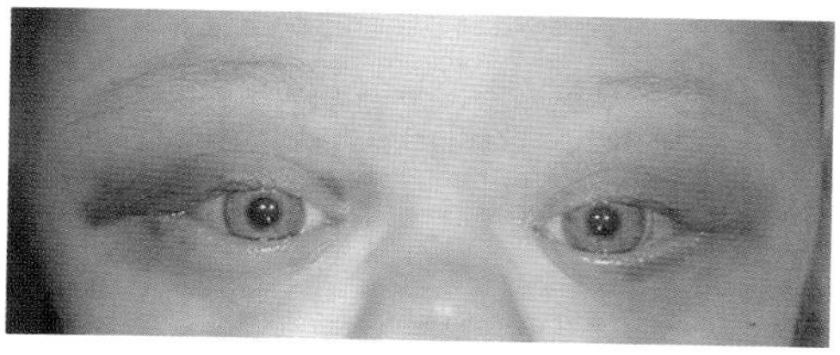

图 28–29 神经母细胞瘤的双眼眶转移，2 岁女童，表现为眶周淤血。

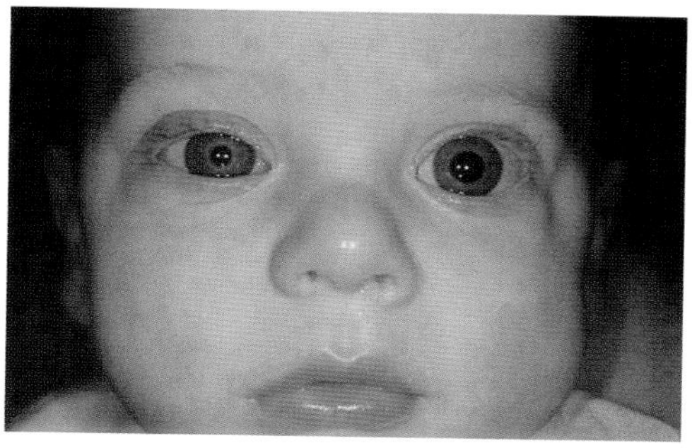

图 28–30 右 Horner 综合征，6 月龄男婴，局限性胸内神经母细胞瘤体征。

视性眼阵挛，特征是眼球快速、多向扫视，是与神经母细胞瘤相关的副肿瘤综合征，与眼眶受累无关。其生存预后良好，但神经性缺陷持续存在。Horner 综合征是原发性颈部或胸顶部神经母细胞瘤，累及交感神经链（图 28–30）。

治疗方式包括手术、化学治疗和放射治疗。1 岁以下儿童出现神经母细胞瘤，比 1 岁以上儿童的预后好。10% 的神经母细胞瘤自发性消退。

（翻译 朱晓鹃 李霞 黄雪 刘添添 // 审校 刘陇黔 蒋宁 石一宁 // 章节审校 石广礼）

Basic Texts

Pediatric Ophthalmology and Strabismus

Brodsky MC. *Pediatric Neuro-Ophthalmology*. 3rd ed. New York: Springer-Verlag; 2016.

Buckley EG, Freedman S, Shields MB. *Atlas of Ophthalmic Surgery, Vol III: Strabismus and Glaucoma*. St Louis: Mosby-Year Book; 1995.

Buckley EG, Plager DA, Repka MX, Wilson ME. *Strabismus Surgery: Basic and Advanced Strategies*. New York: Oxford University Press; 2005.

Coats DK, Olitsky SE. *Strabismus Surgery and Its Complications*. New York: Springer-Verlag; 2007.

Dutton J. *Atlas of Clinical and Surgical Orbital Anatomy*. 2nd ed. Philadelphia: Elsevier; 2011.

Hartnett ME, ed. *Pediatric Retina*. 2nd ed. Philadelphia: Lippincott Williams & Wilkins; 2014.

Helveston EM. *Surgical Management of Strabismus*. 5th ed. Oostende, Belgium: Wayenborgh Publishing; 2005.*

Isenberg SJ, ed. *The Eye in Infancy*. 2nd ed. St Louis: Mosby-Year Book; 1994.

Jones KL, Jones MC, del Campo M. *Smith's Recognizable Patterns of Human Malformation*. 7th ed. Philadelphia: Saunders; 2013.

Katowitz JA, Katowitz WR. *Pediatric Oculoplastic Surgery*. 2nd ed. New York: Springer; 2018.

Lambert SR, Lyons CJ, eds. *Taylor and Hoyt's Pediatric Ophthalmology and Strabismus*. 5th ed. Philadelphia: Elsevier; 2017.

Leigh RJ, Zee DS. *The Neurology of Eye Movements*. 5th ed. New York: Oxford University Press; 2015.

Miller NR, Newman NJ, Biousse V, Kerrison JB, eds. *Walsh and Hoyt's Clinical Neuro-Ophthalmology*. 6th ed. Philadelphia: Lippincott Williams & Wilkins; 2005.

Nelson LB, Olitsky SE, eds. *Harley's Pediatric Ophthalmology*. 6th ed. Philadelphia: Lippincott Williams & Wilkins; 2014.

Parks MM. *Atlas of Strabismus Surgery*. Philadelphia: Harper & Row; 1983.

Parks MM. *Ocular Motility and Strabismus*. Hagerstown, MD: Harper & Row; 1975.

Pratt-Johnson JA, Tillson G. *Management of Strabismus and Amblyopia: A Practical Guide*. 2nd ed. New York: Thieme; 2001.

Rosenbaum AL, Santiago AP, eds. *Clinical Strabismus Management: Principles and Surgical Techniques*. Philadelphia: Saunders; 1999.

Tasman W, Jaeger EA, eds. *Duane's Ophthalmology on DVD-ROM*. Philadelphia: Lippincott Williams & Wilkins; 2013.

Traboulsi EI. A *Compendium of Inherited Disorders and the Eye*. New York: Oxford University Press; 2006.

von Noorden GK. *Atlas of Strabismus*. 4th ed. St Louis: Mosby; 1983.

von Noorden GK, Campos EC. *Binocular Vision and Ocular Motility*. 6th ed. St Louis: Mosby; 2002.*

von Noorden GK, Helveston EM. *Strabismus: A Decision Making Approach*. St Louis: Mosby; 1994.*

* Available online on the Ophthalmic News and Education (ONE®) Network in the Pediatric Ophthalmology Education Center (https:// www. aao. org/ pediatric-ophthalmology-strabismus) and on the Cybersight website (https:// cybersight.org).

参考内容

小儿眼科与斜视

Brodsky MC. *Pediatric Neuro-Ophthalmology*. 3rd ed. New York: Springer-Verlag; 2016.

Buckley EG, Freedman S, Shields MB. *Atlas of Ophthalmic Surgery, Vol III: Strabismus and Glaucoma*. St Louis: Mosby-Year Book; 1995.

Buckley EG, Plager DA, Repka MX, Wilson ME. *Strabismus Surgery: Basic and Advanced Strategies*. New York: Oxford University Press; 2005.

Coats DK, Olitsky SE. *Strabismus Surgery and Its Complications*. New York: Springer-Verlag; 2007.

Dutton J. *Atlas of Clinical and Surgical Orbital Anatomy*. 2nd ed. Philadelphia: Elsevier; 2011.

Hartnett ME, ed. *Pediatric Retina*. 2nd ed. Philadelphia: Lippincott Williams & Wilkins; 2014.

Helveston EM. *Surgical Management of Strabismus*. 5th ed. Oostende, Belgium: Wayenborgh Publishing; 2005.*

Isenberg SJ, ed. *The Eye in Infancy*. 2nd ed. St Louis: Mosby-Year Book; 1994.

Jones KL, Jones MC, del Campo M. *Smith's Recognizable Patterns of Human Malformation*. 7th ed. Philadelphia: Saunders; 2013.

Katowitz JA, Katowitz WR. *Pediatric Oculoplastic Surgery*. 2nd ed. New York: Springer; 2018.

Lambert SR, Lyons CJ, eds. *Taylor and Hoyt's Pediatric Ophthalmology and Strabismus*. 5th ed. Philadelphia: Elsevier; 2017.

Leigh RJ, Zee DS. *The Neurology of Eye Movements*. 5th ed. New York: Oxford University Press; 2015.

Miller NR, Newman NJ, Biousse V, Kerrison JB, eds. *Walsh and Hoyt's Clinical Neuro-Ophthalmology*. 6th ed. Philadelphia: Lippincott Williams & Wilkins; 2005.

Nelson LB, Olitsky SE, eds. *Harley's Pediatric Ophthalmology*. 6th ed. Philadelphia: Lippincott Williams & Wilkins; 2014.

Parks MM. *Atlas of Strabismus Surgery*. Philadelphia: Harper & Row; 1983.

Parks MM. *Ocular Motility and Strabismus*. Hagerstown, MD: Harper & Row; 1975.

Pratt-Johnson JA, Tillson G. *Management of Strabismus and Amblyopia: A Practical Guide*. 2nd ed. New York: Thieme; 2001.

Rosenbaum AL, Santiago AP, eds. *Clinical Strabismus Management: Principles and Surgical Techniques*. Philadelphia: Saunders; 1999.

Tasman W, Jaeger EA, eds. *Duane's Ophthalmology on DVD-ROM*. Philadelphia: Lippincott Williams & Wilkins; 2013.

Traboulsi EI. A *Compendium of Inherited Disorders and the Eye*. New York: Oxford University Press; 2006.

von Noorden GK. *Atlas of Strabismus*. 4th ed. St Louis: Mosby; 1983.

von Noorden GK, Campos EC. *Binocular Vision and Ocular Motility*. 6th ed. St Louis: Mosby; 2002.*

von Noorden GK, Helveston EM. *Strabismus: A Decision Making Approach*. St Louis: Mosby; 1994.*

* Available online on the Ophthalmic News and Education (ONE®) Network in the Pediatric Ophthalmology Education Center (https:// www. aao. org/ pediatric-ophthalmology-strabismus) and on the Cybersight website (https:// cybersight.org).

Basic Texts

Wilson ME, Saunders RA, Trivedi RH, eds. *Pediatric Ophthalmology: Current Thought and A Practical Guide*. Berlin: Springer; 2009.

Wright KW, Strube YJ, eds. *Color Atlas of Strabismus Surgery: Strategies and Techniques*. 4th ed. New York: Springer; 2015.

Wright KW, Strube YJ, eds. *Pediatric Ophthalmology and Strabismus*. 3rd ed. New York: Oxford University Press; 2012.

Wilson ME, Saunders RA, Trivedi RH, eds. *Pediatric Ophthalmology: Current Thought and A Practical Guide*. Berlin: Springer; 2009.
Wright KW, Strube YJ, eds. *Color Atlas of Strabismus Surgery: Strategies and Techniques*. 4th ed. New York: Springer; 2015.
Wright KW, Strube YJ, eds. *Pediatric Ophthalmology and Strabismus*. 3rd ed. New York: Oxford University Press; 2012.

Related Academy Materials

The American Academy of Ophthalmology is dedicated to providing a wealth of highquality clinical education resources for ophthalmologists.

Print Publications and Electronic Products

For a complete listing of Academy products related to topics covered in this BCSC Section, visit our online store at https://store.aao.org/clinical-education/topic/pediatric-ophth-strabismus.html. Or call Customer Service at 866-561-8558 (toll free, US only) or +1 415-561-8540, Monday through Friday, between 8:00 AM and 5:00 PM (PST).

Online Resources

Visit the Ophthalmic News and Education (ONE®) Network at aao.org/onenetwork to find relevant videos, online courses, journal articles, practice guidelines, self-assessment quizzes, images, and more. The ONE Network is a free Academy-member benefit.

Access free, trusted articles and content with the Academy's collaborative online encyclopedia, EyeWiki, at aao.org/eyewiki.

相关学术资料

美国眼科学会致力于为眼科医生提供丰富的、高质量的临床教育资源。

印刷出版和电子读物

若想了解本书中相关主题学术产品的完整列表，请访问我们的在线商店，网址为 https://store.aao.org/clinical-education/topic/pediatric-ophth-strabismus.html. 或者周一至周五，上午 8:00 至下午 5:00（PST）拨打我们的客服电话 866-561-8558（免费，仅限于美国）。

网络资源

访问（ONE®）网站 aao.org/onenetwork，可查找相关视频、在线课程、期刊文章、实践指南、自我评估测验、图片，以及更多资源。DNE® 网站免费对会员开放。

我们与学院合作，打造令大家满意的在线百科全书平台，EyeWiki，帮助大家在 aao.org/eyewiki 获取免费可信的文章和知识。

Study Questions

Please note that these questions are not part of your CME reporting process. They are provided here for your own educational use and identification of any professional practice gaps. The required CME posttest is available online (see "Requesting CME Credit"). Following the questions are a blank answer sheet and answers with discussions. Although a concerted effort has been made to avoid ambiguity and redundancy in these questions, the authors recognize that differences of opinion may occur regarding the "best" answer. The discussions are provided to demonstrate the rationale used to derive the answer. They may also be helpful in confirming that your approach to the problem was correct or, if necessary, in fixing the principle in your memory. The Section 6 faculty thanks the Self-Assessment Committee for providing these self-assessment questions.

1. In testing preliterate children, what optotype has the best calibration and reliability?
   a. HOTV
   b. Tumbling E
   c. Allen figures
   d. Light house chart

2. In what ocular motility abnormality is a comitant deviation present?
   a. nasal wall fracture
   b. infantile esotropia
   c. thyroid orbitopathy
   d. sixth nerve palsy

3. In abbreviations for types of strabismus, the addition of parentheses around the letter Tindicates what characteristic of an ocular deviation?
   a. intermittent
   b. constant
   c. inward
   d. outward

4. The lateral muscular branch of the ophthalmic artery supplies which extraocular muscle(EOM)?
   a. superior rectus
   b. medial rectus
   c. inferior rectus
   d. inferior oblique

5. The orbital layer of an EOM has what unique characteristic?
   a. It inserts on the sclera.
   b. It inserts on the muscle pulley.
   c. It moves the globe.
   d. It is topographically closer to the globe.

测试练习

以下问题不属于 CME 的讲述内容，仅供教学使用以及查缺补漏。CME 的学后测试可在网上查找（见 CME 学分需求），在问题后面的空白处写上答案和讨论。尽管我们已尽量避免产生歧义以及冗杂，但对于最佳答案仍可能有不一致的意见。讨论部分将演绎推导出答案的合理性，这些讨论有助于确认解决问题的方法是否正确，必要时应牢记这些原则。第 6 册编辑组全体人员感谢自我评估委员会提供的这些自我评估问题。

1. 测试学龄前儿童，下列哪种视标有最佳的校准和可靠性？
   a. HOTV 视力表
   b. E 字形视力表
   c. Allen 图片
   d. 灯塔图表

2. 哪种眼球运动异常存在共同性斜视？
   a. 鼻骨骨折
   b. 婴幼儿内斜视
   c. 甲状腺相关眼病
   d. 展神经麻痹

3. 在斜视类型的缩写词中，字母 T 周围加括号表示什么特征的斜视？
   a. 间歇性斜视
   b. 恒定性斜视
   c. 内斜视
   d. 外斜视

4. 眼动脉的外侧肌支供应哪条眼外肌（EOM）？
   a. 上直肌
   b. 内直肌
   c. 下直肌
   d. 下斜肌

5. 眼外肌眼眶部分有什么特点？
   a. 附着于巩膜上
   b. 嵌入肌肉滑车
   c. 转动眼球
   d. 走形上更靠近眼球

6. On left gaze, the medial rectus muscle of the right eye adducts the eye. What term is used to describe this muscle as the eye adducts?
   a. agonist
   b. synergist
   c. antagonist
   d. reciprocal

7. What EOM has only a primary action and no secondary or tertiary action?
   a. lateral rectus
   b. inferior rectus
   c. superior rectus
   d. superior oblique

8. In a complete third nerve palsy, what action of the superior oblique muscle exacerbates the abducted position of the paretic eye?
   a. primary
   b. secondary
   c. tertiary
   d. quaternary

9. What is the primary site in the development of amblyopia?
   a. visual cortex
   b. retinal ganglion cells
   c. nerve fiber layer
   d. lateral geniculate body

10. In the treatment of moderate amblyopia, pharmacologic treatment has been shown to have what level of success compared to patching?
   a. minimal
   b. less
   c. more
   d. equal

11. After laser surgery, a child with retinopathy of prematurity (ROP) demonstrates a 30 prism diopter (Δ) right exotropia on Hirschberg testing. When the left eye is covered, the right eye does not move medially. What is the most likely reason for this finding?
   a. anomalous retinal correspondence
   b. suppression scotoma
   c. positive angle kappa
   d. negative angle kappa

6. 向左注视时，右眼内直肌内转眼球，用什么样的专业术语来描述使眼球内转的这条眼外肌？
   a. 主动肌
   b. 协同肌
   c. 拮抗肌
   d. 配偶肌

7. 哪条眼外肌只有第 1 眼位，没有第 2 和第 3 眼位？
   a. 外直肌
   b. 下直肌
   c. 上直肌
   d. 上斜肌

8. 完全性动眼神经麻痹时，处于哪一眼位使得上斜肌加剧了患眼的外展位置？
   a. 第 1 眼位
   b. 第 2 眼位
   c. 第 3 眼位
   d. 第 4 眼位

9. 弱视发展的主要部位在哪？
   a. 视觉皮质区
   b. 视网膜神经节细胞
   c. 视网膜神经纤维层
   d. 外侧膝状体

10. 在中度弱视的治疗中，与遮盖治疗相比，药物疗法有什么程度的疗效？
   a. 极小
   b. 更差
   c. 更好
   d. 相等

11. 激光术后，患有早产儿视网膜病变（ROP）的儿童在 Hirschberg 测试中表现出 30 三棱镜度（Δ）右眼外斜视，当左眼被遮盖时，右眼不会向内侧移动，这个发现最有可能的原因是什么？
   a. 异常视网膜对应
   b. 中心凹抑制
   c. 正 kappa 角
   d. 负 kappa 角

12. To test for a horizontal deviation using the Maddox rod, in what direction should the cylinders be placed in front of the right eye?
    a. 15° meridian
    b. 45° meridian
    c. 90° meridian
    d. 180° meridian

13. A 6-year-old child presents with a 35Δ intermittent exotropia at distance and a 20Δ intermittent exotropia at near. After the patch test, measurements for this patient are 35Δ exotropia at distance and 30Δ exotropia at near. What is the most likely diagnosis?
    a. pseudodivergence excess intermittent exotropia
    b. divergence excess intermittent exotropia
    c. intermittent exotropia with a high accommodative convergence/accommodation (AC/A) ratio
    d. basic intermittent exotropia

14. A 4-year-old child with an intermittent exotropia has been observed and has had fair control of the deviation. At the most recent visit, a decrease in stereopsis was noted. What most likely explains this finding?
    a. A high AC/A ratio has developed in the patient.
    b. Consecutive esotropia has developed in the patient.
    c. The patient has increased tenacious proximal fusion.
    d. Sensory testing was performed after alignment testing.

15. A 5-year-old child presents with Y-pattern exotropia. What finding can be expected on examination?
    a. Overelevation of the eye is seen on adduction and slight upgaze.
    b. Overelevation is seen on horizontal gaze.
    c. Fundus excyclotorsion is found on fundus examination.
    d. Vertical deviation is noted with head tilts.

16. What is the most appropriate surgery to perform for a V-pattern esotropia with no inferior oblique overaction?
    a. bilateral medial rectus recession with inferior transposition (inferoplacement)
    b. bilateral medial rectus recession with superior transposition (superoplacement)
    c. bilateral lateral rectus resection with inferior transposition (inferoplacement)
    d. unilateral medial rectus recession and lateral rectus resection with inferior transposition (inferoplacement)

17. What pattern strabismus would be most successfully addressed with bilateral weakening of the inferior oblique muscles?
    a. A pattern
    b. V pattern
    c. X pattern
    d. Y pattern

12. 用 Maddox 杆试验检查水平隐斜视，Maddox 杆圆柱应放在右眼前的哪个方位？
   a. 15° 子午线
   b. 45° 子午线
   c. 90° 子午线
   d. 180° 子午线

13. 一名 6 岁的儿童现出现 35 Δ 视远斜视度、20 Δ 视近斜视度的间歇性外斜视，进行遮盖测试之后，该患儿的测量值为 35 Δ 视远斜视度和 30 Δ 视近斜视度，最有可能的诊断是什么？
   a. 假性分开过强型间歇型外斜视
   b. 分开过强型间歇型外斜视
   c. 高 AC/A 型间歇型外斜视
   d. 基本型间歇性外斜视

14. 长期随访一名间歇性外斜视已经得到直接控制的 4 岁儿童，在最近一次随访中发现患儿的立体视觉下降，这一现象最合理的解释是什么？
   a. 患儿出现了高 AC/A 型外斜视
   b. 患儿出现了继发性内斜视
   c. 患儿近端融合增加
   d. 对直试验之后进行了感觉试验

15. 检查一名患有 Y 型外斜视的 5 岁儿童可以发现什么？
   a. 眼球内上转时亢进
   b. 原位眼注视时外斜度数增大
   c. 眼底检查时发现眼底外旋转性斜视
   d. 头部倾斜时发生垂直性斜视

16. 对于下斜肌麻痹的 V 型内斜视最恰当的手术方式是什么？
   a. 双侧内直肌后徙术加下直肌移位术
   b. 双侧内直肌后徙术加上直肌移位术
   c. 双侧外直肌缩短术加下直肌移位术
   d. 单侧内直肌后徙术加外直肌缩短术加下直肌移位术

17. 哪种斜视能通过削弱双下斜肌功能得到成功的控制？
   a.A 型斜视
   b.V 型斜视
   c.X 型斜视
   d.Y 型斜视

18. A 2-year-old child presents with a 30° right head turn. The patient cannot abduct the right eye, and there is narrowing of the palpebral fissure on adduction. What is the most appropriate management?
    a. magnetic resonance imaging (MRI) of the brain and brainstem
    b. lumbar puncture for opening pressure
    c. muscle biopsy and genetics testing
    d. right medial rectus recession

19. With what syndrome has Duane retraction syndrome been associated?
    a. Goldenhar syndrome
    b. Kleinfelter syndrome
    c. Turner syndrome
    d. Waardenburg syndrome

20. What defines type 2 Duane retraction syndrome?
    a. poor adduction and exotropia
    b. poor abduction and esotropia
    c. poor abduction and adduction
    d. poor abduction and exotropia

21. For what condition is botulinum toxin type A most effective?
    a. small-angle esotropia
    b. large-angle exotropia
    c. A-pattern esotropia
    d. chronic sixth nerve palsy

22. A 6-year-old child undergoes bilateral 5-mm medial rectus recession for 35Δ esotropia. One week after surgery, there is a measurement of 30Δ exotropia. What is the most appropriate test to perform next?
    a. test of EOM movements
    b. measurement of stereopsis
    c. measurement of vertical deviations
    d. slit-lamp examination

23. What sort of anomaly is represented by a choroidal coloboma?
    a. agenesis
    b. hypoplasia
    c. hyperplasia
    d. dysraphism

24. For a 5-month-old child with poor visual behavior but no nystagmus, what diagnosis is likely?
    a. retinal dystrophy
    b. cerebral visual impairment
    c. pregeniculate visual impairment
    d. congenital cataract

18. 当一名 2 岁的儿童头部右转 30° 时，右眼不能外转，内转时眼裂变小，接下来最合适的处理是什么？
   a. 脑和脑干的磁共振成像（MRI）
   b. 腰椎穿刺减压
   c. 组织活检和基因检测
   d. 右内直肌后徙术

19.Duane 眼球后退综合征与什么综合征相关？
   a. 戈尔登哈氏综合征
   b. 克氏综合征
   c. 特纳综合征
   d. 瓦尔敦堡综合征

20. II 型 Duane 眼球后退综合征的定义是什么？
   a. 内转受限合并外斜视
   b. 外转受限合并内斜视
   c. 外转受限合并内转受限
   d. 外转受限合并外斜视

21.A 型肉毒素治疗哪种斜视最有效？
   a. 小角度内斜视
   b. 大角度外斜视
   c. A 型内斜视
   d. 慢性展神经麻痹

22. 一名 35Δ 内斜视的 6 岁儿童接受了双侧内直肌 5mm 后徙术治疗，术后 1 周，患儿出现了 30Δ 外斜视，那么接下来应该进行的最恰当的检查是什么？
   a. 眼外肌运动负荷试验
   b. 立体视觉检查
   c. 垂直斜视角度的测量
   d. 裂隙灯检查

23. 脉络膜缺损是（胚裂）发生了哪种异常？
   a. 未发育
   b. 发育不全
   c. 发育过剩
   d. 闭合不全

24. 一个 5 个月大的孩子视力丧失但不伴有眼球震颤，可能的诊断是什么？
   a. 视网膜营养性萎缩症
   b. 脑性瘫痪合并视觉障碍
   c. 外侧膝状体性视觉缺损
   d. 先天性白内障

25. Blepharophimosis-ptosis-epicanthus inversus syndrome is usually inherited in what manner?
   a. autosomal dominant
   b. autosomal recessive
   c. X-linked dominant
   d. X-linked recessive

26. Crouzon syndrome differs from Apert syndrome in that the latter is associated with what finding?
   a. hypertelorism
   b. proptosis
   c. significant syndactyly
   d. inferior scleral show

27. What is the most common type of strabismus associated with craniosynostosis?
   a. A-pattern esotropia
   b. V-pattern esotropia
   c. V-pattern exotropia
   d. A-pattern exotropia

28. A 4-day-old infant presents with chemosis, significant discharge, and corneal ulceration. What is the most likely diagnosis?
   a. chemical conjunctivitis
   b. herpes simplex virus conjunctivitis
   c. *Neisseria gonorrhoeae* conjunctivitis
   d. chlamydial conjunctivitis

29. What is an early ocular manifestation of Stevens-Johnson syndrome?
   a. mucopurulent conjunctivitis
   b. symblepharon
   c. corneal vascularization
   d. entropion

30. A child with new-onset ptosis should be examined for what other finding?
   a. cataract
   b. anisocoria
   c. anisometropic amblyopia
   d. astigmatism

31. In a patient with Horner syndrome, instillation of apraclonidine would be expected to have what effect?
   a. dilation of the affected pupil and no effect on the normal pupil
   b. dilation of the normal pupil and no effect on the affected pupil
   c. dilation of both pupils
   d. no effect on the affected pupil when the lesion is postganglionic

25. 睑裂狭小 – 上睑下垂 – 逆向性内眦赘皮综合征通常以什么方式遗传?
 a. 常染色显性遗传
 b. 常染色体隐性遗传
 c. X 染色体显性遗传
 d. X 染色体隐性遗传

26.Crouzon 综合征与 Apert 综合征鉴别之处是什么?
 a. 眼距过宽
 b. 眼球突出
 c. 并指(趾)现象
 d. 下巩膜暴露

27. 与颅缝线早闭相关的最常见的斜视类型是什么?
 a.A 型内斜视
 b.V 型内斜视
 c.V 型外斜视
 d.A 型外斜视

28. 一个出生 4d 的新生儿表现为球结膜水肿，有明显的分泌物和角膜溃疡，最有可能的诊断是什么?
 a. 化学性结膜炎
 b. 单纯疱疹病毒性结膜炎
 c. 淋病奈瑟菌性结膜炎
 d. 衣原体性结膜炎

29.Stevens–Johnson 综合征早期的眼部表现是什么?
 a. 脓性结膜炎
 b. 睑球粘连
 c. 角膜血管翳
 d. 睑内翻

30. 对患有新发生的上睑下垂的儿童应该注意检查以发现其他什么问题?
 a. 白内障
 b. 瞳孔大小不均
 c. 屈光参差性弱视
 d. 散光

31. 对于 Horner 综合征的患者，安普乐定点眼预计瞳孔会产生怎样的变化?
 a. 引起患侧瞳孔扩大，对正常瞳孔没有影响
 b. 引起正常瞳孔扩大，对患侧瞳孔没有影响
 c. 患侧及正常瞳孔均扩大
 d. 神经节后病变对患侧瞳孔无影响

32. Abnormal development of what ocular structure is the pathologic defect in primary congenital glaucoma?
    a. anterior chamber angle tissue
    b. Descemet membrane
    c. iris
    d. optic nerve

33. On gonioscopy, how does the anterior chamber angle of a normal infant eye differ from that of an adult eye?
    a. The trabecular meshwork is more highly pigmented.
    b. The Schwalbe line is often less distinct.
    c. The junction between the scleral spur and the ciliary body is easily seen.
    d. The uveal meshwork is more difficult to see through.

34. Bilateral posterior subcapsular cataract is diagnosed in a 9-year-old child. What aspect of the examination is most likely to reveal the cause of the cataract?
    a. medication list
    b. musculoskeletal examination
    c. family history
    d. review of systems

35. What test is most likely to determine the etiology of anterior uveitis in a child?
    a. antinuclear antibodies
    b. rheumatoid factor
    c. HLA-B27
    d. Lyme serology

36. Tubulointerstitial nephritis is associated with what ocular condition?
    a. bilateral anterior uveitis
    b. cataract formation
    c. serous retinal detachment
    d. papilledema

37. What is an example of type 1 ROP?
    a. zone I, any stage ROP with plus disease
    b. zone I, stage 1 ROP without plus disease
    c. zone II, stage 3 ROP without plus disease
    d. zone I, stage 2 ROP without plus disease

38. Leber congenital amaurosis can be best diagnosed with what test?
    a. A-scan ultrasonography
    b. electroretinography
    c. fluorescein angiography
    d. optical coherence tomography

32. 原发性先天性青光眼基本病理生理缺陷是什么眼结构的异常发育?
    a. 前房角组织
    b. 角膜后弹力层
    c. 虹膜
    d. 视神经

33. 前房角镜检查中，正常婴幼儿眼的前房角与成人有何不同?
    a. 小梁网的色素含量更高
    b.Schwalbe 线通常不明显
    c. 可以很容易看到巩膜突和睫状体之间的连接处
    d. 葡萄膜网状结构较难看清

34. 一名 9 岁的儿童被诊断为双眼后囊下白内障，哪一方面的诊查最有可能明确引起白内障的原因?
    a. 用药史
    b. 肌肉骨骼检查
    c. 家族史
    d. 系统检查

35 哪种检查最有可能明确儿童前葡萄膜炎的病因?
    a. 抗核抗体检查
    b. 类风湿因子检查
    c. HLA-B27 检查
    d. 血清学检测

36. 肾小管间质性肾炎与哪种眼部疾病相关?
    a. 双眼前葡萄膜炎
    b. 白内障的形成
    c. 浆液性视网膜脱离
    d. 视乳头水肿

37. 下列哪一个病例是 1 型 ROP ?
    a. I 区伴有附加病变的任何一期病变
    b. I 区不伴有附加病变的 1 期 ROP
    c. II 区不伴有附加病变的 3 期 ROP
    d. I 区不伴有附加病变的 2 期 ROP

38. 诊断 Leber 先天性黑朦最好的检查是什么?
    a. A 型超声检查
    b. 视网膜电图
    c. 荧光素血管素造影
    d. 光学相干断层扫描

39. What percentage of retinoblastoma cases arise from somatic nonhereditary mutation of both alleles of *RB1* in a retinal cell?
    a. 10%
    b. 40%
    c. 60%
    d. 80%

40. Children with optic nerve hypoplasia should undergo MRI to evaluate for what finding?
    a. bifid septum pellucidum
    b. empty sella
    c. ectopic posterior pituitary bright spot
    d. chiasmal glioma

41. A basal encephalocele is discovered on routine MRI. What is the most likely associated ophthalmic anomaly?
    a. optic nerve hypoplasia
    b. optic nerve pit
    c. optic nerve coloboma
    d. morning glory disc anomaly

42. Spontaneous hyphema can occur with what intraocular lesion?
    a. juvenile xanthogranuloma of the iris
    b. iris nevus
    c. iris capillary hemangioma
    d. iris cyst

43. What is the most common ocular manifestation of abusive head trauma?
    a. corneal abrasion
    b. hyphema
    c. subconjunctival hemorrhage
    d. retinal hemorrhage

44. What condition is associated with an abnormally high number of crossed fibers in the optic chiasm?
    a. ocular albinism
    b. optic nerve hypoplasia
    c. achromatopsia
    d. morning glory disc anomaly

39. 有多少百分比的视网膜母细胞瘤是由视网膜细胞中 RB1 的 2 个等位基因的体细胞非遗传性突变引起的?
a. 10%
b. 40%
c. 60%
d. 80%

40. 视神经发育不全的儿童进行 MRI 检查可有下列哪些发现?
a. 裂成两半的透明隔
b. 空碟鞍
c. 异位垂体后叶亮点
d. 视神经胶质瘤

41. 常规 MRI 显示基底脑膨出，最可能与之相关的眼部异常是什么?
a. 视神经发育不全
b. 视盘小凹
c. 视盘缺损
d. 牵牛花综合征

42. 哪种眼内病变会引起自发性前方积血?
a. 虹膜黄色肉芽肿
b. 虹膜色素痣
c. 虹膜毛细血管瘤
d. 虹膜囊肿

43. 虐待性头颅外伤最常见的眼部表现是什么?
a. 角膜上皮擦伤
b. 前房积血
c. 结膜下出血
d. 视网膜出血

44. 哪种疾病可引起视交叉中出现大量异常的交叉纤维?
a. 眼白化病
b. 视神经发育不全
c. 色盲
d. 牵牛花综合征

Answer Sheet for Section 6 Study Questions

Question	Answer	Question	Answer
1	a b c d	23	a b c d
2	a b c d	24	a b c d
3	a b c d	25	a b c d
4	a b c d	26	a b c d
5	a b c d	27	a b c d
6	a b c d	28	a b c d
7	a b c d	29	a b c d
8	a b c d	30	a b c d
9	a b c d	31	a b c d
10	a b c d	32	a b c d
11	a b c d	33	a b c d
12	a b c d	34	a b c d
13	a b c d	35	a b c d
14	a b c d	36	a b c d
15	a b c d	37	a b c d
16	a b c d	38	a b c d
17	a b c d	39	a b c d
18	a b c d	40	a b c d
19	a b c d	41	a b c d
20	a b c d	42	a b c d
21	a b c d	43	a b c d
22	a b c d	44	a b c d

第 6 册习题答案解析

题号	答案
1	a b c d
2	a b c d
3	a b c d
4	a b c d
5	a b c d
6	a b c d
7	a b c d
8	a b c d
9	a b c d
10	a b c d
11	a b c d
12	a b c d
13	a b c d
14	a b c d
15	a b c d
16	a b c d
17	a b c d
18	a b c d
19	a b c d
20	a b c d
21	a b c d
22	a b c d

题号	答案
23	a b c d
24	a b c d
25	a b c d
26	a b c d
27	a b c d
28	a b c d
29	a b c d
30	a b c d
31	a b c d
32	a b c d
33	a b c d
34	a b c d
35	a b c d
36	a b c d
37	a b c d
38	a b c d
39	a b c d
40	a b c d
41	a b c d
42	a b c d
43	a b c d
44	a b c d

Answers

1. **a.** Various optotypes are available for recognition visual acuity testing in preliterate children. LEA symbols and the HOTV test are reliably calibrated and have high testability rates for preschool-aged children. For a shy child, testability may be improved by having the child point to match optotypes on a chart with those on a hand-held card rather than verbally identify them. Several symbol charts, such as Allen figures and the Light house chart, are not recommended by the World Health Organization and the National Academy of Sciences because the optotypes are considered confusing, culturally biased, or nonstandardized. The Tumbling E Chart is accurate but conceptually difficult for many preschool children.

2. **b.** A comitant deviation is one in which the size of the deviation does not vary by more than a few prism diopters (Δ) in different positions of gaze or with either eye used for fixating. This occurs in infantile esotropia. A restrictive orbitopathy or a paretic process would lead to an incomitant deviation, in which the measurement varies significantly in different positions of gaze.

3. **a.** The addition of parentheses around the T indicates an intermittent tropia.

4. **a.** The muscular branches of the ophthalmic artery provide the most important blood supply to the extraocular muscles (EOMs). The *lateral muscular branch* supplies the lateral rectus, superior rectus, superior oblique, and levator palpebrae superioris muscles; the *medial muscular branch*, the larger of the two, supplies the inferior rectus, medial rectus, and inferior oblique muscles.

5. **b.** The EOMs exhibit a distinct 2-layer Organization: an outer *orbital layer*, which acts only on connective tissue pulleys, and an inner *global layer*, whose tendon inserts on the sclera to move the globe.

6. **a.** There are 3 important terms relating to the muscles used in monocular eye movements: *agonist*, the primary muscle moving the eye in a given direction; *synergist*, the muscle in the same eye as the agonist that acts with the agonist to produce a given movement; and *antagonist*, the muscle in the same eye as the agonist that acts in the direction opposite to that of the agonist.

7. **a.** With the eye in primary position, the horizontal (medial and lateral) rectus muscles move the eye only horizontally and thus have a primary horizontal action but no secondary or tertiary action.

8. **c.** In a complete third nerve palsy, the only functioning EOMs are the lateral rectus and superior oblique. The tertiary action of the superior oblique is abduction that exacerbates the outward position of the eye.

9. **a.** Positron emission tomography has shown that cortical blood flow and glucose metabolism are lower during stimulation of the amblyopic eye compared with the normal eye, suggesting the visual cortex as the primary site of amblyopia.

答案

1. **a.** 学龄前儿童的视敏度测试可采用各种不同的视标。LEA 图形视力表和 HOTV 字母视力表经过可靠的校准，对学龄前儿童具有很高的可测试率。对于害羞的孩子，通过让孩子指出图表上的视标与手持卡上的视标匹配而不是口头识别它们可以改善可测试性。世界卫生组织和美国国家科学院不推荐几个符号图表，如 Allen 图片和灯塔图表，因为这些视标被认为是混淆的、有文化偏见的或非标准化的。E 字视力表图是准确的，但在概念上对许多学龄前儿童来说很难。

2. **b.** 共同性斜视是指在不同的注视方向或用任一眼睛固定注视，大小不会超过几个棱镜屈光度（Δ）的偏差。这发生在婴幼儿内斜视中。限制性眼眶病或麻痹会导致非共同性斜视，在不同的注视位置测量存在显著差异。

3. **a.** 在 T 周围添加括号表示间歇性斜视。

4. **a.** 眼动脉的肌肉分支为眼外肌（EOM）提供最重要的血液供应。外侧肌支供应外直肌、上直肌、上斜肌和上睑提肌；内侧肌支为两者中较大者，供应下直肌、内直肌和下斜肌。

5.**b.** 眼外肌表现出明显的 2 层组织：前眼眶部分，仅作用于结缔组织滑车，以及后球体部分，其肌腱附着于巩膜以移动球体。

6. **a.** 有 3 个与单眼运动中使用的肌肉有关的重要术语：主动肌，沿给定方向移动眼球的主要肌肉；协同肌，与主动肌存在于同一只眼球中，与主动肌一起产生给定的运动；拮抗肌，与主动肌存在于同一只眼球中，在与主动肌相反的方向起作用。

7.**a.** 当眼球处于第 1 眼位时，水平（内侧和外侧）直肌仅在水平方向上移动眼球，因此具有水平的第 1 眼位但没有第 2 或第 3 眼位。

8. **c.** 在完全性动眼神经麻痹中，唯一有功能的眼外肌是外直肌和上斜肌。第 3 眼位时上斜肌起外展作用，加剧了眼球的外展位置。

9. **a.** 正电子发射断层扫描显示，与正常眼相比，刺激弱视眼时皮质区血流和葡萄糖代谢较低，表明视觉皮质区是弱视的主要部位。

10. **d.** Pharmacologic treatment of moderate amblyopia (visual acuity of 20/100 or better) is as effective as patching and may also be successful in more severe amblyopia (visual acuity of 20/125 to 20/400), particularly in younger children.

11. **c.** *Angle kappa* is the angle between the visual axis and the anatomical pupillary axis of the eye. The fovea is usually slightly temporal to the pupillary axis, making the corneal light reflection slightly nasal to the center of the cornea. This is termed *positive angle kappa*. A large positive angle kappa (eg, from temporal dragging of the macula in cicatricial retinopathy of prematurity [ROP]) can simulate exotropia.

12. **d.** In the *Maddox rod test*, a series of parallel cylinders convert a point source of light into a line image perpendicular to the cylinders. To test for horizontal deviations, the Maddox rod cylinders are placed horizontally in front of the right eye (180° meridian). The patient, fixating on a point source of light, sees a vertical line with the right eye and the point source of light with the left.

13. **a.** When the exodeviation at distance is larger than the deviation at near fixation by 10Δ or more but the distance and near measurements become similar after 30–60 minutes of binocular occlusion using a patch (the *patch test*), pseudodivergence excess intermittent exotropia is the likely diagnosis. An intermittent exotropia may become constant after disruption of binocular fusion with patch testing. In true divergence excess intermittent exotropia, the distance–near discrepancy would persist after patch testing. A patient with distance–near discrepancy may have a high accommodative convergence/accommodation (AC/A) ratio, which would be defined by persistence of the distance–near discrepancy after the patch test but resolution of this discrepancy with a +3.00 add. In a patient with basic intermittent exotropia, the measurement of the deviation at distance would be within 10Δ of the deviation measurement at near without patch testing or a +3.00 add.

14. **d.** Because visual acuity and alignment tests are dissociating and may adversely affect assessment of strabismus control, they should be performed after sensory tests for stereopsis and fusion. Stereopsis may decrease with worsening control of the deviation. Development of a high AC/A ratio would imply a decreased exotropia at near. A spontaneous consecutive esotropia would be rare in a patient with intermittent exotropia. Improved tenacious proximal fusion would improve stereopsis.

15. **a.** In patients with a Y pattern, the exodeviation is greater in upgaze, while the deviation is similar in primary position and in downgaze. This is often seen with pseudo-overaction of the inferior oblique muscle. There may be overelevation of the eye on adduction and slight upgaze, as opposed to true inferior oblique overaction, which is seen with overelevation on horizontal gaze. Other findings that would indicate true inferior oblique overaction include fundus excyclotorsion and vertical deviation with head tilts.

10. **d.** 中度弱视（视力为 20/100 或更好）的药物治疗与眼罩一样有效，并且在更严重的弱视（视力为 20/125 至 20/400）中也可能成功，特别是在年幼的儿童中。

11. **c.** kappa 角是视轴和眼球的解剖学瞳孔轴之间的角度。中央凹通常与瞳孔轴略微垂直，使角膜映光点在角膜中心偏鼻侧。这被称为正 kappa 角。大的正 kappa 角［如早产儿视网膜病变（ROP）中的黄斑的颞侧牵拉］形似外斜视。

12. **d.** 在 Maddox 杆试验中，一系列平行圆柱将点状光源转换为垂直于圆柱的带状光。为了测试水平隐斜视，将 Maddox 杆圆柱水平放置在右眼前方（180° 子午线）。投放固定点光源，患者右眼看到垂直线而左眼看到点光源。

13. **a.** 当视远斜视度大于视近斜视度 10Δ 或更多，但在 30~60min 的遮盖后视远、视近时斜视度相似（遮盖测试），拟诊为假性分开过强型间歇性外斜视。在用遮盖测试破坏双眼融合后，间歇性外斜视度数可能不变。在真性分开过强型间歇性外斜视中，遮盖测试后视远、视近的差异将持续存在。视远、视近存在差异的患者可能具有高调节性集合－调节（AC/A）比例，其可表现为遮盖测试后的视远、视近差异仍然存在，但是该差异可通过增加 +3.00D 球镜解决。基本型间歇性外斜视患者，未进行遮盖测试或增加 +3.00D 球镜时视远、视近斜视度测量差异在 10Δ 内。

14. **d.** 因为视敏度和对直试验是分离的并且可能对斜视控制的评估产生不利影响，所以它们应该在立体视觉检查和融合储备力检查之后进行。随着斜视控制的恶化，立体视觉可能会降低。高 AC/A 的发展意味着视近外斜视度降低。在间歇性外斜视患者中，自发性转变为连续性内斜视很少见。坚持提高近端融合将改善立体视觉。

15. **a.** 在 Y 型斜视的患者中，向上注视外斜视度更大，而在第 1 眼位和向下注视时的斜视度相似。这常见于下斜肌的假性功能亢进。其内转和轻微向上注视时可能加剧，与真正的下斜肌功能亢进是截然不同的，真正的下斜肌功能亢进可表现为水平注视时加剧。其他表明真正的下斜肌功能亢进的体征包括眼底外旋转性斜视和头部倾斜时垂直斜视。

16. **a.** In a V-pattern esotropia, the medial rectus muscles can be recessed and moved toward the apex of the deviation, which would be inferiorly in this case. Lateral muscles should be moved away from the apex of the deviation. A useful mnemonic is MALE: *m*edial rectus muscle to the *a*pex, *l*ateral rectus muscle to the *e*mpty space. When horizontal muscle recession-resection is performed, displacement should be in opposite directions, but this will cause symptomatic torsion if the patient has vision in the eye.

17. **b.** Inferior oblique overaction commonly causes a V pattern. A patterns are most commonly caused by superior oblique overaction. X and Y patterns result from pseudo-overaction of the inferior oblique muscles, and weakening them would not collapse the pattern.

18. **d.** The patient described has type 1 Duane retraction syndrome. A medial rectus recession on the affected side would correct the head turn and centralize the field of binocular vision. While limited abduction may be a result of a sixth nerve palsy, globe retraction causing narrowing of the palpebral fissures is diagnostic of Duane retraction syndrome. Magnetic resonance imaging (MRI) is thus not necessary for further evaluation of a sixth nerve palsy. A lumbar puncture to check for elevated intracranial pressure, which may be indicated in the presence of a sixth nerve palsy, is also not indicated. A muscle biopsy for strabismus is used in cases of suspected chronic progressive external ophthalmoplegia (CPEO) to evaluate for ragged red fibers or mitochondrial DNA changes. A child with CPEO would be expected to present with ptosis and limitation of eye movements but not globe retraction.

19. **a.** Duane retraction syndrome has been associated with Goldenhar syndrome (hemifacial microsomia, ocular dermoids, preauricular skin tags, and eyelid colobomas) and Wildervanck syndrome (sensorineural hearing loss and Klippel-Feil anomaly with fused cervical vertebrae). Kleinfelter syndrome (XXY) and Turner syndrome (XO) are chromosomal abnormalities. Waardenburg syndrome is characterized by hearing loss, retinitis pigmentosa, and a white forelock.

20. **a.** Type 1, the most common form of Duane retraction syndrome, is defined as poor abduction and esotropia. A patient may adopt a head turn to establish binocular fusion, and the esotropia may be seen only in primary gaze or with a head turn to the opposite direction. Type 2 is defined by limited adduction and exotropia. Type 3 is defined as poor abduction and adduction; either esotropia or exotropia may result. Poor abduction should not result in an exotropia.

21. **a.** Clinical trials for botulinum toxin show that it is effective in small-angle strabismus, postoperative residual strabismus, and acute paralytic strabismus. It can be used in active thyroid eye disease and as a supplement to rectus muscle recessions for large-angle strabismus. Botulinum toxin injection is not effective as single treatment for large-angle strabismus, A or V patterns, or chronic paralytic strabismus.

22. **a.** The extreme overcorrection suggests that there is a slipped medial rectus muscle. This would be evident by limited adduction in either eye. In this patient, absence of stereopsis would be expected but not helpful diagnostically. Vertical measurements would not be helpful, nor would findings from a slit-lamp examination.

16. **a.** 在 V 型内斜视中，可将内直肌后徙并朝偏斜的尖端方向移位，在本例即向下移位。外直肌要向远离偏斜的尖端移位。一个有效的助记符号为 MALE：内直肌向尖端，外直肌向开口方向移位。当进行水平肌肉后徙 – 缩短时，垂直方向的移位应是相反的，但是可能会导致患者有视力的眼有症状的旋转。

17. **b.** 下斜肌功能亢进通常会导致 V 型斜视。上斜肌功能亢进通常会导致 A 型斜视。X 和 Y 斜视是由下斜肌的假性功能亢进引起的，削弱它们不会使斜视消失。

18. **d.** 所描述的患者具有 1 型 Duane 眼球后退综合征。患侧的内直肌后徙将矫正头位并集中双眼视野。虽然外展受限可能是第 6 神经麻痹的结果，但眼球回退引起睑裂变窄是 Duane 眼球后退综合征的诊断特征。因此，没有必要做磁共振成像（MRI）来进一步评估第 6 神经麻痹。还不确定用于检查颅内压升高的腰椎穿刺能否表明存在第 6 神经麻痹。在疑似慢性进行性眼外肌麻痹（CPEO）的情况下，可使用斜视肌肉活检来评估蓬毛样红纤维或线粒体 DNA 变化。患有 CPEO 的儿童会出现上睑下垂和眼球运动受限但不出现眼球回退。

19. **a.** Duane 眼球后退综合征与 Goldenhar 综合征（半边小脸症，眼部皮样瘤，耳前皮肤悬垂物和眼睑缺损）和 Wildervanck 综合征（感觉神经性听力丧失和伴有颈椎融合的 Klippel-Feil 畸形）有关。Kleinfelter 综合征（XXY）和 Turner 综合征（XO）是染色体异常。Waardenburg 综合征的特征是听力丧失、视网膜色素变性和额部白发。

20. **a.** I 型是 Duane 眼球后退综合征最常见的形式，定义为外转受限和内斜视。患者可以采用头位转向来建立双眼融合，并且仅在第 1 眼位或者向相反方向转头时可以看到内斜视。2 型定义为内转受限和外斜视。3 型被定义为外转和内转受限，可能导致内斜视或外斜视。外转受限不应导致外斜视。

21. **a.** 肉毒杆菌毒素的临床试验表明，它对小角度斜视、术后残余斜视和急性麻痹性斜视有效。它可用于活动性甲状腺眼病，并可作为大角度斜视的直肌后徙术的补充。肉毒杆菌毒素注射对于大角度斜视，A 型或 V 型或慢性麻痹性斜视的单一治疗无效。

22. **a.** 极度过矫表明内直肌滑脱。这可以通过眼球的内转受限来证明。预计这名患者不会出现立体视觉，但在诊断上没有帮助。垂直斜视角度测量没有帮助，裂隙灯检查的结果也没有用。

23. **d.** Dysraphism represents a failure to fuse. Agenesis represents developmental failure, as is found in anophthalmia, whereas hypoplasia is due to developmental arrest. Developmental excess such as that seen with distichiasis is the cause of hyperplasia.

24. **b.** When vision loss is due to pathology posterior to the lateral geniculate nucleus, nystagmus is generally not present. Retinal dystrophy and congenital cataracts represent pathology anterior to the lateral geniculate nucleus and are associated with nystagmus.

25. **a.** Blepharophimosis-ptosis-epicanthus inversus syndrome may occur as a sporadic or autosomal dominant disorder. It consists of blepharophimosis, congenital ptosis, telecanthus, and epicanthus inversus. Surgery may be necessary early in life.

26. **c.** Crouzon and Apert syndromes appear similar clinically. However, Apert syndrome is associated with an extreme amount of syndactyly. Both syndromes are associated with hypertelorism, proptosis, and inferior scleral show.

27. **c.** Patients with craniosynostoses can have various types of horizontal strabismus. V-pattern exotropia is the most common type.

28. **c.** Ophthalmia neonatorum caused by *Neisseria gonorrhoeae* typically presents in the first 3–4 days of life. In severe cases, it is associated with marked chemosis, significant discharge, and a risk of corneal perforation. Chemical conjunctivitis is a mild, self-limited inflammation occurring in the first 24 hours of life due to instillation of silver nitrate. Herpes simplex virus conjunctivitis usually presents later, often in the second week of life. Chlamydialconjunctivitis usually occurs around 1 week of age and is associated with minimal to moderate discharge and possible pseudomembrane formation.

29. **a.** Stevens-Johnson syndrome is a hypersensitivity reaction that affects the skin and mucous membranes. Early ocular involvement may range from conjunctivitis to corneal perforation. Symblepharon, corneal vascularization, and eyelid anomalies such as entropion or ectropion are later sequelae.

30. **b.** Horner syndrome caused by a lesion along the oculosympathetic pathway must be ruled out in a patient with new-onset ptosis. Affected patients have anisocoria that is greater in dim light and ptosis secondary to paralysis of the Müller muscle. In a child, new-onset Horner syndrome can be idiopathic or secondary to trauma, surgery, or neuroblastoma along the sympathetic chain in the chest. Cataract would not cause acute ptosis. Anisometropic amblyopia and astigmatism would not occur with an acute ptosis; they can develop secondary to long-standing, significant ptosis.

31. **a.** Apraclonidine reverses the anisocoria. It causes dilation of the affected pupil but has no effect on the normal pupil. It will dilate the affected pupil regardless of whether the lesion is pre-or postganglionic.

23. **d.** 闭和不全表示融合失败。未发育代表发育失败，如无眼畸形，而发育不全是由于发育停滞。发育过度如双行睫是导致增生的原因。

24. **b.** 视力丧失是外侧膝状体后的病理造成时，通常不存在眼球震颤。视网膜营养性萎缩症和先天性白内障代表是外侧膝状体前的病理，并与眼球震颤有关。

25. **a.** 睑裂狭小 – 上睑下垂 – 逆向性内眦赘皮综合征可能以散发性或常染色体显性疾病的形式出现。它由睑裂狭小、先天性上睑下垂、内眦过宽和逆向性内眦赘皮组成。需早期手术治疗。

26. **c.** Crouzon 和 Apert 综合征在临床上似乎相似。然而，Apert 综合征与极端的并发症有关。两种综合征都与眼距过宽、眼球突出和下巩膜暴露有关。

27. **c.** 颅缝线封闭过早的患者可有各种类型的水平斜视。V 型外斜视是最常见的类型。

28. **c.** 由*淋病奈瑟氏球菌*引起的新生儿眼炎通常在出生前 3~4 d 出现。在严重的情况下，它与明显的结膜水肿、明显的分泌物和角膜穿孔的风险有关。化学性结膜炎是在出生 24h 内由于滴注硝酸银发生的轻度自限性炎症。单纯疱疹病毒性结膜炎出现较晚，通常在出生第 2 周出现。衣原体结膜炎通常发生在 1 周龄左右，有轻度至中度分泌物并可能有假膜形成。

29. **a.** Stevens–Johnson 综合征是一种影响皮肤和黏膜的超敏反应。早期眼部受累可能包括结膜炎和角膜穿孔。后遗症为睑球粘连、角膜血管化和眼睑异常，如睑内翻或外翻。

30. **b.** 对于新发生上睑下垂的患者，必须排除沿着眼交感神经通路病变引起的 Horner 综合征。患者在昏暗的光线下瞳孔大小不等更为明显，因 Müller 肌肉麻痹继发眼睑下垂。在儿童中，新发作的 Horner 综合征可能是特发性或继发于创伤、手术或胸部交感神经的神经母细胞瘤。白内障不会引起急性上睑下垂。急性上睑下垂不会出现屈光参差性弱视和散光，可以继发于长期显著的上睑下垂。

31. **a.** 安普乐定可恢复瞳孔大小不等。它会引起患侧瞳孔扩大，但对正常瞳孔没有影响。无论病变是在神经节前还是节后，都会引起患侧瞳孔扩大。

32. **a.** The basic pathophysiologic defect in primary congenital glaucoma is decreased aqueous outflow due to abnormal development of neural crest–derived tissue of the anterior chamber angle. Although abnormalities of the Descemet membrane, iris, and optic nerve all occur in primary congenital glaucoma, they are secondary effects from the increased intraocular pressure that occurs in this disease.

33. **b.** The anterior chamber angle of a normal infant eye differs from that of an adult's eye in the following ways: The Schwalbe line is less distinct. The trabecular meshwork is less highly pigmented. Because the uveal meshwork is more translucent than in adult eyes, it is more difficult to see through and therefore the junction between the scleral spur and ciliary body is less easily seen.

34. **a.** Posterior subcapsular cataracts (PSCs) are less common in children than in adults. They are usually acquired and often bilateral. PSCs tend to progress. Causes of PSC include corticosteroid use, uveitis, retinal abnormalities, radiation exposure, and trauma. PSCs can be seen in association with neurofibromatosis type 2. A review of the medication list is most likely to be useful in determining the etiology. In the absence of signs of uveitis, a musculoskeletal examination is less likely to be beneficial. As most PSCs are acquired, family history is also less likely to be helpful.

35. **a.** The most common identifiable etiology of anterior uveitis in a child is juvenile idiopathic arthritis, which occurs in 15%–47% of cases. Antinuclear antibody positivity is typically present in these children; rheumatoid factor is typically negative. Although juvenile spondyloarthropathies are associated with anterior uveitis in children, they are less common; thus, HLA-B27 testing is less likely to be beneficial. Infectious etiologies of anterior uveitis in children are less common, and results of serologic testing are less likely to reveal the etiology in these patients.

36. **a.** Tubulointerstitial nephritis and uveitis (TINU) syndrome is kidney disease associated with chronic or recurrent anterior uveitis in adolescents; the median age at onset is 15 years. The renal disease is characterized by low-grade fever, fatigue, pallor, and weight loss. The uveitis is usually bilateral and may occur before, simultaneously with, or after the renal disease. TINU nephritis is not commonly associated with cataract, serous retinal detachment, or papilledema.

37. **a.** Type 1 ROP is zone I, any stage with plus disease; zone I, stage 3 ROP without plus disease; or zone II, stage 2 or 3 ROP with plus disease. Type 2 ROP is zone I, stage 1 or 2 without plus disease; or zone II, stage 3 ROP without plus disease.

38. **b.** Leber congenital amaurosis is a group of hereditary retinal dystrophies that affect both the rod and cone photoreceptors. It is characterized by severe vision loss in infancy, nystagmus, and poorly reactive pupils. An electroretinogram is typically used to make the diagnosis, showing extinguished waveforms. A-scan ultrasonography, fluorescein angiography, and optical coherence tomography would not be helpful in making the diagnosis.

32. **a.** 原发性先天性青光眼的基本病理生理缺陷是，由于前房角神经嵴衍生组织的异常发育导致的房水流出减少。尽管角膜后弹力层、虹膜和视神经的异常都发生在原发性先天性青光眼中，但它们是由于该疾病眼内压升高所致的继发效应。

33. **b.** 正常婴儿眼的前房角与成人眼的前房角在以下方面不同：Schwalbe 线不那么明显。小梁网的色素沉着程度较低。由于其葡萄膜比成人眼睛更透明，更难以分辨，因此不太容易看到巩膜突和睫状体之间的连接。

34. **a.** 后囊下白内障（PSCs）在儿童中比在成人中少见。它们通常是获得性的、双眼的。PSCs 易发展。引起 PSC 的原因包括使用皮质类固醇、葡萄膜炎、视网膜异常、辐射暴露和创伤。PSC 被表明与 2 型神经纤维瘤病相关。药物清单的审查最有可能帮助确定病因。在没有葡萄膜炎迹象的情况下，肌肉骨骼检查不太可能有作用。由于大多数 PSC 是获得性的，家族史也不太可能有所帮助。

35. **a.** 可引起儿童前葡萄膜炎最常见的确切病因是幼年特发性关节炎，其发生率为 15% ~ 47%。这些儿童通常存在抗核抗体阳性、类风湿因子阴性。虽然幼年脊柱关节炎与儿童前葡萄膜炎有关，但它们并不常见，因此，HLA–B27 检测不太可能有益。引起儿童前葡萄膜炎的传染性病因不太常见，血清学检测的结果不太可能揭示这些患者的病因。

36. **a.** 肾小管间质性肾炎和葡萄膜炎（TINU）综合征是与青少年慢性或复发性前葡萄膜炎相关的肾脏疾病，发病年龄中位数为 15 岁。肾病的特征是低烧、疲劳、皮肤苍白和体重减轻。葡萄膜炎通常是双眼的，可能发生在肾病之前、同时或之后。TINU 肾炎通常不伴有白内障、浆液性视网膜脱离或视乳头水肿。

37. **a.** 1 型 ROP 为 I 区伴有附加病变任一期的病变，I 区不伴有附加病变的 3 期 ROP 或 II 区伴有附加病变的 2 期或 3 期 ROP。2 型为 I 区不伴有附加病变的 1 期或 2 期 ROP 或 II 区不伴有附加病变的 3 期 ROP。

38. **b.** Leber 先天性黑朦是一组遗传性视网膜营养不良疾病，影响视杆和视锥光感受器。其特征是幼年时严重视力丧失、眼球震颤及瞳孔对光反射迟钝。通常用视网膜电图显示熄灭的波形进行诊断。A 型超声、荧光素血管造影和光学相干断层扫描对诊断没有帮助。

39. **c.** Retinoblastoma occurs when both copies of *RB1*, a tumor suppressor gene, have mutations. Approximately 60% of retinoblastoma cases arise from somatic nonhereditary mutations of both alleles of RB1 in a retinal cell. These mutations generally result in unifocal and unilateral tumors. In the other 40% of cases, a germline mutation in 1 of the 2 alleles of RB1 either is inherited from an affected parent (10% of all retinoblastoma cases) or occurs spontaneously in 1 of the gametes.

40. **c.** Optic nerve hypoplasia is characterized by a decreased number of optic nerve axons. It is associated with absence of the septum pellucidum, not a bifid septum pellucidum; with agenesis of the corpus callosum; and with pituitary gland abnormalities. MRI reveals an ectopic posterior pituitary bright spot at the upper infundibulum. This finding is associated with pituitary hormone deficiencies. Optic nerve hypoplasia is not associated with an empty sella on MRI. Chiasmal gliomas are associated with optic nerve elevation, not optic nerve hypoplasia.

41. **d.** Morning glory disc anomaly typically appears as a funnel-shaped excavation of the posterior fundus that incorporates an enlarged optic disc with elevated surrounding retinal pigment epithelium and an increased number of blood vessels looping at the edges of the disc. It is sometimes associated with a basal encephalocele, PHACE (*p*osterior fossa malformations, *h*emangiomas, *a*rterial lesions, *c*ardiac and *e*ye anomalies) syndrome, and moyamoya disease. Optic nerve hypoplasia is associated with pituitary abnormalities and septo-optic dysplasia, not basal encephalocele. An optic nerve pit is not associated with encephalocele or other midline defects. Optic nerve coloboma is associated with CHARGE (coloboma, heart defects, choanal atresia, mental retardation, genitourinary abnormalities, and ear abnormalities) syndrome, but not encephalocele.

42. **a.** Although trauma is the most common cause of hyphema in children, spontaneous hyphemas can occur in juvenile xanthogranuloma of the iris, retinoblastoma, leukemia, and blood dyscrasias. Iris nevus, iris capillary hemangioma, and iris cyst are not associated with spontaneous hyphema formation.

43. **d.** The most common ocular manifestation of abusive head trauma (AHT), present in approximately 80% of cases, is retinal hemorrhage. These hemorrhages can be seen in all layers of the retina and may be unilateral or bilateral. They are found most commonly in the posterior pole but can also be present peripherally. The anterior segment and ocular adnexa are often normal. Hyphema, corneal abrasion, and subconjunctival hemorrhages are less commonly seen in AHT.

44. **a.** Ocular albinism is associated with iris transillumination, foveal aplasia or hypoplasia, and decreased retinal pigmentation. Both human and animal studies have shown an abnormally high number of crossed fibers in the optic chiasm, which precludes stereopsis and is associated with strabismus. Optic nerve hypoplasia and morning glory disc are not associated with abnormalities in the crossed fibers of the optic chiasm. Achromatopsia is not typically associated with optic nerve abnormalities.

39. **c.** 视网膜母细胞瘤发生在肿瘤抑制基因 RB1 的 2 个拷贝都有突变时。大约 60%的视网膜母细胞瘤病例来自视网膜细胞中 RB1 的 2 个等位基因的体细胞非遗传突变。这些突变通常导致单侧单病灶肿瘤。在另外 40%的病例中，RB1 的 2 个等位基因中的 1 个存在种系突变，要么是从患病的亲本遗传（占所有视网膜母细胞瘤病例的 10%），要么是在 1 个配子中自发性的突变。

40. **c.** 视神经发育不全的特征在于视神经轴突的数量减少。它与透明中隔缺如有关，非透明隔裂；与胼胝体发育不全有关，并伴有脑垂体异常。MRI 显示上漏斗部的异位脑垂体后叶亮点。这一发现与垂体激素缺乏有关。视神经发育不全与 MRI 上的空蝶鞍无关。视神经胶质瘤与视神经胶质细胞增殖有关，而不是视神经发育不全。

41. **d.** 牵牛花综合征通常表现为眼底后极部的漏斗形深凹陷，包括具有扩大的视盘周围视网膜色素上皮细胞增加及在视盘边缘处环绕的血管数量增加。它有时与基底脑膨出、PHACE（后颅窝畸形、血管瘤、动脉病变、心脏和眼异常）综合征和烟雾病有关。视神经发育不全与垂体异常和椎间盘发育不良相关，而非基底脑膨出。视盘小凹与脑膨出或其他中线缺陷无关。视盘缺损与 CHARGE（先天性虹膜缺损、心脏缺陷、后鼻孔闭锁、精神发育迟滞、泌尿生殖系统异常和耳部异常）综合征有关，但与脑膨出无关。

42. **a.** 虽然创伤是儿童前房积血的最常见原因，但在虹膜幼年黄色肉芽肿、视网膜母细胞瘤、白血病和血液恶病质均可发生自发性前房出血。虹膜色素痣、虹膜毛细血管瘤和虹膜囊肿与自发性前房积血形成无关。

43. **d.** 在大约 80%的病例中，最常见的虐待性头颅外伤（AHT）的眼部表现是视网膜出血。出血可见于视网膜的所有层，可以是单侧或双侧。最常见于后极部，但也可以存在于周边部。眼前段和眼附属器通常是正常的。在 AHT 中较少见到前房出血、角膜擦伤和结膜下出血。

44. **a.** 眼白化病与虹膜透光、中央凹未发育或发育不全有关，并且视网膜色素沉着减少。人类和动物研究均显示视交叉中大量异常的交叉纤维，这妨碍了立体视觉并且与斜视相关。视神经发育不全和牵牛花综合征与视交叉的交叉纤维异常无关。色盲通常与视神经异常无关。

（翻译 刘未择 // 审校 方严 石一宁 // 章节审校 石广礼）

后　记

美国眼科学会“基础与临床科学教程（Basic and clinical science course，BCSC）”第6册《小儿眼科与斜视（*Pediatric Ophthalmology and Strabismus*，2019-2020）》”中英文对照版即将出版，在此付印之际，有幸邀请到国内外多位专家为此书作序，其中有1990年主持BCSC第一个中文完整翻译版的Dr Mark Tso、2012年主持《眼科临床指南》（Preferred Practice Pattern，PPP）中文完整翻译版的赵家良教授、我敬仰的小儿眼科领域的资深专家刘陇黔教授、张丽军教授，青年专家钱学翰教授、刘虎教授，还有健康快车ICO考试中心的朱丹教授、布娟教授、以及为支持中国眼科教育国际化的方黄吉雯女士和Dr David Taylor，最后还是要特别提一下与我在中国近视防控工作中并肩作战的挚友、我十分尊敬的方严教授。

每每读着他们的一字一句，我就感同身受，就好像我们在共同回眸着过去的二三十年，犹如一道划过天空的彩虹、一道美丽的风景线，在人生最灿烂的年华舞动，这是每一个医生修炼三四十年的果！

他们的字里行间透着肯定和鼓励，给了我信心，使我在寂静、孤独的夜路上继续执着地走！

每每深夜挑灯熬油时，片片雪花、柔和春风、夏日热浪、初秋凉意，一阵阵从窗前掠过，我们坚守一年又半载，2020初至今的世界性疫情延缓了工作进程，终于在这西安最美丽的秋季可以呈现给大家了！

我常常扪心自问，《临床光学》一书出版之后，何以“节外生枝”地出《小儿眼科与斜视》一书？从眼底病跨界反串到小儿眼科？

现行的医疗体制，无论公立医院还是民营，都是治末病，属下医，而近视防控、儿童眼健康应该是初级眼保健的眼科预防学科，属上医，要治未病。

我的好友，一位眼科医院的院长，谈到眼科医院的学科建制时深感困惑，成人斜视分诊到小儿眼科，因为其中涵盖了眼肌专业，如果病人反问“我是成年人”该怎么回答呢？儿童白内障却需要在白内障科就诊、手术，家长就会质疑“为什么不在小儿眼科呢？”。

中国眼肌/斜视学组初始的设立，弱视诊断标准泛化，历经近20年的“矫枉”，依然不能“过正”，反而被弱视治疗产品的“伪专利”充斥，陷入市场化、商业化的泥沼，迄今衍生了 90% 以上的近视人群、30% 以上的高度近视，国家无兵可招、无驾驶员可用，举目远眺 20 年，中国将进入病理性近视的大爆发流行时代！

眼肌组演变为斜视弱视学组，进而更名斜视与小儿眼科专业，但在医院的学科建制中和实际日常临床工作中，大家并没有意识到小儿白内障应纳入小儿眼科，因为一旦婴儿白内障收入成人普通白内障病房，“专家”不去鉴别婴儿胚胎期的风疹感染，手术可能导致毁灭性的双眼球萎缩！婴幼儿先天性青光眼除了滤过手术因瘢痕化而失败外，更严重的是最终会形成高度近视，视网膜专科医生并不能完美地处理好早产儿的视网膜病变问题，儿童上睑下垂即使不遮盖瞳孔的 1/2，手术指征不足，也会诱发散光、近视的快速发展，儿童的斜视手术不考虑屈光不正，手术医生很难理解孩子可能从内斜矫正演变为外斜视、单眼眼球震颤、散光、眼球运动受限。

从早年的屈光学组更替到视光学组、视光专业，又冠以中国特色的“眼”，终难以掩盖“医学眼”的空壳，视光领域“士、师”与“医师”的混淆，更令人无法企及视光与小儿眼科的完美结合。视光学专业的学生若不了解屈光状态与屈光成分的匹配基础知识，则无从理解屈光状态与眼底各组织结构的解剖生理关系。

所以，中国儿童眼健康、近视防控首先是小儿眼科的正确定位，儿童弱视的诊断与近视的鉴别诊断，18 岁以下的屈光不正、视力低常的检测与干预都应在标准的医疗体系下进行，相关行业应该具有医疗属性，其行为均属涉医，医疗应该是社会公益和福利、民生行业。

由于相关主管部门的忽视，主流医疗机构的少为，使得坊间许多自诩的“眼保健”机构频现，它们没有坚实的医学基础，再加上快餐式即学即用型商家的加盟或商业促销培训，它们不仅将自己的孩子调治成病理性近视，还在向社会的亲朋好友传播错误的理念。为了商机，它们恪守低于 1.0 的 6 岁以下孩子就只是“弱视”、就是“弱智”的逻辑，“升视力、降度数”，将无数正常发育的儿童推向了未来三五年眼轴 25mm 的高度近视深渊。家长无法理解三五岁的不正常视力提高到 1.0 之后又会下降，并且一直在下降，其实此“不正常”非彼“不正常”也！

家长获得的暂时安慰一方面是源于医院的冷漠，但更本质的原因是科学发展的严重滞后。国际上迄今没有真正的循证医学，明确近视的有效治疗，提出确切的治疗方法，包括中国流行的“三板斧”和 PPP 提及的 5 个方面。但这并不等于说可以自我臆想“专利”、创造神秘妙方。

医学是一种终身学习的行业，是一种经验科学，需要不断修正、不断探索，通过一个个成功与失败的个案，逐步升华到具有共性的科学。

从国际近 200 年的近视研究史，中医千年来的探索中，我们得出了关于中国近视防控、眼健康工作遵循的 3 句话：近视防控的连续性思想、个性化设计、综合性措施（即连续性思想的 3 个阶段、10 部曲，个性化的 6 种状态 10 道防线，以及综合性的 5 个方面，每天必做

10 项措施）。我们需要从儿童眼发育、屈光成分发育入手，根据婴幼儿、儿童青少年的生理发育特点、病理学特征，为孩子保障未来三五十年的眼健康！

对于儿童眼的系统医学知识的补充，这是每一个近视防控工作者和每一位家长急需补上的一课！这是做好近视防控、眼健康工作的基石！

此书献给热爱孩子、热爱健康、热爱未来的人们！

石一宁

2020 年 8 月 31 日

开学前夜于西安新城石一宁诊所